RECREATIONAL THERAPY HANDBOOK OF PRACTICE

ICF-Based
Diagnosis and Treatment

Heather R. Porter
joan burlingame

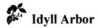 Idyll Arbor

Idyll Arbor, Inc

39129 264th Ave SE, Enumclaw, WA 98022 (360) 825-7797

Idyll Arbor, Inc. Editor: Thomas M. Blaschko

ISBN 1-882883-53-5
ISBN-13 9781-882883-53-0

This book is dedicated to all of the clients, therapists, colleagues, and professors who inspire us every day without knowing and to my family whose love and support mean more then they can ever realize...to my grandmothers for always believing in me, to my mom and dad for always being there for me, to my husband who unwaveringly stands beside me, and to my children (Hannah, Cary, and Guy) who continue to teach me more about the joys of life then any other.
~ HRP

This book is dedicated to the students who are learning to help others enjoy life despite their challenges. One of my mentors, when I asked him how I could pay him back for all of his assistance helping me get through undergrad, said that I was to "pay forward" to repay him. He challenged me to help those just starting out as a way to thank him. This book is one of my ways to thank him for his help. I now challenge those who find this book helpful to pay forward.

~ jb

Contents

Foreword

The World Health Assembly unanimously approved the ICF in 2001. Since then, this is the first commercially available book about the ICF and with ICF in the title. As such, it represents a major milestone for the ICF. It also represents a major milestone for the field of Recreation Therapy (RT), since it will put RT in the lead among other professional associations. They should soon follow suit in developing discipline-specific, ICF-based manuals for their members. This book is organized like the ICF, translates the RT field to the ICF, and even has the 1,494 codes in the appendix! I am pleased to enthusiastically endorse this book for anyone interested in the ICF.

A bit of ICF history will better allow us to place this new and important achievement in perspective. On May 22, 2001, the 189 countries in the Fifty-fourth World Health Assembly (WHA) in the World Health Organization unanimously approved the adoption of the International Classification of Functioning, Disability and Health (ICF). The ICF is a classification that covers human functioning and is based on a universal, integrative, and interactive model, which integrates the social and environmental aspects of disability and health. Resolution WHA54.21 states:

The Fifty-fourth World Health Assembly,

(1) ENDORSES the second edition of the International Classification of Impairments, Disabilities and Handicaps (ICIDH), with the title International Classification of Functioning, Disability and Health, henceforth referred to in short as ICF;

(2) URGES Member States to utilize the ICF in their research, surveillance and reporting as appropriate, taking into account specific situations in Member States, and, in particular, in view of potential future revisions;

(3) REQUESTS the Director General to assist Member States at their request, making use of ICF.

In the five years subsequent to this 2001 resolution, much progress has been made in implementing the tenets of this resolution, including the giant leap forward represented by Porter and burlingame's book. A number of U.S. professional associations have held ICF training sessions, developed important ICF documents, and/or published special journal issues on the ICF. The Spring 2003 issue of *Health Care Financing Review* includes six articles on functional status and the ICF. The June 2003 issue of *Disability and Rehabilitation* included 16 articles on ICF. The June 2004 issue of *Advances in Speech-Language Pathology* included six articles on the ICF, as did a series of 2004 issues of *Perspectives in Neurophysiology and Neurogenic Speech and Language Disorders*. The March 2005 issue of *Rehabilitation Psychology* included five ICF articles, and Volumes 2 and 3 of the 2005 journal *Rehabilitation Education* contained ten ICF articles. Next year the American Psychological Association (APA) will publish *The Manual for Clinical Implementation on ICF*, which may turn out to be the second book on ICF with ICF in its title. The APA Manual and this book by Porter and burlingame are complementary, since this book is discipline-specific, whereas the Manual is about how to code, based on input from many professional disciplines.

Importantly, the American Therapeutic Recreation Association has strongly endorsed the ICF. At the annual American Therapeutic Recreation Association (ATRA) conference held October 7-11, 2005 in Salt Lake City, the ATRA Board of Directors approved a press release which included the following ATRA position statement on the ICF: "The concepts and terminology of the ICF are compatible with recreational therapy practice. ATRA supports the use of ICF language and terminology in recreation therapy practice guidelines, standards of practice, curriculum development, public policy, international relations, and research. ATRA also acknowledges the significance of the use of the ICF classification and coding system as a vehicle to clarify and enhance practice and research in recreation therapy." It closes with this statement by ATRA President Dr. Bryan McCormack: "Our association is pleased to endorse the International Classification of Functioning and sees it as a valuable tool in our treatment services." I hope that the 15,000 U.S. and Canadian members of ATRA will embrace this book, and that university-based instructors adopt it as the basic RT textbook.

ATRA is in good company. Other eminent organizations have also endorsed the ICF definition of functioning, including the World Bank, Disabled Peoples' International, the National Council on Disability, the International Society of Physical and Rehabilitation Medicine, and the United Nations.

At least five U.S. government activities have also advanced the implementation of the ICF. First, in July 2001, the U.S. National Committee on Vital and Health Statistics approved this statement in its final report on collecting functional status information in health records. It states: "Based on its extensive hearing and deliberations over a period of

18 months, the Subcommittee on Populations concluded that a promising candidate as a code set—and the only viable one at present—is the International Classification of Functioning, Disability and Health." Second, the National Institute on Disability Rehabilitation and Research headed by Steven Tingus has adopted the ICF definition of disability, and has funded several multi-million dollar projects which have major ICF components. Third, the Office of Special Education Programs within the U.S. Department of Education has implemented an ICF-based Early Intervention Data Handbook. Fourth, the Office on Disability of the U.S. Department of Health and Human Services headed by Dr. Margaret Giannini has established the ICF Subcommittee of the New Freedom Initiative, and this group has the goal of exploring ICF applications with HHS agencies. Fifth, the Centers for Disease Control and Prevention has funded many developmental ICF projects, including hosting annual North American Collaborating Center ICF conferences, developing contracts for ICF development, and disseminating monthly ICF Clearinghouse messages.

Fortunately, it has become easier professionals to keep up with rapid advancements in ICF. Just four websites will suffice to keep the reader abreast of the ICF world. The first is the WHO Homepage: www3.who.int/icf/icftemplate.cfm. The second is the ICF Clearinghouse website at www.cdc.gov/nchs/about/otheract/icd9/icfhome.htm. As Senior Statistician at the National Center for Health Statistics (now retired) and now as an independent ICF consultant, I have had the professional pleasure of researching and writing these monthly and bi-monthly messages for over four years. All of the information in this preface comes from this source. The third website is www.icfconference.com. The North American Collaborating Center housed at the National Center for Health Statistics Annual sponsors annual ICF meetings and places conference papers and information about the upcoming ICF meeting on this site. I am pleased to have attended more of these conferences than anyone else (11 of the 12 held so far), and the 13th Annual NACC meeting on ICF will be held

in June 2007 in Buffalo, New York. The fourth essential website is cirrie.buffalo.edu/icf/cop/, which has the new ICF Community of Practice. There you will find an ICF Discussion Forum and Bulletin Board, and it includes a Forum message by Heather Porter seeking feedback on this book.

What is the future of ICF? Looking into my crystal ball, I see these issues on the horizon:

1. Investigations into the adequacy and sufficiency of the current set of Environmental Factors for application by health professional.
2. Further attempts to clarify the delineation between "Activities and Participation."
3. More studies looking at ICF in relation to other WHO classifications such as ICD-10.
4. Discussions of ICF in the forthcoming 2nd edition of *Disability in America.*
5. A linkage of ICF with U.N. Declarations on the Rights of Persons with Disabilities.
6. More Governmental programmatic and policy applications of the ICF.

Frankly, I admit to being an ICF enthusiast, aficionado, and downright junkie. I want universal implementation now, because the ICF is a social good for persons with disabilities. To move to this goal, we must move from demonstrations to evidence-based studies, and from there to clinical and administrative applications. That is why this book is so important. It is a handbook for RT clinical application designed to implement the ICF now. It will standardize communication, research, and therapy in the RT field and allow clearer communication with other disciplines. I salute Heather Porter and joan burlingame for this excellent manual. It is a model for other professional groups to follow in their own fields, within the U.S. and internationally.

Paul J. Placek, Ph.D.
ICF Consultant
And
Formerly, Senior Statistician
Office of the Center Director
National Center for Health Statistics

Acknowledgements

We want to thank the following contributors who helped us with the Handbook by providing techniques in their areas of expertise: Magdalena Blaise and Laura Eide. Robert S. Eliot's wife gave us permission to include Dr. Eliot's Quality of Life Index, which we hope will be useful for both readers and clients. We especially want to thank Phyllis Coyne for allowing us to use parts of her book, *Social Skills Training: A Three-Pronged Approach.* As we say in the note at the end of the introduction, we hope to have many more contributors to the next edition of the Handbook.

We want to express sincere gratitude and admiration for the many recreational therapy professionals who have come together to actively advance and promote the ICF as part of recreational therapy practice through their involvement with the American Therapeutic Recreation Association's Public Health — World Health Organization Team. They include Missy Armstrong, Cari Browning, Ann Houston, David Howard, John Jacobson, Youngkhill Lee, Bryan McCormick, Sharon Nichols, John Shank, and Marieke Van Puymbroeck. The authors, who are also involved with this team, are honored to work with such a good group of people.

We would also like to acknowledge the many people who have graciously offered their time and knowledge to review the draft of this book and offer us valuable insights.

Lynn F. Bufka, Ph.D.
Assistant Executive Director
Practice Research and Policy
American Psychological Association
Washington, DC

David Howard, Ph.D., MSW, CTRS
Assistant Professor
Department of Recreation and Sport Management
Indiana State University
Chair of ATRA Public Health — WHO team
Terre Haute, Indiana

Don Lollar, Ed.D.
Senior Research Scientist
Centers for Disease Control/NCBDDD
Atlanta, GA 30333

Bryan McCormick, Ph.D., CTRS
ATRA President
Associate Professor
Department of Recreation and Park Administration
Indiana University
Bloomington, IN

Jessica Rickard, CTRS
SCI Unit Team Leader
Magee Rehab
Philadelphia, PA

John Shank, Ph.D.
Chair
Department of Therapeutic Recreation
Temple University
Philadelphia, PA

Barbara Wilhite, Ed.D., CTRS
Clinical Associate Professor
Department of Therapeutic Recreation
Temple University
Philadelphia, PA

A special thank you to all of the Temple University students in the TR 355 classes over the past few years who have used drafts from the diagnoses section of this book to supplement their learning.

We would also like to offer our heartfelt thanks to Dr. Paul Placek who offered voluntarily to write the forward to this book. Dr. Placek has worked on ICF development and implementation for the past 12 years of his 30-plus-year career at the National Center for Health Statistics and has been acknowledged for this work in the ICF code book. His recent work includes writing the ICF Clearinghouse messages, developing ICF projects, helping plan the annual NACC meetings on ICF, participating in the annual WHO conferences of the Family of International Classifications, and encouraging ICF research. We are grateful for his contribution to this book and are honored to have it recognized by an ICF leader.

Paul J. Placek, Ph.D.
ICF Consultant
Formerly, Senior Statistician, Office of the Director, National Center for Health Statistics

Finally, I would like to personally thank Idyll Arbor for providing me with this opportunity. With special thanks to joan burlingame who had the foresight to base the book's content on the ICF and to Tom Blaschko whose editing and guidance throughout this process has been invaluable.

— Heather R. Porter

Section 1: Introduction

The *International Classification of Functioning, Disability, and Health* (ICF) from the World Health Organization represents a major shift in health care. It looks at health, not from the perspective of disease, disorder, or injury, but from the perspective of how a person's health fits in with the rest of his or her life, the kinds of things the person does, and the environment the person lives in.

It says what recreational therapists have been saying all along.

The *Recreational Therapy Handbook of Practice* was written to bring together the ideas that are already well understood in recreational therapy practice and the new model of health care represented by the ICF. Some of the terminology is different and there are a few differences in perspective, but if recreational therapists take the time to understand and use the ICF, we believe that they will find it to be an excellent tool both for improving practice and for demonstrating the importance of the work we do.

Introduction to the Book

This is not a book that will sit on your shelf and become dusty. It is full of practical information. So, let us share with you what is in the book and how you can best use it.

Section 1: Introduction to the ICF

This section tells you about the ICF (what it is, how it will affect you as a recreational therapist, answers to common questions). It will also tell you a bit about how to score the ICF codes. The nitty-gritty of how to score the codes can be found in Section 3.

Section 2: Diagnoses

This section lists over 30 major diagnoses such as stroke, brain injury, mental retardation, and fibromyalgia. Each diagnosis is described with information about incidence/prevalence, predominant age, causes, systems affected, prognosis, secondary problems, assessments, anticipated findings from an RT assessment, treatment approaches for the whole team and recreational therapy, and specific recreational therapy interventions. Each set of interventions refers you to topics in the Techniques section and specific ICF codes for detailed information on treatment. Many books tell you about what is recommended or suggested to do with a particular client. This book includes detailed information about recreational therapy techniques and how they fit within the ICF model.

Section 3: Treatment and the ICF Model

In section 1, you learned about the ICF. In this section, all of the ICF chapters (Body Structures, Body Functions, Activities and Participation, and Environmental Factors) are reviewed in detail. Each ICF component has an introduction section that explains how to score the ICF codes within the component. Each code within the component is reviewed in detail (how to assess it, document it, treat it, and adapt for it). If there is a specific technique that relates to the code, you will be referred to the technique in the Techniques section.

Section 4: Recreational Therapy Treatment Issues

This section is broken down into four subsections: equipment, concepts, techniques, and assessments.

The Equipment section describes adaptive equipment, along with specific information on how to use the device and where you can get it.

Concepts that are directly related to the ICF codes are discussed in the Concepts section.

The Techniques section reviews over 40 techniques that directly relate to recreational therapy practice and the ICF. Each technique provides a description of what it is, how to use it, how to document it, and adaptations for different types of clients and situations. Some of the techniques even provide worksheets and handouts that you can use in your practice.

The Assessment section provides a brief review of many of the recreational therapy assessments that are mentioned in the ICF code discussions and Techniques section to give you a better understanding of what they are and how you can get a copy of them.

Appendices

The appendices contain a complete list of the ICF codes without their description. This will allow you quick assess to codes without having to go through the meat of the book. There is also a list of common therapy abbreviations, along with a description of anatomical positioning to help with documentation and understanding of terms.

Glossary

The glossary provides definitions of common terms used throughout the book.

Index

The index will be helpful for finding specific ICF codes, concepts, techniques, and assessments. The index also has a list of common recreational therapy terms that refers the reader to the related ICF terms.

Introduction to the ICF

The *International Classification of Functioning, Disability, and Health* (called the ICF for short) was released by the World Health Organization (WHO) in May 2001. It provides a consensual, meaningful, and useful framework that governments, providers, and consumers can use to describe a person's health and health-related domains including body functions, body structures, activities and participation, and the person's interactions with the environment.

Much of our current health care system uses the World Health Organization's *International Classification of Diseases, 10ᵗʰ edition* (ICD-10) to classify health problems. When a person is diagnosed with a disease, disorder, or injury, it is recorded in the health care system as a code (e.g., S62.7 Multiple Fractures of Fingers). This type of classification reflects a medical model based on disease.

Recreational therapists need to understand the ICD-10, but they are not the ones who code the diagnosis. When a person sees a doctor, the doctor assigns a diagnosis to the client that is entered into a computerized health care system. The ICD-10 codes are primarily used by governments for the purpose of reimbursement and gathering statistics (e.g., how many people were diagnosed with breast cancer in 2004) about the country's health status and needs.

The ICF is an additional classification system to complement, not replace, the ICD-10. Instead of just coding the disease, disorder, or injury, the ICF provides codes that health professionals score on a Likert scale to reflect a client's level of impairment with a body structure and function (e.g., moderate impairment of the frontal lobe, severe difficulty with short-term memory) the level of difficulty that a client has with a specific life activity (e.g., mild difficulty carrying out a daily routine), and barriers and facilitators that affect impairment and difficulty (e.g., attitude of family is a moderate facilitator, financial assets are a severe barrier). The development of a database that describes people's functioning in addition to their disease, disorder, or injury will give us a much greater understanding of the relationship between a client's health problems and a client's level of functioning.

Within the next few years recreational therapists, as well as other health care professionals, will be using the ICF to describe their clients functioning. Professional organizations such as the American Psychological Association, the American Therapeutic Recreation Association, and the American Occupational Therapy Association are currently working on how to incorporate the ICF into current clinical practice and introducing their professions to the new terminology and guidelines in preparation for the implementation of this new classification system. As professional organizations review the classification, recommendations for revisions will be made and some of those recommendations may be implemented prior to using the ICF in our health care system.

Overview of the ICF

The ICF is printed in hardback and is available on a CD. To give you an idea of the mass of this classification system, the book (excluding the index) is 265 pages. The *Recreational Therapy Handbook of Practice* was written to describe the basics of the ICF, how it operates, how recreational therapists will be using the ICF, and the codes that relate to the practice of recreational therapy.

The ICF is divided into two parts as shown in Table 1. Part One is called Functioning and Disability and it has two components called "Body Functions and Structures" and "Activities and Participation." Although Body Functions and Structures are grouped together in the overview figure, they are really separate components in the ICF so we will discuss them separately.

- *Body Functions (BF)*: Body Functions are the physiological and psychological functions of the body. It is a component of the ICF that recreational therapists will need to become familiar with since many of the codes in this component fall into the scope of recreational therapy practice. EXAMPLE: A client had a heart attack and became anoxic (lack of oxygen to the brain). As a result he has short-term memory and attention problems. The recreational therapist finds the code for each of the problems (b1440 Short-Term Memory, b1400 Sustaining Attention), and scores the client's level of difficulty with the function. Body Functions codes all begin with a "b" in lower case.

- *Body Structures (BS)*: Body Structures provides a list of anatomical parts of the body such as organs, limbs, and their components. Typically, a physician or nurse practitioner codes a client's level of impairment in Body Structures. EXAMPLE: If a client had a heart attack, the physician would refer to Body Structures, find code s4100 Heart, and score the level of impairment within the structure. It is not anticipated at this time that recreational therapists will be scoring a person's functioning in this area. A list of Body Structures codes is provided in this book without elaboration. This list is provided for completeness so therapists who are reading a

Table 1: Overview of the ICF

	Part I: Functioning and Disability		Part II: Contextual Factors	
Components	Body Functions and Structures	Activities and Participation	Environmental Factors	Personal Factors
Domains	Body functions Body structures	Life areas (tasks, actions)	External influences on functioning and disability	Internal influences on functioning and disability
Constructs	Change in body functions (physiological) Change in body structures (anatomical)	Capacity: Executing tasks in a standard environment Performance: Executing tasks in the current environment	Facilitating or hindering impact of features of the physical, social, and attitudinal world	Impact of attributes of the person
Positive aspect	Functional and structural integrity	Activities and participation	Facilitators	not applicable
	Functioning			
Negative aspect	Impairment	Activity limitation and participation restriction	Barrier/hindrance	not applicable
	Disability			

(WHO, 2001, p.11)

clinical note that lists Body Structures codes and scores will know what they mean without having to find another source of information. Body Structures codes all begin with the letter "s" in lower case.

- *Activities and Participation (A&P)*: Activities and Participation lists the activities that people commonly perform in real life (e.g., taking care of plants, maintaining health, handling stress, preparing meals, swimming, shopping, using transportation, recreation and leisure, spirituality). The scores assigned by the therapist reflect a client's ability to engage or participate in those activities, thus the title of this component is "Activities and Participation." It is different from Body Functions. Body Functions reflects the function in isolation (a client has moderate difficulty with short-term memory), whereas Activities and Participation reflects the client's ability to do an activity (e.g., client has no difficulty in managing a daily routine). The Activities and Participation component is wonderful because it allows us to look at the level of difficulty that a client has with a specific activity, not just the level of body function impairment. As therapists, we know that impairments do not always mean that there will be difficulty with activities or that the level of difficulty with an activity will be the same as the level of the impairment. This type of coding guides our

current health system into a new way of looking at the health and functioning of people. Recreational therapists predominantly assess and address skills within the context of an activity, so most of the codes that the recreational therapist will use are here. Activities and Participation codes all begin with a letter "d" in lower case.

Part Two of the ICF is Contextual Factors. Contextual Factors is divided into two components called Environmental Factors and Personal Factors.

- *Environmental Factors (EF)*: Environmental Factors are things within the person's environment that affect his/her health and functioning (e.g., adaptive equipment, attitudes of other people, physical structure of buildings and land). Recreational therapy practice has a long history of identifying and addressing environmental factors that pose problems for our clients. We often refer to these problems as barriers. Within the ICF, however, not only will therapists score the extent that the environmental factor is a barrier to a specific activity, but they will also score the extent that the environmental factor is a facilitator for a specific activity. The Environmental Factors codes bring attention to specific factors that are causing a problem (or enhancing) the level of difficulty within an activity in the Activities and Participation codes and provide justification for the environmental factor to be included in the treatment plan. Recreational therapists will routinely attach Environmental Factors codes to Activities and Participation codes to show these connections (e.g., financial assets are a moderate barrier to engagement in arts and culture). How to do this is reviewed in Section 3 of the book in the Activities and Participation and Environmental Factors introductions. Environmental Factors codes all begin with a letter "e" in lower case.

- *Personal Factors (PF)*: Personal Factors are things that have to do with a person's life and living. They are not part of a health problem, but rather attributes of a person and his/her way of life that could affect his/her health and functioning. Examples of Personal Factors identified by the ICF include gender, race, age, other health conditions, fitness, lifestyle, habits, upbringing, coping styles, social background, education, profession, past and current experience, overall behavior pattern and character style, individual psychological assets, and other characteristics. Personal Factors, although recognized by the ICF as being influential on a person's health and functioning, are not coded in the ICF. According to the ICF book, they are not classified because of the large social and cultural variances associated with them. The authors additionally theorize that personal factors are often made into facilitators or barriers by other environmental factors, body structures, body functions, and activities and participation (e.g., attitudes of others impact a woman's participation in activity, not that she is a woman; a person's confidence or functional abilities impact a person's participation in sports, not that he is 75 years old). It is important for therapists to also take this cue and look past the personal factors for environmental factors that may be changed to yield a positive result (e.g., changing attitudes of others) Personal factors cannot (or very seldom can) be changed. It is just as important to identify personal factors that facilitate functioning (e.g., it is good to be a woman in this situation or good to be of a certain age) to heighten awareness of positive outside variables that facilitate activity participation (e.g., characteristics of race are accepted/admired within particular settings/situations).

Clinical Terminology in the ICF

When you look through the ICF codes, you will notice that the terminology is quite simple. For example, health professionals use the term "ambulation" to describe the action of moving from one place to another using the legs assisted or not by other people and/or devices (e.g., The client is able to ambulate 50' with minimal assistance and a rolling walker.). The ICF does not recognize the term "ambulation." It uses the basic term "walking" instead. Therapists need to be aware of the terminology changes so that they can find the correct codes. The language chosen by the WHO was chosen for good reason. The terms are simple so that they can be translated and understood by all cultures, all over the world. To help you make this transition, we have included common therapy terms that will guide you to the ICF term. See Table 2. If you look up a term in the index, it will also tell you the appropriate ICF term.

What if We Aren't Using the ICF Yet?

Incorporation of the ICF into health care is anticipated within the next few years. We recom-

Table 2: Translation of Terms

ambulation	d450 Walking
balance (dynamic)	b755 Involuntary Movement Reaction Functions, d410 Changing Basic Body Position
balance (static)	d415 Maintaining a Body Position
community mobility	d460 Moving Around in Different Locations, d465 Moving Around Using Equipment
direction following	d210 Undertaking a Single Task, d220 Undertaking Multiple Tasks
endurance	b740 Muscle Endurance Functions, b455 Exercise Tolerance Functions
fine motor skills	d440 Fine Hand Use
gross motor skills	d445 Hand and Arm Use, d435 Moving Objects with Lower Extremities, b760 Control of Voluntary Movement Functions
initiation	d210 Undertaking a Single Task, d220 Undertaking Multiple Tasks
leisure skill development	d155 Acquiring Skills
range of motion	b710 Mobility of Joint Functions
sequencing	b176 Mental Functions of Sequencing Complex Movements
standing tolerance	d4154 Maintaining a Standing Position
strength	b730 Muscle Power Functions
transfers	d420 Transferring Oneself

mend that therapists begin to incorporate the ICF into current clinical practice whenever possible to make the transition to ICF easier for staff and to start using the ICF model of health to demonstrate the value of recreational therapy interventions. Suggestions include:

1. *Incorporate ICF terminology into current documentation*: Use the term capacity when talking about a client's ability to do an action or task in a standardized testing environment and the term performance when talking about a client's ability to engage in a life situation. Use the term activity limitation when talking about a barrier to an action or task in a standardized testing environment and use the term participation restriction when talking about a barrier to engagement in a life situation.

2. *Use ICF scaling*: Incorporate the use of ICF scaling whenever possible to describe impairments (no, mild, moderate, severe, complete).

3. *Educate other therapists*: Begin educating other recreational therapists about the ICF so they are aware of the anticipated changes and begin incorporating changes into their current clinical practice as appropriate.

4. *Attend ICF training sessions*: ICF training sessions will begin to pop up at local and national conferences. Make plans to attend and encourage other recreational therapy colleagues to attend as well.

5. *Incorporate the ICF into recreational therapy curriculum*: College and university instructors and professors can begin to incorporate ICF education into the recreational therapy degree curriculum to prepare upcoming clinicians for ICF use.

For more information about the World Health Organization visit their web site at www.who.int/en/. Information specifically about the ICF can be found at www3.who.int/icf/icftemplate.cfm. A copy of the ICF that can be searched by keyword is available on line at www3.who.int/icf/onlinebrowser/icf.cfm.

References

World Health Organization (2001). *International classification of functioning, disability, and health, 10th edition.* Geneva, Switzerland: World Health Organization

ICF Coding

First it is important to note that the ICF is a classification system, not an assessment tool. Therapists and other health professionals will continue to use observation, clinical judgment, and various informal and formal assessment tools to identify the specific problems of a client. Once the problems are identified, the therapist will then need to find the appropriate code and score it.

How do I find the correct code?

When looking at the ICF for the first time, the number of codes can be overwhelming. However, the more you look through it and the more you use it, the more you will understand it and be able to quickly identify the correct code. With that said, there are several ways you can find a specific code.

1. *Thumbing*: Thumb through the ICF component that best fits the problem you would like to code. Remember that the codes you are most likely to use will be found in Body Functions or Activities and Participation. If you are looking for a code to describe a specific impairment (e.g., personality impairment), look in the Body Functions component. If you are looking for a code to describe a problem that a client is having with a specific activity (e.g., shopping, play, walking), look in the Activities and Participation component. And finally, if you are looking for a code to describe an external variable that is affecting a client's level of impairment or difficulty, look in the Environmental Factors component.

2. *Index*: Look for the name of the specific impairment or activity in the index of the book. It will refer you to the location of a code or codes that discuss the term. To help you out even further, we provided a description of each code as it relates to therapy practice, as well as how to assess, document, treat, and adapt for the specific impairment or difficulty.

3. *Specific diagnosis*: There are over 30 diagnoses in the Diagnoses section of this book that will guide you to ICF codes with recreational therapy interventions. For example, if you are working with a client who has multiple sclerosis, look up multiple sclerosis in the index or find it in the Diagnoses section where the diagnoses are listed in alphabetical order. Go to the Recreational Therapy Intervention heading towards the end of the diagnosis. There you will find a list of com-mon interventions and the ICF codes that relate to each intervention.

4. *Specific techniques*: If you want to find a code that relates to a specific intervention, go to the Techniques section of this book. There you will find an alphabetical list of common techniques used by recreational therapists. Each technique will guide you to codes that relate to the specific technique. For example, if you are teaching a client how to conserve her energy during community activities, go to "Energy Conservation Training" in the Techniques section, and it will tell you that the code related to that technique is d2303 Managing One's Own Activity Level.

When will I score the codes?

It is currently unclear how often the therapist will score the ICF codes. It is possible that the therapist will score the ICF

• after each encounter (such as assessment and treatment)
• at admission and again at discharge
• in relation to predefined documentation (e.g., weekly, monthly).

Are there specific ICF code forms?

The World Health Organization (WHO) developed a clinical ICF form that is available, but it does not reflect all of the ICF categories that are pertinent to the scope of recreational therapy practice (as well as other therapies). It is important to note that the clinical ICF form is not a finalized document, but rather a working form that will most likely be adapted to meet the needs of a discipline or a facility. The form can be downloaded by selecting the ICF Checklist option on the left-hand bar on the ICF website:
http://www3.who.int/icf/icftemplate.cfm

How do I score the identified code?

How you score the code will depend on which ICF component it is in. Each component of the ICF (Body Functions, Body Structures, Activities and Participation, and Environmental Factors) is scored differently, although there are some similarities in how they are expressed. See the introduction to each of the components in section 3 for scoring instructions.

Contributors and Feedback

We want you to think of this book as "YOUR BOOK." We want it to be accurate and reflect CURRENT recreational therapy practice. We realize that there are many areas that are not covered, especially in the Diagnosis section. So, we need your help!

We are looking for contributors for the next edition. We are especially looking for seasoned clinicians in pediatrics and mental health. If you are an expert in a particular area of practice or a particular subject, we hope you will consider writing about your area of expertise. If you are interested, please send us a letter of inquiry telling us about your clinical knowledge, along with your resume, to

Heather R. Porter
Idyll Arbor, Inc.
39129 264th Ave SE
Enumclaw, WA 98022.

You can also send this to us by e-mail at editors@IdyllArbor.com.

We are also looking for feedback from anyone who reads this book. Suggestions for additional diagnoses, other treatment techniques, and better organization will be very much appreciated. Send your comments to Heather Porter at Heather@IdyllArbor.com and join the ICF Community of Practice — an organization with a discussion forum, bulletin board, and teleconferencing for people who are interested in using the ICF in their practice. Go to http://cirrie.buffalo.edu/icf/cop/ for more information.

If we incorporate your comments or suggestions we will gladly acknowledge your contribution in the next edition.

We look forward to hearing from you!

Sincerely,
Heather R. Porter

Section 2: Diagnoses

This section looks at diagnoses and conditions that recreational therapists work with. Some of the diagnoses in this section have alternate names. Other sections cover multiple issues. The reference list below suggests places where you will find the diagnosis you are looking for. You can also look in the index for references to a particular diagnosis in other parts of the book, even if it isn't covered in the diagnosis section.

Addiction (see Substance Dependence)
Alzheimer's (see Dementia)
Anorexia Nervosa (see Eating Disorders)
Atherosclerosis (see Cardiac Conditions)
Binge Eating (see Eating Disorders)
Bulimia (see Eating Disorders)
Compulsive Eating (see Eating Disorders)
Congestive Heart Failure (see Cardiac Conditions)
Coronary Artery Disease (see Cardiac Conditions)
Degenerative Joint Disease (see Osteoarthritis)
Depression (see Major Depressive Disorder)
Developmental Disability (see Mental Retardation/Developmental Disability)
Heart Attack (see Cardiac Conditions)
High Cholesterol (see Cardiac Conditions)
Hip Replacement (see Joint Replacement)
Knee Replacement (see Joint Replacement)
Myocardial Infarction (see Cardiac Conditions)
Prosthesis (see Amputation and Prosthesis)
Scars (see Burns)
Skin Breakdowns (see "Skin Breakdown" in the Techniques section)
Total Joint Replacement (see Joint Replacement)

Although clients may be categorized by disability, the treatment needs of clients vary for many reasons including severity, ability to adjust to disability, support and resources available, past medical history, secondary disability, age, developmental stage, beliefs and attitudes, and motivation for therapy. Because of the variability within each diagnosis, it is impossible to stipulate a single, universal treatment plan for each diagnosis. To provide guidance for the therapist, we decided to list the most common treatment interventions implemented by recreational therapists who work with a specific population. The term "most common" is defined by the authors as interventions that are applicable to many clients with a specific diagnosis, Specific behavioral issues, cognitive deficits, physical impairments, and social dysfunctions that *could* result from a specific disability are not always addressed. The therapist will need to identify these needs on an individual basis and implement an appropriate treatment plan to address the identified issues.

Dual diagnoses, secondary disabilities, or past medical histories may require the therapist to refer to the other relevant treatment protocols and integrate them as appropriate. The interventions listed are not meant to be a standard universal treatment plan, nor are they to be recognized as a complete or absolute list; they are merely a guide.

Amputation and Prosthesis

Amputation is the complete loss of all limb elements below a certain point. Amputations may be performed because of limb disease, trauma, birth defects, or frostbite.

Limb disease generally falls into three categories: 1. peripheral arterial disease (e.g., a complication of diabetes), 2. cancer, or 3. sudden blockage of an artery (embolus) causing a lack of oxygenated blood for the tissue. When tissue is deprived of oxygen, bacterial infections follow and tissue dies. The decay of tissue is called gangrene. Gangrene is not curable and the dead, infected tissue must be removed before healing can occur.

Amputations are often described by the percentage of the limb remaining. Table 4 and Table 5 show that terminology.

Incidence/Prevalence in US

A national health interview survey conducted in 1996 by the Office on Disability and Health, National Center for Environmental Health, and Centers for Disease Control and Prevention found that there were approximately 1.2 millions persons in the United States with an amputation. See Table 3.

Predominant Age

Information about the presence of amputations by age group, gender, and race is shown in Table 3.

Causes

In the United States the most common reasons for amputation of the upper extremity are birth defects, trauma, and tumors. Upper extremity amputations are seldom the result of a non-cancerous disease process. In children under the age of 15 years the most common reasons for an amputation are birth defects and tumors. For clients between 15 and 45,

Table 3: Absence of extremity

Age Group
< 18 years 70,000
18-44 years 293,000
45-64 years 305,000
65-74 years 223,000
Gender
Male.. 893,000
Female 392,000
Race
White 1,188,000
Black.. 98,000

trauma is the leading cause of upper extremity amputation. In the United States the most common reasons for lower extremity amputations are disease (70%), trauma (22%), birth defects (4%), and tumors (4%) (Moss Rehab, 2005). Diabetes, vascular disease, and heart disease are the leading causes of amputations because of disease. Clients who smoke, get little exercise, and have poor eating habits are at an increased risk of having an amputation.

System(s) Affected

A client with an upper and/or lower extremity prosthesis requires more cardiopulmonary and muscular energy to perform tasks such as walking, household chores, and recreational activities than someone who has all four limbs. Increased levels of energy consumption (percentage above normal) by amputation level are as follows:
- Below knee unilateral amputation: 10-20%
- Below knee bilateral amputation: 20-40%
- Above knee unilateral amputation: 60-70%
- Above knee bilateral amputation: >200%

It is also common for clients who have had an amputation to experience musculoskeletal changes due to compensation for limb loss. For example, a client who has a right below-knee-amputation (R BKA) may weight bear on his left lower extremity more than his prosthetized right lower extremity when standing and walking. When one leg is favored, musculoskeletal changes can cause pain in the hip and back. This is a common problem for clients who are learning how to walk using a prosthesis because they: 1. fear placing weight on the stump, 2. hurt from pressure on the stump, and 3. can't accurately judge the amount of weight being placed through the stump.

Prognosis

- The level of functioning, independence, and quality of life for clients with amputations depends on variables such as rehabilitation received, level of acceptance and adaptation, other medical issues, barriers such as attitudinal or architectural barriers, and level of support.
- Clients who have foot ulcers due to diabetes have an increased risk of future amputations. A major study indicated that after a client had a foot ulcer that healed, his/her chance of having a second foot ulcer that required an amputation was 3% after one year, 10% after three years, and 12% after five years. The risk of a second

amputation increased for clients with diabetes who had already had one amputation to 13% after one year, 35% after three years, and 48% after five years (Apelqvist, Larsson, & Agardh, 1993).

- Clients with acute limb ischemia (ALI) are at increased risk of amputation. Most, but not all, ALI is caused by atherosclerotic disease, so therapists working with clients with atherosclerotic disease should watch for the "five Ps" of ALI: 1. acute pain, 2. pulselessness, 3. pallor, 4. paresthesia, and 5. paralysis (Katzen, 2002).
- Clients with peripheral vascular disease, who smoke and who have experienced at least one arterial occlusion, are ten times more likely to require a lower extremity amputation than non-smokers in the same category (Health and Aging, 2004).

Secondary Problems

- *Pain*: Pain after amputation is usually divided into four types: 1. acute post-surgical pain from the surgery itself, 2. phantom limb pain where the pain is experiences as if it were located in the amputated limb, 3. psychogenic pain in a non-amputated body part where no physical cause is found, and 4. painful residual limb where the pain in the residual limb has an identified cause (Esquenazi, 2003). See b280 Sensation of Pain for more information on pain. See phantom sensation in this Secondary Problems section for more information on phantom pain.
- *Infection*: Infection is a potential problem at the incision site if it is not well cleaned and cared for after surgery. Once the incision site is fully dry and healed, the entire stump site is at an increased risk for infection if the skin breaks open from prosthesis wear.
- *Skin breakdown*: Skin breakdown is also referred to as ulceration. Although skin breakdown can occur for many different reasons (see "Skin Breakdown" in the Techniques section), clients who have an amputation are at an increased risk of developing skin breakdown on the residual limb from the increased pressure and friction of wearing the prosthesis. The increased pressure and friction can be caused by a poor fitting socket, changes in the volume of the residual limb (e.g., swelling), incorrect number of sock plies (see "Prosthetic Socks" in the Equipment section), incorrect placement of the stump in the prosthetic socket, or wearing the prosthesis beyond the tolerance of the skin. Should ulcers develop, the prosthetic wearing schedule may need to be decreased to allow for healing.

- *Edema*: Edema (or swelling) is usually due to constriction of the stump caused by uneven shrinkage of the stump. After the surgical amputation, an ace bandage is wrapped in a figure eight pattern to help form the stump. If it is not wrapped correctly or not worn routinely, the stump will not develop into a smooth form. Despite proper wrapping of the stump, sometimes the distal end of the stump is smaller than the top. If this happens, there will be a greater amount of space at the bottom of the prosthetic socket than at the top. To fill up the end of the prosthetic socket, the client puts on more sock plies, but this constricts the proximal portion of the stump and restricts blood flow to the distal part of the residual limb causing it to swell. If the swelling (edema) is recognized at an early stage (e.g., discoloration due to ruptured capillaries), the problem can be resolved and ulceration can be prevented. Edema must be resolved prior to wearing a prosthesis again.
- *Contractures*: Contractures are usually the result of inactivity. See "Consequences of Inactivity" in the Concepts section for more information. Inadequate range of motion caused by contractures can affect activity performance.
- *Phantom sensation*: The sensation that an amputated limb is still there is called phantom sensation (no pain, just sensation). There are three theories as to why clients experience phantom limb pain and/or phantom limb sensation. One theory is that the remaining nerves continue to generate impulses. Another is that the spinal cord nerves begin excessive spontaneous firing in the absence of expected sensory input from the limb. The third theory is that there is an altered signal transmission and modulation within the somatosensory cortex.
- *Deconditioning*: Deconditioning is a very likely complication due to decreased activity level. See "Consequences of Inactivity" in the Concepts section for more information.
- *Dermatologic problems*: Contact dermatitis, sebaceous cysts, scar irritation, and excessive sweating are common skin management issues. The liner, socks, and suspension mechanism are the usual culprits for contact dermatitis. The socket is a less likely cause. Treatment requires removal of the offending item and appropriate treatment (e.g., topical cream). Cysts and sweating can be a sign of excessive shear forces and components that are improperly fitted. This should be brought to the attention of the prosthetist (Bodeau & Mipro, 2002).

Assessments

Typical Scope of Team Assessment

The surgical team will determine whether or not the client is medically stable enough to undergo amputation surgery (non-traumatic cause). This is decided upon after extensive lab work, a physical exam, and testing reports. For clients who have had a traumatic amputation, the emergency medical team will evaluate the current situation and respond in the appropriate manner.

Once the amputation is completed, the amputation will be formally classified, as the surgeon can't truly be confident about the extent of the amputation until the site is opened and diseased bodily tissue can be clearly seen. All attempts are made to save as many joints as possible during surgery. Prosthetic joints do not function as well as natural joints, so functional skills and independence are greater for those who able to keep major joints. Amputations are classified by the percent of the remaining limb (See Table 4 and Table 5.)

Not every client will be a candidate for a prosthesis. There are several variables to consider. The client with a lower extremity amputation must have sufficient trunk control, upper body strength, static and dynamic balance, and adequate posture to be

successful with a prosthesis. Once these basic skills are achieved, stability, ease of movement, energy efficiency, and the appearance of a natural gait are possible. Other important areas to assess include the level of amputation, the expected function of the prosthesis, the cognitive level of the client, the client's vocation, the client's avocational interests, the cosmetic importance of the prosthesis, the client's financial resources, and the client's motivation to wear a prosthesis.

Anticipated Findings from RT Assessment

The initial evaluation of a client with a newly acquired amputation will most often reflect the following deficits in both stages of rehabilitation (pre-prosthetic training and prosthetic training):

* *Deconditioning*: This may be due to activity restrictions after surgery and/or lifestyle behavior. Clients who have had an amputation due to a disease process such as diabetes typically have a higher rate of sedentary behavior than the normal population.

Table 4: Classification of Upper Extremity Amputation

The following list contains the classification of upper extremity amputation including the percentage of the residual limb left after surgery.   **Above-Elbow**   • Shoulder disarticulation: 0%   • Humeral neck: 0-30%   • Short above-elbow: 30-50%   • Long above elbow: 50-90%   • Elbow disarticulation: 90-100%   **Below-Elbow**   • Very short below-elbow: 0-35%   • Short below-elbow: 35-55%   • Long below-elbow: 55-90%   • Wrist disarticulation: 90-100%   **Hand**   • Transmetacarpal, proximal: Amputation of hand palm slightly above wrist; may include involvement or sparing of the thumb   • Thenar: Loss of thumb   • Transmetacarpal, distal: Amputation of hand palm slightly below fingers; may include involvement or sparing of the thumb   • Transphalangeal: Loss of fingers; may include involvement or sparing of the thumb

From Kottke, F & Lehmann, J (1990).

Table 5: Classification of Lower Extremity Amputation

• Partial toe: Excision of any part of one or more toes   • Toe disarticulation: Disarticulation at the metatarsal phalangeal joint   • Partial foot/ray resection: Resection of the 3rd, 4th, 5th metatarsals and digits   • Transmetatarsal: Amputation through the midsection of all metatarsals   • Symes: Ankle disarticulation with attachment of heel pad to distal end of tibia. May include removal of malleoli and distal tibial/fibular flares.   • Long below-knee: More than 50% of tibial length   • Below-knee: 20-50% of tibial length   • Short below-knee: Less than 20% of tibial length   • Knee disarticulation: Amputation through the knee joint; femur intact   • Long above-knee: More than 60% of femoral length   • Above knee: 35-60% of femoral length   • Short above-knee: Less than 35% of femoral length   • Hip disarticulation: Amputation through hip joint; pelvis intact   • Hemipelvectomy: Resection of lower half of the pelvis   • Hemicorporectomy: Amputation of both lower limbs and pelvis below L4/5 level

From O'Sullivan, S & Schmitz, T (1988).

- *Impaired sense of self*: A physical piece of the person is gone after an amputation. The client does not look the same. Having an abnormal physical appearance can hinder self-esteem, self-confidence, self-concept, adjustment, and body image. Negative sense of self can be reflected in negative behavior or mood, despair about learning new skills, and poor interactions with others. The client may also verbalize disability myths such as "I'm worthless." Getting used to a new physical appearance is often improved when the client becomes engaged enough in activities that s/he sees himself/herself as a "bridge player" again instead of a one-handed oddity.
- *Lack of awareness and knowledge*: Clients with their first amputation will not know how to use a prosthesis.

Treatment Direction

The therapist is likely to see the client with an amputation in three different situations: pre-prosthetic training, prosthetic training, and community recreation. The needs of the client will be different in each. While the treatment is geared toward the specific functional and emotional needs of the client at each phase, the therapist also has an opportunity to provide continuity in treatment in areas such as balancing leisure activities, increasing resource awareness, and in helping polish the client's problem solving skills. Clients typically receive a total of four to ten hours of recreational therapy during each rehabilitative stay.

Pre-Prosthetic versus Prosthetic Training

Amputation rehabilitation is typically divided into two stays:
- *Pre-prosthetic training*: During this stay, the client is taught how to care for the residual limb and how to function without the limb. The client is then discharged until the incision site is fully healed (about three months). Once the incision site is fully healed, the client is readmitted to rehabilitation for prosthetic training.
- *Prosthetic training*: At this stage the client is able to wear a prosthesis and learns how to incorporate it into functional tasks.

Pre-prosthetic Training

The goal of pre-prosthetic training is to teach the client how to function without a limb.

Whole Team Approach

The client learns how to: function without the limb; perform activities of daily living such as dressing and bathing; develop the skills needed for a form of mobility (typically a wheelchair or crutches for a lower extremity amputation, no device for an upper extremity amputation); develop a home exercise program that promotes and improves active range-of-motion throughout all joints, especially in the residual limb; and gain muscular and cardiopulmonary strength. A program to desensitize the residual limb for the prosthesis is initiated and taught to the client. (The skin on the bottom of the residual limb is very sensitive to pressure. Gentle tapping on the distal end of the residual limb is helpful in desensitizing the residual limb). The client is also taught to massage the residual limb to prevent excessive scar formation and wrap the residual limb with an ace wrap in a figure-eight pattern to control edema and promote the development of a properly shaped distal stump so that it fits correctly into a prosthesis.

Recreational Therapy Approach

The primary focus is on the development of a healthy lifestyle plan for the time between losing a limb and being fitted with a prosthesis. (Some clients may never get a prosthesis, so these interventions need to address their needs, too.) The major goals include having the client maintain an active lifestyle, so that wearing prosthesis will be physically possible. An active lifestyle also promotes emotional health (including motivation, self-confidence, and adjustment to disability), which makes it more likely that the client will choose to go to the effort of learning to use a prosthesis.

Recreational Therapy Interventions

The following interventions are commonly used for clients with amputations before they get a prosthesis:

Functional Skill Development

- *Residual limb care*: Educate the client about the importance of caring for his/her residual limb within activities (e.g., being careful that the residual limb does not get bumped, scraped, or injured during activities). Damage to the skin will lengthen the healing period and prolong the person's waiting period to wear a prosthesis. Skin openings could lead to infection. Score this training as d5702 Maintaining One's Health.
- *Movement and range of motion*: The client must understand the importance of, and participate in, regular physical activities that allow for the range of motion of all joints. The physical activities may be a prescribed set of range of motion exercises or leisure activities that provide

the same result. There are some special issues for lower limb amputations:

o When in a seated position, the residual limb should be supported with the knee straight to prevent knee contractures.

o When supine, the residual limb should be straight, not propped up on pillows to prevent hip contractures.

o Lying in a prone position several times a day for a minimum of 30 minutes will also help prevent hip contractures. Recreational therapists can help clients to identify activities that can be performed lying prone to make the time pass more easily and increase the chance the client will perform the proper exercises.

This is also scored as d5702 Maintaining One's Health. See "Exercise Basics" in the Techniques section for additional information.

- *Mobility*: A client who has had a lower extremity amputation will probably use a wheelchair as his/her primary mode of mobility before s/he gets a prosthesis. "Wheelchair Mobility Skills" in the Techniques section has information on how to teach these skills. A client with an upper extremity amputation will probably be able to walk unless other health conditions are present. The ICF covers these issues in Body Functions Chapter 7 Neuromusculoskeletal and Movement Related Functions and A&P Chapter 4 Mobility.

- *Cardiopulmonary endurance and muscle strength*: Identify forms of physical activity that are realistic for post-discharge participation and develop the skills and the desire so the client will be able to function with a prosthesis. See "Exercise Basics" in the Techniques section and ICF codes b455 Exercise Tolerance Functions and b730 Muscle Power Functions.

- *Activity adaptation*: Adapt activities and develop skills for the activities that the client will be participating in without a prosthesis. Work on activities that are appropriate for the client. If the client is scheduled to be back in three months for a prosthesis, don't teach the client how to do seasonal activities that are six months from now. There is more information in "Activity Pattern Development" in the Techniques section. This can be scored with d155 Acquiring Skills.

Education and Counseling

The issues the client needs to understand for better health include:

- *Inactivity*: Refer to the Concepts section for "Consequences of Inactivity" to help explain

how deconditioning will make walking with a prosthesis difficult.

- *Barriers*: See "Integration" and "Community Accessibility Training" in the Techniques section for ideas on how the help the client and the client's family get around in the community. Participating in an active leisure lifestyle that includes community activities is necessary for emotional health. Feeling stuck in the home and staring at the same four walls every day can have a devastating effect on a client's emotional health.

Prosthetic Training

This portion of the training teaches the client how to use a prosthesis.

Whole Team Approach

The client begins prosthetic training once the incision site is fully dry and healed. Clients typically receive inpatient rehab for initial prosthetic training, followed by several months of outpatient or in-home therapy. Prosthetic training focuses on achieving a proper prosthetic fit and maximizing a client's ability to perform tasks using a prosthesis. Once the client is cleared to weight bear on the stump, a wearing schedule is developed that gradually increases the length of time the prosthesis is worn (e.g., one hour on, one hour off; two hours on, two hours off). This allows the stump to desensitize to the pressure and the skin to toughen. Clients are taught how to care for the prosthesis, as well as proper techniques to: don/doff prosthesis; check residual limb for signs of skin breakdown; perform functional transfers and mobility skills; address psychosocial adjustment issues; and learn the skills and resources necessary to lead an optimally healthy, productive, and fulfilling life. Good skin/stump care is an essential component to maintaining independence. Should skin breakdown occur, the client will not be able to wear the prosthesis for a period of time, possibly resulting in further secondary problems such as deconditioning.

Recreational Therapy Approach

The primary focus is on the development of an optimally healthy lifestyle after prosthetic training for health promotion and disability/illness prevention. To achieve this, the client will require education, training, and counseling related to the use and functional incorporation of the prosthesis into home/community tasks.

Recreational Therapy Interventions

In addition to carrying over interventions from the pre-prosthetic stage, as appropriate, the following interventions are commonly used for clients with amputations after they get a prosthesis:

Functional Skill Development

- *Limb and prosthesis care*: Additional care issues include the parts of the prosthesis, how to operate and maintain a prosthesis (d6504 Maintaining Assistive Devices), how to put on and take off a prosthesis, how to incorporate the prosthesis into functional activities, how to inspect the skin on the residual limb for irritation and breakdown, how to adjust the fit of a prosthesis, how to choose and apply sock plies and other liners, abilities and restrictions related to specific activities, specialized adaptive equipment to enhance activity participation, and problem solving techniques. See "Prosthesis" and "Prosthetic Socks" in the Equipment section for more information. Score this training as d5702 Maintaining One's Health, d155 Acquiring Skills, and under the codes for particular body functions and activities.

- *Bilateral integration*: It can be difficult for a client to use a prosthesis within activities because it feels awkward and cannot be manipulated as easily as intact limbs. Incorporating the prosthesis into activities promotes movement of the residual limb and maintains muscle and joint integrity, as well as contributing to independence and functioning. Examples of working on bilateral integration include walking (using both legs) or making a craft project (using both arms). Bilateral integration includes coordination (b760 Control of Voluntary Reaction Functions), balance (b755 Involuntary Movement Reaction Functions), shifting weight from one lower extremity to the other (d4106 Shifting the Body's Center of Gravity), d430 Lifting and Carrying Objects, d440 Fine Hand Use, d445 Hand and Arm Use, d450 Walking, and specific sports movements (e.g., d4554 Swimming). Also refer to the Techniques section for "Body Mechanics and Ergonomics."

- *Postural control and alignment*: Clients have poor posture when using a prosthesis in functional tasks as a way to compensate for discomfort, awkwardness, and lack of skill. If proper body alignments and postures are not maintained, secondary problems may occur (back/hip pain) and functional abilities may not be fully maximized. Therapists teach the client how to incorporate proper posture into activities.

Scoring can be done under one of the codes in b750-b789 Movement Functions.

- *Sensory awareness and processing*: Prostheses do not provide a full sensory experience. Clients must learn how to integrate all of their senses to fully evaluate a situation (judge the ground surface or weight of an item through sight, feel the pressure on the residual limb warning the client of the need to readjust the fit of the prosthesis). This can be coded with d129 Other Purposeful Sensing.

- *Activity adaptation*: The client is taught how to adapt activities that will be part of the client's lifestyle after discharge (d155 Acquiring Skills).

Education and Counseling

Topics discussed during the pre-prosthetic stage are expanded during this stage to cover the use of the prosthesis. Those topics include inactivity, barriers, finding appropriate activities, and integration back into the community. Other topics during this stage include:

- *Energy conservation*: This is required because cardiopulmonary demands are higher when using a prosthesis. See "Energy Conservation Training" in the Techniques section. The client may need to monitor vital signs and adapt activities. S/he will also need to take increased energy demands into account when selecting a method of mobility (e.g., wheelchair propulsion, walking with lower extremity prosthesis) so that the physical demands don't exceed his/her ability or compromise health. The related ICF code is d2303 Managing One's Own Activity Level.

- *Community problem solving*: Activity-related skills such as readjusting the prosthesis in the community, changing sock plies with increased physical activity, and correlating activities with the wearing schedule. These are scored with d175 Solving Problems.

- *Community mobility skills*: These are discussed in "Walking Techniques" and "Wheelchair Mobility" in the Techniques section.

Community Recreation

The therapist is likely to see a client with an amputation in community-based sports or other recreation activities. The primary purpose of the intervention in the community is twofold: 1. ensuring adequate physical activity levels and 2. helping to improve the client's access to leisure and recreation activities. Clients with lower extremity amputations have a high risk of secondary complications because of inactivity. Often this inactivity is due to the extra energy required for mobility. Leisure activities will be suboptimal unless regular involvement in enjoyable physical activity promoting agility, balance, coordination, endurance, stretching, and strengthening occurs. Regular physical activity can increase cardiovascular endurance, mobility efficiency, and symmetry of gait (James, 1973). Access to leisure and recreation activities often involves helping the client identify activities that match the capabilities of his/her prosthesis or identifying specialty prosthetic devices required for specific activities. Many types of physical activity such as walking, riding a bike, or rowing, do not require specialized artificial limbs. Running and swimming are two activities that require specialized artificial limbs.

Miscellaneous

Amputee Coalition of America
900 East Hill Ave, Suite 285
Knoxville, Tennessee 37915-2568
1-888-AMP-KNOW (267-5669)
www.amputee-coalition.org

TRS, Inc (sport prosthetics)
3090 Sterling Circle, Studio A
Boulder, Colorado 80301-2338
1-800-279-1865
www.oandp.com

References

Apelqvist, J., Larsson, J. & Agardh, C. D. (1993). Long-term prognosis for diabetic patients with foot ulcers. *Journal of Internal Medicine, 233*(6):485-91.

Amputee Coalition of America/National Limb Loss Information Center, 2002; www.amputee-coalition.org on 6/1/02.

Bodeau, V. & Mipro, R. (2002). Lower limb prosthetics. http://www.emedicine.com/pmr/topic175.htm on 1/19/04.

Bodeau, V. & Mipro, R. (2002). Upper limb prosthetics. http://www.emedicine.com/pmr/topic174.htm on 1/19/04.

Esquenazi, A. (2003). C183: Pain management post amputation. http://www.aapmr.org/zdocs/assembly/03handouts/C183_5.pdf.

Health and Aging. (2004). Geriatric medicine in clinical practice syllabus http://www.geriatricsyllabus.com/syllabus/main.jsp?cid=SCC-CVD-6.

James, U. (1973). Effect of physical activity in healthy male unilateral above-knee amputees. *Journal of Rehabilitative Medicine, 5*:71-80.

Katzen, B. (2002). Clinical diagnosis and prognosis of acute limb ischemia. *Rev. Cardiovasc Med, 3*(suppl 2):S2-S6.

Kottke, F. & Lehmann, J. (1990). *Krusen's handbook of physical medicine and rehabilitation, 4th edition*. Philadelphia, PA: W. B. Saunders Company.

Moss Rehab. (2005). Amputation fact sheet. Moss Rehab Resource Net. http://www.mossresourcenet.org/amputa.htm.

O'Sullivan, S. & Schmitz, T. (1988). *Physical rehabilitation: Assessment and treatment, 2nd edition*. Philadelphia, PA: F. A. Davis Company

Apraxia

Apraxia is the inability to carry out movements with which the person is familiar despite having the desire and physical ability to complete the task. It is not a failure of the muscles or skeletal structure. It is also not a problem with the senses or a problem with knowledge of how to perform the task. For example, a person may understand how to push a wheelchair, and have the sensory and muscle control to push the wheelchair, but the neurological connections to demonstrate the task do not work correctly.

While apraxia affects many clients with brain injury and diseases affecting the brain, relatively little attention is paid to it compared to its disabling impact. Jacobs (2004) states that "Apraxia is one of the most important and least understood major behavioral neurology syndromes" (p. 2).

Often apraxia is described as what it is not, instead of what it is. Jacobs (2004) references Heilman's definition of apraxia as "a disorder of skilled movement not caused by weakness, akinesia [unusually limited physical activity often due to paralysis], deafferentation [an impairment in the nerves that send information from the body to the central nervous system], abnormal tone or posture, movement disorders such as tremors [rhythmic, involuntary, and purposeless quivering of muscles] or chorea [involuntary and purposeless rapid motions such as blinking, opening and closing one's hand], intellectual deterioration, poor comprehension, or uncooperativeness (p. 2). [Definition of terms added.]

There are many different categories of apraxia:

- *Buccofacial* (also known as facial-oral): The inability to make facial movements such as whistling, licking one's lips, puckering to blow bubbles, winking, or coughing. Buccofacial apraxia is the most common type of apraxia (National Institute of Neurological Disorders and Stroke, 2001).
- *Conceptual* (also called ideational): The inability to plan and carry out complex motor sequences. For example, a client with ideational apraxia would have an inability to complete leisure (and other) activities that require multiple steps such as making a sandwich, saddling a horse, sewing a dress, or square dancing. The client is still able to complete the different steps of the task but is not able to chain them together. If a client has lost the ability to physically plan the use of a piece of recreation equipment or other tools, it is also considered part of conceptual apraxia. Conceptual apraxia affects the client bilaterally with little difference of performance between the two sides of the body other than what is

normally seen with hand dominance (Zoltan, 1996).

- *Constructional*: The inability to draw or construct simple objects that have two or three dimensions. An example of constructional apraxia is the impaired ability to copy a simple line drawing such as the three-dimensional outline of a house. Another example of constructional apraxia is the inability to duplicate a pattern of dominos.
- *Developmental apraxia of speech*: The impaired ability to plan movements required for speech. The impairment is present at birth. Developmental apraxia of speech is also known as articulatory apraxia, childhood apraxia of speech, and developmental verbal apraxia. Sometimes it may also be referred to as developmental verbal dyspraxia. However, with dyspraxia the muscles are impaired, causing slurred speech and trouble with chewing. Because the two diagnoses are often mixed up, the therapist should confirm the diagnosis through ongoing observation during therapy. Clients with developmental apraxia of speech have trouble with pronouncing sounds and often use the sound "da, da, da" as their means of communication. If the client has progressed past the "da" stage, s/he often continues to have difficulty consistently producing the desired sounds after learning them. If the child is able to progress to short sentences, the child will often leave off the last part of words in the sentence. The longer the phrases or sentences become the greater the problem with clear pronunciation becomes. Clients with developmental apraxia of speech have good vocabularies. Developmental apraxia of speech is often called verbal apraxia in adults (see below).
- *Ideomotor*: The inability to demonstrate a physical movement when verbally asked to make the movement. Ideomotor apraxia is often associated with damage to the left hemisphere of the brain. Clients with ideomotor apraxia retain the neurological memory to perform the physical movements and can do so through habit.
- *Limb-kinetic*: The inability to plan fine hand use. This impairment impacts the client's ability to make precise hand movements including independent finger movements and coordination of simultaneous hand movements. Examples of specific activities that may be difficult include cutting meat with a knife and fork, "fanning" a hand of cards so that each card in the client's playing hand can be seen, many arts and crafts

projects, using a screw driver, and zipping up a jacket to stay warm.

- *Oculomotor*: The impaired ability to move the eyes horizontally in the direction that one wants. Oculomotor apraxia is a congenital disorder that may be genetically based. Because clients cannot control the horizontal movement of their eyes they often turn their head quickly to either the right or the left trying to get at least a short glimpse of the object at which they want to look. There is no known treatment for this type of apraxia although the symptoms seem to decrease over a period of a couple of decades.

- *Verbal*: The impairment of the ability to coordinate the physical movements required to produce speech. There are a variety of ways that verbal apraxia is seen in clients. Some clients consistently have trouble pronouncing longer, more complex words because they have difficulty putting together the sounds and syllables. Other clients will have an inconsistent performance, sometimes being able to put together complex words and sounds and other times being unable to do so. Another typical type of verbal apraxia is errors in prosody. Prosody is the ability to use the correct tone, rhythm, or inflection of speech to help clarify a message. Developmental apraxia of speech is considered to be a type of verbal apraxia. It is discussed separately (above) in this section because it is a common type of impairment addressed in special education.

Incidence/Prevalence in US

Apraxia is not usually considered a primary diagnosis but a symptom of other disorders. Because apraxia is considered to be the result of another diagnosis (such as traumatic brain injury or stroke) reliable national or international incidence data has not been kept (Jacobs, 2004). There have been some studies that have tried to look at the incidence of apraxia. For example, Koski, Iacoboni, & Mazziotta (2002) report that 50% of clients with left hemisphere damage due to a stroke exhibit some type of apraxia during the acute recovery stage, while only 10% of clients with right hemisphere damage due to a stroke exhibit some type of apraxia during the acute recovery stage.

Predominate Age

Motor planning impairments can occur at any age. Because many of the primary diagnoses that are associated with apraxia occur in older adults (e.g., dementia, stroke), the predominate age for clients with apraxia is older adults.

Causes

Apraxia is usually considered to be a symptom of other disorders such as stroke (CVA), traumatic brain injury, dementia, and developmental disabilities.

- Apraxia is one of the four primary symptoms of dementia: "amnesia, aphasia, agnosia, and apraxia" (Buettner, p. 136). In a study done by Della Sala, Spinnler, & Venneri (2004) over 40% of the clients with Alzheimer's disease were found to have gait apraxia, a type of limb-kinetic apraxia.

- There are two primary categories of causes for verbal apraxia: 1. acquired verbal apraxia that usually develops during adulthood (such as with stroke, head injury, infections of the brain, or tumors of the brain) and 2. developmental apraxia of speech (DAS) that originates from birth.

- Developmental apraxia of speech has no clearly identified and known cause. Brain-imaging studies have not found anomalies in the brains of children with DAS. Family histories show a tendency for DAS to run in families so there may be a genetic component to some DAS (NIDCD, 2004).

System(s) Affected

Apraxia is a general term that is used to describe a specific type of loss of function in different parts of the body. The systems affected depend on the type of apraxia.

Prognosis

- While little data is available on the morbidity or mortality associated with apraxia, clients with apraxia tend to be dependent in normal, everyday tasks. Because of this dependency many clients with apraxia require some type of assisted living or nursing home setting.

- The cause of the apraxia gives some insight into the prognosis. If a client has apraxia due to sudden trauma of the brain (such as a car accident or stroke), some recovery of function is likely to occur. If the client has apraxia due to a degenerative disease process (such as dementia or a tumor), recovery of function is less likely.

Secondary Problems

Apraxia is a general term for many different types of impairments of motor planning. However, there are studies that link certain types of apraxia with an inability to complete broader tasks. For example:

- Clients who have difficulty with making copies of simple two- or three-dimensional objects also tend to have problems with dressing themselves and with preparing meals (Neidstadt, 1991).
- Clients who have difficulty with reconstructing two- and three-dimensional objects also tend to have problems with somatognosia (body scheme disorders).
- Clients with apraxia have an increased risk of falling. See the Falls topic in "Precautions" in the Concepts section for precautions that should be taken.
- Clients with apraxia often have difficulty preparing and eating food. The client's weight should be monitored.
- Some clients will develop an involuntarily clinched fist. This is a painful secondary problem associated with the inability to make planned hand movements. If the therapist is working outside of a treatment setting and feels that a client is beginning to develop clenched fist, a referral to the client's physician is appropriate.

Assessments

Typical Scope of Team Assessment

The treatment team, including the recreational therapist, will want to determine the extent and scope of apraxia. Square-Storer (1989) points out that individual, discrete motor functions may have a greater or smaller level of impairment than the client's obvious, overall level of impairment. For example, the client's inability to plan movements for his/her left arm may be greater than the client's overall apraxia. Zoltan (1996) suggests that therapists determine if the client has a difference in motor planning performance: 1. when using different parts of the body (e.g., the left arm compared to the right arm), 2. when manipulating objects (transitive movements) compared to expressing ideas or feelings (intransitive movements), and 3. when initiating an activity compared to continuing an activity (e.g., does the client get "stuck" initiating an activity but then completes the activity once started or does the client have problems with each step of the activity).

The NIDCD (2004) recommends that the treatment team rule out other speech and language problems such as muscle weakness and comprehension problems before determining that a client has apraxia. They also recommend that the assessment of function take place over a number of evaluation sessions that include actual activity participation as a portion of the evaluation.

Anticipated Findings of RT Assessment

While it is common for acquired apraxia to show some spontaneous recovery (recovery not linked to treatment), developmental apraxia of speech seldom improves without direct and often intense therapy. The on-going recreational therapy assessments should have specific enough criteria to note change in performance. Change in performance in children is much more likely to be a direct result of intervention than with adults because of adults' ability for some spontaneous recovery.

A fairly detailed history of the client's daily leisure patterns that shows a fairly dramatic decline in physical activity in older adults may be a good indicator of a slowly progressing apraxia related to dementia and other brain disorders. The recreational therapist may find that the client has lost incentive to engage in leisure activities that were previously important to the client. Even if the rest of the treatment team has not identified apraxia as a diagnosis, the possibility should be explored. For example, if the client sits and watches television all day when s/he was previously active, the therapist and treatment team should explore the possibility of apraxia as being the underlying cause of inactivity.

See b176 Mental Functions of Sequencing Complex Movements for more information about specific recreational therapy tests for apraxia.

Treatment Direction

Treatment for apraxia in covered in b176 Mental Functions of Sequencing Complex Movements. Different kinds of apraxia require different treatments as discussed in that section.

Since apraxia is usually considered a secondary impairment as a result of another diagnosis (such as brain injury or dementia), the therapist should also refer to the treatment interventions for the primary diagnosis or the deficits caused by the primary diagnosis.

References

Buettner, L. (1998). Activities as an intervention for disturbed behaviors on the dementia-specific care unit. In Kaplan, M. & Hoffman, S. *Behaviors in dementia: Best practices for successful management*. Baltimore, MD: Health Professions Press.

Della Sala, S., Spinnler, H. & Venneri, A. (2004). Walking difficulties in patients with Alzheimer's disease might originate from gait apraxia. *J. Neurol Neurosurg Psychiatry, 75*(2):196-201.

Jacobs, D. (2004). Excerpt from *Apraxia and related syndromes*. emedicine. May 6, 2004. http://www.emedicine.com/neuro/byname/apraxia-and-related-syndromes.htm

Koski, L., Iacoboni, M. & Mazziotta, J. (2002). Deconstructing apraxia: Understanding disorders of intentional movement after stroke. *Current Opinion in Neurology, 15*:71-77.

National Institute of Neurological Disorders and Stroke. (2001). NINDS Apraxia information page. www.ninds.nih.gov/disorders/apraxia/apraxia.htm

NIDCD (National Institute on Deafness and Other Communication Disorders). (2004). Apraxia of speech. www.nidcd.nih.gov/health/voice/apraxia.asp

Niestadt, M. (1991). Occupational therapy treatment for constructional deficits. *American Journal of Occupational Therapy 46*(2):141-148 reported in Zoltan, 1996.

Square-Storer, P. (1989). *Acquired apraxia of speech.* New York: Taylor & Francis.

Zoltan, B. (1996). *Vision, perception, and cognition: A manual for the evaluation and treatment of the neurologically impaired adult.* Thorofare, NJ: Slack.

Attention-Deficit/Hyperactivity Disorder

Attention-Deficit/Hyperactivity Disorder (ADHD) is a type of developmental disability in which clients have a decreased ability to attend to tasks and an increased, age-inappropriate level of activity. Often poor social skills are part of the disorder. ADHD is the general term for three types of attention deficit or hyperactivity all of which significantly reduce the client's functional ability in at least two of three settings: 1. home, 2. school, and 3. work. The three types are 1. hyperactivity (attention-deficit/hyperactivity disorder, predominantly hyperactive-impulsive type), 2. inattention (attention-deficit/hyperactivity disorder, predominately inattentive type), and 3. combined hyperactivity and inattention (attention-deficit/hyperactivity disorder, combined type). The most frequently mentioned characteristics of clients with ADHD are "1. hyperactivity, 2. perceptual motor impairment, 3. emotional lability, 4. general coordination deficit, 5. disorders of attention (short attention span, distractibility, perseveration, failure to finish things, inattention, poor concentration), 6. impulsivity (action before thought, abrupt shifts in activity, lack of organization, jumping up in class), 7. disorders of memory and thinking, 8. specific learning disabilities, 9. disorders of speech and hearing, and 10. equivocal neurological signs and EEG irregularities" (Kaplan, Sadock, & Grebb, 1994, p. 1066).

Incidence/Prevalence in US

There are numerous groups that have published prevalence rates. They include the US Surgeon General (1999) 3-5% of school-aged children; Mayo Clinic (2001) 7.5% of school-aged children; Centers for Disease Control and Prevention (2002) 7% of school-aged children between the ages of 6-11 years. The CDC broke the numbers down to ADHD without a learning disability (3.3%) and with a learning disability (3.5%).

Predominate Age

ADHD is most noticeable between the ages of two years and eleven years. It is commonly diagnosed once the child reaches school age and problems are noted by teachers. Symptoms become less severe for the vast majority of clients as they approach twenty years of age. This is probably due in part to the reduction in neurobiological causes (they "grow out of it") and an increase in adaptive skills.

Causes

Currently there is no clearly identified, underlying cause of ADHD. ADHD has a neurobiological basis with heredity having a strong influence in most cases. When the client's biological family does not have ADHD in its history, other factors such as high lead concentrations in the blood, prenatal exposure to tobacco and alcohol, low birth weight, or difficulties during pregnancy are potential risk factors. Research does not support the common myths that ADHD is caused by "excessive sugar intake, food additives, excessive viewing of television, poor child management by parents, or social and environmental factors such as poverty or family chaos" (National Resource Center on AD/HD, 2004). Psychosocial factors also play a role in the development of ADHD: "Children in institutions are frequently overactive and have poor attention spans. These signs result from prolonged emotional deprivation, and they disappear when the deprivation ends, such as through adoption or placement in a foster home. Stressful psychic events, disruption of family equilibrium, and other anxiety inducing factors contribute to the initiation or perpetuation of ADHD. Predisposing factors may include the child's temperament, genetic-familial factors, and the demands of society to adhere to a routine way of behaving and performing. Socioeconomic status does not seem to be a predisposing factor" (Sadock & Sadock, 2003).

System(s) Affected

ADHD affects the brain as measured by abnormal but nonspecific results on EEGs and PETs (positron emission tomography). Cognitive testing often reveals decreased cognitive processing ability related to decreased attention span and impulsivity. Central nervous system involvement is often seen in activity limitations and participation restrictions due to problems with perceptual motor function and coordination. Emotional health may be affected with increased incidences of depression and interpersonal problems that may be a direct result of an organic problem or an indirect result of people's negative reactions to the client's impaired social skills.

Prognosis

- While ADHD is considered to be a chronic disorder, it is common for ADHD to diminish in part or fully between the ages of twelve and twenty years. Approximately 80% of children with ADHD experience a significant reduction in impairment as they reach adulthood and are able to lead productive lives as adults (Kaplan, Sadock, & Grebb, 1994). Of the various impairments associated with ADHD, hyperactivity is usually the first to decline with attention span and impulse control impairments lingering. Adults with ADHD tend to be more accident-prone and more impulsive than the general population.

- Adolescents with a dual diagnosis of ADHD and conduct disorder have a 50% chance of being diagnosed with antisocial personality disorder as adults.
- The lingering secondary effects of ADHD are impaired self-esteem, continued learning problems, and impaired social-emotional development and skills.

Secondary Problems

- *Conduct disorders*: Clients diagnosed as having the hyperactivity-impulsivity subtype of ADHD are more likely to have a dual diagnosis of conduct disorder than clients with attention deficit subtype (Kaplan, Sadock, Grebb, 1994).
- *Aggression*: About 75% of children with ADHD show fairly consistent behaviors of aggression and defiance (Sadock & Sadock, 2003).
- *Social skills*: Often social skills are learned through observation and incidental learning. Because of the nature of their impairment, clients with ADHD are not able to use this method of learning and consequently have impaired social skills. Behavioral issues related to ADHD such as inability to delay gratification, jumping up out of their seat at school, emotional lability (easily set off to laughter or tears), perseveration, and unpredictable mood (explosive, irritated by minor stimuli) also limit the number and quality of peer social interactions, affecting social skills development. The lack of age-appropriate social skills typically causes problems fitting in with peers. Studies have shown that children who have a problem fitting in with their peers are at a higher risk for "anxiety, behavioral and mood disorders, substance abuse, and delinquency as teenagers" (National Resource Center on AD/HD, 2004).
- *Dislike for school*: The acquisition, retention, and display of knowledge are hampered by ADHD and other secondary disorders (e.g., a learning disability, communication disorder). "The adverse reactions of school personnel to the behavior characteristics of ADHD and the lowering of self-regard because of felt inadequacies may combine with the adverse comments of peers to make school a place of unhappy defeat" (Sadock & Sadock, 2003). Antisocial behavior and self-defeating, self-punitive behaviors often occur as a result.

- *Impaired community integration skills*: Clients with ADHD have a higher than normal incidence of functional deficits in their ability to 1. comprehend what they read, 2. use math in everyday situations, and 3. manage perceptual motor coordination.
- *Impaired sense of self*: Often clients with ADHD have IQs within the normal range and can understand, to some degree, that they are "different" from other children. Often the behaviors associated with the disorder cause others to ostracize or "put down" these clients contributing to impaired self-esteem, self-confidence, and self-image. Social-emotional impairment is common.
- *Physical activity deficits*: Perceptual motor deficit and general coordination deficit can make it difficult for children with ADHD to participate in sports and other high-level physical activities. Consequently, children with ADHD may feel like failures in physical as well as intellectual tasks.

Assessments

Typical Scope of Team Assessment

Initial symptoms of ADHD, although recognized most often by parents and teachers, are formally diagnosed by a psychiatrist. The criteria for ADHD are defined in the *DSM-IV-TR*.

Using the criteria from the *DSM-IV-TR* to plan treatment for a client with ADHD is not appropriate. The *DSM-IV-TR* criteria should be used only as a screening tool to determine if further assessment is needed. The American Academy of Child and Adolescent Psychiatry lists the most commonly used assessments to determine the treatment that is required as: 1. Parent-completed *Child Behavior Checklist*, 2. *Teacher Report Form* (TRF) of the Child Behavior Checklist, 3. *Conners Parent and Teacher Rating Scales*, 4. ADD-H: *Comprehensive Teacher Rating Scale* (ACTeRS), 5. *Barkley Home Situations Questionnaire* (HSQ), and 6. *Barkley School Situations Questionnaire* (SSQ).

For recreational therapy, tools such as the *Therapeutic Recreation Activity Assessment* (TRAA), the 22 modules in the *Community Integration Program*, the *CERT-Psych/R*, and the *School Social Behavior Scale* (SSBS) will all help pinpoint specific functional impairments and restrictions that need to be addressed in the therapy treatment plan.

Anticipated Findings of RT Assessment

- Recent research indicates that one of the main impairments related to ADHD is impaired executive function. The three areas of executive function that are impaired are 1. working memory (the ability to hold information that was just presented and integrating it into past memory), 2. basic personal organization (e.g., putting things away so that they can be found later, time management, money management), and 3. sense of time (National Resource Center on AD/HD, 2004).
- The therapist helps determine the subtype of ADHD through observing the client's performance in structured tasks that require continuous performance. For example, clients with hyperactivity make errors of commission. Errors of commission mean that the client repeats the activity or motion many more times than appropriate for the situation. If the activity is for the child to find and circle specific items in a drawing (finding the hidden objects), the client with hyperactivity will circle many more objects than the instructions say should be circled. Clients with impulsivity make errors of omission. Errors of omission mean that the client is not able to attend to the task and does not complete the task even though the client indicates s/he is done. For example, in finding hidden objects, the client will give up on the activity before the task is completed at an age-appropriate level.
- Clients are likely to have impaired abilities in peer relationships (lack basic social skills, inattention to direct and subtle cues from others, poor follow-through on commitments, impulsive actions and emotions that may negatively impact others).
- It is not uncommon for a client with hyperactivity-impulsivity ADHD to have better control in some situations such as one-on-one time with the therapist or watching DVDs. The therapist should document the types of situations in which the client is able to function with less impairment.
- Aggressive or defiant behavior is often found, especially when the client is challenged with a difficult activity or if gratification is delayed.
- Impaired self-esteem, self-confidence, and self-image are evident through conversation and reflection activities (e.g., making each letter in the child's name into a positive attribute).
- Due to struggles with intellectual and physical activities, the client may have an unhealthy leisure balance. Leisure activities that have

instant gratification without much intellectual or gross motor skill are often preferred.

Treatment Direction

Whole Team Approach

The treatment team usually takes a bimodal approach to ADHD. Medication and behavioral interventions are often paired together. Medication reduces the behavior. Behavioral modification interventions teach adaptive skills to help increase functioning within specific environments (e.g., school).

Recreational Therapy Approach

Recreational therapists work with clients with ADHD in many different settings (e.g., community recreation program, school setting, rehab setting with ADHD as a secondary diagnosis). Interventions utilized include those that increase functioning in particular environments (e.g., peer recreation, school), with special attention to psychosocial skills including the development of social skills, a healthy sense of self, and a balanced leisure lifestyle.

Recreational Therapy Interventions

Interventions used by recreational therapists for ADHD will vary depending upon many variables including the setting, the impact of dysfunction on particular life activities, the reason for treatment, age of the client, and the level of family involvement. Behavior modification is the foundation for working on many of the skills listed below. See "Behavioral Manipulation" in the Techniques section for guidelines. Some of the most common interventions include:

- *Time management skills*: See b1642 Time Management.
- *Organization skills*: See b1641 Organization and Planning.
- *Memory training*: See b144 Memory Functions.
- *Attention training*: See b140 Attention Functions.
- *Social skills training*: Specific practice in multiple social skills is necessary for clients to improve social skills. Role modeling, play-acting, and other methods of practicing critical social skills may be necessary. During this type of treatment intervention it is important that the therapist be very concrete about the targeted social skills, providing verbal instructions and demonstrating specific actions to be taken. Clients with ADHD seem to have difficulty transferring learned skills from one setting to

another therefore it is important for clients to have many opportunities to practice applying learned social skills in different settings. Studies have found that even after clients with ADHD learn social skills they often need to be cued to use these skills, so cueing may need to be included in the behavior modification program (National Resource Center on AD/HD, 2004). See Activities and Participation Chapter 7 Interpersonal Interactions and Relationships, *Leisure and Social/Sexual Assessment*, and the Techniques section for "Coping with Stress," "Interpersonal Relationship Activities," and "Social Skills Training."

- *Self-esteem*: See "Self-Esteem" in the Techniques section.
- *Managing aggressive behavior*: See "Anger Management" and "Relaxation and Stress Reduction" in the Techniques section.
- *Healthy leisure lifestyle*: See "Activity Pattern Development" and "Education and Counseling" in the Techniques section. Clients with hyperactivity often have difficulty engaging in leisure activities. They may start, but not finish, activities. Leisure education is often initially directed toward finding activities that match or are just a little beyond the client's attention span. Activities that require a longer attention span or more attention to safety than the client is capable of demonstrating should not be used even if they are more interesting to the client.
- *Money management skills*: See b172 Calculation Functions. See d860 Basic Economic Transactions. Clients with ADHD often have problems with managing their money and benefit from very specific, adaptive techniques for money management. Community outings to malls or other locations that offer many purchasing options may be contraindicated until the client has integrated money management strategies that curb impulsive shopping.

Miscellaneous

Parents are encouraged to provide praise and encouragement, focus on the positive, and instill a healthy sense of self in children who have ADHD.

Reference

Centers for Disease Control and Prevention. (2002). Vital and health statistics. www.help4adhd.org/en/about/causes.

Kaplan, H. I., Sadock, V., & Grebb, J. (1994). *Kaplan and Sadock's synopsis of psychiatry: Behavioral sciences clinical psychiatry, 7th edition.* Philadelphia, PA: Lippincott, Williams & Wilkins.

Mayo Clinic. (2001). *Journal of American Medical Association,* January 2001. www.help4adhd.org/en/about/causes.

National Resource Center on AD/HD. (2004). About AD/HD: Causes and pathophysiology. www.help4adhd.org/en/about/causes.

Sadock, B. & Sadock, V. (2003). *Synopsis of psychiatry, 9th edition.* Philadelphia, PA: Lippincott, Williams & Wilkins.

United States Surgeon General. (1999). *1999 Report of the US Surgeon General on mental health,* chapter 3. www.help4adhd.org/en/about/causes.

Back Disorders and Back Pain

There are many different conditions included in the general category of back disorders and back pain. The ones are described here are acute spasms, chronic strains, herniated disks, spinal stenosis, and degenerative disk disease.

Acute sprain without disk rupture: An acute sprain means that a back muscle, ligament, or capsule of the neural arch joints has been injured. The neural arch joints, also called facet joints, are where facets from the two vertebras hook together with cartilage inside a joint capsule. Acute sprains can occur from an excessive stress on a well-conditioned back (e.g., lifting a car engine), a minor stress on a normal but unprepared back (e.g., lifting an object without bending the knees), or a minor stress on an unconditioned or diseased back. Back pain is often experienced immediately with the task. The pain may then dissipate or "let up" but often becomes more intense within several hours after the event. The pain intensifies when swelling (edema) and inflammation at the site cause pressure and pain. The muscles around the site will typically go into spasm to protect the injury, causing additional pain. The pain may also radiate. Pain is felt with movement (kinetic pain) and with rest (static pain).

Chronic strain without disk rupture: The term "strain" means that the tissues involved have exceeded their endurance capacity and pain occurs with physical stress at the site. It can be caused and aggravated by persistent static positions (sitting or standing for prolonged periods of time) or repeated kinetic movement (especially bending forward repetitively over a long period of time). Prior acute sprains, poor posture, obesity, pregnancy, and general deconditioning are conditions that commonly contribute to this problem.

Static pain: The pain is often felt in an unmoving position (especially prolonged standing or sitting) and eased with frequent positional changes. It is not felt with movement (kinetic pain). The pain is usually described as throbbing and aching or sharp and intense. It may radiate into the buttocks, but it rarely radiates into the legs. People who have an increased lumbar curve (lumbar lordosis) seem to be prone to chronic back strain. Genetics may play a role in lumbar lordosis or it may be caused by continual accentuation of the curve by activities or conditions that pull the curve more forward (e.g., large stomach, wearing high heels, standing sway backed). The excessive curve can often be treated by losing weight, strengthening back muscles, and switching to flat or low heel shoes. If the lordosis is allowed to persist, the back can lose flexibility to bend forward and result in kinetic pain.

Kinetic pain: Strain is caused by too much forward bending (e.g., factory worker, child care worker), lower back stresses that are beyond the person's capacity (e.g., lifting 40 pound boxes when the client is only able to lift 30 pound boxes) and poor body mechanics (e.g., lifting using the back instead of bending the knees and using the legs to bear the weight). It often occurs at the location of prior back sprains, Pain is felt when bending forward and resuming an erect posture. It may also be felt in static standing and sitting positions. People who have this problem often have limited back flexibility. The normal lumbar curve is supposed to round when bending forward and in this case it is not. In addition, if the hamstring muscles are tight, they do not lengthen to allow the back to round, contributing to the limitations in flexibility. As the condition progresses, muscle spasms can occur and cause further limitation on the client's ability to lean forward, creating back rigidity (chronic tightness). Scoliosis (sideways curvature of the spine) can occur if rigidity occurs on one side of the back.

Herniated nucleus pulposus (HNP): Between each pair of vertebra is an intervertebral disk. The intervertebral disk provides a cushion that keeps the vertebras apart so they do not rub against each other. They also help in keeping the connecting ligaments taut. The center of the intervertebral disk is called the nucleus pulposus. It is a gel-like substance. The nucleus pulposus is surrounded by tough collagen fibers called the "annulus." An acute sprain or a long-standing strain problem can cause a tear in the annulus allowing the nucleus pulposus to protrude through it (herniate). When the disk ruptures, it can bulge against the posterior longitudinal ligament that lies outside of the annulus (causing inflammation that then impinges on the spinal nerve) and/or it can bulge somewhat laterally (to the side) and cause direct pressure on the spinal nerve. Pain is worse with movement. The pain is exacerbated by laughing, coughing, or straining bowels.

Spinal stenosis: The spinal canal space is narrowed and the spinal nerves that run through the spinal canal become trapped, squeezed, and impinged resulting in pain. People who have spinal stenosis often have a diminished canal space to begin with (congenital) and then degenerative changes in the spine further diminish the spinal canal space. It may be caused by osteoarthritis, Paget's disease, or spondylolisthesis with edema of the cauda equina (Berkow, 1992). It typically affects people in middle age and older adults. It commonly affects the sciatic nerve causing pain to radiate down through the buttocks and legs and causing numbness, tingling, loss of sensation, and muscle weakness. The pain is felt with walking and is relieved by sitting or flexing the back (bending over). Consequently, people with spinal stenosis find it less painful to walk up hills than down hills because the back is somewhat flexed when walking up a hill.

Degenerative disk disease (DDD): The intervertebral disk gradually dehydrates and the annulus begins to break down (collagen fibers fray) as part of the normal aging process. As a result, the disks begin to collapse, the ligaments become slack (because the intervertebral disk is no longer keeping the ligaments taut), and bony overgrowth invades the disk (osteophytes). Nerve roots can become trapped, squeezed, or impinged. The pressure on the nerves and the lack of mobility in the spine can cause both static and kinetic pain. Mobility is more difficult in trunk extension (standing upright) compared to flexion (bending). Pain can radiate down the buttocks and the legs along with numbness, tingling, loss of sensation, and muscle weakness. The degenerative process can also affect one side of the back and contribute to the development of scoliosis. Interestingly, not everyone experiences pain with this process. It is speculated that people who manage spinal stressors (e.g., do not have a history of acute sprains and chronic strain) and keep muscles well conditioned have a greater chance of going through the DDD process without associated pain.

Fibromyalgia: People with fibromyalgia may experience localized or generalized back pain (see diagnosis of "Fibromyalgia").

Descriptors of Back Pain

See Body Functions Chapter 2 Sensory Functions and Pain for information on pain descriptors (acute, chronic, psychogenic).

Incidence/Prevalence in US

The prevalence of back disorders increases with age, reaching 50% in persons over the age of 60 (Berkow, 1992). Back pain (in any form) affects about 15 million people in the United States (Sadock & Sadock, 2003).

Predominant Age

See above

Causes

The causes of the disorders and pain are described above. Also see b280 Sensation of Pain for more information about pain and its causes.

System(s) Affected

Back disorders and pain primarily affect the muscular system and the spinal system.

Prognosis

The prognosis will vary depending on the extent of the injury, the client's past medical history as it impacts recovery, the client's age, the client's activity level, the client's adherence to treatment direction, the psychological state of the client, and any complications from surgery (if performed). Some clients will recover from single episodes of back injuries with no further complications. Others will have ongoing problems that significantly affect the rest of their lives.

Secondary Problems

Deconditioning from limited mobility is common, as well as secondary complications related to inactivity (see "Consequences of Inactivity" in the Concepts section). Limited back flexibility, activities of daily living (e.g., dressing, bathing, meal preparation), and community activities (e.g., work, school, recreation) can also be negatively affected.

Assessments

See b280 - b289 Pain for information about pain assessment.

Anticipated Findings from RT Assessment

- Recreational therapists who see clients with back problems in an inpatient rehabilitation hospital usually find that the clients have had chronic pain for a long period of time and are there either to rehabilitate from a surgical procedure (e.g., laminectomy) or for general conditioning and pain management.
- Therapists may find that the client has been self-medicating with alcohol or drugs to manage pain levels.
- Clients will typically report a lifestyle of progressive losses associated with chronic pain including loss of activity level, loss of a job, loss of identity through job, loss of a family role, loss of favorite hobbies or recreational activities, loss of internal locus of control (pain controls everything), loss of relationships (divorce, friendship), loss of sexuality and intimacy due to pain and

psychological stressors, loss of sleep, loss of appetite, loss of positive feelings (depression), and loss of positive self-image (e.g., appearance, self-esteem, confidence). Consequently, the therapist will find a multitude of other dynamics that may need to be addressed (e.g., communication skills, self-esteem, sexuality, leisure issues).

- Clients who are unemployed or on workers' compensation, often report increased levels of pain since they stopped working. This could be attributed to further deconditioning due to a decreased activity level and/or an increased awareness and sensitivity to the pain because other stimuli related to work are no longer available.

- Clients with a long-standing history of chronic pain often exhibit signs of learned helplessness.

Treatment Direction

"Any type of back pain may be influenced by psychosocial problems and conflicts; these factors regularly alter the patient's perception, behavior, reporting of structurally mediated pain, as well as the resultant degree of dysfunction, disability, and response to therapy" (Berkow, 1992, pg. 1363).

Whole Team Approach

Acute sprain without disk rupture: In order for the tissue to heal, the client will need to rest the area and seek medical attention. To decrease the muscle spasm the client is to lie down on a bed in a comfortable position with his/her hips and knees flexed. The use of heat, massage, oral analgesics (e.g., aspirin, codeine), and/or muscle relaxants (e.g., diazepam) is also helpful. The client is encouraged to rest, but not to sustain bed rest for long periods of time. Manipulation (chiropractics) may help to relieve the pain if it is due to muscle spasm only. Manipulation can aggravate an arthritic joint or further rupture a disk, so careful consideration of this intervention is essential. The physician may limit the client's activities and prescribe physical therapy if pain does not subside. If the treatment recommendations are not followed, the tissue may not heal correctly. This could weaken the area and predispose it to further injury. It could also cause long-term chronic pain. If the acute sprain was due to pregnancy or obesity, the client should wear a lumbosacral corset (sometimes referred to as a "belly bra" for a pregnant woman) after the acute sprain has subsided to help support the lower back. The lumbosacral corset is not a long-term solution. Once the sprain is healed, lumbosacral flexion exercises are often recommended to lessen lumbar lordosis. Other exercises are often used to strengthen the abdominal muscles to help support the skeletal and muscular structures of the back and decrease the risk of the condition becoming chronic or recurrent.

Chronic low back pain: Treatment is aimed at relieving the cause of the pain. This could include weight reduction for people who are obese, improving muscle strength (especially in the abdomen and back), and improving posture. Pain medication may be prescribed to help manage the pain and increase the client's ability to engage in life tasks. Narcotics are usually avoided (Berkow, 1992), although narcotic medication is considered as a treatment option for severe chronic pain that does not have a correctable source. See the note on narcotics below.

Herniated nucleus pulposus (HNP): Clients are typically instructed to follow treatment recommendations similar to those used for acute and chronic sprains. Unlike a chronic sprain, surgery or site injections may be an option if the pain does not resolve and it significantly impacts the client's ability to engage in life tasks.

Spinal stenosis: Conservative measures are for the client to achieve an ideal body weight, improve his/her posture, and strengthen abdominal muscles to help support the back. If these methods do not help to relieve the pain, surgery may be considered. The usual procedure is called a decompression laminectomy. This surgery opens up the spinal canal by excision of a vertebral lamina (cuts away part of a vertebra to alleviate pressure on the spinal nerve).

Degenerative disk disease (DDD): If pain is present (not everyone with DDD experiences pain), proper conditioning of muscles and use of proper body mechanics should help alleviate some of the pain. Surgery or the use of a corset may also be a viable treatment option if more conservative measures fail.

Notes: Interventions will usually include any precautions or parameters set by the treating physician or surgeon. The instructions may include weight lifting restrictions, specific activity restrictions, specific movement restrictions (e.g., avoid excessive trunk rotation and bending), wearing schedules (e.g., must wear thoracic lumbar sacral orthosis when out of bed), and wearing a specific device (e.g., soft collar, corset). The physician will write an order for the specific precautions and parameters that need to be followed.

Narcotics are often a choice for treating pain, but they have significant side effects with the kinds of pain involved in back problems. They are addictive and clients can build up a tolerance to narcotic medication. A better choice is to focus on alternative therapies. One possibility is to increase the body's endorphin level with therapy programs that focus on promoting endorphin release through exercise, laughter, and positive feelings and mood.

Other therapies that are used for back pain include electrical stimulation of the painful area (transcutaneous electric nerve stimulation, TENS) and acupuncture. Studies to show the effectiveness of these are inconclusive.

Recreational Therapy Approach

Recreational therapy primarily focuses on pain management and resumption of life activities.

Recreational Therapy Interventions

Common interventions for recreational therapy include:

- *Body mechanics and ergonomics*: Clients are taught proper body mechanics and ergonomics as they relate to particular recreational and community activities. See "Body Mechanics and Ergonomics" in the Techniques section and ICF sections d410 Changing Basic Body Positions and d5700 Ensuring One's Physical Comfort.
- *Pain management*: The therapist addresses issues that contribute to pain levels including lack of physical exercise, smoking, distorted and negative thinking patterns, absence of laughter, high levels of stress, and shallow breathing. Some modalities include:
  - o Physical exercise to promote endorphin release, aid in weight reduction, and strengthen the abdomen and back. See "Exercise Basics" in the Techniques section for more information.
  - o Laughter and positive mood in therapy sessions to show a balance of emotions. See b1522 Range of Emotion.
  - o Self-confidence and self-esteem by showing the client s/he can do something to relieve the pain.
  - o Internal locus of control for clients who have let pain control their activities.
  - o Smoking cessation described in "Contributors to Stress" under d240 Handling Stress and Other Psychological Demands.
  - o Relaxation training including progressive muscle relaxation and deep breathing. See "Stress Reduction and Relaxation Training" in the Techniques section and d2401 Handling Stress in the ICF codes.
- *Problem solving and resource awareness*: Resource awareness and community problem

solving (d175 Solving Problems) so the client knows how to access resources to problem solve for barriers. See "Community Accessibility Training" in the Techniques section.

- *Energy conservation techniques*: People with chronic back pain often have a history of progressive inactivity due to the pain. During the time the client is rebuilding his/her conditioning, "Energy Conservation Training" in the Techniques section and d2303 Managing One's Own Activity Level may be useful.
- *Community mobility*: Mobility skills addressed will depend on the needs of the client. Activities and Participation Chapter 4 Mobility discusses these issues.
- *Integration*: If clients have not left their home for a long period of time and have convinced themselves that community activity is impossible they may need some integration training. See "Integration" in the Techniques section for more information. Other issues that are addressed include:
  - o "Community Accessibility Training," "Community Leisure Resource Awareness," "Community Problem Solving," and "Personal Leisure Resources Awareness" in the Techniques section.
  - o "Americans with Disabilities Act Education" in the Techniques section.

Other issues that may be seen include lack of knowledge about issues related to:

- *Sexuality*: See b640 Sexual Functions.
- *Inactivity*: See "Consequences of Inactivity" in the Concepts section.
- *Leisure attitudes and values*: Include how recreation leads to better health. See "Education and Counseling" in the Techniques section.
- *New leisure activities*: See "Activity Pattern Development" in the Techniques section.
- *Anger management*: This is especially important related to coping with pain in a healthy manner. See "Anger Management" in the Techniques section.

References

Berkow, R. (1992). *The Merck manual of diagnosis and therapy*. Rahway, NJ: Merck Research Laboratories.

Eliot, R. (1994). *From stress to strength*. New York, New York: Bantam Books

Sadock, B. & Sadock, V. (2003). *Kaplan & Sadock's synopsis of psychiatry, 9th edition*. Philadelphia, PA: Lippincott Williams & Wilkins

Burns

A burn is damage to body tissue that may be caused by chemicals, electricity, heat (thermal), or radiation. Burns are described, or graded, by a combination of severity and percentage of body injured. For clients with burns significant enough to be hospitalized, the treatment causes them to "get worse" before they get better due to the treatments required to treat the burns and save the client's life.

Incidence/Prevalence in US

- Approximately 50,000 people are admitted to US hospitals a year for burns with around 20,000 being directly admitted or transferred to burn units because of the severity of their burns (American College of Surgeons, 1999).
- On the average in the United States in 2001, someone died in a fire nearly every three hours and someone was injured every 34 minutes (CDC NCIPC, 2004).
- In 2001 fire departments responded to 396,500 home fires in the Untied States, which claimed the lives of an estimated 3,140 people and injured another 15,575. Approximately 85% of all US fire deaths occurred in homes (CDC NCIPC, 2004).
- The United States has the fourth highest fire death rate of all industrialized countries. Residential fires are the most important causes of fire-related mortality (CDC NCIPC, 2004).
- 41,000 heat burns resulted in an average of four lost days of work each. Breakdowns of industrial burns were as follows: 16,500 retail trade; 9,500 manufacturing; 8,600 service industry (such as restaurants) (Burnsurvivor Resource Guide, 2004).
- 15,700 chemical burns resulted in an average of two lost days of work each. Breakdowns were as follows: 5,800 manufacturing (such as chemical manufacturers); 3,200 service industry; 2,600 retail industry (Burnsurvivor Resource Guide, 2004).
- Scalds are the leading cause of accidental death in the home for children from birth to age four and are 40% of the burn injuries for children up to age 14 (Burnsurvivor Resource Guide, 2004).

Predominant Age

Groups at increased risk of fire-related injuries and deaths include: children four years and younger, adults 65 years and older, African-Americans and Native Americans, the poorest Americans, people living in rural areas, and people living in manufac-

tured homes or substandard housing (CDC NCIPC, 2004).

Causes

- Cooking is the primary cause of residential fires; smoking is the leading cause of fire-related deaths (CDC NCIPC, 2004).
- Alcohol use contributes to an estimated 40% of residential fire deaths (CDC NCIPC, 2004).
- Most victims of fires die from smoke or toxic gases and not from burns (CDC NCIPC, 2004).
- The out of doors is the most common location to be burned for clients between the ages of five and 74 (Burnsurvivor Resource Guide, 2004).
- Burns as a form of child abuse are as common as central nervous system damage from abuse and two to three times as frequent as skeletal injury, soft tissue injury, abdominal injury, or sexual abuse (Whaley & Wong, 1991).
- Burns follow seasonal trends. Burns due to heating devices and house fires in general typically occur during the winter. Burns due to barbeques and campfires increase during the summer as do injuries from fireworks (around July 4th in the United States). In 2001, emergency rooms saw 9,500 people with fireworks related injuries; more than half involving burns (CDC NCIPC).

System(s) Affected

Even though a burn may appear to affect only the tissue damaged, a significant burn affects almost all systems of the body. See Signs and Symptoms (below) for more information.

Prognosis

- First-degree burns and all but the most severe of the second-degree burns will heal in one to three weeks without medical intervention. Without medical intervention some of the second-degree burns will heal leaving a skin surface that is normal to slightly pitted and with inconsistent pigmentation of the skin.
- Severe second-degree burns and less severe, small-area third degrees may benefit from elective skin grafts and generally take more than three weeks to heal. Pitted, flat and shiny, unevenly pigmented skin and scar tissue should be expected.
- Most third-degree and fourth-degree burns will not heal well without medical intervention.

- Fifty percent survival can be expected with a 62% body surface area (BSA) burn in ages 0-14 years, 63% BSA burn in ages 15-40 years, 38% BSA burn in ages 40-65 years, and 25% BSA burn in patients over 65 years (Dambro, 1998).

Secondary Problems

It is common for the tissue damaged by the burn to be only one of the life threatening situations caused by the burn. Patients also need to be evaluated for fluid/chemical imbalances that occur as a direct result of the burn, respiratory distress, and the psychological impact of the pain and resulting scaring.

During the first 48 hours after a severe burn, body fluids rapidly go to the affected area causing body-wide chemical imbalances and edema. This is followed by an opposite reaction by the body with the withdrawal of fluids from the site and another swing in body fluid imbalance.

The initial movement of fluids to the burn site causes:

- hypovolemia (a lack of blood volume causing life threatening shock),
- hypoproteinemia (an abnormal amount of protein in the blood that tends to cause abdominal pain, diarrhea, edema, and nausea),
- hyponatremia (an inadequate amount of sodium in the blood that may lead to confusion and memory problems, convulsions, and coma),
- hypokalemia (inadequate amount of potassium in the blood that may cause weakness or flaccid paralysis),
- hypotension (blood pressure so low that the body has trouble getting oxygen to tissues), and
- oliguria (problems with producing and passing urine causing the waste produced by the body to build up in the body) (Anderson, Anderson, Glanze, 1994).

After the initial 48 hours the body starts moving fluids away from the damaged tissue resulting in

- decreased serum electrolytes (serum is the sticky fluid portion of the blood that contains electrolytes but not blood cells, platelets, or fibrinogen and a loss of serum electrolytes decreases the body's ability to contract or relax muscle tissue, including the heart),
- diuresis (an abnormally increased production and secretion of urine),
- Curling stress ulcer (a peptic ulcer in the duodenal that is common in people who have acute, severe burns), and
- increased blood volume.

Around 20-40% of clients with severe burns also have respiratory complications (DeGregorio, 1984). The respiratory complications include (Whaley & Wong, 1991):

- *Inhalation injury*: trauma caused to airway and lung tissue due to heat (usually above the vocal cords) and chemical burns (carbon monoxide or other noxious gases) below the vocal cords.
- *Aspiration in unconscious clients*: the entry of secretions, solids, or fluids into the tracheobronchial passages (airway and lungs) that normally would be blocked if the client was conscious with a functioning gag reflex. Aspiration can lead to pneumonia.
- *Bacterial pneumonia*: due to hematogenous infection (spread by the individual's own blood), nosocomial infection (infectious agents picked up in the hospital after admission), or bacteria inspired as a direct result of the burn.
- *Pulmonary edema*: an overabundance of fluid collecting in the lungs because of re-hydration and the body's inability to deal effectively with fluids.
- *Pulmonary embolus*: a mass of air, tissue, or foreign object that lodges itself in a blood vessel in the lungs.
- *Posttraumatic pulmonary insufficiency*: caused by sepsis (contamination of an area and the resulting infection) and the oozing of protein rich fluid into the interstitial spaces of the lungs.

Because of the scaring and disfigurement that are typical with severe burns, clients often have a body image disturbance. A body image disturbance is a negative, subjective image of oneself; a negative perception of how others think about oneself; and/or an inability to adjust to the perceived or real perceptions. The criteria for body image disturbance are

- *Major criteria* (must be present): Verbal or nonverbal negative response to actual or perceived change in structure and/or function.
- *Minor criteria* (may be present): 1. not looking at body part, 2. not touching body part, 3. hiding or overexposing body part, 4. change in social involvement, 5. negative feelings about body with feelings of helplessness, hopelessness, powerlessness, 6. preoccupation with change or loss, 7. refusal to verify actual change, and 8. depersonalization of part or loss (Carpenito, 1992, p. 719-720).

Assessments

Typical Scope of Team Assessment

Burns are usually classified by using a four level ranking and a percentage of the body involved.

Burns that involving some, but not all, of the layers of skin are called partial thickness burns. Partial thickness burns are divided into two levels: 1. first-degree burns involve only the epidermis (top layer of skin) and look reddish and 2. second-degree burns involve the epidermis and corium (top and middle layer of skin) and have a reddish, blistered, and pealing look. Full thickness burns are also divided into two levels: 1. third-degree burns involve at least all of the layers of the skin. Third-degree burns have discoloration (first-degree), blisters (second-degree), and areas of charred or white (ashen) to blackened tissue and 2. fourth-degree burns involve deep tissue/structure loss.

The percentage system used to determine the percentage of body surface area (BSA) burned is called the *Rule of Nines*. Each body part (except for the head) for adults is estimated to be 9% of the BSA. Each upper extremity is 9% for both children and adults. Each lower extremity is 9% for adults and 7% for children. The anterior (front) portion of the torso is 18% for both children and adults, as is the posterior (back) portion of the trunk. The head and neck is considered to be 10% in adults and 18% in children.

Anticipated Findings from RT Assessment

The typical findings of the therapist include a client's discomfort with how s/he looks after the disfiguration of the burn, inability to understand how to communicate with others about the disfiguration, and impaired range of motion for activities due to tissue loss and scaring.

Other common identified needs relate to siblings/children, lack of understanding of medical procedures, and integrating a child back into school.

Treatment Direction

Whole Team Approach

The majority of clients with severe burns will be treated in a burn unit, a specific area in the hospital that has the specialized staff and equipment necessary to treat severe burns. Because of the broad physiological and psychological impact caused by severe burns, the treatment team addresses the physical, psychological, and vocational needs of clients.

Burn rehabilitation usually consists of four phases. Throughout all phases the treatment team is concerned with preventing infection and reducing the functional loss typically caused by scar tissue.

The first phase lasts from one to three days. During this time the treatment revolves around balancing the client's fluid needs and evaluating other injuries and comorbid conditions.

The second phase usually lasts a few days to a week after the burn and revolves around procedures to remove the damaged tissue that will not regenerate and use temporary, living tissue such as pig skin to provide closure of the burn site(s). The biologic closure usually requires numerous, staged surgeries.

The third phase is the replacement of the temporary wound closures with permanent grafts. At this phase any initial reconstruction of body parts such as hands and facial structures is done. Often this takes numerous surgeries.

The fourth phase is rehabilitation, reconstruction, and community reintegration.

There are three major elements of rehabilitation for burns (other than surgery) that are critical for the therapist to understand. They are debridement procedures, splinting, and pressure garments.

Debridement is the removal of contaminated or foreign material from the burn site. The burn (and, often the entire person) is cleaned a minimum of twice daily to remove caked antimicrobials (antibacterial creams and lotions), to keep the injured area clean, to remove any dead tissue, and to remove bacteria. There are three methods used to remove contaminated or foreign material: 1. mechanical — a scrubbing of the burn site until it is clean, 2. surgical — the cutting away of the excess material, and 3. enzymatic — using enzymes to dissolve the dead tissue and unwanted foreign material. While all of these methods may be used, most clients who are hospitalized are "tubbed" (mechanical removal) in a whirlpool to soften and loosen the unwanted material prior to a physical scrubbing of the area. This is a very painful process that happens twice a day. Clients are usually given morphine or similar pain medication. However, the nerves are so raw in the area that the pain medication is usually inadequate to reduce pain to a tolerable level.

Scarring of the burn site is often significant. Scar tissue has limited stretching ability. If the burn was deep enough, the client most likely also lost some muscle tissue, ligaments, and tendons. Splinting may be used to help immobilize a burn site while newly grafted material adheres to the body. It is critical from an early stage to increase and maintain range of motion through the healing and scar tissue development process. Splinting helps reduce the severity of contractures, prevent deformity, and maximize the flexibility of scar tissue. Splinting is a major component of most treatment for burns on extremities helping maintain desired ligament and skin length and decreasing the incidence of contractures.

There are three phasing of splinting: 1. primary splints, 2. post-graft splints, and 3. follow-up splints (DiGregorio, 1984). Primary static splints (splints without moving parts) are used during the acute and pre-splinting phase to prevent loss of range of motion. These splints are worn at all times except when staff (or the client) is working on range of motion exercises, skin care, or self-care. Post-graft splints are crafted before the grafting surgery and then worn for five to fourteen days after surgery to allow healing of the grafted area. Follow-up splints are worn for up to two years after the burn while the tissues in the burn site mature. Whenever possible (e.g., the clients is able to maintain range of motion without constant wearing of the splint), the splint wearing time may be restricted to sleeping and, eventually discontinued. Follow-up splints may be static or dynamic.

Pressure garments are tight elastic clothing specially designed to restrict blood flow to developing scar tissue and to inhibit the growth of raised scar tissue. After significant burns, normal tissue is replaced with scar tissue. Restriction on the growth of scar tissue helps promote long-term range of motion and limit disfigurement. Clients will wear pressure garments over the burned portion of the body twenty-three hours a day, taking them off only to bathe. Clients should have at least two specially fitted sets of pressure garments, allowing the garments to be washed when they are soiled.

Recreational Therapy Approach

Recreational therapy works with the team approach outlined above. The specific role is to identify and provide opportunities for enjoyable activities to help with pain management (power of distraction, relaxation response), engage the client in appropriate physical activities to minimize scar formation and increase physical function, teach the client relaxation techniques to help with pain management, and address issues and skills related to community integration including issues related to adjustment. Clients often get the feeling that almost every member of the medical staff causes them pain. The recreational therapist may be the rare exception.

Recreational Therapy Interventions

Common recreational therapy interventions when working with clients who have burns include:

- *Coping with treatment pain*: See b280 Sensation of Pain. Also see "Relaxation and Stress Reduction" in the Techniques section.
- *Adjustment to disability*: See "Adjustment to Disability" in the Techniques section.
- *Medical play or role-playing*: It is common for the therapist to use medical play to help children and adolescents work through the anger, misunderstandings, and fear associated with burns. This would most likely be scored under one of the subcategories of b126 Temperament and Personality Functions.
- *Community reintegration*: The therapist helps with a phased reintegration back into society after the injury (disfigurement). All aspects of A&P Chapter 7 Interpersonal Interactions and Relationships, A&P Chapter 8 Major Life Areas, and Chapter 9 Community, Social, and Civic Life need to be covered. This also includes preparing the school and other individuals or community groups as appropriate for the client's return.
- *Leisure opportunities*: Score under specific activities in A&P Chapter 9 Community, Social, and Civic Life.
- *Physical activity*: Many of the parts of Body Functions Chapter 7 Neuromusculoskeletal and Movement Related Functions are involved. Also see "Exercise Basics" in the Techniques section.

References

American College of Surgeons. (1999). Guidelines for the operation of burn units. In *Resources for optimal care of the injured patient.* Chicago: Author.

Anderson, K., Anderson, L., & Glanze, W. (Eds.). (1994). *Mosby's medical, nursing, and allied health dictionary.* (4th Ed.). St. Louis, MO: Mosby.

Carpenito, L. (1992). *Nursing diagnosis; Application to clinical practice.* (4th Ed.). Philadelphia, PA: L. B. Lippincott Company.

Dambro, M. (1998). *Griffith's 5-minute clinical consultant.* Baltimore, MD: Williams & Wilkins.

Burnsurvivor Resource Guide. (2004). Medical care guide: Burn statistics. www.attorneyrobertbrenner.com/guide_medical_statistics.htm.

Centers for Disease Control National Center for Injury Prevention and Control. (2004). Fire deaths and injuries. www.cdc.gov/ncipc/factsheets/fire.htm.

DiGregorio, V. (1984). *Rehabilitation of the burn patient.* New York: Churchill Livingston.

Whaley, L., & Wong, D. (1991). *Nursing care of infants and children.* (4th Ed.). St. Louis, MO: Mosby.

Cancer

Cancer is a broad set of diseases that share the characteristic of having abnormal cells that divide without control. As cancer advances, the cancer cells can invade other parts of the body, spreading to nearby tissue or moving through the blood or lymphatic system. Cancer cells impair the function of normal cells. There are four general categories of cancer:

- *Carcinoma*: Cancers that originate in tissues that cover or protect other body parts such as skin tissue or the tissues that line internal organs.
- *Leukemia*: Cancers that originate in bone marrow (bone marrow contains the tissues that form blood) resulting in a proliferation of immature (non-functional) blood cells traveling through the circulatory system.
- *Lymphoma and multiple myeloma*: Cancers that originate in the immune system.
- *Sarcoma*: Cancers that originate in connective tissues including blood vessels, bone, cartilage, muscle, or other connective or supportive tissues.

Incidence/Prevalence in US

This section will review the basic concepts related to cancer incidence and prevalence in the United States and then provide some overall data and statistics for cancer. The National Cancer Institute, which is part of the United States National Institutes of Health, maintains the database for cancer statistics. Listed below are the key terms related to describing incidence and prognosis.

Definitions Related to Incidence and Mortality.

When talking about the incidence or the mortality of cancer, it is a common practice to talk about the rates (number of cases per 100,000 people) of a specific kind of cancer. Some people are diagnosed with more than one cancer. In these cases each type of cancer is counted separately. It is not a common practice to count a relapse (the cancer returning sometime after the person has been diagnosed as being clear of cancer) in incidence and mortality numbers. If a person has more than one tumor of the same type of cancer, this situation is counted as only one incident.

- *Trends of rates* (annual percent change): The annual percent change trend of rates is used to determine if the total number of people newly diagnosed with cancer is increasing or decreasing.
- *Age-adjusted rates for individual years*: People who are elderly are far more likely to be diagnosed with most types of cancers. Age-adjusted

rates allow people to follow trends based on clients' ages and state in which they live.

- *Age-adjusted rates and 95% confidence intervals*: When cancer rates are reported as a range by the National Cancer Institute it means that 95% of all incidences of cancer will fall between the two numbers.
- *Age-specific rates*: In the United States nineteen age groups are used for statistical purposes. The age groups are: 0 (under one year of age), 1-4, 5-9, 10-14, 15-19, 20-24, 25-29, 30-34, 35-39, 40-44, 45-49, 50-54, 55-59, 60-64, 65-69, 70-74, 75-79, 80-84, and 85+.

Definitions Related to Survival.

- *Relative survival rates*: The relative survival rate is expressed as a ratio that compares the number of deaths due to all causes within a specific age group to the number of deaths specifically due to cancer within the same age group.
- *Five-year relative survival rates*: A five-year survival rate is the most common number given to clients when physicians talk about the client's chance of survival. A five-year relative survival rate is an expression of the percentage of people with that type of cancer who lived at least five years after they were first diagnosed. Survival rate is not the same thing as cure (cancer-free) rate.

Definition Related to Lifetime Risk.

By keeping statistics on the risk of developing cancer by ethnicity, age, and gender, health care professionals can better anticipate the types of tests that might be ordered or the scope of symptoms that might be related to cancer based on the client's background. This type of information helps limit the amount of initial testing necessary.

Probability of Developing or Dying of Cancer:

The chance that a client will develop cancer or die of cancer based on age, ethnic background, and gender.

Predominate Age

The incidence of cancer in the United States varies depending on age at diagnosis. Table 6 shows the percentage of people newly diagnosed with cancer based on age groups using 2003 data. (National Cancer Institute, p. 1: Stat Fact Sheets)

Table 6: Cancer diagnosis rates

Percentage of Individuals with Cancer	Age at Initial Diagnosis (% of the total number of people diagnosed with cancer in 2003)
Under 20 years	1.1%
20-34 years	2.7%
35-44 years	6.0%
45-54 years	13.5%
55-64 years	20.8%
65-74 years	26.3%
75-84 years	22.6%
85+ years	7.3%

Table 7: Cancer mortality rates

Race/Ethnicity	Men	Women
All Races	241.5	163.5
White	237.3	162.8
Black	326.8	191.1
Asian/Pacific Islander	143.3	98.0
American Indian/Alaska Native	150.0	111.1
Hispanic	165.1	108.1

Causes

There are four categories of risk factors (causes).

1. *Behavioral risk factors*: Behavioral risk factors are actions that the client can control that either increase or decrease the chances of developing cancer. For example, smoking (or being around people who smoke) increases your risk of developing cancer, including lung cancer.
2. *Biological risk factors*: Biological risk factors are physical attributes that may increase your chances of developing cancer. You may not be able to change your physical attributes but you can change behaviors and modify your environment to reduce your biological risk factors. Your age, gender, race, and skin complexion are examples of biological risk factors that may place you in an increased (or decreased) risk category.
3. *Environmental risk factors*: Environmental risk factors are elements in the world around you that may increase your chance of developing cancer. For example, having a high level of radon in your home or exposure to pesticides may increase your chance of developing cancer.
4. *Genetic risk factors*: Genetic risk factors are inherited tendencies for cancer. If you have multiple family members who have had cancer, you may have an increased genetic risk to also develop cancer.

Prognosis

The prognosis depends on the type of cancer, the stage that the cancer is in (described in Typical Scope of Team Assessment), the treatment options available to the client, the client's ethnic background and gender, and the client's overall health.

The overall rate of people in the United States who survive cancer for at least five years from the time they were diagnosed is 65%. Between the years 2000 and 2003 the age-adjusted death rate for both men and women was 194.5 per 100,000. The median

age of diagnosis of cancer during that time period was 67 while death due to cancer in the United States was 73 years of age. During their lifetime approximately 40% of people living in the United States will develop cancer (National Cancer Institute, 2006).

The client's age, ethnic background, and gender have a big impact on the prognosis. Table 7 shows the mortality rates in the United States from 2000-2003. The rates are based on the number per 100,000 (National Cancer Institute, 2006a, p. 1).

Many clients with cancer live decades after being diagnosed because the cancer either goes into remission or is active but controlled. In other instances the client's life expectancy may be very short, even weeks.

Assessments

Typical Scope of Team Assessment

Clients tend to receive a diagnosis of cancer because they had symptoms that caused them to go to their physician. During the physical exam the physician decided to conduct additional testing including the use of imaging (CT scans, MRI scans, PET scans, and/or x-rays); laboratory tests (sometimes the presence of cancer causes an imbalance of substances in the body fluids); or pathology reports (analysis of cells or tumors obtained through biopsy or surgical removal of tumors).

Cancer staging is an assessment used by treatment teams that helps determine the appropriate treatment protocols for the client, helps determine the client's prognosis, and helps compare treatment results across different facilities. Most types of cancers have specific stages based on the number of cancer cells and the degree to which the cancer has spread to other parts of the body.

In the United States the National Cancer Institute manages the Surveillance, Epidemiology, and End Results Program (SEER) to help identify the most promising treatment protocols. Clinical data is submitted to SEER using a Summary Staging Scale that has five levels (National Cancer Institute, 2006b, p. 3):

1. *In situ* is early cancer that is present only in the layer of cells in which it began.
2. *Localized* is cancer that is limited to the organ in which it began, without evidence of spread.
3. *Regional* is cancer that has spread beyond the original (primary) site to nearby lymph nodes or organs and tissues.
4. *Distant* is cancer that has spread from the primary site to distant organs or distant lymph nodes.
5. *Unknown* is used to describe cases for which there is not enough information to indicate a stage.

The SEER Staging Scale helps compare data for all types of cancers. The most commonly used, clinical-based staging system for cancers that form tumors is the TNM (tumor size, if the cancer has spread to the lymph nodes, and if the cancer has metastasized or spread to other parts of the body). The TNM Staging System is explained in Table 8

To better communicate the estimated stage of the cancer the TNM has an additional numbering system that is used. The numbering system for TNM Staging is detailed in Table 9.

Anticipated Findings of RT Assessment

Being diagnosed with cancer is often a life-altering event. While the majority of clients diagnosed with cancer will survive, a diagnosis of cancer often causes clients to stop and re-evaluate their lives. The treatment phase of cancer often leaves the client very ill, with limited energy, and limited appetite. Cancer treatment is also time-consuming whether it is given as an outpatient or inpatient. Major activities that normally fill the client's waking hours need to be significantly reduced to accommo-date the number of hours associated with treatment, the lack of energy, and the lack of overall health. Given all of these major changes, the potential for death due to the cancer, and the stress put on relationships important to the client, a secondary diagnosis of depression may also be of concern. Not

all cancers have pain associated with the cancer but some have severe pain. Pain and the treatment for pain (including the use of narcotics) also negatively impact the client's ability to function.

Treatment Direction

There are many different ways that cancer is treated and often more than one method is used. Treatment protocols are developed for specific types of cancers taking into consideration the stage of the cancer, the client's age, and the client's preferences. This section contains a brief explanation of different treatment options.

Angiogenesis inhibitors: Angiogenesis inhibitors are a type of drug that slows or blocks the formation of new blood vessels. Researchers are working with angiogenesis inhibitors to determine methods to reduce the blood flow to cancer cells, thus starving them. The National Cancer Institute reports that angiogenesis inhibitors are being used as a treatment option for AIDS-related Kaposi's sarcoma, leukemias, lymphomas, and brain, breast, cervix, lung, ovary, pancreas, prostate, and stomach cancers.

Biological therapy: Biological therapy is a set of treatment protocols that help boost the cancer-fighting capabilities of the immune system. It helps slow down the growth of cancer cells or outright destroys them by enabling the immune system. Another goal of biological therapy is to strengthen the immune system so that it stops the spread of cancer. Biological therapy is different from chemotherapy because it helps strengthen the body's

Table 8: TNM stages

Stage	Definition
Stage 0	Carcinoma in situ (early cancer that is present only in the layer of cells in which it began).
Stage I, II, and III	Higher numbers indicate more extensive disease: greater tumor size, and/or spread of the cancer to nearby lymph nodes and/or organs adjacent to the primary tumor.
Stage IV	The cancer has spread to another organ.

From National Cancer Institute, 2006b, p. 2

Table 9: Additional TNM grading

Primary Tumor (T)	
TX	Primary tumor cannot be evaluated.
T0	No evidence of primary tumor.
Tis	Carcinoma in situ (early cancer that has not spread to the neighboring tissue).
T1, T2, T3, T4	Size and/or extent of the primary tumor.
Regional Lymph Nodes (N)	
NX	Regional lymph nodes cannot be evaluated.
N0	No regional lymph node involvement (no cancer found in the lymph nodes).
N1, N2, N3	Involvement of regional lymph nodes (number and/or extent of spread).
Distant Metastasis (M)	
MX	Distant metastasis cannot be evaluated.
M0	No distant metastasis (cancer has not spread to other parts of the body).
M1	Distant metastasis (cancer has spread to distant parts of the body).

From National Cancer Institute, 2006b, p. 2

own defenses so that the body itself can fight the cancer. In chemotherapy the drugs take an active and direct role in slowing down or destroying cancerous cells. One of the new areas of study for biological therapy is cancer vaccines. Just because biological therapy boosts the body's own immune system does not mean that there are no side effects that impair the client's ability and desire to function. Side effects of biological therapy include appetite loss, bone pain, chills, fatigue, fever, muscle aches, nausea, vomiting, and serious allergic reactions. Biological therapy is used to help treat a variety of cancers including AIDS-related Kaposi's sarcoma, brain, breast, chronic myeloid leukemia, colon, esophagus, hairy cell leukemia, kidney, leukemia, lung, lymphoma, melanoma, multiple myeloma, non-Hodgkin's lymphoma, ovarian, pancreas, prostate, rectum, and uterus.

Bone marrow transplantation and peripheral blood stem cell transplantation: Both bone marrow transplantation (BMT) and peripheral blood stem cell transplantation (PBSCT) are treatments used to counter severe side effects of other cancer treatments, usually chemotherapy and radiation therapy. High-dose chemotherapy or radiation therapy may be needed to destroy cancer cells, but they also destroy normal blood-producing cells. After treatment with high-dose chemotherapy or radiation therapy bone marrow cells or stem cells are given intravenously to the patient to help replace the destroyed cells. The replacement cells may come either from cells harvested from the patient prior to the high-dose treatment or from a donor. A serious side effect of cells from a donor is graft versus host disease (GVHD); a situation in which the body's immune system thinks that the transplanted material is an invading cell. GVHD may develop years after the transplant and affect the digestive tract, liver, and/or skin. GVHD can be fatal.

Chemotherapy: Chemotherapy is the use of drugs that generally act by destroying cells that multiply quickly. Cancer cells are not the only cells in the body that multiply quickly. There are other normal, healthy cells in the body that divide quickly, such as hair cells. As with other types of cancer treatments, a combination of treatment options is used to cure or control the cancer or to reduce symptoms of the cancer. This could include radiation, biological therapy, or surgery.

Gene therapy: Available through clinical trials (and not yet a standard treatment) gene therapy is the process of introducing genetic material into the client's cells to help fight cancer. There are a variety of roles that introduced genetic material can take including boosting the immune system, replacing defective (cancer causing) genes with healthy genes,

increasing cancer cells susceptibility to chemotherapy, or preventing new blood vessels to tumors from being formed.

Hormone therapy: Some types of cancers require hormones to grow. With hormone therapy the physician may use drugs that stop the body from producing the hormones that allow the cancer to grow or may surgically remove the organ (such as the ovaries or testicles) that produce the hormone.

Hyperthermia: Combined with other cancer treatments, some tumors appear to be more sensitive to heat than normal, healthy tissue. The area in which the tumor is located is heated up to 113°F to help reduce the size of the tumor.

Lasers: Lasers create intense rays of light in a very narrow wavelength band that are capable of cutting tissue. The cuts caused by lasers tend to bleed less, allow a smaller incision, and heal faster than cuts created using other surgical instruments. This also helps decrease the incidence of infection. Lasers are a type of surgical tool.

Photodynamic therapy: Photodynamic therapy uses different types of drugs that cause cells to be photosensitive (easily damaged by light) and then exposes the tumor to light. The photodynamic drugs are injected into the client's bloodstream a few days before treatment. This drug is taken up by all cells but lasts longer in cancer cells than it does in normal, healthy cells. When the photodynamic drugs have worked their way out of the normal, healthy cells the physician directs light containing specific wavelengths at the tumor. Photodynamic therapy tends to work with smaller tumors that are located within a third of an inch of the surface of the skin or the lining of internal organs. Clients receiving photodynamic therapy need to stay out of bright light for six weeks after treatment.

Radiation therapy: About half of the clients with cancer receive radiation therapy, often with at least one other therapy. Radiation therapy, used to treat solid tumors, uses ionizing radiation to weaken or destroy the genetic material of the cancer cells. There are different types of ionizing radiation used, including radioactive materials that may be placed inside the person. In this case the fluids leaving the person could contain low levels of radioactive material. The treatment team will have specific protocols to address body fluids.

Surgery: Surgery is the removal of cells and tissue that appear to be cancerous along with cells or tissue in the immediate proximity of the cancer. If there is a chance that the cancer has spread to lymph nodes, the surgeon may also remove the lymph nodes.

Targeted cancer therapies: Also called molecular targeted drugs, targeted cancer therapies use drugs that interfere with the process of cancer cell growth at the molecular level, stopping or slowing the growth of cancer. At this point most of the research on targeted cancer therapies is in the initial stage (testing on animals). A few of the studies have progressed to clinical studies (testing on humans). This type of cancer treatment appears to be very promising.

Recreational Therapy Approach

The recreational therapy approach will vary depending primarily on the setting (e.g., intensive care, outpatient, summer camp for kids that have cancer), the cancer stage (advanced, remission), treatment side effects, level of support, prognosis, and client wishes. The recreational therapist is not usually involved in the medical aspects, but s/he is vital in supporting the client through the process of dealing with the grief and getting through the therapies. The therapist stays current on what is happening medically and helps explain the process and offers appropriate lifestyle adaptations for the client and the client's family. For children with cancer this can include medical play to reduce the fear of cancer treatments.

Recreational Therapy Interventions

Some of the areas that the recreational therapist may address include:

- *Life evaluation*: When faced with a terminal disease, clients are often confronted with life evaluation. Did I live a good life? How do I want to live my remaining days? Now that I have beat cancer, how do I want to live my life differently? In some cases, clients with cancer place a higher value on leisure (e.g., desire to spend more time with family, participate in the three-day breast cancer walk). Recreational therapists not only explore new leisure values, but also help the client to acquire needed skills and identify resources required to participate in realistic choices. See "Education and Counseling" in the Techniques section for information on existential counseling. The ICF does not currently score subjective satisfaction with life, so d155 Acquiring Skills is the appropriate place to score leisure skill development. Reminiscence therapy (or life review) may also be welcomed by clients and loved ones in the end stages of cancer. The

therapist in this case may educate the client's family about the technique and encourage them to use it as appropriate to help their loved one come to peace with the life s/he lived.

- *Activity balance*: The therapist takes the client's energy level into account and helps the client plan a set of activities that cover the physical, emotional, interpersonal, and cognitive domains. There are several chapters in Activities and Participation that will have relevant codes. The therapist needs to carefully evaluate the life areas that the client wants to stay active in and find ways to make it possible. See "Activity Pattern Development" and "Personal Leisure Resource Awareness" in the Techniques section.
- *Modification of activities*: This may be needed to address changes in body structures and functions as a result of treatment (such as amputation). Refer to the Body Functions code that best reflects the impairment for information on how to treat and adapt for the dysfunction.
- *Stress management*: The ICF code is d2401 Handling Stress. Also see "Coping with Stress" and "Relaxation and Stress Reduction" in the Techniques section.
- *Time management*: Dysfunction related to the cancer itself, as well from the cancer treatments, can severely impact a person's ability to engage in activities. Activities are prioritized based on abilities, supports, health, and meaning. See "Energy Conservation Training" in the Techniques section. "Pie of Life" in the Techniques section can also be a helpful tool in prioritizing activities.
- *Depression and grief*: See "Adjustment to Disability" and "Education and Counseling" in the Techniques section.
- *Pain management*: See b280 Sensation of Pain.

References

Shannon, C. (2005). If the dishes don't get done today, they'll get done tomorrow: A breast cancer experience as a catalyst for changes to women's leisure. *Journal of Leisure Research, 37*(2):195-215.

National Cancer Institute. (2006a). Cancer stat fact sheets. http://seer.cancer.gov/statfacts/html/all.html.

National Cancer Institute. (2006b). Staging: Questions and answers. http://www.cancer.gov/cancertopics/factsheet/Detection/staging.

Cardiac Conditions

This section will cover the cardiac conditions coronary artery disease, myocardial infarction, and congestive heart failure.

Coronary artery disease (CAD): Coronary artery disease is almost always due to atherosclerosis. Atherosclerosis is a buildup of cholesterol and other fatty substances called atheromas or atherosclerotic plaques on the wall of the coronary arteries. The build-up causes a narrowing of the arteries and restricts the amount of oxygenated blood to the heart. Lack of adequate oxygenated blood to the heart can cause myocardial ischemia (also called angina or chest pain) or sudden cardiac death. When an artery becomes severely or completely blocked, oxygenated blood does not reach the area of the heart that the artery feeds causing that part of the heart muscle to die. This is called a heart attack or myocardial infarction (MI). CAD is the most common cause of MI (approximately 90% of all MI cases). Atheromas can also rupture triggering the formation of a blood clot. The blood clot may stay in the place where it was formed in the coronary artery (called a thrombosis) or it may break off and travel until it becomes lodged in another artery (called an embolism).

Myocardial infarction (MI): Myocardial infarction is a medical term for a heart attack. The majority of MIs are caused by CAD (90%), although it is possible for a coronary artery to spasm and disrupt the blood flow to the heart causing a MI. Two out of three people experience worsening angina (chest pain), shortness of breath, and fatigue over the course of several days or weeks prior to an MI. Pain in the middle of the chest is the most common symptom of having a MI, although one third of people who have a MI do not have chest pain and one in five people have only mild symptoms or none at all (Merck Manual Home Edition, 2005c). Therefore, in some cases, a MI goes undetected and only shows up on an electrocardiogram (ECG). Non-white women over the age of 75 who have a history of CHF, diabetes, or stroke are the ones who will most often present without chest pain (Manual Home Edition, 2005c). The chest pain experienced with a MI is more severe than angina pain and it is not relieved by rest or medication (e.g., nitroglycerin). Pain typically occurs in one or more of the following areas: middle of the chest, jaw, back, left arm, or right arm (left arm is most common). Other symptoms may include sudden heavy sweating, shortness of breath, a heavy pounding heart, feeling of faintness, unconsciousness, restlessness or anxiousness, and feet, hands, and lips turning slightly blue (Merck Manual Home Edition, 2005c). Heart murmurs and other abnormal heart sounds can usually be heard (by stethoscope) in the early stages of an MI.

Congestive heart failure (CHF): Congestive heart failure (CHF) occurs when the muscles of the heart become weak and the pumping action of the heart becomes impaired. CHF typically affects both the right and left sides of the heart, although it can be more pronounced on one side. In these cases, CHF is described as being right-sided heart failure or left-sided heart failure. CHF can also be described as being a systolic dysfunction or a diastolic dysfunction. In systolic dysfunction, the heart muscles are unable to adequately pump the blood that is received, so more blood remains in the specific ventricle that is weak. Consequently, organs and tissues are not adequately supplied with oxygenated blood and ventricles can become enlarged. In diastolic dysfunction, the walls of the heart become thick and stiff restricting the heart's ability to stretch to accommodate the amount of blood that it needs to hold. In this case, the blood backs up in the circulatory system causing a variety of problems. It increases pressure in the blood vessels causing fluid to be forced into bodily tissues. If fluid backs up from the left atrium, it is forced into the lungs (pulmonary edema) making it difficult for the airways to expand with inhalation causing shortness of breath. If the fluid backs up from the right atrium it causes edema in the legs and enlargement of organs.

Typically, the first manifestation of CHF in an adult is tachycardia (a rapid beating of the heart, usually describing rates over 100 beats per minute). In infants, signs of pulmonary venous congestion (left-sided CHF) typically include tachypnea (rapid breathing), retractions (respiratory distress), grunting, and difficulty feeding, whereas a common sign of right-sided venous congestion include hepatosplenomegaly (enlargement of the liver and spleen). If left untreated, the infant will fail to thrive. In older children, pulmonary venous congestion (left-sided CHF) manifest in tachypnea, retractions, and wheezing (cardiac asthma), whereas common signs of right-sided venous congestion include hepatosplenomegaly, jugular venous distention, edema, ascites (accumulation of serous fluid in the peritoneal cavity), and/or pleural effusions. If left untreated, the child will fatigue easily and may have significant reductions in energy level, cool extremities, vertigo, and fainting episodes.

Incidence/Prevalence in US

CAD: Affects 5-9% of all Americans over the age of 20. It is the leading cause of death in America.

MI: In the US, approximately 1.5 million people have a myocardial infarction (heart attack) each year. Two thirds of them are men.

CHF: One out of every 100 people in the US has CHF.

Predominant Age

CAD: CAD affects primarily adults. Women often develop CAD at a later age than men because they are protected until menopause by higher levels of estrogen. Although CAD affects both sexes and all races, African-American and Southeast Asian males have the highest rates of CAD.

MI: Although the majority of people who have MIs are 65 years or older, 45% of MIs occur in people who are younger than 65 (Crepeau, Cohn, Boyt Schell, 2003). Although rare, children can have MIs. The two leading causes for children are Anomalous Left Coronary Artery Origin from the Pulmonary Artery (ALCAPA) and Kawasaki Disease. Men are at a greater risk than women until the age of 70 when both sexes have the same incidence. It is believed that estrogen may play a role in protecting women from MI's prior to menopause.

CHF: CHF can occur in people of all ages and races (e.g., birth defect in a child), although it is much more prevalent in older populations.

Causes

CAD: Atherosclerosis is the primary cause of CAD and it is mostly attributed to lifestyle including high cholesterol, high blood pressure, smoking, a high-fat diet, physical inactivity, drinking more than two alcoholic drinks a day, and obesity. People who have type-II diabetes (predominately a lifestyle disease) have a high risk of developing CAD because many have concurrent risk factors such as high blood pressure, high cholesterol, obesity, and physical inactivity. The use of male steroids, whether real or synthetic, could increase a person's risk of CAD because it lowers good cholesterol (HDL), raises bad cholesterol (LDL), and causes high blood pressure — all of which can contribute to CAD and MI.

MI: The most common cause of an MI is a blood clot. Rarely, although possibly, an MI can be caused by a coronary artery spasm that halts the blood flow. It has also been reported that that people with type-A personalities have twice the risk of MI and coronary disease related mortality (Sadock & Sadock, 2003).

CHF: The causes of CHF are numerous. They include:

- *CAD*: decreasing the flow of oxygenated blood to the heart muscle leading to damage to heart muscle.

- *MI*: causes injury to the heart that could cause CHF.
- *Myocarditis* (inflammation of the heart muscle): caused by an infection that damages the heart.
- *Valve stenosis* (narrowing of a valve): can hinder blood flow in the heart. Valves can also leak (regurgitation) putting stress on the heart and eventually enlarging the heart so that it does not pump properly.
- *Birth defects of the heart*: can cause the blood to recirculate in the heart causing the heart to work harder.
- *Disorders*: ones that cause fast or irregular heart rhythms can lead to CHF when they cause the heart to pump improperly.
- *Pulmonary hypertension*: can cause the right ventricle to become enlarged leading to right-sided heart failure.
- *Clots* (small and many or one large): in the pulmonary artery they can cause right-sided heart failure.
- *Anemia*: can affect the amount of oxygen carried by the blood requiring the heart to work harder to provide needed amounts of oxygen throughout the body.
- *Hypothyroidism*: causes muscles to become weak (including the heart).
- *Kidney failure*: can cause CHF because excess fluid builds up in the bloodstream thus requiring the heart to pump more blood. Consequently, the heart is overworked and heart failure ensues.
- *High blood pressure*: makes the heart pump more forcefully because it is harder to pump blood into arteries under high pressure. Consequently the walls of the heart thicken and become more rigid, resulting in chambers that can't stretch to fill completely. As people age, stiffening of the heart's walls is common, contributing to this problem.
- *Infections* (such as amyloidosis): and infiltration of certain parasites can cause heart failure.
- *Constrictive pericarditis*: the sac that surrounds the heart, called the pericardium, can become stiff due to constrictive pericarditis that prevents the heart from filling and pumping normally.

System(s) Affected

CAD, MI, and CHF are problems of the circulatory system. Depending on the cause and extent of the problem, many other bodily systems can be affected directly (e.g., blood backing up from CHF can enlarge organs) or indirectly (e.g., limitations of activity contributing to secondary health problems in other systems, such as the musculoskeletal).

Prognosis

CAD: The client's age, the extent of coronary disease (determined by angiography), the severity of symptoms, and ventricular function are the four major factors that influence the client's prognosis (Berkow, 1992). In general, a 1.4% rate of death occurs annually for people with angina and no history of an MI, 7.5% for those with CAD and systolic hypertension, 8.4% for those with CAD and an abnormal ECG, and 12% for those with systolic hypertension and an abnormal ECG (Merck Manual Home Edition, 2005a).

MI: The extent of heart damage and residual function after an MI, in addition to age and past medical history, are variables that affect prognosis. 50,000 of the 1.5 million people in the US who have an MI every year die (Wegner et al., 1995); and half of these deaths occur before reaching the hospital. Ten percent of MI survivors die within the first year after an MI and approximately 50% of people who have an MI are re-hospitalized within a year after a MI event (Garas & Zafari, 2004).

CHF: On average, up to 70% of people with CHF die within 10 years, 50% of people with mild CHF live at least 10 years, and 50% of those with severe heart failure live at least 2 years (Merck Manual Home Edition, 2005b). Death from CHF can occur quickly and without warning.

Secondary Problems

Cardiac conditions in general: Five to 10% of people with cardiac problems have anxiety disorders (particularly panic attacks, and phobias) and 10-15% have mood disorder (predominantly depressive episodes, minor depression, or dysthymia) (Sadock & Sadock, 2003).

Issues related to sexuality: People with cardiac problems may experience problems with impotence, premature or delayed ejaculation, and reduced libido due to medication, depression, and/or fear of causing a cardiac event. The average heart rate during sexual intercourse is 120 beats per minute. People with cardiac conditions should be encouraged to experiment with sexual positions that are less strenuous than the traditional missionary position (e.g., side to side).

CAD: CAD, as previously described, is a major contributor to MI. People with CAD often have a very poor lifestyle leading to secondary problems including decreased energy level, increased stress on the skeletal system (particularly the knees, hips, and back), decreased strength, and possible decreases in cognitive processing from poor nutrition.

MI: There are a variety of secondary problems related to MI.

- *Major depressive disorder* (MDD): MDD has been found to occur in 15-20% of people following myocardial infarction (Sadock & Sadock, 2003). See MDD in the Diagnosis section for more information.
- *Sudden cardiac death*: "High levels of anxiety symptoms are associated with a tripling of risk of sudden cardiac death and also raise the risk of future coronary events in patients with myocardial infarction by two to five times that for non-anxious patients who have had heart attacks" (Sadock & Sadock, 2003, p 829). The cardiovascular system is very sensitive to stress.
- *Abnormal heart rhythms*: 90% of people who have a MI have arrhythmias for a few days after the event making it difficult for the heart to pump properly and increasing their risk for cardiac arrest (Merck Manual Home Edition, 2005c).
- *Scar tissue*: Dead heart tissue is replaced with scar tissue that does not contract like normal heart tissue causing CHF. If more than 50% of the heart is damaged or replaced with scar tissue severe disability or death is likely (Merck Manual Home Edition, 2005c). "Beta-blockers and angiotensin-converting enzyme (ACE) inhibitors can reduce the extent of these abnormal areas by reducing the workload of and the stress on the heart. Thus, these drugs help the heart maintain its shape and function more normally" (Merck Manual Home Edition, 2005c).
- *CHF*: In addition to CHF being caused by scar tissue, CHF can also result from abnormal heart rhythms. If the heart does not pump out adequate amounts of blood from the chamber, the blood can remain in the chamber causing it to become enlarged. Abnormal rhythms are more likely to occur in an enlarged heart and abnormal rhythms make cardiac arrest and MIs more likely.
- *Ruptured heart muscle*: When heart muscle is weak it can rupture from the force of the pumping. This usually occurs from one to ten days after a MI (Merck Manual Home Edition, 2005c). Depending on the location and extent of the rupture, death can occur suddenly.
- *Ventricular aneurysm*: This is when a bulge (aneurysm) forms on the wall of the ventricle (heart chamber). It can cause abnormal heart rhythms, impair the heart's ability to pump properly, and increase the risk of developing blood clots (because blood moves more slowly). In some cases, ventricular aneurysms may be surgically repaired.
- *Blood clots*: Approximately 50% of people who have had a MI develop blood clots in the coronary arteries. Embolisms (traveling blood clots)

occur in up to 5% of these people thus increasing their risk for a cerebrovascular accident (stroke). Prescription of anticoagulants such as heparin and Coumadin help to prevent the formation of blood clots. A daily aspirin tablet is typically prescribed for the rest of a client's life to help prevent clots.

CHF: Secondary complications from CHF will vary greatly depending on the extent and location of heart failure. See the description of causes for CHF above.

Assessments

Typical Scope of Team Assessment

In a rehabilitation setting, therapists receive a written order from the physician indicating the cardiac precautions or parameters that the client must stay within (e.g., blood pressure and heart rate not to rise more than 20 in activity from resting baseline). Within these guidelines, therapists assess the client's ability to engage in functional tasks (e.g., transferring, walking, leisure activities). Heart rate, oxygen saturation levels, blood pressure, and respiration are monitored during activity. In addition the therapist watches for feelings of vertigo (dizziness), nausea, skin color changes, level of pain reported by the client, client's perceived level of exertion (e.g., BORG scale), cool extremities, or feeling faint. See "Vital Signs" in the Techniques section for information on how to assess vital signs. A baseline of functioning is determined and goals are established that stay within the cardiac precaution or parameters set by the physician.

Anticipated Findings from RT Assessment

It is difficult to identify common findings among this population due to the diversity of cardiac damage and functioning. However, since the majority of MIs are due to CAD, therapists will commonly see lifestyle issues that need to be changed (e.g., diet, exercise, stress). The causes of CHF on the other hand are numerous and, therefore, the presentation of the client will vary. In a rehabilitation facility the therapist will probably find poor endurance and strength as key indicators for therapy. Limitations will be imposed on physical exertion by cardiac precautions, parameters, and MET levels. Depression and anxiety are common psychological issues in this population, so therapists should look for these issues.

Treatment Direction

Whole Team Approach

This section is divided into three parts. First, the whole team approach by cardiac diagnosis is reviewed, followed by cardiac rehabilitation, and then therapeutic lifestyle changes.

Team Approach by Cardiac Diagnosis

Common surgical interventions: Surgical interventions for coronary problems include angioplasty (reconstruction of a blood vessel), coronary bypass where another blood vessel is added to go around the occlusion, and a heart transplant. Pharmacological interventions and lifestyle changes are also implemented.

CAD: People with CAD are instructed to make therapeutic lifestyle changes to decrease atherosclerosis. They are not typically seen in a rehabilitation center until a cardiac event occurs (e.g., MI).

Acute MI: If a client thinks s/he is having a heart attack, an ambulance should be called immediately. The client is to chew an aspirin immediately. If a clot is causing the MI, the aspirin will help to reduce the size of the clot and increase the client's chances of survival. Clopidogrel is an alterative to aspirin for people who are allergic to aspirin (trade name Plavix). Another medication, called a beta-blocker, slows down the client's heart rate. Oxygen is administered to increase the amount of oxygen available to the heart. If the MI is being caused by a clot in a coronary artery, a thrombolytic drug is administered intravenously to dissolve the clot. If this is done within six to twelve hours of the onset of symptoms, it will increase blood flow in 60-80% of the people (Merck Manual Home Edition, 2005c). (After this time period, administration of a thrombolytic drug will probably not have an effect.) Aspirin or heparin may be prescribed to enhance the effectiveness of the drug. Morphine may be used to minimize pain and decrease anxiety. Nitroglycerin dilates blood vessels. The goal of all of these measures is to prevent damage to the heart by reducing the amount of work the heart has to do and increase the amount of oxygen it is receiving. Contraindications for the thrombolytic drug are severely high blood pressure, history of stroke, internal bleeding, or recent surgery. The thrombolytic drugs, along with aspirin or heparin, reduce the ability to form blood clots. Excessive bleeding is considered too high a risk in these cases. Surgery (angioplasty or coronary bypass) is used when other measures are ineffective.

During the initial days after having a MI, the client is guarded from physical exertion and stress because they put an increased workload on the heart.

This is why visitors are typically limited and the client may not watch television programs that could cause emotional stress. Smoking is prohibited. Stool softeners are commonly prescribed to prevent constipation and eliminate the need to strain with bowel movements. Anti-anxiety or anti-depressants may be prescribed if anxiety or depression becomes significant enough to impact care and recovery. A MI has the potential to enlarge the heart causing CHF, so angiotensin-converting enzyme (ACE) inhibitors are typically prescribed to limit enlargement of heart muscle and improve survival rate. Once the client is medically stable, s/he is discharged from acute care to home without therapy, to home with outpatient therapy, or to a rehabilitation center.

CHF:

- Diuretics are commonly prescribed to eliminate extra fluid as urine. Since the medication increases the amount of urine that the body produces, people taking diuretics will need to use the bathroom more frequently with increased risk of urinary incontinence.
- Sodium causes fluid retention (and the goal is to reduce fluids) so clients with CHF have restricted sodium intake (typically less than 2,000 milligrams a day). Clients with CHF may be asked to weigh themselves at the same time each day to determine if there is a change in body weight. An increase of more than two pounds per day indicates signs of fluid retention. If this trend continues (two pounds every day or more days than not), it is a sign that CHF is worsening (Merck Manual Home Edition, 2005b). Clients who retain fluid will often have swollen legs despite medication and sodium control. Legs should be raised to drain the fluid out of them and help the body reabsorb the excess fluid. Support stockings may be prescribed to minimize lower extremity swelling. If fluid accumulates in the lungs, sleeping with the head elevated can make nighttime breathing easier.
- ACE inhibitors are commonly prescribed to dilate arteries and veins. The kidneys then excrete extra fluid, decreasing the workload of the heart. A variety of other forms of pharmacology are considered depending on the specific cardiac dysfunction.
- Surgical procedures include the implanting a defibrillator (to correct abnormal heart rhythms), a pacemaker, or heart transplant.

Cardiac Rehabilitation

Singh & Schocken (2004) identify five major goals of cardiac rehabilitation: 1. curtail the pathophysiologic and psychosocial effects of heart disease, 2. limit the risk of reinfarction or sudden death, 3. relieve cardiac symptoms, 4. retard or reverse the atherosclerosis by instituting programs for exercise training, education, counseling, and risk factors alteration, and 5. reintegrate heart disease patients into successful functional status in their families and societies. Singh & Schocken (2004) report that current cardiac care has advanced so much

> that exercise training as an isolated intervention may not be able to cause significant reduction in the morbidity and mortality. Nonetheless, exercise training has the potential to act as a catalyst for promoting other aspects of rehabilitation, including risk factor modification through therapeutic lifestyle changes (TLC) and optimization of psychosocial support. Therefore, the outcome measures of cardiac rehabilitation now include improvement of quality of life, such as the patient's perception of physical improvement, satisfaction with risk factor alteration, psychosocial adjustments in interpersonal roles, and potential for advancement to work commensurate with the patient's skills (rather than simply return to work) (web page).

Additional measures for cardiac rehabilitation, especially for older clients, include functional independence, prevention of premature disability, and reduction in need for custodial care (Singh & Schocken, 2004).

Cardiac rehabilitation is not appropriate for all clients who have a cardiac condition. A list of indications and contraindications for cardiac rehabilitation identified by Singh & Schocken (2004) include:

- *Indications*: recent MI, coronary bypass, valve surgery, coronary angioplasty, cardiac transplant, angina, and compensated CHF. A written exercise prescription is made by the treating physician with directions to follow general cardiac precautions or specific parameters (blood pressure, pulse, oxygen saturation levels).
- *Contraindications*: severe residual angina, uncompensated heart failure, uncontrolled arrhythmias, severe ischemia, left ventricle dysfunction or arrhythmia during exercise testing, poorly controlled hypertension, any hypertensive systolic blood pressure response to exercise, or unstable concomitant medical problems (e.g., poorly controlled or "brittle" diabetes, diabetes prone to hypoglycemia, ongoing febrile illness, active transplant rejection).

Cardiac rehabilitation in a general sense can be described in terms of four phases (Doherty, 2003). Each is reviewed below.

Phase 1: This is when the client is in the acute care hospital. Physical exertion is restricted to transfers (bed to/from chair), basic self-care activities (e.g., brushing teeth, combing hair), and slow paced walking. Orthostatic hypotension (drop in blood pressure with change into more upright position) and tachycardia (rapid heartbeat) are typically apparent in these activities.

Phase 2: This phase begins when the client is discharged from the acute care hospital and lasts for a period of 12 weeks. The focus is on endurance training, activity tolerance, and general reconditioning. Isometric exercises are prohibited.

Phase 3: Strength training is initiated to induce physiological adaptations to exercise and to lower blood pressure and heart rate to decrease the workload of the heart.

Phase 4: This phase focuses on the development of maintenance exercise habits.

Activities within cardiac rehabilitation are carefully prescribed so that injury is prevented and progressive improvement is achieved. All activity places a demand on the heart. The extent of this demand is measured in terms of its metabolic equivalent (MET) as described in "Metabolic Equivalents" in the Concepts section.

Therapeutic Lifestyle Changes

This is a list of common lifestyle changes that are encouraged for clients with coronary problems.

- *Quit smoking*: If a client quits smoking, the risk of developing CAD is cut in half, their risk for having an MI decreases, and, if the client requires coronary bypass surgery, it decreases his/her risk of death after surgery. After one year of smoking cessation, the risk of having a coronary event decreases by 50% (Garas & Zafari, 2004).
- *Control blood pressure*: Uncontrolled hypertension is a risk factor for cardiac disease.
- *Engage in regular physical activity*: Clients who have cardiac conditions must receive approval from their physician prior to starting any exercise program. It will typically include specific cardiac precautions or parameters that must be followed during exercise to decrease risks of a coronary event.
- *Reduce cholesterol*: High cholesterol increases the risk of developing atherosclerosis.
- *Maintain a healthy weight*: Weight loss of 10-20 pounds can decrease the risk for CAD. Extra body weight places an extra workload on an already compromised heart.
- *Eat a healthy diet*: A low-fat diet rich in fruits, vegetables, and fiber is recommended to reduce cholesterol levels and decrease risks for CAD and MI. Eating no more than 10-35% of daily

calories from fat, five servings of fruits and vegetables, and dietary fiber from such sources as oat bran, oatmeal, beans, rice, and citrus fruits is recommended to decrease risks for CAD and MI. Foods high in folic acid (e.g., tomatoes, grains) may also be helpful.

- *Reduce stress*: Stress is a normal part of everyone's lives, but prolonged periods of high stress are dangerous to the cardiovascular system. It increases risk of MI and puts a higher workload on the heart, thus worsening CHF.
- *Limit alcohol*: There is a decreased risk of stroke and MI with mild alcohol consumption (Garas & Zafari, 2004). Despite the benefits of drinking red wine, the American Heart Association does not recommend that non-drinkers begin drinking alcohol.
- *Stop drug use*: Quit using drugs, especially male steroids and drugs that increase blood pressure (e.g., cocaine).
- *Control diabetes*: Controlling blood glucose levels may decrease risks of CAD.

Recreational Therapy Approach

Recreational therapy focuses on cardiac recovery, prevention, and general health promotion. Cardiac precautions or parameters as ordered by the physician are monitored during activity to ensure safety. Additionally, the therapist helps the client to identify and change lifestyle habits that increase the risk of further cardiac dysfunction and teaches the client how to adapt activities so an unsafe cardiac load is avoided. Psychosocial issues and other barriers that hinder participation in life activities are also addressed.

Recreational Therapy Interventions

Interventions that are frequently implemented with clients who have a cardiac condition include:

Functional Skill Development

- *Relaxation training and stress management*: Feelings of excitement, fear, or anger can provoke coronary spasm in clients who have atherosclerotic coronary arteries resulting in myocardial ischemia (Sadock & Sadock, 2003). Chest pain (angina) can also occur in clients who do not have heart problems from high levels of acute mental stress that cause coronary artery spasms. Relaxation training and stress management are effective tools in reducing the impact of stress and preventing heart problems. See ICF code d2401 Handling Stress and "Relaxation and Stress Reduction" in the Techniques section for specific interventions.

- *Physical exercise*: Exercise programs designed within cardiac precautions have all of the benefits described above. The recreational therapist can work with the client to find an exercise program that is satisfying for the client, increasing the chances that the client will actually do the exercises. Aquatic therapy and water exercises can be especially appropriate. See "Exercise Basics" in the Techniques section and ICF codes d5701 Managing Diet and Fitness and b4550 General Physical Endurance.
- *Activity adaptation*: Recreational therapists look for adaptations for activities that require physical exertion above the client's limitations. However, not all activities can be adapted and new leisure pursuits may be required. See "Activity Pattern Development" in the Techniques section.

Education/Counseling

- *Heart-related education*: Provide education on 1. recognition of physical exertion related to specific activities for informed activity choices, 2. self-monitoring of heart rate and blood pressure within activity (see "Vital Signs" in the Techniques section), 3. ability to recognize symptoms of cardiac exertion above limitations during activity and how to make activity accommodations, including signs of fatigue, 4. knowledge of the warning signs of a coronary event, and 5. how to monitor environmental conditions that could put extra stress on the heart (e.g., humidity, pollution levels, temperature extremes). This information would be coded with ICF code d5702 Maintaining One's Health.
- *Energy conservation*: Refer to the Techniques section for "Energy Conservation Training" to decrease the risk of injury.
- *Stopping smoking*: See Contributors to Stress under d240 Handling Stress and Other Psychological Demands for information on assisting clients with smoking cessation.

Integration

- *Activity modification*: Incorporate therapeutic lifestyle changes into life situations. Recreational therapists show how lifestyle issues are part of leisure activities such as smoking while playing cards or eating chips when watching a Sunday football game (Mobily & MacNeil, 2002) and address issues related to changing these habits.

Also see "Activity Pattern Development" in the Techniques section for ideas on how to find appropriate activities.

- *Community reintegration*: See "Integration" in the Techniques section for information on getting the client back into community activities.

References

Berkow, R. (1992). *The Merck manual of diagnosis and therapy*. Rahway, NJ: Merck & Co., Inc.

CDC. (1998). National vital statistics report: Acute myocardial infarction. Nov 1992. 47(9). Available at: http://www.disastercenter.com/cdc/aacutcar.html. Accessed July 12, 2002.

Crepeau, E. B., Cohn, E. S., & Boyt Schell, B. A. (2003). *Willard & Spackman's occupational therapy, 10th edition*. Philadelphia, PA: Lippincott Williams & Wilkins.

Doherty, R. F. (2003). Chapter 41: Cardiopulmonary dysfunction in adults; In *Willard & Spackman's occupational therapy, 10th edition*. Philadelphia, PA: Lippincott Williams & Wilkins.

Garas, S. & Zafari, A.M. (2004). Myocardial infarction. Accessed via website www.emedicine.com.

Johnson, N. A. & Heller, R. F. (1998). Prediction of patient non-adherence with home-based exercise for cardiac rehabilitation: The role of perceived barriers and perceived benefits. *Preventative Medicine, 27*:56-64.

Merck Manual Home Edition (2005a). Coronary artery disease. Accessed via website http://www.merck.com/mmhe/index.html.

Merck Manual Home Edition (2005b). Heart failure. Accessed via website http://www.merck.com/mmhe/index.html.

Merck Manual Home Edition (2005c). Myocardial infarction. Accessed via website http://www.merck.com/mmhe/index.html.

Mobily, K. & MacNeil, R. (2002). *Therapeutic recreation and the nature of disabilities*. State College, PA: Venture Publishing, Inc.

Pflieger, K. (2004). Myocardial infarction in childhood. Accessed via website www.emedicine.com.

Sadock, B. & Sadock, V. (2003). *Synopsis of psychiatry, 9th edition*. Philadelphia, PA: Lippincott, Williams & Wilkins.

Satou, G. & Herzberg, G. (2004). Heart failure, congestive. Accessed via website www.emedicine.com.

Singh, V. & Schocken, D. (2004). Cardiac rehabilitation. Accessed via website www.emedicine.com.

Wegner, N. K., Froelicher, E. S., Smith, L., Ades, P., Berra, K., & Blumenthal, J. (1995). *Cardiac rehabilitation as secondary prevention* [Clinical Practice Guideline No. 17, AHCPR Publication No. 96-0673]. Rockville, MD: US Department of Health and Human Services.

Cerebrovascular Accident

A cerebrovascular accident (CVA), also referred to as a stroke due to its sudden onset, is the result of a blockage or rupture in the blood vessels that supply the brain. When the flow of blood that carries the oxygen and nutrients to the brain is interrupted, damage to the brain occurs that results in neurological impairments. The exact impairments depend on the part of the brain that is damaged.

Often medical attention is not sought right away. The result of the delay is more severe damage since early treatment decreases the severity. The National Stroke Association gives the warning signs of CVA as:
- Sudden trouble walking, dizziness, loss of balance or coordination.
- Sudden severe headache with no known cause.
- Sudden nausea, fever, and vomiting distinguished from a viral illness by the speed of onset (minutes or hours vs. days).
- Brief loss of consciousness or period of decreased consciousness (fainting, confusion, convulsions, or coma).

A newer test, called the SAS (Smile Arms Sentence) test, which is easier for laypeople to give, involves the following three parts:
- Ask the individual to smile.
- Ask him or her to raise both arms.
- Ask the person to speak a simple sentence coherently.

Indications of stroke are an unbalanced smile with one side higher than the other, inability to raise the arms and keep them up (especially if one side is weaker than the other), and the inability to speak a sentence clearly and coherently. If any of the indications are present, medical help should be called immediately.

If the symptoms resolve within a 24-48 hour period and there are no or very minimal residual effects, the incident is referred to as a transient ischemic attack (TIA), otherwise known as a "ministroke." This is often a warning or precursor to a CVA.

CVAs can be classified by the side of the brain affected, the major cerebral vessel involved, and the reason for the interruption of blood flow (blockage or hemorrhage). There are six major vessels that may be used as descriptors for diagnosis. Below is a list of the arteries and the corresponding effects (Crepeau, Cohn, & Schell (2003):

- *Internal carotid*: contralateral hemiplegia, sensory problems, aphasia (usually left hemisphere), and hemianopsia.
- *Anterior cerebral*: contralateral hemiplegia, cognitive deficits, sensory deficits, and aphasia (usually left hemisphere).
- *Middle cerebral*: contralateral hemiplegia (primarily the upper extremity), contralateral hemianopsia, sensory deficits, and language deficits.
- *Posterior cerebral*: contralateral hemiplegia, ataxia, visual deficits (e.g., field cuts, cortical blindness, and problems with normal pursuit eye movements).
- *Basilar*: double vision, facial paralysis, visual deficits, and balance or vestibular disturbances.
- *Cerebellar*: vertigo, difficulties in swallowing, ipsilateral ataxia, and changes in sensation.

The side of the brain that is damaged by the CVA affects the symptoms that the client shows:
- *Left CVA*: right hemiplegia, language deficits, slow and cautious behavior style.
- *Right CVA*: left hemiplegia, visual deficits, quick and impulsive behavior style.

Incidence/Prevalence in US

About 700,000 Americans have a stroke each year. It is one of the leading causes of death in the US and it is a leading cause of severe, long-term disability. There are about 4.8 million stroke survivors alive today (American Stroke Association, 2004).

Predominant Age

According to the National Stroke Association, stroke can affect anyone, but there are several risk factors that increase the chances of having a stroke:
- The chances of having a stroke go up with age. Two-thirds of all strokes happen to individuals over age 65. Stroke risk doubles with each decade past age 55.
- Males have a slightly higher stroke risk than females. However, there are more female stroke survivors over of age of 65 than males because women in the United States live longer.
- African-Americans have a higher stroke risk than most other racial groups.
- Risk is higher for people with a family history of stroke or TIA.

- People with diabetes have a higher stroke risk. This may be due to circulation problems caused by diabetes.

Causes

There are three primary flaws or problems within the vascular system that cause CVA.

1. *Thrombosis*: a blood clot that originates in a brain vessel and blocks blood flow.
2. *Embolism*: a blood clot that originates somewhere else in the vascular system (often the heart), breaks free, and then travels to a cerebral vessel, where it becomes lodged and interrupts blood flow.
3. *Hemorrhage*: a blood vessel that ruptures. It is often caused by a sustained increase in blood pressure.

Stroke is largely preventable. Hypertension, heart disease, high cholesterol, sleep apnea, personal history of a TIA, smoking, alcohol use, and body weight above the recommended Body Mass Index (BMI) all have lifestyle components that if changed would significantly reduce CVA risk.

System(s) Affected

Stroke primarily affects motor, cognitive, sensory, language, and visual functions. The areas include:

- *Motor*: hemiplegia, motor planning, coordination.
- *Cognitive*: consciousness functions, orientation, attention, concentration, problem solving, organizing, planning, perceptual dysfunctions, time management, judgment, insight, sequencing, safety.
- *Sensory*: sensory awareness and processing.
- *Language*: expression and reception of language (aphasia, dysarthria).
- *Visual*: field cuts, neglect, double vision, depth perception.

Strokes can also affect emotions (especially lability), personality, sexual function, and bowel and bladder function. The extent of dysfunction depends on the severity and location of brain damage, client's motivation for and participation in rehabilitation, the brain's innate recovery process, and the level of support and encouragement.

Prognosis

According to the National Stroke Association general recovery guidelines show:

- 10% of stroke survivors recover almost completely.
- 25% recover with minor impairments.
- 40% experience moderate to severe impairments requiring special care.
- 10% require care in a nursing home or other long-term care facility.
- 15% die shortly after the stroke.

Recovery of function can occur for six months to one year (and sometimes longer). However, most of the recovery will occur during the first six weeks after the event.

Secondary Problems

Secondary problems mostly relate to inactivity. Inactivity can result from loss of function, inadequate coping mechanisms, and barriers that hinder involvement in a healthy activity pattern. See "Consequences of Inactivity" in the Concepts section for more information. Activity performance in life tasks can also be substantially affected, such as involvement in work, school, community, recreational pursuits, driving, and relationships.

Assessments

The American Heart Association developed a global classification system called the Stroke Outcome Classification to summarize the neurological impairments, disabilities, and handicaps that occur after stroke (Kelly-Hayes et al, 1998). Since it is a summary score, it is recommended that health care professionals support their rating decision with standardized assessment instruments whenever possible. The American Heart Association hopes that the classification lets health care professionals reliably assess recovery, measure responses to treatment, and describe the long-term impact of stroke on survivors.

Typical Scope of Team Assessment

The rehab team evaluates the client's abilities and limitations via a variety of assessments relevant to their field of expertise. A full analysis is also conducted on the environment of the client to identify available support, limitations of support, adaptations and changes that need to be made to the client's home environment to promote independence and function, etc.

Anticipated Findings from RT Assessment

The RT initial evaluation will often reflect a past medical history of uncontrolled stroke risk factors (e.g., poorly managed diabetes, unrecognized hypertension, smoking, overweight, lack of regular physical exercise, high cholesterol).

Treatment Direction

Whole Team Approach

The whole team approach to CVA rehab is to 1. enhance independence, 2. restore functional skills and adapt for functional losses, 3. prevent secondary complications, 4. encourage and facilitate a healthy adjustment to disability, and 5. train family or an identified caregiver to assist the client after discharge. Because neurological recovery varies and its pathways are variable, the team often focuses on task and skill repetition with familiar activities that evoke a spontaneous reaction (e.g., picking up a ringing telephone, singing the alphabet, typical spontaneous speech like "hello" and counting, simple recreational activities with an inherent repetitive component that was part of the client's premorbid activity pattern such as hammering a nail, kneading dough). This type of action helps to facilitate neuromotor re-training. See "Neuroplasticity" in the Techniques section for more information.

Recreational Therapy Approach

CVA therapy, although rooted in facilitation of neurological recovery mechanisms, is a complex art. The therapist must also evaluate and address psychosocial adjustment issues; resource awareness; CVA risk education; family training; activity adaptation; community integration training; and exploration, identification, and development of skills relevant to lifestyle changes to reduce CVA risk (e.g., regular exercise routine, stress management techniques). How these areas are evaluated and addressed depends on the impairments of the client (e.g., instead of doing CVA risk education with a client who is unable to retain the information presented, information is reviewed with the client's primary caregiver).

What to address first, second, simultaneously, etc., depends on the needs of the client. For example, one client with symptoms of depression may respond best to recreational activities that focus on functional skill development while another client with the same symptoms may be motivated by CVA risk education. No two clients or treatment plans will be exactly the same, yet all treatment plans will be moving towards the same outcome of optimal functioning. The therapist is like a guide who helps the client navigate through the jungle.

The primary goal of recreational therapy is for the client to lead a healthy lifestyle that incorporates CVA prevention activities (e.g., exercise), Therefore

the therapist must balance intervention methods of restoration and adaptation so that activities can be designed by the client and family post discharge to meet their situational and emotional needs.

Recreational Therapy Interventions

CVA is a very complex disability that can result in a range of dysfunction. Interventions that are frequently implemented with clients who have had a CVA include:

Functional Skill Development

- *Cognitive impairment*: See "Neuroplasticity" for information on Cognitive Retraining for restoration of cognitive skills. Specific impairments in mental functioning are discussed throughout Body Functions Chapter 1 Mental Functions. Performance of cognitive skills is discussed throughout A&P Chapter 1 Learning and Applying Knowledge. Also see d210 Undertaking a Single Task and d220 Undertaking Multiple Tasks.
- *Upper extremity function*: See Constraint Induced Movement Therapy in "Neuroplasticity" in the Techniques section for information on how to implement forced use techniques to promote restoration of upper extremity function. The related ICF codes are d440 Fine Hand Use, d445 Hand and Arm Use.
- *Left neglect*: Refer to ICF code b2101 Visual Field Functions for information on how to address left neglect.
- *Other mobility functions*: Address development of mobility functions in the clinic as it relates to what the client needs in particular life situations. See Body Functions Chapter 7 Neuromusculoskeletal and Movement Related Functions and A&P Chapter 4 Mobility for specific deficits.

Education/Counseling (includes family training)

Refer to the following techniques in the Techniques section: "Americans with Disabilities Act Education," "Community Accessibility Training," "Community Problem Solving," "Emergency Response Training," "Energy Conservation Training," and "Lifestyle Alteration Education" as appropriate for each client. Also see "Consequences of Inactivity" in the Concepts section.

Integration (includes family training)

Clients are integrated into their real-life environments. Recreational therapists assess a client's ability to carry over learned skills into real-life environments and teach new or re-designed skills as needed (learned skills do not always transfer into real-life situations). In addition to the previously mentioned interventions, therapists include:

- Language use especially for people who have had a left CVA. The goal is to use the techniques learned in speech therapy in real-life settings. Body Functions Chapter 3 Voice and Speech Functions has more information.
- Community mobility skills as described in A&P Chapter 4 Mobility.
- "Integration" in the Techniques section.
- "Transitioning a Client from Inpatient Rehabilitation to a Communal Environment" in the Techniques section.

Health Promotion after Discharge

See "Activity Pattern Development" in the Techniques section.

Miscellaneous

National Stroke Association
9707 E. Easter Lane
Englewood, CO 80112
1-800-STROKES (787-6537) or (303) 649-9299
www.stroke.org

References

American Stroke Association. (2004). Impact of stroke. http://www.strokeassociation.org/presenter.jhtml? identifier=1033 on 3/5/04.

Crepeau, E., Cohn, E., & Schell, B., (2003). *Willard and Spackman's occupational therapy, tenth edition.* Philadelphia, PA: Lippincott Williams & Wilkins.

Kelly-Hayes, M., Robertson, J., Broderick, J., Duncan, P., Hershey, L., Roth, E., Thies, W., Trombly, C. (1998). The American Heart Association Stroke Outcome Classification. *Stroke 29*:1274-1280.

Chronic Obstructive Pulmonary Disease

People who have Chronic Obstructive Pulmonary Disease (COPD) have one, or a combination of, chronic bronchitis, asthma, and emphysema. All of these interfere with the normal functioning of the lung (see Table 10 below) by obstructing or interfering with part of the breathing system. Consequently, people who have one or more of these diseases may be labeled as having COPD.

- *Chronic bronchitis*: Chronic bronchitis is chronic inflammation of the bronchial tubes with an increase in mucus and mucus secreting cells. The mucus obstructs the bronchioles causing air to become trapped, making it difficult to breathe in and out. The person coughs to try to clear the mucus and becomes short of breath with exertion. Chronic bronchitis is associated with prolonged exposure to bronchial irritants. Smoking is the most common cause of chronic bronchitis.

- *Emphysema*: In emphysema, the walls of the alveoli begin to break down and the lung loses its elasticity. So instead of having many small alveoli, only a few large air sacs remain. To picture this, think about two bubbles touching each other. Each bubble has its own outer surface, just like the alveoli. In alveolar wall breakdown, the wall that keeps the two bubbles separate breaks down and makes one large bubble. Within the lung, less alveoli and bigger air sacs cause a problem. There is less surface area for the exchange of oxygen and carbon dioxide. When combined with the loss of lung elasticity, air can become trapped in the large alveoli leading to poor air exchange and shortness of breath. Chronic bronchitis is often the cause of emphysema.

Table 10: Normal Functioning of the Lung

> **Lung Functioning**
>
> Think of the lungs as an upside down tree. When a breath is taken in by the mouth or nose it travels down the trachea (the tree trunk) and branches into large tubes (heavy branches called "bronchi") and small tubes (thin branches called "bronchioles"). At the end of the small tubes are alveoli, something like the leaves on a tree. These are small air sacs with very thin walls. In these walls are capillaries. When air is taken into the alveoli the capillaries in the air sac walls capture the oxygen and carry it into the bloodstream. The airways (trachea, bronchi, and bronchioles), the lung tissue itself, and the alveoli are elastic. The lung expands when a breath is taken in and contracts/collapses when air is exhaled.

- *Chronic asthmatic bronchitis*: This occurs in people who have an underlying asthmatic problem that results in persistent airway obstruction despite anti-asthmatic therapy.

Incidence/Prevalence in US

COPD is the fourth leading cause of death in the United States and it is projected to jump to the third leading cause of death by 2020. In 2001, 12.1 million people age 25 and older reported being diagnosed with COPD. Interestingly, however, an additional 24 million people in 2001 reported impaired lung function leading the National Institutes of Health to believe that COPD is probably under-diagnosed (National Institutes of Health, 2003).

Predominant Age

COPD is usually diagnosed in young middle age.

Causes

The primary cause of COPD is smoking. This includes all smoked tobacco products (cigarettes, pipe, cigars). Only a small number of people develop COPD from other air allergens (e.g., prolonged exposure to fumes, chemicals, secondhand smoke). In rare cases, COPD can be caused by alpha 1 antitrypsin deficiency. This is a gene-related disorder in which low levels of alpha 1 antitrypsin lead to deterioration of the lung. People who have this deficiency and smoke are instructed to stop smoking, since smoking causes the disease to progress more rapidly.

System(s) Affected

COPD primarily affects the lungs, although other systems may occur as discussed in "Secondary Signs and Symptoms" later in this diagnosis.

Prognosis

Most people can be stabilized with medications. Oxygen therapy may also be needed depending on the severity of the disease (see "Oxygen" in the Techniques section for more information about the use of oxygen). COPD is not reversible. The damage cannot be undone. The progression of the disease, however, can be halted with smoking cessation. The prognosis (years of life, quality of life, functional abilities) depends upon the severity of the disease. People with COPD usually die from complications from the disease. Such complications include infections (pneumonia, the flu), heart failure, and respiratory failure. In the year 2000, COPD contributed to 119,000 deaths in the US (National Institutes of Health, 2003).

Secondary Problems

People with COPD may have poor nutrition, poor muscle strength and endurance, skeletal disease (e.g., decreased bone density), psychosocial issues (depression, anxiety, learned helplessness, loss of internal locus of control), trouble sleeping, and sensory problems. Many of these problems are due to frequent hospitalizations, decreased activity level, deconditioning, medications, lack of sufficient oxygen, and poor adjustment and coping strategies.

Assessments

Typical Scope of Team Assessment

The physician takes a medical history, listens to the client's lungs, and performs a breathing test to confirm the diagnosis of COPD. A common breathing test is the spirometry test. The client blows breath into a tube that measure the amount of air the lungs can hold and how fast the client can exhale. Results of the test help the physician to determine the severity of the disease (at risk, mild, moderate, severe). Other tests may include a chest x-ray and an arterial blood gas test (to determine how much oxygen is in the blood). The treatment team evaluates the client's current level of functioning in all domains and develops a treatment plan that predominantly reflects exercise training and education.

Anticipated Findings from RT Assessment

The recreational therapist will commonly find that the client has been leading a lifestyle that has become increasingly isolative and homebound. Recreational activities are usually limited, with the majority of the client's time being spent watching television, napping, reading, or engaging in other activities that requires little or no physical exertion. It is not uncommon for people with moderate to severe COPD to remain in the home for weeks or months at a time. There is often high anxiety surrounding any activity that requires physical exertion and feelings of depression are commonly reported from lack of social contact and having to cope with a chronic disease that greatly limits the client's ability to participate in activities that s/he once enjoyed. Some clients can become quite bitter and angry about their situation contributing to the distancing of friends and family. A history of falls and complaints about loss of balance are common due to deconditioning (weakened muscles, loss of flexibility, poor

endurance). Clients are typically unaware of the connection between exercise and pulmonary health or dismiss suggestions to exercise with comments like, "The doctor just doesn't understand that I can't do that." Learned helpless and external locus of control are also common findings.

Treatment Direction

Whole Team Approach

The rehabilitation team works on the treatments described below.

Exercise training: Exercise training is a cornerstone of pulmonary rehabilitation. Exercise training consists of endurance, strength, and flexibility training. Endurance training is predominantly addressed through walking. Strength training may include lifting weights, unsupported arm exercises, and therabands. Flexibility training is addressed through range of motion and stretching exercises. The benefits derived from exercise training are evident within a very short time, but they are only maintained for as long as exercise is continued. "Therefore, efforts at improving long-term adherence with exercise training at home are necessary for the long-term effectiveness of pulmonary rehabilitation" (Sharma & Arneja, 2003, p. 16). The benefits of exercise in pulmonary rehabilitation include

- *Reduced shortness of breath.*
- *Increased appetite*: This is important because many people who have COPD are malnourished due to loss of appetite and inability or difficulty in obtaining food.
- *Decreased stress and anxiety*: Feelings of stress and anxiety can bring on attacks of shortness of breath, so reduced stress can reduce attacks of shortness of breath.
- *Stronger and more flexible muscles*: Weak muscles require more oxygen to perform a task and poor flexibility can lead to falls.
- *Increased quality of sleep*: Adequate sleep helps with energy level.
- *Reduced need for oxygen therapy*: Both less time using oxygen and lower oxygen flows are possible.

Self-image changes: The incorporation of exercise into the client's daily routine after discharge can be very difficult for clients on many different levels. It is a new way of thinking and behaving. People who are seen in inpatient rehabilitation for COPD typically have moderate to severe COPD and have mostly adapted to the COPD by giving up activities that cause shortness of breath, specifically activities that require physical exertion. This results in staying at home more; having fewer social contacts; deconditioning from lack of exercise; experiencing feelings of depression, anxiety, and/or isolation; lack of outside stimulation with possible disorientation; and difficulties in obtaining supplies from the community (e.g., prescriptions, groceries). Energy is typically reserved and spent only on necessary self-care activities (e.g., bathing, dressing, simple meal preparation). Breaking this long-term cycle of behavior can be difficult and adopting a different view of pulmonary care through exercise may not be easily accepted. Although clients experience the pulmonary benefits of exercise firsthand while at the rehabilitation center and may verbalize their intention to follow an exercise program after discharge, carryover is often poor. It sometimes seems as if the clients choose to keep their disease because it is more comfortable for them. To increase the likelihood of exercise carryover, problem solving, resource awareness, education, and development of a positive self-image must be included in the rehabilitation program.

Medications and oxygen therapy: Inhaled steroids or bronchodilators may be prescribed to open up the airways to make it easier to breathe. Oxygen therapy may be provided as needed (PRN) or throughout the day. Lack of adequate oxygen can damage organs, decrease alertness, induce feelings of fatigue, and cause shortness of breath. See "Oxygen" in the Techniques section for more information.

Education: Health professionals educate clients with COPD on the following:

- *COPD*: People with COPD need to be educated about the disease and their role in managing it with the hope that it will increase compliance with recommendations.
- *Energy conservation and work simplification*: This if often referred to as the five Ps: prioritize, plan, pace, position, and pounds. See "Energy Conservation Training" in the Techniques section for detailed information.
- *Medication*: People with COPD are educated about the types of medication they are taking, their action, side effects, proper dosage, and proper use. Special training on the use of oxygen therapy may also be needed.
- *Living will*: The case manger or social worker is typically the person who addresses this issue with the client. The client is made aware of a thing called a living will. A living will stipulates what interventions are acceptable and unacceptable (e.g., artificial life support, resuscitation) should the client be unable to make the decision. This is a delicate issue that is addressed routinely with clients who enter a hospital setting so that the client's wishes are respected.

- *Vaccines*: It is typically recommended that the client receive flu and pneumococcal vaccines to decrease risks of developing illnesses.
- *Smoking cessation*: Clients who smoke are told to quit smoking. This will slow down the progression of the disease. Smoking cessation assistance may be offered if needed (e.g., nicotine patch, nicotine gum, counseling).
- *Pollutants and allergens*: Clients are to stay away from air pollutants and allergens that can affect lung function.

Adaptive equipment: The prescription of adaptive equipment (e.g., walking aid, adaptive recreation equipment) can help decrease the amount of energy used for specific tasks. This may include a mobility aid such as a cane, walker, or wheelchair; a self-care piece of equipment such as a dressing stick or a reacher; or a recreational aid such as lightweight gardening tools or adaptive computer aids to help with maintaining proper body mechanics and ergonomics.

Psychosocial and behavioral intervention: This includes individual or group therapy that focuses on stress management and relaxation training, techniques for managing anxiety and panic to help reduce shortness of breath, techniques for managing feelings of depression, and discussions about healthy coping techniques. Ongoing support groups can be helpful for people with COPD and their families.

Breathing techniques: There are two types of breathing techniques that can be helpful when the client feels short of breath:

- *Pursed-lip breathing* (PLB): Pursed lip breathing is used when the client feels short of breath from activity, stress, or anxiety. Short and rapid breathing patterns are common in people who have COPD. PLB makes the client focus on a slower breathing pattern. When the lips are pursed while exhaling, pressure within the airway increases, which helps to keep the airway open. When inhaling with the lips pursed, the major portion of the work is transferred from the diaphragm to the ribcage muscles. Resting the diaphragm also helps to reduce shortness of breath. Technique: The client is instructed to purse his/her lips (as if to whistle or blow out a candle) and slowly exhale for four to six seconds.
- *Leaning forward posture*: Leaning forward postures are helpful to reduce shortness of breath because it reduces respiratory effort. A client who is short of breath should sit down and lean forward (e.g., rest arms on a tabletop) and then perform PLB to open up the airway.

Nutritional counseling: Approximately 50% of the people who are hospitalized with COPD have protein and calorie malnutrition (Sharma & Arneja, 2003). Consequently, progressive weight loss is common. People with COPD often do not have an adequate dietary intake. They also burn more calories with minimal activities (increased resting energy expenditure), have difficulty obtaining food from the market (e.g., walking, transporting bags of groceries), and may lack a healthy adaptation for this problem. Poor nutritional intake also affects the client's energy, which makes it even harder to obtain food. The treatment team educates clients with COPD about the importance of maintaining a proper weight and receiving adequate nutrition to maintain strength. This is also coupled with problem solving and resource awareness to help with carryover. On the opposite spectrum, obesity can also affect respiratory function. Extra body weight puts a greater strain on the respiratory system, especially for activities that require the client to stand or walk. Clients who are overweight are encouraged to decrease body fat. Issues that surround the person's ability to obtain healthy food (e.g., ability to go to the supermarket instead of eating home delivery fast food) need to be addressed and counseling sessions with a nutritionist are recommended to develop healthy meal plans.

Recreational Therapy Approach

The recreational therapy approach addresses many of the topics described in the team approach. The difference is that the recreational therapist puts a much stronger focus on integration of these skills into the client's real-life environment.

Recreational Therapy Interventions

Interventions that are commonly implemented with clients who have COPD include:

Functional Skill Development

- *Exercise training*: See b455 Exercise Functions and "Exercise Basics" in the Techniques section.
- *Adaptive equipment and techniques*: Recreational therapists recommend (and may fabricate) adaptive equipment to minimize exertion for tasks. Equipment recommendations should be lightweight (more weight equals more exertion) and of simple construction (more complexity equals more exertion). Adaptive techniques to minimize exertion in specific recreational activities are also recommended. Equipment is discussed in Environmental Factors Chapter 1 Products and Technology. Teaching the client how to use the equipment may be scored with

d155 Acquiring Skills, d570 Looking after One's Health, or the code for the specific task the adaptation addresses.

Education/Counseling

- *Lifestyle changes*: ICF code d240 Handling Stress and Other Psychological Demands has a lot of information on how the client can be taught new ways to handle the stress of having COPD.
- *Smoking cessation*: See Contributors to Stress under d240 Handling Stress and Other Psychological Demands for information on assisting clients with smoking cessation.
- *Other education*: As needed, refer to the Concepts section for information on "Consequences of Inactivity" and the Techniques section for "Community Accessibility Training," "Lifestyle Alteration Education," "Activity Pattern Development," "Education and Counseling" (for leisure education and counseling), "Energy Conservation Training," "Body Mechanics and Ergonomics," "Relaxation and Stress Reduction" (to help to decrease feelings of stress and anxiety that can bring on attacks of shortness of breath), "Personal Leisure Resource Awareness," "Community Leisure Resource Awareness," and "Self-Esteem" (to work on locus of control).

Integration

- *Community reintegration*: See "Integration" in the Techniques section for ways to get the client back into the community again.
- *Social support*: Social support is helpful to reduce feelings of depression and isolation. People who have a good social support system are also healthier and appear to have better coping skills. Interaction, in and of itself, provides opportunities for learning, sharing, and self-expression. All of this is beneficial for health promotion. See A&P Chapter 7 Interpersonal Interactions and Relationships and A&P Chapter 9 Community, Social, and Civic Life.

References

National Emphysema Foundation. (2004). COPD and exercise. http://www.emphysemafoundation.org/pulhthex.aspx on 10/1/04.

National Institutes of Health. (2003). *Chronic obstructive pulmonary disease*. NIH publication # 03-5229. Bethesda, MD: NHLBI Health Information Center.

Sharma, S. & Arneja, A. (2003). Pulmonary rehabilitation. www.emedicine.com on 10/1/04.

Dementia

Dementia is a general term to describe multiple disorders in which the client experiences decreased cognitive function while not losing consciousness. Dementia is a long-term, usually progressive, process often lasting ten years or more. The long-term, fairly steady decline is what distinguishes dementia from other cognitive impairments such as delirium, mental retardation, and schizophrenia. While continued deterioration of memory (learning and retrieving information) is the classic symptom, there are other common cognitive impairments associated with dementia. These include:

- Declining ability to recognize one's relationship to others and things; orientation (b114).
- Declining ability to understand and integrate information; intellectual functions (b117).
- Impaired ability to solve problems (b1646).
- Decreased ability to identify and comprehend the meaning of sensory stimulation; perceptional ability (b156).
- Impaired mental functions related to language (b167).
- Impaired ability to weigh different options for actions and increasing inability to form opinions; judgment (b1645).
- Declining ability to act in a socially and contextually appropriate manner in relationships (d7).
- Declining ability to focus attention on the task at hand while losing the ability to filter out distracting noises and movements (d160).

There are many types of dementia, often associated with the underlying, suspected cause of the disease. All types of dementia have a significant decline in multiple cognitive abilities that include a decline in memory and at least one of the following: 1. aphasia 2. apraxia, 3. agnosia, and 4. decline in executive function. The five most recognized types of dementia are

- *Alzheimer's type*: A broad-based loss of cognitive function that is gradual and progressive. It is associated with plaque in the cortex and fibrillary degeneration in the pyramidal ganglion cells.
- *Vascular dementia*: A general decline in cognitive function that is accompanied by specific neurological symptoms such as an exaggerated deep tendon reflex, weakness of an extremity, or abnormal gait patterns indicative of multiple, small strokes or damage to the cortex of the brain.

- *Dementia due to other general medical conditions*: A general decline due to a medical condition other than Alzheimer's or cerebrovascular. Some of the possible causes are tumors, diabetes, hypothyroidism, vitamin B12 deficiency, and infection.
- *Substance-induced persisting dementia*: The general decline in cognitive function linked to persisting effects of substances including alcohol, a drug of abuse, or medication.
- *Dementia due to multiple etiologies*: A general decline in cognitive ability that is likely due to multiple causes such as vascular lesions in the cortex and chronic use of alcohol.

While 75% of clients with dementia are living at home, the primary reason for admission to a nursing home is dementia (Burke & Morgenlander, 1999).

Incidence/Prevalence in US

Just over 1% of adults over the age of 65 have dementia. This rate significantly increases to almost 25% for adults over the age of 85. Dementia of the Alzheimer's type accounts for close to 50% of all types of dementia. Vascular dementia accounts for up to 30% of clients with dementia (Sadock & Sadock, 2003).

Predominate Age

The vast majority of clients with dementia are over the age of 60 with the notable exception of clients with dementia caused by AIDS or Down syndrome.

Causes

Dementia is a term that describes an outcome (loss of cognitive function but not consciousness). There are many different disorders or situations that can lead to this outcome, as described above.

System(s) Affected

The primary body system affected by dementia is neurological related to mental functions. As the disease progresses, many of the other body functions are affected either directly by the disease process or due to the client's decreased physical activity and ability to take care of himself/herself.

Prognosis

Dementia is a terminal disease. Research results disagree on how long a client is likely to live after being diagnosed with dementia. The average is stated as being anywhere between three and eight years with an outside range of ten to twenty years.

It is estimated that up to 15% of clients with dementia can improve or reverse the dementia if early and appropriate treatment is taken (Sadock & Sadock, 2003).

Secondary Problems

- *Agitation and aggression*: These are secondary problems for about half of the clients with dementia (Burke & Morgenlander, 1999). The agitation and aggression may be seen in combativeness, hyperactivity, or disinhibition related to socially acceptable behaviors.
- *Decubitus ulcers* (skin breakdowns, pressure sores): often due to inactivity or compulsive scratching, picking, or itching.
- *Depression*: a common secondary diagnosis in dementia affecting up to 20% of the clients (Burke & Morgenlander, 1999). The depression is often caused by an organic problem such as a left cerebral hemisphere stroke; neurological deterioration that is part of the mental deterioration of dementia; or because of neurological damage due to Parkinson's disease, AIDS, or other medical disorders. Apathy is a common side effect of depression.
- *Pacing*: almost continuous and compulsive walking is a common characteristic of dementia.
- *Psychosis*: Delusions (false, fixed beliefs) and hallucinations (the perception of something that does not really exist) are secondary problems with some clients with dementia. It is fairly common for clients with dementia to suspect that a family member, staff person, or other client is stealing from him/her. Hallucinations often include seeing or hearing someone from the client's past or perceiving that s/he is in a home that s/he used to occupy.
- *Sleep disturbance*: This is one of the most common reasons that a client is institutionalized. While the client's sleep cycle may be broken up because of medical reasons, such as the need to urinate more frequently, part of the problem may be due to the inordinate amount of napping done throughout the day.

Assessments

Typical Scope of Team Assessment

Clients with dementia receive a complete physical exam to establish the likely cause of the progressive cognitive impairment. There are numerous classification systems that help group clients with patterns of functional loss. Some of the classification systems have three stages (early, mid, and late), some four stages (mild, moderate, moderately severe, and severe), and some have seven stages (no impairment, very mild decline, mild decline, moderate decline, moderately severe decline, severe decline, and very severe decline). The Alzheimer's Association (2005) has combined the three sets of classifications in their "Stages of Alzheimer's Disease."

Stage 1: *No Cognitive Impairment.* Unimpaired individuals experience no memory problems and none are evident to a health care professional during a medical interview.

Stage 2: *Very Mild Cognitive Decline.* Individuals at this stage feel as if they have memory lapses, especially in forgetting familiar words or names or the location of keys, eyeglasses, or other everyday objects. But these problems are not evident during a medical examination or apparent to friends, family, or co-workers.

Stage 3: *Mild Cognitive Decline.* (Early-stage Alzheimer's can be diagnosed in some, but not all, individuals with these symptoms.) Friends, family, or co-workers begin to notice deficiencies. Problems with memory or concentration may be measurable in clinical testing or discernible during a detailed medical interview. Common difficulties include:
- Word- or name-finding problems noticeable to family or close associates.
- Decreased ability to remember names when introduced to new people.
- Performance issues in social or work settings noticeable to family, friends, or co-workers.
- Reading a passage and retaining little material.
- Losing or misplacing a valuable object.
- Decline in ability to plan or organize.

Stage 4: *Moderate Cognitive Decline.* (Mild or early-stage Alzheimer's disease) At this stage, a careful medical interview detects clear-cut deficiencies in the following areas:
- Decreased knowledge of recent occasions or current events.
- Impaired ability to perform challenging mental arithmetic, for example, to count backward from 100 by 7s.
- Decreased capacity to perform complex tasks, such as planning dinner for guests or paying bills and managing finances.
- Reduced memory of personal history.
- The affected individual may seem subdued and withdrawn, especially in socially or mentally challenging situations.

Stage 5: Moderately Severe Cognitive Decline. (Moderate or mid-stage Alzheimer's disease) Major gaps in memory and deficits in cognitive function emerge. Some assistance with day-to-day activities becomes essential. At this stage, individuals may:

- Be unable during a medical interview to recall some important personal history.
- Become confused about where they are or about the date, day of the week, or season.
- Have trouble with less challenging mental arithmetic, for example counting backward from 40 by 4s or from 20 by 2s.
- Need help choosing proper clothing for the season or the occasion.
- Usually retain substantial knowledge about themselves and know their own name and the names of their spouse or children.
- Usually require no assistance with eating or using the toilet.

Stage 6: Severe Cognitive Decline. (Moderately severe or mid-stage Alzheimer's disease) Memory difficulties continue to worsen, significant personality changes may emerge, and affected individuals need extensive help with customary daily activities. At this stage, individuals may:

- Lose most awareness of recent experiences and events as well as of their surroundings.
- Recollect their personal history imperfectly, although they generally recall their own name.
- Occasionally forget the name of their spouse or primary caregiver but generally can distinguish familiar from unfamiliar faces.
- Need help getting dressed properly.
- Experience disruptions of their normal sleep/waking cycle.
- Need help with handling details of toileting.
- Have increasing episodes of urinary or fecal incontinence.
- Experience significant personality changes and behavioral symptoms, including suspiciousness and delusions, hallucinations, or compulsive, repetitive behaviors such as hand wringing or tissue shredding.
- Tend to wander and become lost.

Stage 7: Very Severe Cognitive Decline (Severe or late-stage Alzheimer's disease) This is the final stage of the disease when individuals lose the ability to respond to their environment, the ability to speak, and, ultimately, the ability to control movement.

- Frequently individuals lose their capacity for recognizable speech, although words or phrases may occasionally be uttered.
- Individuals need help with eating and toileting and there is general incontinence of urine.

- Individuals lose the ability to walk without assistance, then the ability to sit without support, the ability to smile, and the ability to hold their head up. Reflexes become abnormal and muscles grow rigid. Swallowing is impaired.

Anticipated Findings of RT Assessment

The majority of clients with dementia also have a behavioral diagnosis of one type or another. Review the *Secondary Problems* section above for suggestions of what to look for during the assessment.

Many clients with dementia also have pain as a secondary problem that can greatly impact the client's ability to benefit from therapy. See b280 Sensation of Pain for more information.

Treatment Direction

Whole Team Approach

The initial goal of the treatment team is to find a treatment that will reduce the deficits of the clients by finding and treating a medical cause. In the majority of cases this is not possible. The overall approach to untreatable dementia is to support the remaining functions of the client and to make the client comfortable. Some ideas include:

- Providing orientation materials (large clock, calendars, etc.).
- Ensuring plenty of time for tasks so the client does not feel rushed.
- Tolerating non-harmful activities such as pacing in ways that keep the client from getting lost or leaving the facility and prevent the client from getting into other client's rooms.
- Providing limited amounts of psychotropic medications for depression while watching for side effects.
- Using validation techniques instead of cognitive arguments about hallucinations or delusions.
- Re-establishing a healthy sleep routine for clients with dementia by offering activities that require handwork such as crafts activities and simple housework instead of television watching, which frequently leads to long naps.
- Providing daily physical exercise involving movement and stretching of all extremities as well as walking (when the client is able to walk) at a consistent time each day.
- Providing adequate daytime light. The rooms that are used by clients during the daytime should have good light, preferably natural light.

Recreational Therapy Approach

Recreational therapists support the team approach, especially in the areas of orientation, physical exercise, activities that that clients can do, and validation training for other staff.

Despite the stage of dementia, there are several general guidelines for setting up the environment for activity when possible:

- Because the client has a decreased ability to filter extraneous sensory input, the environment should have limited stimulation. The therapy room (or activity room) should not be cluttered. Traffic through the room should be limited or avoided during the therapy session. There should be no other activities with other clients going on within visual or auditory proximity. Any other external noises should be extinguished whenever possible (e.g., turning off the TV, talking with a supervisor about removing the communication speaker from the therapy room).

- One of the greatest methods to assist clients with dementia is to create an environment that is supportive. This includes adequate lighting because the eye has a decreased ability to take in light as it ages; eliminating glare off of shiny floors, furniture, and metal objects through the use of carpet and dull/soft finishes; and providing safe areas for the client to walk including stable chairs with arms so the client can sit and rest safely.

Recreational Therapy Interventions

Interventions that are frequently implemented with clients who have dementia include:

- *Sensory stimulation*: See b156 Perceptual Functions and "Sensory Stimulation" in the Techniques section.
- *Orientation*: See b114 Orientation Functions.
- *Standard routine*: Create a standard routine to reduce disorientation and agitation, as well as promote internal locus of control, self-efficacy, and predictability. See d230 Carrying Out a Daily Routine and "Activity Pattern Development" in the Techniques section.
- *Stress reduction techniques*: These can reduce agitation. See d240 Handling Stress and Other Psychological Demands and "Relaxation and Stress Reduction" in the Techniques section.
- *Leisure time physical activity*: See d920 Recreation and Leisure and "Exercise Basics" in the Techniques section.
- *Compensatory strategies for memory loss*: See b144 Memory Functions and Cognitive Retraining in "Neuroplasticity" in the Techniques section.

References

Alzheimer's Association. (2005). Stages of Alzheimer's Disease. http://www.alz.org/AboutAD/Stages.asp#stage1.

Burke, J. & Morgenlander, J. (1999). Managing common behavior problems in dementia. *Postgraduate Medicine Online*. October, 1999.

Sadock, B. & Sadock, V. (2003). *Synopsis of psychiatry* (9th ed.). Philadelphia, PA: Lippincott, Williams & Wilkins.

Diabetes Mellitus

Diabetes mellitus (DM) is a complex disease that occurs when insulin production is too low (or lacking entirely) or when the body is unable to effectively use the insulin it produces because of defects in the insulin receptors. The result is that the body does not metabolize carbohydrates, protein, or fat correctly, leading to severe complications and death if it is not treated.

The body, in its normal state, manufactures insulin to transport sugar (also called glucose) into cells. The cells use the sugar for energy. In diabetes, the body does not properly produce or use insulin. Therefore, glucose builds up in the blood causing a variety of health problems. Many cases of DM go undetected because the symptoms mimic symptoms of other problems. The symptoms include excessive thirst, extreme hunger, frequent urination, unusual weight loss, increased fatigue, irritability, and blurry vision. It is often not until a person experiences a health problem (e.g., circulation problem, wound that won't heal) that s/he seeks medical attention and is given the diagnosis of DM.

There are four primary classifications of diabetes (Centers for Disease Control and Prevention, 2003).

- *Type 1 Diabetes* (T1D): Insulin dependent diabetes mellitus (IDDM) and juvenile-onset diabetes are now called type 1 diabetes. Type 1 diabetes develops when the body's immune system destroys the pancreatic beta cells that make insulin. It primarily occurs in children and young adults. Risk factors for type 1 diabetes include autoimmune, genetic, and environmental factors.

- *Type 2 Diabetes* (T2D): Non-insulin dependent diabetes mellitus (NIDDM) and adult-onset diabetes are now called type 2 diabetes. It is the most common form of diabetes. The body does not produce enough insulin or the cells cannot use the insulin properly so there is a build-up of glucose it the bloodstream. If glucose levels are not reduced, damage can occur to many body systems including the eyes, kidneys, nerves, and heart. Type 2 diabetes is associated with older age, obesity, family history of diabetes, prior history of gestational diabetes, impaired glucose tolerance, physical inactivity, and race/ethnicity. Clients who have type 2 diabetes can usually control their blood glucose by following a special diabetic diet, participating in a regular exercise program, achieving and maintaining ideal body weight, and taking oral medication. Insulin may also be needed.

- *Gestational Diabetes* (GD): During pregnancy some women develop gestational diabetes, a form of glucose intolerance. Gestational diabetes occurs more frequently among African-Americans, Hispanic/Latino Americans, and Native Americans. It is also more common among obese women and women with a family history of diabetes. During pregnancy, gestational diabetes requires treatment to normalize maternal blood glucose levels to avoid complications in the infant.

- *Pre-diabetes*: Pre-diabetes is a condition that occurs when a person's blood glucose levels are higher than normal but not high enough for a diagnosis of T2D.

Incidence/Prevalence in US

- In the year 2002, DM was the fifth leading cause of death by disease in the US (Diabetes Care, 2003). Most of these deaths are related to diabetes-associated cardiovascular disease (Healthy People 2010).

- Approximately 800,000 people are diagnosed with diabetes every year (Clark, 1998).

- Approximately 90-95% of Americans diagnosed with diabetes have T2D (ADA, Diabetes Symptoms, 2004).

- From 1995 to 2025, the number of adults with diabetes is projected to increase by 122%, from 135 million to 300 million (King, Aubert, & Herman, 1998).

- The Third National Health and Nutrition Survey in the US showed that 40-50% of people with diabetes have poor control of glucose levels (Harris et al, 1999). Poor control is a significant risk factor for diabetic complications. Control of glucose levels is achieved through pharmacology and compliance with healthy lifestyle behaviors.

- Almost 90% of all people with newly diagnosed T2D are overweight (ADA, Weight Loss Matters, 2004).

- African-Americans, Hispanic/Latino Americans, Native Americans, and some Asian Americans, Native Hawaiian, or other Pacific Islanders have a greater incidence of T2D than other groups (CDCP, 2003).

Predominant Age

DM affects men and women equally (about 8.7% of each gender). The approximate number of people in the US with DM is 206,000 people under age 20 (0.25% of all people in this age group); 18 million people 20 to 59 (8.7% of all people in this age group); and 8.6 million people 60 and older (18.3% of all people in this age group). Approximately one in every 400 to 500 children and adolescents has T1D. T2D (which used to be seen only in adults) is increasingly being diagnosed in children and adolescents (CDCP, 2003).

Causes

There is no known cause of DM, but genetics, environmental factors, and lifestyle factors such as obesity and lack of exercise appear to play dominant roles (ADA, 2004, All About Diabetes).

System(s) Affected

See Secondary Problems below.

Prognosis

- *T1D*: Clients who have T1D will need to take insulin via an insulin pump or injections for their entire life. There are no known methods to prevent or cure T1D.
- *T2D*: The prognosis for people who have T2D will vary depending on the level of glucose control that client is able to maintain. In some cases if the client loses enough weight, T2D will go away.
- *GD*: After pregnancy, 5-10% of women with gestational diabetes have type 2 diabetes. Women who have had gestational diabetes have a 20-50% chance of developing diabetes in the next 5-10 years (ADA, The Metabolic Syndrome, 2004; CDCP, 2003).
- *Pre-diabetes*: Clients with pre-diabetes can prevent the development of type 2 diabetes through diet and exercise. Thirty minutes a day of moderate physical activity and a 5-10% reduction in body weight produces about a 58% reduction in diabetes, as the glucose levels return to normal ranges (ADA, 2004, How to Prevent Pre-Diabetes).

Secondary Problems

Hypoglycemia: This is when blood sugar becomes too low. Symptoms include shakiness, dizziness, sweating, hunger, headache, pale skin color, sudden moodiness or behavior changes, clumsy or jerky movements, seizure, difficulty paying attention, confusion, and tingling sensations around the mouth. If hypoglycemia occurs, blood sugar can be raised by taking three glucose tablets, ½ cup of fruit juice, or five to six pieces of hard candy. Clients are taught to carry blood sugar testing supplies and a form of sugar at all times to manage

hypoglycemia. Clients are encouraged to check their blood sugar level as soon as they feel low blood sugar coming on. After blood sugar is tested and treatment implemented, blood sugar should be rechecked at 15-20 minutes to see if it went back up. If blood sugar is still low and symptoms persist, treat it again (more sugar) and wait another 15-20 minutes and recheck the blood sugar. If blood glucose levels do not rise, the client could pass out. If this occurs, immediate treatment is required, such as an injection of glucagon or emergency treatment in a hospital. The client is educated on how to self-inject glucagon and told to train others (e.g., family, friends, coworkers) on how to inject it if s/he passes out. If glucagon is not available, the client will need to be taken to the closest emergency room for treatment of low blood sugar (ADA, Hypoglycemia, 2004).

Hyperglycemia: This is when blood sugar becomes too high. This could be caused by injection of too little insulin or when the body is not using the insulin effectively. The signs and symptoms of hyperglycemia include high levels of sugar in the urine, frequent urination, and increased thirst. Exercising can often lower blood sugar, however if the blood sugar is above 240 mg/dl, the urine must be checked for ketones with a urine stick. If ketones are present, exercise is contraindicated because it will increase the ketone level and can further raise the blood sugar level. Any time blood sugar levels stay high, the client will need to seek further treatment (ADA, Hyperglycemia, 2004).

Ketoacidosis: This is a serious condition where excess ketones and acidosis develop because of faulty carbohydrate metabolism. When carbohydrates can't be used for fuel, the body metabolizes proteins instead. The waste products include so many ketones that the body can't get rid of all of them in the urine. It mostly occurs in clients who have T1D and can rarely occur in clients with T2D (ADA, 2004, Diabetes Symptoms). Ketoacidosis usually develops slowly, but when vomiting occurs, the condition can develop within a few hours. The first symptoms of ketoacidosis are thirst or a very dry mouth, frequent urination, high blood sugar levels (detected using a Glucometer), and high levels of ketones in the urine (detected by a urine stick). Next, other symptoms occur: constantly feeling tired, dry or flushed skin, nausea, vomiting, abdominal pain, difficulty breathing, a fruity odor on the breath, a hard time paying attention, or confusion. Ketoacidosis is life threatening and requires immediate treatment (ADA, 2004, Ketoacidosis).

Secondary problems that can occur from uncontrolled blood glucose levels include (CDCP, 2003):
- *Heart disease and stroke*: Heart disease is the leading cause of diabetes-related deaths. Adults

with diabetes have heart disease death rates that are two to four times higher than adults without diabetes. The risk for stroke is two to four times higher among people with diabetes. About 65% of deaths among people with diabetes are due to heart disease and stroke.

- *Blindness*: Diabetes is the leading cause of new cases of blindness among adults 20-74 years old. Diabetic retinopathy causes from 12,000 to 24,000 new cases of blindness each year.
- *Kidney disease*: Diabetes is the leading cause of treated end-stage renal disease (ESRD), accounting for 43% of new cases. In 2000, 41,046 people with diabetes began treatment for ESRD and a total of 129,183 people with diabetes underwent dialysis or kidney transplantation.
- *Nervous system disease*: About 60-70% of people with diabetes have mild to severe forms of nervous system damage. The results of such damage include impaired sensation or pain in the feet or hands, slowed digestion of food in the stomach, carpal tunnel syndrome, and other nerve problems. Severe forms of diabetic nerve disease are a major contributing cause of lower-extremity amputations.
- *Amputations*: More than 60% of non-traumatic lower-limb amputations in the United States occur among people with diabetes. From 2000 to 2001, about 82,000 non-traumatic lower-limb amputations were performed each year on people with diabetes.
- *Dental disease*: Almost one-third of people with diabetes have severe periodontal diseases with loss of attachment of the gums to the teeth measuring five millimeters or more.
- *Complications of pregnancy*: Poorly controlled diabetes before conception and during the first trimester of pregnancy can cause major birth defects in 5-10% of pregnancies and spontaneous abortions in 15-20% of pregnancies. Poorly controlled diabetes during the second and third trimesters of pregnancy can result in excessively large babies, posing a risk to the mother and the child.
- *Other complications*: Uncontrolled diabetes often leads to biochemical imbalances that can cause acute, life-threatening events, such as diabetic ketoacidosis and hyperosmolar (nonketotic) coma. People with diabetes are more susceptible to many other illnesses and, once they acquire these illnesses, often have worse prognoses than people without diabetes.
- *Hyperosmolar hyperglycemic nonketotic syndrome* (HHNS): HHNS can take days or weeks to develop. It occurs in both T1D and T2D, although it is most common in T2D. It is usually brought on by an illness or infection. In HHNS, the blood sugar levels rise and the body tries to get rid of the excess sugar through the urine. At first, the body makes lots of urine and later the amount of urine becomes less and very dark. The client may become very thirsty from so much loss of fluid. Even if the client is not thirsty, s/he is to drink lots of liquids because of the chance of becoming dehydrated. Severe dehydration will lead to seizures, coma, and eventually death. Warning signs of HHNS include blood sugar level over 600 mg/dl, dry and parched mouth, extreme thirst (although this may gradually disappear), warm and dry skin that does not sweat, high fever (over 101°F), sleepiness or confusion, loss of vision, hallucinations, and weakness on one side of the body.

Assessment

Typical Scope of Team Assessment

There are two tests that determine if a client has pre-diabetes or diabetes. One is the fasting plasma glucose test (FPG). A fasting blood glucose level between 100 and 125 mg/dl signals pre-diabetes and greater than 126 mg/dl confirms diabetes. The second test is the oral glucose tolerance test (OGTT). The client has to fast and then drink a glucose-rich beverage. Two hours after drinking the beverage, a blood glucose level is taken. A level between 140 and 199 mg/dl signals pre-diabetes and a level greater than 200 mg/dl confirms diabetes.

Clients are admitted to a rehabilitation facility when disabling complications from DM occur (e.g., amputation). The health care team assesses the past and present management of the disease to plan future treatment.

Anticipated Findings from RT Assessment

If the client is seen in a rehabilitation facility with a secondary diagnosis of DM and a primary diagnosis of a complication of DM, it can be suspected that blood glucose levels have not been effectively managed via medication, insulin, and/or lifestyle changes. Analysis of the client's lifestyle should be made to find areas where the client can make healthier choices.

Treatment Direction

Whole Team Approach

Once diagnosed with DM, the physician seeks to control the client's glucose levels through pharmacology and lifestyle recommendations. The client is educated and counseled about lifestyle changes to manage glucose levels and prevent secondary complications. The treatment team or Diabetes Self-Management Education programs, as described by Mensing (2004) can provide the education. Healthy People 2010 reports that only 45% of all people with diabetes in the year 1998 received formal diabetes education. Patient education is critical. It has been found that people who do not receive diabetes education show a fourfold increased risk of a major complication (Nicolucci et al, 1996).

Some of the specific educational components include:

Proper nutrition: Adhering to a diabetic diet will help with glucose control and reduce central body fat to help cells respond better to insulin.

Regular physical activity: Thirty minutes a day of moderate physical activity can: 1. build and maintain muscle mass that burns calories and increases glucose uptake, lowering blood glucose levels, 2. improve the body's response to insulin, 3. reduce or even eliminate the need for diabetes medication by lowering blood glucose levels, 4. lower cholesterol and reduce blood pressure, 5. improve circulation, and 6. reduce the risk for heart disease and stroke (ADA, Physical Activity, 2004). Weight loss and exercise are the most important "modifiable" lifestyle behaviors in managing diabetes (Horton, 1998). Regular physical activity has also been associated with positive changes in self-efficacy, self-esteem, and psychological stress (Castaneda, 2000).

Cardiovascular disease: The risk of cardiovascular disease can be lowered with diet, weight loss, exercise, and stopping smoking. Improved control of cholesterol and lipids can reduce cardiovascular complications by 20-50%.

Blood pressure: Blood pressure control can reduce cardiovascular disease (heart disease and stroke) by approximately 33-50%, and can reduce microvascular disease (eye, kidney, and nerve disease) by approximately 33%. In general, for every 10 mm Hg reduction in systolic blood pressure, the risk for any complication related to diabetes is reduced by 12%.

Smoking: Smoking compromises the cardiovascular system and increases the risk for diabetic complications such as amputation and myocardial infarction. Smoking may even have a role in the development of type 2 diabetes (Diabetes Care, 2004).

Glucose level awareness: Clients are taught to be aware of the symptoms of too much or too little glucose in the blood, as described earlier. Depending on their level of competence, they or their caretakers will be taught how to check for blood sugar levels and related measures. The team will make sure that the client always has a source of sugar available for hypoglycemia and understands the need to get treatment for hyperglycemia and immediate treatment for ketoacidosis.

Tight glucose control: Clients may be taught to control glucose level in a narrow range. This usually is between 90 and 130 mg/dl before meals and less than 180 mg/dl two hours after starting a meal (ADA, 2004, Tight Diabetes Control). This is referred to as "tight control." The medical team is responsible for deciding if tight control is appropriate and showing the client how to do the testing. In general, for every 1-point reduction in A1C (a blood test that measures the average blood glucose level over the past two to three months), the risk of developing microvascular diabetic complications (eye, kidney, and nerve disease) is reduced by up to 40%.

Preventive care practices: Detection and treatment of diabetic eye disease with laser therapy can reduce the development of severe vision loss by an estimated 50-60%. Comprehensive foot care programs can reduce amputation rates by 45-85%. Detection and treatment of early diabetic kidney disease can reduce the development of kidney failure by 30-70%.

Despite pharmacological and lifestyle interventions, DM is not always easily controlled. Although controlling DM decreases the risk of developing problems from the disease, it does not guarantee that the disease will not affect other systems.

Recreational Therapy Approach

Therapists addressing DM focus on education about diabetes and its complications and how they will affect the client's level of independence, functioning, and quality of life. Education in the clinic is not enough. Therapists also teach clients how to manage diabetes in real-life settings through integration training (see "Integration" in the Techniques section). This helps to increase feelings of self-efficacy and leads to better outcomes (Jack, 2003).

Recreational therapists also look for lifestyle changes that the client can make to improve his/her prognosis. Helping a client find better exercise and eating patterns is part of what recreational therapists do. The therapists can also work on raising the level of self-efficacy of the client so that the client has the ability and desire to follow through on a healthier lifestyle.

There are several tests that clients with DM need to have available. Any recreational therapist who works with clients who have diabetes should know how to give the tests on outings. Basic blood sugar and ketone tests are a minimum.

Recreational Therapy Interventions

Interventions that are frequently implemented with clients who have DM include:

- *Education*: The therapist teaches the client about diabetes as it relates to involvement in activity (e.g., monitoring glucose levels in a community setting) and how to minimize the risks of complications from the disease through lifestyle changes in the areas of nutrition, exercise (see "Exercise Basics" in the Techniques section), smoking cessation (see Contributors to Stress under d240 Handling Stress and Other Psychological Demands), blood pressure control (see "Vital Signs" in the Techniques section), and weight control (see "Obesity" in the Diagnoses section). These can be scored with ICF code d570 Looking After One's Health.
- *Physical exercise*: Skeletal muscles are responsible for burning 70-85% of the glucose in the bloodstream (Cartee, 1994), so an exercise program that decreases body fat and increases muscle mass is ideal (Castaneda, 2000). For people with diabetic retinopathy and/or neuropathy, sustained isometric muscle contractions increase the risk for retinal detachment and vitreous hemorrhage so they should be avoided. Light weights and high repetitions with exercises that are adapted for the client's abilities and limitations are usually all right. Clearance by the client's physician is required. Foot injuries should be avoided with proper footwear, adequate fluids are required, and glucose levels will need to be monitored any time the exercise routine is modified. Also be sure to find exercises the client will continue to do after discharge. Otherwise everything else you have done will be for nothing. See ICF codes d5701 Managing Diet and Fitness and b455 Exercise Tolerance Functions and "Exercise Basics" in the Techniques section.
- *Community problem solving*: Teach clients how to maintain proper glucose levels in community settings (e.g., eating out), as well as how to problem solve for diabetic complications (e.g., low blood sugar). Score these interventions with d175 Solving Problems and d570 Looking After One's Health.
- *Stress management and relaxation training*: Stress can alter glucose levels, precipitate involvement in unhealthy lifestyle choices, and cause bodily changes, all of which can affect glucose control. Identify sources of stress for the client and work to remove stressors, minimize stressors, and change the way the client reacts to stressors to a more positive response. See d2401 Handling Stress and "Relaxation and Stress Reduction" in the Techniques section.

Miscellaneous

Special Note about Insulin

Insulin can be stored at room temperature for about a month before it expires, however it can last much longer if stored in the refrigerator. It cannot be placed in extreme heat (glove compartment of a car) or exposed to freezing temperatures. Therefore, clients who need to take insulin into the community must be educated on its correct storage (e.g., purse, carrying case).

Depending on where insulin is injected (thigh, upper arm, or abdomen), it enters the bloodstream at different speeds (ADA, 2004, Tight Control). Insulin shots given in the abdomen work the fastest, followed by the upper arms, and then the thighs and buttocks. Clients should be consistent with the area of injection (e.g., abdomen injection before breakfast every time and upper arm injection before dinner every time) to have more reliable insulin results. Injections are to be in the same area but not the same spot because hard lumps or fatty deposits could develop that would affect insulin action.

National Certification Board for Diabetes Educators
330 East Algonquin Road, Suite 4
Arlington Heights, Illinois 60005
Voice 847-228-9795
Fax 847-228-8469
Email info@ncbde.org
http://www.ncbde.org

American Diabetes Association
ATTN: National Call Center
1701 North Beauregard Street
Alexandria, VA 22311
1-800-DIABETES
e-mail: AskADA@diabetes.org
http://www.diabetes.org

References

American Diabetes Association. (2004). All about diabetes. http://www.diabetes.org/about-diabetes.jsp.
American Diabetes Association. (2004). Diabetes symptoms. http://www.diabetes.org/diabetes-symptoms.jsp.
American Diabetes Association. (2004). How to prevent pre-diabetes. http://www.diabetes.org/diabetes-prevention/how-to-prevent-diabetes.jsp.

American Diabetes Association. (2004). Hyperglycemia. http://www.diabetes.org/type-2-diabetes/hyperglycemia.jsp.

American Diabetes Association. (2004). Hypoglycemia. http://www.diabetes.org/type-2-diabetes/hypoglycemia.jsp.

America Diabetes Association. (2004). Ketoacidosis. http://www.diabetes.org/type-1-diabetes/ketoacidosis.jsp

American Diabetes Association. (2004). Physical activity. http://www.diabetes.org.

American Diabetes Association. (2004). Tight diabetes control. http://www.diabetes.org/type-2-diabetes/tight-control.jsp.

American Diabetes Association. (2004). The metabolic syndrome. http://www.diabetes.org/weightloss-and-exercise/weightloss/metabolicsyndrome.jsp.

American Diabetes Association. (2004). Type 2 diabetes. http://www.diabetes.org/type-2-diabetes.jsp.

American Diabetes Association. (2004). Weight loss matters. http://www.diabetes.org/weightloss-and-exercise/weightloss.jsp.

Cartee, J. D. (1994). Influence of age on skeletal muscle glucose transport and glycogen metabolism. *Med Sci Sports Exercise, 26*:577-585.

Castaneda, C. (2000). Type 2 diabetes mellitus and exercise. *Nutrition in Clinical Care, 3*(6):349-358.

Centers for Disease Control and Prevention. (2003). National diabetes fact sheet: General information and national estimates on diabetes in the United States, 2002. Atlanta, GA: US Department of Health and Human Services, Centers for Disease Control and Prevention. http://www.diabetes.org/diabetes-statistics/national-diabetes-fact-sheet.jsp.

Clark, C. (1998). How should we respond to the worldwide diabetes epidemic? *Diabetes Care 21*:475-476.

Diabetes Care (2003). Economic impact of diabetes in the US, 2002. *26*:917-932. http://care.diabetesjournals.org/cgi/content/full/26/3/917.

Diabetes Care (2004). Smoking and diabetes: Position statement. *A27*:S74-75. http://care.diabetesjournals.org/cgi/content/full/27/suppl_1/s74

Harris, M. I., Eastman, R. C., Cowie, C.C., Flegal, K. M., & Eberhardt, M. S. (1999). Racial and ethic differences in glycemic control of adults with type 2 diabetes. *Diabetes Care 22*:403-408.

Healthy People 2010 accessed via www.health.gov/healthypeople/.

Horton, E. (1988). Exercise and diabetes mellitus. *Med Clin North America, 72*:1301-1321.

Jack, L. (2003). Diabetes self-management education research: An international review of intervention methods, theories, community partnerships, and outcomes. *Dis Manage Health Outcomes, 11*(7):415-428.

King, H., Aubert, R. E., & Herman W. H. (1998). Global burden of diabetes, 1995-2025: Prevalence, numerical estimates, and projections. *Diabetes Care, 21*:1414-1431.

Mensing, C. (2004). National standards for diabetes self-management education. *Diabetes Care, 27*:Sup 1.

Nicolucci, A., Cavaliere, D., Scorpiglione, N., Carinci, F., Capani, F., Tognoni, G., & Benedetti, M. M. (1996). A comprehensive assessment of the avoidability of long-term complications of diabetes. *Diabetes Care, 19*:927-933.

Eating Disorders

Eating disorders are part of a group of disorders that share a common, underlying attribute: the client's interaction with food causes an unhealthy, even life-threatening, situation. Commonly three disorders are included in this group: anorexia nervosa, bulimia nervosa, and binge eating disorder. There are two other disorders that are often classified as eating disorders: Prader-Willi syndrome and pica.

- *Anorexia nervosa*: A client of any age whose body weight is 15% less than a normal, healthy weight. The low weight is directly related to a refusal (behavioral actions) to maintain body weight. The underlying psychological cause of this refusal is an impaired perception of self that convinces the client that s/he is too fat, accompanied by a strong fear of gaining weight. Behaviorally, clients with anorexia nervosa often engage in extensive exercise activities, dwell on food (cognitively reinforcing a fear of eating "too much"), and hold a remarkably inaccurate perception of what their body looks like.

- *Binge eating disorder*: Recurring and regular episodes of eating an unusually large amount of food in a relatively short period of time while lacking a sense of control over how much or what is eaten. For overeating behaviors to be considered binge eating at least three of the following five actions must be present: 1. the client consumes the food at a rate greater than normal, 2. the client continues to eat to the point of physical discomfort, 3. the client starts eating even when s/he is not hungry, 4. the client often eats alone to avoid others seeing how much s/he is eating, 5. the client feels depressed and/or ashamed about how much s/he eats.

- *Bulimia nervosa*: Bulimia nervosa is a type of binge eating where the client engages in unhealthy behaviors to avoid weight gain. The behaviors used to get rid of the excess calories include self-induced vomiting; alternating bingeing and fasting; use of laxatives, diuretics, enemas or other medications to reduce the body's absorption of calories; or excessive exercise. When a diagnosis of bulimia nervosa is determined, it is usually classified as either "purging type" or "non-purging type."

- *Prader-Willi syndrome*: Unlike the three previous types of eating disorders, which are believed to have their roots in maladaptive emotional responses to stressful situations (although probably partially based in genetics), Prader-Willi syndrome is a set of impairments clearly caused by a genetic disorder. Typically clients with Prader-Willi syndrome start the first three years of life with failure to thrive (low body weight) which then transitions into a compulsive eating disorder. The compulsion is so strong that locks have to be placed on refrigerators, food cabinets, and trashcans. One unusual aspect of this syndrome is that it appears that the more weight the client gains, the more his/her IQ drops. IQ is not regained with weight loss, so it is very important for these clients to maintain a healthy weight.

- *Pica*: Pica is the compulsive eating of things that would normally be considered non-edible. Pica is almost always associated with mental retardation. Because clients with pica do not learn new information or behaviors easily, the therapist's task is to provide a safe environment to reduce the ingestion of non-edible objects.

Incidence/Prevalence in US

- *Anorexia nervosa*: The incidence of anorexia nervosa in the United States is 0.3% for females. The ratio of females to males diagnosed with anorexia nervosa is 9:1. There does not seem to be an agreement across studies as to whether the incidence of anorexia nervosa is increasing.

- *Binge eating disorder*: Approximately 2% of Americans are thought to have a binge eating disorder (around four million adults) with the ratio of women to men being three women to two men (National Institutes of Health, 2004).

- *Bulimia nervosa*: Bulimia nervosa (full syndrome) is estimated to affect 1% of women in the United States. Currently the ratio of women to men with bulimia is 9:1. However, the literature expresses concerns that the diagnostic criteria used for bulimia are gender-biased so that more women are diagnosed than men. A less gender-biased diagnostic criterion will likely be developed. Some studies have identified a partial bulimia nervosa syndrome with an estimate that the partial syndrome affects 5.4% of the population (Agency for Healthcare Research and Quality, 2006).

Predominate Age

- *Anorexia nervosa*: Studies have identified that the typical age at diagnosis is between 15 and 19 years of age with some studies suggesting an increasing number of pre-pubertal children and mid-to-late-life onsets.

- *Binge eating disorder*: Binge eating disorder is a newly recognized disorder. Because of this, there is not a base of research or literature to document the predominate age of clients with the disorder.
- *Bulimia nervosa*: Typically bulimia nervosa is first diagnosed in adolescence or early adulthood.

Causes

- *Anorexia nervosa*: Anorexia nervosa appears to be caused by familial (genetic) and environmental factors; although the actual interaction and causes from these two factors have not been clearly identified (Agency for Healthcare Research and Quality, 2006).
- *Binge eating disorder*: Over half of the clients with binge eating disorder were experiencing depression at the onset. It is not clear whether the depression contributed to the development of binge eating or if the depression is caused by binge eating. (It is probably a little of both to varying degrees, depending on the client.) There is also the debate of whether yo-yo dieting (dieting, gaining back the weight, dieting again, and so forth) causes some clients to develop binge eating disorders or whether yo-yo dieting is just a common symptom of binge eating disorder. Similar to anorexia and bulimia, there is increasing evidence that familial (genetic) sources may be a partial cause of binge eating.
- *Bulimia nervosa*: Similar to anorexia nervosa, research is increasingly pointing to familial (genetic) roots in addition to the previously identified environmental factors.

System(s) Affected

Since many eating disorders seem to develop during adolescence, the disorder interferes with normal adolescent growth and development including the development of appropriate social skills.
- *Anorexia nervosa*: Psychological impairments may include compulsive behaviors, anxiety, and depression. Physiological functioning impairments may include damage to the heart and other organs, reproductive complications, and osteoporosis.
- *Binge eating disorder*: Cardiovascular impairment due to obesity. Psychological impairments include depression, low self-efficacy, and low self-esteem.
- *Bulimia nervosa*: Gastrointestinal impairment (consequences of purging), potential permanent loss of normal bowel function, and damage to teeth from vomiting. Electrolyte abnormalities are also common. Psychological functioning is commonly impaired leading to a secondary diagnosis.

Prognosis

A review of the literature by the (US) Agency for Healthcare Research and Quality (2006) found that treatment outcomes were the same across gender, age at time of treatment, ethnicity, or cultural group for anorexia nervosa, binge eating disorder, and bulimia nervosa. No mention was made in this review related to socioeconomic status at time of treatment.
- *Anorexia nervosa*: There is a relatively high morbidity and mortality associated with anorexia nervosa; estimated to be 0.56% per year or twelve times the mortality rate of their peers who do not have anorexia nervosa (Sullivan, 1995). Anorexia nervosa is one of the two top psychiatric disorders for increased risk of premature death (substance abuse is the other leading cause of premature death). Regaining and maintaining normal weight does not necessarily constitute a remission from this disorder. For clients who responded to treatment, studies found that ten years after initial treatment approximately half of the clients were within normal weight ranges, but many of that group continued to exhibit depression and "to suffer from a variety of personality disorders, obsessive-compulsive disorder, Asperger syndrome, and autism spectrum disorders" (Agency for Healthcare Research and Quality, 2006, p. 4). Lower levels of depression and compulsivity during initial treatment are indicators of increased chances for good treatment outcomes while a history of alcohol or substance use disorders are indicators for increased mortality.
- *Binge eating disorder*: The diagnostic criteria for binge eating disorder are new enough that a baseline from which to establish a prognosis has not been established.
- *Bulimia nervosa*: Unlike anorexia nervosa, bulimia nervosa is not associated with an increased risk of death but frequently is associated with a secondary psychiatric diagnosis. Secondary medical problems often persist. These are listed in the next section.

Secondary Problems

Typically treatment for eating disorders includes cognitive and/or behavioral therapy along with medications, often second-generation antidepressants. AHRQ's *Management of Eating Disorders* (2006) documented the harm associated with treatment for eating disorders as well as the strengths. Within each diagnostic group, side effects of medications were clearly identified as one of the negative aspects of treatment. For example, up to 90% of patients with anorexia nervosa experienced at least one undesirable medication side effect with between 6-14% of patients discontinuing the medication because of the side effects. The side effects caused 24% of the clients with binge eating disorder taking tricyclic antidepressants to discontinue the medication.

Clients with eating disorders tend to exhibit, to a pathological extreme, one or more of three personality traits that are based on biochemical factors, environmental factors, and genetic roots. The three are novelty seeing, harm avoidance, and reward dependence. Table 11 lists the characteristics of each of the three personality traits. The therapist will need to consider the specific cluster of the characteristics when s/he is developing the treatment program for each client.

- *Anorexia nervosa*: Clients with anorexia nervosa tend to have personality types that include anxiety, harm avoidance, low self-esteem, obsessive behaviors, and perfectionism. Clients are often diagnosed with depression and anxiety at the onset of the disorder. The anxiety may decrease with treatment, but depression seems to persist after recovery and achieving normal weight.

- *Binge eating disorder*: Most, but not all, clients who have binge eating disorder are overweight or obese. Clients with binge eating may exhibit numerous secondary problems including impaired self-esteem and impaired feelings of self-worth, increased level of suicidal thoughts (compared to peers), difficulties handling stress, increased weight leading to high blood pressure, high blood cholesterol levels, heart disease, type 2 diabetes, and trouble sleeping.

Table 11: Personality Traits

Personality Trait	Characteristics
Novelty Seeking	<ul><li>Distractible</li><li>Easily bored</li><li>Exploratory</li><li>Impulsive</li><li>Neglects details</li><li>Promptly tries new things</li></ul>
Harm Avoidance	<ul><li>Cautious</li><li>Easily fatigable</li><li>Inhibited</li><li>Shy</li><li>Tense</li><li>Worries</li></ul>
Reward Dependence	<ul><li>Eager to please others</li><li>Sensitive to social cues</li><li>Sympathetic listener</li><li>Warm personality</li></ul>

- *Bulimia nervosa*: Around 80% of clients with bulimia nervosa will be diagnosed with another psychiatric disorder during their life (Agency for Healthcare Research and Quality, 2006). Clients with bulimia nervosa tend to have harm avoidance and novelty seeking personality traits. Clients who purge using frequent vomiting "may experience electrolyte abnormalities, metabolic alkalosis, erosion of dental enamel, swelling of the parotid glands, and scars and calluses on the back of their hands" (Agency for Healthcare Research and Quality, 2006, p. 16). Clients who purge using laxatives may have electrolyte imbalance and potentially have a permanent loss of normal bowel functions.

Assessments

Typical Scope of Team Assessment

Because eating disorders are psychiatric diagnosis that usually have significant, secondary medical implications, a broad medical and psychological assessment is standard. Medical tests evaluate body functions such as blood pressure, blood chemistries, urine specific gravity and fluid intake/output, weight, electrocardiograms, and bone density. Emotional and cognitive functioning is also evaluated including standardized tests such as the *Beck Depression Inventory*, *Body Shape Questionnaire*, and *State-Trait Anxiety Inventory*.

A nutritional assessment is completed for each client. This assessment evaluates whether the client is receiving adequate nutrition and calories. It also looks at the patterns around eating including eating alone or with others, food that may have been totally eliminated from the client's diet, who prepares the client's food, specific food rituals used by the client, and the types of food most likely to be inappropriately used during crisis.

Increasingly health care is using the Body Mass Index (BMI) as a basis for assessing weight, specifically whether a client is underweight, normal, or overweight.

A note should be made about assessment and binge eating disorder. It seems that the professionals working with clients who have eating disorders have determined that binge eating disorder is a specific, distinct diagnosis. However, the *DSM-IV-TR* does not describe a specific set of criteria for binge eating disorder so practitioners must list the client's diagnosis as "Eating Disorders Not Otherwise Specified"). Because more than one type of "other" eating disorder is grouped into this category, research to measure outcomes of treatment has been hampered.

Anticipated Findings of RT Assessment

When working with clients diagnosed with eating disorders the recreational therapist will tend to focus on three areas for skill development: leisure functioning, stress management, and social functioning. Because the vast majority of clients with eating disorders also have a second disorder or disease (comorbidity or dual diagnosis) the therapist's assessment should also evaluate potential strengths and areas of impairment due to the other diagnosis. Specific areas to assess for each of the diagnoses include:

Anorexia Nervosa:
- Body image disturbance
- Compulsive exercise
- High need to be in control
- Impaired ability to cope with stress
- Impaired leisure skills
- Impaired self-esteem
- Impaired social skills

Binge Eating:
- Alcohol and/or substance abuse
- Feeling isolated, not feeling a part of the community
- Impulsive behavior with feelings of being out of control and not in charge of his/her life

Bulimia Nervosa:
- Harm avoidance
- Impaired cooperativeness
- Impaired leisure skills
- Impaired self-directedness
- Impaired self-esteem
- Impulsivity
- Novelty seeking

Treatment Direction

Whole Team Approach

A summary of the studies reviewed by the Agency for Healthcare Research and Quality (2006) found that the best long-term outcomes occurred when the treatment team created a therapeutic milieu based on: 1. an environment set up to mimic elements of a supportive community, 2. sound clinical management, and 3. supportive psychotherapy. A non-community-based, cognitive behavioral therapy, and nutritional counseling protocol was not as effective.

Recreational Therapy Approach

The recreational therapist works with the treatment team to provide:

- *Emotional support*: The recreational therapist is one of the few people a client with an eating disorder comes in contact with who is offering pleasant options.
- *Activities*: alternative choices for non-food-centered activities.
- *Social and coping skills*: more effective ways to interact with others.

Recreational Therapy Interventions

The field of recreational therapy has a book addressing the assessment and treatment of clients with eating disorders: *Eating Disorders: Providing Effective Recreational Therapy Interventions* by Miller and Jake (2001). For therapists working with these clients the information in that book covers most of what the therapist needs. The recreational therapist's treatment usually focuses on the following areas:

- *Self-worth, self-esteem, and personal boundaries*: Helping the client develop a sense of "who they are" (working on self-worth and self-esteem through the identification of positive attributes not related to weight or body image) and strengthening personal boundaries. See "Self-Esteem" and "Boundaries" in the Techniques section and ICF codes b122 Global Psychosocial Functions, d710 Basic Interpersonal Functions, and d720 Complex Interpersonal Functions.
- *Stress management techniques*: Helping the client identify his/her own unique physiological, emotional, and behavioral responses to increased stress levels and then learning specific, positive stress management techniques to reduce the level of stress. See "Relaxation and Stress Reduction" in the Techniques section and d240 Handling Stress and Other Psychological Demands.
- *Body image distortion*: Clients with eating disorders almost always have a distorted view of how they look to others. Their perceptions of the actual attributes of their bodies are not based on fact or reality. Changing these very entrenched and distorted views is a difficult task and one that clients will probably struggle with their entire life. The therapist may want to start with activities that increase the client's skills of observation, but not observation related to the client's own physical characteristics. For example, drawing a simple still life that requires the client to realistically see an object and then attempt to recreate the image of that object through fine motor activity. ICF code b1142 Orientation to Person is one place to code this

type of intervention, as well as b1801 Body Image.

- *Leisure education*: Clients with eating disorders have historically spent excessive amounts of time, thought process, and activity on their attention to food, self-image, and exercise. The therapist is likely to find that the client has a deficit related to a balanced repertoire of leisure activities. These are covered in "Activity Pattern Development" in the Techniques section.

- *Social skills and interpersonal relationships*: Social isolation, anxiety, and underlying depression are critical areas for the therapist to address by teaching new, concrete social skills. Often the client has spent an inordinate amount of time obsessing on his/her body image and isolated himself/herself from activities that involve food. Because of this, the basic skills needed to create and nurture friendships may be lacking. Wanting to help others, a common social pattern for clients with eating disorders, is often not the type of social skill that needs to be developed. Instead, working on the basic skills of mutual respect and assistance (accepting help while also

offering help), basic give and take during conversation ("us" centered conversations), and being sensitive to the feelings of others (correctly "reading" the other person's body language and spoken word instead of wondering how the other person is perceiving him/her, especially body image) are good places to begin developing appropriate social skills. ICF codes in A&P Chapter 7 Interpersonal Interactions and Relationships cover these issues.

References

Agency for Healthcare Research and Quality. (2006). *Management of eating disorders*: Evidence Report/Technology Assessment Number 135. Rockville, MD: Author.

Miller, D. and Jake, L. (2001). *Eating disorders: Providing effective recreational therapy interventions*. Ravensdale, WA: Idyll Arbor, Inc.

National Institutes of Health. (2004). *Binge eating disorder*: NIH Publication No. 04-3589. Bethesda, MD: Author.

Sullivan PF. (1995). Mortality in anorexia nervosa. *American Journal of Psychiatry, 152*(7):1073-4.

Fibromyalgia

Fibromyalgia (FM) is a form of soft-tissue rheumatism. Unlike other forms of rheumatic disease, inflammation is not present. The word "myalgia" means pain and "fibro" means in the muscles, ligaments, and tendons. FM is characterized by chronic widespread pain in the muscles, ligaments, and tendons that has lasted for more than three months. Involvement includes both the left and right sides of the body, above and below the waist, and pain located in the head and trunk.

People with FM have multiple tender point sites. Tender points are quarter size areas on the body that produce pain when pressure is applied. In addition to a history of widespread pain that has lasted over three months, a person must also have at least 11 tender point sites out of a possible 18 for a diagnosis of FM. Because the tender spots are small, many people are only aware of a few tender points although more are identifiable through digital palpitation (applying

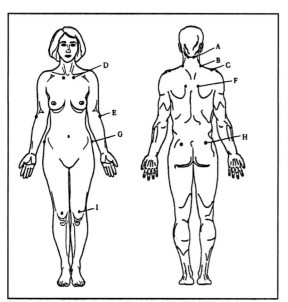

Figure 1: Locations of tender points
A. Either side of the back of the neck just below the hairline
B. Either side at the base of the neck in back
C. Either side of the upper back between the neck and shoulder
D. Either side of the chest, top of the breastbone below the clavicle
E. The inside of the forearms just below the elbow joint
F. Either side of the upper back near the inside of the shoulder blades
G. Either side of the lower back just below the waist
H. The right or left buttocks under the hipbones
I. Just above either kneecap

pressure with the fingers). Tender point sites are shown in Figure 1. Currently, there are no blood work markers or other forms of medical technology that can diagnose FM. It is diagnosed through client report, a physical exam that includes a tender point evaluation, and a physical with a full blood workup to rule out other possible medical conditions.

In addition to pain and tender points, people with FM experience many other symptoms. Some people with FM do not experience these symptoms and those that do, experience them at different severities. The report of these symptoms helps the rheumatologist confirm a diagnosis of FM, although they are not required. Approximately 90% of people with FM complain of profound fatigue, sleep disturbances related to and sometimes unrelated to pain, and feelings of anxiety and depression. It is unknown if these symptoms are related to the FM process or they are a result of coping with FM. For example, feelings of anxiety and depression could arise from struggling to cope with FM. Poor sleep could be caused by anxiety or pain and profound fatigue could be attributed to constant lack of quality sleep. Whether or not these symptoms are part of the disease or are secondary problems is difficult to determine. However, the high percentage of people who experience these problems shows that they are probably connected to the syndrome of FM.

Another common problem associated with FM is referred to as "fibro-fog." Fibro-fog describes a group of cognitive problems that are typically experienced by people with FM. These include feelings of confusion, lapses in memory (especially short-term memory), word finding problems, word or name mix-ups (calling something a wrong name), and difficulty concentrating. These problems, like the ones previously discussed, could be caused by anxiety, depression, and lack of sleep; they could be directly connected to the FM process; or they could be a separate medical condition. Irritable bowel syndrome (also referred to as spastic colon) is also seen with FM. It is characterized by abdominal pain, bloating, and alternating constipation and diarrhea. Other common symptoms of FM include migraine and tension headaches, tingling limbs, restless leg syndrome, dizziness, pain in the temporomandibular joint (TMJ), and a heightened sensitivity to weather and noise.

Because it is difficult to determine whether the symptoms seen with FM are related or part of another disease process, a full medical workup is commonly conducted to rule out other medical conditions. Conditions that must be ruled out before a diagnosis of FM is given include hypothyroidism and other rheumatic diseases. FM may also be present in association with chronic fatigue syndrome, depressive disorders, systemic lupus, osteoarthritis, and rheumatoid arthritis.

Incidence/Prevalence in US

FM affects approximately 3.5 million Americans. Women are seven times more likely to develop FM than men. Almost 20% of people with rheumatic diseases, such as systemic lupus, osteoarthritis, or rheumatoid arthritis, also have fibromyalgia (Arthritis Foundation, 2006a).

Predominant Age

FM usually affects women in childbearing years, but it can also affect children and older adults.

Causes

A primary cause of FM has not been identified. It may be caused by different factors, alone or in combination, such as an infectious illness, physical trauma, emotional trauma, hormonal changes, muscle abnormalities, or neurotransmitters (Arthritis Foundation, 2006b).

Clients with FM show elevated levels of substance P, which initiates pain signals after injury, and low levels of serotonin, which tones down the intensity of pain signals. The stress response, a communication mechanism between the brain and body that helps a client respond to physical and emotional challenges, is also impaired. Whether these abnormalities are a cause or a result of fibromyalgia is unknown.

Stress often precipitates FM and exacerbates FM symptoms. Stress "causes localized arterial spasm that interferes with perfusion of oxygen in the affected areas" (Sadock & Sadock, 2003, p. 837) resulting in pain. In other words, when stress occurs, an area or areas of the body respond with arterial spasm. The artery, which carries oxygenated blood to the muscles, is unable to transfer the oxygen effectively to the muscle. The muscle, when deprived of oxygen, is damaged, often showing up as a muscle spasm, and pain ensues.

System(s) Affected

FM affects the muscular system, although other systems could possibly be involved including psychological-emotional, circadian rhythm (sleep cycle), and the hormonal system.

Prognosis

FM may remit spontaneously (in milder cases) with decreased stress but can become chronic or recur at frequent intervals (exacerbate and remit). FM symptoms can last for weeks or months and can be brought on by emotional or physical stress or they can appear without reference to a direct stressor. The functional prognosis (ability to participate in life activities and lead a quality life) is usually favorable with a comprehensive, supportive program, although some degree of symptoms tends to persist (Berkow, 1992). Studies have reported disability rates as high as 44% in people with FM (Arthritis Foundation, 2006a). Pain can become disabling leading to problems with walking. Cognitive problems can affect work performance. On a positive note, a Norwegian study followed 33 women who were diagnosed with FM over a period of six to eight years and found that in the long run FM is more likely to get better than worse and that women who have had FM "for quite some time" tend to manage quite well (Arthritis Foundation, 2002).

Secondary Problems

The secondary problems associated with FM vary greatly depending on the severity of FM symptoms, the perception of control that the person has in managing the symptoms (client's control over symptoms versus disease process that controls symptoms), and the client's initiation and maintenance of proactive steps in managing the symptoms. Pain, lack of quality sleep, depression, anxiety, irritable bowel, migraine and tension headaches, tingling limbs, restless leg syndrome, and dizziness can all have an impact on the client's ability to participate in life tasks, perform self-care, engage in recreational opportunities, care for others, exercise, and socialize. Secondary problems that arise from these issues often lead to inactivity (see "Consequences of Inactivity" in the Concepts section).

Assessments

Typical Scope of Team Assessment

See the Description on how FM is diagnosed. Therapists assess the type and extent of FM symptoms and how they impact the client's ability to engage in tasks and lead a quality life. The assessment tools used to determine a baseline of functioning will vary depending on the facility and therapist preference.

Anticipated Findings from RT Assessment

The anticipated findings will vary depending on the type and extent of FM symptoms. A list of common anticipated findings includes:

- Clients often lack participation in a regular exercise program due to pain or fear of exacerbating FM symptoms.
- Clients who have had long-term chronic FM pain show a steady decrease in their activity level. Clients gradually give up activities that are not viewed as being necessary (e.g., recreational activities, social activities).
- Stress, anxiety, and depression are common. Clients may lack effective coping strategies.
- Clients may be experiencing poor quality sleep and problems related to poor quality sleep (e.g., irritability, "fibro-fog").
- Clients may be experiencing mild to severe cognitive problems that interfere with life tasks. Some may report cognitive problems that come and go completely or are constant but vary in severity.

Treatment Direction

Whole Team Approach

Since a specific cause of FM has not been identified, current treatment revolves around symptom management. Medication may be prescribed to help manage pain. Narcotics are usually avoided. Although FM does not have inflammation, some clients report pain relief from non-steroidal anti-inflammatory drugs (NSAIDs). Injections of an anesthetic (e.g., procaine) into the affected area may be helpful for clients who are experiencing severe pain. Other medications may be prescribed to aid in better sleep, reduce feelings of anxiety and/or depression, control irritable bowel problems, and relieve headaches. Clients are educated about FM, the role that stress plays on FM symptoms, and their role in helping to manage FM symptoms. A physical exercise program is initiated and specific physical impairments are addressed (e.g., limited range of motion).

Recreational Therapy Approach

The FM cycle of stress, pain, and lack of sleep leading to more stress needs to be broken. RT focuses on helping people with FM to make lifestyle changes that affect the severity of all of symptoms. The amount or relief from lifestyle changes will vary.

Recreational Therapy Interventions

Interventions that are frequently implemented with clients who have fibromyalgia include:

Functional Skill Development

- *Handling stress*: Reducing stress and learning healthy ways to manage stress improve sleep and decrease pain. Relaxing the muscles increases oxygen flow and reduces pain. Decreased pain improves the client's quality of sleep. Better sleep helps with cognitive problems. Reduction of all of the other issues will also reduce feelings of anxiety, depression, and fatigue leading to less stress. See ICF code d2401 Handling Stress.
- *Physical exercise*: Participation in a regular exercise program helps the client achieve a deeper and more restful sleep; decreases feelings of anxiety, depression, and fatigue; strengthens muscles that have become weakened from disuse; increases oxygen intake to muscles; and promotes the release of endorphins (the body's natural pain killers) to aid in pain reduction. Clients begin with a gentle exercise program that focuses on deep breathing and range of motion (e.g., yoga, stretching program, walking, water exercise) rather than a high impact exercise program (e.g., running on the treadmill) that can exacerbate FM symptoms. Clients who respond well to gentle exercise programs and desire to increase the intensity of their exercise program should receive clearance from their physicians before beginning. If a more vigorous exercise program is undertaken, clients need to watch for changes in FM symptoms and adjust their exercise program accordingly. Gentle exercises that promote deep breathing and range of motion should never be discontinued since they are the basis for managing FM symptoms. Therapists monitor the client's response to exercise, document reported changes (e.g., change in pain level, pain location, symptoms), and adjust the exercise program accordingly. "Exercise Basics" in the Techniques section and ICF code d5701 Managing Diet and Fitness provide more information for treatment and coding.
- *Compensatory strategies for cognitive problems*: Hopefully, achieving better quality sleep and decreasing feelings of anxiety, depression, and fatigue will have a positive impact on cognitive problems associated with FM. If the problems are not resolved, therapists teach clients compensatory strategies for each cognitive deficit noted. Body Functions Chapter 1 Mental Functions and A&P Chapter 1 Learning and Applying Knowledge discuss cognitive

functioning. Also look at the Compensation Approach under Cognitive Retraining in "Neuroplasticity" in the Techniques section.

Education and Counseling

- *Handling stress*: Refer to the Techniques section for "Relaxation and Stress Reduction," "Coping with Stress," "Education and Counseling" (for information on changing distorted thinking patterns through CBT), and "Energy Conservation Training" (for fatigue management).
- *Physical activity*: Refer to "Consequences of Inactivity" in the Concepts section.
- *Sleep improvement*: Identify aids to help with amount, onset, maintenance, and quality of sleep as discussed in ICF code b134 Sleep Functions.
- *Smoking cessation*: Smoking increases pain levels so see smoking cessation in d240 Handling Stress and Other Psychological Demands for information on assisting clients with smoking cessation.
- *Diet*: Caffeine and sugar are stimulants that should be avoided since they can affect the client's ability to achieve a sound sleep and may contribute to feelings of anxiety. ICF code d5701 Managing Diet and Fitness discusses related issues.

Integration

- *Community reintegration*: See "Integration" in the Techniques section for ways to get the client back out into the community.
- *Social support*: People with FM need opportunities for social support, as well as the skills and the resources to access such support. Isolation contributes to feelings of depression. Social support helps to deal with stress (e.g.,

another person to confide in, sharing of ideas, sources of laughter and enjoyment). Therapists educate clients on the importance of social support in the management of FM symptoms and identify opportunities for social support after discharge. Therapists identify and address skills related to being able to follow through with this recommendation. If clients need assistance in developing social skills refer to "Social Skills Training" in the Techniques section. See A&P Chapter 7 Interpersonal Interactions and Relationships for other aspects of social interactions.

- *Community mobility skills*: See A&P Chapter 4 Mobility.

Health Promotion after Discharge

See "Activity Pattern Development" in the Techniques section for suggestions on finding activities that are interesting to clients to promote follow through after discharge.

References

Arthritis Foundation. (2006a). Delivering on the promise in fibromyalgia. http://www.arthritis.org/research/Research_Program/Fibromyalgia/default.asp.

Arthritis Foundation. (2006b). Fibromyalgia. http://www.arthritis.org/conditions/DiseaseCenter/Fibromyalgia/fibromyalgia_diagnosed.asp.

Arthritis Foundation. (2002). Fibromyalgia: Long-term outcome looks up. *Journal of Rheumatology, 28*(9), http://www.arthritis.org/resources/arthritistoday/2002_archives/2002_03_04_Research_Fibro.asp.

Berkow, R. (1992). *The Merck manual of diagnosis and therapy*. Rahway, NJ: Merck & Co, Inc.

Sadock, B. & Sadock, V. (2003). *Kaplan & Sadock's synopsis of psychiatry*. Philadelphia, PA: Lippincott Williams & Wilkins.

Generalized Anxiety Disorder

Generalized Anxiety Disorder (GAD) is one of twelve anxiety disorders classified by the American Psychiatric Association in the *Diagnostic and Statistical Manual of Mental Disorders*. It is characterized by excessive and uncontrollable worry about everyday things more days than not for at least six months. "The intensity, duration and frequency of the worry are disproportionate to the issue and interfere with the performance of tasks and ability to concentrate" (American Anxiety Association of America, 2004). The anxiety also manifests in physical symptoms, often including muscle tension, sweating, nausea, gastrointestinal problems, jumpiness, fidgeting, trembling, inability to relax, being easily startled, trouble sleeping, and feeling "on edge." The source of worry can vary (e.g., finances, job, responsibilities, and relationships).

Some anxiety is normal. In fact, it is a healthy emotion that alerts us to internal or external threats. "It prompts a person to take the necessary steps to prevent the threat or to lessen its consequences" (Sadock & Sadock, 2003, p. 592). Some examples of everyday events that increase anxiety are running to catch the last bus, trying to find the car keys when you're running late for an appointment, or preparing for a tough exam. Whether or not an event is perceived as stressful, thus heightening feelings of anxiety, "depends on the nature of the event and on the person's resources, psychological defenses, and coping mechanisms" (Sadock & Sadock, 2003, p. 592).

Anxiety, not GAD, can be described as being mild, moderate, or severe (Pary et al, 2003). Mild anxiety, as previously discussed, is normal and healthy. However, moderate or severe anxiety interferes with daily functioning and, if it persists more days than not over a period of six months, may warrant a diagnosis of GAD. Pary et al (2003) delineates the severity of anxiety through these definitions:

- Mild anxiety sharpens the senses and expands the perceptual field, preparing us for action. Learning and problem-solving skills are enhanced.
- Moderate anxiety levels decrease the perceptual field. Sight, hearing, touch, taste, and smell are limited and the ability to think is impaired. Problem solving and the ability to mobilize resources can be hindered.
- Severe anxiety levels constrict the perceptual field so that an individual's focus is limited to one specific detail. Completing a task or processing new information is compromised, and

behavior and attention are directed toward the anxiety.

People who have GAD feel like they are "losing control" of themselves and/or the situation during periods of extreme anxiety. For example, Sarah states that when she is trying to get out the dorm building to get to class on time, her friends often delay her with conversation. When this occurs, her anxiety begins to heighten and she experiences somatic symptoms (heart pounding, shaking). She then becomes hyper fixated on "getting out the door" and becomes short-fused and easily agitated. Because this situation occurs frequently, Sarah starts worrying about this problem hours before her class ("I know what's going to happen as soon as I step out of my room. Jim is going to be out there and will start asking me a ton of questions about the weekend."). This "negative running tape" is destructive because it heightens anxiety about a situation before it even occurs. Negative and anxious thinking also heighten somatic symptoms, which, in turn, increase anxiety until the feedback between the way the body feels and the anxiety it causes spirals out of control. Anxious thoughts and feelings do not have to be in the context of an interaction with another person, they can result from internal cues by themselves.

Incidence/Prevalence in US

GAD is one of the most prevalent anxiety disorders. Throughout a lifetime of GAD occurs in approximately 5% of the general population (Wittchen & Hoyer, 2001). The ratio of women to men with the disorder is about two to one, but the ratio of women to men who are receiving treatment is about one to one.

Predominant Age

In most people, GAD develops gradually during adolescence and reaches clinical significance during young adulthood (Leger et al, 2003). A diagnosis of GAD, however, is generally uncommon before the age of 25 (Carter et al, 2001). Approximately 10% of women older than 39 years of age will have GAD over the course of their lifetime (Wittchen & Hoyer, 2001). A specific age of onset is difficult to determine because 1. many people when diagnosed with GAD report that they have been anxious throughout their entire life and 2. one third of people with GAD do not seek psychiatric treatment but rather seek out medical specialists (e.g., cardiologists) for somatic symptoms of GAD (Anxiety Disorders Association of America, 2004).

Causes

Anxiety disorders may develop from a complex set of risk factors, including genetics, brain chemistry, personality, and life events (Anxiety Disorders Association of America, 2004). About 25% of first-degree relatives of people with GAD are also affected (Sadock & Sadock, 2003). Cognitive-behavioral therapy (a school of psychology) believes that people with GAD incorrectly or inaccurately perceive dangers. "The inaccuracy is generated by selective attention to negative details in the environment. This is caused by distortions in information processing and by an overly negative view of the person's own ability to cope. Psychoanalytic therapy believes that anxiety is a symptom of unresolved unconscious conflicts" (Sadock & Sadock, p. 632). Psychological trauma occurring in childhood and other stressful life events may also trigger or contribute to the development of GAD.

System(s) Affected

GAD affects various systems in the body through the influence of the client's emotional state. When anxiety is resolved or minimized, systems typically recover. Anxiety affects the client's motor functioning (shakiness, restlessness, headaches), gastrointestinal system (diarrhea, constipation, pain, nausea, feeling of "butterflies" in the stomach), cardiovascular system (heart palpitations), respiratory system (shortness of breath), autonomic system (excessive sweating), mood (irritable, easily startled), cognition (trouble concentrating, difficulty learning new information and behaviors, misperception of events and situations, poor short-term memory, difficulty with abstract thinking), and social functioning (difficulty forming and maintaining relationships).

Prognosis

Because of the high incidence of comorbid mental disorders in clients with GAD (having another mental disorder in addition to GAD), the clinical course and prognosis of the disorder are difficult to predict. However, GAD is a chronic condition that may well be lifelong (Sadock & Sadock, 2003). People with an anxiety disorder are three to five times more likely to go to the doctor and six times more likely to be hospitalized for psychiatric disorders than non-sufferers (Anxiety Disorders Association of America, 2004). Pharmacological

treatment of GAD is typically a six to twelve month treatment, however about 25% of clients relapse in the first month after discontinuing medication, and 60-80% relapse over the course of the next year. Therefore, if pharmacological interventions are successful in managing GAD, long-term use of medication may be necessary (Sadock & Sadock, 2003). Many individuals who undergo psychotherapy for GAD report that they continue to have anxiety after discharge. However, they are better able to "use the anxiety symptoms as a signal to reflect on internal struggles and to expand their insight and understanding" (Sadock & Sadock, 2003, p. 634-35).

Secondary Problems

A fundamental characteristic of GAD is comorbidity with other psychiatric conditions (Pary et al, 2003): 62.4% major depression, 39.5% dysthymia (chronic depressed mood), 37.6% alcoholism, 35.1% simple phobia, 34.4% social phobia, 27.6% drug abuse, and 23.5% panic disorder.

Comorbid GAD in elderly patients is associated with a more severe presentation of depressive illness and possible suicidal preoccupation (Lenze et al, 2000).

Assessments

Scope of Team Assessment

The criteria for GAD are defined in the *DSM-IV-TR*. They include excessive anxiety about a number of events that occurs during more than half of the days in a six-month period. It is difficult for the client to control the worry and it is associated with physical and mental symptoms including being keyed up, fatigued, irritable, and tense. The client may have difficulty sleeping and concentrating. The anxiety may be about anything and must cause the client significant distress in some function. Anxiety caused by substances, a medical condition, or some other defined disorder is not considered GAD.

Even if anxiety is not classified as GAD, it can still be treated with some of the techniques shown below. Some of the medical conditions that may cause symptoms of anxiety include (Longe, 2001):

- adrenal tumor
- AIDS
- alcoholism
- carcinoid syndrome (symptoms including flushing, labored breathing, and heart palpitations as a result of a carcinoid tumor)
- central nervous system degenerative diseases
- chronic obstructive pulmonary disease (COPD) (a chronic and progressive disease of the lungs

causing difficulty getting air into and out of the lungs)

- coronary insufficiency (impaired flow of oxygenated blood to the blood vessels around the heart)
- Cushing's disease (metabolic disorder)
- delirium (cognitive processing impairment due to acute illness)
- diabetes
- fibromyalgia
- hyperthyroidism (an overactive thyroid gland)
- hypoglycemia (too little glucose in the blood)
- Meniére's disease (early stages) (inner ear disease that causes vertigo)
- mitral valve prolapse (incomplete closure of the heart valve causing problems with blood flow)
- postconcussional syndrome (a grouping of problems that occur after a head injury including dizziness, poor concentration, and anxiety)

Medication and other substances can also induce anxiety including excessive caffeine use, drug or alcohol withdrawal, substance abuse (cannabis, LSD, PCP, amphetamines, cocaine, ephedrine), and some prescription medication (antihistamines, antidepressants, benzodiazepines) (Longe, 2001; Zuckerman, 2000).

Anxiety may be a symptom of another psychiatric disorder. The treatment team will want to determine if the symptoms of anxiety are because of mood disorders (such as depressive disorder with anxiety), phobias, panic disorder, obsessive-compulsive disorder, adjustment disorder with anxiety, hypochondriasis, adult-attention deficit/hyperactivity disorder, somatization disorder, or any other personality disorder.

If an anxiety disorder is thought to be present, an evaluation from a mental health professional is sought. The general clinician may explore the nature and extent of the anxiety to better understand its impact on life tasks by asking questions about what situations or memories cause anxiety, how the anxiety feels, and what helps to relieve the anxiety.

People experiencing severe anxiety can be at increased risk for suicide. Therefore, it is important to ask highly anxious individuals about suicidal and/or homicidal ideation (Pary et al, 2003).

Anticipated Findings from RT Assessment

- Heightened and prolonged anxiety can affect learning and development of healthy coping mechanisms, so maladaptive coping strategies may be apparent.
- A client with GAD is typically easily discouraged, indecisive, mildly depressed,

apprehensive, impatient, irritable, easily distracted, and spends a considerable amount of time worrying about impending disasters (Mobily & MacNeil, 2002). Consequently, some clients may manage the anxiety by reducing their involvement in life tasks leading to social isolation and loss of a social support system. Other clients may try to take on too many tasks, trying to handle everything they worry about, leading to exhaustion and perceived loss of control.

Treatment Direction

Whole Team Approach

An eclectic approach (a combination of therapy techniques) is more effective than using a single technique when treating GAD. Techniques that are commonly used include identification and alteration of anxiety producing thoughts, development of healthy coping strategies, teaching relaxation training, gradual exposure to anxiety provoking situations, opportunities to talk about the anxiety, and modeling. The therapist who provides a listening ear and models calm, confident, and empathetic behavior can be very powerful. The simple act of listening is very effective in deescalating a highly anxious client. Reflecting behaviors that the therapist desires to instill in the client can be an effective tool in modifying behavior.

Recreational Therapy Approach

RT utilizes the same approach as the whole team approach. However, RT focuses on control of GAD within functional activities (e.g., eating in a crowded restaurant, getting on an elevator).

Recreational Therapy Interventions

Common recreational therapy interventions for GAD include:

- *Reducing anxiety-evoking thoughts*: Some clients are able to verbalize specific situations that increase their anxiety, but individuals with GAD generally are anxious in many situations and are unable to identify specific triggers that increase their anxiety to an unhealthy level ("I just feel anxious all the time."). Therapists still need to help clients identify situations. Art therapy is often a useful modality, especially for children and for clients with suppressed events. See ICF codes b1522 Range of Emotion, and d175 Solving Problems.
- *Coping strategies*: GAD is a long-term disorder that rarely resolves completely. Consequently,

clients must be taught how to cope with GAD. Strategies that decrease the focus on anxiety and increase the focus on mastery and success foster and strengthen the client's internal locus of control. The family of the client may also benefit from training on how to assist their family member in the management of GAD. See "Coping with Stress" and "Self-Esteem" in the Techniques section.

- *Relaxation training*: Therapists utilize a variety of formal and information relaxation techniques. See d2401 Handling Stress and "Relaxation and Stress Reduction" in the Techniques section.
- *Appropriate activities*: Activities and Participation Chapter 9 Community, Social, and Civic Life covers lifestyle changes the clients can make to add more appropriate activities. Activities that promote abdominal breathing, noncompetitive, process-oriented activities, and self-paced, repetitive, and rhythmical activities can be helpful in reducing stress (Mobily & MacNeil, 2002).
- *Exposure to anxiety-evoking situations*: The goal is to expose the client to situations slowly so s/he can learn to handle them. Small tasks in the facility such as asking the client to buy a small item at the gift shop shortly before his/her next scheduled therapy session can start the process. Role-playing anxiety-producing situations and community integration will raise the potential for anxiety. See b1522 Range of Emotion, d175 Solving Problems, and d2401 Handling Stress.

In all of these interventions, the goal is to work with the client when the anxiety level is under control. Communication with a severely anxious person must be brief, simple, and direct. At panic level, the perceptual field is so diminished that people no longer effectively interpret outside stimuli. Communication and activities are dysfunctional and self-absorbed. Feelings of anger, fear, and helplessness may emerge explosively and be directed toward self or others in a fight-or-flight reaction. When severe anxiety is present, the therapist must get the client to a safe place physically and emotionally before continuing with therapeutic interventions.

Miscellaneous

Anxiety Disorders Association of America
8730 Georgia Avenue, Suite 600
Silver Spring, MD 20910
Voice (240) 485-1001
Fax (240) 485-1035
www.adaa.org

References

American Anxiety Association of America. (2004). Generalized anxiety disorder. http://www.adaa.org/AnxietyDisorderInfor/GAD.cfm on 3/20/04

Anxiety Disorders Association of America. (2004). Brief overview of anxiety disorders. http://www.adaa.org/AnxietyDisorderInfor/OverviewAnxDis.cfm on 3/20/04

American Psychiatric Association. (2000). *Diagnostic and statistical manual of mental disorders, 4th edition, text revision*. Washington, DC: American Psychiatric Association.

Carter R. M., Wittchen H. U., Phister H., & Kessler R. C. (2001). One-year prevalence of subthreshold and threshold DSM-IV generalized anxiety disorder in a nationally representative sample. *Depression and Anxiety 13*:78-88.

Corey, G. (1996). *Theory and practice of counseling and psychotherapy, 5th edition*. Pacific Grove, CA: Brooks/Cole Publishing Company.

Leger, E., Ladouceur, R., Dugas, J., & Freeston, M. (March 2003). Cognitive-behavioral treatment of generalized anxiety disorder among adolescents: A case series. *Journal of the American Academy of Child and Adolescent Psychiatry, 42*(3):327-330.

Lenze, E. J., Mulsant, B. H., Shear, M. K., Schulberg, H. C., Dew, M. A., & Begley, A. E. (2000). Comorbid anxiety disorders in depressed elderly patients. *American Journal of Psychiatry, 157*:722-728.

Longe, J (2001). *The Gale encyclopedia of medicine, 2nd edition*. Farmington Hills, MI: Gale Group. http://search2.webfeat.org:5554/ on 3/20/04

Mobily, K. & MacNeil, R. (2002). *Therapeutic recreation and the nature of disabilities*. State College, PA: Venture Publishing, Inc.

Newmark, C. (1996). *Major psychological assessment instruments, 2nd edition*. Needham Heights, Massachusetts: Allyn & Bacon.

Pary, R., Matsuchka, P., Lewis, S., Caso, W., & Lippmann, S. (2003). Generalized anxiety disorder. *Southern Medical Journal, 96*(6).

Sadock, J. & Sadock, V. (2003). *Kaplan & Sadock's synopsis of psychiatry, 9th edition*. Philadelphia, PA: Lippincott Williams & Wilkins.

Sue, D., Sue, D., & Sue, S. (1997). *Understanding abnormal behavior*. New York, NY: Houghton Mifflin Company.

Wittchen, H. U. & Hoyer J. (2001). Generalized anxiety disorder: Nature and course. *Journal of Clinical Psychiatry, 62*(Suppl 11):15-19.

Guillain-Barré Syndrome

Guillain-Barré (ghee YAN-bah RAY) syndrome (GBS) is an illness in which the body attacks its own nerve cells. GBS affects the peripheral nervous system (nerve roots that exit the vertebral column to muscles and organs) and not the nerves in the brain or spinal cord. It is characterized by symmetrical muscle weakness (and/or paralysis) that begins in the legs and rises upward (ascending paralysis). People often report feelings of weakness, loss of balance (feeling unsteady), pain, and/or paresthesia. In children, pain is often the most prominent symptom. Reflexes are absent (areflexia) and autonomic dysfunction is frequently affected (e.g., fluctuations in heart rate, blood pressure). In severe cases, weakness can progress into the respiratory, facial, and esophageal muscles leading to problems with respiration, speech, and swallowing. Weakness and paralysis is usually at its maximum three to four weeks after initial symptoms.

The percentage of people who experience respiratory failure and require intubation is unclear; findings indicate anywhere from 5-30% (Beers & Berkow, 2004; Mack, 2004; Cha-Kim, 2004). Weakness typically begins to surface from five days to three weeks after an infectious illness, surgery, or immunization (Beers & Berkow, 2004). The most common bacterium associated with GBS is Campylobacter jejuni, which normally only causes diarrhea. Although the connection to these events is unclear, there appears to be a significant correlation.

GBS has many other names including acute inflammatory demyelinating polyneuropathy, acute febrile polyneuritis, acute idiopathic polyneuritis, infections polyneuritis, and Landry's ascending paralysis. There have been numerous underlying illnesses or infections identified as leading to GBS, which may be one of the reasons this disease is known by so many different names.

Incidence/Prevalence in US

Within the United States, approximately three out of every 100,000 adults are diagnosed with GBS and one out of every 100,000 children is diagnosed with GBS (Mack, 2004; Cha-Kim, 2004).

Predominant Age

GBS affects both males and females at any age and without regard to race or ethnicity. However, it does appear that there are a greater percentage of older people than younger people diagnosed with GBS (Mack, 2004).

Causes

The cause of GBS is unknown; however it is believed "that the mechanism of the disease involves an abnormal T-cell response precipitated by a preceding infection" (Mack, 2004).

System(s) Affected

GBS affects motor functioning more than sensory functioning. The number of systems affected depends upon the progression of the disease and the time lapse before medical intervention (how high up the body the disease progresses before it is halted by medical intervention). At the very least the peripheral nervous system, the muscular system, autonomic functioning, and reflexes are affected. If the disease is severe, it can additionally affect bowel and bladder functioning, speech, respiration, swallowing, and vision.

Prognosis

Approximately 75-85% have complete or good recovery, 15-20% have moderate residual impairments, and 1-10% have significant permanent disability (Cha-Kim, 2004). Mortality rates range from 2-12%. Deaths are typically a result of autonomic instability, pneumonia, respiratory distress, and pulmonary emboli. People who are over the age of 40 and who have rapid progression to quadriparesis or underlying malignancy have a poorer prognosis (Mack, 2004). Return of function can vary from several weeks to several years. Recovery should begin within two to four weeks after the progression of the disease ceases (Cha-Kim, 2004). Reoccurrence of GBS is rare in children, although approximately 5% of adults have another bout of GBS years after the first occurrence (Mack, 2004). Some people may continue to have chronic reoccurrences of GBS, referred to as chronic inflammatory demyelinating polyradiculoneuropathy (CIDP).

Secondary Problems

Complications from inactivity and bed rest (deep vein thrombosis, skin breakdown, muscle contractures), and issues related to pain management (medication, heat, transcutaneous electrical nerve stimulation, relaxation training) are common areas that require attention in addition to the ones already reviewed.

Assessments

Typical Scope of Team Assessment

A diagnosis of GBS is made mostly by observing symptoms (ascending tract weakness and areflexia) and taking a history of recent infectious illness, surgery, or immunization. Various lab work and imaging studies are used to confirm the diagnosis. Once the client is stabilized in the acute care setting, s/he may be transferred to an inpatient acute care rehabilitation center. The rehabilitation team assesses the client's baseline level of functioning using discipline-specific diagnostic tools to assess muscle strength, range of motion, sensation, mobility, speech, swallowing, respiration, autonomic functioning, and ability to perform specific daily activities (e.g., transfers, dressing, eating).

Anticipated Findings from RT Assessment

The anticipated findings will vary depending upon the extent of the dysfunction, the age of the person, and the person's prior medical history. In general, however, a therapist can anticipate:

- *Anxiety*: The person is commonly in an anxious state. People with GBS often report that the weakness seemed to "come out of nowhere" and progress rapidly. There is often little time to prepare for hospitalization so affairs are often in disarray (e.g., who is going to care for the person's children and pets, finances) causing anxiety and loss of internal locus of control. Anxiety, worry, and fear of the prognosis are common for an adult with GBS and for the parents of a child with GBS. If the client is a child, anxiety is often expressed in relation to the child's developmental level.
- *Pain*: Complaints of pain and need for pain management interventions are common.
- *Autonomic dysfunction*: The client may have orthostatic hypotension, high blood pressure, tachycardia, trouble breathing (may have a ventilator), and absent reflexes.
- *Lack of Leisure*: Leisure is often not a voiced priority for adults, compared to children who often desire to play. However, participation in leisure activities may help reduce the perceived level of pain and re-direct the client from anxiety-producing thoughts.
- *Lower extremity weakness*: In order to be admitted to an inpatient rehabilitation hospital, the extent of weakness or paralysis must significantly impair the person's functioning. The client will have the minimum of moderate to severe weakness or paralysis of the lower extremities.

Treatment Direction

Whole Team Approach

Plasmapheresis or intravenous immunoglobulin (IVIG) is typically administered in the early stages of the disease because it can shorten the course of the disease and hospitalization, as well as reduce mortality and incidence of permanent paralysis (Beers & Berkow, 2004). Vital signs are taken frequently to monitor the need for assisted breathing. Fluids are pushed to decrease risks of urinary tract infection and kidney stones. Precautions are adopted to decrease risks of developing skin breakdown. Passive range-of-motion exercises are necessary to prevent contractures and activity is encouraged within safe parameters. Heparin is commonly prescribed to prevent blood clots from forming as a secondary complication from increased bed rest. Paralyzed extremities are protected from trauma (e.g., bed rails to protect the arm from falling off the side of the bed). In general, therapy aims to 1. improve the muscular system; 2. enhance ability to perform life tasks; and 3. educate the person and the family about the disease, the anticipated course that it will take, and how to prevent secondary complications that are caused by a decreased level of activity.

Recreational Therapy Approach

The approach used by the recreational therapist focuses on four areas: 1. aspects of the client's lifestyle that will reduce long-term secondary impacts, 2. psychosocial adjustment, 3. adaptation of activity to allow a more normal lifestyle, and 4. addressing specific symptoms that result from GBS.

Recreational Therapy Interventions

Interventions that are frequently implemented with clients who have GBS include:

- *Psychosocial adjustment*: Participation in recreation, leisure, play, and community activities can help with psychosocial adjustment. Consider referring and helping clients integrate into formal and informal community groups to aid with social support. Cha-Kim (2004) notes that "psychosocial functional health status can be impaired even years after the GBS event [and that] psychosocial performance does not seem to correlate with the severity of residual physical function. Poor conditioning and easy fatigability may be contributory factors. Therefore, providing long-term attention and support is important" (p. 8). Places for more information and codes to use can be found in d240 Handling Stress and

Other Psychological Demands; A&P Chapter 9 Community, Social, and Civic Life; and "Integration," "Education and Counseling," and "Coping with Stress" in the Techniques section.

- *Movement and mobility*: Recreational therapy seeks to improve areas of difficulty. These will vary from client to client although most revolve around the muscular system including: d410 Changing Basic Body Position, d415 Maintaining a Body Position, d420 Transferring Oneself, d440 Fine Hand Use, d445 Hand and Arm Use, d450 Walking, and d460 Moving Around in Different Locations. Also see "Walking Techniques" and "Wheelchair Mobility Skills" in the Techniques section.
- *Physical exercise*: See "Exercise Basics" in the Techniques section.
- *Pain*: Therapists use the anxiety and stress management interventions reviewed previously to help with pain management. See b280 Sensation of Pain.
- *Lifestyle and secondary impacts*: Refer to the Concepts section for "Consequences of Inactivity."
- *Adaptation*: Recovery from GBS can range from several weeks to several years, so in many cases the recreational therapist teaches the client how to adapt for areas of impairment and difficulty to promote independence and functioning within

activities and life situations. See d155 Acquiring Skills; "Energy Conservation Training," "Integration," and "Activity Pattern Development" the Techniques section; and "Neuroplasticity" in the Techniques section for how to balance CIMT recovery challenges with adaptations.

Miscellaneous

Guillain-Barré Syndrome Foundation International
PO Box 262
Wynnewood, PA 19096
Fax: 610-667-0131
Voice: 610-667-7036
www.Guillain-Barré.com

References

Beers, M. & Berkow, R. (2004). *Merck manual internet edition*. Guillain-Barré syndrome. www.merck.com on 11/21/04.

Cha-Kim, A. (2004). Guillain-Barré syndrome. www.emedicine.com on 11/22/04.

Centers for Disease Control. (December 10, 2003). Questions & answers: Guillain-Barré syndrome. http://www.cdc.gov/flu/about/qa/gbs.htm.

Guillain-Barré Syndrome Foundation International. (2002). What is Guillain-Barré? www.Guillain-Barré.com on 11/23/04.

Mack, K. (2004). Guillain-Barré syndrome in childhood. www.emedicine.com on 11/22/04.

Joint Replacement

Total joint replacement is the removal of a diseased or damaged joint and the implantation of an artificial joint called a prosthesis. This procedure can be done for any joint of the body including knees, hips, ankles, toes, fingers, wrist, elbows, and shoulders. This section covers total joint replacements of the hip and knee since they are the most common in the rehabilitation setting.

The typical client has a history of osteoarthritis, rheumatoid arthritis, or traumatic joint injury and presents with severe joint pain during activity and rest (affecting the client's sleep). The client's ability to perform daily life tasks is also substantially impaired due to the pain. Other symptoms may include disabling stiffness, swelling, locking, and giving way. All conservative treatment measures (medication, assistive devices, therapy, bracing, weight loss) are exhausted before considering total joint replacement (Palmer, 2004).

Clients who have a hip or knee replacement will need to follow specific precautions (see "Precautions" in Concepts section). However, there are other common surgeries that a therapist will see in a rehabilitation setting that may also have to follow these precautions (even though they are not total hip or knee replacements). To clarify the differences in these surgeries, a description of four primary hip and knee surgeries are provided (Crepeau, Cohn, & Schell, 2003).

- *Hip fracture with closed reduction*: This is a break in any portion of the femur that can be manipulated into its natural position without major surgery. The client must follow weight-bearing precautions established by the surgeon and total hip precautions (THP).
- *Total hip replacement* (THR) or *total hip arthroplasty* (THA): This is the surgical removal of a diseased or injured hip joint, which is replaced with a prosthetic appliance. If the articular surfaces of both the acetabulum and the femur are replaced, the prosthesis is considered a total hip arthroplasty. If the femoral head is replaced and the acetabulum is not altered, the prosthesis is considered a hip hemiarthroplasty. The client must follow weight-bearing precautions and total hip precautions.
- *Hip fracture with open reduction and internal fixation* (ORIF): This is a surgical procedure that uses wires, screws, or pins applied directly to the fractured bone segments to keep them in place. This rehab therapist must clarify if THP, modified THP, or weight-bearing restrictions were ordered by the surgeon.

- *Total knee replacement* (TKR) or *total knee arthroplasty* (TKA): This is the implantation of a device to substitute for damaged joint surfaces. Related terms come from the type of prosthesis. Unicompartment or hemiarthroplasty is partial replacement of the joint. Hemiarthroplasty replaces the diseased component. Typically, active movement of the knee is encouraged during all activities after the surgery. Twisting motions that put undue stress on the joint should be avoided. Weight-bearing restrictions may also be prescribed.

Components of the Replacement

Components of the total hip arthroplasty include the acetabulum component that is held in place by screws, spikes, a special cement, or cementless design (as described later in this section). It is typically made out of plastic and may have a metal backing. The second component of the prosthesis is the femoral stem that is also held in place with cement or has a cementless design. It is typically made out of metal or ceramic.

During a total knee replacement, the end of the femur bone is removed and replaced with a metal shell (femoral component). The end of the lower leg bone (tibia) is also removed and replaced with a channeled plastic piece with a metal stem (tibial component). Depending on the condition of the kneecap portion of the knee joint, a plastic "button" may also be added under the kneecap surface (patellar component). The components are typically made out of plastic and metal. They are held in place with cement or have a cementless design.

Cemented vs. uncemented prosthesis (Rasul, 2002).

- Cemented joint replacement is a procedure in which bone cement or polymethylmethacrylate (PMMA) is used to fix the prosthesis in place. It is most frequently used for older adults who are less active. It is also used for those who have osteoporosis. Pain relief and enhanced joint mobility are noticeable immediately after surgery. The cement can loosen over time and sometimes bits of cement break off and cause further pain or joint damage.
- Ingrowth or cementless joint replacement is done by pressing the prosthesis into place so it holds with friction. The prosthesis is covered with a textured metal or special bone-like substance, which allows bone to grow into the prosthesis, thus negating the need for cement to hold it in place. This procedure is based on a fracture-

healing model. It may last longer than a cemented prosthesis because there is no cement that can loosen. It is used frequently in younger, active clients. There is extended recovery time, however, when compared to the cemented prosthesis, because of the length of time for the natural bone to grow and attach to the prosthesis.

Primary vs. revision surgery:
- Primary joint replacement or arthroplasty refers to the first replacement surgery.
- Revision refers to a second or succeeding surgery performed usually for an unstable, loose, or painful joint replacement.

Contraindications for undergoing a hip or knee replacement (NIH, 1994; NIH, 2003; Palmer, 2004):
- Active local or systemic infection or other medical conditions that preclude safe anesthesia and the demands of surgery and rehabilitation.
- Severe vascular disease.
- Obesity, a relative contraindication because of a higher mechanical failure rate in heavier patients and increased risk of delayed wound healing and perioperative infection.
- Some neurological impairments.
- Skin conditions within the field or surgery.

Incidence/Prevalence in US

Approximately 267,000 total knee replacements (American Association of Orthopaedic Surgeons, 2001a) and 168,000 total hip replacements (American Association of Orthopaedic Surgeons, 2001b) are performed each year in the US.

Predominant Age

THR: Two-thirds of all THR procedures are performed in individuals who are older than 65. The rate of THR increases for patients up to 75 and then declines. The highest age-specific incidence rates of THR are between 65 and 74 years of age for men and 75 and 84 years of age for women. Recent comparisons of rates of THR reveal that more are being done in the young and in the older patients. Among the older patients, there has been an increase in THR in patients with more comorbidity. In regards to gender, 62% of all THR procedures in the US are performed on women.

TKR: In the past, patients between 60 and 75 years of age were considered to be the best candidates for TKR. Over the past two decades, however, the age range has been broadened to include more elderly patients (e.g., octogenarians and beyond), many of whom have a higher number of comorbid conditions, and younger patients, whose

implants may be exposed to greater mechanical stresses because of higher levels of physical activity over an extended time period.

Causes

Rheumatoid arthritis, osteoarthritis, or a traumatic joint injury can cause severe joint damage resulting in pain and limited function. When non-surgical interventions fail to manage these issues, a total joint replacement may become a viable option.

System(s) Affected

The primary system affected is the musculoskeletal system. However other bodily systems can be affected positively as a secondary effect of surgery (e.g., increased activity due to decreased joint pain may result in increased cardiopulmonary endurance).

Prognosis

THR

Women have significantly worse preoperative functional status than men and are 35% more likely to report the use of a walking aid at the time of surgery. These differences persist even after adjustment for other demographic and clinical characteristics. "The benefits of a long-term therapeutic exercise program for patients who have undergone THR have not been clearly demonstrated to improve mobility or hip stability. There appears to be insufficient appreciation for the role of exercise in THR rehabilitation; however, there is evidence that hip weakness persists up to two years after surgery in the presence of a normal gait" (National Institutes of Health, 1994). Mobility and stability issues may remain unresolved.

More than 90% of individuals will never need revision surgery. However, because more young clients are having hip replacements and wearing away of the joint surface becomes a problem after 15 to 20 years, revision surgery is becoming more common. A 3% prevalence of prosthetic loosening is observed at 11 years and a 1% prevalence of prosthetic infection (Jacobson, 2002).

TKR

There appears to be rapid and substantial improvement in pain, functional status, and overall health-related quality of life in about 90% of clients, and 85% of clients are satisfied with the results of surgery. Kneeling is usually uncomfortable, but it is not harmful (NIH, 2003). The client may feel a soft clicking of the metal and plastic with knee flexion or walking. These usually diminish over time (American

Association of Orthopaedic Surgeons, 2001). The best predictor of range of motion following total knee replacement is the preoperative range of motion. Long-term studies of cemented TKR show a 91-96% prosthesis survival rate at 14-15 years of follow-up. Cementless designs do not have the same length of follow-up, but studies at 10-12 years report a 95% prosthesis survival rate (Crepeau, Cohn, & Schell, 2003).

The proportion of patients with good-to-excellent outcomes declines with each successive revision. Reports vary from 10% (NIH, 2003) to 20% (MedicineNet) in the number of clients who require revision surgery after ten years. Factors that increase a client's risk of needing revision surgery include being 55 years of age or younger, male gender, diagnosis of OA, obesity, and presence of comorbid conditions (NIH, 2003). Obesity puts the replaced knee at an increased risk of loosening or dislocation and younger clients, who are more physically active than older adults, increase the risk of trauma and stress to the replaced knee.

Both THR and TKR

The client must be cleared by the surgeon to resume driving. The surgeon bases this decision on muscle control to provide adequate reaction time for braking and accelerating, joint flexion and extension to comfortably sit in the car and operate brake and gas pedal, and stability of joint surgery. Many surgeons do not want the client to be in a vehicle for several weeks (typically six weeks) after surgery.

Clients need to avoid excessive physical activity as defined by their surgeon. Excessive activity or weight may accelerate this normal wear and cause the replacement to loosen and become painful (American Association of Orthopaedic Surgeons, 2001).

* *Expected activity after surgery*: recreational walking, swimming, golf, driving, light hiking, recreational biking, ballroom dancing, normal stair climbing.
* *Activity exceeding usual recommendations after surgery*: vigorous walking or hiking, skiing, tennis, repetitive lifting exceeding 50 pounds, repetitive aerobic stair climbing.
* *Dangerous activity after surgery*: jogging or running, contact sports, jumping sports, high impact aerobics.

Metal components of the joint replacement may activate metal detectors at airports and other buildings that require such security. The client should request a card from his/her surgeon that verifies joint replacement surgery and alert security personnel prior to going through a metal detector.

Clients with joint replacements should alert their doctors and dentists that they have an artificial joint. These joints are at risk for infection by bacteria introduced by any invasive procedures such as surgery, dental or gum work, urological and endoscopic procedures, as well as from infections elsewhere in the body.

Sexual activity may be contraindicated until the two-month follow-up appointment with the surgeon.

Secondary Problems

There is less than a 1% mortality rate for knee and hip replacement surgery. Some of the possible complications from surgery include deep vein thrombosis and pulmonary emboli, wound healing problems, wound and deep tissue infection often associated with diabetes mellitus and obesity, pneumonia, myocardial infarction, joint instability or malalignment, hip dislocation if THP are not maintained, urinary tract infection, nausea and vomiting (usually related to pain medication), nerve damage, blood vessel injury, infection, and loss of appetite. Associated risks of anesthesia include heart, lung, kidney, and liver damage. Long-range complications of joint replacement surgery include prosthetic loosening and wear.

Secondary problems from surgery (Palmer, 2004):
* *Pain*: Reduced by long-acting narcotic analgesics. Attention to side effects is imperative.
* *Bowel and bladder functions*: Constipation caused by decreased mobility, post-anesthesia effects, or a side effect of narcotic analgesics is a frequent complaint.
* *Nutrition and hydration*: Elderly clients are at risk for malnutrition and dehydration due to physical limitations and/or cognitive deficits. Dehydration can lead to acute metabolic or renal problems.

Assessments

Prior to approval and acceptance of joint replacement surgery, the orthopedic surgeon conducts an assessment (Rasul, 2002; American Association of Orthopaedic Surgeons, 2001a, 2001b).
* A medical history, in which the orthopedic surgeon gathers information about general health and the extent of hip or knee pain and how it affects the ability to perform daily activities.
* A thorough physical examination that includes the assessment of the hip's or knee's mobility, strength, and alignment.
* X-rays to determine the extent of damage or deformity in the hip.

- Blood tests or other tests to determine the condition of the bone and soft tissues of joint

Typical Scope of Team Assessment

Clients who receive inpatient rehabilitation services are evaluated primarily in the following areas: replaced joint range of motion without breaking precautions, functional abilities to perform life tasks, knowledge and application of joint and weight-bearing precautions, and adjustment to situation.

Discharge is recommended only when wound healing is satisfactory, knee flexion of 90° has been achieved, the patient is considered to be safe and supported in the home environment, and no complications are present. Anti-clotting medication is often continued at home for a period of time.

Not all clients who undergo a THR or TKR will receive inpatient rehabilitation services. Some clients skip inpatient rehab and receive in-home and outpatient therapy services only. These clients typically are younger clients who do not have a significant past medical history that requires close monitoring, do not present with any mental or cognitive deficits that would impact their ability to adhere to precautions and exercise regime, and do possess the motivation and initiative to follow through with the surgeon's directions.

Anticipated Findings from RT Assessment

History of progressive inactivity: clients adapt their lifestyle to meet the challenges of living with joint pain and limited joint function. Some of the complications of this type of adaptation include:
- Pulmonary, cardiac, and muscular deconditioning
- Increased weight
- Poor nutrition
- Depression
- Loss of a healthy leisure lifestyle
- Social isolation

Treatment Direction

All care must take into account surgical precautions related to keeping the surgery site protected. These include no immersion in water, bandages to prevent irritation from clothing, support stockings to decrease the risk of deep vein thrombosis, and observation of the site to detect early signs of infection. Ice is used to reduce swelling, heat to increase range of motion. Appropriate diet promotes proper tissue healing. Exercise programs are established by physical therapists to restore muscle strength and reduce scarring.

TKR

The surgeon prescribes specific weight-bearing precautions, a knee immobilizer, and a schedule to wear a continuous passive motion (CPM) machine. The knee immobilizer is a soft Velcro brace from the ankle to the middle thigh. The patient wears it after a TKR until quadriceps strength is regained. In certain situations, careful resistive or gradual ROM exercises are initiated (Rasul, 2002). The CPM machine is placed on the affected leg when the client is in bed to gently bend and straighten the knee without the assistance of the client. It can assist with managing edema (swelling), enhancing range of motion, and improving venous circulation thus decreasing risks of deep vein thrombosis.

THR

The surgeon prescribes specific weight-bearing precautions, total hip precautions, and an abduction wedge pillow.

Whole Team Approach

Due to the short-length of stay, the team's primary focus is on increasing range of motion in the replaced joint within precautions, restoring functional skills to complete life tasks, walking, educating the client on how to maintain precautions after discharge through adaptation and modification of activities, increasing the client's awareness of the benefits of exercise in achieving optimal outcomes, developing a home exercise program, and identifying resources to solve problems with life tasks.

Recreational Therapy Approach

Therapists address the issues noted in the whole team approach using the modalities of leisure and recreation. Finding enjoyable activities that the client actually does will help the goals of increasing strength and range of motion. Activities also aid in better sleep, reduction of pain, maintenance of a positive attitude, and healthy weight loss. Therapists also focus on the systemic issues (environmental and personal factors) that affect the client's ability to continue involvement post discharge.

Recreational Therapy Interventions

The following interventions are commonly used for clients with joint replacements.
- *Benefits of leisure*: Clients are educated about the importance of active leisure for recovery and health promotion with particular attention to enhancing range of motion and muscle strength. See "Consequences of Inactivity" in the Concepts section.

- *Physical leisure activity*: Exercise options are reviewed and explored for recovery and long-term health promotion. See "Activity Pattern Development," "Exercise Basics," and "Integration" in the Techniques section. Also see d920 Recreation and Leisure and d570 Looking After Oneself.
- *Functional mobility skills*: RTs address the development of mobility skills within specific recreational and community activities that will be part of the client's lifestyle after discharge. Include all of the aspects d4 Mobility that apply to the client's current and future condition. Also see "Integration" in the Techniques section.
- *Community problem solving and resource awareness*: Resource awareness education goes hand-in-hand with community problem solving since knowledge of resources and how to access them are essential skills to problem solve for barriers. The information reviewed will vary depending on the needs of the client. Possibilities include "Community Accessibility Training," "Energy Conservation Training," "Personal Leisure Resource Awareness," and "Community Leisure Resource Awareness" in the Techniques section. ICF codes include d175 Solving Problems; e140 Products and Technology for Culture, Recreation, and Sport; and d940 Human Rights.

Miscellaneous

Blood clot prevention is important following joint replacements. Warning signs include increasing pain in the calf, tenderness or redness above or below the knee, and increasing swelling in the calf, ankle, and foot. Warning signs that the clot has traveled to the lung include sudden increased shortness of breath, sudden onset of chest pain, and localized chest pain with coughing. Immediate medical attention is required (American Association of Orthopaedic Surgeons, 2001a, 2001b).

Joint prostheses are especially prone to harbor infections that may not be treatable. Bacteria enter the bloodstream during dental procedures, urinary tract infections, or skin infections. Bacteria can lodge around the joint replacement and cause an infection. A client with a joint replacement should take antibiotics prior to dental work or any surgical procedure that could allow bacteria to enter the bloodstream. Immediate medical attention is required

if there is an infection. Warning signs of a possible joint replacement infection are

- Persistent fever (higher than 100°F orally)
- Shaking and chills
- Increasing redness, tenderness, or swelling of the joint wound
- Drainage from the joint wound
- Increasing joint pain with both activity and rest (American Association of Orthopaedic Surgeons, 2001a, 2001b).

A fall in the first few weeks after surgery can damage the joint replacement and may result in a need for further surgery. Stairs are particularly hard until the hip or knee joint is strong and mobile. An assistive device should be used for walking until balance, flexibility, and strength are restored.

Falls prevention is an important issue. See falls precautions under "Precautions" in the Concepts section.

References

American Association of Orthopaedic Surgeons. (2001a). Total knee replacement. http://orthoinfo.aaos.org/booklet/thr_report.cfm?thread_id=9&topcategory=knee on 1/18/04

American Association of Orthopaedic Surgeons. (2001b). Total hip replacement. http://orthoinfo.aaos.org/booklet/thr_report.cfm?thread_id=2&topcategory=hip on 1/18/04

Crepeau, E., Cohn, E., Schell, B. (2003). *Willard and Spackman's occupational therapy, tenth edition*. Philadelphia, PA: Lippincott Williams & Wilkins.

Jacobson, J. (2002). Hip replacement. http://www.emedicine.com/radio/topic830.htm on 3/22/04

MedicineNet. (NA). Total knee replacement http://www.medicinenet.com/script/main/ques.asp?qakey=9622 on 3/22/04.

National Institutes of Health. (1994). NIH consensus statement on total hip replacement. *12*(5), http://consensus.nih.gov/ cons/098/098_intro.htm on 3/20/04.

National Institutes of Health. (2003). NIH consensus development conference on total knee replacement. http://consensus.nih.gov/cons/117/117cdc_statementFINAL.html on 3/21/04.

Palmer, S. (2004). Total knee arthroplasty. http://www.emedicine.com/orthoped/topic347.htm on 3/22/04.

Rasul, A. (2002). Total joint replacement rehabilitation. http://www.emedicine.com/pmr/topic221.htm on 3/23/04.

Major Depressive Disorder

Major Depressive Disorder (unipolar depression), or MDD, is one of two depressive mood disorders classified by the American Psychiatric Association in the *Diagnostic and Statistical Manual of Mental Disorders*. (The other depressive mood disorder is dysthymic disorder.) MDD is characterized by two or more weeks of depressive symptoms that significantly interfere with the ability to function and complete life tasks. Such symptoms include trouble sleeping, unwanted weight gain or loss, loss of pleasure, difficulty concentrating, feelings of hopelessness or worthlessness, and suicidal ideation.

In children and adolescents, the clinical characteristics are the same as in adults, but the prominent characteristics differ. "In children, symptoms of anxiety (including phobias and trouble separating from caretakers), physical complaints, and behavioral problems seem to occur more frequently. Adolescents tend to have more sleep and appetite disturbances, psychosis (hallucinations or delusions), and impairment of functioning than younger children" (Birmaher & Axelson, 1998).

Incidence/Prevalence in US

MDD is the leading cause of disability in the US and worldwide (World Almanac and Book of Facts, 2004). It occurs in about 10-25% of women and 5-12% of men within the course of their lifetime (Sadock & Sadock, 2003), affecting an estimated 13-14 million people (World Almanac Book of Facts, 2004). "The reasons for the difference [in the ratio of women to men] have been hypothesized to involve hormonal differences, the effects of childbirth, differing psychosocial stressors for women and for men, and behavioral models of learned helplessness" (Sadock & Sadock 2003, p. 535). The prevalence of depression (both MDD and dysthymic disorder) in children and adolescents is not well studied, but it appears to occur in approximately 2% of children and 6% of adolescents (Ford-Martin, 2001). Depression is more common in rural areas than in urban areas (Sadock & Sadock, 2003).

Predominant Age

"The mean age of onset for MDD is about 40 years, with 50% of all clients having an onset between the ages of 20 and 50" (Sadock & Sadock, 2003, p. 536). However, younger people seem to be more at risk for depression, as evidenced by an NIH study that found within a one-year period, three times as many persons aged 18 to 29 experienced depression as those over the age of 60 (World Almanac and Book of Facts, 2004).

Causes

There are many variables that are thought to contribute to the development of MDD.

Hormones: Hormones are thought to play a role in the development of depression due to a correlation between childbearing or menopause and depression. Childbearing years are marked by the highest rates of depression, followed by the years prior to menopause (World Almanac and Book of Facts, 2004).

Drugs and alcohol: Individuals who abuse alcohol or illicit drugs have higher incidence of depression (Gartside, 2003).

Genetics: Clinical depression seems to run in families. First-degree relatives of individuals with major depressive disorder are two to three times as likely to have major depressive disorders (Sadock & Sadock, 2003; Ford-Martin, 2001).

Environmental triggers (negative events): A lack of support, family conflict, aversive experiences in early childhood (such as abuse and neglect), death, divorce, and medical illnesses may predispose a person to develop clinical depression.

- *Traumatic separation*: Traumatic separation in childhood predisposes one to depression. Adult losses are said to revive the traumatic childhood loss and so precipitate adult depressive episodes (Sadock & Sadock, 2003).
- *Impaired sense of self*: When a child does not receive a positive sense of self-esteem and self-cohesion from his/her parents, there is a massive loss of self-esteem that presents as depression (Sadock & Sadock, 2003).
- *Stressful events*: One of the greatest causes of depression is stressful events. Research has shown that experiences that negatively affect a person's self-esteem are more likely to produce episodes of depression than events that don't negatively impact self-esteem. Because of the different ways that people look at events based on their past experiences, seemingly minor negative events may have large impacts on some people.
- *Loss of parents or significant others*: "The most compelling data indicate that the life event most often associated with development of depression is losing a parent before age 11. The environmental stressor most often associated with the onset of an episode of depression is the loss of a spouse. Another risk factor is unemployment — persons out of work are three times more likely

to report symptoms of an episode of major depression than those who are employed" (Sadock & Sadock, 2003, p. 541).

Physical illness: Many physical illnesses, including cardiovascular disease and cancer, as well as neurological disorders (e.g. head injury, stroke, Parkinson's disease, Huntington's disease, dementias), are associated with an increased risk of depression. This may be due to stresses of lifestyle change or changes in the brain's pathology (Gartside, 2003). A condition referred to as "vascular depression" occurs mostly in older adults when interrupted blood flow causes subtle damage to nerve pathways involved in mood and motivation (Miller, 2004). This is a more likely cause of late-onset depression (over age 60) than genetic or developmental influences (Ford-Martin, 2001).

Medication: Depression can be a side effect of some commonly prescribed medications (e.g., beta-blockers, antiviral medications, and calcium channel blockers) (Gartside, 2003).

Other mental disorders: People with obsessive-compulsive disorder, histrionic personality disorder, and borderline personality disorder are at a greater risk for developing depression than people with other personality disorders such as antisocial personality disorder and paranoid personality disorder. People with other forms of depressive disorders (cyclothymic disorder, dysthymic disorder) are at risk for developing MDD or bipolar I disorder (Sadock & Sadock, 2003).

Inability to meet goals: Depression may occur when a person becomes aware of the discrepancy between extraordinarily high ideals and the inability to meet those goals (Sadock & Sadock, 2003).

Living life for another or ideal: When clients realize that they have been living their life for someone else rather than for themselves and that the person or ideal for which they have been living is never going to respond in a manner that will meet their expectations, depression may occur (Sadock & Sadock, 2003).

System(s) Affected

MDD affects appetite, behavior, concentration, energy level, mood, relationships, sleep, suicidal thoughts, and cognition.

Prognosis

A MDD episode usually lasts six to nine months. Half of all clients diagnosed with an MDD episode will have another MDD episode within three years, and three quarters will have another MDD episode within ten years (Reus, 2000). The risk of suicide increases with each successive MDD episode — 50% after one episode, 70% after two episodes, and 90% after three episodes (Ford-Martin, 2001).

In children and adolescents each MDD episode lasts approximately seven to nine months with about 90% of recurrent major depressive episodes ending by one and a half to two years after the onset of depression. Six to ten percent of MDD episodes become chronic. Interestingly, 20-40% of adolescents with MDD develop bipolar disorder within five years after the onset of depression. Children and adolescents with clinical depressions (MDD and dysthymic disorder) are at a high risk for suicide, homicide, abuse of alcohol/drugs, physical illnesses, and poor academic and psychosocial functioning. Adolescents diagnosed with MDD who receive group cognitive-behavioral therapy, relaxation training, and group problem-solving therapy may prevent recurrences of depression for 9-24 months after treatment (Birmaher & Axelson, 1998).

Secondary Problems

- Depression is associated with increased risk of cardiac morbidity and mortality and increased susceptibility to cancer. This may be due to an altered immune system from depression (Reus, 2000).
- Risk of suicide. See "Suicide and Suicidal Ideation" in he Diagnosis section for more information
- Behavioral, cognitive, social, and physical symptoms of MDD can result in secondary conditions such as decreased physical activity, lack of social support, and difficulty concentrating and attending to life tasks.

Assessments

Typical Scope of Team Assessment

The American Psychiatric Association sets the criteria used to diagnose a MDD episode. Either 1. depressed mood or 2. loss of interest or pleasure must be present. Other symptoms include weight loss or gain, too much or too little sleep, psychomotor agitation or retardation observed by others, fatigue, feelings of worthlessness or guilt, diminished ability to concentrate or think, and recurrent thoughts of death or suicidal ideation. There must be at least five symptoms, on an almost daily basis, during a two-week period. The symptoms must cause significant distress or impairment in functioning. MDD is not a correct diagnosis if the symptoms are caused by medication, medical condition, or bereavement during the first two months after the loss.

MDD is described as "recurrent" when two or more major depressive episodes occur with a break of at least two consecutive months in which criteria are not met for a major depressive episode.

Tests used to make the diagnosis of MDD include the *Hamilton Depression Scale* (HAM-D), *Child Depression Inventory* (CDI), *Geriatric Depression Scale* (GDS), *Beck Depression Inventory* (BDI), and the *Zung Self-Rating Scale for Depression* (Ford-Martin, 2001).

Children and adolescents: It can be difficult to diagnose a child or adolescent with MDD because the depressed and irritable mood often limits conversation, thus making exploration of feelings limited. Additionally, parents and teachers often attribute behavioral changes to issues other than depression (e.g., "He is just still mad about being grounded last month."). Common behavioral changes that may signal signs of depression include: 1. withdrawn, whiny, or moody behavior, 2. anger or tearfulness over little things, 3. negative or overwhelming views of many situations, 4. limited interaction with others, 5. withdrawal from favorite activities, and a 6. decline in school performance (grades, skipping classes, getting into trouble at school). It is important for parents to be aware of the signs of depression, especially once the child is diagnosed with a single MDD episode, and for the mental health professional to gather data from outside sources (e.g., ask parents about child's behavior) as part of the clinical assessment. Additionally, mental health professionals must be aware of the differential diagnosis of depression since 40-70% of children and adolescents with clinical depression also have other coexisting psychiatric diagnoses, such as disruptive behavior disorders (conduct disorder, oppositional-defiant disorder, and attention deficit/hyperactivity disorder), anxiety disorders, abuse of drugs and/or alcohol, and eating disorders (bulimia and anorexia). The incidence and severity of suicide attempts also increase after puberty; therefore the assessment of depression must always include a screening for suicidal ideation (Birmaher & Axelson, 1998).

Older adults: In older adults, symptoms of depression are often manifested in disorientation, memory loss, and distractibility (APA, 2000). Mental health professionals must be aware of medical conditions that may contribute to these depressive symptoms including vascular depression or dementia. Generally, dementia is characterized by a steady decline in cognitive function, rather than a sudden onset. However, events such as a cerebrovascular accident can cause a sudden onset of cognitive impairment.

Anticipated Findings from RT Assessment

- Behavioral, physical, social, and cognitive changes due to MDD, as described in the team assessment section.
- Lack of desire to participate in pleasurable or recreational activities (anhedonia).
- Suicide precautions. Restrictions may be placed on community reentry training and the availability and use of specific recreational supplies.
- Limited social skills and lack of social support.
- Poor self-esteem and loss of internal locus of control.
- Possible presence of another mental disorder, as described in the team assessment section.
- Individuals with depression may score significantly lower than non-depressed clients on scales measuring pleasure from activity involvement (Mobily & MacNeil, 2002, p. 80).

Treatment Direction

Whole Team Approach

There are many single and combined approaches to the treatment of MDD.

- *Antidepressant medication.*
- *Cognitive-behavioral therapy* (CBT): This helps clients identify and change negative and distorted thinking patterns that may be contributing to depression (Reus, 2000; Sadock & Sadock, 2003). Common cognitive distortions include: 1. arbitrary inference, 2. specific abstraction, 3. overgeneralization, 4. magnification and minimization, 5. personalization, 6. absolute dichotomous thinking (Sadock & Sadock, 2003). See "Education and Counseling" in the Techniques section for more information on CBT.
- *Interpersonal therapy*: focuses on changing unhealthy personal relationships that contribute to depression.
- *Family therapy, social skills training, and group therapy*: Usually for children and adolescents. The primary goals are to reduce depressive symptoms and improve coping skills, problem solving skills, academic functioning, and parent-child and peer relationships. Family therapy focuses on the dynamics that occur within the family system, rather than focusing solely on the individual with the mental disorder.
- *Electroconvulsive therapy* (ECT): has been found effective in treating 80-90% of cases of severe depression, but the exact reasons why the positive changes occur are not fully understood (Reus, 2000; Sadock & Sadock, 2003). The client typically receives six to eight session of ECT over a two-week period. Transient memory

loss and confusion are common side effects that do not persist long-term (Reus, 2000).

- *Phototherapy*: Exposure to high intensity, full spectrum light. This is commonly used for seasonal depression (e.g., winter blues).
- *Sleep deprivation*: "The only therapeutic intervention that has antidepressant benefit within 24 hours, although the response is usually transient and occurs in only half of subjects" (Reus, 2000).

Recreational Therapy Approach

Recreational therapy aims to alleviate symptoms of depression through encouragement of team interventions and promotion of healthy activities to facilitate positive change.

Recreational Therapy Interventions

The following interventions are commonly used for clients with major depressive disorders.

- *Physical exercise*: Regular, moderate physical activity is known to decrease symptoms of depression. See "Exercise Basics" in the Techniques section for information on beginning an exercise program. Also see ICF topics d920 Recreation and Leisure and b455 Exercise Tolerance Functions.
- *Leisure education*: The therapist educates clients about the benefits of recreational activity in alleviating symptoms of depression and preventing relapse. See "Consequences of Inactivity" in the Concepts section and d5702 Maintaining One's Health in the ICF.
- *Initiation*: The therapist designs and implements structured recreational activities and gradually progresses clients into unstructured or self-initiated recreational activities. See "Personal Leisure Resource Awareness" and "Community Leisure Resource Awareness" in the Techniques section). ICF sections b1301 Motivation and b1265 Optimism are also relevant.
- *Social skills training*: Social skills training is a strong component of the recreational therapy program fostering healthy interaction patterns and developing skills needed to initiate and benefit from social support from others. See "Social Skills Development" in the Concepts

section and "Social Skills Training" in the Techniques section for more information. In the ICF more information can be found in Activities and Participation Chapter 7 Interpersonal Interactions and Relationships.

- *Changing distorted thinking patterns*: Cognitive-behavioral techniques are discussed in b1601 Form of Thought and "Education and Counseling" in the Techniques section.
- *Stress management and relaxation training*: See "Relaxation and Stress Reduction" in the Techniques section.
- *Self-concept and self-esteem*: Improving self-concept and self-esteem can help with depressive symptoms. See codes b1266 Confidence and b1800 Experience of Self. Also see "Self-Esteem" in the Techniques section.
- *Family training*: Family training is helpful, especially when working with children and adolescents, to teach family members how to best help their loved one after discharge. For adult clients, the therapist must not break the client's right to confidentiality.

References

American Psychiatric Association. (2000). *Diagnostic and statistical manual of mental disorders, 4th ed., text revision.* Washington, DC: American Psychiatric Association.

Birmaher, B. & Axelson, D. (1998). Depression. *The Gale encyclopedia of childhood and adolescence* http://69.0.144.8/ on 3/12/04.

Ford-Martin, P. (2001). Depressive disorders. *The Gale Encyclopedia of Medicine, 2nd edition* http://69.0.144.8/ on 3/11/04.

Gartside, S. (2003). Affective disorders. *Encyclopedia of life sciences.* http://69.0.144.8/ on 3/9/04.

Miller, M. (2004). Mind and moods: Accepting life's limits. *Newsweek*, p.66. http://69.0.144.8/ on 3/13/04.

Mobily, K. & MacNeil, R. (2002). *Therapeutic recreation and the nature of disabilities.* State College, PA: Venture Publishing, Inc.

Reus, V. (2000). Mood disorders. *Encyclopedia of life sciences.* http://69.0.144.8/ on 3/11/04.

Sadock, J. & Sadock, V. (2003). *Kaplan & Sadock's synopsis of psychiatry, 9th edition.* Philadelphia, PA: Lippincott Williams & Wilkins.

World Almanac and Book of Facts. (2004). Depression. http://69.0.144.8/ on 3/10/04.

Mental Retardation/Developmental Disability

Both mental retardation and developmental disability are broad terms that encompass a similar set of chronic disorders. The difference between the two terms is often just one of semantics and the affiliation of the individual using the term. Because there is so much overlap, most people use "MR/DD" (mental retardation/developmental disability) to describe the broad scope of disorders and impairments.

Mental retardation and developmental disabilities are similar in that they both include limitations in communication, self-care, social situations, school or work activities, and independent living. Both diagnoses coexist with other conditions including cerebral palsy, seizure disorders, vision impairment, hearing loss, and attention-deficit/hyperactivity disorder (ADHD). If someone is trying to distinguish between MR and DD, they usually look at the following differences: Mental retardation is usually regarded as existing from birth. (By definition it must appear prior to the age of 18.) There must be IQ results that show an intellectual impairment.

People with mental retardation can and do learn new skills, but they develop more slowly than people with average intelligence and adaptive skills. There are different degrees of mental retardation, ranging from mild to profound. A person's level of mental retardation can be defined by their intelligence quotient (IQ), or by the types and amount of support they need.

The levels of mental retardation are shown below. The reason for the range in some score limits is that the two organizations (AAMR and APA) primarily involved in defining MR have set slightly different IQ limits for the categories.
- *Mild mental retardation*: IQ range of 50-55 to 70. This category accounts for the majority of clients with mental retardation (approximately 75%). Clients with mild mental retardation can be expected to reach a cognitive functional level of approximately sixth grade and can often live in the community with some community support.
- *Moderate mental retardation*: IQ range of 35-40 to 50-55. This category accounts for approximately 20% of clients with mental retardation.
- *Severe mental retardation*: IQ range of 20-25 to 35-40.
- *Profound mental retardation*: IQ range below 20-25.

Knowing the client's measured IQ provides the therapist with a partial understanding of the client's ability to learn new skills. Many other factors also impact a client's ability to function in his/her community.

The American Association on Mental Retardation (AAMR) does not consider mental retardation to be a medical or mental disorder. Instead, AAMR considers mental retardation to be a state of impaired functioning that starts when the individual is a child. This state of functioning has impairments in both intelligence and the ability to adapt to the environment.

The AAMR has five essential assumptions:
- Functioning levels must be compared to similar ages, peers, and cultures and include the community context.
- Cultural and linguistic differences in communication, sensory, motor, and behavioral factors must all be considered during assessment.
- Limitations and strengths often coexist.
- Limitations are described to explain needed supports.
- With appropriate personalized supports over a sustained period, the life functioning of the person with mental retardation generally will improve (AAMR, 2002).

Developmental disabilities tend to include a broader range of causes. Onset may occur (by definition) up to the age of 22. Low IQ scores are not required. Deficits in functioning are sufficient for a diagnosis of DD. See the causes section for some of the possible reasons for later onset of DD.

Table 12 shows some of the more common genetic syndromes and diseases associated with MR/DD.

The schools have another, similar definition for clients who qualify for special education opportunities. The United States' law governing special education is titled Individuals with Disabilities Education Act (IDEA). IDEA's definition for clients who qualify for special services is

> …significantly sub average general intellectual functioning, existing concurrently with deficits in adaptive behavior and manifested during the developmental period, that adversely affects a child's educational performance. [34 *Code of Federal Regulations* §3000.7(c)(6)]

IDEA lists mental retardation as only one of the many possible types of developmental disabilities including disabilities in which the client may have an average or above average IQ.

Table 12: Syndromes and Diseases Associated with MR/DD

Name	Commonly Found Functional Limitations and Commonly Found Physical Attributes
Apert	MR; premature fusion of skull, finger, and toe bones
Bardet-Biedl	Mild to moderate MR; loss of night vision which progresses to blindness; obesity; extra or fused fingers or toes
Beckwith-Wiedemann	Occasionally mild to moderate MR; large body and tongue; defect in abdominal wall
Cornelia de Lange	MR; small, possibly malformed feet, hands; continuous eyebrows
Cri du Chat	Severe MR; degenerating to profound; decreased muscle tone and cardiac disorders are common; small head; cries like a catcall when young; wide set eyes; receding chin
Down Syndrome	MR; decreased muscle tone; congenital heart disease; small stature, atlantoaxial dislocation condition
Ehlers-Danlos	Increased risk management required during activities; poor healing of wounds; hypertension of joints
Ellis-van Creveld	Occasional MR; cardiac defects; short extremities
Erb's Palsy	Decreased abduction of arm; decreased flexion of forearm; injury to 5th and 6th cervical nerves due to injury during delivery
Fetal Alcohol Syndrome	Delayed development; possible MR; possible hyperactivity; small head, large space between nose and upper lip
Fetal Hydantoin	Borderline to mild MR; cleft lip; depressed nasal bridge; widely spaced eyes; due to prenatal exposure to anticonvulsants (e.g., Dilantin)
Fragile X	Possible autistic like behaviors; MR; large head; prominent ears
Goldenhar	Possible deafness; occasional MR; ear deficits; lateral cliff-like extension of edge of mouth; cleft palate
Hurler	Impaired vision due to cloudy corneas; severe MR; decreased muscle tone; short stature; excessive body hair
Klinefelter	Potential osteoporosis; obese trunk with long legs; poor verbal skills and other learning disabilities; may not develop until adolescence; immature sex organs
Lowe	Impaired vision due to cataracts; MR; hyperactivity; kidney abnormalities
Menkes	Progressive cognitive deterioration; MR; seizures; kinky hair; feeding difficulties
Prader-Willi	Borderline to moderate MR; compulsive eating disorder; poor muscle tone; small body stature; rounded face
Riley-Day	Decreased sensory awareness; decreased pain awareness; increased risk of choking; emotional lability; MR;
Rubinstein-Taybi	MR; small head; slanted eyes; broad thumb
Sanfilippo	MR with deteriorating cognitive ability; stiffness of joints; coarse facial features
Seckel	Moderate to severe MR; short stature; small head
Sjogren-Larrson	Difficulty with ambulation due to spasticity in lower extremities; MR; dry, rough, scaly skin
Smith-Lemli-Opitz	Irritable; MR; difficulty with eating; droopy eyelids; upturned nose
Trisomy 18	MR; poor fine motor skills due to hand clenched as part of the syndrome; narrow eyes; small head; early death
Tuberous Sclerosis	Seizures; occasional MR; non-malignant tumors of the brain; brownish as well as white patches on skin
Turner	IQ usually low normal with impaired verbal scores; left-right disorientation; difficulty drawing pictures of people; and tendency to remain socially immature; webbing of neck and short stature
Waardenburg	Deafness; white hair lock; widely spaced eyes
Williams	Mild MR; usually good social skills, poorer motor skills; small stature

Used with permission. burlingame, j. (2001). *Idyll Arbor's therapy dictionary*. (2nd ed.). Ravensdale, WA: Idyll Arbor, Inc. pp. 208-210

Incidence/Prevalence in US

- In developed countries mental retardation affects 1-3% of the population (Sebastian, 2002). In the United States this represents about 125,000 additional cases of mental retardation a year.
- Mental retardation is more prevalent in males than females (1.5:1.0) (Silka & Hauser, 1997).

Predominate Age

Because mental retardation and developmental disabilities are, by definition, chronic disorders that start in childhood, both are found throughout the lifespan.

Causes

Since MR/DD is a diagnosis based on observed outcome (functional ability that is limited because of problems with cognitive ability), there are many causes that can lead to that outcome. The ARC (2004) lists five general categories of causes of mental retardation:

- *Genetic conditions*: Abnormalities of genetic material that are inherited from the client's parents; errors in the combining or grouping of genes; damage to the client's genetic material during pregnancy because of overexposure to X-rays, toxic chemicals, infections, or other factors.
- *Poverty and cultural deprivation*: Exposure to disease-producing conditions, inadequate health care, and malnutrition. Children in impoverished conditions often lack exposure to healthy, stimulating environments required for proper neurological development.
- *Problems after birth*: Infections, injuries, or lack of oxygen during the child's earlier years. Some of the causes include
  - *Chicken pox*: Highly contagious viral infection caused by a herpes virus.
  - *Encephalitis*: Inflammation of the brain that may be caused by an infection, exposure to toxins in the environment, or bleeding in the brain.
  - *Exposure to lead, mercury, and other toxins*: Lead toxicity may cause a coma, convulsions, cortical blindness, delirium, and/or mania. Mercury poisoning may cause a wide range of problems including irritability, slurred speech, tremors, staggering, and renal failure. All have long-term effects that cause loss of functional abilities.
  - *Hib disease*: A bacterial disease that usually affects children under the age of five with two-thirds of the exposures coming from day care settings.
  - *Measles*: A highly contagious viral infection that, in some cases, can lead to encephalitis.
  - *Meningitis*: An inflammation or infection of the covering of the brain or the spinal cord often with sudden and severe onset with a severe headache, irritability, and stiffness of the neck.
  - *Near drowning*: A situation in which the client's body functions, including breathing and heartbeat, have ceased due to prolonged submersion in water.
  - *Shaken baby syndrome*: A tearing of cerebral blood vessels and bleeding because

the child was shaken violently by a caretaker.
  - *Whooping cough*: Also known as pertussis — a respiratory disease with a pronounced cough followed by a whooping sound when the air is taken back into the lungs. A lot of mucus is produced during coughing spasms that may happen five to fifty times a day for eight or more weeks. Young children may choke on the mucus, causing a lack of oxygen in the brain.
- *Problems at birth*: Medical conditions at birth that cause damage to the brain including low birth weight, premature delivery, and inability to assimilate oxygen after delivery.
- *Problems during pregnancy*: Prenatal exposure to alcohol or drugs, toxins found in cigarette smoke, malnutrition of the mother during pregnancy, and serious illness of mother during pregnancy.

System(s) Affected

Mental retardation affects the nervous system (cognitive functioning) although it is common for the client to have numerous systems affected because of the frequency of secondary problems. Developmental disabilities (that are outside the scope of mental retardation) may affect any of the body's systems depending on the underlying cause of the developmental disability.

Prognosis

- For clients with mild mental retardation and without a mental illness dual diagnosis that significantly impacts function, the client should be able to live in the community with some support systems in place.
- For clients with moderate mental retardation and without a mental illness dual diagnosis that significantly impacts function, the client is likely to benefit from a group home or other residential setting that provides daily and on-going support.
- For clients with severe mental retardation with or without a mental illness dual diagnosis that significantly impacts function, the client is likely to benefit from a group home or other residential setting that provides significant daily and on-going support.
- For clients with profound mental retardation, with or without a mental illness dual diagnosis that significantly impacts function, the client is likely to benefit from a group home or other residential setting that provides daily and on-going support. Clients at this level often have significant medical complications and often need

to reside where nursing care is available 24 hours a day.

- The prognosis for clients is best anticipated by evaluating their functional ability rather than their measured IQ.
- Certain types of mental retardation or developmental disabilities are degenerative in nature. Clients with Down syndrome, Prader-Willi syndrome, Duchene's muscular dystrophy, and fragile X syndrome all show loss of function as they age.
- Significantly shorter life span than average. About 20 years shorter for adults with Down syndrome. About 10 years shorter for other MR/DD diagnoses.

Secondary Problems

Mental illness is a relatively common secondary diagnosis for clients with mental retardation. The rate of mental illness for clients with mental retardation is many times higher than for normal populations with estimates that up to two thirds of the clients with mental retardation also qualify for a mental illness diagnosis (Sadock & Sadock, 2003). The type of mental illness often depends on the level of cognitive impairment. Clients with mild mental retardation are more likely to have disruptive and conduct-disorder behaviors while clients with severe mental retardation are more likely to have SIB (self-injurious behavior) or autism. Clients with profound mental retardation are the least likely to exhibit mental illness. Also, the percentage of clients with mental retardation who develop a mental illness increases with age (ARC, 1993). The information presented below will help explain the broad-based impact that mental illness has on clients with mental retardation:

- 50% of clients with mental retardation have a mood disorder as measured on standardized testing tools. (Because testing tools that measure mood disorders have not been standardized for clients with mental retardation, this percentage should be seen as a general indication of prevalence and not a firm figure.) (Sadock & Sadock, 2003).
- 41% of school-aged children with mental retardation were diagnosed with at least one type of mental illness (Sadock & Sadock, 2003).
- 30% of clients with severe or profound mental retardation have behavioral symptoms of aggression, which is one of the primary reasons for this diagnostic group to be placed on psychotropic medications (Barnhill, 1999).
- 2-3% of clients with mental retardation meet the criteria for schizophrenia (Sadock & Sadock, 2003).

Clients with a dual diagnosis of mental illness and mental retardation are often the most difficult ones to successfully integrate into a community setting, even with extensive support systems in place (Bongiorno, 1996).

Criminal behavior: People with MR/DD are more likely to be in prison than people without MR/DD. The ARC, ACLU, and Amnesty International have identified this disproportionate number of people with MR/DD in prison populations as an area of concern.

Assessments

Typical Scope of Team Assessment

MR/DD is assessed in four dimensions:
- Dimension I (Intellectual Functioning and Adaptive Skills).
- Dimension II (Psychological/Emotional Considerations).
- Dimension III (Physical/Health/Etiology Considerations).
- Dimension IV (Environmental Considerations).

The American Association on Mental Retardation outlines a three-step procedure for diagnosing, classifying, and determining the support needed by people with mental retardation.

The first step determines if the person is eligible for support. A person is eligible if his/her IQ is 70 to 75 or below and if s/he has significant disabilities in two or more adaptive skill areas and if the age of onset was below age 18. Adaptive skill areas are assessed to determine the supports needed.

The second step identifies the strengths and weaknesses and the need for support by describing the person's strengths and weaknesses, psychologically and emotionally, by describing the person's overall physical health, and by describing the individual's current environmental placement as well as the optimal environment that would facilitate his/her continued growth and development.

The third step identifies the kind and intensity of support needed for each of the four dimensions. In general, the level of support the person needs parallels the person's limitations. Therefore, this third step requires the interdisciplinary team to determine the general intensities of needed support across all four dimensions. The four possible intensities of support are intermittent, limited, extensive, and pervasive. A person classified as needing intermittent support on one or more of the four dimensions does not always need the support or needs short-term support during life-span transitions such as an acute medical crisis. A person classified as needing limited support on one or more of the four dimensions needs time-limited consistent supports, usually requiring fewer staff members than the more intense levels of support. A person classified as needing extensive support on one or more of the four dimensions needs support characterized by regular involvement (for example, daily) in at least some environments (such as work or home), which is not time limited. A person classified as needing pervasive support on one or more of the four dimensions needs constant, high-intensity support provided across environments (Fletcher, 1996).

In the United States it is not customary to diagnose a child as having mental retardation until s/he has reached the chronological age of three years. This custom is probably because most standardized tests that measure IQ are not written for children younger than 3½ years. Another reason may be that federal and state educational funding for testing and treatment is not available for individuals under the age of 36 months (Public Law 94-142 and Public Law 101-476).

An additional comment should be made about IQ scores. In 2003 the *Science Daily Magazine* (December 6) reported that IQ scores rise five to twenty-five points each generation. This is called the "Flynn effect." For this reason IQ tests are updated every ten to twenty years allowing the average IQ to remain at 100. For clients who are fairly high functioning, the publication date of the IQ test they are taking may make a difference in qualifying for services (if the test is fairly new and thus more difficult).

> A score from a test taken at the end of one cycle can vary widely from a score derived from a test taken at the beginning of the next cycle, when the test is more difficult, says Stephen J. Ceci, professor of human development at Cornell. Among children, the researchers found nearly a six-point difference between those taking the two tests. "This variance can make the difference between a child being diagnosed as mentally retarded or not," Ceci says. "This study shows for the first time that two children in the same classroom with the same cognitive ability could be diagnosed differently simply because different test norms were used for each child" (*Science Daily Magazine*, 2003).

Anticipated Findings of RT Assessment

- *Lack of diversify of leisure skills*: Many clients will need a broadening of leisure activities for which the client has the basic, minimum skills required to engage in the activity. Carter (2002) documents this problem and the resulting health issues by stating, "What is known is that these individuals tend to participate in sedentary leisure, the most common being watching television or listening to the radio with family and friends. As a consequence, their leisure patterns don't help them maintain their health and fitness levels. This scenario is exacerbated by a lack of coordinated community preventative health care, thereby resulting in secondary health conditions such as high blood pressure and cholesterol, heart disease, diabetes, obesity, chronic skin problems and hygiene-related issues" (p. 1).

- *Specific leisure skill deficits*: Schleien (1991) points out that clients with mental retardation/developmental disabilities tend to have serious skill deficits. He suggests that recreational therapists work on skill development in two areas: 1. increased skills related to interacting with people and 2. increased skills related to using and interacting with objects. It may take some clients years to learn a few basic leisure skills. The recreational therapist may want to work on one new skill every three to six months, gradually increasing the clients' skill levels.

- *Opportunities for collateral skill development*: As clients increase their functional leisure skills it is not unusual to find that other collateral skills, such as social interactions and attention span, increase at the same time (Vandercook, 1987). The opposite is also true. When a client's social or basic cognitive skills are lower than his/her potential, the client's leisure skills will also be below potential. The recreational therapist is likely to find that many skills need to be improved to achieve any level of independence in leisure activities. For this reason, especially with this population group, recreational therapists coordinate their interventions with the rest of the treatment team. Various authors have listed specific collateral skills that can be acquired within the context of functional leisure skill development, including (from Coyle, Kinney, Riley, & Shank, 1991):
  - Communication and language skills (Rogow, 1981; Bates & Renzaglia, 1982).
  - Cooperation, relationship building, taking turns, and sharing materials (Kibler, 1986; Schleien & Wehman, 1986).
  - Appropriate manipulation of materials and motor skills (Orelove & Sobsey, 1987; Sherrill, 1986).
  - Increased body image and self-image (Verhoven, Schleien, & Bender, 1982).

- *Impaired ability to generalize skills*: The generalization of skills refers to the ability to take a skill learned during one activity and, with some modification, use a similar skill in a new activity. For example, if a client has developed the basic skill of holding a pencil, it does not mean that the client will generalize and modify that skill to allow him/her to hold a paintbrush. Overlearning a skill helps a client improve his/her ability to generalize skills. It is difficult to determine the difference between when someone has learned a skill and when someone has overlearned a skill. A client is generally considered to have integrated a skill well enough into normal patterns when s/he can complete the task twenty times in a row without errors.

- *Impaired social skills*: It is common for clients with developmental disabilities to have impaired social skills. In almost all cases the recreational therapist will be working formally or informally on social skills with clients.
- *Age-inappropriate leisure interests*: Many clients with mental retardation, and some with other developmental disabilities, will express interest in leisure activities that are age-inappropriate (activities that are generally geared toward clients who are younger). Much of this mismatch between age and activity interest is because a client's developmental level is delayed and the activities that s/he chooses may be well matched to his/her skill level, but not to his/her chronological age. Part of the recreational therapist's challenge is to help the client learn leisure activities that s/he will personally enjoy that also help her/him fit better into the community.
- *Impaired community integration skills*: One of the primary barriers to leisure activities in the community for clients with MR/DD is a lack of skills related to using resources in the community.

Treatment Direction

The types of treatment depend on the client. Possible types of treatment are shown below for clients with MR. Clients with DD will have similar limitations depending on the extent of the disability.

- *Mild mental retardation*: The common types of training or learning objectives for clients in this category include ADLs (A&P Chapter 5 Self-Care), basic community safety skills (d135 Rehearsing), community integration skills ("Integration" in the Techniques section), independent leisure skills (d155 Acquiring Skills), personal safety skills (d135 Rehearsing), prevocational skills, and social skills (A&P Chapter 7 Interpersonal Interactions and Relationships). Identification of clients with mild mental retardation is often not diagnosed before

the child has been in elementary school for a couple of years (when the academic requirements increase).

- *Moderate mental retardation*: The common types of training or learning objectives for clients in this category include basic community safety (d135 Rehearsing), basic sensory stimulation ("Sensory Stimulation" in the Techniques section), development of leisure skills to be used with staff support/structure (d155 Acquiring Skills), development of skills to use basic play/recreation objects (d155 Acquiring Skills), environmental awareness (d110-d129 Purposeful Sensory Experiences), and social skills (A&P Chapter 7 Interpersonal Interactions and Relationships).
- *Severe mental retardation*: The common types of training or learning include basic community safety skills (d135 Rehearsing), basic sensory stimulation ("Sensory Stimulation" in the Techniques section), development of leisure skills to be used with staff support/structure (d155 Acquiring Skills), development of skills to use basic play/recreation objects (d155 Acquiring Skills), and environmental awareness (d110-d129 Purposeful Sensory Experiences).
- *Profound mental retardation*: The common training or learning objectives include development of leisure skills to be used with staff support/structure (d155 Acquiring Skills), development of skills to use basic play/recreation objects (d155 Acquiring Skills), basic sensory stimulation ("Sensory Stimulation" in the Techniques section), and environmental awareness (d110-d129 Purposeful Sensory Experiences).

Recreational Therapy Interventions

The primary impacts of mental retardation on an individual's ability to engage in life situations are

- *Age-inappropriate behaviors*: It takes a long time for an individual with mental retardation to develop appropriate skills. The therapist will need to ensure that any skill that the individual is learning will be appropriate for him/her for the next 15 years. Code this as d155 Acquiring Skills.
- *Activities of daily living*: Lack of ability to tend to basic daily living needs significantly impacts the client's ability to engage in activities outside of the home. Especially for residents in supportive living situations, emphasis should be placed on skills required for activities of daily living (ADLs) in the community (using public restrooms, washing hands, donning and doffing

coats, etc.) as described in A&P Chapter 5 Self-Care.

- *Initiation*: Lack of initiation tends to be caused by: 1. lack of knowledge of how to participate in an activity and 2. lack of permission to start an activity. (Many individuals who live in facilities are used to being cued to do anything or used to being required to get permission prior to starting an activity.) d210 Undertaking a Single Task and d220 Undertaking Multiple Tasks look at these issues.

- *Safety awareness*: Frequently individuals with mental retardation are at increased risk of harm due to a general lack of judgment (b1645 Judgment). Specific training programs that replace the need for making a judgment are frequently helpful (e.g., training individuals that the first step to riding a bike is to put on a bike helmet, never cross a road without a "walk" sign). See d135 Rehearsing.

- *Balance of leisure*: Especially for individuals who live in facilities, the opportunity for leisure in all domains (fine and gross motor, cognitive, and social) tends to be at the whim of the house staff. The therapist can assist in the maintenance of a balanced leisure lifestyle by providing in-services for house staff, by providing written instructions, and by monitoring actual participation patterns. The *Recreation Participation Data Sheet* (RPD) is a good method of monitoring this balance. Codes in A&P Chapter 9 Community, Social, and Civic Life can be used to score this intervention.

- *Psychiatric complications*: Specific interventions to address the behaviors that negatively impact the individual's ability to integrate into the community should be addressed first, possibly prior to specific skill development. At times there will be clients who are dangerous to people in the community and should not be integrated. These individuals will need to be taught a balanced set of skills that can be used while residing inside the grounds of the facility.

References

Alexander, D. (1998). Prevention of mental retardation: Four decades of research. *Mental Retardation and Developmental Disabilities Research Reviews. 4*:50-58.

American Association on Mental Retardation. (2002). Definition of mental retardation. http://www.aamr.org/Policies/faq_mental_retardation.shtml.

American Psychiatric Association. (1994). *Diagnostic and statistical manual of mental disorders* (4th ed.). Washington, DC: American Psychiatric Association.

Anson, C. & Shepherd, C. (1990). A survey of post-acute spinal cord patients: Medical, psychological, and social characteristics. *Trends: Research News from Shepherd Spinal Center.*

Arieti, S. (2004). Schizophrenia. *Encyclopedia Americana* http://search2.webfeat.org:5554/ on 4/47/04.

Ascher-Svanum, H. & Krause, A. (1991). *Psychoeducational groups for patients with schizophrenia: A guide for practitioners.* Gaithersburg, MD: Aspen Publications.

Barnhill, J. (1999). The relationship between epilepsy and violent behavior in persons with mental retardation. *NADD Bulletin Archive, 2,* #3. Kingston, NY: National Association for Dually Diagnosed.

Berryman, James, and Trader (1990). The benefits of therapeutic recreation in physical medicine. In Coyle, C., Kinney, W., Riley, B. & Shank, J. (Eds.). (1990). *Benefits of therapeutic recreation: A consensus view.* Ravensdale, WA: Idyll Arbor, Inc.

Bongiorno, F. (1996). Dual diagnosis: Developmental disability complicated by mental illness. http://www.sma.org/smj/96dec2.htm.

Brier, N. & Demb, H. (1978). *Adolescence in the developmentally disabled: Stage or syndrome.* Manuscript submitted for publication.

Brown, A. & Murphy, L. (date unknown). *Aging with developmental disabilities: Women's health issues.* http://www.thearc.org/faqs/whealth.html. accessed 10/21/04.

Carter, M. (2002). Inclusive fitness strategies: Building wellness among developmentally disabled adults. *Parks & Recreation Journal,* Dec. 2002.

Carter, M., Van Andel, G. & Robb, G. (1985). *Therapeutic recreation: A practical approach.* St. Louis: Time Mirror/Mosby.

Coyle, P., Kinney, W., Riley, B., & Shank, J. (Eds.). (1991). *Benefits of therapeutic recreation: A consensus view.* Ravensdale, WA: Idyll Arbor, Inc.

Denkowski, G. & Denkowski, K. (1985). The mentally retarded offender in the state prison system: Identification, prevalence, adjustment, and rehabilitation. *Criminal Justice and Behavior, 12*(1):53-70.

Dew, M., Lynch, K., Ernst, J., & Rosenthal, R. (1983). Reaction and adjustments to spinal cord injury: A descriptive study. *Journal of Applied Rehabilitation Counseling, 14*(1):32-39.

Duvall, E. (1971). *Family development.* Philadelphia, PA: Lippincott.

Gold, M. (1978). *Try another way.* Sacramento, CA: The California Project.

Goldstein, A., Sprafin, R., Gershaw, N., Klein, P. (1980). *Skillstreaming the adolescent: A structured learning approach to teaching prosocial skills.* Champaign, IL: Research Press Company

Grimm, N. (1979). Falling through the cracks: Characteristics of a community mental health population with both mental-emotional disturbances and mental retardation. Paper presented at Northwest Pacific Society of Neurology and Psychiatry. Harrison Hot Springs, British Columbia, June 1, 1979.

Hartl Chambliss, C. (1988). *Group involvement training: A step-by-step program to help chronic mentally ill patients.* Oakland, CA: New Harbinger Publications.

Hutchinson, M. & Lloyd. (1975). Maximizing transfer benefits of special programs. *Journal of Leisureability, 2*(4):2-7.

Liberman, R, P. (November 2002) Keys to recovery from schizophrenia. University of California, Los Angeles. http://my.webmd.com/content/article/55/65603.htm.

Luckey, R. & Shapiro, I. (1974). Recreation: An essential aspect of habilitative programming. *Mental Retardation, 12*(5), 33-35.

Mobily, K. & MacNeil, R. (2002). *Therapeutic recreation and the nature of disabilities.* State College, PA: Venture Publishing, Inc.

Panda, K. (1971). Social reinforcement: Theoretical issues and research implications. *Psychological Studies 26*:319-339.

Pauulsson, K. (1980). Integration of physically handicapped pupils in schools in Sweden. Paper presented at the 1980 World Congress of Rehabilitation Interactions, Education Seminar, June 17, 1980.

Reld, F. & Wineman, D. (1952). *Controls from within.* New York, NY: Freeman Press.

Rinck, C. et al., (1989). The adolescent with myelomeningocele: A review of parent experiences and expectations. *Adolescence, 24*(95):699-710.

Roder, V., Jenull, B., & Benner, H. (1998). Teaching schizophrenia patients recreational, residential, and vocational skills. *International Review of Psychiatry, 10*(1).

Sadock, B. & Sadock, V. (2003). *Synopsis of psychiatry* (9th ed.). Philadelphia, PA: Lippincott Williams & Wilkins.

Schleien, S. (1991). Severe multiple disabilities. In D. Austin & M. Crawford (Eds.). *Therapeutic recreation: An introduction.* (pp. 189-223). Englewood Cliffs, NJ: Prentice Hall.

Sebastian, C. (2002). Mental retardation. eMedicine, http://www.emedicine.com/med/topic3095.htm#section~author_information.

Silka, V. & Hauser, M. (1997). Psychiatric assessment of the person with mental retardation. *Psychiatric Annals, 27*:3.

Soder, M. (1980) School integration of the mentally retarded. In *Research and development concerning integration of handicapped pupils in the ordinary school system.* Stockholm: National Swedish Board of Education.

Spearing, M. (1999). Schizophrenia. National Institute of Mental Health http://www.nimh.nih.gov/publicat/schizoph.cfm#schiz3 on 4/25/04.

Sue, D., Sue, D., & Sue, S. (1997). *Understanding abnormal behavior.* New York, New York: Houghton Mifflin Company.

The ARC. (1993). Mental illness in persons with mental retardation. http://www.thearc.org/faqs/mimrqa.html.

The ARC (accessed 2004). *Introduction to mental retardation.* http://www.thearc.org/faqs/mrqa.html.

Vandercook, T. (1987). Generalized performance of community leisure skills with peers. Unpublished manuscript, University of Minnesota, reported in Coyle, P., Kinney, W., Riley, B., & Shank, J. (Eds.). (1991). *Benefits of therapeutic recreation: A consensus view.* Ravensdale, WA: Idyll Arbor, Inc.

Walker, H. (1980). Development of a model social behavior survival (SBS) program for mainstreaming handicapped children into less restrictive educational settings. Paper presented at the CEC Conference, Eugene, OR, February 29, 1980.

Zoerink, D. (1989). Effects of a short-term leisure education program upon the leisure functioning of young people with spina bifida. *Therapeutic Recreation Journal, 22*(3):44-52.

Multiple Sclerosis

Multiple sclerosis (MS) seems to be an autoimmune disease. The body's own defense system attacks the fatty substance (myelin) that surrounds and protects the nerve fibers of the brain, optic nerves, and spinal cord. The damaged myelin may form scar tissue (sclerosis). Sometimes the nerve fiber is damaged or destroyed, causing nerve impulses to and from the brain to be distorted or interrupted (National Multiple Sclerosis Society, 2006).

As the damage occurs, the myelin covering of the nerves becomes inflamed, swollen, and detached from the fibers. Eventually, the myelin is destroyed. Scar tissue forms over the nerve fibers in place of the myelin. Nerve impulses do not travel as fast or as accurately across the scarred areas, so impulses are blocked or delayed from traveling to or from the brain. Our bodies rely on the timing and strength of many different nerve impulses to help us interpret the environment. When some of the impulses are sent incorrectly, it can lead to an array of uncomfortable sensations in addition to straightforward sensory loss and loss of motor control. Ultimately, this process leads to degeneration of the nerves themselves, which probably accounts for the permanent disabilities that develop in MS (Mayo Clinic, 2006).

Multiple sclerosis usually takes one of four disease courses as identified by that National MS Society (2006):
1. *Relapsing-remitting (RRMS)*: This is the most common type of MS. MS symptoms flare up (exacerbate) and then subside (remit, not remission). Exacerbations usually last several days to several weeks. The client may have total or only partial recovery. Around 70-75% of clients with MS initially begin with this course.
2. *Secondary-progressive (SPMS)*: When exacerbations become steadily progressive and only partial recoveries are achieved with each exacerbation, the course of the disease is described as SPMS. Of the 70-75% who start with RRMS, more than 50% will develop SPMS within 10 years, 90% within 25 years.
3. *Primary-progressive (PPMS)*: PPMS is a steady progression of symptoms without signs of remitting.
4. *Progressive-relapsing (PRMS)*: A steady progression of symptoms with obvious acute attacks. Approximately 6-10% of people with MS appear to have PRMS.

Making a diagnosis of MS is not a simple process. MS symptoms are often attributed to other health problems and consequently misdiagnosed. Often clients will wait years after developing symptoms before they are diagnosed with MS. The most helpful test to identify demyelination is magnetic resonance imaging (MRI). However not all lesions can be detected by the MRI and the presence of lesions does not confirm an MS diagnosis. Lesions can be caused by many other health issues (aging process with no clinical significance, stroke). MRI scans can be helpful in tracking disease progression once a positive MS diagnosis is obtained. A conclusive diagnosis requires evidence of multiple patches of scar tissue (lesions) in different parts of the nervous system (brain, spinal cord), and at least two separate attacks of the disease (exacerbations or flare-ups).

Incidence/Prevalence in US

MS is two to three times more common in women than in men. Approximately 330,000 Americans have MS. Of the various ethnic groups, MS is most common amongst Caucasians.

Predominant Age

MS generally occurs between the ages of 20-30 (early onset), however some clients do not experience symptoms until after the age of 50 (late onset).

Causes

Why the body's defenses attack the myelin sheath is unknown. However, there are several scientific theories about the causes of MS (National MS Society, 2006):
- *Immunologic*: MS is an autoimmune process where the body's immune system attacks its own central nervous system destroying the myelin sheath.
- *Environmental*: Epidemiology studies suggest that early exposure to an environmental agent might be a triggering factor in people who are predisposed by genetic factors to develop MS. The frequency of MS increases for clients who live farther away from the equator. MS seems to appear more frequently in states above the 37th parallel. The 37th parallel extends from Newport News, VA to Santa Cruz, CA, running along the northern border of North Carolina to the northern boarder of Arizona and including most of California. If a person moves from a higher risk area to a lower risk area, the risk is lowered only if the move occurs prior to adolescence. Certain

outbreaks or clusters of MS have been identified, but their significance is unknown.

- *Viral*: A virus is the triggering agent that causes demyelination and inflammation. Some suggest that mycobacteria, which have some virus-like qualities, might be the cause.
- *Genetic*: Although MS is not hereditary, a genetic marker has been shown to increase the chances of developing MS. If a person has a genetic predisposition to MS and is exposed to a triggering environmental agent, an autoimmune response is more likely to develop.

System(s) Affected

MS is a disease of the central nervous system (brain and spinal cord); therefore any system that is directly related to the CNS has the possibility of being affected. The term "possibility" is used because the course and symptoms of MS vary in severity. The *primary symptoms* are the direct result of demyelination: weakness, numbness, tingling, tremor, visual problems (double, blurry), pain, paralysis, poor balance, bowel and bladder dysfunction, slurred speech, decline in cognitive functioning (reasoning, memory, processing), and dysphagia.

MS symptoms can be aggravated by external variables unrelated to the internal MS disease process. The most common things that aggravate MS symptoms include heat, fatigue, and stress.

- *Heat*: Heat from any source (sunbathing, hot tubs, opening the oven door, hot shower, hot weather) worsens MS symptoms. The problems aggravated by heat usually disappear once the heat is removed and the body's core temperature is brought down. Interestingly, the National MS Society says that the cost of an air conditioner may be tax deductible if a physician writes a prescription. Heat and humidity cause the myelin sheath to conduct electricity less efficiently. Cold temperatures can also cause problems (spasticity), while cool weather (60s, 70s) seems to provide an optimal environment. In addition, involvement in an aquatics program in a cool pool has been found to help with nerve conduction, thus improving functioning.
- *Fatigue and stress*: Fatigue is one of the major complaints of MS making it both a symptom and something that makes the other symptoms worse. MS fatigue is not like a healthy person's fatigue. It is an extreme fatigue that affects motivation and the ability to perform daily activities, not to mention significantly impacting the person's desire and ability to participate in recreation and leisure activities. It is not the typical fatigue that

a person experiences after a long day. This type of fatigue seems to be unique to clients who have MS. It typically occurs every day and gets worse as the day progresses, despite the activity level of the day. Researchers are still not sure if the fatigue is due to the MS process or another variable such as lack of proper nutrition, lack of adequate sleep, medication, depression, or stress.

Prognosis

The functional impact that MS has varies due to the wide range of dysfunction (mild to severe), as well as the unpredictability to the disease. Although MS can be defined by four disease courses, it can be difficult to know when exacerbations will occur and how much function will be lost or regained. For a client with MS, the disease makes planning of any kind difficult. It is estimated that approximately 95% of clients with MS have a normal life expectancy. If a client with MS dies early, it is often due to secondary problems of the disease (e.g., pneumonia, cardiovascular disease). At the present time, MS does not have a cure, although cases of spontaneous remyelination have been seen and medication has helped in slowing down exacerbations or decreasing the duration of the attack.

Secondary Problems

Secondary symptoms: These are complications that result from the primary symptoms. They include:

- *Bowel and bladder dysfunction*: kidney stones, urinary tract infections, coded with b610-b639 Urinary Functions.
- *Sexual dysfunction*: b640 Sexual Functions.
- *Muscle atrophy*: see "Consequences of Inactivity" in the Concepts section.
- *Poor postural alignment and trunk control*: b760 Control of Voluntary Movement Functions.
- *Muscle contractures and loss of range of motion*: b710 Mobility of Joint Functions.
- *Osteoporosis and fractures*: see "Osteoporosis" in the Diagnoses section.
- *Respiratory problems*: shallow breathing, as discussed in b440-b449 Functions of the Respiratory System.
- *Decubitus ulcers*: see "Skin Breakdown" in the Techniques section.
- *Deep vein thrombosis*: see "Consequences of Inactivity" in the Concepts section.
- *Decreased cardiovascular endurance and increase in cardiovascular disease*: b455 Exercise Tolerance Functions.
- *Orthostatic hypotension*: see b420 Blood Pressure Functions and "Vital Signs" in the Techniques section.

- *Pneumonia*: see "Consequences of Inactivity" in the Concepts section.
- *Spasticity*: see b735 Muscle Tone Functions.

Tertiary symptoms: These are the social, vocational, emotional, and psychological problems caused by the other symptoms. They include problems with relationships, driving, and working. Clients also find MS challenges their ability to cope and adjust because of the unpredictable nature of the disease. Emotional and psychological issues that commonly arise include depression, anxiety, and changes in personality and behavior. These changes may be a direct result of the lesions or from inadequate adaptive coping mechanisms.

Assessments

Typical Scope of Team Assessment

The first strep is to confirm the diagnosis of MS, as described earlier. After that the rehab team evaluates the course of the disease and the impact of the primary, secondary, and tertiary symptoms on life tasks. The types of assessments vary depending upon observed losses. Typically clients are not admitted to an inpatient stay unless they have moderate to severe loss of function. Clients with minimal dysfunction are usually seen on an outpatient basis (or not at all) and rarely have access to recreational therapy services.

Anticipated Findings from RT Assessment

The RT initial evaluation will typically reflect:
- *Patterns of decreased physical activity*: As dysfunction and fatigue advance, completing everyday tasks requires more time and energy. The client is forced to prioritize activities because of limited energy and function. Consequently, basic self-care, work, and homemaking skills are most often chosen, while recreational pursuits, community tasks, and maintaining relationships are sacrificed.
- *Tremors of the upper extremity*: These significantly impair the client's ability to perform functional tasks of writing, typing, fine crafts, and small object manipulation (e.g., buttons).
- *Fatigue*: Even simple tasks may cause fatigue that greatly impacts the client's ability to participate in community activities.
- *Stress*: Caused by the unknown nature of the disease course and loss of ability. Since there is a progression of dysfunction, the client constantly has to make adjustments to work, family role, self-care, leisure/recreation, and other life tasks.

The anticipation of further dysfunction, along with current life stressors, often results in anxiety and depression expressed through behavior, verbalizations, or physical symptoms.
- *Cognitive dysfunction*: Memory, word finding, reasoning, and processing information may be affected. This impacts the client's ability to perform instrumental activities of daily living, such as using the telephone, balancing a checkbook, and using reference materials.
- *Safety concerns*: Initiation and participation in complex community activities may cause safety concerns, which the client may or may not understand because of cognitive dysfunctions.
- *Lack of participation*: Affects the client's activity level, thus exacerbating secondary problems.
- *Resource awareness deficit*: For many clients this may be their first therapy experience even though they have had MS for a number of years. Therefore, their level of resource awareness may be minimal in the area of personal and community resources.

Treatment Direction

Whole Team Approach

The team's focus is to maximize the client's abilities. The goal is to increase the client's skills and abilities in functional life tasks (activity performance) by restoring lost function and teaching adaptive techniques when necessary.

Recreational Therapy Approach

Therapists follow the team approach and address prevention of secondary and tertiary complications. Given the time constraints often associated with providing treatment and the progressive nature of MS, the therapist often prioritizes adaptation and prevention. Clients typically have a two to three week stay and receive a total of six to nine hours of recreational therapy.

Recreational Therapy Interventions

Interventions that are frequently implemented with clients who have MS include:

Functional Skill Development

- *Mobility*: Mobility skills addressed with this population will vary depending upon mobility limitations and activities. Therapists address mobility skills as they specifically relate to participation in life situations. This most commonly includes transfers, lifting and carrying objects, fine hand use, hand and arm use, walking, moving around in different locations, moving around using equipment, and using transportation. See, as required, the topics in A&P Chapter 4 Mobility and Body Functions and Chapter 7 Neuromusculoskeletal and Movement Related Functions.

- *Memory*: Short-term memory loss is a common problem associated with MS. Therapists seek to improve short-term memory function through neuroplasticity interventions. Short-term memory loss can also be addressed with compensatory strategies. Cognitive Retraining in "Neuroplasticity" in the Techniques section and b144 Memory Functions have more details.

- *Vision*: Blurry and/or double vision (diplopia) are common visual problems associated with MS. Therapists typically wait a few days to see if the problem resolves or minimizes before addressing adaptations since it may be transient. If the problem appears to be permanent, an ophthalmologist consult is sought for further evaluation. Unresolved visual problems will require adaptations. The therapist helps the client identify, develop, and integrate compensatory strategies for vision as they relate to participation in specifically identified activities (e.g., needlework, reading, completing daily responsibilities). In addition to the ICF codes b210-b229 Seeing and Related Functions, see e240 Light for information on compensatory strategies for vision.

- *Lifestyle changes*: The use of energy conservation techniques, getting adequate sleep, involvement in a cardiovascular exercise program, avoiding heat, eating a healthy diet, assessing the impact of medications with a physician, and managing stress may assist with fatigue management. It is also important to pay attention to emotional health since MS fatigue may be associated with depression and stress. Refer to the Techniques section for "Energy Conservation Training" (for fatigue management), "Community Accessibility Training," "Community Problem Solving," "Lifestyle Alteration Education," "Relaxation and Stress Reduction," "Coping with Stress," and "Exercise Basics."

- *Community, social, and civic life*: Social relationships are often sacrificed due to energy limitations and health issues related to MS. Social relationships, specifically formation and participation in friendships, are important for health. By identifying the client's interests, compatible social groups can be identified (e.g., church group, special interest group). Integration training that incorporates learned skills is ideal in many situations to facilitate engagement. See "Activity Pattern Development" and "Integration" in the Techniques section. This intervention can be coded with d7200 Forming Relationships or the appropriate code in A&P Chapter 9 Community, Social, and Civic Life.

Miscellaneous

The National Multiple Sclerosis Society provides helpful information on new research, techniques, and resources. This organization provides newsletters, information on a variety of help topics, current research, support groups, and much more. It also provides information on additional MS resources and web-links.

National Multiple Sclerosis Society
733 Third Avenue
New York, NY 10017
1-800-FIGHT-MS (344-4867)
www.nationalmssociety.org

References

Mayo Clinic. (2006). Multiple Sclerosis. http://www.mayoclinic.com/health/multiple-sclerosis/DS00188.
National Multiple Sclerosis Society. (2006). About MS: What Is Multiple Sclerosis? http://www.nationalmssociety.org/What%20is%20MS.asp.

Obesity

Obesity is defined as excess body fat. It is the second leading cause of preventable death after smoking (American Obesity Association, 2002). A client is defined as obese if his/her body weight is more that 20% above the desirable body weight for the client's age, sex, height, and body build.

For adults (age 20 and older), the Body Mass Index (BMI) is the most commonly used instrument to determine the appropriateness of a client's body weight for both males and females. The intersection of a client's body weight and height indicates a client's BMI which correlates with specific BMI categories: healthy weight (BMI of 18.5-24.9), overweight (BMI of 25-29.9), obesity class 1 (BMI of 30-34.9), obesity class 2 (35-39.9), or severe obesity class 3 (40 or more).

Despite its common use, the BMI is not a perfect instrument. Some athletes may have a high BMI due to muscle mass (not excess fat) whereas people who have low muscle mass and a high fat percentage may score low on the BMI. Although the BMI is still commonly used in individual health care, it is a better indicator of risk of disease within a population rather than for a specific client. To better determine a client's health risks, it is recommended that waist circumference be used in conjunction with the BMI. Waist circumference is determined by wrapping a measuring tape around a client's waist (just above the hipbones and below the rib cage). Women who have a waist circumference of 35" or more and men who have a waist circumference of 40" or more along with a BMI greater than 25 have a greater risk for developing Type 2 Diabetes, hypertension, and cardiovascular disease (American Obesity Association, 2002). Abdominal fat is associated with a higher risk of these conditions than peripheral fat (e.g., fat on the legs, buttocks, or hips). If a client's BMI is in the healthy weight range but his/her waist circumference is greater than what is recommended, the client is still a risk for the conditions mentioned above due to the high percentage of fat in the abdominal area.

For children, the BMI is measured through a pediatric growth chart. Overweight is defined as greater than or equal to 95th percentile of the age- and sex-specific BMI. There is not a formalized obesity category for children or teenagers.

Incidence/Prevalence in US

The 1999-2002 National Health and Nutrition Examination Survey (NHANES) estimated that 34% of US adults are overweight (BMI of 25-29.9) and that an additional 31% of US adults are obese (BMI greater than 30). Less than half of the US adult population is a healthy weight (35%). Overweight children and teenagers are a rising concern. The 1999-2002 NHANES found that approximately 16% of children ages 6-19 were overweight. This is almost triple the amount from previous NHANES studies. NHANES studies in the 1960s, 1970s, and 1980s indicated that approximately 4-7% of children ages 6-19 were overweight. This number jumped to 11% in the late 1980s/early 1990s and has now jumped again to 16% in the latest survey. Approximately 80% of people who are obese have a family history of obesity (Sadock & Sadock, 2003). African-Americans, American Indians, Hawaiians, and Hispanic Americans have higher rates of overweight and obesity than Caucasian Americans. Although overweight and obesity affect people at all levels of education, those with less education have higher rates of overweight and obesity.

Predominant Age

American adults have a greater percentage of overweight and obesity than children under the age of 19 as reviewed in Incidence/Prevalence.

Causes

Obesity can be influenced by genetics, environment, and behavior. Some clients seem to have a genetic predisposition to gain weight and store fat. It is estimated that eight to thirty genes may be responsible for influencing obesity. A client's environment can also be very influential in the amount of caloric intake and physical activity. This may be related to cultural practices or familial patterns of behavior (e.g., promotion of unhealthy food or large portions, sedentary leisure behaviors, learned eating behaviors to cope with anxiety and stress). Eating excessively large portions of food at one time (bingeing) has been found to release natural opiates in the brain in some clients, providing a feeling of pleasure that perpetuates the overeating behavior. Medical conditions that contribute to weight gain, independent of eating and physical activity patterns, include hypothyroidism, Prader-Willi syndrome, pseudohypoparathyroidism, Bardet-Biedl syndrome, Cohen syndrome, Down syndrome, Turner syndrome, Cushing syndrome, growth hormone deficiency or resistance, leptin deficiency, precocious puberty, polycystic ovarian syndrome, prolactin-secreting tumors, Frohlick's syndrome (Freemark, 2004; Sadock & Sadock, 2003). Certain medications can also cause clients to gain weight such as antipsychotics (e.g., Zyprexa, Clozaril, Seroquel), mood stabilizers (e.g., Eskalith, Depakene, Tegretol), cortisol, Megace, sulfonylureas, monoamine oxidase inhibitors (MAOIs), oral contraceptives, insulin (in excessive doses), thiazolidinediones, risperidone, and clozapine (Freemark, 2004; Sadock & Sadock, 2003).

Systems Affected

Overweight and obesity affect all major bodily systems including the heart, lungs, muscles, and bones (AOA, 2002). It lowers cardiovascular and pulmonary endurance and lowers mobility.

Prognosis

Overweight and obesity cause approximately 300,000 deaths per year in the United States and cost about $100 billion (AOA, 2002). It is estimated that approximately 26-41% of preschoolers with obesity and 42-63% of school-aged children with obesity will have obesity as adults (Freemark, 2004). Long-term management of obesity class 2 and 3 in adulthood is rarely successful due to the many obstacles that the client must manage on a daily basis. It is estimated that 90% of clients who lose a significant amount of weight eventually gain all of it back (Sadock & Sadock, 2003). Consequently, prevention of obesity in children should be the first line of defense in preventing this disease.

Secondary Problems

Overweight and obesity are risk factors for various medical conditions including diabetes, hypertension, osteoarthritis, cerebrovascular accident, heart disease, various cancers (rectum, prostate, breast, uterus, cervix), depression, and sleep apnea. Obesity can also carry a negative social stigma that affects the development of social relationships, education, and employment. "Among teens and young adults who were tracked after seven years, overweight females were found to have completed less schooling, were less likely to have married, and had higher rates of household poverty compared to their non-overweight peers. For overweight males, the only adverse outcome was a decreased likelihood of being married" (Freemark, 2004, p 5). Once a client attains a normal weight, signs of a mental disorder may surface because s/he no longer has the coping strategy for stressors of overeating (Sadock & Sadock, 2003).

Assessments

Typical Scope of Team Assessment

Underlying medical conditions are treated or ruled out and appropriate referrals made (e.g., psychiatrist/psychologist consult for eating disorder of bingeing, depression). Height, body weight, and waist circumference are measured and documented to determine a baseline to note regression or progression. A diet and physical activity history is taken and evaluated to determine needs.

Anticipated Findings from RT Assessment

Sedentary lifestyle: Clients who are overweight or obese (outside of weight gain from medical complications) are likely to have a sedentary lifestyle. The more sedentary a client is, the fewer calories s/he needs to maintain his/her body weight. Extra calories are stored as fat. For example, a physically active 25-year-old adult may burn 2,400 calories a day compared to a sedentary 25-year-old adult who consumes the same 2,400 calories yet only burns off 1,500 calories a day resulting in the body storing the extra 900 calories. (This is referred to as energy balance, comparing the calories coming into the body versus calories being expended.) Sedentary leisure preferences begin in childhood and are often reinforced through parental modeling. Sedentary leisure behaviors do have merit, but active leisure behaviors are also important for a healthy lifestyle.

Social isolation: Clients who are overweight or obese may feel ostracized within their peer group thus limiting the development and maintenance of social relationships. Distancing from social interactions may be the choice of the client due to poor self-esteem/self-confidence and/or the result of other peers avoiding socializing with over-weight/obese peers. Social relationships are a necessary component of health promotion for their supportive function. They need to be part of the client's activity pattern.

Poor eating habits: Clients who are overweight or obese (outside of the effects of a medical condition) typically have poor eating habits that have resulted in increased weight. This is often the result of food choices (high fat and calorie foods) and portion sizes. Fast food and processed foods have become more common in the American diet and portion sizes have dramatically increased over the past decade. Eating habits begin in childhood and can be very difficult, but not impossible, to change in adulthood.

Poor cardiovascular endurance: Extra body weight puts more stress on the heart, lungs, and muscles requiring a greater amount of energy for a task. Poor cardiovascular endurance limits a client's ability to engage in physical activities and often becomes a primary barrier to continued participation in physical activity.

Treatment Direction

Whole Team Approach

If there is an underlying medical condition that is causing weight gain, appropriate treatment for the condition is recommended and implemented. If weight gain is a consequence of a sedentary lifestyle and poor eating habits, interventions are designed and implemented to assist the client in making lifestyle changes. Health behavior changes in the areas of diet and exercise can be difficult to make and there are a variety of approaches to assist clients in overcoming obstacles. The outcome goals, however, are the same: to achieve and maintain a healthy, well-balanced diet that supports healthy weight loss and to engage in physical activity at least five days per week for a determined amount of time and intensity. The amount of time and intensity will vary depending on the abilities and limitations of the client. Specific parameters may be established by the treating physician (e.g., blood pressure, heart rate, oxygen saturation level) and medical clearance for physical activity may be needed for obese clients who have other medical conditions.

- Healthy People 2010 recommends that healthy adults participate in at least 30 minutes of moderate intensity physical activity on most days of the week to reduce their risk of chronic disease. To prevent gradual, unhealthy weight gain in adulthood, physical activity should be increased to 60 minutes of moderate to vigorous intensity that does not exceed caloric intake. To sustain weight loss in adulthood, the recommendations further increase to 60-90 minutes of daily moderate intensity physical activity that does not exceed caloric intake. The most common barrier identified for failure to be physically active is lack of time. Interestingly, several short bouts of exercise (e.g., three to six 10-minute bouts of exercise over the course of a day) that equal the recommended time for engaging in physical activity is just as effective as continuous activity (United States Department of Health and Human Services and United States Department of Agriculture, 2005). Healthy children should engage in physical exercise at least 60 minutes a day to maintain health and prevent unhealthy weight gain.
- An exercise program should include cardiovascular conditioning, stretching exercises for flexibility, and resistance exercises for muscle strengthening and endurance (United States Department of Health and Human Services and United States Department of Agriculture, 2005).
- Examples of moderate physical activity include light gardening and yard work, dancing, golf (walking and carrying clubs), bicycling (< 10 mph), walking (3.5 mph), weight lifting (general light workout), and stretching. Examples of vigorous physical activity include running or jogging (5 mph), bicycling (>10 mph), swimming (slow freestyle laps), aerobics, walking (4.5 mph), heavy yard work (chopping wood), weight lifting (vigorous effort), and basketball (vigorous) (United States Department of Health and Human Services and United States Department of Agriculture, 2005).

A consult with a nutritionist is typically ordered to assist clients in identifying healthy food choices and appropriate portion sizes that fit within their lifestyle. Diets that are high in protein, low in carbohydrates, and low in fat may provide fast initial results, but the US Department of Health and Human Services along with the US Department of Agriculture do not recommend their long-term use due to the risk of nutrient deficiencies. The focus should be on a healthy balance of various foods including fruits, vegetables, whole grains, and lean proteins. Whenever possible, clients who are overweight or obese should avoid high-risk environments that lead to poor eating habits. Keeping a food diary can be helpful to obtain a true assessment of caloric intake.

Family involvement is a crucial component of weight loss. Often the entire family needs to change its eating and exercise habits. If the family does not operate as a cohesive unit, one person will find it difficult to change when everyone else in the home is engaging in unhealthy behaviors.

Smoking cessation, or prevention, should be a part of the treatment plan. Smoking tobacco is commonly known for decreasing appetite to prevent or limit weight gain (Freemark, 2004). The serious and life threatening secondary complications caused by smoking tobacco do not warrant the use of this product for weight control.

It is important to note that the focus for an adult who is overweight or obese is to loss weight, while the focus for a child is to slow down the rate of weight gain while achieving normal growth and development (United States Department of Health and Human Services and United States Department of Agriculture, 2005). A loss of 5-20% of an adult's total body weight can reduce many of the health risks associated with obesity in adults (Freemark, 2004).

Typically a last resort to weight loss in markedly obese clients is bariatric surgery (e.g., the stomach is made smaller by transecting or stapling one of the stomach curvatures).

Recreational Therapy Approach

The recreational therapy approach is the same as the team approach. A description of recreational therapy specific interventions related to the team approach follows.

Recreational Therapy Interventions

Interventions that are frequently implemented with clients who are obese include:

- *Nutrition*: Particular attention is paid to making healthy food choices in real life. Recreational therapists assess how food is a part of leisure activities, such as eating high fat popcorn at the movie theatre, and address issues related to changing these habits. Clients are taught how to recognize environmental or emotional cues that trigger poor eating habits (e.g., watching television; when stressed, anxious, or depressed). Keeping a food diary is helpful to increase the client's awareness of these situations or emotional states. Clients are encouraged to follow a dietician-prescribed diet rather than the current diet fad, to eat slowly, to not engage in any type of activity while eating that will distract the client from realizing how much food is consumed or trigger continuous eating, and to not eat when on the run. Reinforcing success through non-food rewards can be helpful when established goals are met (e.g., buying a new outfit, going to see a play). Social support is also very valuable (e.g., friends, weight loss group meetings). Code this with d5701 Managing Diet and Fitness.
- *Exercise training*: Clients who are overweight or obese and are cleared to engage in physical exercise are engaged in physical leisure activities as part of the recreational therapy treatment plan. Physical leisure activities are chosen based on client interest, needs, and realistic continuance after discharge. If a client can find something that s/he enjoys doing (A&P Chapter 9 Community, Social, and Civic Life) and reaps the physical benefits of exercise as a secondary benefit, then the client is more likely to continue with the activity (belonging to a walking club where "chit-chat" is plentiful may be a fantastic motivator to participate in club walks). Barriers to participation are identified and assistance is given to remove them (d175 Solving Problems). See Interest Exploration in "Activity Pattern Development" and "Exercise Basics" in the Techniques section. Code the exercise training with b455 Exercise Functions and d5701 Managing Diet and Fitness.
- *Social support*: Social support is a vital component of maintaining behavior changes. Healthy social relationships reduce feelings of depression and isolation and promote learning, sharing, and self-expression. Clients may need to learn how to form friendships and identify places to meet new people. The therapist finds the strengths of the client (e.g., good singer, good listener, artistic) and places that the client can exhibit those skills (e.g., choir, volunteer work at a nursing home, art class). This increases the client's likelihood of success to boost self-esteem and confidence, as well as providing an environment where people share a common interest. Having a common interest promotes conversation and conversation is a doorway to the development of a friendship. See A&P Chapter 7 Interpersonal Interactions and Relationships and "Self-Esteem" in the Techniques section.
- *Sense of self*: Self-esteem, body image, self-confidence, openness to experiences, and positive outlook may be affected in clients who are overweight or obese. See ICF codes b1800 Experience of Self, b1801 Body Image, b1266 Confidence, b1264 Openness to Experience, b1265 Optimism, and "Self-Esteem" in the Techniques section

References

Agency for Healthcare Research and Quality. (2005). Screening for obesity. http://www.ahrq.gov/clinic/2ndcps/obesity.pdf on 4/28/05.

American Obesity Association. (2002). Health affects of obesity. www.aoa.com.

Centers for Disease Control. (2005). Prevalence of overweight and obesity among adults. http://www.cdc.gov/nchs/products/pubs/pubd/hestats/obese/obse99.htm on 5/26/05

Feldman, S. S. & Elliott, G. R. (1990). *At the threshold: The developing adolescent*. Harvard University Press: Cambridge, MA.

Freemark, M. (2004). Obesity. www.emedicine.com on 4/28/05

Harter, S. (1989). Causes, correlates, and the functional role of global self-worth: A life-span perspective. In J. Kolligian & R. Sternberg, eds., *Perceptions of competence and incompetence across the life span*. Yale University Press: New Haven. CT.

James, W. (1982). *Psychology: The briefer course*. Holt, Rinehart, & Winston: New York, New York.

Sadock, B. J. & Sadock, V. A. (2003). *Kaplan and Sadock's synopsis of psychiatry*. New York, New York: Lippincott Williams & Wilkins.

United States Department of Health and Human Services and United States Department of Agriculture (2005).

Dietary guidelines for Americans 2005. http://www.health.gov/dietaryguidelines/ dga2005/document/ on 4/30/05

Osteoarthritis

Osteoarthritis (OA), or degenerative joint disease (DJD), is the most common type of arthritis. Unlike other forms of arthritis, it occurs asymmetrically and does not affect internal organs. Cartilage, which is the tissue that cushions the ends of bones in a joint, slowly wears away and spurs grow from the edge of the bone. Bare bone ends begin to rub against each other, causing steady or intermittent pain, swelling, tenderness, and loss of motion in the joint. A crunching feeling or sound may be present. Bits of bone (called osteophytes) or cartilage may break off and float inside the joint space causing even greater pain and damage. Joint pain and stiffness result. It primarily affects the thumb, fingers, neck, lumbar section of the spine and weight-bearing joints (knees and hips).

- *Hands*: OA in the hands (thumb and fingers) tends to run in families. It affects more women than men. Small, bony knobs may appear on the distal joints of the fingers called Heberden's nodes. Similar knobs, called Bouchard's nodes, can appear on the middle joints of the fingers. Fingers can become enlarged and gnarled, and they may ache or be stiff and numb. The base of the thumb joint is also subject to OA.
- *Knees*: Knees are primary weight-bearing joints and are most commonly affected. They may be stiff, swollen, and painful making life tasks difficult (walking, climbing stairs). If not treated, OA in the knees can lead to disability.
- *Hips*: OA of the hip, like OA of the knee, can cause pain, stiffness, and severe disability.
- *Spine*: Stiffness and pain in the neck or lower back from OA can cause weakness or numbness in the arms or legs.

Incidence/Prevalence in US

Approximately 20.7 million adults in the United States have OA. Most persons over the age of 75 are affected with OA in at least one joint, making this condition a leading cause of disability in the US (Rush University Medical Center, 2004).

Predominant Age

OA first appears asymptomatically in the second to third decades and becomes universal by age 70. Almost all persons by age 40 have some pathologic changes in weight-bearing joints, although relatively few people are symptomatic. Men and women are equally affected, but onset is earlier in men (Berkow, 1992).

Causes

The exact cause is unknown, but a combination of multiple variables is suspected to contribute to the development of OA. This includes being overweight, the aging process, joint injury, stresses on joints from certain jobs and sports activities, and genetics.

System(s) Affected

OA primary affects the musculoskeletal system. Secondary complications from pain and inactivity may result.

Prognosis

There are varying degrees of disability and functional compromise. Appropriate exercise and care can often keep symptoms in check and allow the client to live a normal life. Significant pain in weight-bearing joints is one of the major causes for joint replacement.

Secondary Problems

- *Muscle atrophy*: Loss of muscle strength is often a consequence of decreased activity levels.
- *Psychological changes*: Depression, anxiety, and feelings of helplessness are common in clients who live with chronic disease.
- *Cardiopulmonary endurance*: Decreased involvement in cardiopulmonary conditioning due to primary symptoms (pain, stiffness) and secondary symptoms (fatigue, depression) often results in compromised endurance.
- *Pain*: Painful joints may impact the client's ability to perform life tasks.
- *Sexual dysfunction*: Pain, limited range of motion, limited endurance, and psychological changes can affect the client's ability to participate in physical sexual activity.
- *Upper and lower extremity weakness and numbness*: Upper extremity impairments may occur from OA in the neck and lower extremity impairments may occur from OA in the lower back.
- *Sedentary lifestyle*: Other secondary problems may result due to a sedentary lifestyle including pneumonia, urinary tract infection, decubitus ulcers, deep vein thrombosis, cardiovascular disease, obesity, hypertension, and contractures.

Assessments

A client with OA often learns to manage the disease via education from his/her physician and literature from various organizations. If pain begins to hinder the client's ability to complete basic life tasks (e.g., dressing, bathing, walking), the individual is often referred to outpatient occupational and physical therapy services. Since OA is not reversible, should impairments become disabling, elective joint replacement surgery may be performed. Total joint replacement (TJP) is the most frequent admitting diagnosis for inpatient physical rehabilitation for those who have OA. Therapists may also see clients in an inpatient setting with OA as a secondary admitting diagnosis.

Typical Scope of Team Assessment

Although OA is frequently a secondary admitting diagnosis, it still requires attention and treatment. The treatment team assesses the present, as well as the past course and management of the disease. This includes evaluation of activity limitations and participation restrictions that hinder the client's activity performance, functional joint limitations in range of motion and strength, knowledge and skills related to life task adaptations (what techniques has client implemented in the past), knowledge and functional application of joint protection and energy conservation techniques, available resources for assistance, and psychosocial adjustment.

Anticipated Findings from RT Assessment

- *Depression*: Depression is a common psychological issue for individuals with chronic disease.
- *Secondary disability*: Conditions that directly relate to a sedentary and inactive lifestyle (e.g., hypertension, obesity, muscle atrophy).
- *Impaired mobility*: This can be a result of OA in the hip, knee, or lower back or a secondary complication from a sedentary lifestyle (e.g., hip contractures).
- *Activity limitations and participation restrictions*: Activity limitations are often a result of the primary symptoms of the disease (pain, limited range of motion) and participation restrictions are often associated with environmental and personal factors (transportation, finances, adapted devices).
- *Pain, fear, and anxiety*: Clients often report that fear and anxiety of having or causing pain is a pivotal factor in choosing, initiating, and participating in life tasks (recreational activities, household chores, social events).

- *Past involvement in highly physical activities*: This includes a physically demanding job (e.g., manufacturing work) and/or sporting activities (e.g., skiing, running).
- *Obesity*: Being overweight is known to aggravate the development of OA.

Treatment Direction

Primary treatment goals for OA are to improve joint care through rest and exercise, maintain ideal body weight, control pain, and achieve a healthy lifestyle. Approaches include medication, alternative therapies, surgery, pain relief techniques, rest and joint care, exercise, and weight control.

Whole Team Approach

- *Exercise*: Research shows that exercise is one of the best treatments for OA. Exercise can improve mood and outlook, decrease pain, increase flexibility, improve the cardiovascular system, maintain a healthy body weight, and promote general physical fitness. The amount and form of exercise will depend on which joints are involved, how stable the joints are, and whether or not the joint has been replaced with a prosthesis. Interestingly, strengthening the thigh muscle (quadriceps) has been found to relieve symptoms of knee osteoarthritis and prevent more damage. In addition, individuals with knee OA who are active in a regular exercise program report feeling less pain and functioning better.
- *Psychological health*: Developing a positive outlook is vitally important in the management of chronic disease to assist with motivation, initiation, and participation in life tasks that contribute to quality of life.
- *Rest and joint care*: Joints can become painful from excessive activity or prolonged sedentary states. The client must learn to monitor his/her activity level to manage pain and functioning. Splints may be prescribed, especially for OA in the hands, to minimize pain and allow joints to rest and maintain neutral positions when sleeping. They are not used extensively since stiffness and pain can also result from immobilization.
- *Stress management and relaxation training*: These help to manage pain and relax muscles.
- *Pain management*: Moist heat (warm towels, hot packs, warm shower) may be helpful to reduce pain.
- *Weight control*: Less weight means less stress on weight-bearing joints. Exercise helps with weight loss. Moreover, individuals who are overweight and who do not have symptomatic

OA may reduce their risk of developing symptoms by losing weight.

- *Surgery*: Surgery may be performed to relieve pain and disability of OA. Surgery may be performed to remove loose pieces of bone and cartilage from the joint (if they are causing mechanical symptoms of buckling or locking), resurface (smooth out) bones, or reposition bones. However, joint replacement surgery is the most common (80% of all OA surgeries).

Recreational Therapy Approach

To manage OA, outside of joint replacement surgery (discussed separately in the Joint Replacement diagnosis), the therapist focuses on the general treatment directions to manage joint care through rest and exercise, maintain ideal body weight, control pain, and achieve a healthy lifestyle. Therapists also address psychological issues.

Recreational Therapy Interventions

Interventions that are frequently implemented for clients who have OA include:

- *Physical exercise*: Exercise aids in better sleep, reduction of pain, maintenance of a positive attitude, and healthy weight loss. Water exercises are especially beneficial because they provide range of motion, endurance, and strength building with less stress on joints than land-based exercise. See "Exercise Basics" in the Techniques section and ICF code b455 Exercise Tolerance Functions for details on designing and monitoring an exercise program. RT focuses on not only the specific form of exercise but also the environmental and personal factors that affect the client's ability to continue exercising after discharge (transportation, finances, carryover of skills into a community environment, etc.). Other components of RT treatment are problem solving (d175 Solving Problems), resource awareness (see "Personal Leisure Resource Awareness" and "Community Leisure Resource Awareness" in the Techniques section), and integration training (see "Integration" in the Techniques section). Therapists may need to educate the client on the benefits of exercise for OA and the complications and disabilities that can arise from leading a sedentary lifestyle as discussed in "Consequences of Inactivity" in the Concepts section. Leisure interest exploration and testing may be helpful in identifying exercise options that interest and satisfy the client (discussed in Interest Exploration in "Activity Pattern Development" in the Techniques section).

- *Joint care*: Clients are taught joint protection techniques (as discussed in b710 Mobility of Joint Functions and "Fine Hand Use Ergonomics" in the Techniques section), energy conservation techniques ("Energy Conservation Training" in the Techniques section), and proper body mechanics ("Body Mechanics and Ergonomics" in the Techniques section) to prevent further joint damage. Therapists must be sure clients follow the instructions for when to wear splints, as well as donning and doffing them correctly. Clients are taught how to adapt and modify life tasks to incorporate techniques. This may include prescription and training about adaptive equipment. This instruction can be scored using ICF codes d155 Acquiring Skills, d570 Looking After One's Health, and d2303 Managing One's Own Activity Level.

- *Pain and stress management*: Stress management and relaxation training techniques are taught to the client and then monitored for effectiveness in managing pain. Therapists also address negative and distorted thought processes through cognitive-behavioral therapy (CBT) interventions that positively correlate with managing stress and pain levels. See ICF codes b280-b289 Pain, d240 Handling Stress and Other Psychological Demands, and d570 Looking After One's Health. More information may also be found in "Relaxation and Stress Reduction" and "Education and Counseling" in the Techniques section.

- *Healthy lifestyle*: The development of a healthy activity pattern that accounts for activity limitations and participation restrictions is a vital component of therapy because the client needs to learn how to balance exercise and rest (see "Activity Pattern Development" in the Techniques section). These interventions can be coded with d5702 Maintaining One's Health and d230 Carrying Out Daily Routine. Therapists often should include the topic of sexuality when addressing re-involvement in life tasks since pain, limited range of motion, limited endurance, and psychological changes can affect the client's ability to participate in physical sexual activity (see b640 Sexual Functions, d7702 Sexual Relationships).

- *Integration training*: Carryover of learned skills into a "real-life" environment is essential to promote follow through with a designed activity pattern (e.g., transition client to aquatics program at YMCA). See "Integration" in the Techniques section and score the specific activity within the real-life setting such as d6200 Shopping, d9204 Hobbies, d4701 Using Private Motorized

Transportation and/or the specific skills within the integrated setting, e.g., d465 Moving Around Using Equipment.

Miscellaneous

Research shows that clients with OA who take part in their own care report less pain and make fewer doctor visits. They also enjoy a better quality of life (NIH, 2002).

Research shows that adding patient education and social support is a low-cost, effective way to decrease pain and reduce the amount of medicine used (NIH, 2002).

References

Arthritis Foundation. (2004). Osteoarthritis. http://www.arthritis.org/ AFStore/StartRead.asp?idProduct=3328 on 3/14/04.

Berkow, R. (1992). *The Merck manual of diagnosis and therapy*. Rahway, NJ: Merck & Co, Inc.

National Institutes of Health. (2002). Handout on health: Osteoarthritis. http://www.niams.nih.gov on 3/13/04.

Rush University Medical Center. (2004). Arthritis statistics. http://www.rush.edu/rumc/page-P07502.html on 3/14/04.

Osteoporosis

Osteoporosis is a chronic, progressive bone disease. Bone tissue deteriorates and bone mass is lost. Bones become porous and brittle. Consequently, bones become fragile and break easily. Osteoporosis affects almost the entire skeletal system. Fractures of the wrist, spine, and hip are the most common result.

Bones are important. They provide structural support for muscles, protect vital organs, and store calcium that is essential for bone mass density and strength. Bones are living tissues that are constantly changing. Inside the bone are osteoblasts and osteoclasts. Osteoblasts form new bone and osteoclasts absorb and remove old bone. It is an ongoing process where old bone is removed and new bone is developed.

Up until about the age of 30, the body builds and stores bone efficiently. After the age of 30, bones begin to break down faster than they can be rebuilt. Bone mass in women begins to diminish even faster after menopause when the ovaries stop producing the hormone estrogen. Although genetics play a dominant role in the development of osteoporosis, people before the age of 30 can help protect themselves from developing osteoporosis in later life by following several suggestions from the National Osteoporosis Foundation (see Prognosis). Children, adolescents, and young adults can develop strong bones by eating a balanced diet that is rich in calcium and vitamin D, participating in regular weight-bearing exercise, and abstaining from smoking and excessive alcohol intake.

Specialized tests called bone density tests measure bone mineral density (BMD). They can detect osteoporosis and low bone mass density, help predict chances of fracturing, and be used to monitor the effects of treatment. The World Health Organization has established definitions of osteoporosis based on bone mass density measurements in white women. These scores are helpful in making treatment decisions, but they are not the sole determinant.

- *Normal*: Bone density no lower than one standard deviation (SD) below the mean for young adult women (T-score above -1).
- *Low bone mass* (osteopenia): Bone density 1.0 to 2.5 SD below the mean for young adult women (T-score between -1 and -2.5).
- *Osteoporosis*: Bone density 2.5 SD or more below the mean for young adult females (T-score at or below -2.5).

There are four types of osteoporosis:

1. *Juvenile osteoporosis*: Usually begins between the ages of eight and fourteen and is commonly detected when the child complains of bone pain and/or has a fracture.
2. *Type I osteoporosis* (postmenopausal osteoporosis): This occurs in women between the ages of 50 and 70. It is marked by a rapid decrease in bone density. Fractures in the distal forearm (wrist) and vertebral bodies are common.
3. *Type II osteoporosis*: This occurs in people over the age of 70. In addition to wrist and vertebral fractures, hip fractures are common.
4. *Secondary osteoporosis*: This is when osteoporosis occurs because of an underlying disease process. Osteoporosis is a common secondary disability that could result from sickle cell anemia, hemophilia, hyperthyroidism, diabetes mellitus, Cushing syndrome, pregnancy, estrogen deficiency, malnutrition, anorexia nervosa, alcoholism, liver disease, myeloma, leukemia, lymphoma, metastatic disease, medications (heparin, steroids, Dilantin), immobility, and weightlessness (as in space).

Incidence/Prevalence in US

About eight million men and women in the United States have osteoporosis, and nearly 22 million more have low bone mass, placing them at increased risk for osteoporosis and fractures (National Osteoporosis Foundation, 2004). Women are four times more likely to develop osteoporosis than men. White women have the highest prevalence of osteoporosis. One in every two white women will have an osteoporosis-related fracture in her/his lifetime (National Osteoporosis Foundation, 2003).

Predominant Age

Osteoporosis is most common in women after menopause (around 50), and the chance of having osteoporosis increases as the client gets older.

Causes

Risk factors for developing osteoporosis include: being female (especially a white female), being over the age of 50 (the risk increases with increasing age), having a fracture after the age of 50, having low bone mass (as determined by a bone density test), having a primary relative (e.g., parent, sibling) who has a history of fractures, being thin and/or having a small frame, having a family history of osteoporosis, having an estrogen deficiency as a result of menopause (especially if it is early or surgically induced), having abnormal absence of menstrual periods (amenorrhea), having a history of anorexia nervosa, having a low lifetime calcium intake, having a vitamin D deficiency, using particular medications, such as corticosteroids and anticonvulsants that can affect bone density, the presence of certain chronic medical conditions (see Secondary Osteoporosis), having a low testosterone level (if male), leading an inactive lifestyle, cigarette smoking, excessive use of alcohol, and prolonged bed rest.

System(s) Affected

Osteoporosis primarily affects the skeletal system, but complications from osteoporosis can affect many other body systems. Fragility of bones makes fracturing easy, so clients often limit their activities to avoid fracturing. Limiting activity levels (depending on the extent) can affect the cardiopulmonary system and the muscular system. The kidneys can be affected because increased calcium in the urine may cause kidney stones. Osteoporosis also affects psychological systems including social relationships, social roles (caregiver now the recipient of care), and emotional health (depression, loss of self-esteem and confidence, anxiety, coping with pain and loss of function).

Prognosis

Once osteoporosis is detected, clients are encouraged to participate in regular weight-bearing exercise, increase calcium and vitamin D intake, stop smoking, limit alcohol intake, and eat a healthy diet. Clients may need to take prescription medication that can halt the disease process. The damage that has occurred from osteoporosis cannot be reversed, but it can be halted. People do not usually realize they have osteoporosis until they have a fracture.

Secondary Problems

Over 300,000 hip fractures, 700,000 vertebral fractures, and 250,000 wrist fractures annually are due to osteoporosis in the US (National Osteoporosis Foundation, 2004). Vertebral compression fractures and hip fractures cause the most concern.

Vertebral compression fractures: Fractures can occur from very minimal stressors such as coughing, lifting, or bending. Some spinal fractures occur over time and do not produce a severe onset of symptoms thus not alerting the person to the injury. When a fracture does occur, the person will experience severe back pain and spasms. Spasms subside with decreased movement, so people who have a vertebral fracture often remain in bed to avoid moving and

causing another muscle spasm. Spinal deformities such as kyphosis or stooped posture (also called hunchback) can occur over time causing problems with reaching and bending. If multiple thoracic fractures occur, restrictive lung disease could develop. If multiple lumbar fractures occur, the anatomy of the abdomen can become affected leading to constipation, abdominal pain, distention, reduced appetite, and premature satiety (feeling full when not fully nourished).

Hip fractures: Hip fractures in people with osteoporosis occur from falls, especially falls onto the side of the hip because there is not a lot of tissue there to protect the bone. Sometimes falls are blamed for causing fractures, when what has really happened is that a fracture occurred first and caused the fall.

Assessments

Typical Scope of Team Assessment

If osteoporosis is suspected or the person is over the age of 65, a bone density test is conducted. If osteoporosis is confirmed, the physician will make appropriate recommendations to halt the disease process. If a vertebral or hip fracture occurs, the client will be sent to an acute care hospital to confirm the fracture and perform surgery if needed. Inpatient or outpatient therapy is commonly prescribed for rehabilitation. Once in the rehab setting, therapists evaluate the functional abilities of the client while maintaining vertebral or hip precautions as outlined by the surgeon.

Anticipated Findings from RT Assessment

Recreational therapists usually see clients who have been admitted to rehabilitation centers for a vertebral or hip fracture. Recreational therapists also see clients who have a secondary diagnosis of osteoporosis or a high risk for developing it. For clients who have osteoporosis as a primary or secondary diagnosis, the recreational therapist will usually find that the client has been leading a predominantly sedentary lifestyle. Secondary complications of leading such a lifestyle will also be evident (see "Consequences of Inactivity" in the Concepts section).

Treatment Direction

Whole Team Approach

Rehabilitation: Physical medicine and rehabilitation can reduce disability, improve physical function, and lower risk of subsequent falls in patients with osteoporosis. Components of such a program frequently include a goal-oriented exercise regimen, appropriate diet, modalities for pain relief, psychosocial support, and various assistive devices (National Osteoporosis Foundation, 2003).

Pain management: The first step is to minimize pain associated with fractures. Vertebral fractures cause severe pain that can last from one to two weeks and may require bed rest in the supine position (on the back). Narcotic medication is considered as a treatment option for pain relief. Clients are monitored for reactions to narcotic pain medication.

Falls prevention: See Falls Precaution in "Precautions" in the Concepts section.

Exercise: Restoration of muscular activity to the osteoporotic bone is done in carefully graduated steps to avoid further fractures. Clients can become very fearful of moving and participating in activity because they are afraid of causing a fracture. Activities to avoid are those that require good balance, physical contact, and participation in a crowded environment where bumping might occur. Clients who have had a vertebral fracture are taught how to do deep breathing to open up the chest wall, perform prescribed exercises to strengthen abdominal and back muscles to support the spine (isometric exercises are helpful to strengthen the abdominal wall and prevent kyphosis), and apply techniques for conserving their backs. Flexion forces (bending) increase the risk of fracturing vertebra so clients are encouraged to stand in an upright position during activity whenever possible or adapting the activity to encourage an upright position (e.g., putting a small step stool on a table top to increase the height of an item rather than bending over the table).

Clients who have an unhealed vertebral fracture and are wearing a thoracic orthosis should avoid activities that require more than slight bending (flexion of the trunk) or twisting (rotation of the trunk). They should also avoid lifting heavy items that stress the spine (weight limits will vary and are set by the treating physician). These precautions are also followed after the vertebral fracture is healed to prevent further vertebral fractures.

Weight-bearing exercises (such as standing and walking) are implemented by physician's order to promote the development of bone mass. Weight-bearing precautions will be ordered by the physician (see Weight-bearing Precautions in "Precautions" in the Concepts section). Not only does participation in exercise activities help the bones absorb calcium, it also aids in maintaining a healthy body weight. Extra weight that puts increased stress on the skeletal system should be avoided.

Nutrition: A healthy diet must include adequate intakes of calcium and vitamin D. Good sources of calcium include dairy products, broccoli, figs, almonds, and fortified foods (e.g., cereals, orange juice). Good sources of vitamin D include fatty fish, fortified foods, and skin production with sunlight exposure. Clients are also encouraged to stop smoking and reduce alcohol intake (no more than one to two drinks per day).

Controlling underlying disease processes: People who have underlying conditions that increase their risk for developing osteoporosis should seek to eliminate the condition.

Medication: For individuals who have been diagnosed with osteoporosis, a variety of prescription medications are available to halt the disease.

Fluid intake: Clients are encouraged to drink lots of fluids (1.5-2 liters of water a day) to dilute the urine and prevent kidney stone formation.

Care of paralyzed limbs: It should be assumed that osteoporosis is present in limbs that are paralyzed and precautions must be taken to prevent falls and fracturing whether or not a diagnosis of osteoporosis exists.

Surgery: In some cases, surgery may be indicated (severe pain persisting longer than six months, condition threatens to cause or has caused neurological damage, or gross spinal deformity).

Recreational Therapy Approach

Recreational therapy follows the whole team rehabilitation approach described above.

Recreational Therapy Interventions

Interventions that are frequently implemented with clients who have osteoporosis include:

- *Pain management*: Refer to the Techniques section for "Relaxation and Stress Reduction" (especially deep breathing since it also helps to open up the chest wall — an issue for people who have had vertebral fractures and are at risk for developing restrictive lung disease). Pain may also be heightened by outside variables (e.g., feelings of anxiety or depression, shallow breathing, self-destructive thinking patterns, increased focus on pain). See Generalized Anxiety Disorder or Major Depressive Disorder for techniques to manage feelings of anxiety or depression. See "Education and Counseling" in the Techniques section for information on changing distorted thinking patterns (the ABC personality theory helps to explain how an increased focus on pain heightens the level of pain). ICF codes that apply to this part of treatment include b280-b289 Pain, d2401 Handling Stress, b152 Emotional Functions, and d175 Solving Problems.

- *Falls prevention*: See Falls Precaution in "Precautions" in the Concepts section. Code this as d570 Looking After One's Health.
- *Exercise*: The goal of exercise for recreational therapy is that the client identifies and participates in safe physical activities after discharge that will provide weight bearing and muscle pull. Swimming and aquatic exercises help people who have osteoporosis because they promote chest expansion, spinal extension, balance, coordination, and cardiopulmonary fitness (Slipman, 2003). Other forms of exercise to promote weight bearing and muscle pull include walking and seated range of motion exercises. Refer to the Techniques section for "Exercise Basics" and "Energy Conservation Training." Code this intervention as b455 Exercise Tolerance Functions, d570 Looking After One's Health, or a code related to the specific goal of a particular exercise.
- *Smoking and alcohol*: Clients with osteoporosis are encouraged to quit smoking and decrease alcohol intake since it affects the development of bone. See d240 Handling Stress and Other Psychological Demands for information on assisting clients with smoking cessation and social drinking.
- *Psychological, emotional, and social health*: A chronic disease that causes pain with activity can have a significant impact on a client's psychological, emotional, and social health. See ICF code d240 Handling Stress and other Psychological Demands and relevant parts of A&P Chapter 7 Interpersonal Interactions and Relationships and A&P Chapter 9 Community, Social, and Civic Life. In addition to the ICF codes, refer to the Techniques section for "Education and Counseling" and "Adjustment to Disability."

Miscellaneous

National Osteoporosis Foundation
1232 22nd Street NW
Washington, DC 20037
http/www.nof.org.

References

National Osteoporosis Foundation. (2003). *Physician's guide for treatment and prevention of osteoporosis*. Washington, DC: National Osteoporosis Foundation.

National Osteoporosis Foundation. (2004). About osteoporosis. www.nof.org.

Stolov, W. & Clowers, M. (1981). *Handbook of severe disability*. Washington, DC: US Government Printing Office.

Slipman, C. (2003). Osteoporosis. www.emedicine.com.

Parkinson's Disease

Parkinson's disease (PD) is a progressive, degenerative neurological disorder. The neurons in the basal ganglia (called substantia nigra) die or are damaged causing a slow degeneration of the nervous system. The result is a depressed production of dopamine and poor connections among neurons in the basal ganglia. This causes:

- *Tremors* that affect a client's coordination and proprioception. The tremors tend to increase when the client tries to attempt a purposeful activity (intention tremor). Around 70% of clients with PD also have involuntary rhythmic resting tremors (Vargas, 2004).
- *Poor coordination.*
- *Increased muscle tone* (rigidity).
- *Slowed or reduced movement* (bradykinesia).
- *Impaired balance.*
- *Stiff facial expression* (appears as if starring because of decreased eye blinking).
- *Shuffling gait and stooped posture* (head and shoulders hang forward).
- *Muffled speech*, characterized by a soft (hypophonia) and monotonous tone as well as stuttering because of muscular problems related to forming words.
- *Sweating abnormalities.*
- *Sexual dysfunction* (Merck Manual Home Edition, 2004; National Parkinson Foundation, 2004).

Symptoms typically begin on one side of the body (asymmetric) and progress to the other side (symmetric). Mild symptoms progress to more severe symptoms and extreme fatigue can exacerbate the symptoms. The symptoms appear when approximately 80% of the substantia nigra is affected (National Parkinson Foundation, 2004). A client must have two out of three cardinal features to be diagnosed with PD. This includes an asymmetric resting tremor (tremors when the limb is not being used), rigidity of muscles (determined by resistance to passive range of motion of a joint), and bradykinesia (slowed, reduced movement). A fourth cardinal sign, postural instability (loss of balance) typically emerges eight or more years into the disease process (Hauser & Pahwa, 2004). Other common problems of PD include:

- *Depression*: About 30% of clients with PD have depression (Sadock & Sadock, 2003). This may be directly related to chemical changes in the brain from PD; but it can also be a secondary problem of PD related to psychosocial adjustment.
- *Sense of smell*: Clients with PD may complain of a decreased sense of smell. This may be caused by difficulty breathing in enough air required for sniffing or it may be caused by degeneration of neurons involved in the sense of smell. An impaired sense of smell can affect appetite and possibly contribute to an increased risk of malnutrition (Merck Manual Home Edition, 2004). The sense of smell is also very important for safety (e.g., smell of gas or rancid food).
- *Falls*: Clients with PD often report having problems initiating a first step (called "start-hesitation"). Once the first step is initiated, sometimes clients just halt walking without any warning, feeling as if their feet are glued to the floor (called "freezing"). It can also be difficult to stop, turn, and maneuver around obstacles. A short, shuffling gait with a hanging head and shoulders, and limited arm swing can also increase the client's risk for falls, especially if it becomes a short stumbling run with a pronounced forward lean (festinating gait). This type of gait can result in a fall and injury, especially since clients with PD have difficulty making a quick forward hand movement to break the fall.
- *Dementia*: Fifteen to 30% of clients with PD develop dementia late in the disease process (Hauser & Pahwa, 2004).
- *Swallowing*: The muscle rigidity in the face can make swallowing difficult causing the person to drool or choke. Malnutrition and dehydration can also occur as a result of swallowing dysfunction.

Incidence/Prevalence in US

It is estimated that 1.5 million Americans have PD (National Parkinson Foundation, 2004).

Predominant Age

One out of every 250 people over the age of 40 and one out of every 100 people over the age of 65 have PD (Merck Manual Home Edition, 2004). It commonly begins between the ages of 50 and 79 and is twice as common among Caucasians as African-Americans (Merck Manual Home Edition, 2004). Although the numbers are small, people under the age of 40 can have PD. It is estimated that 5-10% of people with PD are under the age of 40 (National Parkinson Foundation, 2004). Parkinson's disease is also about 1.5 times more common in men than women (Hauser & Pahwa, 2004).

Causes

There is no identified cause of PD, although researchers believe that a person's genes and the environment play a role. Environmental issues include the use of pesticides, living in a rural environment, consumption of well water, exposure to herbicides, and proximity to industrial plants or quarries (Hauser & Pahwa, 2004).

When the brain sends a message to a muscle for movement (e.g., raise an arm), the message passes through the basal ganglia. The basal ganglia are located deep in the brain at the base of the cerebrum. The collection of neurons helps to smooth out and coordinate muscle movements. As an impulse travels through the basal ganglia, the neurons release a neurotransmitter called dopamine. Dopamine allows the neurons in the basal ganglia to communicate with each other. Parkinson's disease impairs nerve impulses. This, in turn, causes the symptoms seen.

System(s) Affected

PD affects the neuromuscular system.

Prognosis

Literature on prognosis is varied. One report states that clients with PD are expected to live a nearly normal life span with pharmacological interventions (Gancher, 2004), while another report says that clients with PD live several years longer than before the invention of new medications, which was 15 years (Blackmer, 2004). Good management of symptoms, however, usually only lasts four to six years with pharmacological interventions. After that the disease progresses despite medical interventions (Hauser & Pahwa, 2004). Clients tend to have a "rollercoaster effect" with short plateaus of improved function and decreased symptoms followed by increased impairment (Vargas, 2004). When measuring outcomes, specific treatment interventions should have long enough trial periods to determine the significance of the intervention. Shorter trial periods may have false outcomes because of the rollercoaster effects.

Secondary Problems

Secondary problems from PD include:
- *Psychological issues*: Depression, as reviewed in the description, may occur from trying to cope with a chronic, progressive disability or it may be a primary symptom of PD due to changes in brain chemicals. Feelings of anxiety, loss of internal locus of control, and poor frustration tolerance may also occur.

- *Decreased activity*: Movement dysfunction from PD limits physical activity that could lead to secondary complications from inactivity such as cardiac deconditioning, skin breakdown, and pneumonia.
- *Increase risk of falls*: The neurological impairment leaves the client at an increased risk of falling and a decreased ability to catch the fall to reduce injury. Fractures and contusions result.

Assessments

Typical Scope of Team Assessment

A diagnosis of PD is made by evaluating the client's symptoms. There is no test that confirms the diagnosis. Consequently, clients typically refuse to believe that they have PD and consult various health professionals before accepting the diagnosis. In the rehabilitation setting, evaluation of the client's dysfunction is made with discipline-specific tools.

Anticipated Findings from RT Assessment

The anticipated findings will vary depending upon the severity of the disease. Possible findings include:
- *Decreased activity level*: caused by movement limitations.
- *Decreased involvement*: fewer social or community activities and increased isolative behaviors.
- *Depression*: loss of internal locus of control, poor frustration tolerance level, and feelings of anxiety.
- *Tremors and coordination problems*: including resting tremors, muscle rigidity, and bradykinesia.
- *Falls*.
- *Changes in life roles*: may or may not be well accepted by the client.
- *General deconditioning*.

Treatment Direction

Whole Team Approach

Treatment goals are prioritized based on management of symptoms, involvement in life tasks that are important to the client, and activities that promote health and optimize quality of life. Restoration of function may be a goal if function was lost from deconditioning rather than the disease process.

Recreational Therapy Approach

Same as the whole team approach.

Recreational Therapy Interventions

Recreational therapy interventions for clients with Parkinson's include:

- *Physical leisure activity*: Identify safe forms of exercise that the client enjoys and develop participation skills. See b455 Exercise Tolerance Functions, d5701 Managing Diet and Fitness, d155 Acquiring Skills, and "Exercise Basics" in the Techniques Section.
- *Aquatic therapy*: aquatic therapy techniques, specifically protocols from Bad Ragaz and Watsu, are becoming a standard intervention due to their success mitigating symptoms. See Vargas (2004).
- *Socialization*: Increase opportunities for socialization and identify opportunities for socialization after discharge. Identify social reservations of the client (e.g., embarrassment, difficulty speaking) and problem solve to overcome barriers. Existential therapy techniques may be helpful. See "Education and Counseling" in the Techniques section for information on existential therapy. Code using d9205 Socializing and d175 Solving Problems.
- *Relaxation training*: Relaxation training can help to reduce muscle tension related to stress and anxiety that is not part of the physiological process of the disease. Added muscle tension from stress and anxiety could impact functional abilities. See "Coping with Stress" and "Relaxation and Stress Reduction" in the Techniques section. Code with d240 Handing Stress and Other Psychological Demands.
- *Locus of control and productivity*: Focus on activities that increase locus of control and feelings of productivity including b1266 Confidence and b1265 Optimism.
- *Exploration of life activities*: Explore the client's life priorities. What life activities can be adapted? What activities can be substituted? And what life activities may need to be given up entirely? Adapting, substituting, or giving up activities is not easy for some clients for a variety of reasons (e.g., not accepting progression of the disease, refusing to participate in an adapted activity). Don't try to force changes, but do provide information, resources, and instruction on adapted activities (d155 Acquiring Skills) for future reference. See "Adjustment to Disability" and "Education and Counseling" in the Techniques section for more information.
- *Falls prevention and safety*: Talk about issues related to falls and being safe in the home and the community (e.g., general falls prevention education, specific education about falls prevention in particular activities). See d5702 Maintaining One's Health and Falls Precautions in "Precautions" in the Concepts section.
- *Adjustment*: Suggest participation in a Parkinson's support group to help with adjustment to the disease. Some clients find it helpful to talk with other people who are going through the same things that they are. It can be uplifting and motivating to talk with other clients who have made adaptations and continue to live meaningful and fulfilling lives. See "Adjustment to Disability," as well as "Coping with Stress" in the Techniques section.
- *Energy conservation and community integration*: Extreme fatigue can exacerbate the symptoms of PD, so the therapist needs to be careful not to over-fatigue the client. Attention is also given to the amount of physical exertion required to participate in life activities so adaptations to minimize fatigue may be recommended. The therapist educates the client about energy conservation techniques with particular emphasis on engagement in community and recreational activities. See "Energy Conservation Training" in the Techniques section. Community integration training can be helpful to assess the client's ability to apply techniques in a real-life setting. See "Integration" in the Techniques section.

Miscellaneous

National Parkinson Foundation, Inc.
1501 NW 9th Avenue / Bob Hope Road
Miami, Florida 33136-1494
Telephone: 1-800-327-4545
Fax: (305) 243-5595
www.parkinson.org

References

Blackmer, J. (2004). Parkinson disease. www.emedicine.com on 12/12/04.

Gancher, S. (2004). Parkinson disease in young adults. www.emedicine.com on 12/12/04.

Hauser, R. & Pahwa, R. (2004). Parkinson disease. www.emedicine.com on 12/12/04.

Merck Manual Home Edition. (2004). Parkinson disease. www.merckhomeedition.com on 12/12/04.

National Parkinson Foundation. (2004). About Parkinson disease. www.parkinson.org.

Sadock, B. & Sadock, V. (2003). *Kaplan & Sadock's synopsis of psychiatry*, 9th edition. Philadelphia, PA: Lippincott Williams & Wilkins.

Vargas, L. (2004). *Aquatic therapy: Interventions and applications*. Ravensdale, WA: Idyll Arbor, Inc.

Rheumatoid Arthritis

The National Institute of Arthritis and Musculoskeletal and Skin Disorders (NIAMSD), a division of the National Institutes of Health, describes RA in the following way (NIH, 2004):

> In rheumatoid arthritis, the immune system, for unknown reasons, attacks a person's own cells inside the joint capsule[1]. White blood cells that are part of the normal immune system travel to the synovium and cause a reaction. This reaction, or inflammation, is called synovitis, and it results in the warmth, redness, swelling, and pain that are typical symptoms of rheumatoid arthritis. During the inflammation process, the cells of the synovium grow and divide abnormally, making the normally thin synovium thick and resulting in a joint that is swollen and puffy to the touch. As rheumatoid arthritis progresses, these abnormal synovial cells begin to invade and destroy the cartilage and bone within the joint. The surrounding muscles, ligaments, and tendons that support and stabilize the joint become weak and unable to work normally. All of these effects lead to the pain and deformities often seen in rheumatoid arthritis. Doctors studying rheumatoid arthritis now believe that damage to bones begins during the first year or two that a person has the disease. This is one reason early diagnosis and treatment is so important in the management of rheumatoid arthritis.

RA affects primarily wrist joints and finger joints closest to the hand; however it can also affect the neck, shoulders, elbows, hips, knees, ankles, and feet. It presents in a symmetrical pattern, meaning that it affects the same joints on the right and left sides. Clients typically complain of feeling pain and stiffness that lasts for more than 30 minutes upon awakening in the morning or after a long rest. Joints become swollen, reddened, and painful during and after excessive use. Some additional symptoms and problems that a client may experience with RA include (NIH, 2004):

- *Anemia*: A decrease in the normal number of red blood cells.
- *Depression*: Most experience some degree of depression, anxiety, and feelings of hopelessness.
- *Fatigue.*
- *Functional limitations*: related to life tasks.
- *Malaise.*
- *Impaired range of motion.*

- *Joint deformity.*
- *Fever*: occasional.
- *Neck pain.*
- *Dry eyes and mouth*: although less common.
- *Rheumatoid nodules*: Bumps under the skin that often form close to the joints affecting about one fourth of people with RA.
- *Sensory changes*: especially in the hands and feet.
- *Inflammation*: Other parts of the body including blood vessels, lining of the lungs, and the sac enclosing the heart.

RA varies from person to person. For some, symptoms may last a few months or years and then disappear without causing any noticeable damage. Others may have a mild or moderate disease, with periods of worsening symptoms, called flares, and periods when they feel better, called remissions. Still others have a severe disease that is active most of the time, lasts for many years, and leads to serious joint damage and disability (NIH, 2004).

Incidence/Prevalence in US

RA affects approximately 2.1 million Americans (NIH, 2004; Rush University Medical Center, 2004).

Predominant Age

The average onset for rheumatoid arthritis is between the ages of 20 and 45 years old, however it can also affect young children and teenagers. Juvenile rheumatoid arthritis (JRA) occurs in children sixteen years of age or younger. RA affects two to three times more women than men. RA occurs in all races and ethnic groups (NIH, 2004; Rush University Medical Center, 2004).

Causes

RA is believed to be caused by the following factors, either alone or in combination. Research is still being conducted (NIH, 2004):

1. *Genetic factors*: Specific genes may play a role in whether a person develops RA and how severe the disease will become. However, some clients possess these genes and don't develop RA, while others don't have these genes and develop RA. Therefore, one's genetic make-up is believed to be one of many variables in the development of RA.
2. *Environmental factors*: It is believed that an environmental factor, such as a virus, bacterium,

---

[1] A joint (the place where two bones meet) is surrounded by a capsule that protects and supports it. The joint capsule is lined with a type of tissue called synovium, which produces synovial fluid that lubricates and nourishes joint tissues.

or mycobacterium may trigger the disease process. The exact agent is unknown.

3. *Hormones*: Deficiencies or changes in certain hormones may promote the development of RA in genetically susceptible clients who have been exposed to an environmental triggering agent.

System(s) Affected

RA predominantly affects the musculoskeletal system, but sensory changes, internal organ involvement (heart, lungs, blood vessels), energy levels, and psychological issues may be present.

Prognosis

As many as 75% of clients improve somewhat with conservative treatment during the first year of disease; but 10% are eventually disabled despite full treatment (Berkow, 1992). Studies have shown that people who are well informed and participate actively in their own care experience less pain and make fewer visits to the doctor than other people with rheumatoid arthritis (NIH, 2004).

Secondary Problems

- *Cardiopulmonary endurance*: Decreased involvement in cardiopulmonary conditioning due to the primary symptoms (pain, stiffness, limited range of motion) and secondary symptoms (fatigue, depression) often results in compromised endurance.
- *Fatigue*: Fatigue is a common problem because of the increased time and effort required to complete life tasks.
- *Joint deformity*: Joint deformity occurs as a result of changes in the joint.
- *Muscle atrophy*: Loss of muscle strength is often a consequence of decreased activity levels.
- *Osteoporosis*: Many older women are at risk for osteoporosis, and rheumatoid arthritis increases the risk further, particularly if they are taking corticosteroids such as prednisone that affect bone density (NIH, 2004).
- *Pain*: Joints become tender and painful during and after excessive use, impacting the client's ability to perform life tasks.
- *Psychological changes*: Depression, anxiety, and feelings of helplessness are common in clients who live with chronic disease.
- *Sexual dysfunction*: Pain, limited range of motion, resultant inflammation from activity, limited endurance, and psychological changes can affect the client's desire to participate in sexual activity.

- *Bone loss*: Women with RA are at an increased risk of bone loss and fracture in the areas immediately surrounding the affected joints due to the development of osteoporosis for several reasons (NIH, 2003):
    1. Medications prescribed for the treatment of RA can trigger significant bone loss.
    2. Pain and loss of joint function caused by the disease can result in inactivity, further increasing osteoporosis risk.
    3. Bone loss in rheumatoid arthritis may occur as a direct result of the disease.
    4. Women, a group already at increased osteoporosis risk, are two to three times more likely than men to have RA.

Assessments

Typical Scope of Team Assessment

A client with RA often learns to manage the disease through education from his/her physician and literature from various organizations. If joint deformity, inflammation, and pain begin to hinder the ability to complete basic life tasks, the client is often referred to outpatient therapy services. A client is only admitted to an inpatient physical rehabilitation center if the RA has substantially affected his/her ability to complete life tasks and a more comprehensive approach to treatment is needed. Therapists may also see clients in an inpatient setting with RA as a secondary admitting diagnosis.

Since most clients with RA have adopted techniques for managing the disease prior to their inpatient rehab admission, the treatment team assesses the present, as well as the past course and management of the disease. This includes evaluation of activity limitations and participation restrictions that hinder the client's participation in life situations. Specific areas of assessment include the extent of joint deformity; the process of the disease (time lines between flares and remissions); functional joint limitations in the areas of range of motion, strength, and coordination; ability to perform life tasks and skills; knowledge and skills related to life task adaptations (techniques the client has implemented in the past); knowledge and functional applications of joint protection and energy conservation techniques; available resources for assistance; and psychosocial adjustment.

Anticipated Findings from RT Assessment

- *Depression*: Depression is a common psychological issue for many clients with RA. A change in premorbid recreational activities (inability to participate in favorite activities due to RA), lack of control over his/her lifestyle, and unpredictable pain and/or unexpected functional limitations may affect the client's ability to cope with the disease and lead to depressive symptoms (Smith & Yoshioka, 1992).

- *Impaired mobility*: This can be a result of RA in the hip, knee, or ankle joints or a secondary complication from a sedentary lifestyle (e.g., hip contractures).
- *Pain, fear, and anxiety*: Clients often report fear and anxiety of having or causing inflammation and the resultant pain is a pivotal factor in choosing, initiating, and participating in life tasks.
- *Secondary disabilities*: Disabilities caused by inactivity as discussed in "Consequences of Inactivity" in the Concepts section.

Treatment Direction

Whole Team Approach

Focus is on management of symptoms and prevention of secondary disability. The goals of treatment are to relieve pain, reduce inflammation, slow down or stop joint damage, and improve the client's sense of well being and ability to function. Medical interventions to address these issues include (NIH, 2004):

- *Medication*: To control pain, decrease inflammation, or slow down the course of the disease.
- *Surgeries*: To reduce pain, improve joint function, and improve functional performance in life tasks.
- *Joint replacement*: To remove a damaged joint and replace it with a prosthetic joint.
- *Tendon reconstruction*: Tendons (tissues that attach muscle to bone) are reconstructed by attaching an intact tendon to the damaged tendon. This is most frequently done to the hand to increase hand function.
- *Synovectomy*: This is the removal of the inflamed synovial tissue as part of tendon reconstructive surgery. Synovectomy is seldom performed by itself anymore because not all the tissue can be removed, and it eventually grows back.

Recreational Therapy Approach

"Therapeutic recreation specialists should seek to intervene with orthopedic impairments by managing pain, decreasing depression while increasing self-esteem, and preventing secondary disabilities" (Mobily & MacNeil, 2002). These suggestions can easily be absorbed into the three stages of the disease. Trombly (1989) recommends specific goals that can

be adopted by many allied health professionals. Clients are taught prior to discharge the rationale for stages of treatment and educated on the importance of maintaining mobility and protecting joints throughout their lives.

Acute Stage: Synovial Inflammation and Proliferation

The overall approach is to: prevent joint deformity and pain by resting the affected joints (splints, positioning), assist the client to cope with the unpredictable nature of the disease, and begin energy conservation education. Recreational therapists follow prescriptive splint-wearing schedules as established by the occupational therapist and physician. The recreational therapist may need to assist the client in donning and doffing the splint. The therapist can monitor the inflammation process by asking the client to rate his/her pain level prior, during, and after activity (see b280 Sensation of Pain for information on how to rate pain levels). Within the acute stage, activity should be minimized (explore activities that do not aggravate inflammation). Passive or very gentle active-assisted motion is done by the occupational or physical therapist to each joint daily to maintain mobility.

Subacute Stage: Post-Inflammation

The general approach is to maintain or increase mobility, strength, and endurance; maintain or increase functional abilities; prevent deformity by use of splinting and joint protection techniques; develop problem-solving skills relative to energy conservation and joint protection; and assist in psychosocial adjustment to chronic pain and disability.

Chronic Stage: Burn Out of Disease

At this stage, inflammation has fully subsided and resultant deformity is evident. The therapist's approach at this stage is a continuation of stage two's approach with a stronger focus on preparation for discharge and long-term health promotion. Premorbid leisure activities may need to be replaced if they cause pain, are incompatible with joint protection techniques, or if the client does not desire to participate in an adaptive form of the activity. Prescription and training on the use of adaptive equipment is a common need. The development of healthy activity patterns that account for activity limitations and participation restrictions is a vital component of therapy at this stage, as the client needs to learn how to balance exercise and rest. The more active a patient is in planning and controlling his/her own care, the greater the chance of successful compliance (Hasselkua, 1987). Frequent short rests are recommended over long bed rests due to the increased risk of secondary complications from prolonged sedentary activity. Since depression is a common psychological issue experienced by clients with RA, the activity pattern should have activities that help manage the symptoms of depression (social opportunities, activities that reflect strengths of the client to promote self-esteem and confidence) and energy conservation techniques to avoid fatigue and resulting frustration. Therapists should be careful to include the topic of sexuality when addressing re-involvement in life tasks since pain, limited range of motion, resultant inflammation from activity, limited endurance, and psychological changes may have affected the client's ability to participate in sexual activity. Carryover of learned skills into a "real-life" environment is essential to promote follow through with activity patterns (e.g., transition client to an aquatics program at the YMCA).

Recreational Therapy Interventions

The following techniques are often used to implement the recreational therapy programs during the three stages of RA:

- *Activity adaptations*: See d175 Solving Problems and d155 Acquiring Skills.
- *Joint protection*: See b710 Mobility of Joint Functions.
- *Adaptations to function*: See "Fine Hand Use Ergonomics" and "Body Mechanics and Ergonomics" in the Techniques section.
- *Energy conservation*: See "Energy Conservation Training" in the Techniques section.
- *Emotional health*: Discussed and scored in d240 Handling Stress and Other Psychological Demands and "Coping with Stress," "Adjustment to Disability," "Relaxation and Stress Reduction," and "Self-Esteem" in the Techniques section.
- *Exercise and mobility*: See b455 Exercise Tolerance Functions and many specific codes in A&P Chapter 4 Mobility. Other topics in the Techniques section include "Integration" "Exercise Basics," and "Walking Techniques." Recreational therapy focuses not only on the specific form of exercise but the systemic issues that surround the client's ability to continue involvement in exercise after discharge. Also see

"Consequences of Inactivity" in the Concepts section.
- *Sexuality*: See b640 Sexual Functions.
- *Leisure education*: See "Activity Pattern Development" in the Techniques section.

Miscellaneous

RA often improves during pregnancy, although the reason is not clear. Results of one study suggest that the explanation may be related to differences in certain special proteins between a mother and her unborn child. These proteins help the immune system distinguish between the body's own cells and foreign cells. Such differences, the scientists speculate, may change the activity of the mother's immune system during pregnancy (NIH, 2004).

National Institute of Arthritis and Musculoskeletal and Skin Diseases
877-22-NIAMS
www.niams.nih.gov

References

Berkow, R. (1992). *The Merck manual of diagnosis and therapy*. Rahway, NJ: Merck & Co, Inc.

Hasselkua, B. R. (1987). Emerging trends in geriatric care. *OT Week*, Feb 19, 1987, 5-6.

Mobily, K. & MacNeil, R. (2002). *Therapeutic recreation and the nature of disabilities*. State College, PA: Venture Publishing, Inc.

National Institutes of Health. (2004). Rheumatoid arthritis. http://www.niams.nih.gov/hi/topics/arthritis/rahandout.htm on 3/17/04

National Institutes of Health. (2003). What is rheumatoid arthritis? http://www.governmentguide.com/govsite.adp?bread=*Main&url=http%3A//www.governmentguide.com/ams/clickThruRedirect.adp%3F55076483%2C16920155%2Chttp%3A//www.nih.gov/ on 3/17/04.

Rush University Medical Center. (2004). Arthritis statistics. http://www.rush.edu/rumc/page-P07502.html on 3/14/04.

Smith, S. & Yoshioka, C. (1992). Recreation functioning and depression in people with arthritis. *Therapeutic Recreation Journal, 26*(4):21-30.

The Arthritis Foundation (2004). Rheumatoid arthritis. http://www.arthritis.org/conditions/DiseaseCenter/ra.asp on 3/15/04.

Trombly, C. (1989). *Occupational therapy for physical dysfunction, 3rd edition*. Baltimore, MD: Williams & Wilkins.

Schizophrenia

Schizophrenia is a complex disorder in which clients are out of touch with reality because of a brain dysfunction. The impairments include impaired thinking, delusions, emotional instability, and hallucinations. Many health professionals believe that schizophrenia is not a single disorder, but a variety of combined disorders that are often seen together. For a client to be diagnosed with schizophrenia, s/he must meet the basic criteria of the disorder, which includes having two or more symptoms (hallucinations, disorganized speech, grossly disorganized or catatonic behavior, and negative symptoms such as a flattened affect) lasting for a period of at least six months that significantly impacts occupational and social performance.

- *Hallucinations*: Auditory hallucinations are the most common, although any of the five senses can be affected. Hallucinations are not based on real images or sensations (e.g., a client hears voices when no other person is present). The voices are usually threatening, obscene, accusatory, or insulting and they may converse among themselves or comment on the client's life or behavior. Visual hallucinations are the second most common. Other types of hallucinations include tactile (feeling stimulation with no external cause), olfactory (smelling something that isn't there), and taste (tasting a flavor that is not present).

- *Disorganized thought and speech*: Thought disorders found in clients with schizophrenia are commonly reflected in their actions and speech. The client may verbalize very strange ideas or beliefs, exhibit garbled and incoherent speech that is not understandable to the listener or have no verbalizations at all (mutism), have flights of ideas that quickly change and do not relate to one specific topic, demonstrate problems attending and concentrating on physical or cognitive tasks, or complain of "thought control" or "thought broadcasting."

- *Catatonic behavior*: compulsive and motiveless resistance to all requests to change any behavior or posture.

- *Flattened affect*: an on-going lack of emotion in facial and verbal expression.

Other symptoms that often present in schizophrenia include odd tics (rapid, sudden, and non-rhythmic motor movements or vocalizations that the client has little control over) or mannerisms (deep-seated, involuntary, and habitual movements such as continually stroking the jaw with the thumb), echopraxia, poor hygiene, odd clumsiness, and uncoordinated movements. Some experienced clinicians report a perceived inability to establish a comfortable interaction with clients with schizophrenia: one that is unrestrained and mutually accepting on which to build a therapeutic relationship. This perception, called a precox feeling, has not been proven through research, but is a commonly held perception among practitioners (Sadock & Sadock, 2003).

Clients who meet the basic criteria for schizophrenia are also assigned a prominent type. There are four prominent types of schizophrenia (Sadock & Sadock, 2003):

1. *Paranoid type*: delusions (often of grandeur or persecution) and/or auditory hallucinations; can be very aggressive and hostile; late onset.
2. *Disorganized type* (formally called hebephrenic): very active, but aimless and "silly" behavior; poor contact with reality and poor self-care; inappropriate social and emotional responses.
3. *Catatonic type*: marked disturbance in motor function, with extremes of excitement and stupor; resistance to having body parts moved by someone else; mutism, malnutrition, exhaustion, and self-injurious behavior.
4. *Residual type*: emotional blunting, eccentric behavior, illogical thinking, social withdrawal, and mild loosening of associations.

Incidence/Prevalence in US

Schizophrenia affects 1% of the US population (American Psychiatric Association, 1994). Each year, it is estimated that clients with schizophrenia account for 20-25% of public mental health hospital admissions and 16% of all psychiatric clients who receive any type of treatment. However, clients with schizophrenia make up about 50-55% of the resident population in mental health hospitals, more than any other disease (Arieti, 2004), because of their frequent long hospital stays (Sadock & Sadock, 2003).

Predominant Age

Schizophrenia usually begins before the age of 25; however it can occur any time from puberty to the age of 45. After the age of 45, the risk of developing this illness sharply decreases. Schizophrenia has been reported to have been seen in childhood, but psychiatrists disagree on whether such cases belong in the same clinical category as adult schizophrenia. Although schizophrenia affects both men and women equally, there is a significant difference in the age of onset. The peak age of onset for men is 10 to 25 years old, while women peak between the ages of 25 and 35 years old. About 90% of clients in treatment for schizophrenia are between age 15 and 55.

Causes

The cause of schizophrenia is unknown, but it is believed to be a combination of many factors that may include (Sadock & Sadock, 2003):

- *Chemical changes in the brain.*
- *Social stressors in urban settings*: Urban social stressors are believed to affect the development of schizophrenia in at-risk persons.
- *Genetics and hereditary*: First-degree biological relatives of persons with schizophrenia have a ten times greater risk for developing the disease than the general population. Also supported in studies of twins.
- *Social class*: People in lower socioeconomic classes have higher rates of schizophrenia.
- *Recent immigrant to the US*: Some studies report a high prevalence of schizophrenia among recent immigrants, a finding implicating abrupt cultural change as a stressor involved in the cause of schizophrenia.

Psychopathology (the study of mental disorders) also includes some other theories as to the origin or schizophrenia:

- *Psychoanalytic theory*: Schizophrenia is believed to be "an adaptive method to avoid panic, terror, and disintegration of the sense of self." It is a result of cumulative traumas during early development (Sadock & Sadock, p. 483).
- *Learning theory*: Learning theory proposes that children learned irrational behaviors and broken thought processes from their parents and the environment.
- *Diathesis-stress model of schizophrenia*: When clients with poor information processing, attention, coping mechanisms, and social skills experience stress, their inability to handle the stress may lead to a schizophrenic episode. This, in turn, causes more stress, which perpetuates the cycle (Sue, Sue, & Sue, 1997).

System(s) Affected

Schizophrenia affects the client's cognition, emotions, relationships, basic self-care, and physical skills. Deficits in these areas affect secondary life areas as discussed in "Secondary Problems" below.

Prognosis

While the majority of clients with schizophrenia seen by the recreational therapist will become progressively worse over time, there are still a significant number of clients who are able to function without the help of the health care system. These clients participate in community recreation opportunities without the recreation leaders realizing that they have schizophrenia. Ascher-Svanum and Krause (1991) talk about the "Rule of Thirds": "one-third of all people diagnosed with schizophrenia will recover completely, one-third of all people diagnosed with schizophrenia will improve but need occasional hospitalizations, and one-third of all people diagnosed with schizophrenia will not improve" (p. 79).

Sadock & Sadock (2003) report that specific characteristics are thought to be indicators of a good or poor prognosis in schizophrenia. A client is more likely to have a good prognosis if s/he has 1. a late onset of schizophrenia; 2. stressful precipitating life events prior to the onset of schizophrenia; 3. a current acute onset of symptoms; 4. a healthy social, sexual, and work history; 5. symptoms of a depressive mood disorder and a family history of mood disorders; and 6. a marriage that includes a good support system. A client is more likely to have a poor prognosis if s/he has 1. a young onset; 2. no obvious precipitating life stressors; 3. an insidious onset (very slow and subtle development so a beginning date is hard to identify); 4. no marriage (single, widowed or divorced) and a poor support system; 5. an unhealthy social, sexual, and work history; 6. withdrawn and autistic behavior; 7. a family history of schizophrenia; 8. neurological signs and symptoms; 9. a history of perinatal trauma; 10. had no remissions within a three year period of time or many relapses; 11. negative symptoms; and 12. a history of assault.

The first five years after receiving the diagnosis of schizophrenia generally dictate the course of the disease. Sometimes people with schizophrenia have a long period of remission after the first exacerbation of symptoms and are able to return to their prior level of functioning. However, exacerbations and remissions are common and subsequent schizophrenia exacerbations do not usually remit completely. More frequent exacerbations suggest a poorer prognosis. The inability for a client with schizophrenia to fully recover from the exacerbation is what sets mood disorders apart from schizophrenia.

Other aspects of the prognosis include (Sadock & Sadock, 2003):

- About 75% of clients with severe schizophrenia cannot work and are unemployed.

- In families with high levels of expressed emotion, the relapse rate is high.
- Post-psychotic depression may follow a psychotic episode.
- The severity of disability due to the secondary symptoms of the disease usually rises over time.
- The ability to lead a socially integrated life occurs in about one third of the clients.

Secondary Problems

- *Higher mortality rate*: Persons with schizophrenia have a higher mortality rate from accidents and natural causes than the general population.
- *Suicide*: About 50% of all clients with schizophrenia attempt suicide and approximately 15% of all clients with schizophrenia die from suicide.
- *Cigarette smoking*: More than three fourths of all clients with schizophrenia smoke cigarettes compared with less than half of psychiatric clients as a whole.
- *Drug and alcohol use/abuse*: It is estimated that 15-25% of clients with schizophrenia use cannabis, 5-10% use cocaine, and 30-50% abuse or are dependent on alcohol. Drug and alcohol use/abuse is commonly associated with a poor prognosis.
- *Homelessness*: It is estimated that one-third to two-thirds of people who are homeless have schizophrenia.
- *Eye movement dysfunction*: The ability to visually follow objects is impaired in 50-85% of clients with schizophrenia (Sadock & Sadock, 2003). In normal populations the percentage is below 10%. Clients with schizophrenia also have a high blink rate.
- *Violence*: Suicidal or homicidal violence may occur in response to auditory or visual hallucinations commanding the client to act, but the risk of homicidal violence in people with schizophrenia is no greater than that of the general public.
- *Tardive dyskinesia*: Clients who use antipsychotic drugs for long periods of time are at an increased risk of developing tardive dyskinesia (Mobily & MacNeil, 2002).

Assessments

Typical Scope of Team Assessment

There is no laboratory test for schizophrenia although various tests (laboratory tests for blood chemistry, urinalysis for drugs and alcohol, and EEGs) are usually conducted to rule out other causes when the symptoms first appear. Recent advancements in the use of brain imaging (CAT scans, MRIs,

and fMRIs) have shown noticeable differences in the brain structure of clients with schizophrenia compared to normal populations. However, the diagnosis is still usually based on clinical interview, observation, and family reports. Information should always be verified from additional sources. The *DSM-IV-TR* establishes a set of criteria for diagnosing schizophrenia (and the particular type of schizophrenia) based on symptoms, level of dysfunction, and duration.

Psychological testing: Clients with schizophrenia often perform poorly on neuropsychological testing, especially in the areas of vigilance, memory, attention, problem solving, and concept formation.

Premorbid signs and symptoms: There may be signs and symptoms prior to the development of schizophrenia. They may include a history of schizoid personality characterized by quiet, passive, and introverted behavior resulting in few or no friends, dates, or involvement in team activities (Sadock & Sadock, 2003). Adolescents may show a sudden onset of obsessive-compulsive behavior and/or somatic complaints followed by a decrease in ability to perform functional tasks. The client may also develop an increased interest in abstract concepts including philosophy, the occult, religion, and other "improvable" ideas.

Differential diagnosis: Other disorders that may cause symptoms of schizophrenia need to be ruled out. These include:
- Schizophreniform Disorder
- Brief Psychotic Disorder
- Schizoaffective Disorder
- Borderline Personality Disorder
- Substance Induced Disorders

Anticipated Findings from RT Assessment

An in-depth initial assessment is appropriate for the first time the therapist sees a client. While leisure interests and patterns are important, more critical is the need to establish a baseline of functional community skills: using the phone; making change; endurance, coordination, and muscle power for activities; relationships with staff in the local parks and recreation district making it easier for the client to participate in community recreation activities.

The typical findings on the recreational therapy assessment are likely to be
- *Structured settings*: The client does best in a structured setting. This may mean that the group activity is structured but it also means that the process for engaging in any activity should be structured.
- *Poor stress management*: A deficit in stress management skills and an increased stress level.

- *Social skill atrophy*: with reduced support systems and difficulty participating in leisure activities with others.
- *Poor self-efficacy*: Feeling powerless and passive.
- *Poor survival skills*: Lacking basic survival skills, especially if the client is homeless.

Clients are usually not admitted until they are in an acute psychiatric crisis, often because they failed to take their medications. It will take a few days of making sure that the clients take their medications and experience reduced symptoms before the therapist can obtain good assessment results. Conducting the recreational therapy assessment within the first few days of admission may produce interesting results, but it will not provide the therapist with a realistic idea of the client's functional level.

For clients in long-term residential facilities a broad baseline of skills should be assessed when the client is not in an acute crisis.

Treatment Direction

Whole Team Approach

A variety of approaches are utilized in the treatment of schizophrenia, including:
- *Antipsychotic medication and psychotherapy*: Only effective if the client takes his/her medication regularly.
- *Coping skills*: Especially those that help the client respond to, and recover from, stressful events.
- *Communication skills building*: Overlearning helps when the client is dealing with an acute crisis.
- *Cognitive-behavioral therapy*: Discussed in "Education and Counseling" in the Techniques section.
- *Social skills training*: Discussed in the Techniques section.
- *Family therapy*: Especially useful if it lowers the level of expressed emotion in the household.
- *Vocational therapy*: Obtaining and maintaining employment mostly in sheltered workshops, job clubs, and part time or transitional employment programs.
- *Hospitalization*: For diagnostic purposes, stabilization of medications, stress reduction, safety concerns because of suicidal or homicidal ideation, grossly disorganized or inappropriate behavior, and/or an inability to obtain basic needs. Treatment must be coordinated with after care facilities.

Recreational Therapy Approach

Because clients with schizophrenia are frequent users of the mental health inpatient system, the therapist should plan on establishing an ongoing program that can be carried out across multiple admissions. The starting point is to establish a baseline and continue with ongoing assessments of the client's functional level in fine hand movements, interpersonal skills, community skills, and functioning in small groups. In subsequent admissions the therapist can track changes in the baseline and relate them to other aspects of the client's treatment, including medication and life outside of the facility.

Recreational therapists provide therapy to achieve the goals in the whole team approach. They are especially responsible for working on coping skills, social skills, and finding appropriate leisure opportunities for the client. A leisure education program that works well with clients who are frequently admitted to inpatient psychiatric units is the *Leisure Step Up* program by Dehn (1995). *Leisure Step Up* is an eleven-step leisure education program that is very basic and practical. It may take the client two to six admissions to complete any step of the program. The therapist will need to maintain a set of files on each client to facilitate the continuity of treatment. See "Participation" in the Concepts section for more information on the *Leisure Step Up*.

Clients with schizophrenia who reside in state institutions tend to be very impaired. While it is important for the therapist to encourage the client to make decisions about his/her leisure, it is the therapist's responsibility to ensure that the client gets frequent moderate physical exercise most days of the week (as long as the client has his/her physician's clearance). This moderate exercise should be enjoyable and varied enough that the client is able to maintain a balance of leisure interest as his/her functional level decreases as time goes by. A method of increasing participation in leisure activities for clients who are very impaired with schizophrenia in a residential setting is to structure the recreation programming so that clients must "earn" points or tickets to be able to attend their favorite activity. Among the ways of earning points is going to new activities, with the goal of making the new activities familiar to the client.

Recreational Therapy Interventions

Most clients with schizophrenia will receive recreational therapy services either in a long-term placement setting (such as a state psychiatric hospital) or in a short-stay psychiatric unit (average stay between three and twelve days). Clients with schizophrenia who live in group homes often do not receive the services of a recreational therapist because of government caps on health care funding.

Recreational therapy treatment for clients with schizophrenia generally falls under the "Five Ss": 1. structure, 2. stress management skills, 3. social skill development and/or maintenance, 4. self-efficacy training, and 5. survival skills.

- *Structure*: This is critical for the client to function well. Ad lib activities, arts and crafts activities that stress creativity instead of following a set of steps, or recreation activities where the clients can just "hang out" often create so much stress for clients with schizophrenia that their functional ability drops. Structure is also important in teaching the client different skills. Writing out the steps (or using pictures to show the steps) and then making sure that the order is followed each time is important. Toward discharge the client will seem to need less structure. However, the therapist should continue to encourage a more rigid following of the steps than s/he would with other populations. Clients are very likely to start losing function soon after discharge and need to rely on rote memory for tasks to maintain as much function as possible. This type of treatment can be scored using d210 Undertaking a Single Task and d220 Undertaking Multiple Tasks.

- *Stress management skills*: Clients benefit from being able to identify two or three symptoms of stress such as tension in the shoulder muscles, trouble concentrating or sleeping, worrying, and depression. Some clients will not be able to state the specific event that caused their stress to increase, so basic education on events that cause stress may also be appropriate. Techniques to reduce stress are discussed in "Relaxation and Stress Reduction" in the Techniques section. Clients with schizophrenia should avoid techniques that use visualization as these may feed into developing hallucinations or delusions. These issues are discussed in d240 Handling Stress and Other Psychological Demands.

- *Basic social skills*: See "Social Skills Training" in the Techniques section and individual codes in A&P Chapter 7 Interpersonal Interactions and Relationships.

- *Self-efficacy skills*: While many self-efficacy programs emphasize a client's increased cognitive awareness of his/her feelings and teach the client how to speak for himself/herself, self-efficacy skills for clients with schizophrenia should emphasize practical competence over intellectual insight (Hartl Chambliss, 1988). ICF codes

b1266 Confidence and d177 Making Decisions address these issues. The worksheets in *Leisure Step Up* also help clients develop the practical competence skills needed to participate in community leisure (even if the "community" is a state institution). Self-efficacy for clients with schizophrenia revolves around the ability to make their own decisions because of self-sufficiency. By learning how to "follow regular schedules, to keep appointments, to recognize explicit rules and procedures, and to join in planning activities" a client is better able to control his/her life (Hartl Chambliss, 1988, p. 30).

- *Basic survival skills*: Basic survival skills are not only skills related to shopping for food, being able to make change, simple budgeting, and preparing meals. Since many clients with schizophrenia will be homeless at some point in their lives, the recreational therapist may need to teach some very basic survival skills to some clients. These skills relate to keeping warm and dry, knowing where the community drinking fountains and bathrooms are located, how to find food (including what native plants are not toxic), transportation options, etc. The types of techniques taught by groups such as Outward Bound but modified for urban environments provide the therapist with an appropriate skill development course. These interventions can be scored using d155 Acquiring Skills, d570 Looking After One's Health, and d175 Solving Problems.

References

American Psychiatric Association. (1994). *Diagnostic and statistical manual of mental disorders* (4th ed.). Washington, DC: American Psychiatric Association.

Arieti, S. (2004). Schizophrenia. *Encyclopedia Americana* http://search2.webfeat.org:5554/ on 4/47/04.

Ascher-Svanum, H. & Krause, A. (1991). *Psychoeducational groups for patients with schizophrenia: A guide for practitioners*. Gaithersburg, MD: Aspen Publications.

burlingame, j. & Blaschko, T. (2002). *Assessment tools for recreational therapy and related fields, third edition*. Ravensdale, WA: Idyll Arbor.

Dehn, D. (1995). *Leisure Step Up*. Ravensdale, WA: Idyll Arbor.

Hartl Chambliss, C. (1988). *Group involvement training: A step-by-step program to help chronic mentally ill patients*. Oakland, CA: New Harbinger Publications.

Sadock, B. & Sadock, V. (2003). *Synopsis of psychiatry* (9th ed.). Philadelphia, PA: Lippincott Williams & Wilkins.

Sue, D., Sue, D., & Sue, S. (1997). *Understanding abnormal behavior*. New York, New York: Houghton Mifflin Company.

Sickle Cell Anemia

Sickle cell anemia is caused by a recessive genetic disorder that is chronic in nature, has cycles of painful "crises" followed by remissions, and increases the client's susceptibility to infection. In sickle cell anemia normal hemoglobin is replaced by a hemoglobin variant. There are five primary types of sickle cell disease with the most prominent one seen in the United States being sickle cell anemia. The other types of sickle cell are not considered anemia but other types of blood hemoglobin diseases.

Clients with sickle cell disease (including sickle cell anemia) have abnormally formed hemoglobin that, when stressed, develops crystals along the edge of the red blood cells and changes their shape to become a crescent or sickle shape. The change is called sickling. The crescent shape makes it harder for the red blood cells to travel through veins and arteries, causing a partial or complete blockage. The blockage, in turn, causes cell death and pain. Some clients who do not have sickle cell anemia but are genetic carriers of the trait (called sickle cell trait) may also experience sickling under extreme conditions, many of which might occur during recreational activities. The conditions that aggravate sickle cell disease are

- *Dehydration*: This can occur because of excessive loss of water from the body from sweating or other methods. The client should make sure that s/he takes in fluids equal to the amount lost through activity.
- *Cold temperatures*: When the body is exposed to cold temperatures, the blood supply system in the arms and legs tends to constrict. The stress from the cold and the reduced blood flow may trigger a sickle cell crisis.
- *Increased body temperature* (usually over 101°F): The client should seek immediate medical help if s/he develops a fever. The client should also avoid hot tubs, saunas, and other activities that might increase his/her body temperature to 101°F or higher.
- *Infection*: Pneumococcal sepsis and Salmonella osteomyelitis are the most common. One of the biggest positive impacts of treatment for decreasing the mortality rate of sickle cell is the prophylactic use of daily doses of penicillin (or similar antibiotics).
- *Strenuous physical exercise*: Any time someone engages in strenuous physical exercise, s/he temporarily depletes the blood of available oxygen. Moderate exercise is important for people with sickle cell anemia but they should avoid getting winded.

Incidence/Prevalence in US

Sickle cell anemia is found predominately in Black Americans, with one in 500 having sickle cell disease and slightly fewer than 10% carrying the genetic trait. A small percentage of clients with Mediterranean heritage also carry the recessive sickle cell trait. The disease affects an equal number of females and males (Danbro, 1998).

Predominate Age

Since sickle cell anemia is a chronic, hereditary disorder that is found in all ages of clients. The first symptoms usually develop after six months of age.

Causes

Sickle cell anemia goes through cycles of remission and acute crisis (flare-ups of the disease) caused by factors in the environment and the client's activity choices, including overexertion, exposure to cold temperatures, exposure to infections, increased body temperature, significant emotional stress, and dehydration.

System(s) Affected

Tissue ischemia (a decrease in the supply of oxygenated blood to cells causing pain and decreased function of the affected tissue/organ) and necrosis (death of body tissue) are major concerns, as they affect many different body systems including:

- *Blood*: The premature death of red blood cells exceeds the body's ability to produce new red blood cells, especially when the client is in crisis.
- *Bones*: Through multiple crises the bones are weakened with the potential of bone rarefaction (decrease in the density) and osteoporosis, which increases the client's potential for fracturing bones. Other skeletal deformities may also develop including lordosis (a spinal deformity that causes the lumbar spine to have an excessive curve backwards) and kyphosis (a spinal deformity that causes the thoracic portion of the spine to curve forward causing rounded shoulders and impairs lung capacity).
- *Central nervous system*: Because of the potential for blockage of vascular system, clients have an increased risk of a cerebrovascular accident. One author (Swift, 1989) found that children with sickle cell anemia scored one standard deviation lower than their siblings on cognitive tests. The

assumption is that this difference is due to brain damage from ischemia and necrosis.

- *Heart*: Clients with sickle cell anemia often have heart damage due to ischemia and necrosis. A lack of appropriate levels of physical activity and the emotional stress associated with sickle cell disease may also play a factor.
- *Kidney*: Tissue ischemia and necrosis of the kidney causes enuresis (wetting the bed), hematuria (blood in the urine), inability to concentrate urine, and nephritic syndrome (inflammation of the kidneys).
- *Liver*: Multiple crises cause necrosis of liver tissue, which means healthy liver tissue is replaced with fibrotic (scar) tissues. The liver produces bile that helps the body digest fats in the small intestine; balances the body's level of bilirubin (if not balanced, jaundice that produces the yellow discoloration of the skin and eyes occurs); secretes fats, glucose, proteins, and vitamins (all necessary for feeding the cells in the body); processes hemoglobin to allow the body to use its iron; and converts poisonous ammonia produced as a by-product of cell function into urine.
- *Physical stature and maturation*: Clients with sickle cell anemia tend to physically mature more slowly than their peers. This causes additional stress for adolescents, who, as a group, already have a lot to cope with as they move through the teenage years. Due to ongoing pain (even at times when their body is not in crisis), clients are not inclined to participate in activities as much as their peers. Anorexia (low body weight) may also be a problem, further compounding body image issues.
- *Spleen*: The spleen cells become enlarged with sickled cells during a crisis, destroying cells. The destroyed cells are replaced with fibrotic tissue. The spleen filters bacteria in the body so it helps fight infection.

Prognosis

A lot of progress has been made in the treatment of clients with sickle cell anemia over the last quarter century. Currently about 85% of the clients with sickle cell anemia live to adulthood. There are a variety of subtypes of sickle cell anemia. For clients with sickle cell the average age of death for males is 42 years and females 48 years. Quite a few clients are now living 70+ years with a large segment of adults with sickle cell anemia being in their 50s (BlackHealthCare.com, 2000).

Secondary Problems

- *Pain*: Crisis events (times when the hemoglobin have sickled and blocked the flow of the blood).
- *Aseptic necrosis*: The client may have a decreased range of motion in joints, especially his/her hips.
- *Scleral icterus* ("yellow eyes"): Yellowing of the whites of the eyes because of damage to the liver.
- *Increased risk of infections*: Good hand washing, especially after being in public places, is an important habit for clients with sickle cell anemia to develop.
- *Delayed physical and sexual maturation*: Youth and adolescents with sickle cell anemia tend to have delayed physical and sexual maturation. Because their development is delayed (they catch up with their peers when they are in their twenties), clients receive teasing from their peers. Secondary problems often are based on the client's inability to cope with the teasing and poor body image.

Assessments

Typical Scope of Team Assessment

Clients are usually diagnosed with sickle cell disease by the time they are two years old. The earliest symptoms usually occur around the age of six months. Laboratory tests are usually done to confirm the diagnosis with CAT scan or MRI imaging to rule out a stroke and a bone scan done to rule out osteomyelitis. Ongoing assessment is used to track the status of the client's organs that are damaged during crises.

Anticipated Findings of RT Assessment

- *Impaired knowledge of leisure opportunities*: Leisure education is appropriate for the client and family to help the client have as normal of a life as possible with a variety of leisure activities appropriate for the client's interest and activity limitations.
- *Inadequate coping mechanisms*: The client will likely need additional skills in coping with pain, activity limitations, and frequent separation from friends during sickle cell crises that result in hospitalization.
- *Adolescent power struggles*: It is normal for adolescents to want to go their own way and not comply with the structure imposed by adults. For adolescents with sickle cell disease this power struggle could place the client in a life-threatening situation. The recreational therapist works

with the client, family, and team members to identify areas that the client can have real and reasonable control over life issues while agreeing to comply with necessary treatment limitations.

Treatment Direction

Whole Team Approach

The whole team works first on solving the acute problems of a sickling crisis. When the client is stabilized, the team provides education on how to avoid future events, adaptations for deficits, and general health information related to the disease.

Recreational Therapy Approach

Clients with sickle cell anemia are likely to be seen through numerous admissions. The areas that recreational therapists frequently address with clients with sickle cell anemia include: 1. normalization of the developmental process that is negatively impacted by inpatient stays, 2. development of skills to cope with pain and stress, 3. development of leisure activities that do not make the sickle cell disease worse, 4. self-esteem bolstering, and 5. locus of control issues (especially with teenagers).

Providing education related to recreational activities is a major portion of the recreational therapist's responsibility. The important topics include information about:

- *Exposure to cold*: Clients need to avoid getting cold. That includes dressing appropriately for the weather, including ensuring appropriate protection from rain.
- *Increased body temperatures*: Clients should avoid activities that have the potential to raise their internal body temperatures above 101°F including hot tubs, saunas, and exercising in hot weather.
- *Competitive sports*: It is usually not appropriate for clients with sickle cell to engage in competitive sports (BlackHealthCare.com, 2000). Competitive sports usually require individuals to push themselves physically and often expose them to a variety of severe weather. Youth are also susceptible to peer pressure if they are "pulled" because of potential risks, not completing the game or workout.
- *Hypoxia* (lack of oxygen reaching the cells): While normal levels of activity tend to be okay for clients with sickle cell, excessive levels of activity, or even increased activity levels at one time in multiple activities that use oxygen, can precipitate a sickle cell crisis. The types of activities to avoid are strenuous physical exercise, emotional stress, and activities in high

altitudes (e.g., flying in a plane without controlled cabin pressure or driving or hiking over mountain passes). Scuba diving is also contraindicated.

- *Hydration*: It is normal for clients to be given a minimum amount of fluid to drink each day. The recreational therapist should work with the rest of the medical team to develop guidelines of when the minimum amount should be increased. The therapist should provide basic information such as the location of the drinking fountains in regularly used parks or recreation facilities and the types of foods available at concession stands that count toward hydration (soups, Jell-O, puddings, frozen popsicles, Slurpies). Avoiding environmental causes of dehydration (sun exposure and hot temperatures) is another important part of leisure activity planning.
- *Lower extremity injuries*: Clients with sickle cell disease are at an increased risk of developing skin ulcers in their lower extremities (BlackHealthCare.com, 2000). The recreational therapist who is working with clients in a community setting should look for possible ulcerations of the lower extremity to encourage prompt medical attention. In inpatient settings nursing staff will often notice cuts and ulcerations on the lower extremities during their normal physical exam. If the therapist sees a problem developing on the lower extremities, or if the client cuts, bruises, or develops a blister on his/her lower extremities during activities, the therapist should report it immediately to the person in charge of the child's health care.
- *Infection control*: The client should be encouraged to wash his/her hands frequently as the main defense against infection. While it is important for clients to avoid hot temperatures or chill from cold or wet weather, being outside usually reduces the exposure to infection.
- *Photosensitivity*: Clients under the age of five years often receive daily prophylactic doses of antibiotics to prevent infections. Often the antibiotics prescribed cause the client to be hypersensitive to sunlight. When working with a client to develop a balanced leisure repertoire, the therapist needs to make sure that direct, unprotected exposure to sunlight is limited.
- *Renal diuresis* (increased rate of the formation of urine causing an increased rate of urination): Clients usually have an increased rate of renal diuresis causing them to need to use the bathroom more frequently. It also increases the chance of enuresis (bedwetting). In planning recreational activities the therapist should ensure adequate and frequent breaks to use the restroom.

Also, for camping activities, sensitivity to the likelihood that clients may wet the bed is needed. Extra sleeping bags and quietly waking the child or youth in the middle of the night to use the restroom are appropriate modifications to activity. It is not appropriate to suggest that the client drink less before going to bed, as the enuresis is not because the client drank too much fluid but because the body processed the fluid faster than normal. Travel by motor vehicles and trains have not been found to increase the risk of crisis (BlackHealthCare.com, 2000). When trips are planned, ensure that adequate stops for restroom use and stretching are scheduled.

Recreational Therapy Interventions

Some of the common recreational therapy interventions for clients with sickle cell anemia include:

- *Education*: Covering the topics discussed above would be scored as d570 Looking After One's Health.
- *Exercise*: It is extremely important for clients to get regular, moderate exercise on a daily basis. Twenty minutes a day of moderate exercise that avoids exposing the client to increased body temperatures or cold temperatures is important. In bad weather a moderate workout at the local gym or walking the mall is appropriate. The recreational therapist should work with the client to find appropriate kinds of exercise as discussed in d920 Recreation and Leisure and "Activity Pattern Development" in the Techniques section. See "Exercise Basics" in the Techniques section
- *Self-esteem*: Self-esteem is important for a client with sickle cell disease because there are many limitations caused by the disease. The recreational therapist needs to make sure the client also understands that there are still things s/he can do to control the disease and activities that s/he can still participate in. See "Self-Esteem" in the Techniques section.

References

BlackHealthCare.com. (2000). Sickle cell anemia — Case management. www.blackhealthcare.com/BHC/SickleCell/CaseManagement.asp.

Swift, A. (1989). Neuropsychological impairment in children with sickle cell anemia. *Pediatrics 84*(6):1077-1085.

Spinal Cord Injury

A spinal cord injury (SCI) damages the spinal cord (and may or may not include damage to the bony structures of the spinal column). The spinal cord is a set of nerves that provides communication between the brain and the rest of the body. When there is damage to the spinal cord, communication is interrupted. Spinal cord injuries may be partial or complete, temporary or permanent.

Classification of Injury

Spinal cord injuries are broadly defined as tetraplegia, paraplegia, or spinal fracture. Since 1990 the most frequent neurological category is incomplete tetraplegia (30.8%), followed by complete paraplegia (26.6%), incomplete paraplegia (19.7%), and complete tetraplegia (18.6%). Trends over time indicate an increasing proportion of clients with incomplete paraplegia and a decreasing proportion of persons with complete tetraplegia.

- *Tetraplegia*: a spinal cord injury that ranges from C1 to T1. Clients experience a loss of feeling and/or movement in their head, neck, shoulder, arms, and/or upper chest. Fifty-one percent of clients with spinal cord injury have tetraplegia (National Spinal Cord Injury Association, 2004). Previously called quadriplegia.
- *Paraplegia*: the general term describing lost feeling and/or impaired ability to move the lower parts of the body. The body parts that may be affected are the chest, stomach, hips, legs, and feet. A client with level T2 to S5 spinal cord injuries has paraplegia. Approximately 45.9% of clients with spinal cord injury have paraplegia.
- *Spinal fracture*: A person can "break their back or neck" yet not sustain a spinal cord injury if the bones around the spinal cord (the vertebrae) are damaged, but the spinal cord is not affected. In these situations, the client will not experience paralysis unless damage to the spinal cord occurs because the bones are not stabilized.

The classification system broadly used in rehab medicine classifies injuries by 1. level of injury (e.g., C-2), 2. type of injury (e.g. incomplete), 3. *American Spinal Injury Association Impairment Scale* (e.g. AIS D), and by 4. syndrome, where applicable (e.g. central cord syndrome).

Level of Injury

To determine the level of injury, loss associated with sensation, muscle movement, and muscle strength are tested. An X-ray shows where the damage occurred to the vertebrae. The site of injury, however, does not always determine the extent of the injury. For example, a client may have a T4 damage, yet secondary damage from edema results in presentation of a T3 level injury.

To determine the extent of injury, several tests are administered. A "pin prick" test determines intact, diminished, and/or extinguished sensation (feeling). This is also referred to as assessing dermatomes, which are the areas of skin supplied with nerve fibers by a single spinal nerve root. Diminished or absent sensation in a particular dermatome will identify the nerve damaged. The client is instructed to move each limb/joint in all available ranges to determine motor function loss. Finally, a strength test is administered to determine the extent of motor dysfunction and graded according to the *Manual Muscle Examination (MME)*. See b730 Muscle Power Functions for more information about the MME. Based on the results of these tests a level of injury is determined (e.g., T2).

Type of Injury

Complete: Complete spinal cord lesions result in no function, sensation, or voluntary movement below the level of the injury. Both sides of the body are equally affected.

Incomplete: With the advances in acute treatment of SCI, incomplete injuries are becoming more common. Incomplete spinal cord lesions are characterized by preservation of some sensory and/or motor function below the level of injury. They are typically the result of a partial transection of the spinal cord or contusions (bruises) to the spinal cord caused by displaced bone. If the source of pressure can be identified, surgery or traction can decompress the cord. The relief of pressure and subsequent resolution of edema (soft tissue swelling from injury) may result in return of function. Early return of function is a good sign, although recovery is variable and unpredictable. If partial dysfunction remains despite decompression, spinal cord damage can be tracked to a specific area of the spinal cord (anterior, posterior, central, lateral) by evaluating the clinical presentation of the client through the tests described earlier. Damage to a specific area of the spinal cord results in a typical presentation of sensory and motor function, as explained below.

Incomplete Lesion Syndromes

When the spinal cord is not completely severed, the deficits depend on which part of the cross-section of the spinal cord is damaged.

Anterior cord syndrome: Damage to anterior portion of cord and/or vascular supply to the anterior portion of the cord results in loss of motor power, loss of pain and temperature sensations, with preservation of position, vibration, and touch sense. This is typically a result of compression due to fracture dislocation or cervical disk protrusion.

Central cord syndrome: Damage to the central area of the cord produces greater neurological impairment in the upper extremities (cervical tracts more centrally located) than in the lower extremities (lumbar and sacral tracts more peripheral). Many clients have normal sexual, bowel, and bladder function. Most develop the ability to walk and may have some remaining distal arm weakness or dysfunction. This is commonly caused by hyperflexion injuries in the cervical region, congenital injuries, degenerative narrowing of the spinal canal, or compressive forces resulting in hemorrhage and edema.

Posterior cord syndrome: Damage to the posterior area of the cord and/or its vascular supply causes loss of position, vibration, and deep touch, with preservation of motor power, pain, and temperature. The sense of proprioception (the awareness of a limb's position in space) is lost, which can limit the client's potential for developing a functional gait. A wide-based gait pattern is typical. This type of injury is commonly caused by posterior impact injuries or when hyperextension forces compress or traumatize the posterior (sensory) cortex of the spinal cord along with the posterior columns.

Brown-Sequard syndrome: Damage to one lateral side of the cord, usually seen as a result of a stab wound, results in the loss of voluntary motor control, sensation, and decreased reflexes at the corresponding dermatome level on the same side (ipsilateral) as the cord damage. There is also a lack of superficial reflexes, clonus, and a positive Babinski sign. On the opposite side (contralateral) there is loss of sense of pain and temperature several dermatome segments below the level of injury.

American Spinal Injury Association Impairment Scale

A classification system developed by the American Spinal Injury Association classifies the extent of spinal cord injury, as shown in Table 13. On admission to rehab, the transfer note from the acute care hospital may provide an initial AIS classification of the client (e.g., AIS,A; AIS,C). To understand the implications of a client's AIS score, the recreational therapist must know how to score muscle strength on the standard six-level scales from normal to no strength as shown in b730 Muscle Power Functions.

Incidence/Prevalence in US

Approximately 450,000 people in the US have spinal cord injuries. There are about 10,000 new SCIs every year (National Spinal Cord Injury Association, 2004).

Predominant Age

The majority of spinal cord injuries (82%) involve Caucasian males between the ages of 16-30 who are single and employed. African-Americans, however, are at a higher risk than whites. The percentage of cases occurring among African-Americans has been increasing in recent years (National Spinal Cord Injury Association, 2004).

Causes

- *Trauma*: Since 1990, motor vehicle accidents account for 41% of the SCI cases reported. The next largest contributor is falls followed by acts of violence (primarily gunshot wounds), and recreational sporting activities (National Spinal Cord Injury Association, 2004).
- *Tumor*: If the tumor and the resulting pressure are removed, motor and sensory function may be restored depending on the amount of damage to the spinal cord.
- *Transverse myelitis* (TM): TM is an acute inflammatory process affecting both sides of the spinal cord. It is a rare disease that affects one to four people per million. There is no single etiology for TM but in many cases it is the result of damage to neural tissues by an infectious agent and/or the immune system. It affects people at any age, but there are clusters between the ages of 10-19 years and again between 30-39 years. It is not gender specific and does not seem to have a hereditary influence. Approximately one third

Table 13: American Spinal Injury Association Impairment Scale

A: Complete. No motor or sensory function is preserved in the sacral segments S4-S5.
B: Incomplete. Sensory but not motor function is preserved below the neurological level and includes the sacral segments S4-S5.
C: Incomplete. Motor function is preserved below the neurological level, and more than half of key muscles below the neurological level have a muscle grade less than 3.
D: Incomplete. Motor function is preserved below the neurological level, and more than half of key muscles below the neurological level have a muscle grade of 3 or more.
E: Normal. Motor and sensory function is normal.

of clients recover fully or have mild impairment in function, one third are left with moderate dysfunction, and one third have severe dysfunction that does not resolve. When the client has a clear and unexplained disruption in sensorimotor function, a spinal MRI and lumbar puncture are often prescribed to determine if there is acute inflammation causing the loss of function (Kerr, 2001).

System(s) Affected

Spinal cord injury affects motor and sensory systems below the level of injury. Clients who sustain a C1, C2, or C3 injury (ventilator dependent) will have additional respiratory, voice, and speech system dysfunction. Depending on the level and extent of the injury and the client's lifestyle habits, secondary systems can be affected. These may include bowel and bladder, sexual function, skin, lungs, heart, muscles, joints, bones, and hematological systems. Consequently the client may have specific precautions and parameters to follow: sitting schedule, blood pressure monitoring, pulse monitoring, activity limitation, oxygen saturation level, ventilator time, out of bed schedule, equipment parameters (e.g., client wearing a "clam shell" may have to wear it at all times when out of bed).

Prognosis

Life expectancies for clients with SCI are slightly below life expectancies for clients without a spinal cord injury. Mortality rates are significantly higher during the first year after injury than during subsequent years, particularly for clients with severe injuries. The complications that cause early death are pneumonia, pulmonary emboli, non-ischemic heart disease, and septicemia (infection in the blood). The most common hospitalizations after rehab are for urinary tract infections, skin breakdowns, autonomic dysreflexia, pneumonia, depression, and substance abuse (National Spinal Cord Injury Association, 2004).

Currently there is no cure for SCI, although pharmacology advances have been made. Clinical trials have shown that the administration of methylprednisolone (a high dose steroid) improves recovery by about 20% when given within eight hours after injury. Methylprednisolone is helpful in decreasing swelling, a source of secondary damage. Swelling not only causes secondary damage, but it can also mask a client's true functional level. Edema impinges on nerves by compressing them, resulting in an impairment of function. It can take days to weeks for edema to dissipate, but once it subsides further function may be revealed.

Six months is the average time for return of function, but with many injuries, especially incomplete injuries, the client may recover some functioning as late as 18 months after the injury. In very rare cases, people with SCI will regain some functioning years after the injury. Only a very small fraction of clients recover all functioning.

Secondary Problems

In addition to the problems listed below, a person with a SCI is at risk of all the secondary problems reviewed in "Consequences of Inactivity" in the Concepts section.

- *Respiratory problems*: Clients who have a spinal cord injury above T4 are at a higher risk for developing respiratory problems, including pneumonia, atelectasis (total or partial collapse of the lung), and aspiration. This can be the result of poor cough reflex and poor sitting posture that decreases the depth of the client's breathing. Air passages start to shut down and bacteria begin to grow.
- *Heterotopic ossification* (HO): HO is the overgrowth of bone in primary joints that frequently occurs after a fracture. It causes pain and decreases movement, often resulting in joint fusion. Surgery may be necessary. Preventative measures include active and passive range of motion programs and activities that promote functional range (e.g., adaptive Tai Chi).
- *Spasticity*: Nerve cells below the level of injury are partially or fully disconnected from the brain. When nerves below the level of injury are stimulated (pain, stretching, annoying external stimuli), the sensation is transmitted to the spinal cord. Because of the disconnection with the brain, spinal cord reflexes will cause muscles to contract. Spasticity is also triggered by bladder or kidney infection and skin breakdown. Minor stimulation can cause severe spasticity in a client who has limited flexibility. Prevention measures include a regular range of motion exercise program and avoiding triggers (e.g., bladder/kidney infection, skin breakdown). Medication may be necessary to control spasticity. Spasticity, however, also has an up side. It helps to maintain muscle size, bone strength, and circulation. Spasticity can also help with performing certain tasks where increased rigidity can be advantageous (e.g., performing transfers), as well as serve as a warning sign for other problems (e.g., bladder or kidney infection, skin breakdown). Therefore, spasticity is only treated when it interferes with the client's ability to perform func-

tional tasks or interferes with basic needs (e.g., sleep).

- *Autonomic dysreflexia* (AD): Clients who have a spinal cord injury at or above the T6 level are at risk for experiencing AD. Because of the disconnection between the brain and the spinal cord, stimuli can cause severely high blood pressure resulting in a stroke. Any stimulus that causes pain or discomfort below the level of injury can trigger AD. Most common are full bladders, bowel impaction, annoying external stimuli, bladder infections, pressure sores, and medical tests or procedures. Clients who are experiencing AD will complain of symptoms that are directly related to the rise in blood pressure such as severe headaches and vision problems. The client will become flushed and sweat profusely or develop goose bumps. Should a client experience AD, the therapist should immediately call for assistance and begin a search to find the cause of the problem (e.g., kinked catheter line, tight belt) and remove it if possible. Because of the potential severity of the situation, medical assistance and corrective actions must be immediate. A recreational therapist who takes clients into the community must know the proper procedures for dealing with AD including how to catheterize and evacuate a client's bowels. Waiting until an ambulance comes or until returning to the unit may be too late. Clients should be taught how to take preventative measures (e.g., regular bowel and bladder routine, awareness of external stimuli, regular skin checks), as well as how to recognize AD signs and access medical assistance. AD is not often seen by paramedics, so the client should carry a card that states his/her susceptibility to AD, the causes, and treatment procedures.
- *Neuropathic/spinal cord pain*: Clients can experience nerve-generated pain (aching, sharp stabbing pain, phantom limb pain). Medication and nerve block procedures can be helpful. Other alternative approaches have also been found to be somewhat helpful (e.g., relaxation techniques).
- *Bowel and bladder dysfunction*: See b610-b639 Urinary Functions. See b525 Defecation Functions.
- *Sexual dysfunction*: See b640 Sexual Functions.
- *Sweating*: Spinal cord injury paralyzes sweating in dermatomes below the injury level. Consequently, clients must be very careful to maintain their body temperatures, avoiding getting too hot. In contrast to loss of sweating below the injury site, many people with spinal cord injury may have abnormal increases of sweating above

the injury site, often in their upper torso and face. This is a form of autonomic hyper-excitability or spasticity. It is not unusual for people to sweat profusely on one side of the face and not the other. Such abnormal sweating responses may develop early or late after injury.

Assessments

Typical Scope of Team Assessment

The client's level and type of injury are re-evaluated on a regular basis to determine the client's most current functional level. Each rehab team member conducts an assessment of the client. Outcomes from each assessment are discussed with the team and a team treatment plan is developed to maximize the client's independence, quality of life, and function.

Anticipated Findings from RT Assessment

Spinal cord injuries are generally a result of accidents; so the therapist can assume that the client and family are unaware of the physical, emotional, financial, and social problems associated with these injuries. The client often reports feelings of being on overload. There are large amounts of information to learn in a short length of time when the client has barely begun to come to grips with what has happened and how s/he is going to deal with all these changes. It is normal for the client to exhibit signs of grieving and difficulty coping. Consequently behavioral issues (due to poor coping skills) and clinical features of depression and anxiety are common. Assess whether the client knows about adaptive equipment, recreational activities, accessibility, resources, community services, transportation options, etc. Also assess the client's perceptions of disability, such as feeling worthless, unproductive, or unlovable, making it difficult to identify and solve barriers.

Treatment Direction

Whole Team Approach

The primary purpose of treatment is to
- stabilize the client
- enhance function though skill development and adaptive equipment
- reduce the chance of secondary medical problems.

By achieving these three goals the client is likely to have an improved quality of life. The average length of stay for inpatient rehabilitation varies from three to six weeks.

The spinal cord injury team must function as a cohesive group due to the amount of information and skills that must be addressed and incorporated into real-life settings. Many SCI teams have a checklist of information that must be reviewed, taught, and mastered by the client. Therapists are assigned particular areas from the checklist. These areas then become the responsibility of the therapist to complete prior to the client's discharge. The goal is for the client to return home and be able to function safely.

Recreational Therapy Approach

Same as Whole Team Approach with specific interventions listed below. It is not uncommon for a recreational therapist to have 10-15 objectives to accomplish in only nine to twelve contact hours.

Recreational Therapy Interventions

Interventions that are frequently implemented for clients who have had a SCI include:

Functional Skill Development

- *Stress*: See d240 Handling Stress and Other Psychological Demands and "Relaxation and Stress Reduction" and "Coping with Stress" in the Techniques section.
- *Movement and mobility*: The client must stay active to keep fitness levels, deep breathing, and range of motion. See Body Functions Chapter 7 Neuromusculoskeletal and Movement Related Functions, A&P Chapter 4 Mobility, and "Activity Pattern Development" in the Techniques section.
- *Adaptive skills*: Clients learn basic adaptation and modification skills for recreational, home, and community activities as they relate to their functional abilities. See d155 Acquiring Skills.

Education/Counseling

Many lifestyle topics may need to be covered with the client. They include:

- "Community Problem Solving," "Americans with Disabilities Act Education," "Lifestyle Alteration Education," "Emergency Response Training," "Relaxation and Stress Reduction," "Coping with Stress," and "Skin Breakdown" in the Techniques section.
- "Consequences of Inactivity," "Self-esteem," and "Maslow's Hierarchy of Needs" in the Concepts section.
- b640 Sexual Functions for sexuality education.

Integration

Clients are integrated into their real-life environments. Recreational therapists assess a client's ability to carry over learned skills into real-life environments and teach new or re-designed skills as needed. In addition to the above topics, therapists include the development of social skills (A&P Chapter 7 Interpersonal Interactions and Relationships), self-care in community settings (A&P Chapter 5 Self-Care), d610 Acquisition of Goods and Services, d910 Community Life, and d920 Recreation and Leisure.

Miscellaneous

American Spinal Injury Association
345 East Superior Ave, Room 1436
Chicago, IL 60611
312-238-1242
http://www.asia-spinalinjury.org

National Spinal Cord Injury Association (NSCIA)
870 Georgia Ave, Ste 500
Silver Spring, MD 20910
800-962-9629
nscia2@aol.com
http://www.spinalcord.org

National Spinal Cord Injury Hotline
2200 Kernan Dr.
Baltimore, MD 21207
800-526-3456
SCIHOTLINE@aol.com
http://scihotline.org

Paralyzed Veterans of America
801 18th St NW,
Washington, DC 20006
800-424-8200
info@pva.org
http://www.pva.org

References

Crepeau, E., Cohn, E., & Schell, B. (2003). *Willard and Spackman's occupational therapy*. Philadelphia, PA: Lippincott Williams & Wilkins.

Kerr, D. (2001). "Transverse myelitis" in *Current therapy in neurologic disease*, (6th ed.). Mosby Press: NA http://www.myelitis.org/Kerr-Current%20therapy%20chapter%20with%20figures.pdf on 2/28/04.

National Spinal Cord Injury Association. (2004). http://www.spinalcord.org on 2/28/04.

O'Sullivan, S. & Schmitz, T. (1988). *Physical rehabilitation: Assessment and treatment*, (2nd ed.). Philadelphia, PA: F.A. Davis Company.

Young, W. (2003). *Acute spinal cord injury*. Rutgers University: http://carecure.rutgers.edu/spinewire/Articles/AcuteSCI/AcuteSCI.htm on 2/28/04.

Substance-Related Disorders

Substance-related disorders are a broad category of related medical problems caused by substances such as alcohol or drugs. In health care, substance-related disorders are divided into four primary categories: 1. substance intoxication, 2. substance withdrawal, 3. substance abuse, and 4. substance dependence.

- *Substance intoxication*: The ingestion of an intoxicating substance in high enough quantities to cause measurable changes in functional behavior as a result of the substance's impact on the client's central nervous system. Intoxication is usually relatively short-lived (hours or days). The functional changes include impairment of emotional regulation, decreased ability to cognitively process information, impaired executive function, and decreased social and occupational capability.
- *Substance withdrawal*: Symptoms associated with reducing the intake of a substance that has been used heavily and for a relatively long period of time. The symptoms must be significant enough to negatively impact function in one or more areas. The length of time and amount of substance use needed to experience withdrawal is influenced by the type of drug and the client's physiology. In some cases substance withdrawal can be a life-threatening situation.
- *Substance abuse*: A maladaptive pattern of substance use that leads to at least one of the following: 1. significant negative impact on major areas of living such as school, work, or home life; 2. on-going use of the substance when use could cause injury (such as drinking and driving); 3. multiple legal problems as a result of substance use; or 4. continued use of the substance when it causes problems with relationships (such as a spouse filing for divorce).
- *Substance dependence*: A maladaptive use of a substance that results in a clinically significant impairment with at least three of the following also evident: 1. physical tolerance to the substance so that an increased amount is needed to obtain the same results as before, 2. withdrawal symptoms occur when amount of substance is reduced, 3. larger amounts are used than the client intended to use, 4. there is a persistent desire for the substance, 5. a great deal of time is spent related to use of the substance, 6. important activities are given up because of the substance, and 7. the client continues to use the substance even though s/he knows it makes things worse.

The World Health Organization no longer recognizes the term addiction, having dropped the term in 1964. The therapist working in a health care setting should use the term "substance dependence" instead.

In addition to the four categories listed above, the American Psychiatric Association lists nine other substance-related disorders that it categorizes under other headings. The first four are the most common, so a description is provided. These diagnoses are identified on a client's chart only when the symptoms are severe enough to require medical intervention.

- *Substance intoxication delirium*: A change of consciousness (often seen as a noticeable decrease in a client's ability to pay attention or shift attention as the situation dictates) and a change in cognition (often seen as a relatively sudden decrease in memory function) that occurs over a short period of time and seems to be related to substance use. The decreased function tends to fluctuate and develops over a matter of hours or days. One of the key criteria for substance intoxication delirium is that the loss of consciousness and cognition is greater than would be expected from the substance alone.
- *Substance withdrawal delirium*: A type of delirium associated with the body's response to withdrawal of a substance. The symptoms are the same as described under substance intoxication delirium; the cause of the delirium is different.
- *Substance-induced persisting dementia*: A dementia that is linked to substance abuse and remains long after the client has stopped using and no longer has physiological effects of withdrawal. It is not related to delirium. The client has a persisting memory deficit and at least one other cognitive impairment. Some improvement may be seen after abstaining from substance use. However, the prognosis is not good for significant return of cognitive ability. Substance-induced persisting dementia is usually seen in clients who have a long history of substance use.
- *Substance-induced persisting amnestic disorder*: A history of substance abuse and the inability to remember new information or recall past information (amnestic disorder), which are likely related to each other, is considered substance-induced persisting amnestic disorder. This inability to remember or recall is not related to dementia or delirium. The impairment must be significant enough to cause the client to not be

able to function independently at work, home, or in the community. Substance-Induced Persisting Amnestic Disorder is often known by two other names: Wernicke's encephalopathy and Korsakoff's syndrome. Wernicke's encephalopathy is an acute, early stage substance-induced disorder that, with treatment, offers a good chance of some recovery. Symptoms include unsteady gait, problems with balance, and abnormal eye movements. Treatment includes abstaining from substance use, daily doses of thiamine, and good nutrition. Korsakoff's syndrome is considered to be a progression from Wernicke's. The symptoms become chronic, usually irreversible and lead to death.

- *Substance-induced psychotic disorder*
- *Substance-induced mood disorder*
- *Substance-induced anxiety disorder*
- *Substance-induced sexual dysfunction*
- *Substance-induced sleep disorder*

There are some other key phrases that are often used as part of the diagnosis and treatment documentation. These are listed below.
- With physiological dependence
- Without physiological dependence
- Early full remission
- Early partial remission
- Sustained full remission
- Sustained partial remission
- On agonist therapy
- In a controlled environment
- Codependence
- Enabling
- Denial

The United States Government collects data on drug trends in eleven different drug categories as part of the National Institute on Drug Abuse (NIDA) Epidemiologic Trends in Drug Abuse report.

Incidence/Prevalence in US

In a 2000 survey (Substance Abuse and Mental Health Services Administration, 2000) approximately 40% of the US population reported using one or more illicit substances in their lifetime, 15% reported using illicit substances within the past year, and 6.3% (or 14 million people) reported using illicit substances at least once during the 30 days before the 2000 survey interview.

The survey found that almost half (46.6% or 104 million Americans age 12 and older) reported being current drinkers. Men are more likely to be binge drinkers than women. Men also have higher rates of alcohol dependency. The higher the educational

level, the more likely the current use of alcohol. Ten percent of those surveyed said that they had driven a vehicle under the influence of alcohol (Sadock & Sadock, 2003).

Among illicit substances, marijuana was found to be the most commonly used (59% of all users reported using marijuana only, 17% of all users reported using marijuana and another illicit substance, and the remaining 24% of users reported using illicit substances other than marijuana). The lower the level of education, the more likely is the current use of illicit drugs (Substance Abuse and Mental Health Services Administration, 2000).

Predominant Age

- *Illicit drug use*: Approximately 23% of individuals age 12 to 17 use illicit drugs, compared to 48% of individuals age 18-25, 53% of individuals age 26-34, and 29% of individuals age 35 or older.
- *Alcohol use*: Approximately 39% of individuals age 12-17 use alcohol, compared to 84% of individuals age 18-25, 90% of individuals age 26-34, and 88% of individuals age 35 or older. Approximately 7% of individuals age 12-17 reported binge drinking within the previous month, compared to 32% of individuals age 18-25, 23% of individual 26-34, and 11% of individuals age 35 and older.

Causes

- *Psychodynamic theories*: Substance use may be related to depression, poor coping skills, and/or societal and cultural pressures. Psychodynamic approaches are mostly used with clients with substance abuse rather than clients with alcohol abuse. "In contrast to alcoholic patients, clients with polysubstance abuse are more likely to have had an unstable childhood, more likely to self-medicate with substances, and more likely to benefit from psychotherapy" (Sadock & Sadock, 2003, p. 387). Considerable research links personality disorders with the development of substance dependence.
- *Behavioral theories*: Substances produce a positive effect that acts as a positive reinforcement for substance-seeking behavior. Alcohol may be used as a coping mechanism for dealing with stress, anger, or pain. Alcohol consumption may also be socially encouraged in some environments.
- *Genetic factors*: A child who has a parent with an alcohol use problem has a four times greater risk of having an alcohol use problem even if the

child is not raised by the parents and is exposed to different environmental factors.

- *Neurochemical factors*: Particular neurotransmitters, neurotransmitter receptors, and pathways of the brain are affected by substance use. Defects in neurotransmitter functions may make the client more prone to illicit drug dependence.

Systems Affected

Alcohol intoxication can cause irritability, violent behavior, feelings of depression, and, in rare instances, hallucinations and delusions. It also interferes with sleep quality (multiple awakenings during the sleep cycle resulting in decreased deep sleep). Longer term, escalating levels of alcohol consumption can produce tolerance as well as such intense adaptation of the body that stopping can cause a withdrawal syndrome marked by a minimum of insomnia, evidence of hyperactivity of the autonomic nervous system, and feelings of anxiety. Long-term alcohol abuse can result in worse symptoms, as discussed above.

The blood alcohol level is used as an international standard for alcohol intoxication (Sadock & Sadock, 2003).

- At a level of 0.05% alcohol in the blood thought, judgment, and restraint are loosened and sometimes disrupted.
- At 0.1% voluntary motor actions usually become perceptible clumsy.
- In most states, legal intoxication ranges from 0.08-0.15% blood alcohol level.
- At 0.2% functions of the entire motor area of the brain are measurably depressed and the parts of the brain that control emotional behavior are also affected.
- At 0.3% a person is commonly confused or may become stuporous (slow to react and in a confused state).
- At 0.4-0.5% the person falls into a coma. At higher levels, the primitive centers of the brain that control breathing and heart rate are affected, and death ensues secondary to direct respiratory depression or the aspiration of vomit.
- Clients with long-term histories of alcohol abuse can tolerate much higher concentrations of alcohol than alcohol-naïve persons. Their alcohol tolerance may cause them to appear less intoxicated than they really are.

Systems affected by the abuse or dependence on illicit drugs can include all body structures, functions, and life activities depending upon the substances and the extent of their use. For further information see *A Primer of Drug Action: A Concise, Non-technical Guide to the Actions, Uses, and Side Effects of Psychoactive Drugs, 6th edition* written by Robert M. Julien, MD.

Prognosis

Alcohol

- Alcohol abuse reduces life expectancy by about 10 years.
- Approximately 10-40% enter a formal treatment program during the course of their alcohol dependence. About 60% of those who enter and complete rehabilitation will maintain abstinence for one or more years if they meet the following criteria: no antisocial personality disorder, no other substance abuse or dependence, no severe legal problems, general life stability, a job, close family contacts, motivation to stay sober, and a good support system (Sadock & Sadock, 2003).

Illicit Drugs

- The prognosis for recovery or improved functioning for people with illicit drug abuse or dependence is not clear. Outcomes are influenced by many variables such as the type of program, quality and comprehensive nature of the program, client's readiness to change, extent of dependency, other health conditions of the client, job skills, level of life satisfaction, coping mechanisms, and environmental factors such as level of support (Sadock & Sadock, 2003).

Secondary Problems

Codependence: Often clients cannot continue to survive in the community without unhealthy support (pathological interdependencies) from family members and friends. Family members and friends share certain characteristic behaviors that enable the client to remain dependent on substances. This may include lying for the client in order to 1. protect him/her or 2. shelter other family members.

Physical, mental, and social health: Substance abuse or dependence can affect many body structures and functions, as well as activities and participation. The extent of dysfunction will depend on the specific substance and the extent of its use.

Antisocial personality disorder: Approximately 35-60% of clients with substance abuse or substance dependence also meet the diagnostic criteria for antisocial personality disorder. If a person has substance abuse and antisocial personality disorder, the person is more likely to use illegal drugs, have more psychopathology, have less life satisfaction, and be more impulsive, isolated, and depressed than people with antisocial personality disorder alone.

Depression and suicide: About 40% of clients diagnosed with alcohol abuse or dependence and about 30-50% of those with opioid abuse or dependence meet the criteria for Major Depressive Disorder within their lifetime. This is more than double the average prevalence of around 15%. Clients who abuse substances are 20 times more likely to die by suicide than the general population. About 15% of clients with alcohol abuse or dependence commit suicide. See "Suicide and Suicidal Ideation" in the Diagnosis section for more information.

Assessment

Typical Scope of Team Assessment

The *DSM-IV-TR* has specific criteria for dependence, abuse, intoxication, withdrawal, and specific substance induced disorders for many substances including alcohol; amphetamines; caffeine; cannabis; cocaine; hallucinogens; inhalants; nicotine; opioids; phencyclidine; sedative, hypnotic, or anxiolytic drugs (such as benzodiazephines, barbiturates); anabolic steroids; and other substance-related disorders. The team will assess the strength of the substance-related disorder and other physical, social, and emotional deficits caused by the disorder.

Anticipated Findings from RT Assessment

The findings will vary depending upon the specific substance used, the presentation of the client, and identified goals. In general, therapists will see impaired physical and mental health, impaired social skills, unhealthy leisure choices that revolve around substance use, and maladaptive coping mechanisms.

Treatment Direction

Not everyone with a substance abuse or dependence disorder needs intensive therapy. However, clients who have a severe substance abuse or dependence that impacts their ability to function usually require a high degree of professional intervention. "The best treatment programs combine specific procedures and disciplines to meet the needs of the individual patient after a careful assessment" (Sadock & Sadock, 2003, p. 388).

Whole Team Approach

A general and broad approach to treatment of substance abuse or dependence includes three steps: intervention, detoxification, and rehabilitation.

- *Intervention*: An intervention is a process that makes it clear to the client that his/her substance use is causing harm to self and others. The intervention may be social, legal, medical, or psychiatric. A formal intervention enlists the enablers of the substance user to show the user the harm his/her use causes and collapse the support system. The related idea of a "confrontation" is not as effective at breaking through the user's defenses or at removing the supports that allow continued substance use (Lucas, 2005). Family members and friends must learn to allow the client to suffer the consequences of substance use to give the client the energy and the motivation necessary to stop.
- *Detoxification*: The process for detoxification will vary depending on the specific substance, but the end result is to have the client's body free and clean of the substance.
- *Rehabilitation*: The depth and length of a rehabilitation program will vary depending on the needs of the client (e.g., short-term outpatient, several month inpatient). The goal of rehabilitation is to teach the client needed skills to stay substance free and successfully integrate into the community as a functioning person. One important form of rehabilitation is involvement in a 12-step program such as Alcoholics or Narcotics Anonymous. Other programs to provide a healthy, substance-free community for the client can also be used.

Recreational Therapy Approach

Recreational therapists who work in community settings such as the Boys and Girls Club may participate in an intervention. The usual role is in rehabilitation.

Recreational Therapy Interventions

Common recreational therapy interventions for clients with substance abuse/dependence include:
- *Social skills training*: Often people who abuse or become dependent on substances feel that they cannot relate to other people unless they are using a substance. They may also lack appropriate social skills, which may have been a motivator for substance use (e.g., "If I drink, people will like me"). Social skill development is often retarded by substance use, so clients will need to learn the skills that they missed. These issues are covered in A&P Chapter 7 Interpersonal Interactions and Relationships. and some of the ideas in "Social Skills Training" in the Techniques section.

- *Coping with stress*: Start by looking at d240 Handling Stress and Other Psychological Demands. Therapists may use a variety of the approaches described there. The therapist will also want to be sure that the client is involved in activities that meet client needs (A&P Chapter 9 Community, Social, and Civic Life). Activities that may be well accepted include those that offer a feeling of excitement such as adventure-based activities that can be realistically carried over into the client's real life.

- *Temperament and personality functions*: People who abuse or have become dependent on substances often lack the skills of cooperation (b1261 Agreeableness) and trust (b1267 Trust-worthiness). These skills are essential for recovery and sobriety in order to initiate, engage, and fully benefit from social support (from people and/or higher power). Being confident, self-assured, and assertive (b1266 Confidence) is also important to assist with saying "No," avoiding slippery situations, and empowering the client to seek out and engage in more positive leisure experiences. Specific interventions are described under b126 Temperament and Person-ality Functions.

- *Spirituality*: Spirituality as discussed in 12-step programs can be a helpful intervention for recreational therapy. See d930 Religion and Spirituality for details. A search to find purpose and meaning in life may help. See Existential Counseling in "Education and Counseling" in the Techniques section.

- *Social support*: Social support is a vital component for long-term rehabilitation. Thera-pists assist the client in identifying people in his/her life that can offer positive social support and teach the client needed social skills to actively seek out assistance when needed. See A&P Chapter 7 Interpersonal Interactions and Relationships. Therapist should also consider recommending involvement in a 12-step pro-gram as appropriate for support.

- *Environmental changes*: The therapist assists clients in finding external factors that promote use of substances (e.g., groups of friends, environmental triggers) and problem solves for how to avoid these temptations. Solving prob-lems can be scored under d175 Solving Prob-lems. The use of Environmental Factors codes in Chapter 3 Support and Relationships and Chapter 4 Attitudes can be helpful.

- *Healthy leisure*: A person who has a history of substance abuse or dependence often has a pattern of leisure activities that revolves around substance use (e.g., going to the bar, hanging out on the corner). A new understanding of leisure and leisure values will need to be addressed (see "Education and Counseling" in the Techniques section). Exploration and identification of healthy leisure activities that fit in the client's real life, along with the development of skills for successful participation, are required. See "Personal Leisure Resource Awareness," "Community Leisure Resource Awareness," and "Activity Pattern Development" in the Techniques section for more information. When addressing leisure skill development, score d155 Acquiring Skills. When addressing issues related to leading a healthy leisure lifestyle, score d570 Looking After One's Health.

- *Self-esteem*: Some clients may find that they do not like themselves when not under the influence of a substance because they think a substance user is who they are. They need to learn to be another type of person. See "Self-Esteem" in the Techniques section.

References

Bailey-Spielman, M. & Blaschko, T. (1998). Healthy caring. In F. Brasile, T. Skalko, & j. burlingame. *Perspectives in recreational therapy; Issues of a dynamic profession.* Ravensdale, WA: Idyll Arbor, Inc.

burlingame (2001). *Idyll Arbor's therapy dictionary, 2nd edition.* Ravensdale, WA: Idyll Arbor, Inc.

Deiser, R. & Voight, A. (1998). Therapeutic recreation and relapse prevention intervention. *Parks & Recreation, 33*(5).

Hood, C. (2003). Women in recovery from alcoholism: The place of leisure. *Leisure Sciences, 25*:51-79.

Julien, R. (1992). *A primer of drug action: A concise, non-technical guide to the actions, uses, and side effects of psychoactive drugs, 6th edition.* New York, New York: W. H. Freeman and Company.

Lucas, K. (2005). *Outwitting your alcoholic: Keep the loving and stop the drinking.* Ravensdale, WA: Idyll Arbor, Inc.

Malkin, M. & Benshoff, J. (1996). Therapeutic recreation interventions in substance abuse treatment programs. *Parks and Recreation, 31*(10): 26-29.

Nation, J., Benshoff, J., & Malkin, M. (1996). Therapeutic recreation programs for adolescents in substance abuse treatment facilities. *Journal of Rehabilitation,* Oct/Nov/Dec 1996, 10-16.

Sadock, B. & Sadock, V. (2003). *Kaplan & Sadock's synopsis of psychiatry, 9th edition.* New York, New York: Lippincott Williams & Wilkins.

Substance Abuse and Mental Health Services Administration. (2000). National Survey on Drug Use & Health. http://oas.samhsa.gov/nsduh.htm.

Suicide and Suicidal Ideation

Suicide is the act of killing oneself and suicidal ideation is the perseveration of thought of killing oneself. Suicide is often associated with mood disorders and is most prevalent in adolescents and the elderly. Suicidal ideation may be a passing impulse or a phenomenon that is long-standing with the individual having spent a lot of thought about potential actions. Suicidal ideation is similar to, but not the same as, suicidal gestures or attempts.

Incidence/Prevalence in US

The Centers for Disease Control (2004) report:
- Suicide took the lives of 29,350 Americans in 2000.
- More people die from suicide than from homicide. In 2000, there were 1.7 times as many suicides as homicides.
- Overall, suicide is the 11th leading cause of death for all Americans.
- For young people, 15-24 years old, suicide is the third leading cause of death, behind unintentional injury and homicide.
- Males are more than four times as likely to die from suicide as females. However, females are more likely to attempt suicide than males.
- 57% of suicides in 2000 were committed with a firearm.
- Suicide rates among the elderly are highest for those who are divorced or widowed.
- Risk factors for suicide among older clients differ from those among the young. Older clients have a higher prevalence of depression, more social isolation, and are more likely to use highly lethal methods. They also make fewer attempts per completed suicide, have a higher-male-to-female ratio than other groups, have often visited a health-care provider before their suicide, and have more physical illnesses.
- In 2000, more than 264,000 persons were treated for nonfatal, self-inflicted injuries in hospital emergency departments; 60% were probable suicide attempts.

Predominant Age

- Suicide rates increase with age and are highest among Americans aged 65 years and older. The ten-year period, 1980-1990, was the first decade since the 1940s that the suicide rate for older clients rose instead of declined.
- Persons under age 25 accounted for 15% of all suicides in 2000. From 1952 to 1995, the incidence of suicide among adolescents and young adults nearly tripled.

Causes

Often the cause is a combination of psychiatric distress or mental illness and circumstances associated with social situations or relationships. For example, 50% of completed suicides are associated with major depression or bipolar disorders, 25% of completed suicides are associated with substance abuse disorders, and 10% of completed suicides are associated with schizophrenia and other psychotic disorders (Dambro, 1998).

Systems(s) Affected

N/A

Prognosis

Around 15% of individuals who are suicidal with an underlying depression will end up being successful in killing themselves.

Signs and Symptoms

Suicide can be prevented. In most cases, there are warning signs that someone is contemplating a suicide attempt. The most effective way to prevent suicide is to recognize the warning signs, take them seriously, and know how to respond to them.

The warning signs are
- Talking about suicide.
- Always talking or thinking about death.
- Making comments about being hopeless, helpless, or worthless.
- Saying things like "It would be better if I wasn't here" or "I want out."
- Depression (deep sadness, loss of interest, trouble sleeping and eating) that gets worse.
- A sudden, unexpected switch from being very sad to being very calm or appearing to be happy.
- Having a "death wish," tempting fate by taking risks that could lead to death, like driving fast or through red lights.
- Losing interest in things the person used to care about.
- Visiting or calling people to say goodbye.
- Putting affairs in order, tying up lose ends, changing a will.

Be especially concerned if a person is exhibiting any of these warning signs and has attempted suicide in the past. According to the American Foundation for Suicide Prevention, 20-50% of people who commit suicide have had a previous attempt (The Cleveland Clinic, 2004).

Assessments

Typical Scope of Team Assessment

If an individual is thought to be suicidal, additional screening should take place. The health care community often uses a variety of methods to decide if an individual is at risk of taking his/her own life. This includes directly asking the individual if s/he is considering suicide and using a scale such as the SAD PERSON risk assessment. An individual should be considered at a high risk for suicide if s/he has at least five of the following risk factors: **S:** sex, **A:** age, **D:** depression, **P:** previous attempt, **E:** ethanol abuse, **R:** rational thinking loss, **S:** social support loss, **O:** organized plan, **N:** no spouse, **S:** sickness.

Anticipated Findings by RT

- In addition to mental illness or substance abuse risks, individuals who are single (including divorced or widowed), have a recent history of loss (loved one, job, social supports), and have an important date coming up (holiday, anniversary, birthday) are at an increased risk. This type of information often is discovered during the assessment process.
- Clients who are at risk of taking their own lives also tend to demonstrate obvious levels of helplessness, poor problem solving skills, and aggressive behavior while participating in activities.
- While not tested by formal clinical studies, empirical reports indicate that a score of "one" in the subscale "Meaning of Life" on the Free Time Boredom may be an indicator of a risk of suicide.

Treatment Direction

Whole Team Approach

- Provide a reasonable level of safety in the least restrictive environment. This includes removing objects that the individual can use to harm himself/herself and an appropriate level of observation, which may include two- or four-point restraints.
- Address underlying mental illness, substance abuse, or loss of support as appropriate.
- A behavioral contract between the treatment team and the client that states the client will not harm himself/herself.

- Typically an individual who is physically restrained is released from the restraints for ten to fifteen minutes per hour. Treatment may include appropriate types of stretching exercises to music or similar activity during this time. The RT may provide this service or provide ideas and supplies to the staff assigned to supervise the individual during these release times.

Recreational Therapy Approach

Recreational therapy supports the team approach, especially in the areas of protecting the client from hurting himself/herself:
- RT interventions must be fully supportive of the suicide precautions outlined by the physician and treatment team.
- The therapist should ensure that therapy or activity locations do not provide an opportunity to jump. Jumping is the most common method of suicide for individuals hospitalized for depression.
- Any supplies that the client might use to harm himself/herself are contraindicated. Typically any string-like object cannot be more than 7" long. Objects that might be used as a means to cut the skin or impale the body or objects that can be used to choke are prohibited.

Recreational Therapy Interventions

- *Coping skills*: See "Coping with Stress" and "Adjustment to Disability" in the Techniques section. Code with d240 Handling Stress and Other Psychological Demands.
- *Anger management trio*: Teach 1. relaxation techniques, 2. cognitive therapy, and 3. skill development. See "Anger Management," "Relaxation and Stress Reduction," and "Education and Counseling" in the Techniques section.
- *Physical exercise*: Engaging in physical exercise can help alleviate feelings of depression. Code with d240 Handling Stress and Other Psychological Demands and d5701 Managing Diet and Fitness.
- *Problems solving*: Teach what to do if feelings of suicide arise after discharge from the program. Code as d175 Solving Problems.

Miscellaneous

Suicide is not a random act but an action based on what the client perceives as his/her best course of action given the circumstances. The client often feels an intense and unbearable need to escape from the situation and can see only a narrow set of options available. Most often when a person is suicidal, s/he appears very depressed, sad, and often lethargic. However, this is not always the case.

In some individuals, once they have selected a course of action, the intense feeling of helplessness lifts and they appear happier even though they still fully intend to kill themselves. More than once, a physician has released a client for an outing with the recreational therapist, only to have the client successfully carry out the suicide plan on the outing. When taking clients who have been recently released from suicide precautions on outings, the therapist should still informally implement some precautions such as one-on-one supervision, avoiding locations that provide the opportunity to jump, and eliminating the availability of sharp objects.

References

Centers for Disease Control, National Center for Injury Prevention and Control. (2004). www.cdc.gove/ncipc/factsheets/sicfacts.htm, 1/15/04

Dambro, M. R. (1998). *Griffith's 5 minute clinical consultant*. Baltimore, MD: Williams & Wilkins.

The Cleveland Clinic. (2004). http://www.clevelandclinic.org/health/health-info/docs/3300/3342.asp?index=11352.

Traumatic Brain Injury

A traumatic brain injury occurs from a direct trauma to the brain. This includes penetrating or missile injuries (e.g., gunshot wound) and non-penetrating brain injuries (closed head injury). Health care professionals sometimes misuse the term "head injury" when they are really talking about a traumatic brain injury. Head injury is when there is an injury to a client's head (e.g., laceration of the forehead) and traumatic brain injury is when there is an injury to a client's brain caused by a traumatic event (e.g., motor vehicle accident resulting in diffuse brain injury). There may or may not be a TBI from a head injury. One confusing term is "closed head injury." It means a non-penetrating brain injury. (Cerebrovascular accidents are another kind of injury to the brain, but they are very different from TBIs.) The most common types of TBIs include:

Depressed skull fracture: Bony fragments of the skull press against the brain causing damage to a focal area of the brain.

Acceleration-deceleration injury or shearing injury: This type of injury is caused when the body is traveling at a high speed and then comes to an abrupt stop (e.g., motor vehicle accident, fall). It results in a widespread brain injury to many of the axons in many parts of the brain. (See "Nervous System" in the Concepts section for a discussion of brain structure.) Injury to axons leads to a breakdown of communication within the brain and less effective processing for the connections that remain. There are three reaction movements that occur during acceleration-deceleration events:

- The direct impact of the brain and skull (e.g., from when the head hits the dashboard) causes a focal (localized) brain injury. This is usually a contusion on the frontal lobes of the brain.
- The impact bounces the brain around within the skull causing more contusions.
- After the brain tissue slams against the inside of the skull at impact, a bounce-back motion occurs. This motion throws the head and brain in the opposite direction, causing a second bruise on the opposite side of the brain. This is referred to as a "coup-contrecoup" injury (one side to the other side). This results in bruising with a great deal of local damage along with tearing and stretching throughout the rest of the brain.

Shaken baby syndrome: When a baby is forcibly shaken, it causes coup-contrecoup damage to the brain.

Concussion: This is when a client loses consciousness or feels dazed and confused after a blow to the head. Concussion can be mild or severe and symptoms of brain injury might not show up for days after the injury. Impairments can be subtle or they can require urgent attention. Signs of concussion include: headaches that get worse; numbness, weakness, and decreased coordination; repeated vomiting; difficulty with cognition; cannot be awakened; one pupil larger than the other; blurry vision; convulsions or seizures; slurred speech; and restlessness, agitation, and confusion. If the client is a child, also look for crying that won't subside, refusal to eat or nurse, inability to be consoled, listless behavior, change in play or school behavior, lack of interest in favorite toys, loss of new skills (using the toilet), or change in sleep patterns.

The criteria established by the Traumatic Brain Injury Model Systems states that for someone to have a TBI, one of the following has occurred (Novack, 1999a):

- A documented loss of consciousness. The length of time is not indicated. It can be brief or long.
- Amnesia of the event. This means they cannot recall the actual traumatic event.
- A Glasgow Coma Scale (GCS) score of less than 15 during the first 24 hours. See "Glasgow Coma Scale" in the Assessment section for more information.

Incidence/Prevalence in US

It is estimated that 2.5 to 6.5 million Americans are living today with a TBI-related disability. Approximately 1.5 to 2 million people a year sustain a TBI. TBI is the leading cause of long-term disability for children and young adults (NIH, 1998).

Predominant Age

National Institutes of Health (1998) state that the highest incidence of TBI occurs between 15 and 24 years of age and over 70, with an additional, less striking incidence in children five and under. Males are twice as likely as females to experience a TBI.

Causes

There are no bodily warning signs to indicate that a traumatic brain injury is about to occur since it is caused by an outside force. However, a keen awareness of safety may alert a client to the increased possibility of injury and therefore be encouraged to take an action (e.g., child riding bike on bumpy ground without a helmet, adult instructs child to put on a helmet). Traumatic brain injury is largely preventable.

- Half of all TBIs are related to alcohol use.
- Fifty percent of all TBIs are due to motor vehicle accidents, bicycle, or pedestrian-vehicle incidents.
- Falls are the second greatest cause of TBI for older adults and young children. For older adults, falls are typically due to medication, osteoporosis, or alcohol. For young children, falling out of strollers, walkers, or shopping carts are leading causes of TBI.
- Approximately 20% of TBIs are violence related. Clients between the age of 15 and 24 are at the highest risk for both firearm and non-firearm assaults.
- Seventy-five percent of TBIs of children five and under are unintentional. However, abuse is a factor that needs to be considered. This includes "shaken baby syndrome" and other physical abuse.
- Three percent of TBIs are due to sporting injuries. It is estimated that 90% are mild TBIs, so this number may be severely underestimated because many injuries go undetected or untreated. Clients between the age of five and 24 are at greatest risk. Boxing is known to cause brain damage from repeated blows. Currently, soccer is being looked at because of its head-drills (hitting the ball with the head) that may cause repeated small TBIs leading to problems with attention, concentration, problem solving, and reasoning. Although it is unproven, therapists who work in sports should be aware of these issues and keep abreast of new research and literature (www.headinjury.com is a good source).

System(s) Affected

The brain controls and regulates voluntary and involuntary body functions, so there can be a wide spectrum of dysfunction. Outside of the array of physical impairments (e.g., coordination, strength, balance), cognitive, social, and emotional impairments arise. These include problems with alertness, arousal, impaired vision, processing of auditory information, attention, concentration, word-finding, explaining complex ideas in a logical fashion, judging distances, memory, reasoning, problem solving, restlessness, agitation, frustration tolerance, lability, irritability, confabulation, insight, impulsivity, socially inappropriate behavior, initiative, flat affect, paranoia, blaming others for negative events, depression, and anxiety (Novack, 1999b).

Prognosis

The depth and length of a coma, and the length of post-traumatic amnesia are used as a general predictor of the long-term outcomes of brain injury. There are two types of post-traumatic amnesia (PTA): anterograde PTA is impaired memory of events that happened after the TBI and retrograde PTA is impaired memory of events that happened before the TBI. As a general rule, the longer one remains in a coma or state of post-traumatic amnesia, the more severe the brain injury. Additionally, the client's abilities six months after injury are a good indication of the eventual outcome one year or several years after injury (Sandel, 1994). However, due to advances in medical technology and training, more clients are surviving severe injuries and return of function has been noted even several years after the initial injury. Other factors that influence prognosis are extent of injury, age of client, and location of injury.

In addition to the above prognostic variables, the brain's ability to adapt to injury must be considered. The brain may find different pathways to send and receive information or create new pathways. The brain will try to recover, but in order for that to happen it has to be stimulated (Novack, 1999b). In the right environment, recovery can continue for years. "Neuroplasticity" in the Techniques section has more information.

Secondary Problems

Secondary problems of a traumatic brain injury include:
- *Anoxic injury*: No oxygen getting to the brain due to heart or lung failure at the time of injury resulting in brain damage.
- *Hypoxic injury*: Reduced oxygen getting to the brain due to heart or lung dysfunction at the time of injury resulting in brain damage.
- *Hematomas*: A collection or pooling of blood that can increase intracranial pressure (ICP). Three types of hematomas can cause injury to the brain: epidural, subdural, and intracerebral hematoma. Epidural means "outside the dura," or covering of the brain (bleeding between the skull and the dura). "Subdural" means "under the dura" (bleeding between the dura and arachnoid membrane). Intracerebral means bleeding within the brain itself. ICP is controlled by surgery.
- *Infections*.
- *Edema*: swelling of the brain.

Assessment

Typical Scope of Team Assessment

Two common scales of assessment used for brain injury are the *Glasgow Coma Scale* and the *Rancho Los Amigos Scale of Cognitive Functioning*.

The *Glasgow Coma Scale* is a brief assessment of the level of consciousness and the duration of a coma. The highest possible score is a 15 and the lowest possible score is a three. A score of 13-15 is considered a mild brain injury, 9-12 a moderate brain injury, and eight or less a severe brain injury. A score of eight or less indicates that the client is in a coma. There are three subcategories in the GCS: 1. Eyes Open (EO), 2. Best Verbal Response (BVR), and 3. Best Motor Response (BMR). The score is written so that each function is described (e.g., EO4+BMR6+VR4=14). See *Glasgow Coma Scale* in the Assessment section.

The *Rancho Los Amigos Scale of Cognitive Functioning* is an eight-level scale that helps identify the cognitive level of functioning after a traumatic brain injury. It was designed to measure and track a client's recovery through behavioral observation. Rancho Los Amigos Hospital is currently testing the validity of a ten-level scale to replace the eight-level scale. Rancho Los Amigos Hospital recommends that the revised scale not be used until further validity and reliability of the tool are established (Burton, 2003).

Other assessment tools used by health professionals will vary depending upon the state of consciousness of the client. Often clinicians use observational methods within the context of an activity for evaluation, especially with clients who are agitated and restless. The *Community Integration Program* (Armstrong and Lauzen, 1994) and the *CERT-Psych/R* (Parker, 1990) are appropriate, standardized recreational therapy assessments to use for observation of a client's skills.

Anticipated Findings from RT Assessment

- Physical, cognitive, social, and emotional impairments that affect the client's ability to function optimally in a work, school, home, and community environment.
- Clients between the ages of 15 and 24 may have a history of high-risk activities.
- Overlearned leisure, social, language, and self-care skills may present outside of anticipated abilities. Overlearned skills may "shine through" even though the client has deficits in this area. Because it is overlearned, it is more automatic. For example, a client who has been involved in the hobby of woodworking for many years has problems with sequencing. Yet when presented

with a simple wood project, he is able to sequence the steps involved. A client who has expressive aphasia is able to say curse words clearly. A client who was a salesperson prior to his injury and has social skills deficits still puts out his hand for someone to shake it.

Treatment Direction

Whole Team Approach

During the initial weeks of inpatient rehabilitation, the team primarily focuses on restoration of skills through graduated tasks and repetition based on the theories of brain plasticity. The last weeks of the client's rehabilitation stay focus on transitioning the client into his/her discharge environment (e.g., community living program, at home with spouse). This includes teaching the client and caregiver (as appropriate) compensatory strategies and techniques to facilitate the recovery process post discharge.

Recreational Therapy Approach

Recreational therapy supports the team approach with the interventions described below.

Recreational Therapy Interventions

An outline of the *Rancho Los Amigos Cognitive Levels of Functioning* grouped into four different stages, along with the general treatment guidelines that accompany each stage is shown below. Note that the suggested interventions only relate to cognitive functioning. Additional treatment will need to be added for physical, visual, language, social, and/or psychological impairments. Modalities used to address dysfunction should always be activities that are going to be part of the client's activity pattern after discharge because clients with TBI often have difficulty transferring learned skills into a new context. Cognitive retraining strategies are used to promote restoration of the cognitive skills reviewed below (see Cognitive Retraining in "Neuroplasticity" in the Techniques section).

Rancho 1 (coma stage): The client at this level does not respond to sounds, sight, touch, or movement. Although it is unclear if it helps to improve cognitive function at this stage, therapists often use sensory stimulation as an intervention with clients at this level to monitor progression to the next stage.

Interventions for this stage:
- b110 Consciousness Functions.
- b156 Perceptual Functions.
- "Sensory Stimulation" in the Techniques section.

Rancho II, III (low arousal stage): Clients begin to respond to sensory stimulation. Therapists try to elicit purposeful responses and one-step direction following by providing stimuli to invoke spontaneous responses (e.g., hand a client a deck of cards to encourage "shuffling" response). Therapy is done in a quiet environment with minimal distractions.

Interventions for this stage:
- b110 Consciousness Functions.
- b156 Perceptual Functions.
- b114 Orientation Functions.
- b140 Attention Functions.
- d2100 Undertaking a Simple Task.

Rancho IV, V, VI (post-traumatic amnesia stage): Clients are disoriented and may be agitated and restless. Therapy is provided in a quiet environment with minimal distractions. The goal is to gradually improve the client's basic cognitive processes in the areas of attention, memory, and orientation. Therapy sessions start out short (e.g., two 15-minute sessions) and get longer (e.g., one 30-minute session). The therapist gently redirects the client back to the task at hand should s/he become distracted. Modalities chosen reflect the client's interests to maximize attention, motivation, and willingness to participate in the task. The therapist should be flexible within the specific modality (e.g., cards: sort cards, build a card tower, count cards, Blackjack) and change modalities as required to keep the client's attention.

Interventions for this stage:
- b114 Orientation Functions.
- b140 Attention Functions.
- d2100 Undertaking a Simple Task.
- b144 Memory Functions.
- Community Integration, especially Modules 1A — Environmental Safety, 1B — Emergency Preparedness, and 1C — Basic Survival Skills of the Community Integration Program (Armstrong & Lauzen, 1994) for clients at Levels V and above.

Rancho VII, VIII (post-confusional stage): Clients are oriented x3 (person, place, time) and do not exhibit agitation or restless behavior. Clients typically have problems with higher-level cognitive skills (problem solving, reasoning, organizing, planning, referencing, decision making) and become overloaded (decompensate) in stressful situations. The therapist addresses restoration of these skills through graduated tasks and repetition, teaching the client and family compensatory strategies to manage impairments (e.g., use of a memory book, a daily activity schedule). Integration training, family training, and social skills training are emphasized.

Interventions for this stage:
- b164 Higher Level Cognitive Functions.
- b144 Memory Functions.
- d155 Acquiring Skills.
- d160-d179 Applying Knowledge.
- d230 Carrying Out a Daily Routine.
- d710-d729 General Interpersonal Interactions
- Community Integration, After the client has completed the modules listed above (Modules 1A-1C) the client can move on to Module 3B — Grocery Store, a transportation module for the type of transportation the client will be using, and Module 5C — Leisure Activities. Module 2B — Restaurant is an especially good module to add because it helps the therapist gauge the client's response to noisy environments and measure community reading skills.

Other skills that will be helpful at this stage include "Coping with Stress" and "Relaxation and Stress Reduction" in the Techniques section.

Miscellaneous

Head Injury Hotline
212 Pioneer Bldg
Seattle, WA 98104-2221
206-621-8558
www.headinjury.com

References

Armstrong, M. & Lauzen, S. (1994). *Community integration program, 2nd ed.*, Ravensdale, WA: Idyll Arbor.

Burton, W. (2003). *Comments on the revision of the Rancho Los Amigos cognitive levels of functioning scale.* Downey, CA: Rancho Los Amigo National Rehabilitation Hospital.

Centers for Disease Control and Prevention. (2004). Epidemiology of traumatic brain injury. www.cdc.gov.

Centers for Disease Control and Prevention. (2004). Brain injury and concussion. www.cdc.gov on 3/13/04.

National Institutes of Health. (2002): Traumatic brain injury: Hope through research. http://www.ninds.nih.gov/health_and_medical/pubs/TBI.htm on 3/12/04.

National Institutes of Health. (1998). NIH consensus report: Rehabilitation of persons with traumatic brain injury. *16*(1). http://odp.od.nih.gov/consensus/cons/109/109_intro.htm on 3/13/04.

Novack, T. (1999a). Recovery after traumatic brain injury. http://www.neuroskills.com/ on 3/10/04.

Novack, T. (1999b). What to expect after traumatic brain injury. Presented at the Recovery after TBI Conference 9/99. http://www.neuroskills.com/ on 3/10/04.

Sandel, E. (1994). Traumatic brain injury: Causes and consequences. Chapter from *Family articles about traumatic brain injury*. Tucson, AZ: Communication Skill Builders.

Section 3: Treatment and the ICF Model

Each code is listed and described as it appears in the official ICF book. We also provide a further description of each code as it relates to recreational therapy practice, along with information on how to assess, treat, adapt, and document related to the particular code. A complete list of all ICF codes without descriptions is available in Appendix A.

Body Functions

Body functions include physiological and psychological functions that are used to indicate the extent of a client's impairments in these areas.

Scoring

Recreational therapists will routinely score Body Functions codes in most practice settings.

Body functions are the physiological functions of body systems (including psychological functions).

Impairments are problems in body functions or structures representing a significant deviation or loss.

To score a Body Functions impairment the therapist first identifies the appropriate code to score using the General Coding Guidelines shown to the right.

The code is written down in its entirety. This includes the letter and number (all Body Functions codes begin with the letter "b"). A decimal point is placed after the code. After the decimal point the extent of the client's impairment is recorded. This is called the first qualifier.

The scoring scale for Body Functions is shown in Table 14. There is only one qualifier.

Example: A client has moderate short-term memory problems. The code for short-term memory is b1440. The appropriately written code would look like this: b1440.2

Body Functions Code	1st Qualifier (Extent of Impairment)
b1440.	2

General Coding Guidelines

1. Choose the appropriate codes that best reflect the client's functioning as it relates to the purpose of the encounter.
2. Only choose codes that are relevant to the context of the health condition. For example, if a person has impairments with involuntary movement functions (e.g., b6653 Tremors), but is being evaluated for cognitive functioning, only cognitive functioning should be coded.
3. Do not make inferences (assumptions) about a client's functioning in other areas based on a Body Functions impairment. Each function should be evaluated and then scored separately. For example, just because a person has a moderate impairment with b1641 Organization and Planning, it does not mean that the client will have difficulty with d230 Carrying Out Daily Routine.
4. Only choose codes that reflect the specific predefined timeframe. Functions that relate to a timeframe outside of the predefined timeframe should not be coded.
5. Use the most specific code whenever possible. For example, if a client has an impairment with sustaining attention, score the specific code of b1400 Sustaining Attention rather than the broader code of b140 Attention Functions.

Table 14: Body Functions Qualifier

Scoring for First Qualifier		
0 NO impairment	(none, absent, negligible…)	0-4%
1 MILD impairment	(slight, low…)	5-24%
2 MODERATE impairment	(medium, fair…)	25-49%
3 SEVERE impairment	(high, extreme…)	50-95%
4 COMPLETE impairment	(total)	96-100%
8 not specified		
9 not applicable		

Chapter 1 Mental Functions

This chapter is about the functions of the brain: both global mental functions, such as consciousness, energy, and drive, and specific mental functions such as memory, language, and calculation mental functions.

Global Mental Functions (b110-b139)

b110 Consciousness Functions

General mental functions of the state of awareness and alertness, including the clarity and continuity of the wakeful state.

Inclusions: functions of the state, continuity and quality of consciousness, loss of consciousness, coma, vegetative states, fugues, trance states, possession states, drug-induced altered consciousness, delirium, stupor

Exclusions: orientation functions (b114); energy and drive functions (b130); sleep functions (b134)

- *b1100 State of Consciousness*
  Mental functions that when altered produce states such as clouding of consciousness, stupor, or coma.
- *b1101 Continuity of Consciousness*
  Mental functions that produce sustained wakefulness, alertness, and awareness and, when disrupted, may produce fugue, trance, or other similar states.
- *b1102 Quality of Consciousness*
  Mental functions that when altered effect changes in the character of wakeful, alert, and aware sentience, such as drug-induced altered states or delirium.
- *b1108 Consciousness Functions, Other Specified*
- *b1109 Consciousness Functions, Unspecified*

Treatment for Consciousness Functions

The therapist observes the client's reaction to single and multimodal stimuli in order to determine a baseline of consciousness functioning. (Multimodal stimuli mean stimulation using more than one sense at a time, e.g., sense of touch and sense of hearing.) Once a baseline level of functioning is determined, the therapist focuses on an approach that increases the client's ability in this area. If a client's consciousness skills are not fully recovered, the therapist will then change his/her approach to an adaptation approach that focuses on identifying specific adaptations and modifications that will maximize the client's independence, function, and safety.

The therapist begins with clinical observation. The therapist presents the client with single or multimodal stimuli and observes the client's response. Stimuli can be tactile (e.g., touching the client's hand, rubbing the client's upper arm), visual

(e.g., therapist standing in view of the client, showing the client pictures of family members, handing the client a piece of artwork), auditory (e.g., saying hello and addressing the client by his/her given name, a loud clap, music), gustatory (e.g., ice chips, lemonade), and/or olfactory (e.g., holding a small bottle of scented oil under the client's nose, spraying a room freshener). If a client is in a coma, sensory stimulation techniques as briefly described above are helpful in monitoring changes in the state of consciousness (see "Traumatic Brain Injury" in the Diagnosis section). For example, if a client is in a coma (Rancho Los Amigos Level I), an eye opening response to stimuli may represent a positive change in the client's status to a Rancho Los Amigos Level II.

The therapist measures the client's response by

- Specific response observed (e.g., opens eyes on command, no reaction to loud noise or light touch).
- Length of time the behavior was observed (e.g., client's continuity of consciousness was five consecutive minutes within a 30-minute session).
- Level of assistance that the client required to invoke a response to stimuli in relation to a specific task (e.g., client requires maximum assistance using many types of cues to open his eyes and turn his head in the direction of therapist).

There are many factors that can influence the client's level of consciousness. For example, clients tend to become harder to arouse in the afternoon and even more so in the evening because of fatigue. Clients who are depressed may also be difficult to arouse. Consequently, the therapist must be consistent when measuring consciousness to be able to accurately reflect changes. For example, if a therapist assesses the client's baseline for continuity of consciousness in the late morning, then her follow-up assessments should also be conducted in the late morning.

The therapist has one standardized testing tool that fits well with this type of therapy intervention and documentation. The *FOX* measures six areas in what it terms the "social" domain. The six areas are 1. the client's reaction to others, 2. the client's interactions with objects, 3. the client's seeking attention from others to manipulate the environment, 4. the client's interactions with objects, 5. the client's concept of self, and 6. the client's interactions with others. For more details see the discussion of the *FOX* in the Assessment section.

Once the baseline is determined, the therapist uses specific strategies to facilitate neuroplasticity. Strategies are graduated in complexity and length to provide realistic functional challenges for the client (see "Neuroplasticity" in the Techniques section for information on graduated tasks and techniques). For example, the therapist begins treatment in a non-distracting environment and then gradually works the client up to functioning in a minimally distracting environment. She then challenges the client further by upping the distraction in the room to a moderate level with the goal of progressing the client to a normally distracting environment (no intervention needed to alter environment).

Other ideas can also be useful for treatment of consciousness functions. Below is a list of enhancements recommended by O'Sullivan and Schmitz (1988) to promote arousal or consciousness.

- Implement short periods of stimulation (5-10 minutes) and intersperse them throughout the day to balance rest with activity.
- Use different types of stimulation (auditory, visual, tactile, olfactory, gustatory) by themselves or in combination, e.g., provide an auditory stimuli of saying "hello" and stating the client's name or provide auditory and tactile stimuli together by saying "hello," stating the client's name, and touching the client's shoulder.
- Use activities that are important to the client (e.g., a recreational task that is attractive to the client). Activities that are important and attractive to the client increase motivation and initiation skills.
- Avoid over-stimulating the client. If the client is over-stimulated by an overwhelming amount of stimuli in the environment, s/he may react in one of two ways: shut down by withdrawing inwardly or express over-stimulation through behavioral expression of agitation (e.g., outbursts). Agitated clients who demonstrate excessive levels of arousal also benefit from a controlled application of sensory techniques. Frequently, sources of stimulation from the environment precipitate bouts of agitation and disorganization. The client is generally unable to process stimuli effectively and is similarly unable to control responses, which are often bizarre and combative.
- Careful assessment can reveal the offending stimuli and those that have a calming influence. Therapists should 1. eliminate or reduce irritating stimuli, 2. use a quiet non-distracting environment and gradually build up the client's toler-

ance to a more stimulating environment, 3. minimize unexpected surprises since they can precipitate outbursts, 4. establish a predictable routine and structure to the day (e.g., therapies are held on the same day, at the same locations within the facility, and as much as possible involve the same task or activity), 5. if a new activity is used, the therapist carefully explains the activity to the client before it is attempted and provides verbal reassurance and manual guidance during the execution of the new activity, and 6. if an agitated outburst occurs, the therapist calmly redirects the client's attention away from the cause of irritation. Often selection of a task over which the client has some control will help the client regain composure. The therapist should provide a model for calm, controlled behavior (speak slowly and calmly at a moderate volume that conveys understanding and control) and reward each successful effort with positive reinforcement (e.g., "You handled that really well.").

- Verbal explanations should be kept brief and to the point to keep the client focused on the specific stimuli.
- Keep a 24-hour record of the types of sensory stimuli used, the individuals who applied them, and the client's responses.

Some clients, especially those with severe brain injury, may be unarousable initially. They are not in a coma, but just very low functioning. The client typically won't open his/her eyes, respond physically to a stimuli (e.g., turn his head toward the stimuli), or even acknowledge the presence of a stimuli in any manner (e.g., shooing away the therapist with an arm, looking away, leaning forward toward stimuli). Since the client at this level is unable to engage in a task, the therapist is to provide stimulation to invoke a response with the goal for the client to show simple signs of arousal (e.g., eye opening). Some techniques that have been helpful with this type of client include:

- Rubbing a cold washcloth on the back of the client's neck (the back of the neck is sensitive to temperature).
- Turning the lights off and then on again.
- Clapping loudly.
- Changing your voice tone when giving a command (e.g., say "open your eyes" sweetly, commandingly, or matter-of-factly).
- Using touch alone or in conjunction with another stimulus (e.g., squeeze the client's hand, touch the client's upper back, and say the client's name).
- Calling the client by his/her name. Some clients may respond better to a nickname if it was

commonly used by friends and family (e.g., client may respond to "Nick" but not to "Nicholas"). Some clients, however, respond to formal names better (commands more attention) despite having been commonly addressed by a nickname (e.g., Mr. Jones, Nicholas).

- Using fresh air (especially cold or cool air). Cool or cold fresh air commonly invokes an eye opening response (e.g., open an outside door so that the client gets a burst of cold air, use an air-conditioned room that is kept cooler than the rest of the facility).

If a client does not fully recover consciousness functions, the therapist will have to adapt or modify the client's environment and tasks to maximize functioning. The therapist shifts from a restorative approach to an adaptation/modification approach. For example, the therapist will need to educate the client's caregivers on how to stimulate the client (or reduce environmental stimulation if the client is easily over-stimulated) to promote further recovery of consciousness functions after discharge.

b114 Orientation Functions
General mental functions of knowing and ascertaining one's relations to self, to others, to time, and to one's surroundings.
Inclusions: functions of orientation to time, place, and person; orientation to self and others; disorientation to time, place, and person
Exclusions: consciousness functions (b110); attention functions (b140); memory functions (b144)

- *b1140 Orientation to Time*
  Mental functions that produce awareness of day, date, month, and year.
- *b1141 Orientation to Place*
  Mental functions that produce awareness of one's location, such as one's immediate surroundings, one's town or county.
- *b1142 Orientation to Person*
  Mental functions that produce awareness of one's own identity and of individuals in the immediate environment.
  - o *b11420 Orientation to Self*
    Mental functions that produce awareness of one's own identity.
  - o *b11421 Orientation to Others*
    Mental functions that produce awareness of the identity of other individuals in one's immediate environment.
  - o *b11428 Orientation to Person, Other Specified*
  - o *b11429 Orientation to Person, Unspecified*
- *b1148 Orientation Functions, Other Specified*
- *b1149 Orientation Functions, Unspecified*

Treatment for Orientation Functions

The therapist is to challenge the client with an orientation task in each sphere (person, place, and time) by asking the client several questions. The therapist must already know the answers to the questions to be able to determine the accuracy of the client's answers.

Person: What is your name? How old are you? Are you a grandfather (social roles)? Do you have any brothers, sisters, or children? What are their names? How old are they? Show the client pictures of his/her family and ask the client to tell you who they are.

Place: What city and state are we in? What is the name of this facility? What floor are you on? What is your room number? Topographical orientation (also known as spatial orientation) is a form of orientation to place. Although it is not defined by the World Health Organization, it is a common form of orientation that is assessed and addressed in a rehabilitation setting. Topographical orientation is the mental function that produces awareness of where one is in relation to the environment using both visual and non-visual input to understand the layout of one's world. For example, if a client is standing in front of the hospital cafeteria, she should be able to form a "mental map" of where she is in relation to her room.

Time: What time of day is it? Which meal did you just eat? What activity are you going to next? What day of the week is it? What month is it? What season is it? What is the year?

The therapist should also observe the client's behavioral responses to assess orientation, especially for clients who are unable to speak or whose expression of speech is impaired (e.g., Does the client seem to be aware of being a separate individual? Does the client get lost easily when walking around the hospital floor and/or is the client unable to find his/her room? Does the client attempt to put on a heavy coat when it is 80°F outside? Does the client's facial expression look puzzled or fearful when someone in his/her immediate family is standing in front of him/her?). Orientation to self is the most basic function. (See "Basic Awareness of Self as Part of Socialization" in the Concepts section.) Orientation to person seems to come back before orientation to place. And orientation to place seems to come back before orientation to time. Orientation to person is a retrograde memory function (client's ability to remember information that occurred before the injury), while orientation to place and time require the client to learn, retain, and recall new information. Problems with retrograde memory may resolve due to the normal healing process of the brain, whereas the ability to learn, retain, and recall new information are more complex skills that take longer to recover.

The most common method of measuring orientation is the scale called *orientation x3*. As burlingame (2002) points out, the protocols for determining orientation x3 are not well developed, so the scores should always be taken as a general measurement of orientation and not as specific orientation. Similarly to consciousness, variability in orientation is seen as the day progresses. In addition to noting the time of day that the therapist is measuring orientation, the therapist should measure the client's response in the following ways:

- *Terms of sphere* (e.g., "client is oriented to person without cueing, but is not oriented to time"; "client is alert and oriented x3 [oriented in all three spheres]"). If a client is not alert, it is very hard for him/her to be oriented.
- *Percentage of orientation* (e.g., client is oriented to place at 50% — this means that the client was able to answer only 50% of the orientation questions about place or that the client was observed being disoriented to place about half the time through behavioral observation).
- *Level of assistance needed* (e.g., client requires moderate verbal cues to orient to place).
- *Relation to task dysfunction* (e.g., client requires moderate verbal cues to locate the cafeteria secondary to poor topographical orientation).

Once a baseline level of functioning is determined, the therapist focuses strategies to enhance the client's functioning. If a client's orientation is not fully recovered, the therapist also includes an adaptation approach that identifies specific adaptations and modifications that will maximize the client's independence, functioning, and safety.

Therapists enhance the skills of orientation by challenging the client with orientation tasks. This is done in accordance with cognitive retraining strategies (see "Neuroplasticity" in the Techniques section). Some of the techniques commonly used include:

Asking the client one specific orientation question (e.g., What is the name of this facility?). If the client says, "I don't know" or gives a wrong answer, provide the client with cues to identify the right answer (e.g., It's a rehab hospital in Malvern. It begins with the letter "B."). The therapist should refrain from giving the client the specific answer whenever possible to promote cognitive restructuring.

Developing and adhering to a daily routine for the client. A structured and consistent routine will help to orient the client because it will be predictable and repetitive. For example, the client always goes to speech therapy at nine in the morning, followed by recreational therapy at ten in the morning. As a result of this schedule, the client may begin to associate therapy with a specific time (thus increasing the client's attention to time). In addition, the client will travel the same route, the client's room to the speech clinic, the speech clinic to the recreational therapy clinic, the recreational therapy clinic back to the client's room. A consistent travel pattern will assist the client in remembering the environmental layout (the environment can be confusing if you are always coming and going from different places and from different directions), thus helping to orient him/her to the environment (orientation to place, including topographical orientation).

Organizing the client's personal environment so that it consistently enhances orientation (e.g., shoes are always inside the closet on the floor, orientation materials are always kept in a binder on the side of the wheelchair).

Making and posting clear signage for specific locations (e.g., a big arrow and a picture of a toilet that points to where the bathroom is located and then a big picture of a toilet on the outside of the bathroom door).

Teaching the client to look for landmarks (e.g., notice the large painting of the night sky on the wall, notice the lobby area, notice the pool).

Using orientation materials such as a calendar on the wall in the client's room (have the client cross off the day after dinner), using maps (e.g., a simple map of the client's floor, a map of the client's neighborhood), using pictures with labels (e.g., pictures of each family member with the name written on the picture), making sure the client has (and promoting the use of) a watch and a clock, and/or using a memory book (also called a log book) as described in "Neuroplasticity" in the Techniques section.

Using a daily orientation group that focuses on cognitive remediation techniques for orientation. Many facilities run a reality orientation group first thing in the morning (either before or after breakfast) to orient clients to the day and to help them prepare their orientation materials for the day (e.g., review each client's therapy schedule and make sure it is put in the memory book, check the correctness of the calendar inside the memory book).

Using cognitive remediation techniques to orient the client at the beginning of each treatment session. For example, ask the client what his/her name is, what therapy s/he is now attending, what is typically done at this therapy, what the name of the hospital is, what time of day it is.

If a client does not fully recover orientation functions, the therapist will have to adapt or modify the client's environment and tasks to maximize functioning. The therapist shifts from a restorative approach to an adaptation approach. In addition, the therapist will need to educate the client's caregivers on how to promote further recovery of orientation after discharge. Adaptation and modification of the client's environment are very important for the client's safety, functioning, and emotional health. If the client is not properly oriented, injury could result. For example, the client could become lost (topographical orientation). Another consideration is that of functioning. If a client is not properly oriented to time (e.g., time of day), then the client's sleep cycle could become disturbed and activities might be initiated at inappropriate times (e.g., client thinks that it is morning when it is evening and attempts to get ready for work). Finally, disorientation can affect the emotional health of clients. Being told, "No, you're wrong. That's not right." can take a toll on the client's self-esteem and self-confidence, possibly leading to depression.

Compensatory strategies for disorientation are not very different from what a therapist uses to enhance the skills of orientation. Compensatory strategies used during treatment are kept and carried over into the client's daily routine outside of the hospital setting. The therapist is responsible to assess assimilation of the compensatory strategies into the client's "real life" and make changes as necessary to promote best functioning. Changes should be as minimal as possible. For example, a client may have used a large binder to hold reference papers for orientation in the hospital setting, but now finds it difficult to constantly carry around the large binder for community tasks such as grocery shopping, hiking with the kids, and bike riding. The therapist may suggest using a backpack to carry the binder so that the client's hands are free for activity. If the client is able to alter the shape and content of the "memory book" (without additional disorientation) to a smaller date book organizer, then it would fit in a waist pack, back pants pocket, or pocket book. It is not unusual for a client to have a large binder in the home environment and a small date book organizer in the community environment.

b117 Intellectual Functions

General mental functions, required to understand and constructively integrate the various mental functions, including all cognitive functions and their development over the life span.
Inclusions: functions of intellectual growth; intellectual retardation, mental retardation, dementia

Exclusions: memory functions (b144); thought functions (b160); higher-level cognitive functions (b164)

Treatment for Intellectual Functions

This refers to the normal healthy growth and maintenance of integrative cognitive processes. Disabilities like mental retardation, dementia, and other disabilities that affect intellectual functioning are described by the ICF as having impairments in "intellectual functions."

Document impairments in intellectual functions in terms of:

- *Stage of functioning* (e.g., Client is performing at Piaget's sensorimotor stage.)
- *Type of deficit* (e.g., Client's intellectual abilities are seriously compromised by dementia). Specific deficits should be scored in the relevant category.
- *Level of assistance* (e.g., Client is expected to progress to some concrete reasoning ability through training with Montessori materials.)

Therapists' work with intellectual functions falls into two broad categories: helping in the development and mitigating loss.

Helping in the development of intellectual functioning occurs primarily in school settings and with MR/DD populations. It may also apply in some psychiatric situations. In these cases the therapist's goal is to follow the normal course of intellectual development and provide challenges that allow the client to progress to higher levels of functioning. This can be done in group or individual settings by using activities that teach more mature thought processes. The therapist can present situations, such as appropriate touching, and lead a discussion about how a person decides what is appropriate. At one level there are rules to be followed. At a higher level there are reasons for the rules. A therapist in this case would explain the concept of looking for the reasons behind the rules, give the clients practice in finding reasons for the things they do, and teach ways to use the reasons to come up with appropriate rules in novel situations. Similarly the therapist can teach concepts from the next developmental stage in any of the areas covered by intellectual functioning.

Therapists mitigate the loss of intellectual function when there is damage to the brain. This includes TBI, stroke, and dementia. Losses may also occur from psychological trauma. If it is possible to improve the intellectual function, the process is similar to helping the development as described above. The additional complication in the case of loss is dealing with the client realizing that some ability has been lost. See the Techniques section for "Adjustment to Disability" for more information. When intellectual function is not expected to be restored, as in the case of dementia, the therapist's responsibility is to find adaptations that the client or the client's caregivers can use to reduce the harmful effects of the loss. This includes appropriate restrictions on the client's activities (e.g., they may no longer be allowed to make investment decisions) and dealing with the feelings of loss that accompany these restrictions. It is important to support the client as much as possible in making decisions and not take away choices when it is not necessary. Finding the appropriate balance of autonomy and support for the client's current (and changing) mental abilities is the goal of this treatment.

b122 Global Psychosocial Functions

General mental functions, as they develop over the life span, required to understand and constructively integrate the mental functions that lead to the formation of the interpersonal skills needed to establish reciprocal social interactions, in terms of both meaning and purpose.
Inclusions: such as in autism

Treatment for
Global Psychosocial Functions

See the treatment descriptions in "Activities and Participation Chapter 7 Interpersonal Interactions and Relationships."

b126 Temperament and Personality Functions

General mental functions of constitutional disposition of the individual to react in a particular way to situations, including the set of mental characteristics that makes the individual distinct from others.
Inclusions: functions of extraversion, introversion, agreeableness, conscientiousness, psychic and emotional stability, and openness to experience; optimism; novelty seeking; confidence; trustworthiness
Exclusions: intellectual functions (b117); energy and drive functions (b130); psychomotor functions (b147); emotional functions (b152)

- *b1260 Extraversion*
  Mental functions that produce a personal disposition that is outgoing, sociable, and demonstrative, as contrasted to being shy, restricted, and inhibited.
- *b1261 Agreeableness*
  Mental functions that produce a personal disposition that is cooperative, amicable, and accommodating, as contrasted to being unfriendly, oppositional, and defiant.

- *b1262 Conscientiousness*
  Mental functions that produce personal dispositions such as in being hard-working, methodical, and scrupulous, as contrasted to mental functions producing dispositions such as in being lazy, unreliable, and irresponsible.
- *b1263 Psychic Stability*
  Mental functions that produce a personal disposition that is even-tempered, calm, and composed, as contrasted to being irritable, worried, erratic, and moody.
- *b1264 Openness to Experience*
  Mental functions that produce a personal disposition that is curious, imaginative, inquisitive, and experience-seeking, as contrasted to being stagnant, inattentive, and emotionally inexpressive.
- *b1265 Optimism*
  Mental functions that produce a personal disposition that is cheerful, buoyant, and hopeful, as contrasted to being downhearted, gloomy, and despairing.
- *b1266 Confidence*
  Mental functions that produce a personal disposition that is self-assured, bold, and assertive, as contrasted to being timid, insecure, and self-effacing.
- *b1267 Trustworthiness*
  Mental functions that produce a personal disposition that is dependable and principled, as contrasted to being deceitful and antisocial.
- *b1268 Temperament and Personality Functions, Other Specified*
- *b1269 Temperament and Personality Functions, Unspecified*

Treatment for
Temperament and Personality Functions

Temperament and personality are common descriptors used by recreational therapists in documentation, as well as common areas for treatment goals. Impairments in temperament and personality are seen in mood disorders (e.g., bipolar disorder, major depressive disorder), personality disorders (e.g., borderline personality disorder, paranoid personality disorder), organic disorders (e.g., dementia), childhood disorders (e.g., autism), drug and alcohol abuse, childhood abuse, and learned behavior.

Therapists who note a change or oddity in a client's temperament or personality functions should request an evaluation by a psychologist, psychiatrist, or neuropsychologist as appropriate.

In addition to studying the extent of temperament and personality impairment observed by other members of the treatment team, the recreational therapist documents additional information including:
- The specific function and extent of impairment (e.g., client has severe distrust in others; the

client's psychic stability is moderately compromised secondary to dementia).

- The impact of the impairment on activity (e.g., client's extreme shyness prevents her from forming friendships thus limiting her circle of support; client's lack of optimism is seriously limiting her ability to participate in therapy sessions).
- Functionality of the subcategory on performance (e.g., client exhibits confidence in his approach to outdoor community walking).
- Effect of treatment on impairment (e.g., client has shown a 50% increase in optimistic verbalizations since initiation of journaling therapy; child has become more conscientious of caring for play toys as evidenced by putting them away correctly at the end of the day).

Once a root cause of the problem has been identified, treatment is prescribed. Treatment may include:
- *Medication*: e.g., medication for psychic stability.
- *Specially designed experiences*: e.g., use of "new games" or adventure therapy to facilitate development of trust; activities that will facilitate feelings of success to promote confidence.
- *Journaling*: e.g., writing three positive things that happened each day in a journal to promote optimism.
- *Behavior modification*: e.g., positive reward for conscientious behavior. See "Behaviour Manipulation" in the Treatment section.
- *Group work*: e.g., using a jigsaw approach in a group project that requires the individual to cooperate with another to complete a task, do not give the client all of the resources to complete the project on his/her own so that it forces the person to interact and cooperate with others to complete the task.
- *Social skills*: Working on the development of a particular social skill and providing opportunities to apply learned skills (e.g., teach a client techniques on how to make a friend and then provide small group opportunities for the client to practice making a new friend). Making friends is a social skill that contributes to several of the personality functions. See Activities and Participation Chapter 7 Interpersonal Interactions and Relationships and "Social Skills Training" in the Techniques section.
- *Opportunities for leadership*: Be sure success is highly likely (e.g., to enhance extraversion, confidence, and openness to experience).
- *Challenges*: to promote openness to experience (e.g., participation in new activities, socializing with a different peer group, activities that require imagination and creativity, projects that encourage the client to seek answers to questions).
- *Role-playing*: e.g., practice reacting to situations in a more positive and healthy manner such as responding to constructive criticism.

A positive and reinforcing approach is best in most situations. Situations where there is a risk of failure are typically avoided until the client has built up a basic faith in his/her abilities. Risk is slowly increased so that the client can continue to have an overall sense of being able to recover from failure and try the activity again.

Despite interventions, temperament and personality functions may not change or fully resolve. Health care professionals who are working with clients who have organic changes, such as dementia, that impair temperament and personality functions may need to alter the client's environment (e.g., removing things that affect psychic stability such as obnoxious stimuli), educate caregivers about the cause of the impairment (e.g., brain injury) and how to best respond to temperament and personality that is not typical of their loved one (e.g., teach parents how to deescalate their daughter when she becomes paranoid of others; how to raise a spouse's self-confidence), and put safety measures in place when appropriate (e.g., suicide prevention, cancel or place a hold on credit cards when client becomes manic).

b130 Energy and Drive Functions
General mental functions of physiological and psychological mechanisms that cause the individual to move towards satisfying specific needs and general goals in a persistent manner.
Inclusions: functions of energy level, motivation, appetite, craving (including for substances that can be abused), and impulse control
Exclusions: consciousness functions (b110); temperament and personality functions (b126); sleep functions (b134); psychomotor functions (b147); emotional functions (b152)
- b1300 Energy Level
  Mental functions that produce vigour and stamina.
- b1301 Motivation
  Mental functions that produce the incentive to act; the conscious or unconscious driving force for action.
- b1302 Appetite
  Mental functions that produce a natural longing or desire, especially the natural and recurring desire for food and drink.
- b1303 Craving
  Mental functions that produce the urge to consume substances, including substances that can be abused.

- *b1304 Impulse Control*
  Mental functions that regulate and resist sudden intense urges to do something.
- *b1308 Energy and Drive Functions, Other Specified*
- *b1309 Energy and Drive Functions, Unspecified*

Treatment for Energy and Drive Functions

These descriptors have to do with a client's mental functions that impact energy level, motivation, appetite, craving, and impulse control. Mental functions that control these issues can be affected by injury (e.g., traumatic brain injury), disease processes (e.g., chronic fatigue syndrome, cancer), and physiological changes in the body that alter chemical and hormonal balance (e.g., depression, prescription medications, illegal substance abuse). A client's behavior can also alter the chemical make-up of the body affecting mental functions (e.g., lack of exercise, lack of sleep, lack of proper nutrition).

Energy Level

Low energy should be expected and allowed for when a client has a major illness or disability. Changes in sleep, eating, and exercise patterns are commonly affected by low energy, as well as psychological and physiological changes related to illness (e.g., adjustment issues, medications). When the immune system is compromised by illness, energy levels are directed to healing rather than to outside activity.

Therapists carefully evaluate the client's history and behavioral patterns to identify modifiable variables (e.g., exercise, nutrition, sleep, coping skills), underlying disorders (e.g., depression, chronic fatigue syndrome, multiple sclerosis, reduced energy level from chemotherapy for cancer), and current medications and substances (e.g., substance abuse such as alcohol, drowsiness as a side effect of a medication) that could be affecting energy levels. Baselines of functioning are determined and goals are established.

Low energy levels are commonly a result of the interaction of many factors (e.g., client experiences fatigue from multiple sclerosis but also does not exercise regularly, adapt adequately for energy-demanding tasks, and get good quality sleep). Therapists should refer to the specific diagnoses for more specific information about the problems contributing to low energy levels.

Energy level can be measured by amount of time (e.g., participated in social activity for 15 minutes prior to fatigue), descriptors of poor, fair, good, and excellent (e.g., exhibited poor motivation for therapy), and level of assistance (e.g., requires moderate encouragement to perform task).

Treatment for energy level issues is usually done in conjunction with the rest of the treatment team. There are times when a client's energy will be low as a result of the illness or treatment. The therapist needs to make sure that other issues discussed in this set of functions, especially a lack of motivation, are not being mistaken for a lack of energy.

The therapist can work on making sure that the client has adequate nutrition, sleep, and time to rest during activities. Activities themselves can be energy enhancing as discussed in the *Vitality through Leisure* assessment.

Motivation

"Motivation is a state of being that produces a tendency toward action. The state may be one of deprivation (e.g., hunger), a value system, or a strongly held belief (e.g., religion). In the mediation of learning and perception, biological mechanisms play an important role in motivating behavior. An organism tries to maintain homeostasis or internal balance against any disturbance of equilibrium (e.g., a thirsty animal is motivated to find water and drink). Social motives, such as the need for recognition and achievement, also account for behavioral patterns (e.g., studying to get good grades). But the intensity of motivation to master any task in a particular situation is determined by at least two different factors: the achievement motive (desire to achieve) and the likelihood of success" (Sadock & Sadock, 2003, p 148).

People's motivation for goals and objects vary according to the value that they place on different things (e.g., one person may strongly value academics, another may strongly value social status within a peer group, and yet another may value restoring his/her level of independence). Understanding what motivates a client is important to identify activities and life events to address in therapy (e.g., returning to school, roller skating, walking outdoors, gardening, automotive maintenance). Therapists are aware that clients may have motivations that stay constant for long periods of time (e.g., client desires to finish school, get a job at a major law firm, and buy a home on Society Hill), but they are also aware that motivators fluctuate as a person's views, situations, and life experiences change. For example, a person currently attending college full time may highly value graduating with a high grade point average in the hope of landing a good job. However, if she just had a skiing accident and damaged her spinal cord, a high grade point average (although still important to her) may take second place to achieving independence in self-care activities.

One of the most challenging issues for recreational therapists is motivating a client to address issues that the client is not fully ready to embrace. For example, often when a recreational therapist walks into a client's room and proceeds to talk with the client about his/her lifestyle, the response is, "I'm not really interested in that right now. I just want to be able to walk, use the bathroom, and get back home." Abraham Maslow has created a hierarchy of needs that help in understanding this situation. The basic idea is the people will be motivated by basic physiological needs such as hunger and thirst until those needs are satisfied. After that they care about safety, love and belonging, self-esteem, and self-actualization. Getting back to normal life takes top priority. The recreational therapist should acknowledge that and work on issues that will help the client reach his/her immediate goals. For more information on Maslow see "Maslow's Hierarchy of Needs" the Concepts section.

Once people have met the needs in the first two levels of Maslow's hierarchy, their motivations become more complex. There are several ways for the therapist to evaluate the client's motivation.

Motivation can be assessed through a client interview (e.g., What do you value in your life? What is important to you right now? What would you like to accomplish when you're here? If you could do anything you wanted to do, what would it be?), as well as observation of the client's verbalizations and behavior (e.g., client's concern of being able to care for her children, client asking when he can play golf again). One of the most common methods is to identify the leisure interests of the client through brainstorming.

The therapist should also consider formal assessments including the *Leisure Interest Measure, Leisure Satisfaction Measure, Leisure Motivation Scale, Leisurescope Plus,* and the *Free Time Boredom* measure. Each of these assessments measures some aspect of what motivates a client to pursue leisure and recreational activities.

Once the therapist determines the motivational level of the client, the therapist verbally reflects to the client an understanding of his/her situation and validates the client's concerns and feelings. This in turn shows the client that the therapist truly understands the "place" where s/he is and facilitates the development of the client-therapist relationship.

Therapists may go on to talk about the importance of these activities (e.g., walking outside to get the mail each day) or the need to further develop or alter activities to positively affect the client's health

condition (e.g., "You are really lucky that your stroke was so mild. To decrease your risks of having another stroke, which could be a lot worse, we really need to get some exercise into your schedule.").

When therapists establish goals with their clients, the focus needs to be on what motivates the client. Establishing small incremental goals that are success driven will help keep up the motivation. For example, if a client is finding it difficult to perform floor to chair transfers (requires moderate assistance) and does not believe that he will ever be independent, his motivation for the task is low and his perceived level of success is low. Knowing that the client is motivated by spending time with his children and that one of the activities that the client enjoys doing with his children is fishing on a lake in a small boat, the therapist incorporates the activity into the task of a chair to floor transfer. The therapist validates the client's value of spending time with his children and fishing and sets a one-foot tall block in front of the chair. The client is to transfer onto the block (a smaller task than directly onto the floor) and then from the block onto the floor, all the while visualizing that the goal of the transfer is not to merely get down onto the floor but onto a boating dock so that the client can then transfer into the boat. The goal of achieving this skill is turned into a goal that has personal value to the client.

If the client does not feel that his/her values are being addressed, the client may become non-compliant with therapy. A re-evaluation of the client's values is conducted if this is suspected and goals are re-established as appropriate (e.g., A client in a rehabilitation hospital values being able to walk and therefore refuses all therapy except physical therapy. The recreational therapist discusses the RT treatment plan with the client and puts added focus on walking during functional activities both in the home and in the community). Other factors can also contribute to or influence non-compliance (e.g., behavior issues, disorientation, delusions, depression, fear, and anxiety). A holistic view of the client's motivation will help the therapist during treatment.

Appetite

A person's appetite can fluctuate depending on various factors:
- Discomfort or pain with eating or digesting food.
- Prescription medications.
- Illegal drugs.
- Psychological issues that suppress or stimulate appetite such as depression, mania, and stress.
- Personal perception of certain foods, such as "food looks unappetizing."
- Level of physical activity.

- Likes and dislikes of certain foods.
- Availability of foods.
- Influences of perceived consequences of consuming foods such as those associated with anorexia and bulimia.
- Injury to the area of the brain that controls appetite.
- Learned eating behaviors and patterns.
- Psychiatric diagnosis of anorexia, bulimia, and binge eating.
- Psychiatric diagnosis of which an eating disorder is a common comorbid diagnosis such as intermittent explosive disorder and obsessive-compulsive disorder.

A healthy appetite can be defined by calories consumed and balance of food consumed. The number of calories and the balance of different foods will vary depending on the needs and health of the client (e.g., calorie restricted for weight loss, avoidance of certain foods secondary to irritated bowel).

Therapists document the health of a client's appetite by noting the amount of food eaten at a given time (e.g., client ate 50% of breakfast), the type of foods eaten (e.g., client reports having eaten only a piece of celery for the entire day), the number of meals eaten (e.g., client ate two complete meals today), reaction to foods eaten (e.g., client vomited after eating half a turkey sandwich), client's behavior related to food (e.g., client angry at being watched during meals), and general reports of the client about his/her appetite (e.g., Client reports having a poor appetite/ravenous appetite).

Treatment involves addressing the underlying conditions that affect appetite (e.g., detoxification from drugs, medication to control mental illness, nutrition education, increased physical activity level, counseling to address body image). Referrals to other healthcare disciplines are initiated as needed (e.g., nutritionist, psychologist, gastroenterologist). Where health is severely compromised, as in anorexia, the treatment team will need to work together on a plan and each member of the team will need to observe the client carefully when in charge of the client's treatment to make sure the plan is being carried out.

Craving

Craving is defined as the mental functions that produce an urge to consume substances such as tobacco products, illegal drugs (e.g., cocaine, heroin, ecstasy, marijuana), and legal drugs (e.g., narcotic pain medication, alcohol). A craving is more than a mere thought. The craving for a substance can be strong enough that it takes priority over other life activities. Cravings can be mild (e.g., client reports a slight craving for a cigarette when wearing a nicotine patch) to severe (e.g., meeting basic hygiene, nutrition, and sleep needs take a backseat to finding and using heroin).

Impulse Control

Mental dysfunction related to impulse control is most commonly seen in clients with traumatic brain injury, dependencies and addictions (substance, gambling, sexual, etc.), schizophrenia (impulse to act on hallucinations), kleptomania (impulse to steal), mania (impulse to assault or threaten), delusional disorders (impulse to act on delusion), depression (impulse to commit suicide), bingeing (impulse to overeat), and/or anger management problems such as intermittent explosive disorder (impulse to act on feelings of rage). See separate diagnoses of traumatic brain injury, substance use, schizophrenia, major depressive disorder, and eating disorders for more information.

Impulse control problems are believed to be related to neurobiological mechanisms, psycho-dynamic factors, and psychosocial factors. Biologically, parts of the brain that control a person's ability to not act on an impulse may be impaired (such as in traumatic brain injury). Psychodynamically, a person may act on impulses to avoid emotional pain (e.g., impulsive action becomes a coping mechanism such as in kleptomania or bingeing). Impulse control problems may also be related to psychosocial issues (e.g., such as in learned behavior from improper role modeling or violence in the home). Whether or not psychodynamic and psychosocial issues truly affect the mental functions of the brain to control impulses is difficult to say, however it cannot be excluded.

Impulse control is commonly measured by the amount of times that an impulse is experienced, the amount of times the client is able to resist the impulse, and the intervention used by the therapist and/or client to reduce or extinguish each impulse (e.g., Client decreased from six to three episodes of impulsive walking away from the treatment session resulting in a 50% reduction. Therapist stated the remaining time of the treatment session to the client when signs of impulsiveness appeared. On two occasions the client self-initiated looking at the clock and self-controlled the impulse to walk away from the treatment session.).

Fatigue, over-stimulation, and psychological trauma can lower a person's ability to control impulses (Sadock & Sadock, 2003). Therefore, therapists should seek to minimize these issues whenever possible. Treatment to minimize or extinguish unhealthy impulses may include the use of pharmacology, social support, and behavior modification interventions. (See "Behavior Manipulation" in the Techniques section.) If a specific disability or illness is identified, the therapist should refer to the diagnosis for more specific interventions.

b134 Sleep Functions

General mental functions of periodic, reversible, and selective physical and mental disengagement from one's immediate environment accompanied by characteristic physiological changes.

Inclusions: functions of amount of sleeping, and onset, maintenance, and quality of sleep; functions involving the sleep cycle, such as in insomnia, hypersomnia, and narcolepsy

Exclusions: consciousness functions (b110); energy and drive functions (b130); attention functions (b140); psychomotor functions (b147)

- **b1340 Amount of Sleep**
  Mental functions involved in the time spent in the state of sleep in the diurnal cycle of circadian rhythm.
- **b1341 Onset of Sleep**
  Mental functions that produce the transition between wakefulness and sleep.
- **b1342 Maintenance of Sleep**
  Mental functions that sustain the state of being asleep.
- **b1343 Quality of Sleep**
  Mental functions that produce the natural sleep leading to optimal physical and mental rest and relaxation.
- **b1344 Functions Involving the Sleep Cycle**
  Mental functions that produce rapid eye movement (REM) sleep (associated with dreaming) and non-rapid eye movement sleep (NREM) (characterized by the traditional concept of sleep as a time of decreased physiological and psychological activity).
- **b1348 Sleep Functions, Other Specified**
- **b1349 Sleep Functions, Unspecified**

Treatment for Sleep Functions

The ability to initiate sleep, maintain a healthy amount and quality of sleep, and keep to a healthy sleep-wake rhythm is influenced by many factors including chemical changes within the brain. Behavior can influence chemical changes within the brain. Inadequate amount and quality of sleep can affect energy levels, attention, concentration, and mood (e.g., irritability). Sleep is also needed to promote healing. When sleeping, the body is able to direct more energy to healing.

Sleep functions are affected by

- *Schedules.*
  o *Jet lag.*
  o *Changes in work schedule* (e.g., changing from a day shift to a night shift).
- *Psychological issues and disorders.*
  o *Stress and anxiety*: can cause difficulty in relaxing to allow for sleep.
  o *Night terrors*: can be caused by psychological stress, medications, withdrawal from substance use, or posttraumatic stress disorder.
  o *Avoidance behavior*: excessive sleeping may be an avoidance behavior.
  o *Depression*: insomnia, multiple awakenings, and hypersomnia (excessive sleeping) are common symptoms of depression.
  o *Mania*: a decreased amount of time sleeping is a common symptom of mania.
- *Neurological disorders*: including dementia and Parkinson's.
- *Environment*:
  o *Environmental changes*: such as sleeping in a new room, needed nursing care during the night, common noises at bedtime are absent such as the sound of a fan, and room temperature. Although many of these issues are related to things that are outside of the brain, it is important to note that these things can influence the chemicals within the brain that help to regulate sleep.
  o *Noise* (e.g., nurses in the hallway, construction).
- *Pregnancy*: can cause sleep function problems due to hormonal changes and discomfort.
- *Substances*:
  o *Stimulants*: such as caffeine and cocaine that keep the person awake outside of normal sleep patterns thus impacting a person's circadian rhythm.
  o *Depressants and muscle relaxants*: cause drowsiness and may induce sleep outside of typical sleep patterns.
  o *Alcohol withdrawal*: Insomnia is a common problem associated with alcohol withdrawal. It can last for several weeks or longer. Medication to aid with sleep is to be avoided due to addictive tendencies.
  o *Withdrawal from psychoactive drugs*: resulting in extremely vivid and frightening dreams.
  o *Smoking*: High doses of nicotine can interfere with sleep onset. Nicotine withdrawal can cause either drowsiness or arousal.
- *Urinary incontinence* or urgency during the night.

Therapists may document:

- *Ability to fall asleep*: e.g., client fell asleep in 10 minutes after relaxation exercises.
- *Number of sleep hours*: e.g., six hours of continuous sleep.
- *Clock time slept*: e.g., 10:00 P.M. to 6:00 A.M.
- *Number of times woken during the night*: e.g., client reports waking up at 1:00 A.M. and 3:00 A.M. during the night with night terrors.
- *Techniques used*: what was tried to assist with healthy sleep (e.g., As per client report, client independently initiated relaxation training exercise of progressive muscle relaxation at 10:00 P.M. and was able to fall asleep by 10:30 P.M.).

Therapists identify variables that affect a client's sleep and aim to reduce or eliminate the problems. This may include helping the client develop a consistent routine. This is a very common problem for people who are adjusting to life changes. For example, prior to injury the client woke up at 7:00 A.M. and went to bed at 10:00 P.M. to be able to work during the day. After a disability or life changing event where the normal events of the day are disrupted, sleep is often affected (e.g., doesn't have to wake up at 7:00 A.M. to go to work so sleeps in to 10:00 A.M. and stays up to 2:00 A.M.). Maintaining sleep cycles in a health care setting is very important for infants and toddlers to promote healthy development. Therefore therapists should coordinate therapy sessions to allow appropriate breaks for rest and sleep periods.

Therapists can alter the environment to help the client fall asleep and maintain sleep (e.g., turning on a fan if that is what the client is used to listening to at bedtime, playing soft music, darkening the room, shutting the door to minimize noise, having an appropriate number of covers and pillows available). Therapists can recommend that clients who have difficulty falling asleep avoid caffeinated drinks and foods (e.g., coffee, colas, chocolate), alcohol, and tobacco for at least six hours before bedtime. Stress management and relaxation training may be helpful. See the Techniques section for "Relaxation and Stress Reduction."

Other recommendations that can help sleep functions include management of underlying causes of sleep impairments (e.g., antidepressant medication for major depressive disorder, extinguishing sources of anxiety), keeping a consistent daily sleep-wake schedule (e.g., wake up and go to sleep at the same time every day), only lying in bed when it is time to sleep (e.g., do not use the bed to do work or watch television), avoiding daytime naps, exercising regularly in the morning, avoiding stimulation prior to bedtime (e.g., going for a run, work activities), engaging in relaxing activities prior to bedtime (e.g., leisure reading, needlecrafts), a long hot shower or bath before bedtime, no nighttime snacking, and making the bedroom a quiet and comfortable space to help induce relaxation.

b139 Global Mental Functions, Other Specified and Unspecified

Specific Mental Functions (b140-b189)

b140 Attention Functions

Specific mental functions of focusing on an external stimulus or internal experience for the required period of time.

Inclusions: functions of sustaining attention, shifting attention, dividing attention, sharing attention; concentration; distractibility

- *b1400 Sustaining Attention*
  Mental functions that produce concentration for the period of time required.
- *b1401 Shifting Attention*
  Mental functions that permit refocusing concentration from one stimulus to another.
- *b1402 Dividing Attention*
  Mental functions that permit focusing on two or more stimuli at the same time.
- *b1403 Sharing Attention*
  Mental functions that permit focusing on the same stimulus by two or more people, such as a child and a caregiver both focusing on a toy.
- *b1408 Attention Functions, Other Specified*
- *b1409 Attention Functions, Unspecified*

Treatment for Attention Functions

The therapist observes all of the attention functions of the client in both a non-distracting and distracting environment. The therapist will need to have a clear view of a clock or be wearing a watch to note the time when attention to the task begins and when it ends to determine a total length of time that the client was able to attend to the task. For example, give the client a wood project that needs to be sanded. Provide the client with only the piece of wood and one piece of sandpaper. Observe the client's ability to remain focused on the task at hand (sustained attention). Next, give the client the written directions that go with the woodworking project. Observe the client's ability to shift his attention between the directions and the project (shifting attention). Next, have the client perform a physical skill that is part of the client's treatment plan while working on the wood project. For example, have the client stand while working on the wood project and direct him to pay attention to his posture (standing tall, maintaining desired weight bearing on a lower extremity, etc.). Observe the client's ability to pay attention to two things at the same time (dividing attention). Lastly, assist the client with a portion of the wood project (e.g., assembling the pieces) and observe the client's ability to attend to the project appropriately with the therapist (sharing attention, does the client notice that the therapist has a piece of the project that he is looking for, does the client exhibit behavioral changes when sharing a task, etc.).

The therapist measures the client's response in terms of:

- *Length of time*: e.g., client is able to sustain attention to a task for 30 minutes in a highly distracting environment.
- *Percentage of task*: e.g., client is able to sustain attention to a simple task at 50% — meaning that the client was able to sustain attention to 50% of the task or sustain attention to the task 50% of the time.
- *Level of assistance*: e.g., client requires moderate verbal cues to shift attention from one task to another in a minimally distracting environment.
- *Dysfunction related to task*: e.g., client requires moderate tactile cues for grooming at the bathroom mirror secondary to poor divided attention skills.

There are a variety to issues that affect a client's attention functions including stimulus intensity, novelty, past experience, memory, motivation, expectancy, complexity of task demands, distractions, and fatigue (O'Sullivan and Schmitz, 1988). The therapist should be aware of these issues and try to account for these issues within sessions:

1. Choose a treatment time when the client is not fatigued.
2. Vary the complexity of the task to observe attention changes. Does the client's ability to focus on a task vary depending on the complexity of the task? For example, a client is asked to sand a piece of wood and he is able to attend to the task for 30 minutes. However, when he is asked to do a task that involves reading (e.g., read instructions for the wood project), he is highly distracted and requires moderate verbal cues to attend to the task. The therapist needs to explain the variability in the amount of the assistance needed. In this example, reading is a more complex task than sanding a piece of wood. Reading requires the individual to be able to read words, remember the previous sentences to be able to see the whole concept of the material, have good vision, and have adequate attention functions for reading. Therefore, therapists must be aware of the inherent characteristics of each

task and tease out the specific problem or problems for the client.

3. Choose tasks that are attractive to the client (e.g., a recreational interest).
4. Consider the inherent stimulus of the activity. A stimulus that has an action component is inherently easier to attend to (e.g., a toy that sings and dances will draw attention more than a piece of wood that sits on the table and does nothing).

The therapist works on increasing a client's attention functions by designing treatment sessions that slightly challenge the client beyond his/her current level. Some recommendations are to:

- Use graduated tasks. The therapist chooses activities that require slightly more skill than the client's current baseline. For example, if the client's baseline for sustained attention is five minutes, then the therapist should choose modalities that inherently require an increased length of attention of 10 minutes. More than 10 minutes is not advised in this case because the therapist risks frustrating the client by asking for something far beyond the client's ability. It could also cause the client to feel inadequate or angry and possibly affect the client-therapist relationship and the client's motivation to attend and participate in therapy. Tasks should not be simple. They should be possible to accomplish, but progressively more challenging. (In cases, such as dementia, where functions are being lost, the therapist must progressively reduce the complexity of tasks to level appropriate for the client.)
- Manipulate the environment (e.g., start out in a quiet and non-distracting environment and gradually increase the distractions from the environment).
- Choose activities initially that are familiar and enjoyable to the client and gradually transition to advanced activities of daily living that are not as attractive or familiar to the client yet are realistic parts of the client's activity pattern after discharge (e.g., begin with gardening activities and progress to finding phone numbers in the phone book or reading a letter from an insurance company).
- Choose simple repetitive activities and increase the complexity by adding activities that require more diverse skills and increased attention functions. For example, sanding a wood project is a simple repetitive physical motion that requires less sustained attention than the task of reading directions about which parts to sand.
- Use treatment sessions of an appropriate length. Treatment sessions may need to be short and

multiple rather than one long session, especially if the client's attention span is shorter than five minutes (e.g., schedule three 10-minute sessions rather than one half-hour session).

- Use a variety of interventions to help the client maintain attention (verbal cues, demonstration, pictorial illustrations, videos, gestural cues, computer software programs, etc.).
- Provide the client with immediate positive feedback (e.g., "You are doing a wonderful job. Do you know that you paid attention to the game for 20 minutes without me saying a word! Yesterday you were only able to pay attention for 15 minutes.").
- Encourage the client to maintain eye contact during social tasks (e.g., conversations, discussions within a group) to help with paying attention to the task and being able to divide attention.
- Structure or limit information presented to the client. Good verbal commands using adequate volume and inflection can provide an effective means of directing attention. Clearly identify the key task elements (e.g., there are five business names on the list, find each one in the phone book and then write each phone number down on this piece of paper).
- Break the task into simple components if the task is complex. As learning progresses, the whole task and its component parts should be practiced, as well as the provision of increased distractions to promote the development of advanced skills.

Some clients with severe attention function deficits "perseverate" on one action, verbalization, or thought. This means that the client gets stuck on a particular action (e.g., snapping fingers, tapping hand on table), verbalization (e.g., a name, curse word), or a thought (e.g., Client asks, "Where is my mom? She said she would be here." Therapist replies, "She is coming at 3:00 P.M." Two minutes after this conversation the client asks the therapist the same question again.). The problem of perseveration is caused by deficits in attention functions and memory functions. O'Sullivan and Schmitz (1988) give suggestions on how to best work with this type of client:

> Patients with severe attentional deficits are unable to attend to important stimuli and often appear erratic in thought and action. Consistency must become the hallmark of treatment. The treatment schedule, setting, procedures, verbal instructions, and therapist should be consistent from day to day. Activities that work within the limitations of the patient's attention span should be planned. ... Key factors in achieving success in treatment are the establishment of a daily routine and the prompt reinforcement of desired behaviors. Patients who perseverate appear to get stuck on a thought or action plan and persist in repeating themselves over and over again. These patients should be guided gently into a new activity. Use of interesting activities can help refocus attention, and use of well-defined sequences of activities can help limit perseveration episodes. Successful completion of each part of the sequence should be positively reinforced (p. 261).

If the client's attention functions are not fully recovered or do not reflect the appropriate developmental level of the client, the therapist will need to adapt activities to maximize the client's functioning, independence, and safety. Some recommendations include:

- Teach the client's caregivers how to manipulate the client's environment to reduce distractions, provide appropriate cueing to redirect the client back to a task (see "Behavior Manipulation" in the Techniques section), and use adaptive aids such as a recorder that plays a general verbal cue to encourage attention to a simple repetitive task (e.g., a tape recorder that plays, "Nancy, keep eating, you're doing a good job" every three minutes might allow the caregiver time to get dressed in the morning without having to continually cue the client to eat her breakfast).
- Zoltan (1996) recommends additional adaptations for attention function deficits: 1. The client prepares himself/herself to attend to a task via statements spoken internally or out loud (e.g., "I have to really concentrate on this and read this sentence."); 2. The client vocalizes step by step what s/he is doing as s/he performs the task ("First, I am going to open up the checkbook. Now I am going to find the right page," etc.); 3. Caregivers and friends speak slowly and in short phrases and sentences with pauses to allow time for processing; 4. The client paraphrases what s/he just heard and the speaker repeats the information if needed; 5. The client learns to cue others to speak more slowly and request repetition; 6. Distractions in the external and internal environment of the client are reduced: External — remove clutter and reduce noise level; Internal — reduce hunger, pain, anger, fatigue, etc. (e.g., adjust room temperature, provide rest periods, teach the client how to shelve emotional internal distracters through techniques such as visual imagery); 7. Tasks are modified so that the elements of information processing are emphasized or highlighted. For example, underline an important part of written directions, or make important elements visually bigger or a

different color. This will help the client discriminate different components of the learning task.

Because of the kind of tasks s/he is concerned with, the recreational therapist is in a very good position to help the client with real-world attention functions. The therapist's ability to increase attention skills in the client will help all of the members of the treatment team in their work with the client.

b144 Memory Functions
Specific mental functions of registering and storing information and retrieving it as needed.
Inclusions: functions of short-term and long-term memory, immediate, recent, and remote memory; memory span; retrieval of memory; remembering; functions used in recalling and learning, such as in nominal, selective, and dissociative amnesia
Exclusions: consciousness functions (b110); orientation functions (b114); intellectual functions (b117); attention functions (b140); perceptual functions (b156); thought functions (b160); higher-level cognitive functions (b164); mental functions of language (b167); calculation functions (b172)

- **b1440 Short Term Memory**
  Mental functions that produce a temporary, disruptable memory store of around 30 seconds duration from which information is lost if not consolidated into long-term memory.
- **b1441 Long Term Memory**
  Mental functions that produce a memory system permitting the long-term storage of information from short-term memory and both autobiographical memory for past events and semantic memory for language and facts.
- **b1442 Retrieval of Memory**
  Specific mental functions of recalling information stored in long-term memory and bringing it into awareness.
- **b1448 Memory Functions, Other Specified**
- **b1449 Memory Functions, Unspecified**

Treatment for Memory Functions

Zoltan (1996) defines the memory process in sequential phases:

1. *Sensory memory*: This is when the individual selectively attends to stimuli in the environment. Information at this first stage of processing is distorted.
2. *Working memory*: Information acquired in "sensory memory" is retained by mental repetition (rehearsal). Information is encoded and consolidated (integrated into the client's current memory schema or framework) in long-term memory. The consolidation process can take minutes to hours and may be stored for months or a lifetime. The deeper "working memory"

processes information, the better it is remembered.
3. *Retrieval of stored information*: The mind searches for the information and then it directs the appropriate verbal or motor response.

The therapist challenges the client's memory functions and assesses the client's response. There are many ways to test memory functions. Some examples include:

- *To test short-term memory functions*: Short-term memory is also referred to as "working memory" because it stores information that is currently being used (e.g., looking up a phone number and then dialing it without looking at it again). It is difficult to put a time limit on how long information stays in short-term memory; however the ICF defines it as having a 30-second duration. One way that therapists can test short-term memory is to tell the client three one-word items (e.g., house, flower, dog) and ask the client to immediately repeat them.
- *To test long-term memory*: 1. The therapist asks the client to tell him/her the three items used to test short-term memory at a later time (e.g., after five minutes, after 30 minutes, the next day). 2. The therapist asks the client long-term memory questions (therapist must know the correct answer) such as where did you go for vacation last year, what is your birthday. The first method tests the client's ability to form long-term semantic memories. The second method looks at the ability to create autobiographical memories of past events.
- *To test retrieval of memory*: Teach the client a new task and ask the client to perform the new task at a later date (e.g., the next treatment session). Note that the tests of long-term memory (above) also test the retrieval functions. It is nearly impossible to test for long-term memory without using the retrieval process.

Memory can be measured by:
- *Scales* (e.g., poor, fair, good, excellent).
- *Percentage of memory function* (e.g., client's immediate recall is 60% of material presented).
- *Ratio* (e.g., client is able to recall 4:6 [four out of six] items after five minutes).
- *Level of assistance* (e.g., client requires moderate verbal cues to recall family members).
- *Dysfunction related to task* (e.g., client requires minimal verbal cues to gather needed items at the grocery store secondary to poor memory functions).

The therapist enhances memory functions through repetition, graduated tasks, and cueing. (See "Neuroplasticity" and "Behavioral Manipulation" in the Techniques section.) Zoltan (1996, pp. 140-141) lists 11 treatment principles when remediating memory functions:

1. The remediation of short-term memory will have limited effect in early stages of recovery.
2. Attentional processes and sensory memory should be addressed first.
3. Attention training results in improved memory in many clients.
4. Along with attention and concentration, rehearsal is a necessary antecedent of memory retraining.
5. The client must relearn rehearsal skills before any other form of working memory training can work. The therapist must evaluate how many rehearsals are required to bring the client's memory to average levels.
6. Teach the client to rehearse information in a manner that will ensure that it transfers to long-term memory so that it can be retrieved at a later time.
7. Effective encoding of information is required for future recall. If the material is well analyzed, recall at a later time will be easier.
8. Identify and characterize client's preserved memory abilities and build memory-retraining strategies around them.
9. Research has shown that it is possible to teach a client with severe memory loss different kinds of domain specific learning that can be applied to activities of daily living. This is only accomplished if the procedure is consistent, the job is broken down into component steps, and the client is taught each component directly.
10. Organization facilitates recall. The client with brain damage may lose the ability to organize automatically.
11. Straight repetitive drills do not appear to generalize to untrained memory or functional memory outside the clinic. Repetition with the use of vanishing cues, however, has been shown to be effective. Computer software with vanishing cues built into the program is especially helpful.

Use an indirect, direct, or domain-specific approach depending on the client's awareness of memory loss, strategy used, and recall status.

If the client's memory functions are not adequate, adaptations need to be developed. This may include the use of:

- *External aids* (organizer, schedules, logs, lists, pictures, recorder, directions, audio tape, watches, alarms, labels).
- *Training in active listening skills.*
- *Chunking or grouping*: Provide a way of organizing information to be recalled. For example, the client can put things into categories (write shopping list items under specific categories). It doesn't have to be written. For example, the client might remember that she needs to buy purple flowers at the store by repeating to herself that the top of the letter "P" in purple is round, just like a flower, and also like the container that she wants to plant them in. Therefore, she is using the shape of a circle to help her remember what she needs to buy at the store. Items and information can be grouped by color, size, shape, function, origins, etc.
- *Mental retracing*: This is when you retrace steps in your mind (e.g., I can't find my keys. I thought they were on the table. Let me think. When I came home, I took the mail out of the mailbox and then opened the door. I walked inside and put the mail down on the hutch. Oh, I put the keys down with the mail on the hutch.).
- *Visual imagery*: Client closes his/her eyes and pictures in the mind's eye the information, the task, or the action (e.g., the client pictures herself in the locker room at the YWCA and walks through the process of re-dressing to help her to remember all of the items she needs to take with her — hairdryer, towel, change of clothes, lock for the locker, soap, etc.).
- *Story method*: The client forms a story about the words or phrases s/he is to remember. For example, if a client has to remember to call his friend Dave, buy dog food, and call the water department, he might remember it by making up a story. (Dave ate the dog food and then needed a drink of water.)
- *Association*: Two new pieces of information can be associated or new information can be associated with old information. Associations can be gained from all sensory modalities. An emotional association can also assist in recall. For example, remembering a name can be easier if the client thinks about all of the other people she knows with the same name and associates the new person with the other people.
- *Pegging*: Develop a word from the first letters of things that need to be recalled (e.g., DEEP: D: deep breathing, E: eat right, E: exercise, P: play).

b147 Psychomotor Functions
Specific mental functions of control over both motor and psychological events at the body level.
Inclusions: functions of psychomotor control, such as psychomotor retardation, excitement and agitation,

posturing, catatonia, negativism, ambitendency, echopraxia and echolalia; quality of psychomotor function

Exclusions: consciousness functions (b110); orientation functions (b114); intellectual functions (b117); energy and drive functions (b130); attention functions (b140); mental functions of language (b167); mental functions of sequencing complex movements (b176)

- *b1470 Psychomotor Control*
  Mental functions that regulate the speed of behaviour or response time that involves both motor and psychological components, such as in disruption of control producing psychomotor retardation (moving and speaking slowly, decrease in gesturing and spontaneity) or psychomotor excitement (excessive behavioral and cognitive activity, usually nonproductive and often in response to inner tension as in toe-tapping, hand-wringing, agitation, or restless-ness).

- *b1471 Quality of Psychomotor Functions*
  Mental functions that produce nonverbal behaviours in the proper sequence and character of its subcomponents, such as hand and eye coordination, or gait.

- *b1478 Psychomotor Functions, Other Specified*
- *b1479 Psychomotor Functions, Unspecified*

Treatment for Psychomotor Functions

See "Activities and Participation Chapter 4 Mobility" for a discussion of treatment for deficits in psychomotor functions.

b152 Emotional Functions

Specific mental functions related to the feeling and affective components of the processes of the mind.

Inclusions: functions of appropriateness of emotion, regulation, and range of emotion; affect; sadness, happiness, love, fear, anger, hate, tension, anxiety, joy, sorrow; lability of emotion; flattening of affect

Exclusions: temperament and personality functions (b126); energy and drive functions (b130)

- *b1520 Appropriateness of Emotion*
  Mental functions that produce congruence of feeling or affect with the situation, such as happiness at receiving good news.

- *b1521 Regulation of Emotion*
  Mental functions that control the experience and display of affect.

- *b1522 Range of Emotion*
  Mental functions that produce the spectrum of experience or arousal of affect or feelings such as love, hate, anxiousness, sorrow, joy, fear, and anger.

- *b1528 Emotional Functions, Other Specified*
- *b1529 Emotional Functions, Unspecified*

Treatment for Emotional Functions

The appropriateness, regulation, and range of emotion are affected by changes in the brain (e.g., traumatic brain injury, stroke), life experiences (e.g., taught through childhood not to show emotion), culture (e.g., Italians often have a colorful and dramatic show of emotions), psychological trauma (e.g., abused child has a restricted range of emotions), psychological illness (e.g., major depressive disorder, bipolar personality disorder), and the current social situation (e.g., being at a funeral, a special social occasion that requires the individual not to engage in conflicts with others).

If emotional deficits are suspected, the therapist can further assess the client by observing:

- *Appropriateness of emotion*: The therapist observes the congruence among the client's verbalization, behavioral actions, and the current situation. The therapist should also ask the client, as appropriate, to confirm whether or not s/he perceives congruence. For example, a client is talking about a happy occasion, yet her affect expresses sadness. The therapist shares his observation with the client by saying, "Your words denote happiness about the occasion, yet you sound so sad. Are you sad?" The client responds, "No, I'm not sad." The therapist probes, "Are you aware that you sound sad?" Client answers, "No."

- *Regulation of emotion*: The therapist observes the client as previously described in "appropriateness of emotion." A client who has problems regulating emotion may or may not be aware of this occurrence. For example, a client may scream loudly when communicating in a quiet room with the therapist, while another client will be unable to control the constant variability in emotional expression (e.g., switches from sadness, to paranoia, to excitability, to anger).

- *Range of emotion*: The therapist observes the client as previously described in "appropriateness of emotion." Clients with limited range of emotion are unable, or have difficulty with, the full spectrum of emotional expression. Clients may not be able to show or express love, anger, etc.

Emotional functions can be measured by:

- *Description of incongruence* (e.g., "Client's emotional expression is not congruent with verbalizations. Client's words express sadness, yet affect is upbeat and cheerful.")

- *Percentage* (e.g., "Client is able to regulate emotional responses within treatment sessions 75% of the time.")
- *Level of assistance* (e.g., "When verbally distracted from the current situation, the client is able to halt emotional lability events.") Some clients who become emotionally labile (begin crying, and sometimes laughing, out of context) as a result of a brain injury can be cued out of the perseverative-like event through distraction.
- *Dysfunction related to task* (e.g., "Client requires moderate verbal cues to express emotion of anger within a conflict.")

A therapist can utilize a variety of approaches to help a client enhance emotional functioning. The following ideas have proven to be successful for clients who are ready to improve their emotional functions.

1. *Drama*: Client portrays a character that expresses the emotional function goals of the client. For example, a client who lacks the ability to show sadness portrays a client who is sad about the loss of her sister. Psychodrama is a type of drama therapy that enables the client to act out a specific interaction that holds psychological meaning. It allows the client the opportunity to try out new behaviors within a safe therapeutic environment. For example, the therapist portrays the abusive parent and the client portrays himself within the context of a typical interaction that the client has with the parent. Roles are often reversed (therapist plays the client and client portrays the parent). Giving a client a safe environment to explore and express emotions that had negative consequences attached can be helpful to increase the client's emotional range.
2. *Social skills training*: See "Social Skills Training" in the Techniques section.
3. *Other creative arts*: Like drama, creative arts such as music, dance, writing, clay, painting, and crafts provide an alternative form of emotional expression, thus providing the client with the psychological benefits of such expression. It may also prove helpful in leading the client to vocal expression of the emotion (e.g., easier to write about anger than to talk about it). For more information about the creative arts see Nathan and Mirviss (1998) *Therapy Techniques Using the Creative Arts*.
4. *Direct feedback*: Providing the client with direct and immediate feedback about his/her emotional expression may increase the client's awareness of the behavior, thus allowing the client to incorporate techniques to change his/her emotional response. For example, if a client is screaming a conversation in a quiet room with the therapist, the therapist should say to the client, "Do you realize that you are screaming loudly?" Once the client becomes aware of the behavior in a therapy setting, the therapist can teach him how to become aware of the behavior in other settings (e.g., look at the response from the other person) and how to decrease his/her speech volume (e.g., take a deep breath and talk softly as if a child were sleeping or any other association that the client is able to use to bring down his volume to a normal conversational level). Repetitive use of a technique within functional tasks can increase the learning process of the compensatory strategies.

Therapists need to be aware, though, that the above approaches are not appropriate for all clients. There may be other issues that need to be resolved before the client is ready to allow himself/herself to have a full range of emotions again. There may also be physical causes, such as brain injury, that need time to heal before the client can be expected to display a normal range of emotions. Clients who have continued to have a flat affect, who are emotionally labile, who are unable to regulate their emotions, or who have a limited range of emotions despite interventions may benefit from the following adaptations.

- *Pharmacology* (medication): Certain medications can be helpful in controlling mood, thus increasing the client's appropriateness, regulation, or range of emotions (e.g., a depressed client is prescribed an antidepressant from the psychiatrist and is now able to experience feelings of pleasure and joy).
- *Distraction*: Distracting the client for a moment from the conversation or task at hand can be very helpful to halt an emotional lability event. For example, if the client is crying during a game of checkers and you know that the client is emotionally labile (the uncontrollable crying is not due to feelings of sadness), asking the client "What time is it?" may disrupt the event and halt the behavior.
- *Direct feedback*: Teach caregivers how to provide feedback to the client to facilitate awareness of emotional expressions (see "direct feedback" in previous section). Some clients may respond negatively to direct feedback (e.g., increased agitation, violent behavior) and therefore it may be contraindicated. If this is the case, behavior modification techniques may be helpful.

See "Activities and Participation Chapter 7 Interpersonal Interactions and Relationships" for more treatment ideas.

b156 Perceptual Functions

Specific mental functions of recognizing and interpreting sensory stimuli.
Inclusions: functions of auditory, visual, olfactory, gustatory, tactile and visuospatial perception, such as hallucination or illusion
Exclusions: consciousness functions (b110); orientation functions (b114); attention functions (b140); memory functions (b144); mental functions of language (b167); seeing and related functions (b210-b229); hearing and vestibular functions (b230-b249); additional sensory functions (b250-b279)

- *b1560 Auditory Perception*
  Mental functions involved in discriminating sounds, tones, pitches, and other acoustic stimuli.
- *b1561 Visual Perception*
  Mental functions involved in discriminating shape, size, colour, and other ocular stimuli.
- *b1562 Olfactory Perception*
  Mental functions involved in distinguishing differences in smells.
- *b1563 Gustatory Perception*
  Mental functions involved in distinguishing differences in tastes, such as sweet, sour, salty, and bitter stimuli, detected by the tongue.
- *b1564 Tactile Perception*
  Mental functions involved in distinguishing differences in texture, such as rough or smooth stimuli, detected by touch.
- *b1565 Visuospatial Perception*
  Mental function involved in distinguishing by sight the relative position of objects in the environment or in relation to oneself.
- *b1568 Perceptual Functions, Other Specified*
- *b1569 Perceptual Functions, Unspecified*

Treatment for Perceptual Functions

Perception is more than just awareness of sensations. It is an awareness, processing, and integrative skill as O'Sullivan & Schmitz (1988, p. 94) explain:

> Perception cannot be viewed as independent of sensation. However, the quality of perception is far more complicated than the recognition of the individual sensations. Perception is the ability to select those stimuli that require attention and action, to integrate those stimuli with each other and with prior information, and finally to interpret them. The end result of this process enables the individual to make sense out of a complex and constantly changing internal and external sensory environment. Perceptual ability is clearly a

prerequisite for learning, and rehabilitation is largely a learning process.

The categories in this section do not address whether the client has the ability to receive sensory input. Those issues are dealt with in Body Functions Chapter 2 Sensory Function and Pain. The functions described in this chapter deal with the ability to process sensory stimuli once they have reached the brain.

When assessing a client's function within a task, careful attention should be given to sensory and perceptual problems (e.g., client smells a flower and says it smells like a banana, unable to identify a piece of paper). Should sensory or perceptual problems be suspected, further evaluation will be needed. It can be very difficult to tease out perceptual problems from other problems. For example, if the therapist asks a client to pick up a pencil off the table and the client does not respond, the problem could lie in the area of language processing (maybe the client has receptive aphasia — words spoken sound like gibberish), visual object agnosia (unable to identify common objects), visual neglect (pencil is on the left side of the table and the client has left neglect), severe attention problems (unable to follow one-step directions), etc. To do the assessment well the therapist must have: 1. a full knowledge of the deficits associated with specific disabilities (e.g., a client with a right stroke is prone to having left neglect), 2. the ability to rule out other possible deficits (e.g., place the pencil on right side of the table, show the client a picture of a pencil and then put the palms of your hands in the air to express the question of "Where is it?", move the client into a quiet and then a highly distracting environment to find out if distractions play a role in being able to attend to the verbal command of picking up the pencil, etc.), 3. good observational skills, 4. the ability to manipulate environmental factors, and 5. understanding of the findings of other health professionals. (Note that all of these confounding factors should also be documented with the appropriate part of the ICF. When deciding on treatment, they will probably have a higher priority than deficits in perceptual functions.)

Once the therapist knows that sensory function itself is intact and can make the instructions clear to the client, presenting examples of stimuli in any of the sensory modes in this chapter is relatively straightforward. It is mostly a matter of having an appropriate set of examples. A variety of specific testing tools for perceptual problems are clearly reviewed in Zoltan's book *Vision, Perception, and Cognition* (see references). Therapists document the deficits in the following ways:

- *Percentage of behavior* (e.g., Client has visual object agnosia, however client is able to identify common objects through tactile perception at 25% — in other words, when the client is presented with visual objects, the client is able to identify 25% of the objects presented using tactile perception.)
- *Dysfunction related to task* (e.g., Client requires moderate assistance when going up and down stairs due to problems with depth perception; Client requires supervision when traveling to and from school due to inability to successfully compensate for color agnosia.)
- *Descriptors*: Poor, fair, good, excellent (e.g., Client exhibits poor figure-ground perception).
- *Level of assistance* (e.g., Client requires cueing 20% of the time to attend to the light used to signal a phone call.)

Treatment for deficits in perceptual functions consists of trying to increase the client's ability to recognize and correctly interpret sensory stimuli and finding adaptations for functionality that is not currently present.

Increasing abilities is most often done through repeated practice. Techniques for focusing attention are appropriate for all of these deficits because part of the problem is that the brain has lost the ability to focus a particular type of attention. Here are some ideas for the specific modalities discussed in the ICF:

- *Auditory perception*: Practice identifying sounds that are important to the client's lifestyle (e.g., smoke detector, telephone, doorbell, teakettle whistle). If the deficit includes problems with understanding speech, the recreational therapist should work on matching spoken words with objects or pictures to help rebuild an aural vocabulary.
- *Visual perception*: There are several common visual deficits. If the problem is recognizing objects by sight, hand the client objects repetitively in treatment sessions and say the name of the object. Ask the client to repeat the name of the object. Have a label on the object with the name of the object. Have the client try to pick out the object from a variety of objects on a table. See the discussion on form discrimination, below, for more ideas. If the problem is identifying faces, practice matching names with faces that are familiar to the client. If the problem is in seeing the relationship between objects in the whole visual field, practice combining parts of the task into a whole through multimodal cues (verbal, hand over hand). If the problem is identifying colors (which is important in the community for actions like crossing streets), practice naming and identifying colors.
- *Olfactory perception*: Practice with odors that are important for the client. Oil-based olfactory stimuli are usually better than alcohol-based.
- *Gustatory perception*: Practice tastes. Start with simple tastes (salty, sweet) and move on to food tastes (apples, hamburgers).
- *Tactile perception*: Practice identifying shapes and textures without using vision. As always, start with simple forms and textures (wooden blocks, warm water) before moving to more subtle objects.

If the deficits are interfering with advanced activities of daily living or creating a safety issue, the therapist should make adaptations that will help the client deal with the deficit. One of the most important adaptations to consider is the use of a companion animal. Companion animals are usually thought of as appropriate for sensory deficits, but they can help the client with perceptual function deficits as well. Examples of other adaptations include:

- *Auditory perception*: Change sounds to a visual cue (e.g., flashing light on telephone placed in clear view within the home). For speech issues, teach the client how to cue others that they need to speak more slowly and allow more time for the client to process the conversation.
- *Visual perception*: If the problem is recognizing objects by sight, put labels on items that will be used for functional tasks so the client can recognize the object by its name. If the problem is identifying faces, provide names on pictures; teach acquaintances to say their name when greeting the client. If the problem is in seeing the relationship between objects in the whole visual field, simplify the tasks that a client regularly performs into singular components (e.g., a dinner plate with one portion of the meal and one utensil). If the problem is identifying colors, recommend that assistance be provided, especially if the client is unable to judge the color of the traffic light by evaluating traffic patterns or the location of the lights relative to one another.
- *Olfactory perception*: Make sure the client has support so that he does not come to harm by not being able to smell. Two examples are being sure not to eat spoiled foods by mistake and being aware of smoke alarms since the client can't smell smoke.
- *Gustatory perception*: As with olfactory perception, make sure that spoiled foods aren't eaten.
- *Tactile perception*: Use vision as a compensatory strategy. Teach the client to use vision to tell the

shape and texture of items. If heat and cold are an issue, make sure the client is protected from dangerous situations, such as scalding water and hot stoves.

Form Discrimination

Form discrimination (a part of visual perception) is an inability to attend to variations in form (e.g., mistaking a water pitcher for a urinal). Some additional ideas for addressing the deficit include: practice sorting objects (e.g., sort checker pieces and coins), encourage the use of tactile perception to distinguish items (e.g., checker pieces have a raised rough edge and coins are smooth). In addition to using labels on objects, you can also use these ideas for making form discrimination easier. Keep items in the same place as much as possible. The more organized things are, the more familiar the client will become with the items (e.g., hammers are in the top drawer of the toolbox and screwdrivers are in the second drawer of the toolbox). Shapes are best recognized when they are in upright positions, so try to put commonly used items in this position (e.g., hang toothbrushes on the wall, hang the hammer and the screwdriver on the wall, buy "stand up" toothpaste).

Visuospatial Perception

Visuospatial perception is often described in two contexts. Although they are not clearly identified by the ICF, they are commonly assessed and addressed in clinical environments.

1. *Depth perception* (or stereopsis): The ability to perceive the third dimension of depth. This is necessary for actions such as climbing stairs, driving, and grasping objects. To provide therapy for the deficit, have the client utilize tactile perception to identify distances between or among items. For example, if a client is going to make a craft project, line up the supplies perpendicular to the client. Have the client feel each craft supply in its place in line (feel the bottle of glue, then reach behind the glue and feel the scissors, reach behind the scissors and feel stack of paper, etc.). Play computer games that stimulate skills of depth perception (e.g., car racing, any game that has approaching targets). Adaptations include encouraging the client to rely on tactile perception to identify distances (e.g., feel the distance between the wheelchair and the bed before transferring). Use environmental adaptations to promote safety (e.g., place a bright color tape on the edge of steps).
2. *Figure-ground perception*: The inability to distinguish the foreground from the background.

Items in the environment appear to blend together and it is difficult for the client to separate different objects. Practice with attention is one of the best ways to help the client reduce this deficit. Place several objects into a box so that the objects overlap each other. Ask the client to identify what s/he sees. Gradually increase the number of items in the box. Adaptations include keeping the environment neat and organized so that items are clearly delineated from one another. Use high contrast backgrounds whenever possible. For example, if a client wants to paint on a white piece of paper, place a dark colored tablecloth on the table so that the client is able to clearly see the edges of the paper. In addition, paint the handles of the paintbrushes white so that they too stand out on the dark tablecloth. Use a white mug to hold the water, etc.

b160 Thought Functions
Specific mental functions related to the ideational component of the mind.
Inclusions: functions of pace, form, control and content of thought; goal-directed thought functions; logical thought functions, such as pressure of thought, flight of ideas, thought block, incoherence of thought, tangentiality, circumstantiality, delusions, obsessions, and compulsions
Exclusions: intellectual functions (b117); memory functions (b144); psychomotor functions (b147); perceptual functions (b156); higher-level cognitive functions (b164); mental functions of language (b167); calculation functions (b172)

- *b1600 Pace of Thought*
  Mental functions that govern speed of the thinking process.
- *b1601 Form of Thought*
  Mental functions that organize the thinking process as to its coherence and logic.
  Inclusions: impairments of ideational perseveration, tangentiality, and circumstantiality
- *b1602 Content of Thought*
  Mental functions consisting of the ideas that are present in the thinking process and what is being conceptualized.
  Inclusions: impairments of delusions, overvalued ideas, and somatization
- *b1603 Control of Thought*
  Mental functions that provide volitional control of thinking and are recognized as such by the person.
  Inclusions: impairments of rumination, obsession, thought broadcast, and thought insertion
- *b1608 Thought Functions, Other Specified*
- *b1609 Thought Functions, Unspecified*

Treatment for Thought Functions

Thought function impairments are generally seen in mental health disorders such as schizophrenia, bipolar disorder, delusional disorders, phobias, depression, dementia, and obsessive-compulsive disorder, as well as physical disabilities that impair the brain including dementia, traumatic brain injury, and cerebrovascular accident.

Thought can be described as process (ability to put together ideas and associations) and content (specific things the person is thinking about).

Formal thought disorders identified by Sadock and Sadock (2003) include:

1. *Circumstantiality* (trouble getting to the point): When trying to relay an idea, the client lacks the ability to relay the thought in a goal directed manner. Irrelevant thoughts and ideas are unnecessarily explained. The client eventually comes back to his/her main thought.
2. *Clang associations* (rhyming): Thoughts are associated by the sound of words rather than by their meaning, e.g., through rhyming or assonance.
3. *Derailment* (synonymous with loose associations): A breakdown in both the logical connection between ideas and the overall sense of goal directedness. The words make sentences, but the sentences don't make sense.
4. *Neologism*: The invention of new words or phrases or the use of conventional words in idiosyncratic ways.
5. *Perseveration*: Repetition out of context of words, phrases, or ideas.
6. *Tangentiality*: The client loses the thread of the conversation and pursues divergent thoughts that are influenced by internal and external stimuli. The client does not return to the original thought (e.g., A client begins to talk about wanting a specific food. Before telling the therapist the specific food he wants, he thinks about the nurse who brought the food the last time. He begins to talk about the nurse and does not return to telling the therapist the specific food he wants.).
7. *Thought blocking*: A sudden disruption of thought or a break in the flow of ideas. The client may say that s/he is unable to remember what s/he wanted to say or is unable to recall what s/he was talking about.

Common measurement descriptors of thought functions include:

- *Pace of thought*: Typically described as being slow, fast, or hesitant. For example, "Client's hesitant pace of thought impairs his ability to effectively problem solve for simple tasks."
- *Form of thought*: Described by type of formal thought disorders as previously reviewed. For example, "Client's form of thought is tangential."
- *Content of thought*: Described by dominant patterns (e.g., delusions; preoccupations; obsessions; compulsions; phobias; plans, intentions, or recurrent ideas about suicide or homicide; symptoms of hypochondria; and specific antisocial urges) (Sadock & Sadock, 2003). For example, "Client obsessed about washing her hands throughout the 30-minute treatment session."
- *Control of thought*: Described by who or what the person believes is controlling his/her thoughts (e.g., self, a demon, God, the man across the hallway). For example, "Client reports that his thoughts are being controlled by a demon."

Refer to specific diagnoses for information on treatment interventions (e.g., schizophrenia, dementia). In general, pharmacology can be helpful to minimize or extinguish invasive, unhealthy thoughts (e.g., delusions, obsessions). Cognitive behavioral interventions can help to change distorted thought patterns (e.g., phobias, negative thought patterns about the self). Other psychological interventions may be helpful depending upon the level of dysfunction and orientation of the client (e.g., existential counseling for exploration of life meaning may help alleviate feelings of depression thus reducing or eliminating recurrent ideas of suicide). See Activities and Participation Chapter 2 General Tasks and Demands and "Education and Counseling" in the Techniques section for a review of psychological interventions.

b164 Higher-Level Cognitive Functions
Specific mental functions especially dependent on the frontal lobes of the brain, including complex goal-directed behaviours such as decision-making, abstract thinking, planning and carrying out plans, mental flexibility, and deciding which behaviours are appropriate under what circumstance; often called executive functions.
Inclusions: functions of abstraction and organization of ideas; time management, insight and judgment; concept formation, categorization and cognitive flexibility
Exclusions: memory functions (b144); thought functions (b160); mental functions of language (b167); calculation functions (b172)
- *b1640 Abstraction*
  Mental functions of creating general ideas, qualities or characteristics out of, and distinct

from, concrete realities, specific objects, or actual instances.

- *b1641 Organization and Planning*
  Mental functions of coordinating parts into a whole, of systematizing; the mental function involved in developing a method of proceeding or acting.
- *b1642 Time Management*
  Mental functions of ordering events in chronological sequence, allocating amounts of time to events and activities.
- *b1643 Cognitive Flexibility*
  Mental functions of changing strategies, or shifting mental sets, especially as involved in problem-solving.
- *b1644 Insight*
  Mental functions of awareness and understanding of oneself and one's behaviour.
- *b1645 Judgment*
  Mental functions involved in discriminating between and evaluating different options, such as those involved in forming an opinion.
- *b1646 Problem-Solving*
  Mental functions of identifying, analyzing, and integrating incongruent or conflicting information into a solution.
- *b1648 Higher-Level Cognition Functions, Other Specified*
- *b1649 Higher-Level Cognition Functions, Unspecified*

Treatment for Higher-Level Cognitive Functions

Each of the ICF subheadings is discussed below. Note that these functions are intertwined. Reading through all of them will help the therapist understand their complexity and interrelatedness. In addition, ideas in one section will often be useful in evaluating a skill or teaching a technique in another section.

Abstraction

To think abstractly is to conceptualize. It is an integration of skills that requires the client to generate ideas, to compare and differentiate, to recognize relationships, and to categorize. It also has components of memory, attention, cognitive flexibility, and problem solving. A client that is able to think abstractly would be able to recognize that a paintbrush and a jar of paint are both painting supplies or that a sarcastic remark from another client was a consequence of the disagreement they had five minutes ago. Contrasting with thinking abstractly is thinking concretely. The client who is thinking concretely is only able to recognize objects or verbalizations in isolation. He would have no connection to other things or be able to conceptualize a higher level of thinking. For example, a client would see a paintbrush as simply a paintbrush. It

would hold no connection to the other art supplies that surrounded him. And, if a sarcastic remark was directed towards him from another client, he would react to the remark as if it held no connection to the disagreement that just occurred.

If problems with abstraction are thought to be present, the therapist would assess this ability through:

1. Observing the client's verbal responses. Does the client view events in isolation? Is he able to see the consequences of an action or that the event is related to another action? For example, if the client is told that she is not allowed to drive, does she see this limitation as only not being able to operate the car?

2. Observing the client's behavioral responses. For example, ask the client to gather gardening supplies from the closet. If the client looks confused, becomes frustrated or agitated with the task, brings out a variety of items from the closet that are unrelated to gardening supplies (e.g., a hammer, a board game, a broom), or replies to the request by asking for clarification (e.g., "What do you mean?"), then the therapist may suspect that the client has problems with abstraction.

3. Asking the client specific questions to test his/her ability to compare categories (how are a pear and an apple alike?), differentiate (what is the difference between a hammer and a screwdriver?), generalize specific items to abstract categories (a pear is a ___ [fruit], a spoon is a ____ [utensil]), and identify what does not belong within a category (what does not belong: parakeet, swan, crow, poodle?).

Once deficits in abstraction have been identified, the therapist must determine a baseline of functioning. Abstraction functions can be measured in terms of:

- *Descriptors*: poor, fair, good, excellent.
- *Percentage*: e.g., Client is able to categorize items correctly 50% of the time. Client is able to form logical relationships between two items 75% of the time.
- *Level of assistance*: e.g., Client requires moderate verbal cues to separate items into two categories. Client requires moderate verbal cues to form logical relationships between two items.
- *Dysfunction related to task*: e.g., Client required minimal verbal cues to place clothing into appropriate drawers secondary to difficulty with categorization of clothing items. Client requires close supervision in woodworking area secondary to safety issues resulting from poor formation of logical relationships.

To enhance development or restoration of abstraction skills the therapist can:

- *Utilize cognitive remediation techniques*: Challenge the client to sort items into categories, compare and differentiate among items, and form logical relationships (e.g., have the client organize supplies in the woodworking room, have the client organize items that have been purposely put into a box for the client to organize, ask the client to name what does not belong on the table for the task at hand [therapist to purposely place something on the table that is not needed], ask the client to name what is missing to complete the task at hand [provide paintbrush and paper, but no paint]).
- *Provide challenges*: Challenge the client to apply abstraction skills in a functional environment. For example, identify a specific store on the mall directory (the mall directories are often divided into categories), order a complete meal from a menu (has to refer to categories of food items and form relations of food items to one another), prepare a simple meal in a kitchen (challenge the client to know categories of supplies — I need a fork, a fork is a utensil, utensils are in the drawer — as well as form relationships of parts to make a whole — to make a scrambled egg I need milk, salt, pepper, etc.).

If the client does not develop or recover adequate abstraction skill for functional tasks, the therapist can:

- Make up cheat sheets of parts that make a whole for common daily tasks (e.g., recreational supplies needed for a specific activity; ingredients to make a specific recipe and where the supplies are located). The therapist may also find it helpful to develop audiotapes that describe the task (e.g., making scrambled eggs for breakfast).
- Educate caregivers about the client's problem with the skill of abstraction and describe how it will specifically affect the client's functional life skills (e.g., may have trouble finding things at stores, may be missing parts necessary for a task because of difficulties forming associations, may have trouble linking events together and forming consequences or trouble "thinking" about things ["if this happens, then that might happen" thinking]). The therapist should teach the caregivers how to give the client supervision and cueing.

Organization and Planning

Organizing and planning are not isolated skills. They require integration of several skills. Zoltan (1996) explains this integration process, "In order to plan, the individual must be able to conceptualize change from the present situation, relate objectively to the environment, conceive alternatives, weigh alternatives and make a choice, and develop a structure or framework to give direction to the carrying out of the plan" (p. 157). Clients must also possess the skills of abstraction, cognitive flexibility, and memory, in addition to processing strategies. The client "must be able to estimate the degree of task difficulty, then an appropriate plan or strategy can be developed. If this understanding or awareness is lacking, then the [client's] strategies will be ineffective" (p. 157).

The therapist can best assess organization and planning functions through clinical observation. Zoltan (1996) gives the therapist a working outline for assessing this function through clinical observation and activity analysis.

General guidelines for evaluation:

1. Determine whether the client is aware that he has a planning deficit. Defective planning often can be revealed by asking the client what he intends to do.
2. Observe the client in a number of settings and activities during the day. Can the client plan for activities requiring two-step operations? Three-step? More complex operations?
3. Give the client a complex task without instructions. If the client begins the task without a plan, ask him to create one and begin the task again. The client's plan can then be evaluated for organization and completeness.
4. Establish functional baseline measures. Consider the duration and frequency of the problem. Select relevant functional tasks as the basis of evaluation and reassessment.

Specific areas and questions to consider and evaluate:

1. Is the client logical and consistent in his/her approach to the task?
2. How reliable is his/her chosen method?
3. Is there a common problem or consistently faulty planning strategy that is generalized to several activities?
4. Can the client conceptualize change (as evidenced through verbal or other means of communication) from the present?
5. Can the client present alternatives and make a choice based on his/her judgments?

6. Can s/he weigh alternatives and make a choice based on his/her judgments?
7. Does s/he appear to have a framework for the plan or direction s/he is demonstrating for task completion?
8. Can s/he accurately estimate task difficulty?

Note that questions and observations such as these can be applied to both functional and cognitive perceptual motor tasks. For example, inability to complete block designs and layout of graphic designs can be indicative of poor planning and task organization.

These and similar questions can be incorporated into a checklist or used in conjunction with a frequency rating scale (e.g., always, sometimes, rarely, never). To improve validity, rule out decreased attention, poor memory, decreased mental flexibility and abstraction, impaired problem solving, and aphasia as causes of poor performance.

Once deficits in organization and planning have been identified, the therapist must determine a baseline. Organization and planning can be measured in terms of:
- *Percentage*: e.g., Client is able to complete 50% of a three-step organization and planning task.
- *Level of assistance*: e.g., Client requires minimal assistance for planning and organizing simple tasks.
- *Dysfunction related to task*: Client requires moderate assistance to develop next semester's college course schedule secondary to difficulty with organizing information.

To enhance planning and organizing functions the therapist can:
1. Start with simple planning tasks that require only two or three steps and gradually progress to more complex tasks using graduated tasks.
2. Ask the client to verbalize the sequential steps of a task before it is performed.
3. Pose questions to the client to help him/her develop organizational and planning skills (e.g., what do we need next, how are we going to do that, what should we do if X happens, what are we trying to accomplish).
4. Repeat organizational and planning skills to improve processes.
5. Teach the client organizational and planning skills by helping the client to identify and break down main categories (e.g., To plan a two-day trip to the shore, we have to find out when the shore house is available, make reservations, pack, and then drive there. Let's look at each one separately. The first one is to find out when the shore house is available, so let's make a list of

what we have to do to find this out. What do you think should go here? Find the realtor's phone number, call the realtor, and ask for availability of two consecutive days in June.).

If the client does not fully develop or recover adequate organization and planning functions for functional tasks, the therapist can:
- Educate the client's caregivers about the client's deficits in this area and the type and amount of assistance needed.
- Identify specific compensatory strategies to maximize the client's independence and functioning. This may include the use of lists, day planners, calendars, and specific task worksheets. For example, if the client has to travel often (e.g., a child who has divorced parents and often travels back and forth between two houses), the therapist may help the client develop a checklist of tasks before each trip including a packing list (e.g., before I leave I have to feed the hamster and take out the trash, in my suitcase I have to put...). Students should be encouraged to use day planners and to make notations to help with planning and organizing class requirements. For example, the student should not only mark down when a paper is due, but should also make notations of when to begin research for the paper and when to begin typing the paper, etc.

Time Management

Many of the ideas described in organization and planning also apply to time management. The three basic requirements for time management are to understand how long a task is going to take, to create a schedule that has enough time for each of the tasks the client plans to do, and to allow appropriate amounts of time for transitioning between tasks.

Deficits in time management can be measured in terms of:
- *Descriptors*: poor, fair, good, excellent.
- *Percentage*: e.g., Client allows enough time for transitioning between tasks 20% of the time.
- *Level of assistance*: e.g., Client requires moderate assistance for scheduling a day with four or more tasks.
- *Dysfunction related to task*: e.g., Client expects to be able to do two tasks at the same time in different locations.

Teaching time management requires techniques similar to teaching organization and planning:
1. Help the client analyze the requirements of a task, specifically looking at how long each step is going to take.

2. Plan parts of a day, working up to a full day, to teach how to allow time for each task and how to estimate the time for transition between tasks. (Getting dressed and seeing a friend for breakfast requires time for dressing and travel time between home and the restaurant, as well as the time spent eating and getting to the next activity.)
3. Teach the client how to use a day planner to schedule events. (This is *not* an adaptation because it is normal for people to use day planners to keep track of their activities.)
4. Teaching the client how to estimate transition times, including how long a drive will take at different times of the day.

Adaptations include detailed activity sheets as described in Organization and Planning that include the time to complete an activity, help from caregivers in filling in a day planner, and lists of tasks that need to be done on a regular basis (buy food, wash clothes) so they can be added to the client's schedule.

Cognitive Flexibility

Cognitive flexibility refers to the ability of the client to change strategies and shift mental mindsets, especially as involved in problem solving. Zoltan (1996, p. 167) explains that "the [client] with poor mental flexibility will have difficulty releasing a particular stimulus from his attention. The [client's] behavior appears perseverative and an appropriate set of responses may be followed by a set of inappropriate responses. This occurs because the [client] continues to respond to prior cues that are no longer relevant. The [client] may show poor association ability and have difficulty in evaluating the relevance of the result obtained from a given problem. This stimulus-bound or perseverative behavior makes it difficult for the [client] to generalize knowledge for future problem solution." A client who has difficulty shifting mental mindsets and changing strategies in accordance with a changed mindset will have difficulty solving problems, theorizing concepts, and seeing things from a different point of view. Clients may also have problems forming and maintaining social relationships.

If problems with cognitive flexibility are suspected, the therapist should explore further testing by:
• Choosing a task that can be manipulated to test the client's cognitive flexibility. For example, give the client a "word search" puzzle (horizontal and vertical letters evenly spaced over the page — the goal is to find predetermined words

within the puzzle). The puzzle is not to be used in this way. Ask the client to cross out all of the "A's", about a quarter of the way through the puzzle, ask the client to stop crossing out the "A's" and begin crossing out the "D's", and so on. Evaluate whether or not the client is able to shift from one task to another.
• During a conversation with the client, abruptly switch topics of conversation to evaluate the level of difficulty with cognitive flexibility (e.g., when talking about the goals of the session the therapist says, "Oh, I forgot, I wanted to ask you about your therapy schedule for tomorrow. What is your schedule like?").
• Ask the client to sort a pile of change by type of coin. After the client begins to do this task, change the request often to evaluate the client's ability to shift from one task to another (e.g., now begin sorting the change into piles of seven cents, now take one cent from each of the piles of seven cents).

The therapist can document cognitive flexibility with:
• *Dysfunction*: e.g., Client was unable to change tasks three times without frustration. Client took 10 seconds to answer a question not related to the current task.
• *Level of assistance*: e.g., Client required a question not related to task to be repeated twice before answering.

The above-mentioned tasks can be used to further enhance cognitive flexibility, although using real-life tasks and situations is better. Some ideas include changing tasks within a home environment (e.g., making a sandwich while giving directions to another person on setting the table; reading a map or written directions while keeping track of the road signs; appropriately engaging in social conversation while following directions for a craft project). It can be difficult to differentiate between divided attention, shifting attention, and cognitive flexibility. Attention to a task does not equal understanding of a task, whereas cognitive flexibility requires the client to understand and respond to the changing task or situation.

Clients who continue to have difficulty with cognitive flexibility will typically show better outcomes in less stimulating environments. Written responses that the client can reference might also be helpful for common, everyday activities. Family members should be educated not to bombard the client with multiple tasks and to provide the client with one request or topic of conversation at a time. Adequate time should be provided after the end of one task or situation to allow the client to "clear" for the next task or situation. It is recommended that the client and family seek to minimize common tasks or situations that compete for the client's attention (e.g., let the answering machine take the phone calls and respond to phone calls at a later time as appropriate, plan and organize the morning routine to make it as simple as possible so that multiple tasks do not have to be completed simultaneously).

Insight

Insight is the client's awareness of himself or herself. A client who is insightful recognizes his/her strengths and weaknesses, whereas a client who lacks insight has a diminished or absent awareness of abilities and limitations. Consequently, the client who lacks insight may not recognize (and adamantly deny) that deficits are present, thus putting himself/herself at an increased risk for injury and negative outcomes. Clients with impaired insight about their deficits can become hostile and agitated when confronted about an observed problem, have a very low frustration/tolerance level for tasks that challenge deficit areas, exhibit impulsive behavior, have poor safety awareness, have an inability or diminished ability to compensate for deficits depending on the extent of impaired insight, exhibit poor social skills and defiant personality, blame an observed problem on an external source (e.g., "I can't remember what you told me because it wasn't important. I only remember things that are important."), and/or refuse to attend or participate in therapy ("because nothing is wrong with me"). The client who experiences difficulty achieving self-established goals (e.g., "I want to live by myself.") may blame failure on others (displaced failure — "They think I'm dumb, but I know better. My mom doesn't want me living in my own apartment because she wants to see me more.") or internalize failure due to other variables (e.g., "No one likes me. That's why they are sending me to live at the nursing home.") that could lead to the development of other psycho-emotional issues (e.g., low self-esteem, lacking internal locus of control, poor self-confidence, depression, anger).

Barco et al (1991) suggests that there are three levels of awareness (insight) that form a basis for evaluation and treatment.

1. *Intellectual awareness*: the cognitive capacity of the client to understand to some degree that a particular function is diminished from premorbid levels.
2. *Emergent awareness*: the ability of clients to recognize a problem when it is actually occurring.

3. *Anticipation awareness*: the ability to anticipate that a problem is going to happen because of some deficit.

If problems with insight are thought to be present, the therapist can assess the client's awareness by:

*   *Intellectual awareness*: Ask the client a general question during the evaluation that gives the client an opportunity to convey his/her deficits. For example, "Tell me what you notice is different about yourself since you had the motorcycle accident."
*   *Emergent awareness*: Observe how the client reacts while in the midst of a problem. Does she recognize that there is a problem? Does she attempt to fix or solve the problem? Is she able to identify the source of the problem? At what level is the client aware (if aware) of her deficits that are affecting the situation? Does the client become angry, agitated, or hostile? Does the client blame poor performance on an external source? Does the client deny having the problem?
*   *Anticipatory awareness*: Ask the client questions about what types of problems s/he thinks may occur within specific tasks (e.g., "Do you think you will have any trouble balancing the checkbook?" can be directed to a client who lacks insight into his problems with math; "Do you think you will have any trouble getting into the house?" can be directed to a client who lacks insight into problems with walking up and down steps; "How do you plan on doing the grocery shopping when you get home?" can be asked of a client who is not allowed to return to driving and who used to drive back and forth to the grocery store).

Documenting insight can be done in the following ways:

*   *Dysfunction*: e.g., Client is not aware of problems with time management even when he has missed an appointment.
*   *Level of assistance*: e.g., Client requires prompting to anticipate problems with tasks, especially when supplies are running out.
*   *Reaction to dysfunction*: e.g., Client blames failure with his bus trip for a community outing on therapist's incomplete instructions. Client becomes angry when left-side neglect is pointed out.

The therapist can assist the client in developing greater insight by using the strategies reviewed below:

1. Develop a list of the strengths and weaknesses of the client and review them at each session.
2. Providing direct, clear, and concrete feedback about the client's performance ("There is a mistake in the checkbook. Can you find it?" Give the client adequate time to review the work. Give the client a clue as to where the problem is located — "It is on the second line of the checkbook." Again, give the client adequate time to review the work. If the client is unable to identify the problem, point out the specific problem — "Right here the addition is wrong. Two plus six is eight. You wrote down a seven." Observe the client's reaction to the feedback. Give the client measurable feedback — "So far, we have found six errors on one page. Last session, you had 15 errors to a page. You are doing much better, but you are still having some trouble with math. Do you agree? Do you think that mistakes in balancing your checkbook will cause any problems?" If the client is not able to anticipate problems, the therapist must tell the client what problems could occur — "If your checkbook is misbalanced you may overdraw your account. An important check might bounce. You will have to pay additional fees not only to the bank for the bounced check but possibly to the company who you wrote the check to because it would be documented as being late. If these incidents continue to happen regularly, let's think worst case scenario and say your rent check bounces continually, your landlord may terminate your lease.").
3. Teach the client how to deal with feelings of anger in a healthy way by teaching anger management strategies. (See "Anger Management" in the Techniques section.) Have the client practice applying these techniques in treatment sessions when feelings of frustration surface.
4. Provide positive feedback to the client when insight is displayed.
5. Consider the use of videotaping or role-playing to provide a different type of feedback to the client about his/her performance.

If the client has absolutely no insight into his or her deficits, the strategies described above are not appropriate. However the therapist should continue to monitor the client for a positive change in insight. For clients who are unable to demonstrate adequate insight into deficits, the therapist shifts his/her focus from a development or restorative approach to an adaptive approach. Adaptations for insight include:

- Educating caregivers about the client's impaired insight into his/her deficits. This can be a hard concept for caregivers to understand. They may need education about the injured brain.
- Teaching caregivers how to manipulate the environment to ensure the client's safety (e.g., lock up the car keys).
- Teaching the caregivers how to continue to facilitate insight by implementing strategies that the therapist found helpful during treatment.

Judgment

Judgment is the ability to discriminate between and evaluate different options. Judgment, like many other of the higher-level cognitive skills, is not an isolated skill. Judgment also includes the use of the skills of cognitive flexibility, problem solving, shifting attention, and thinking. Additionally, coming to a conclusion includes the skill of decision-making.

To assess judgment, present the client with a problem and ask the client to weigh the available choices and form a decision. Problems can be simple, moderate, or complex. For example, "You would like to visit with both your friends and your parents. Your friends and your parents are only available to visit you at the hospital on Wednesday evening at 6:00 P.M. You prefer to visit with your family separate from your friends. What choices do you have? What would you decide to do and why?" Evaluate the client's thought process in comparing and discriminating ideas. Prompt the client with alternatives if needed (e.g., If you choose your family, what affect do you think this would have on your friends? If you choose your friends, are there alternative ways to visit with your family? What if you needed to see your family on Wednesday night because they were bringing you a new pair of shoes for therapy?).

The skill of judgment can be described and measured in terms of:

- *Complexity of the problem*: The type of problems that the client can handle (simple, moderate, complex).
- *Client's comprehensiveness*: How well the client can consider and discriminate options (e.g., no difficulty, mild, moderate, severe difficulty).
- *Related cognitive functions*: Other things that impair the client's ability to make judgments (e.g., difficulty sustaining attention or shift attention, difficulty solving problems).

Client's who have difficulty weighing options and making decisions (judgment) should be encouraged to seek out assistance from others who have the best interest of the client at heart (e.g., asking spouse to look over a contract before it is signed, asking mother about ideas for re-organizing the kitchen). The environment should be free of distractions, as much as possible, to promote concentration and attention to thinking. It can be helpful for the client to write the question or problem at the top of a piece of paper. Ask the client to brainstorm possible ideas/solutions and number them down the side of the paper (do not think about the idea/solution, just write it down). After the client has exhausted his/her ideas, go back and evaluate each brainstormed idea individually and make notations after each suggestion for reference. Once all of the suggestions are considered, evaluate the totality of ideas and choose the best option. As previously discussed, the client may also benefit from asking another person to offer suggestions/ideas for the list and assist with weighing the options and coming to a decision.

Problem Solving

Problem solving, like many of the other functions described in this section, is not an isolated skill. It is the integration of many skills that form the client's ability to solve problems.

> Problem solving is not a single function, but rather the integration of several cognitive skills. It requires attention, the ability to devise and initiate a plan, information access (both sensory from the environment and memory) and a feedback system, which give information on the effectiveness of the solution and the need for revision. Additional prerequisites for problem solving include good impulse control, the ability to organize and categorize, mental flexibility, and reasoning skills. Problem solving is an active process and breakdown can occur at any stage. In addition, the client's reasoning ability can determine the quality of the manner in which a problem will be formulated and the strategies applied for problem solutions (Zoltan, 1996, p. 160).

A client who has difficulty solving problems will most likely lack the ability to think abstractly (client thinks concretely), appear impulsive with the task (quickly tries to rush through it), exhibit confusion as to where to begin and how to solve the problem, and have trouble learning from mistakes and successes. Interestingly, "unless the client has some degree of problem-solving skills, s/he will be unable to apply newly learned skills to new situations" (Zoltan, 1996, p. 161). Therefore, problem solving is more than just the ability to solve a cognitive problem like "What would I do if...?", but will also affect the client's ability to generalize newly learned skills (motor skills, cognitive skills, social skills) into other tasks.

If there seems to be a deficit in problem-solving skills, the therapist can best assesses the skill through clinical observation. The therapist presents the client with a problem and observes the client's ability to solve it. This includes:

1. The client's ability to acknowledge that the problem is indeed a problem. Some clients may not see something as a problem even though the therapist sees it as a problem. This could be due to the client's coping mechanisms or personality. Therefore, the therapist should pose several questions and problems and look for patterns of response. Examples of questions:
    a. What would you do if you were driving on a two-lane country back road with no intersecting streets and someone was driving very fast and very close to the back of your car?
    b. What would you do if someone was knocking on your door and you didn't know who it was?
    c. What would you do if you were lost?
2. The ability of the client to fully appreciate and understand the complexity of the problem. Is the client able to see the problem from multiple perspectives? Does the client appreciate all of the elements of the problem (e.g., only recognizes two out of the possible four elements of the problem)?
3. The ability of the client to identify solutions to the problem. Is the client aware of personal or community barriers related to solving the problem (e.g., are the solutions realistic given the resources available)? Is the client able to compare this problem to past learning experiences (e.g., client experienced this problem in the morning and is now facing the same problem again)?

Evaluation of a client's problem-solving skills can also be assessed via an action task. For example:

1. Use the game Parquet. Chose a simple block design of four or six pieces. Show the design to the client and ask the client to replicate it. Observe how the client solves the problem. Is it thoughtful (does the client study the picture, does he organize the blocks needed, does he refer to the picture after placing each block) or disorganized (quickly grabs block pieces, doesn't refer to the picture of the design, says that he is done when the block design is incorrect, does not refer to the picture upon completion to check his work, etc.)?
2. Observe the client's behavior within a complex functional task (e.g., transferring from a wheelchair to the bed). Does the client follow the proper sequential steps (see "Transfers" in the Techniques section) or does the client appear

impulsive and disorganized (e.g., attempts to transfer from the wheelchair to the bed without removing his feet from the foot pedals and placing them on the floor)?

Once deficits in problem solving have been identified, the therapist must determine a baseline of functioning. Problem-solving functions can be measured in terms of:
- *Descriptors*: poor, fair, good, excellent.
- *Percentage*: e.g., Client is able to problem solve for simple tasks 35% of the time.
- *Level of assistance*: e.g., Client requires occasional verbal cues to problem solve for complex tasks.
- *Dysfunction related to task*: e.g., Client requires supervision at all times when in a community environment secondary to poor problem-solving skills related to safety.

Once a baseline of functioning is determined, the therapist facilitates the development or restoration of problem-solving skills primarily through the use of functional activities that are going to be part of the client's lifestyle after discharge (e.g., meal planning, driving directions, dealing with kid's schedules that overlap, developing a college course schedule that works around other responsibilities). Once functional activities have been identified, the therapist is to:
- Challenge the client with problem-solving tasks and provide the appropriate cueing to facilitate acknowledgement of a problem, the appreciation and understanding of the problem, and the ability to identify effective solutions. Tasks should be graduated (simple to complex). Cueing is often done in the form of leading questions (e.g., What do you think would happen if you don't ask for directions? How do you think your daughter would react to that solution? What is the first thing you should do when you want to transfer from the wheelchair to the bed?) and general verbal cues to refocus the client on the problem-solving process (e.g., Did you check the picture of the design to make sure it is right?).
- Provide the client with immediate feedback about his/her performance. Don't wait until the client is finished with the process and then go back and correct it. Feedback is to be given within the task. If a client is moving on to the next step in the process without fully completing the first step, the therapist is to stop the client and provide cueing to assist the client in completion of the first step of the task. For example, the therapist makes up an activity schedule that reflects conflicts among the kids' schedules (soccer award dinner and ballet recital time

overlap). If the client acknowledges that the mock activity schedule shows a problem but fails to acknowledge the total complexity of the problem (e.g., doesn't take into account feelings of the children), the therapist should halt the client before she attempts to go on to identifying solutions. The therapist might review the whole scope of the problem again because "I think we might be missing something." The therapist would then pose leading questions to help the client identify the parts of the problem that she missed.
- Teach the client basic activity analysis skills. Meaning, teach the client how to break down and look at the individual parts of the activity. For example, ask the client to look at the components of taking a two hour drive — transferring into the car, having someone load the wheelchair into the car trunk, putting on the seatbelt, performing weight shifts in the car every 30 minutes, opening, reading, and closing a map, etc. The development of analytical skills will help the client with problem-solving functions.

If the client is unable to demonstrate adequate problem-solving skills, the therapist shifts his/her focus from a development or restorative approach to an adaptive approach. Adaptations for problem-solving skills include:
- Providing references for solutions to common problems (e.g., make a flow chart that helps the client find a solution to overlapping schedules of children's activities)
- Provide worksheets for common planning needs (e.g., develop a "going to the shore" vacation checklist that categorically reflects all of the items that must be packed and taken care of in order to go on a shore vacation).
- Educate the client's caregivers about the client's problems in this area and teach them how to cue the client to facilitate further development of problem-solving skills.
- Teach the client to recheck his/her work at least two times before finalizing a solution.

Tell the client that it is appropriate to ask for help with problem-solving tasks from people that s/he trusts. Receiving help is not an "easy way out," but rather a compensatory strategy to minimize complications.

b167 Mental Functions of Language
Specific mental functions of recognizing and using signs, symbols, and other components of language.
Inclusions: functions of reception and decryption of spoken, written, or other form of language such as

sign language; functions of expression of spoken, written, or other forms of language; integrative language functions, spoken and written, such as involved in receptive, expressive, Broca's, Wernicke's and conduction aphasia

Exclusions: attention functions (b140); memory functions (b144); perceptual functions (b156); thought functions (b160); higher-level cognitive functions (b164); calculation functions (b172); mental functions of complex movements (b176); Chapter 2 Sensory Functions and Pain; Chapter 3 Voice and Speech Functions

- *b1670 Reception of Language*
  Specific mental functions of decoding messages in spoken, written, or other forms, such as sign language, to obtain their meaning.
  - o *b16700 Reception of Spoken Language*
    Mental functions of decoding spoken messages to obtain their meaning.
  - o *b16701 Reception of Written Language*
    Mental functions of decoding written messages to obtain their meaning.
  - o *b16702 Reception of Sign Language*
    Mental functions of decoding messages in languages that use signs made by hands and other movements, in order to obtain their meaning.
  - o *b16708 Reception of Language, Other Specified*
  - o *b16709 Reception of Language, Unspecified*
- *b1671 Expression of Language*
  Specific mental functions necessary to produce meaningful messages in spoken, written, signed, or other forms of language.
  - o *b16710 Expression of Spoken Language*
    Mental functions necessary to produce meaningful spoken messages.
  - o *b16711 Expression of Written Language*
    Mental functions necessary to produce meaningful written messages.
  - o *b16712 Expression of Sign Language*
    Mental functions necessary to produce meaningful messages in languages that use signs made by hands and other movements.
  - o *b16718 Expression of Language, Other Specified*
  - o *b16719 Expression of Language, Unspecified*
- *b1672 Integrative Language Functions*
  Mental functions that organize semantic and symbolic meaning, grammatical structure, and ideas for the production of messages in spoken, written, or other forms of language.
- *b1678 Mental Functions of Language, Other Specified*
- *b1679 Mental Function of Language, Unspecified*

Treatment for
Mental Functions of Language

The codes in this section relate to the reception, expression, and integration of language functions for communication.

Difficulty with reception of spoken, written, or sign language can be due to a variety of things such as lack of knowledge (doesn't know sign language, doesn't understand the Spanish language), difficulty learning, and hand dysfunction. If the cause of difficulty is knowledge or learning, the therapist would use the codes listed in Activities and Participation Chapter 2 Learning and Applying Knowledge. If the cause of difficulty is related to hand dysfunction, the therapist would refer to specific hand functions in s7302. If the cause of difficulty is related to mental impairments that cause the person to have difficulty understanding, expressing, or integrating language functions, the therapist would use the mental function codes in this section. Common causes of mental function impairments related to language include damage to the language areas of the brain from stroke, traumatic brain injury, and developmental disability.

Verbal language impairments are typically divided into the two main categories of receptive aphasia and expressive aphasia. Receptive aphasia is difficulty understanding spoken language. Expressive aphasia is difficulty expressing verbal language. A common expressive language impairment is called dysarthria. Dysarthria is a loss of function in the muscles used for speech and voice production making it difficult to understand (increased speech rate, decreased speech volume, slurred speech — see Body Functions Chapter 3 Voice and Speech Functions for more information about dysarthria). All other language and comprehension skills are intact. Another common expressive language problem is word finding (can't find the word to say). If a person has both receptive and expressive aphasia it is called global aphasia. In global aphasia, severe deficits are found in all language processes, including speech production, auditory comprehension, reading, and writing.

Further delineations of language impairments include fluent and non-fluent aphasia (definitions from *Idyll Arbor's Therapy Dictionary*, burlingame, 2001). In fluent aphasia (also called Wernicke's aphasia), the person's speech is fluent (it has a natural grammatical flow) with paraphasic errors (words may be unrelated to the current topic or unintelligible). Auditory comprehension, reading comprehension, and writing comprehension are impaired. In non-fluent aphasia (also called Broca's aphasia), speech is effortful and halting. Auditory comprehension is relatively good but not perfect. Reading comprehension is better than written output.

To assess a client's expressive language skills, challenge and observe the client in communication (e.g., sign a question, ask a verbal question, engage in conversation, ask client to write and read).

Document the observations in terms of:

- *Type of deficit*: e.g., Client exhibits global aphasia.
- *Degree of impairment*: none, mild, moderate, severe.
- *Percent of impairment*: e.g., exhibits word-finding problems in 25% of verbal conversation.
- *Level of assistance*: e.g., requires moderate verbal cues to incorporate compensatory strategies for dysarthria in social conversation.
- *Dysfunction related to task*: e.g., requires moderate verbal cues when requesting assistance from store employee secondary to word-finding difficulty.

To assess a client's receptive language skills, challenge the client with a receptive language task and observe the results (e.g., verbalize/sign a question such as "What is your name?" or "How are you today?"). Problems with hearing must be ruled out if asking a question verbally.

Document the observations in terms of:

- *Type of deficit*: e.g., Client exhibits receptive aphasia, but little expressive aphasia.
- *Extent of impairment*: e.g., no, minimal, moderate, severe.
- *Percent of impairment*: e.g., appears to understand approximately 40% of one-step verbal commands.
- *Level of assistance*: e.g., requires moderate gestural cues to increase receptive language abilities from baseline of 50-75%.
- *Dysfunction related to task*: e.g., requires moderate gestural cues from friends in social conversation secondary to poor receptive language skills.

Expressive Language Techniques

To enhance a client's expressive language functions a variety of techniques can be employed. Clients who have difficulty expressing needs through one form of language will often seek another form of communication (e.g., has difficulty with verbal expression so points to needed objects instead). This is a good compensatory strategy but it does not encourage neuroplasticity to promote recovery if language impairments are caused by a brain injury. Consequently, clients with expressive language difficulties who are in the recovery stage should be

encouraged to vocalize, write, and read. Therapists need to provide clients with increased time to communicate, provide praise, and acknowledge frustration. Common sounds, words, and signs are repetitively drilled to promote recovery. Alternative communication techniques to use with language production (e.g., pointing, gesturing, demonstrating, writing, drawing) are taught to decrease the client's frustration and increase successful communication.

If a client has word finding problems, provide cues to enhance word finding (it starts with the letter R, it is the color of your shirt, it's the color of a valentine, it starts with the sound "RRR"). The goal is for the client to identify the correct word/sign and then produce it. Saying the word that the client is trying to express will minimize frustration and increase speed of communication, but it will not enhance neuroplasticity in the recovery phase. See "Neuroplasticity" in the Techniques section.

Receptive Language Techniques

If a client has global aphasia, the use of pictures and demonstrative and gestural cues are most helpful for communication. Clients with global aphasia who are in the recovery phase should be briefly re-assessed daily for positive changes (e.g., able to verbalize, sign, write, or read a word) and then build upon the skill.

When working with clients who have receptive language problems, 1. limit the number of words/signs used in a communication to decrease complexity of communication, 2. limit the number of directions given at one time and gradually increase as appropriate, 3. utilize a variety of cueing techniques to ascertain the types of cues that are most helpful for the client (demonstrative, gestural, tactile), 4. provide hand over hand assistance with verbal action words (e.g., push).

Also see Activities and Participation Chapter 3 Communication for information on application of language in activities.

b172 Calculation Functions
Specific mental functions of determination, approximation, and manipulation of mathematical symbols and processes.
Inclusions: functions of addition, subtraction, and other simple mathematical calculations; functions of complex mathematical operations
Exclusions: attention functions (b140); memory functions (b144); thought functions (b160); higher-level cognitive functions (b164); mental functions of language (b167)

- *b1720 Simple Calculation*
  Mental functions of computing with numbers, such as addition, subtraction, multiplication, and division.

- *b1721 Complex Calculation*
  Mental functions of translating word problems into arithmetic procedures, translating mathematical formulas into arithmetic procedures, and other complex manipulations involving numbers.
- *b1728 Calculation Functions, Other Specified*
- *b1729 Calculation Functions, Unspecified*

Treatment for Calculation Functions

Number processing is different from calculation. Number processing includes the recognition and comprehension of numbers (verbal, written, Roman numerals). Calculation is the identification and understanding of arithmetic symbols (e.g., +, -, x) and words (e.g., plus, divide, difference), as well as the ability to recall and apply arithmetic facts to mathematical problems (e.g., algebra facts such as how to find "x").

Calculation is an important life skill as it is needed to be able to balance a checkbook, figure out pay, add up prices of food items at a grocery store to stay within a budget, cook and bake from a recipe, figure out taxes, and figure out a schedule (e.g., leave at 9:00 A.M. to be at a destination by 9:30 A.M. because it takes 30 minutes to drive there), just to name a few.

Difficulty with calculation functions can be a consequence of knowledge and learning or mental dysfunction. If the problem lies in knowledge and learning, refer to Activities and Participation Chapter 1 Learning and Applying Knowledge (d172 Calculating). If the difficulty is due to mental impairment (e.g., brain injury), then calculation functions in this section would be appropriate. The mental function impairment of having difficulty with calculations is referred to as acalculia.

Assess a client's ability to recognize written numbers (e.g., "12"), spoken/signed numbers (e.g., hold up two fingers, say the number two), and numbers written in the form of words (e.g., "twelve"). Assess the client's ability to identify both symbolic and written out arithmetic symbols (e.g., +, addition, -, subtraction) and perform simple calculation functions (e.g., 2+6, eight subtracted from twelve) and complex calculation functions (e.g., balance three checkbook transactions).

Document outcomes in terms of:

- *Extent of impairment*: e.g., moderate difficulty with simple calculations.
- *Percent of impairment*: e.g., 50% of checkbook math correct.
- *Level of assistance*: e.g., independent with addition of double digits, moderate cueing required to multiply single digits.

- *Dysfunction related to task*: e.g., requires moderate assistance for purchasing art supplies secondary to moderate difficulty with simple calculations.

To enhance number or calculation functions, begin at the client's baseline of functioning (e.g., able to add double-digit numbers correctly at 80%) and use repetitive number or calculation tasks at (and slightly above) the client's level of functioning (e.g., some single but mostly double-digit addition problems). Problems should be directly related to life activities that are common for the client (e.g., adding up price tags). If number or calculation functions do not improve, evaluate the need for adaptive devices (e.g., calculator). Identification of someone to assist the client with calculations may be needed (e.g., someone to help the client balance the checkbook, understand a bill).

b176 Mental Functions of Sequencing Complex Movements
Specific mental functions of sequencing and coordinating complex, purposeful movements.
Inclusions: impairments such as in ideational, ideomotor, dressing, oculomotor, and speech apraxia
Exclusions: psychomotor functions (b147); higher-level cognitive functions (b164); Chapter 7 Neuromusculoskeletal and Movement Related Functions

Treatment for Mental Function of Sequencing Complex Movement

Sequencing complex movement is a function required in almost every kind of activity from walking to talking to watching a tennis match. Apraxia is the inability to sequence certain movements in the absence of loss of motor power, sensation, or coordination. In other words, the client has the motor power, sensation, and coordination necessary to perform movement, but lacks the ability to perform these movements due to impaired neurological connections. For more details about specific types of apraxia see "Apraxia" in the Diagnosis section.

Assessing problems in sequencing complex movement involves the whole treatment team, but the recreational and occupational therapists are especially important in the assessment because they work with clients when the clients are performing complex tasks. Some simple ways for the recreational therapist to test for problems with sequencing complex movements are

- Asking the client to write out a list of activities that s/he used to like. If the client has difficulty writing, or even holding the pen, then apraxia may be present.

- Asking the client to pantomime using a specific piece of equipment (e.g., pair of scissors) for an activity that s/he has done in the past. If the client is not able to make the arm and hand movements to pretend that s/he has the equipment and to pantomime through the actions of using the equipment, then ideomotor apraxia may be present. The therapist should expect fairly crisp and clear movements from the client during this test. If these movements are "fuzzy," out of order, or inappropriate, further testing for apraxia is indicated.
- Placing in front of the client a variety of common pieces of equipment used in leisure activities (e.g., scissors, paintbrush, ping-pong paddle, a few playing cards). Ask the client to pick up each item one at a time and pantomime using each item. Clients who are not able to pick up the items (and who don't have limb weakness or paralysis) may have limb-kinetic apraxia. Clients who incorrectly pantomime the use of items may have conceptual apraxia.
- Asking a client to blow bubbles (demonstrate how to). If the client cannot blow bubbles, there is a chance that s/he has buccofacial apraxia.

Another test in a community setting to differentiate buccofacial apraxia from dyspraxia is to ask the client to lick his/her lips. If the client can lick his/her lips upon command, s/he probably does not have buccofacial apraxia. If the client does not lick his/her lips on command, place something sweet and sticky (such as jam or honey) on the person's tongue. Then let the client know that you are going to put some jam on his/her lips but *do not* ask the client to do anything with it. If the client licks the jam off his/her lips without your asking him/her to do so (and the person could not lick his/her lips earlier on command), then the client probably has apraxia. If the client does not automatically lick the jam off without you instructing him/her to, then the person probably has dysarthria (Zoltan, 1996).

If the therapist suspects that the client may have apraxia, it is appropriate to have the client engage in one-on-one activity with the therapist to determine the client's ability to physically prepare a meal, prepare for and go for a walk, and go shopping. If the client is not able to be independent in these activities but still performs relatively well in other therapy groups, the discharge location or date may need to be adjusted. The therapist works with the client in a one-on-one situation so that the client's performance is not impacted by watching others perform the same task.

Clients with developmental apraxia of speech may also have problems with fine hand use and acting out behavior. The therapist will want to observe the client's functional level of fine hand use and to document the client's coping techniques (or impairments) as the client engages in activity.

The treatment for lack of function in sequencing complex movements usually involves treating the cause of the apraxia, if it is known. Developmental apraxia of speech is the type of apraxia that most commonly has a separate treatment, usually led by the speech pathologist. For the other types of apraxia, the therapist is looking for adaptations that will help reduce the number of problems the apraxia causes. The adaptations depend on the kind of apraxia the client has. Specific treatment directions for different types of apraxia are listed below.

Buccofacial Apraxia

The speech pathologist will probably be responsible for designing the treatment for buccofacial apraxia. The recreational therapist should be aware that the client will not be able to perform actions with the lips and face on command. Visual cues may be more effective.

Conceptual Apraxia

Clients with conceptual apraxia are able to function better if the activity takes place in context (engaging in gardening activities in a garden or greenhouse instead of at a table in the therapy room).

Constructional Apraxia

The type of impairment seen in constructional apraxia tends to be different depending on the side of the brain that is affected. For clients with damage to the right hemisphere of the brain the impairments tend to be related to placing the object in the correct location in space, duplicating an object with correct proportions and perspective, and analyzing the relationship between parts. Clients with right hemisphere impairment do not seem to benefit from having a model close by or having part of the picture already drawn in for them to complete. In fact, Zoltan (1996) indicates that presenting the client with a partially completed construction only confuses the client more, decreasing functional ability.

For clients with damage to the left hemisphere of the brain the impairments tend to be related to initiating and planning the correct sequence of actions needed to reconstruct an object. It is not uncommon for clients with damage to the left hemisphere to also have visual cuts (visual neglect) which can have an added impact on the client's ability to reconstruct an object. Clients with left hemisphere impairments do tend to benefit from having the model close by, benefit from having a portion of the drawing started for them, and improve with practice.

If the recreational therapist finds that a client has constructional apraxia during arts and crafts projects, the therapist should also consider exploring the client's potential impairment related to meal preparation, dressing correctly for the activity and weather, and other activities that involve self-care in preparing for or engaging in activity.

Developmental Apraxia of Speech

Clients have difficulty communicating. It is not uncommon to see young children with developmental apraxia of speech act out by pushing, hitting, kicking, and otherwise disrupting other children's play. This behavior is thought to be a result of stress and frustration at not being able to communicate ideas, needs, and feelings. As children enter middle school, coping responses to impaired communication caused by apraxia often include being passive or shy and often answering questions with, "I don't know." Clients with developmental apraxia of speech often have decreased functional ability when they are under stress. Age-appropriate stress reduction skill training is often an important part of recreational therapy intervention and should be part of the client's Individual Education Program (IEP).

Clients with developmental apraxia of speech often improve to the point of having basic, functional communication skills after frequent and long-term speech therapy. This usually means two to three times a week for at least two years. The recreational therapist will want to use the same techniques suggested by the speech pathologist. Often the client will be able to get the intent of his/her message across even though the sentence structure, words, and pronunciation are incorrect. The recreational therapist should repeat the client's sentence while role modeling the correct form. For example, "Yes, I agree that the kitten looks funny as it chases the string."

Clients with developmental apraxia of speech often have a good vocabulary but are not able to "find" the words to pronounce. Sign language and picture boards are good methods of increasing the client's ability to communicate.

Ideomotor Apraxia

Clients can often perform a motor planning task if the therapist does not use a verbal command. For example, if the therapist is playing checkers with a client, the client will be able to move a checker piece without cueing. If the therapist cues the client to move the checker piece, the client often becomes confused and will not be able to execute the task. If the client is distracted and is not taking his/her turn, it is far more effective if the therapist cues the client by pointing to the checkerboard instead of using a verbal cue.

There are two forms of ideomotor apraxia (Zoltan, 1996). The first form occurs when there is damage to the portion of the brain that stores visuokinesthetic motor information. If there is damage to this portion of the brain, the client is unlikely to self-correct performance because s/he does not recognize impairment in performance. The therapist can see that a client has this type of ideomotor impairment when s/he observes that the client is not noticing a problem with his/her performance. This type of impairment increases the therapist's need to structure the environment for increased safety when the client is learning a new activity. The second type of ideomotor apraxia is when the client has the ability to identify problems with his/her motor performance. Clients with this kind of ideomotor apraxia often improve with practice during therapy and activity. Visual cues or physical cues (prompting, manipulation, or hand-over-hand) may increase client performance. Verbal cues tend to have little positive impact and may cause the client's performance to worsen. Ideomotor apraxia may be either unilateral (one side of the body) or bilateral (both sides of the body).

Limb-Kinetic Apraxia

Leisure planning for clients with limb-kinetic apraxia will probably need to include activities that allow the assistance of others, as this type of apraxia has the greatest impact on the ability to be independent. "The presence of limb apraxia, more than any other type of neuropsychological disorder, correlates with the level of caregiver assistance required six months after stroke" (Koski, Iacoboni, & Mazziotta, 2002).

Oculomotor Apraxia

As would be expected with the inability to control the visual senses, clients with oculomotor apraxia have trouble with reading skills. Social skills may also be delayed, as the client tends to miss subtle gestures and facial expressions. This lack of sensory information in social situations makes it harder for the person to correctly interpret what is going on. Treatment includes helping the client enhance his/her other sensory inputs allowing a fuller understanding of his/her environment.

Verbal Apraxia

Clients with verbal apraxia tend to be far better at understanding language than communicating and using language. This impairment of language often overlaps with other impairments including being able to read, write, and use math. The therapist will want to observe the client's actual skills for integration and activities skills related to reading restaurant menus, determining how much money is needed to go swimming at the community pool, keeping a bowling score, etc.

b180 Experience of Self and Time Functions

Specific mental functions related to the awareness of one's identity, one's body, one's position in the reality of one's environment and of time.
Inclusions: functions of experience of self, body image, and time

- *b1800 Experience of Self*
  Specific functions of being aware of one's own identity and one's position in the reality of the environment around oneself
  Inclusions: impairments such as depersonalization and derealization
- *b1801 Body Image*
  Specific mental functions related to the representation and awareness of one's body.
  Inclusions: impairments such as phantom limb and feeling too fat or too thin
- *b1802 Experience of Time*
  Specific mental functions of the subjective experiences related to the length and passage of time.
  Inclusions: impairments such as jamais vu and déjà vu
- *b1808 Experience of Self and Time Functions, Other Specified*
- *b1809 Experience of Self and Time Functions, Unspecified*

Treatment for Experience of Self and Time Functions

Treatment ideas for this category will be separated into the three subcategories because we feel that they present significantly different issues for the recreational therapist.

Experience of Self

Like orientation to person, experience of self includes a person's awareness of his/her identity. At the most basic level, it requires awareness of self as a separate entity. (See "Basic Awareness of Self as Part of Socialization" in the Concepts section.) Experience of self, however, includes an additional descriptor of having an awareness of one's position in the reality of the environment around oneself. This includes the impairments of depersonalization (the

feeling that the body or the personal self is strange and unreal) and derealization (the perception of objects in the external world as strange and unreal).

Questions that can be asked to determine depersonalization include "Do you or have you ever felt detached/unattached/divorced from yourself?", "Did you ever act in so strange a way you considered the possibility that you might be two different people?", "Are you always certain who you are?", "Ever feel like you were/your mind was outside/watching/apart from your body?" (Zuckerman, 2000, p. 52).

Questions that can be asked to determine derealization include, "Did you ever get so involved in a daydream that you couldn't tell if it were real or not?", "Did you ever feel that things around you/the world were/was very strange/remote/unreal/changing?", "Do things seem natural and real to you, or does it seem like things are make-believe?", "Do things or objects ever seem to be alive?" (Zuckerman, 2000, p. 53).

Causes of depersonalization and derealization include neurological disorders such as epilepsy, migraine, brain tumors, cerebrovascular disease, cerebral trauma, encephalitis, dementia of the Alzheimer's type, and Huntington's disease; toxic and metabolic disorders such as hypoglycemia, hyperparathyroidism, carbon monoxide poisoning, hyperventilation, and hypothyroidism; idiopathic mental disorders such as schizophrenia, depressive disorders, manic episodes, conversion disorder, anxiety disorders, obsessive-compulsive disorder, personality disorders, and phobic-anxiety depersonalization syndrome. In normally healthy persons it may be caused by exhaustion; boredom; sensory deprivation; emotional shock; and substance use including alcohol, barbiturates, benzodiazepine, marijuana, and any other hallucinogenic substance such as PCP (Sadock & Sadock, 2003).

Documentation of the condition should include:
- *Length/persistence of episode*: e.g., Client felt objects were unreal 2/3 of the day.
- *Strength of the feeling*: e.g., Client expressed concern about not being able to feel like part of the group due to fatigue associated with chemotherapy treatment.

The underlying disorder causing depersonalization or derealization is treated accordingly. Refer to the specific diagnosis for treatment recommendations. Approximately 50% of people with depersonalization and/or derealization are believed to have long-lasting conditions (Sadock & Sadock, 2003).

Body Image

Body image is the specific mental functions that allow one to conceive a representation and awareness of one's body. This includes impairments such as phantom limb (feeling that an amputated limb is still there) and feeling too fat or too thin, such as body image distortions that are common in anorexia and bulimia.

Impairments in body image are identified through verbalizations and behavior of a client (e.g., "I fell when I stood out of bed because I thought my leg was still there. I could have sworn my leg was still there"; A 90-pound girl who is 16 years old says, "I am so fat it makes me sick to my stomach to look at myself.").

Measurement of body image distortion is typically described with:

- *Descriptors*: such as healthy, unhealthy, distorted, aware, and unaware (e.g., Client has a healthy body image.)
- *Severity*: e.g., Client's body image is distorted; client believes that she is grossly obese at 5' 2" and 75 pounds.

See the diagnoses of amputation and eating disorders for more information about body-image-specific assessments.

Treatment under this code of the ICF relies mainly on cognitive retraining. The goal is to present enough experiences and examples to change the way the client thinks about the situation. For example, a client who tries to use an amputated limb needs many experiences with having the limb not there before he will understand not to rely on it. These need to be done safely. A client with anorexia needs many examples of healthy bodies (including medical information about nutrition and the need for some fat to be healthy). Miller and Jake (2001) have many examples of recreational therapy techniques to use in *Eating Disorders: Providing Effective Recreational Therapy Intervention*. (See "Education and Counseling" in the Techniques section for more information.)

One important consideration for therapists dealing with eating disorders is that the client will not be able to process well cognitively until s/he is stabilized medically. Document treatments for medical conditions, such as arrhythmia or malnutrition, with the appropriate ICF codes.

Experience of Time

Orientation to time (b1140) is an awareness of the day, date, month, and year. This is different from experience of time (b1802) that includes déjà vu (the illusion of having already experienced something actually being experienced for the first time, a repetition of a situation) and jamais vu (false feeling of unfamiliarity with a real situation that a person has experienced).

Both of these impairments fall under the classification of paramnesia, which is the falsification of memory by distortion of recall. A feeling of déjà vu once in a while in a normal, healthy person is not considered an impairment. Disturbances in memory can be caused by a variety of neurological impairments, substance use, and medical conditions.

Documentation of the specific impairment and its occurrence is noted in the client's medical chart (e.g., client reports feelings of déjà vu almost daily).

There are no specific treatment recommendations for either déjà vu or jamais vu. Therapists should treat the underlying condition, which will vary depending on the cause of the memory disturbance.

b189 Specific Mental Functions, Other Specified or Unspecified

b198 Mental Functions, Other Specified

b199 Mental Functions, Unspecified

References

Barco, P. P., Crosson, B., Bolesta, M. M., Werts, D., & Stout, R. (1991). Training awareness and compensation in postacute head injury rehabilitation. In Kreutzer, J. S. & Wehman, P. H. *Cognitive rehabilitation for persons with traumatic brain injury*. Bisbee, AZ: Imaginart Press.

burlingame, j. (2001). *Idyll Arbor therapy dictionary*. Ravensdale, WA: Idyll Arbor.

burlingame, j. & Blaschko, T. M. (2002). *Assessment tools for recreational therapy and related fields, third edition*. Ravensdale, WA: Idyll Arbor, Inc.

Feldman, S. & Elliott, G. (1990). *At the threshold: The developing adolescent*. Cambridge, MA: Harvard University Press.

FOX. (1988). Ravensdale, WA: Idyll Arbor.

Koski, L., Iacoboni, M. & Mazziotta, J. (2002). Deconstructing apraxia: Understanding disorders of intentional movement after stroke. *Current Opinion in Neurology, 15*:71-77.

Miller, D. & Jake. L. (2001). *Eating disorders: Providing effective recreational therapy intervention*. Ravensdale, WA: Idyll Arbor.

Nathan, A. & Mirviss S. (1998). *Therapy techniques using the creative arts*. Ravensdale, WA: Idyll Arbor.

O'Sullivan, S. & Schmitz, T. (1988). *Physical rehabilitation: Assessment and treatment*. Philadelphia, PA: F.A. Davis Company.

Ragheb, M. G. (2005) *Vitality through leisure assessment*. Ravensdale, WA: Idyll Arbor.

Sadock, B. & Sadock, V. (2003). *Kaplan & Sadock's synopsis of psychiatry, 9th edition*. Philadelphia, PA: Lippincott Williams & Wilkins.

Zoltan, B. (1996). *Vision, perception, and cognition: A manual for the evaluation and treatment of the neurologically impaired adult*. Thorofare, NJ: Slack.

Zuckerman, E. (2000). *Clinician's thesaurus, fifth edition*. New York: Guilford Publications.

Chapter 2 Sensory Functions and Pain

This chapter is about the functions of the senses, seeing, hearing, tasting, and so on, as well as the sensation of pain.

Seeing and Related Functions (b210-b229)

b210 Seeing Functions
Sensory functions related to sensing the presence of light and sensing the form, size, shape, and colour of the visual stimuli.
Inclusions: visual acuity functions; visual field functions; quality of vision; functions of sensing light and color, visual acuity of distant and near vision, monocular and binocular vision; visual picture quality; impairments such as myopia, hypermetropia, astigmatism, hemianopia, color blindness, tunnel vision, central and peripheral scotoma, diplopia, night blindness, and impaired adaptability to light
Exclusions: perceptual functions (b156)

Treatment for
Seeing Functions

Visual impairments are due to genetics (e.g., astigmatism), injury to the visual center of the brain (e.g., stroke, traumatic brain injury, multiple sclerosis), injury to the structures of the eye (e.g., damage to the retina), and the normal aging process. Seeing functions decline as people grow older. This includes "a decreased ability to focus on close objects or to see small print, a reduced capacity to adjust to changes in light and dark, and diminished ability to discriminate color. The aged eye requires about 3-4 times more light than the young eye to see well" (burlingame, 2001, p. 312). Therefore, therapists working with older adults should routinely evaluate visual skills with this population.

There are various visual impairments that affect multiple seeing functions. Some of the most common include:

- *Cataract*: A progressive disease of the eye where the lens of the eye becomes opaque. Cataract surgery is approximately 98% successful in removing the damaged lens and replacing it with an artificial lens.
- *Macular degeneration.*
- *Diabetic retinopathy*: Damage to the small blood vessels that provide blood to the eye. Blindness can occur.

Therapists need to be aware of visual functions as they affect normal activity. If an impairment is noted, the therapist scores the extent of the visual impairment along with the related Activities and

Participation categories that are affected by the visual impairment (e.g., d166 Reading, d170 Writing).

More information on visual function is given in the following sections on acuity, field, and quality of vision.

- *b2100 Visual Acuity Functions*
  Seeing functions of sensing form and contour, both binocular and monocular, for both distant and near vision.
  - *b21000 Binocular Acuity of Distant Vision*
    Seeing functions of sensing size, form, and contour, using both eyes, for objects distant from the eye.
  - *b21001 Monocular Acuity of Distant Vision*
    Seeing functions of sensing size, form and contour, using either right or left eye alone, for objects distant from the eye.
  - *b21002 Binocular Acuity of Near Vision*
    Seeing functions of sensing size, form and contour, using both eyes, for objects close to the eye.
  - *b21003 Monocular Acuity of Near Vision*
    Seeing functions of sensing size, form and contour, using either right or left eye alone, for objects close to the eye.
  - *b21008 Visual Acuity Functions, Other Specified*
  - *b21009 Visual Acuity Functions, Unspecified*

Treatment for
Visual Acuity Functions

Common conditions that affect a person's ability to see far and near are
- *Myopia* (near sightedness): A person is able to see things up close but has difficulty seeing things that are at a distance.
- *Hyperopia* (far sightedness): A person is able to see things at a distance but has difficulty seeing things that are close.
- *Astigmatism*: In the normal, healthy eye, light rays enter the eye and converge at a single point resulting in a clear picture. In astigmatism, the light rays that enter the eye do not converge at a single point because of distortion in the lens or the shape of the eyeball resulting in a blurry picture.
- *Amblyopia* (lazy eye): There is a decreased acuity of vision (also referred to as a dimness of vision) in one eye. No physical defect or disease accounts for the impairment. Most people have a dominant eye. In amblyopia the non-dominant

eye has become so much less dominant that the brain-eye connection has weakened enough to result in less visual acuity.

- *Diplopia* (double vision): This is usually the result of decreased range of motion in one eye although it may also be related to amblyopia.
- *Depth perception problems*: The client has difficulty determining the distance of objects by using binocular vision.
  (Note that the last three conditions may be the result of problems with the external muscles of the eye. If this is the case, the problem should also be scored as b2152 Functions of the External Muscles of the Eye.)
- *Total blindness*: No sight
- *Legally blind*: Visual acuity of less than 6/60 or 20/200 or visual field restriction of 20° or less.
- *Glaucoma*: A disease of the eye that increases intraocular fluid pressure. If left untreated over time, the optic disk becomes damaged, the eyeball can harden, and partial to complete loss of vision can occur, starting with a loss of peripheral vision, which should be noted in b2101 Visual Field Functions.
- *Macular degeneration*: Damage to the macula of the retina that causes blindness in the center of the visual field. It is caused by several different diseases. In severe cases complete loss of vision may occur in the macular region. This may be coded under visual field function (b2101).

Visual acuity is a measurement of how clearly a person is able to see at various distances. "Visual acuity is measured by stating '20/__,' with the value placed in the blank space representing how far/close a person must be to an object to perceive it as clearly as a person with normal vision would at 20 feet. In other words, if a client had a visual acuity of 20/200, the client could see clearly at 20 feet what most people can see clearly at 200 feet" (burlingame, 2001, p 312). The definition for legal blindness of "6/60" is a measure of near vision that means the person can see as well at six feet as a normal person can see at 60 feet.

In addition to the extent of impairment, a therapist will score the Activities and Participation codes that are affected by visual acuity impairments and make additional notes within their own documentation including compensatory techniques, equipment, and/or assistance needed (e.g., Secondary to myopia, client wears prescription lenses at all times in community settings to clearly see signage). The therapist may also note the extent of the visual acuity impairment (no, mild, moderate, severe, complete) as it affects the client's ability to participate in activities (e.g., client reports mild

impairment with binocular acuity of near vision when sewing).

Treatment for myopia, hyperopia, astigmatism, and legal blindness generally requires prescription lenses, although laser surgery is becoming a popular option. If a person has amblyopia, the strong eye may be patched for short periods of time to strengthen the lazy eye.

If double vision (diplopia) is a problem, clients are often instructed to wear an alternating patch over one eye (i.e., wear the patch on the right eye one day and then the left eye the next day). This eliminates one of the two images, but it adds a new problem of not having depth perception. Range of motion exercises for the eye along with the use of the alternating patch may resolve the problem. If the problem does not resolve, the client is referred to an ophthalmologist for further evaluation and recommendations. Diplopia is typically caused by damage to the brain due to traumatic brain injury, stroke, or multiple sclerosis.

If depth perception is a problem, the person will have difficulty determining the distance of objects, posing a challenge to reaching out and accurately grasping an object, judging the distance of traffic, and walking up and down stairs. People who have depth perception problems can often learn how to judge the correct distance of objects but it requires practice. The therapist should provide a sufficient number of situations for the client to feel comfortable in a real-world situation on his/her own.

Glaucoma is treated with eye drops that helps to decrease the pressure of the eye or with surgery to create a bleb (seen as a lump above the iris) that helps in draining the aqueous humors in the eye and, thereby, reducing the pressure.

Therapists who have clients with any of these conditions need to encourage their clients to follow the appropriate procedures. This ranges from coming up with strategies to keep glasses from being lost to devising ways to make sure the client wears a patch at appropriate times and takes eye drops as required. Other adaptations that might be required include large print books, larger calendars, special screen settings on computers to allow larger font sizes, and larger signage. For some situations the client can carry a magnifier (ranging from eyeglasses to a closed circuit television system) to help with activities.

If a person is legally blind or totally blind, the person is taught how to use other senses (e.g., listening for the clicking noise at the traffic light and the sound of the traffic to sense when the light has changed, reading Braille), adaptations (e.g., pinning socks together before throwing them in the wash; keeping one dollar bills flat, folding five dollar bills in half, and folding ten dollar bills in quarters), assistance from others (e.g., seeing eye dog, spouse), technology (e.g., talking watch, computer program that reads aloud what is scanned), and mobility equipment for safety (e.g., walking stick). See "Canes" in the Equipment section for more information.

- *b2101 Visual Field Functions*
  Seeing functions related to the entire area that can be seen with fixation of gaze.
  Inclusions: impairments such as in scotoma, tunnel vision, anopsia

Treatment for Visual Field Functions

Common visual field impairments include:
- *Visual neglect*: A lack of awareness of one side of the environment (right or left neglect/hemianopsia). Left neglect is very common in individuals who have a right cerebrovascular accident (CVA). The person neglects the left side of his/her environment from the midline over (bumps into things on the left, is not aware of items that are on the left side of the table). Seeing functions in the both eyes are usually intact, but neither eye is capable of processing information from the left half of its visual field. It is a brain problem rather than an eye problem that is affecting the person's vision. Unlike other kinds of visual function problems, a person with visual neglect can't see objects in the left half of his/her visual field *and* she also loses the awareness that there is *anything on* the left side of his/her body. Neglect can be very dangerous. A client with neglect doesn't have the proper brain function to realize that there may be a car coming down the road from the left when attempting to cross the street. It is also difficult to use environmental cues: When walking down a hallway, a client who has left neglect will have no awareness of what is on the left side of the hall. On the return trip, the client will report that there is nothing familiar about the hallway because he didn't see the left side of the hallway on the way there and can't see the original right side of the hallway (which he was watching on the first trip) on the way back.
- *Field loss*: A person's visual field is described as the total area that the person is able to see without moving his/her head. "The normal monocular field of vision is approximately 60° upward, 60° inward, 70-75° downward, and 100-110° outward" (Zoltan, 1996, p 33). Field loss is actually loss of visual function in a certain visual field quadrant of the eye. Each eye is divided

into four quadrants (upper and lower, left and right). Field loss is often the result of brain injury (e.g., client has visual field cut in the right upper quadrant of the left eye). Some of the terms used are
  - o *Homonymous hemianopsia*: loss of the outer half of the visual field from one eye and the inner half of the visual field of the other eye. See visual neglect, above.
  - o *Circumferential blindness*: No vision around the circumference of each eye's visual field.
  - o *Bitemporal hemianopsia*: Loss of the outer vision of both eyes
  - o *Homonymous inferior quadrantanopsia*: loss of vision in right or left lower quadrant of both eyes
- *Visual spatial inattention*: Visual neglect of particular quadrant(s) of the eye. It is inattention due to a brain dysfunction, rather than a vision loss due to damage of the eye.

Visual neglect may resolve with neuroplasticity. Although in many cases it does not. Clients are taught how to compensate for neglect by turning their head to the neglected side to scan the neglected side of the environment. Visual cues, often referred to as anchors, can be helpful. These are brightly colored lines that are placed on the far side of the neglected environment as a visual cue so that the client knows when s/he has turned his/her head far enough to see the neglected environment (e.g., stick a piece of red tape along the neglected side of the computer monitor frame, place a neon colored ruler on the neglected side of a book page).

In addition to an anchor, the therapist uses multi-modal cues to prompt the client to turn his/her head to the neglected side (e.g., verbal cues such as "do you see the pen, keep turning your head to the left until you see the pen," gestural cues such as pointing to the left side of the client's neglected environment, auditory cues such as tapping on the left side of the table to cue the client to turn his/her head to the neglected left side).

The ultimate goal is for the client to independently scan the neglected environment using a consistent rhythmic approach (e.g., while walking the client turns his head to the left to scan the neglected left side of the environment with every other step taken, while reading the client routinely turns her head to the left to scan the neglected left side after reaching the right side of the page).

If the client is unable to independently compensate for visual neglect, precautions must be taken to ensure the safety of the client. Such adaptations/precautions include the use of mirrors. Placing mirrors on the unaffected visual side can cue the client to look towards the neglected side or, at the very least, provide a reflection of the neglected environment within the unaffected visual field (e.g., placing a mirror on the opposite wall directly across from the bathroom door so that when the client is walking down the hallway and the bathroom door is on the person's neglected side, the image in the mirror alerts the client to the bathroom door). Another technique is to use bicycle mirrors. Place a pair of prescription or non-prescription glasses on the client and clip a bicycle mirror (small round mirrors about one to two inches around) onto the outer edge of the frame of the glasses on the unaffected side. Play around with the positioning of the bicycle mirror so that when the client looks straight ahead s/he sees a reflection of the neglected side in the unaffected visual field (e.g., when the client with left neglect looks straight ahead, he sees the right side of the environment and a reflection of the left side of his environment). There are no studies on the effectiveness of mirrors and left neglect but they are commonly used in rehabilitation facilities as a technique for accommodation. Mirrors are not helpful for all clients, especially those who are unable to identify that the reflection is of the opposite side.

Teaching clients how to compensate for field loss and visual spatial inattention is the same as visual neglect. The client needs to learn how to move his/her head into a position that allows him/her to see in the area of field loss. Mirrors however are not usually used. Since the client only needs to compensate for a small piece of visual field loss/inattention (different from neglect that is an entire side of vision) the use of mirrors can become confusing, bothersome, and ineffective.

In addition to the extent of impairment, a therapist will score the Activities and Participation codes that are affected by visual field loss and make additional notes in their own documentation including the type of visual field loss (neglect, quadrants of field loss, quadrants of visual spatial inattention), amount of assistance needed (e.g., moderate verbal cues to scan left side of environment), compensatory strategies taught (e.g., use of an anchor for reading), the client's ability to utilize compensatory strategies (e.g., client independent with utilization of anchor to compensate for left neglect when reading), and safety concerns related to visual field problems along with recommended safety precautions (e.g., should not use power tools, cross streets alone).

- *b2102 Quality of Vision*
  Seeing functions involving light sensitivity, color vision, contrast sensitivity, and the overall quality of the picture.

  o *b21020 Light Sensitivity*
    Seeing functions of sensing a minimum amount of light (light minimum), and the minimum difference in intensity (light difference).
    Inclusions: functions of dark adaptation; impairments such as night blindness (hyposensitivity to light) and photophobia (hypersensitivity)
  o *b21021 Colour Vision*
    Seeing functions of differentiating and matching colours.
  o *b21022 Contrast Sensitivity*
    Seeing functions of separating figure from ground, involving the minimum amount of luminance required.
  o *b21023 Visual Picture Quality*
    Seeing functions involving the quality of the picture.
    Inclusions: impairments such as in seeing stray lights, affected picture quality (floaters or webbing), picture distortion, and seeing stars or flashes
  o *b21028 Quality of Vision, Other Specified*
  o *b21029 Quality of Vision, Unspecified*

Treatment for Quality of Vision

Quality of vision can be affected by night blindness (hyposensitivity — decreased sensitivity to light making it difficult to see when it is dark), photophobia (hypersensitivity — increased sensitivity to daylight making it difficult to see during the day), color blindness (partial or total inability to distinguish certain colors, usually red from green, or a total inability to see colors), floaters, stray lights, and seeing stars or flashes.

Documentation of quality of vision is usually done by another member of the treatment team, but the recreational therapist may be one of the first to notice changes in vision that show up during activities. In many cases early detection and reporting to the rest of the team can limit the amount of damage that occurs.

The recreational therapist will document Activities and Participation codes that are affected by visual impairments (e.g., d630 Preparing Meals) and additional notes in their own documentation including the specific quality of vision dysfunction (e.g., client has floater that distracts him when reading), the extent that the impairment interferes with specific activities (e.g., difficulty seeing the card rack causes a moderate impairment with card playing), compensatory strategies taught and implemented (e.g., client educated about adaptations for night blindness), effectiveness of compensatory strategies (e.g., client independently matched and coordinated an outfit using clothing labels that have the color of the piece of clothing written on the clothing label), and amount of assistance (if any) to maximize vision quality (e.g., requires moderate assistance to read menu in a dark restaurant).

Treatment may be performed in part by the therapist, but it is more likely that the therapist will be responsible for appropriate adaptations. The adaptations for particular conditions follow:

People who have hyposensitivity (night blindness) should avoid driving at night and have adequate lighting in the home when it becomes dark. Bright nightlights can be especially helpful if s/he needs to get up in the middle of the night. If nightlights are not sufficient, turning on a table lamp before getting out of bed during the night may be an adaptation that is necessary for safety. It is normal for people to require more light to see as they get older because the retina gets thicker. Therapists working with older adults should be sure that they provide adequate lighting in their environment for all of their activities, especially ones requiring fine visual discrimination, including reading.

If photophobia is present, the person would benefit from wearing protective sunglasses and staying out of direct sunlight (e.g., sit in the shade, wear a brimmed hat). The therapist needs to make sure that sunglasses are available and used as appropriate.

Depending on the colors that are indistinguishable, people who are color blind will need to make accommodations to assist with dressing (e.g., pinning matched socks together before putting them in the wash, labeling clothes with the name of their color, watching for the location of traffic lights to determine which color is lit).

Other treatment and adaptations may be required for contrast sensitivity and overall picture quality. Often practice will improve the client's ability to work around the vision problems. Adaptations include learning to take second and third looks to be sure of what was actually seen and making sure that adequate lighting is always available. Some of the devices described for low visual acuity functions (b2100) may also be helpful.

b215 Functions of Structures Adjoining the Eye
Functions of structures in and around the eye that facilitate seeing functions.
Inclusions: functions of internal muscles of the eye, eyelid, external muscles of the eye, including voluntary and tracking movements and fixation of the eye, lachrymal glands, accommodation, papillary reflex; impairments such as in nystagmus, xerophthalmia, and ptosis
Exclusions: seeing functions (b210); Chapter 7 Neuromusculoskeletal and Movement-Related Functions

- *b2150 Functions of Internal Muscles of the Eye*
  Functions of the muscles inside the eye, such as the iris, that adjust the shape and size of the pupil and lens of the eye.
  Inclusions: functions of accommodation; papillary reflex
- *b2151 Functions of the Eyelid*
  Functions of the eyelid, such as the protective reflex.
- *b2152 Functions of External Muscles of the Eye*
  Functions of the muscles that are used to look in different directions, to follow an object as it moves across the visual field, to produce saccadic jumps to catch up with a moving target, and to fix the eye.
  Inclusions: nystagmus; cooperation of both eyes
- *b2153 Functions of the Lachrymal Glands*
  Functions of the tear glands and ducts.
- *b2158 Functions of Structures Adjoining the Eye, Other Specified*
- *b2159 Functions of Structure Adjoining the Eye, Unspecified*

Treatment for Functions of Structures Adjoining the Eye

Nystagmus, as well as fixation and tracking problems, can impact many activities including walking and fine motor activities. Eyelid functioning can affect wetness of the eye (may require eye drops if the eyelid does not blink). If the eyelid does not open, depth perception problems will be present. Therapists may score one of the preceding categories if an impairment is noted (e.g., papillary reflex is absent after a blow to the head in a sporting activity). Other common problems that a therapist may note are impairments of nystagmus (jumpy vision), fixation and tracking of the eye, and eyelid functioning (unable to open eyelid, absence of blinking reflex). Problems with the pupil and iris muscles will be scored here, but they may also cause problems with vision that should also be scored in the earlier codes for visual functioning. For example, if the iris is damaged so the pupil cannot close, the client will almost certainly have some photophobia (b21020). The therapist will be mainly responsible for reporting how these functional deficits impact activity with Activity and Participation codes.

Treatment and adaptations will generally be in activities supporting the goals of other team members including encouraging the client to work on strengthening and controlling eye movements through range of motion exercises and using eye drops as appropriate.

b220 Sensations Associated with the Eye and Adjoining Structures
Sensations of tired, dry, and itching eye and related feelings.
Inclusions: feelings of pressure behind the eye, of something in the eye, eye strain, burning in the eye; eye irritation
Exclusions: sensation of pain (b280)

Treatment for Sensations Associated with the Eye and Adjoining Structures

If a client has problems with any of the sensations mentioned above, the therapist scores this code as it relates to the extent of the impairment. Therapist may not have a direct intervention for these problems (e.g., eye drops are given by nursing), however therapists need to be aware of these problems as they impact participation in activities (e.g., irritation of the eye impacts ability to focus on the computer screen 30 minutes as required for writing a letter).

Some of these conditions, especially sensations of pressure or burning, may be indications of serious conditions. Sudden onsets should be reported to the medical team immediately.

b229 Seeing and Related Functions, Other Specified and Unspecified

Any other seeing or related functions not mentioned in the previous categories are scored under this code. Therapists make a notation of the problem to the right of the scored code.

Hearing and Vestibular Functions (b230-b249)

b230 Hearing Functions
Sensory functions relating to sensing the presence of sounds and discriminating the location, pitch, loudness, and quality of sounds.
Inclusions: functions of hearing, auditory discrimination, localization of sound source, lateralization of sound, speech discrimination; impairments such as deafness, hearing impairment, and hearing loss
Exclusions: perceptual functions (b156) and mental functions of language (b167)

- *b2300 Sound Detection*
  Sensory functions relating to sensing the presence of sounds.
- *b2301 Sound Discrimination*
  Sensory functions relating to sensing the presence of sound involving the differentiation of ground and binaural synthesis, separation, and blending.
- *b2302 Localization of Sound Source*
  Sensory functions relating to determining the location of the source of sound.

- *b2303 Lateralization of Sound*
  Sensory functions relating to determining whether the sound is coming from the right or left side.
- *b2304 Speech Discrimination*
  Sensory functions relating to determining spoken language and distinguishing it from other sounds.
- *b2308 Hearing Functions, Other Specified*
- *b2309 Hearing Functions, Unspecified*

Treatment for Hearing Functions

Therapists score hearing functions codes to note the extent of the specific hearing impairments. If hearing functions are impaired, therapists will also score Activities and Participation codes that are affected by hearing impairments (e.g., d350 Conversation, d115 Listening, d7600 Parent-Child Relationships). If hearing functions are impaired, the person should receive further evaluation from relevant health professionals (e.g., ear, nose, and throat physician; audiologist) to determine the specific problems and interventions needed (e.g., intercochlear implant, hearing aid).

Loss of hearing functions is a common problem associated with the aging process so therapists who work with this population should evaluate hearing function on a basic level (e.g., ability to accurately hear conversation in a small group, respond appropriately to auditory stimuli in the environment such as a ringing telephone). It is possible that the therapist may become aware of hearing problems before the rest of the treatment team, especially those related to activities such as localization or lateralization of sound. If the therapist notes a problem, s/he should request a referral as needed for further evaluation.

Hearing impairments can be a safety concern (e.g., doesn't hear smoke detector, doorbell, oven timer) and therefore adaptive equipment may need to be explored and taught to the client (e.g., flashing light on the telephone, flashing light by the door to signal a ringing doorbell). The therapist is responsible for assisting the client in learning how to use hearing equipment in real-life settings.

Clients who are deaf or significantly hearing impaired will benefit from learning sign language along with exploration of other forms of communication (e.g., augmentative communication devices, verbalizations, writing, gesturing, body language, TTY for using the telephone).

b235 Vestibular Functions
Sensory functions of the inner ear related to position, balance, and movement.
Inclusions: functions of position and positional sense; functions of balance of the body and movement

Exclusion: sensation associated with hearing and vestibular functions (b240)

- *b2350 Vestibular Function of Position*
  Sensory functions of the inner ear related to determining the position of the body.
- *b2351 Vestibular Function of Balance*
  Sensory functions of the inner ear related to determining the balance of the body.
- *b2352 Vestibular Function of Determination of Movement*
  Sensory functions of the inner ear related to determining movement of the body, including its direction and speed.
- *b2358 Vestibular Functions, Other Specified*
- *b2359 Vestibular Functions, Unspecified*

Treatment for Vestibular Functions

Vestibular impairments may be deduced by a therapist by ruling out other problems that can cause difficulty with positioning, balance, and movement such as brain injury, loss of strength, impaired flexibility, and impaired motor planning. However, vestibular impairments are best determined by specific testing/evaluation of the inner ear. Consequently, the health professional who confirms a vestibular problem (e.g., physician, audiologist) would most likely be the one to score the preceding codes rather than a therapist. Therapists are more likely to use codes in the Activities and Participation Chapters that are affected by vestibular impairments (e.g., d4602 Moving Around Outside the Home and Other Buildings, d415 Maintaining a Body Position).

Additional notes that therapists may make in their documentation related to vestibular impairments include the extent that it interferes with specific activities (e.g., vestibular problems with balance cause a moderate impairment with walking), and compensatory strategies taught and implemented (e.g., client educated about safety precautions to decrease risk of falls from vestibular balance problems).

Vestibular impairments may or may not be able to be corrected. Much of the treatment will be medical, but the therapist is involved in providing activities that help in the retraining of stability, position, and balance. Often vestibular problems are only a part of balance issues. (See b7603 and "Balance" in the Techniques section for additional information.) The therapist can provide valuable exercises that help other parts of the problem such as strength and proprioception from nerve pathways besides the inner ear. For more information about appropriate exercises, see "Motor Learning and Training Strategies" in the Techniques section and the books, *Exercises for Frail Elders* and *FallProof! A Comprehensive Balance and Mobility Training*

Program. If vestibular problems remain, therapists prescribe equipment (e.g., walking devices such as a cane) and adaptations (e.g., decreasing speed of movement, availability of physical support) to minimize risk of injury.

b240 Sensations Associated with Hearing and Vestibular Functions

Sensations of dizziness, falling, tinnitus, and vertigo.
Inclusions: sensations of ringing in ears, irritation in ear, aural pressure, nausea associated with dizziness or vertigo
Exclusions: vestibular functions (b235); sensation of pain (b280)

- *b2400 Ringing in Ears or Tinnitus*
  Sensation of low-pitched rushing, hissing, or ringing in the ear.
- *b2401 Dizziness*
  Sensation of motion involving either oneself or one's environment; sensation of rotating, swaying, or tilting.
- *b2402 Sensation of Falling*
  Sensation of losing one's grip and falling.
- *b2403 Nausea Associated with Dizziness or Vertigo*
  Sensation of wanting to vomit that arises from dizziness or vertigo.
- *b2404 Irritation in the Ear*
  Sensation of itching or other similar sensations in the ear.
- *b2405 Aural Pressure*
  Sensation of pressure in the ear.
- *b2408 Sensations Associated with Hearing and Vestibular Function, Other Specified*
- *b2409 Sensations Associated with Hearing and Vestibular Function, Unspecified*

Treatment for Sensations Associated with Hearing and Vestibular Functions

If an impairment with hearing or vestibular sensation is evident, the therapist scores the extent of impairment, along with the Activities and Participation codes that are affected by the impairments (e.g., d9200 Play, d640 Doing Housework, d4553 Jumping). Some, but not all, of these sensations are inquired about by the therapist. It is more common that therapists rely on the client to tell the therapist about feeling such sensations and only inquire about these sensations when they are suspected (e.g., loss of balance, pressing on the ear, doubling over).

In addition to scoring the impairment and related Activities and Participation codes, the therapist may make additional notes in his/her own documentation related to sensations associated with hearing and vestibular functions including the specific sensation impairment (e.g., ringing in the ears), the extent that it interferes with specific activities (e.g., feelings of nausea on long car rides is a barrier to visiting son who lives three hours away), compensatory strategies taught and implemented (e.g., client educated about techniques to decrease aural pressure when flying in an airplane), effectiveness of compensatory strategies (e.g., client able to independently perform techniques to decrease aural pressure), and amount of assistance (if any) to minimize sensation problems (e.g., requires moderate cues to ask for assistance from another when having difficulty hearing a sound due to tinnitus).

Sometimes the impairments are correctable with pharmacology. If impairments persist, therapists assist the client in identifying adaptations to minimize risk of injury and maximize functional performance (e.g., avoiding activities that stimulate sensation impairment such as riding in a car for a prolonged period of time, increase attention to or ask another's opinion about a sound or noise if unable to hear it correctly due to ringing in the ears such as trying to distinguish between two similar sounds of a car motor).

b249 Hearing and Vestibular Functions, Other Specified and Unspecified

Any other impairment related to hearing and vestibular functions not described would be scored using this code.

Additional Sensory Functions (b250-b279)

b250 Taste Function

Sensory functions of sensing qualities of bitterness, sweetness, sourness, and saltiness.
Inclusions: gustatory functions; impairments such as ageusia and hypogeusia

Treatment for
Taste Function

Therapists score this code if there is taste function impairment. This is different from the Activities and Participation code d120 Other Purposeful Sensing, which is intentionally using the sense of taste to experience stimuli.

There are four broad classifications of taste including sweet, sour, bitter, and salty. Each taste is sensed by receptors on a particular portion of the tongue. The taste buds on the tongue transmit their information to the medial temporal lobe. The combination of the signals from these receptors form part of what we call taste. The rest of what we call taste is made up of a combination of other senses including the sense of smell, touch, vision, and

hearing. This code deals only with the part that comes directly from the mouth.

In documentation, the therapist should note how impaired the client's sense of taste is (e.g., not able to taste and identify bitter foods). In addition to noting the extent of the impairment, therapists may make additional notes about taste impairments such as level of assistance required (e.g., independent in identifying expiration dates on food items), and impact on activity (e.g., Client reports loss of pleasure in eating secondary to taste function impairment. Consequently, client has been consuming fewer calories and has lost 20 pounds within the last month).

Treatment for taste impairments is the responsibility of other members of the medical team. People who have taste impairments are instructed to be alert to food expiration dates and food labels (e.g., eating a salty food but doesn't realize it is a salty food from taste when client should not eat salty foods because of high blood pressure). The recreational therapist can help with these adaptations by showing the client how to read sodium levels on food packages and explaining other ways besides taste to identify foods the may not still be edible (e.g., checking expiration dates).

b255 Smell Function

Sensory functions of sensing odors and smells.
Inclusions: olfactory functions; impairments such as anosmia or hyposmia

Treatment for
Smell Function

Therapists score this code if there is smell function impairment. This is different from the Activities and Participation code d120 Other Purposeful Sensing, which is intentionally using the sense of smell to experience stimuli.

It is estimated that people can discriminate among 10,000 different odors (Sadock & Sadock, 2003). Once an odor enters the nose it stimulates communication to the olfactory bulb in the brain where it is interpreted.

People who are unable to smell or have difficulty discriminating odors need to take adaptive precautions for safety (e.g., smoke detectors) and be alert to dangerous situations that are normally discovered by smell (e.g., do not leave food unattended on the stove top, have gas heater checked regularly for leaks).

Therapists should note the extent of the impairment and make additional notes in their documentation about smell impairments such as specific problems (e.g., unable to identify the smell of smoke), recommendations (e.g., instructed to install and maintain smoke detectors within the home), level of assistance (e.g., requires minimal verbal cues to recall safety precautions for smell impairments), and impact on activity (e.g., Client reports loss of interest in cooking secondary to smell impairments. Consequently, client has been eating packaged heat-up meals that are not meeting her nutrition needs.).

Treatment of problems with the sense of smell is usually the responsibility of other members of the medical team. The recreational therapist is responsible for teaching adaptations that will keep the client safe in the home and community.

b260 Proprioceptive Function
Sensory functions of sensing the relative position of body parts.
Inclusions: functions of statesthesia and kinaesthesia
Exclusions: vestibular functions (b235); sensations related to muscles and movement functions (b780)

Treatment for
Proprioceptive Function

Proprioceptive functioning is the ability to identify where a limb is in space without vision. It includes both position (statesthesia) and movement (kinesthesia). To evaluate statesthesia, the client should close his/her eyes and the therapist should slowly move one of the client's limbs (e.g., slowly move right arm from client's lap out laterally). Ask the client to describe where the limb is located. To evaluate kinesthesia, ask the client to close his/her eyes and then passively and slowly move a client's limb into a different position. Ask the client to describe what movements the therapist made with the limb (e.g., lowered the left arm).

Although the function of proprioception is coded as an isolated skill in this chapter, the function of proprioception is required for many skills requiring physical movement (e.g., d450 Walking, d420 Transferring Oneself, d4554 Swimming). Impairments in functioning in other areas should be noted using the relevant codes.

The therapist should assess the extent of the proprioceptive impairment, including specific proprioceptive impairments (e.g., client has problems with kinesthesia), the extent that it interferes with specific activities (e.g., difficulty jumping over obstacles when eyes are fixed on a target), compensatory strategies taught and implemented (e.g., client educated about use of vision to compensate for proprioceptive impairments), effectiveness of compensatory strategies (e.g., client able to independently compensate for proprioceptive impairment using vision when playing a video game by glancing down at the controller before moving thumb/fingers to another button), and amount of assistance (if any) to minimize proprioceptive problems (e.g., requires moderate cues to look at video game controller when moving thumb/fingers to another button to increase accuracy).

If proprioception impairments do not fully resolve, clients are taught how to compensate for the deficits by using the sense of vision.

b265 Touch Function
Sensory functions of sensing surfaces and their texture or quality.
Inclusions: functions of touching, feeling of touch; impairments such as numbness, tingling, paraesthesia, and hyperaesthesia [Note: these inclusions overlap with b2702]
Exclusions: sensory functions related to temperature and other stimuli (b270)

Treatment for
Touch Function

Therapists score this code if there is touch function impairment. This is different from the Activities and Participation code d120 Other Purposeful Sensing, which is intentionally using the sense of touch to experience stimuli. It is unclear why there is an overlap in the inclusions for b265 and b2702. We suggest that the therapist be aware of the overlap and score functions where the client has functional difficulties sensing a surface or an object using this code. Dysfunctions in sensing passive touch should be scored with codes included in b2702.

Therapists commonly evaluate sensation of light touch and stereognosis as it pertains to the client's ability to perform life tasks (e.g., identify a house key when standing outside the house at night; ability to experience pleasure from light touch in intimacy).

To evaluate light touch the therapist asks the client to close his/her eyes. The therapist then gently touches the client with various items (e.g., cotton ball, Q-tip) and asks the client to tell the therapist what the object feels like. To evaluate stereognosis, ask the client to close his/her eyes and place a common item in the hand (e.g., hairbrush, paintbrush, key) and ask the client to identify the item by touch.

Documentation should include the type and extent of the touch impairment and related Activities and Participation codes that are affected by touch impairment (e.g., d770 Intimate Relationships). The therapist should document the specific touch impairment (e.g., light touch absent in the right upper extremity), the extent that it interferes with specific activities (e.g., poor stereognosis impairs client's ability to identify the light switch in the dark), compensatory strategies taught and implemented (e.g., client educated about using night lights to compensate for stereognosis), effectiveness of compensatory strategies (e.g., client able to independently find his house key on his key ring in the dark by using a keychain light), and amount of assistance (if any) to minimize touch problems.

If touch functions continue to be impaired after treatment, compensatory strategies are taught to minimize injury and maximize safety (e.g., using visual skills to evaluate the texture of something if unable to identify it by feel).

b270 Sensory Functions Related to Temperature and Other Stimuli

Sensory functions of sensing temperature, vibration, pressure, and noxious stimulus.

Inclusions: functions of being sensitive to temperature, vibration, shaking or oscillation, superficial pressure, burning sensation, or a noxious stimulus

Exclusions: touch functions (b265); sensation of pain (b280)

- *b2700 Sensitivity to Temperature*
  Sensory functions of sensing cold and heat.
- *b2701 Sensitivity to Vibration*
  Sensory functions of sensing shaking or oscillation.
- *b2702 Sensitivity to Pressure*
  Sensory functions of sensing pressure against or on the skin.
  Inclusions: impairments such as sensitivity to touch, numbness, hypaesthesia, hyperaesthesia, paraesthesia and tingling [Note: these inclusions overlap with b265]
- *b2703 Sensitivity to Noxious Stimulus*
  Sensory functions of sensing painful or uncomfortable sensations.
  Inclusions: impairments such as hypalgesia, hyperpathia, allodynia, analgesia, and anaesthesia dolorosa
- *b2708 Sensory Functions Related to Temperature and Other Stimuli, Other Specified*
- *b2709 Sensory Functions Related to Temperature and Other Stimuli, Unspecified*

Treatment for Sensory Functions Related to Temperature and Other Stimuli

Temperature

Sensation of temperature is important for safety (e.g., a hot pot, cold weather). If adaptations for loss of temperature sensation are not implemented, the client could experience burns, frostbite, or heat stroke. Bodily processes can also be affected by temperature and have detrimental affects (e.g., extreme heat can increase blood pressure).

Therapists score this code if there is temperature sensation impairment. This is different from the Activities and Participation code d120 Other

Purposeful Sensing that is intentionally using temperature sensing to experience stimuli.

Therapists evaluate a client's ability to distinguish temperatures on the skin and in his/her environment. To distinguish temperatures on specific skin surfaces (e.g., on lower extremities on a client who has paralysis in the legs), use a warm and a cold item. Alternate placing the warm and cold item in different locations on the skin and ask the client to tell you if s/he feels something warm or cold. For a warm and cold item, the therapist can use the corner of a cold washcloth and another washcloth that was warmed in the microwave or capped test tubes filled with warm and cold water.

To evaluate the client's ability to sense temperature in the environment, open a window or door or go outside for a minute and ask the client to describe the temperature. The inability to sense outside temperatures is a common problem in complete spinal cord injury. A person who has a complete spinal cord injury will not have sensation below the level of impairment. Additionally, many people with complete spinal cord injuries do not sweat below the level of injury, so the client may sweat profusely above the level of injury on hot days in an attempt to cool the body. Also, people with tetraplegia or high-level paraplegia may not sweat above the injury level as well. This may give the person a false sense of the temperature (e.g., when wet from sweating a cool breeze may indicate to the person that it is getting cooler outside when the temperature of the day has not gotten cooler; the person may think it is hotter out than it really is due to the profuse sweating).

People who have difficulty determining temperature changes on the skin or in the environment need to learn how to rely on other senses to compensate for the loss. This includes the use of hearing (e.g., listening to the weather station on the radio or television), vision (e.g., looking at others to see how they are dressed for the day, making sure the light is off on the electric stove to indicate that it is cool), and routinely taking precautionary measures when unsure (e.g., using a potholder if the pot may still be hot, not carrying a hot casserole dish on the lap to be able to propel a wheelchair and carry the dish at the same time). People who have a complete spinal cord injury are to also avoid prolonged exposure (greater than one hour) to outside temperatures above 90°F. If a client complains of feeling ill and has had prolonged exposure to high outdoor temperatures, move the client into a cooler environment and utilize cooling techniques (e.g., air conditioning, cool towels on the forehead, around the neck, and under the arms). Symptoms should subside within 30-60 minutes. If a person with a spinal cord injury anticipates having to be outdoors on a hot and humid day, precautions should be taken to keep the core body temperature down (e.g., drink lots of cool water, wear a hat, stay in the shade, wet a towel and place it around the neck, wear loose clothing that breathes).

In addition to scoring the extent of the temperature impairment and related Activities and Participation codes that are affected by the impairment (e.g., d630 Preparing Meals, d5404 Choosing Appropriate Clothing), the therapist may make additional notes related to temperature functions including the specific temperature impairment (e.g., no sensation of temperature from the waist down), the extent that it interferes with specific activities (e.g., Client reports desire to sit on the beach for prolonged periods of time after discharge. Prolonged sun exposure without full temperature sensation increases client's risk for heat stroke and sunburn), compensatory strategies taught and implemented (e.g., Client instructed to wear a 45+ sun block, sit in the shade under a beach umbrella, wear a brimmed hat, and drink cool water when sitting on the beach for prolonged period of time to decrease risk of heat stroke and sunburn), effectiveness of compensatory strategies (e.g., client able to sit outside in the sun using techniques to decrease affects of unrecognized heat for one hour without adverse affects), and amount of assistance (if any) to minimize temperature problems (e.g., requires moderate cues to utilize other senses to assess temperature of items prior to taking action).

Other Stimuli

There are numerous disabilities that cause touch function impairments including spinal cord injury and diabetic neuropathy.

Sensitivity to vibration and pressure are involved in reacting to things in the environment that touch the client. It would include the ability to sense when someone is touching the client on the shoulder to get the client's attention and the ability of the client to realize when s/he has bumped into something that s/he doesn't see. To evaluate the extent of impairment, the therapist can provide a set of stimuli to various areas of the skin. These should include light touch, vibration, and potentially painful stimuli (e.g., a pinprick) to evaluate how well the client can sense the stimuli.

Being able to sense noxious stimuli (b2703) is one of the most important ways we avoid serious injuries. Not being able to feel pain can lead to serious risks for clients in that they can continue with actions that are causing serious injury and not realize that they have a condition that requires immediate medical attention. This is the section we suggest you use to document the inability to sense pain. However, if there are indications that the inability to sense pain is an issue, the therapist should also look at b280 Sensation of Pain for indications that the ability to sense pain is absent.

Documentation should include the type and extent of the touch impairment and related Activities and Participation codes that are affected by touch impairment (e.g., d770 Intimate Relationships, d6500 Making and Repairing Clothes). The therapist should cover the specific touch impairment (e.g., light touch absent in the right upper extremity), the extent that it interferes with specific activities (e.g., lack of pain receptors in leg puts client at risk for injury when in the rose garden), compensatory strategies taught and implemented (e.g., client will scan body for injury when on trail with thorn bushes), effectiveness of compensatory strategies (e.g., pressure releases have reduced decubitus ulcers on legs to only one occurrence in last two weeks), and amount of assistance (if any) to minimize touch problems (e.g., requires moderate cues to scan full environment to identify location of outside touch, such as when someone taps the client on the back to get his attention).

If touch functions continue to be impaired after treatment, compensatory strategies are taught to minimize injury and maximize safety (e.g., weight shifts to decrease decubitus ulcers, using visual skills to scan body for injuries).

b279 Additional Sensory Functions, Other Specified and Unspecified

Additional sensory functions not described in the preceding codes would be scored here. See related diagnosis of "Sensory Deprivation."

Pain (b280 - b289)

b280 Sensation of Pain

Sensation of unpleasant feeling indicating potential or actual damage to some body structure.

Inclusions: sensations of generalized or localized pain, in one or more body part, pain in a dermatome, stabbing pain, burning pain, dull pain, aching pain; impairments such as myalgia, analgesia, and hyperalgesia

- *b2800 Generalized Pain*
  Sensation of unpleasant feeling indicating potential or actual damage to some body structure felt all over, or throughout the body.
- *b2801 Pain in Body Part*
  Sensation of unpleasant feeling indicating potential or actual damage to some body structure felt in a specific part, or parts, of the body.

o   *b28010 Pain in Head and Neck*
Sensation of unpleasant feeling indicating potential or actual damage to some body structure felt in the head and neck.

o   *b28011 Pain in Chest*
Sensation of unpleasant feeling indicating potential for actual damage to some body structure felt in the chest.

o   *b28012 Pain in Stomach or Abdomen*
Sensation of unpleasant feeling indicating potential or actual damage to some body structure felt in the stomach or abdomen.
Inclusions: pain in the pelvic region

o   *b28013 Pain in Back*
Sensation of unpleasant feeling indicating potential or actual damage to some structure felt in the back.
Inclusions: pain in the trunk; low backache

o   *b28014 Pain in Upper Limb*
Sensation of unpleasant feeling indicating potential or actual damage to some body structure felt in either one or both upper limbs, including hands.

o   *b28015 Pain in Lower Limb*
Sensation of unpleasant feeling indicating potential or actual damage to some body structure felt in either one or both lower limbs, including feet.

o   *b28016 Pain in Joints*
Sensation of unpleasant feeling indicating potential or actual damage to some body structure felt in one or more joints, including small and big joints.
Inclusions: pain in the hip; pain in the shoulder

o   *b28018 Pain in Body Part, Other Specified*

o   *b28019 Pain in Body Part, Unspecified*

- *b2802 Pain in Multiple Body Parts*
Unpleasant sensation indicating potential or actual damage to some body structure located in several body parts

- *b2803 Radiating Pain in a Dermatome*
Unpleasant sensation indicating potential or actual damage to some body structure located in areas of skin served by the same nerve root.

- *b2804 Radiating Pain in a Segment or Region*
Unpleasant sensation indicating potential or actual damage to some body structure located in areas of skin in different body parts not served by the same nerve root.

Treatment for Sensation of Pain

This set of codes relates to pain in the body. Therapists score the extent of the pain, along with related Activities and Participation codes that are affected by physical pain (e.g., d2401 Handing Stress, d4105 Bending, d4154 Maintaining a Standing Position, d4300 Lifting, d450 Walking, d4552 Running, d540 Dressing, d6506 Taking Care of Animals).

The manifestation of physical pain can result from a traumatic or non-traumatic injury (e.g., fall, overuse injury) or occur as a secondary disability from another health problem (e.g., walking with a bad knee for years can cause back pain from poor posture and improper weight bearing and shifting on the affected leg). The health problem can also be a result of a congenital disability, the aging process, and other disabilities that commonly have associated body pain (e.g., fibromyalgia).

Physical pain is described as acute or chronic.

Acute: Acute pain is described as having a short duration and is usually from a known cause such as an injury or an acute illness. Recovery is usually expected from acute pain.

Chronic: Chronic pain is described as a persistent pain of long duration (at least several months). It is an expected or unexpected long-term pain (e.g., pain that is a symptom of a chronic progressive disease or pain that persists after the expected healing period). It often results in a severely decreased activity level and consequential disability. Some chronic pain has a source that cannot be identified. Other chronic pain has an identified source, but treatment has not yet succeeded (and may never succeed) in relieving the pain.

In addition to the physical origins of pain, pain can originate from psychological stressors (psychogenic pain). Stressors that are suppressed may manifest in pain. It is difficult to tell whether a pain is psychogenic only, psychogenic pain in conjunction with a physical pain, or a physical pain with an, as yet, unidentified cause. Pain that does not appear to have a physical source should not automatically be described as psychogenic pain. The pain sensors themselves can go awry causing impaired pain sensations without another kind of physical origin.

If possible, the source of the pain is identified though testing and scans (e.g., MRI). The team assesses the location of the pain, the severity of the pain, the duration of the pain, and related activities that cause or exacerbate the current pain. Therapists ask the client how long s/he has been experiencing the pain and what methods and interventions have been employed in the past to help manage the pain (e.g., narcotic medication, exercise, meditation, heat, ice).

Pain can be very difficult to measure because it is subjective and people's pain tolerance varies. Pain tolerance is often affected by mood, personality, and circumstance. A common way to measure pain is to ask the client to rate his/her pain on a scale of zero to ten. Zero equals no pain; a one equals mild pain (doesn't interfere with activities). A five equals moderate pain (present and interferes with activities but is not disabling). A ten equals the severest pain imaginable (disabling, unable to function). Therapists ask the client to rate his/her pain prior to the start of treatment, during various treatment activities, and following treatment to help determine a pain pattern and note progression or regression of pain.

Another common way to measure pain is through face pictures. This is especially useful with children, when there is reduced mental capacity, and when there is a language barrier. There are eleven faces. Each face corresponds with the numbers zero through ten. For example, a happy face is the number zero and a face drawn with eyes wide open and an anguished expression would denote a ten. The client is asked to point to the face that best represents how s/he is currently experiencing pain.

Lastly, a pain map may be drawn. A pain map is an anatomical chart of the front and back of the body. The client makes an "x" in areas where pain is experienced. Next to each area, the client is to chart the dates when pain is experienced, pain descriptors (e.g., burning, throbbing), pain intensity (zero through ten), interference with life activities (e.g., unable to drive the kids to school in the morning), what increases the pain (e.g., dressing activities), and what seems to decrease the pain (e.g., lying down on the bed for about 15 minutes after dressing). Clients are usually asked to do a pain map each day for several days (client is given five anatomical charts and asked to map pain for five days). This helps the therapist to identify patterns of pain and possible interventions to help manage pain. It also helps the client to become more aware of his/her pain. In some instances, however, an increased awareness to pain can backfire. Increased attention and focus on pain can increase the intensity and duration of pain.

To document the pain, the therapist describes the pain rating scales used, pain levels and patterns identified, locations of pain, pain triggers, pain management interventions implemented, effectiveness of pain management interventions, level of assistance the client needs to implement pain management interventions, education provided about manifestation of pain within the body, pain descriptors, and the extent that pain interferes with specific activities. In addition to scoring the pain functions impairment also score related Activities and Participation codes that are affected by the pain.

Treatment for pain will vary depending on the root cause, if it can be identified, the experience of the client in dealing with the pain, and the extent that psychological issues are involved. See the specific diagnosis that is causing the pain for treatment direction. In addition to pharmacology, common interventions include improving psychological processes (see "Education and Counseling" in the Techniques section), using the power of distraction, and relaxation training (see "Relaxation and Stress Reduction" in the Techniques section).

b289 Sensation of Pain, Other Specified or Unspecified

b298 Sensory Functions and Pain, Other Specified

b299 Sensory Functions and Pain, Unspecified

References

Best-Martini, E. and Botenhagen-DiGenova, K. (2003). *Exercises for frail elders.* Champaign, IL: Human Kinetics.

burlingame, j. (2001). *Idyll Arbor's therapy dictionary,* (2nd ed.). Ravensdale, WA: Idyll Arbor, Inc:

Roser, D.J. (2003). *FallProof! A comprehensive balance and mobility training program.* Champaign, IL: Human Kinetics.

Sadock, B. & Sadock, V. (2003). *Kaplan & Sadock's synopsis of psychiatry, 9th edition.* Philadelphia, PA: Lippincott Williams & Wilkins.

Zoltan, B. (1996). *Vision, perception, and cognition: A manual for the evaluation and treatment of the neurologically impaired adult.* Thorofare, NJ: Slack.

Chapter 3 Voice and Speech Functions

This chapter is about the functions of producing sounds and speech.

Recreational therapists need to consider the following issues having to do with voice and speech functions when coding under this section.

Language versus Speech

The concepts of language and speech are often thought of as being the same thing. However, they are quite different. Language (as in b167 Mental Functions of Language) is the method of expression or communication, which may or may not be vocal. Speech (as in Chapter 3 Voice and Speech Functions), on the other hand, is the use of the voice (talking, speaking).

Causes of Voice and Speech Impairments

Common causes of voice and speech function impairments include hearing impairments, mental retardation, cleft lip (incomplete joining of the upper lip), cleft palate (abnormal passageway through the roof of the mouth into the airway of the nose), cerebral palsy, traumatic brain injury, multiple sclerosis, Alzheimer's disease, Parkinson's disease, cerebrovascular accident (CVA), brain tumor, selective mutism (a child chooses or pretends not to be able to talk in certain settings, which may indicate an emotional or psychiatric disturbance in the child possibly caused by child abuse), injury to muscles needed for speech, medication side effects, amyotrophic lateral sclerosis (ALS), throat or tongue cancer, and surgical removal of the tongue or voice box (laryngectomy).

General Treatment of Voice and Speech Functions

In addition to an ear, nose, and throat specialist (ENT), the speech language pathologist (SLP) is the primary allied health professional to evaluate, diagnosis, and treat voice and speech impairments. Depending on the specific voice and speech impairment, recommendations are made for surgery (e.g., repair of cleft palate), medications (e.g., for psychiatric problem), counseling (e.g., for abuse, coping, and adjustment), specialized equipment (e.g., hearing aids, augmentative communication device, picture boards), or therapy interventions (e.g., strengthening facial muscles, learning how to slow down the rate of speech, recommendations for a tailored learning environment for deaf children, learning American Sign Language).

Recreational therapists incorporate recommended speech equipment and techniques into treatment plans to facilitate the development of voice and speech functions into various life tasks (e.g., participating in community, home, work, and school settings). Consequently, recreational therapists must be familiar with common voice and speech impairments, equipment, and techniques to be able to accurately describe impairments when they are observed and effectively facilitate voice and speech skills.

Voice and speech impairments can affect many life tasks (e.g., asking for assistance, interaction with peers, employment, schoolwork) thus having an impact on meeting personal health needs (e.g., feeling confident, having good self-esteem, forming social relationships, and communicating with health professionals). Speech deficits may also reduce the client's ability to attain basic living needs. This may include taking a lower paying job that requires less verbal communication thus impacting personal finances or avoiding certain stores where verbal communication is commonly expected thus impacting the ability to obtain needed items. Additionally, for some individuals, the stress of having to cope with the effect of the impairment on life activities can surface as depression thus limiting participation in life activities even further.

Consequently, therapists need to assess the impact of the impairment on all life activities and create a treatment plan that addresses these issues. For example, the therapist may need to look at educating the teacher on how to best accommodate a child with a stuttering problem, teaching the client alternative communication techniques that are specific to interacting with his/her peer group, facilitating the development of self-esteem through identification of the client's strengths and opportunities for peer recognition of strengths, identifying other forms of communication to more accurately reflect the meaning of the message such as the use of body language, the environment, writing, facial expressions, eye contact, etc. More specific treatment recommendations will be found under each specific voice and speech component.

General Documentation of Voice and Speech Functions

Recreational therapists document voice and speech impairments in their notes as they relate to participation in specific life activities. The extent of the impairment, however, will most likely be scored by a speech language pathologist or other health professional that specializes in speech and voice (e.g., ear, nose, and throat specialist).

Documentation related to speech and voice functions includes the specific impairment (e.g., stuttering), techniques utilized to enhance voice and speech production (e.g., requires minimal verbal cues to increase voice volume), use of equipment/techniques in real-life settings (e.g., able to effectively communicate with peers at school utilizing an augmentative communication device with minimal assistance), ability to use compensatory strategies (e.g., able to sign 50 words independently), and impact of impairment on life tasks (e.g., client reports that dysarthria is a major hindrance to forming social relationships).

b310 Voice Functions

Functions of the production of various sounds by the passage of air through the larynx.

Inclusions: functions of production and quality of voice; functions of phonation, pitch, loudness, and other qualities of speech; impairments such as aphonia, dysphonia, hoarseness, hypernasality, and hyponasality

Exclusions: mental functions of language (b167); articulation functions (b320)

- *d3100 Production of Voice*
  Functions of the production of sound made through coordination of the larynx and surrounding muscles with the respiratory system.
  Inclusions: functions of phonation, loudness; impairment of aphonia
- *b3101 Quality of Voice*
  Functions of the production or characteristics of voice including pitch, resonance, and other features.
  Inclusions: functions of high or low pitch; impairments such as hypernasality, hyponasality, dysphonia, hoarseness, or harshness
- *b3108 Voice Functions, Other Specified*
- *b3109 Voice Functions, Unspecified*

Treatment for Voice Functions

This section of the ICF includes all of the deficits associated with not being able to produce the sounds required for speech. Specific impairments identified by the ICF that fall under this category are listed and defined in the glossary.

Evaluating the deficits in this section consists of two parts. First other professionals will evaluate the physical cause of the problem. Then the recreational therapist evaluates how the problem affects the client's participation in activities. For example, in b310 be sure to observe whether the unusual vocal

characteristics cause negative reactions in people who come in contact with the client. Children with hypernasality, for example, are often perceived as less intelligent than peers who speak normally.

Document as described in the introduction to this chapter.

When treating the deficits of voice production and quality, recreational therapists incorporate specific recommendations from voice and speech specialists into their treatment plans as they relate to the client's participation in life activities. Treatment interventions will vary depending on the specific impairment and level of dysfunction. General treatments for voice and speech functions are included in the introduction.

If voice volume is impaired, it is particularly important to get the client to speak loudly enough so that s/he can be easily heard by another. Providing verbal cues alone may be sufficient, but if this does not increase speech volume to a sufficient level, ask the client to "yell" as if the person was on the other side of the room. Soft voices that can't be heard by other residents are one of the major reasons why residents in long-term care facilities do not interact with one another.

If a person is unable to speak (aphonia) or the quality of voice is poor enough that others can't understand the client, adaptations are required. American Sign Language may be taught along with other forms of direct (e.g., writing, gesturing) and indirect (e.g., body language, eye contact, dress) communication. Other forms of treatment will vary greatly depending on the specific impairment that is causing the problem, so it is particularly important for the recreational therapist to collaborate with the speech and language specialist.

b320 Articulation Functions

Functions of the production of speech sounds.

Inclusions: functions of enunciation, articulation of phonemes; spastic, ataxic, flaccid dysarthria; anarthria

Exclusions: mental functions of language (b167); voice functions (b310)

Treatment for Articulation Functions

Articulation functions can be described as difficulty forming sounds and stringing sounds together. Common articulation problems include substituting one sound for another (e.g., wabbit for rabbit), omitting a sound (e.g., han for hand), and distorting a sound (e.g., ship for sip, incorrect enunciation of phoneme blends such as "bl" or "th").

The specific impairments identified by the ICF that fall under this category are listed and defined in the glossary. Evaluation of deficits in articulation can be done by several professionals on the health care team including the recreational therapist. The causes of the deficits are documented in the Body Structures section of the ICF, but the functionality of articulation is described and coded here. Recreational therapists should note how problems with articulation affect the client in advanced activities of daily living.

Document as described in the introduction to this chapter.

Treatment involves incorporating specific recommendations from voice and speech specialists into recreational therapy treatment plans as they relate to the needs of the client and the hindrances the articulation deficits pose to participation in life activities. Treatment interventions will vary depending on the specific impairment and level of dysfunction. However, there are several intervention techniques that are commonly employed to improve articulation. One involves over-pronunciation of each syllable in a word with a decreased rate of speaking. The therapist can verbally cue the client to slow down the speech rate by asking the client to tap his/her finger on the table in tempo to the speech syllables (e.g., he... went... to... the... kit... chen... to... get... a... bowl ...of... spa... ghet... ti). Other techniques involve speech drills that work on specific problem areas (e.g., saying a set of 12 words that begin with the phoneme blend "bl" three times each) and facial and mouth exercises to improve muscular control, strength, and range of motion (e.g., open mouth wide and then close, stick tongue out and side to side, puff up cheeks). Interventions that are incorporated into the recreational therapy treatment plan are checked with the voice and speech specialist to ensure consistency of approaches and techniques.

Adaptations for articulation functions are similar to those used in b310 Voice Functions. There may be an added complication, though, because many articulation problems are caused by damage to the central nervous system (e.g., stroke). Adaptations, such as the American Sign Language or writing instead of speaking, may also be difficult because of the diagnosis. Training caretakers to anticipate needs may be required when the client in unable to make his/her needs known.

b330 Fluency and Rhythm of Speech Functions
Functions of the production of flow and tempo of speech.
Inclusions: functions of fluency, rhythm, speed, and melody of speech; prosody and intonation; impairments such as stuttering, stammering, cluttering, bradylalia, and tachylalia
Exclusions: mental functions of language (b167); voice functions (b310); articulation functions (b320)

- *b3300 Fluency of Speech*
  Functions of the production of smooth, uninterrupted flow of speech.
  Inclusions: functions of smooth connection of speech; impairments such as stuttering, stammering, cluttering, dysfluency, repetition of sounds, words or parts of words, and irregular breaks in speech
- *b3301 Rhythm of Speech*
  Functions of the modulated, tempo, and stress patterns in speech.
  Inclusions: impairments such as stereotypic or repetitive speech cadence
- *b3302 Speed of Speech*
  Functions of the rate of speech production.
  Inclusions: impairments such as bradylalia and tachylalia
- *b3303 Melody of Speech*
  Functions of modulation of pitch patterns in speech.
  Inclusions: prosody of speech, intonation, melody of speech; impairments such as monotone speech
- *b3308 Fluency and Rhythm of Speech Functions, Other Specified*
- *b3309 Fluency and Rhythm of Speech Functions, Unspecified*

Treatment for
Fluency and Rhythm of Speech Functions

Voice and speech are more than just words; the tone, flow, pitch, and melody of the voice also convey much of the message (e.g., wanting to express feelings of love in a sweet and quiet way, express anger in a quick and explosive manner, or express business competence in a "quick and to the point" manner). This is referred to globally as the fluency and rhythm of speech. When problems occur in this area, messages may not be clear (e.g., trying to convey compassion may come out sounding like insincerity). They may be misinterpreted by the receiver or be a disappointment to the sender when the message doesn't sound the way the person intended it to sound.

The specific impairments identified by the ICF that fall under this category are listed and defined in the glossary.

Other members of the health care team will be doing much of the evaluation of deficits in fluency and rhythm of speech. The recreational therapist evaluates how the deficits affect participation in life activities. Issues such as stammering can cause marked reluctance to participate in normal activities because the client may be embarrassed about the inability to speak clearly. In other instances, the person may not be aware of his/her abnormal speech patterns. For example, someone in the manic phase of bipolar disorder may not be aware that his speech is rapid and pressured (tachylalia). The amount of awareness that the client has is an important part of the evaluation.

Document as described in the introduction to this chapter, paying special attention to whether the client might be able to make changes in the deficits that are observed.

Treatment involves finding ways to improve fluency and rhythm. Fluency and rhythm impairments are commonly accentuated by stress and anxiety. So when there are impairments, therapists should first consider ways that stress can be minimized or eliminated (e.g., deep breathing, planning and organizing ahead of time, and practicing events that produce anxiety). More details on relaxation can be found in "Relaxation and Stress Reduction" in the Techniques section.

When the client is not aware that there is a deficit, education may be necessary. Tape recordings and videotaping will help the client to see how his/her speech patterns are different.

In some cases, such as stammering, the client may not be able to completely control the problem, so adaptations may be required. The therapist can educate the client about other forms of communication to assist with conveying messages effectively including the role of body language (e.g., posturing, eye contact, hand movement, facial expressions), dress (e.g., business, casual, flirty), and environment. Utilization of alternative modes of communication should also be encouraged as appropriate (e.g., written reports in lieu of or in addition to verbal reports, using PowerPoint presentations and videos, chalkboard, dry erase board, e-mail). Relying totally on alternative forms of communication should not be encouraged unless it is absolutely necessary.

Adaptations in the environment are often necessary, too. Educating peers and people in places of authority (e.g., teachers, employers, parents) about the impairment and how they can best assist the person in communication (e.g., allow the person extra time to convey a thought, provide cueing if needed, reiterate points that are clear and ask for clarification of points that are unclear) should also be part of the treatment plan to facilitate further skill development and effective communication.

b340 Alternative Vocalization Functions

Functions of the production of other manners of vocalization.
Inclusions: functions of the production of notes and range of sounds, such as in singing, chanting, babbling, and humming; crying aloud and screaming
Exclusions: mental functions of language (b167); voice functions (b310); articulation functions (b320); fluency and rhythm of speech functions (b330)

- *b3400 Production of Notes*
  Functions of production of musical vocal sounds.
  Inclusions: sustaining, modulating, and terminating productions of single or connected vocalizations with variation in pitch such as in singing, humming, and chanting
- *b3401 Making a Range of Sounds*
  Functions of production of a variety of vocalizations.
  Inclusions: functions of babbling in children
- *b3408 Alternative Vocalization Functions, Other Specified*
- *b3409 Alternative Vocalization Functions, Unspecified*

Treatment for Alternative Vocalization Functions

Deficits in these alternate vocalization functions may not be noticed by other members of the treatment team. They tend to show up more in activities than in diagnostic situations. The recreational therapist needs to be aware of the range of normal functions and note when a client is outside the norms.

Evaluation involves observations of the client in many situations, watching for appropriate alternative vocalizations. Checking the client's ability to sing is one possibility, but the other types of vocalization (or lack of them) will probably be more important for most treatment situations. For infants, deficits in babbling behavior can be one of the first indications of a psychological problem, such as autism.

Documentation should include observations of the client with detailed notes of the situation and what more normal behavior would be. For example, "The three-year-old client fell off the swing and badly skinned her knee, but seemed to be fighting against making any crying sound." This is the kind of deficit that may point toward problems other than voice and speech functions, but documenting this deficit is part of the evidence necessary to demonstrate other problems exist.

In treatment recreational therapists incorporate specific recommendations from voice and speech specialists into their plans as they relate to the needs of the client and the hindrances deficits pose to participation in life activities. Treatment interventions will vary depending on the specific impairment and level of dysfunction. Common interventions to promote alternative vocalizations include addressing underlying issues (e.g., issues of abuse that conditioned a child not to scream), providing sensory stimulation (e.g., tickling the infant and providing bright colored toys and mirrors to promote babbling), and playing games and engaging in recreational activities that promote alternative vocalizations (e.g., a game of echoing sounds to promote the development of sound ranges, singing and humming to music, playing games that encourage the child to scream such as being "it" in the game hide-and-seek and having to say "ready or not here I come").

b398 Voice and Speech Functions, Other Specified

b399 Voice and Speech Functions, Unspecified

Any other voice or speech function not described in the previous components would be noted and scored under this code.

Chapter 4 Functions of the Cardiovascular, Hematological, Immunological, and Respiratory Systems

This chapter is about the functions involved in the cardiovascular system (functions of the heart and blood vessels), the hematological and immunological systems (functions of blood production and immunity), and the respiratory system (functions of respiration and exercise tolerance).

Normally recreational therapists will not do the initial evaluation for most of the codes in this chapter. One important exception is b455 Exercise Tolerance functions. Refer to this code for further information.

During advanced activities of daily living and other RT programming, recreational therapists assess and monitor vital signs that are part of this chapter including pulse (b4100 heart rate, b4101 heart rhythm), blood pressure (b420 blood pressure functions), oxygen saturation levels (b4301 oxygen-carrying functions of the blood), and respiration (b4400 respiration rate, b4401 respiratory rhythm, b4402 depth of respiration). See "Vital Signs" in the Techniques section for information on how to assess and monitor pulse, blood pressure, and respiration. See "Oxygen" in the Techniques section for information on how to assess and monitor oxygen saturation levels.

Vital signs are frequently assessed and monitored by a variety of health professionals, including recreational therapists, in hospital and rehabilitation settings. Vital signs may also be assessed in community recreation programs in response to injury (e.g., blow to the head during a sporting event), an unforeseen health event (e.g., cardiac arrest), or to ensure the safety of a participant (e.g., assessing blood pressure when a client with a T1 complete spinal cord injury appears to be going into autonomic dysreflexia).

See specific diagnoses of "Cardiac Conditions" and "Chronic Obstructive Pulmonary Disease" that require frequent monitoring of vital signs.

Functions of the Cardiovascular System (b410-b429)

b410 Heart Functions
Functions of pumping the blood in adequate or required amounts and pressure throughout the body.
Inclusions: functions of heart rate, rhythm, and output; contraction force of ventricular muscles; functions of heart valves; pumping the blood through the pulmonary circuit; dynamics of circulation to the heart; impairments such as tachycardia, bradycardia, and irregular heart beat as in heart failure, cardiomyopathy, myocarditis, and coronary insufficiency

Exclusions: blood vessel functions (b415); blood pressure functions (b420); exercise tolerance functions (b455)
- *b4100 Heart Rate*
  Functions related to the number of times the heart contracts every minute.
  Inclusions: impairments such as rates that are too fast (tachycardia) or too slow (bradycardia)
- *b4101 Heart Rhythm*
  Functions related to the regularity of the beating of the heart.
  Inclusions: impairments such as arrhythmias
- *b4102 Contraction Force of Ventricular Muscles*
  Functions related to the amount of blood pumped by the ventricular muscle during every beat.
  Inclusions: impairments such as diminished cardiac output
- *b4103 Blood Supply to the Heart*
  Functions related to the volume of blood available to the heart muscle.
  Inclusions: impairments such as coronary ischemia
- *b4108 Heart Functions, Other Specified*
- *b4109 Heart Function, Unspecified*

Treatment for Heart Functions

This section covers all of the functions of the heart and its responsibility for circulating blood throughout the body. Any interruption in the function of the heart is immediately life threatening. Recreational therapists should know how to do cardiopulmonary resuscitation as part of their practice. Malfunctions may or may not be life threatening, but the onset of a malfunction, such as tachycardia, is a significant event that the recreational therapist must know how to handle.

In general, a recreational therapist is not responsible for routine evaluation of heart function, however it is the responsibility of the recreational therapist to monitor heart rate during therapy sessions when:
1. Clients have cardiac precautions or parameters.
2. Clients have specific exercise tolerance issues or goals that need to be monitored to denote current functioning status (e.g., length of time client is able to maintain target heart rate during aerobic exercise, heart rate response to a particular form, length, and intensity of exercise).

3. Heart rate is an indicator of response (e.g., heart rate is monitored to ascertain effect of relaxation training or response to anxiety producing stimuli).
4. Obtaining baseline status to determine next approach when feelings of discomfort are reported by a client or suspected by the therapist (e.g., client reports feeling lightheaded during community integration session).

See "Vital Signs" in the Techniques section for instructions on how to find and monitor pulse (heart rate).

When monitoring a client's heart rate, the recreational therapist may feel a change (or note a concern) with the regularity, speed, or strength of the client's pulse. The therapist records and documents heart rates within discipline documentation, as well as alerting other health professionals to immediate concerns. For example, the therapist may be taking a client's resting heart rate prior to physical activity and note that the pulse is rapid and irregular. The client does not appear to be in distress. The therapist immediately takes the client back to the nursing station, does not leave the client unattended, and verbally alerts the client's primary nurse to the finding to seek confirmation of the problem and determine needed interventions.

In general, treatment of a heart function problem is outside the scope of recreational therapy practice. However, it is not uncommon for recreational therapists to implement a treatment plan in which heart rate is an indicator (e.g., response to activity) or to be part of the treatment team that monitors heart rate for the reasons reviewed previously. Recreational therapists may also teach clients how to find and monitor heart rate, as well as how to best respond to heart rate changes in a community setting (e.g., call emergency response unit, decrease intensity of exercise to lower heart rate).

Adaptations may be required for the client to ensure that physical activity is within safe limits for the client's condition (e.g., changing the intensity of the activity through the use of adaptive equipment or activity modifications). Close evaluation of the activities that the client plans to engage in after therapy is essential for clients with cardiac problems to decrease risk of injury or death (e.g., a client who has had a triple bypass tells the recreational therapist that he plans to go for long walks on the beach every day after he is discharged — walking on sand, as well as walking in heat, increases stress on the heart). Clients may not always understand the level of effort required by some activities, so it is important for the therapist to take a close look at the client's planned activity pattern after discharge and make recommen-

dations. See "Cardiac Conditions" in the Diagnosis section and "Metabolic Equivalents" in the Concepts section for more information.

b415 Blood Vessel Functions
Functions of transporting blood throughout the body.
Inclusions: functions of arteries, capillaries and veins; vasomotor function; functions of pulmonary arteries, capillaries and veins; functions of valves of veins; impairments such as in blockage or constriction of arteries; atherosclerosis, arteriosclerosis, thrombo-embolism, and varicose veins
Exclusions: heart functions (b410); blood pressure functions (b420); hematological system functions (b430); exercise tolerance functions (b455)

- b4150 Functions of Arteries
  Functions related to blood flow in the arteries.
  Inclusions: impairments such as arterial dilation; arterial constriction such as in intermittent claudication
- b4151 Functions of Capillaries
  Functions related to the blood flow in the capillaries.
- b4152 Functions of Veins
  Functions related to blood flow in the veins, and the functions of valves of veins.
  Inclusions: impairments such as venous dilation; venous constriction; insufficient closing of valves as in varicose veins
- b4158 Blood Vessel Functions, Other Specified
- b4159 Blood Vessel Functions, Unspecified

Treatment for Blood Vessel Functions

This section covers all of the functions of the blood vessels, which are responsible for circulating blood throughout the body. As with heart functions, some are immediately life threatening and others are not.

Evaluation of blood vessel function is not normally a recreational therapist's responsibility, but there are some conditions that are more likely to show up during activities and the recreational therapist is responsible for recognizing the existence of a problem. One example is Raynaud's phenomenon. During an episode, the fingers and/or toes can become white or deep blue due to blood vessel constriction. If the vessels in the hands or feet remain constricted until circulation is completely cut off, the fingers or toes will become deformed or gangrene may set in. In this case, the therapist needs be aware of the changes in the hands or feet and get the client medical treatment if the condition persists. Similarly, the therapist needs to be aware of other indications of deficits in blood vessel functions such as the onset of numbness or pain. The diagnosis is not the recreational therapist's responsibility, but noticing that there is a problem is.

Documentation depends on the incident. The most important aspect of the documentation is that the rest of the medical team knows about the incident. In a community recreation setting, it may be the responsibility of the therapist to make sure that medical care is provided for the client.

Treatment is outside the scope of recreational therapy practice.

Adaptations may be required for the client to ensure that the amount of exercise or the type of exercise is within safe limits for the client's condition.

b420 Blood Pressure Functions

Functions of maintaining the pressure of blood within the arteries.

Inclusions: functions of maintenance of blood pressure; increased and decreased blood pressure; impairments such as in hypotension, hypertension, and postural hypotension

Exclusions: heart functions (b410); blood vessel functions (b415); exercise tolerance functions (b455)

- *b4200 Increased Blood Pressure*
  Functions related to a rise in systolic or diastolic blood pressure above normal for the age.
- *b4201 Decreased Blood Pressure*
  Functions related to a fall in systolic or diastolic blood pressure below normal for the age.
- *b4202 Maintenance of Blood Pressure*
  Functions related to maintaining an appropriate blood pressure in response to changes in the body.
- *b4208 Blood Pressure Functions, Other Specified*
- *b4209 Blood Pressure Functions, Unspecified*

Treatment for Blood Pressure Functions

This section covers issues with blood pressure. Many of these issues are evaluated by other medical team members, but the recreational therapist should know how to take an accurate blood pressure reading if his/her clients are subject to blood pressure changes. Clients with complete spinal cord injuries at or above T6 are at risk for autonomic dysreflexia, a life-threatening condition that includes greatly increased blood pressure. Many medications have side effects that increase the risk of postural hypotension (a drop in blood pressure in response to a more upright position — lying to sitting, sitting to standing) and the likelihood of fainting when standing up. Postural hypotension is also common in clients who have been lying in bed for long periods of time. In this instance, postural hypotension will typically dissipate progressively with increased mobility. High blood pressure increases the risks of exercise so the therapist should be aware of limitations on a client with hypertension (e.g., cease

physical activity if blood pressure rises above a set level).

Recreational therapists monitor blood pressure during therapy sessions when:
1. Clients have cardiac precautions or parameters.
2. Clients have specific exercise tolerance issues or goals that need to be monitored to denote current functioning status (e.g., blood pressure response to a particular form, length, and intensity of exercise; response to movement into and out of different positions such as squatting to standing or sitting to standing).
3. Blood pressure is an indicator of response (e.g., response to stress or activity, response to removal of an external stimulus during an episode of autonomic dysreflexia).
4. Obtaining baseline status to determine the next approach when feelings of discomfort are reported by a client or suspected by the therapist (e.g., client reports feeling lightheaded during community integration session, client becomes pale and faint).

See "Vital Signs" in the Techniques section for instructions on how take and record blood pressure.

Blood pressure readings taken by the recreational therapist are recorded in the medical record. Any reading that is abnormal (e.g., extremely low blood pressure in a client whose blood pressure is typically normal) or causes immediate concern (e.g., blood pressure that is outside of parameters and does not respond to therapist's intervention — reduction in activity, deep breathing, change in body position, removal of external stimuli in autonomic dysreflexia) is immediately reported to the appropriate health professional (e.g., attending physician, primary nurse) to determine the next intervention.

In general, medical management of blood pressure functions is outside the scope of practice for recreational therapists (e.g., prescription of medication). However it is not uncommon for recreational therapists to implement a treatment plan:
1. that assists in blood pressure control (e.g., physician cleared physical activity for weight loss to decrease blood pressure, relaxation training, positional changes in therapy sessions to assist in resolving postural hypotension in a client who has been lying in bed for a prolonged period of time),
2. in which blood pressure is an indicator (e.g., response to activity), or
3. to monitor blood pressure for the reasons mentioned previously.

Recreational therapists may also teach clients how to monitor blood pressure with automatic blood pressure cuffs in community settings (e.g., how to monitor blood pressure at the gym), and how to best respond to blood pressure changes in a community setting (e.g., call emergency response unit, change intensity of physical activity, implement relaxation techniques, search for annoying external stimuli if in autonomic dysreflexia).

Adaptations may be required for the client with hypertension or cardiac precautions/parameters to ensure that physical activity is within safe limits for the client's condition (e.g., changing the intensity of the activity through the use of adaptive equipment or activity modifications), as well as to prevent fainting or falling episodes with clients who are subject to hypotension. Close evaluation of the activities that the client plans to engage in after therapy is essential for clients with cardiac problems to decrease risk of complications, injury, or death (e.g., stroke, heart attack, and falls).

Functions of the Hematological and Immunological Systems (b430-b439)

b430 Hematological System Functions
Functions of blood production, oxygen, and metabolite carriage, and clotting.
Inclusions: functions of the production of blood and bone marrow; oxygen-carrying functions of blood; blood-related functions of spleen; metabolite-carrying functions of blood; clotting; impairments such as anemia, hemophilia, and other clotting dysfunctions
Exclusions: functions of the cardiovascular system (b410-b429); immunological system functions (b435); exercise tolerance functions (b455)
- *b4300 Production of Blood*
  Functions related to the production of blood and all its constituents
- *b4301 Oxygen-Carrying Functions of the Blood*
  Functions related to the blood's capacity to carry oxygen throughout the body.
- *b4302 Metabolite-Carrying Functions of the Blood*
  Functions related to the blood's capacity to carry metabolites throughout the body.
- *b4303 Clotting Functions*
  Functions related to the coagulation of blood, such as at a site of injury.
- *b4308 Hematological System Functions, Other Specified*
- *b4309 Hematological System Functions, Unspecified*

Treatment for Hematological System Functions

These functions have to do with the production of blood and the circulation of blood throughout the body. Any deficits in the areas of blood production, oxygen carrying, or metabolite carrying will have significant effects on the energy levels of the client. Issues with clotting functions may require special precautions, such as in the case of hemophilia (a lack of clotting agents in the blood, which can lead to uncontrollable bleeding) or clients who are on blood thinning medications, such as Coumadin, which prevent the blood from clotting.

While recreational therapists do not evaluate these functions, they need to understand the limitations of clients who have deficits in any of these functions (e.g., decrease risk of injury during activity to prevent bleeding or bruising). If one of these functions is the cause of deficits in exercise tolerance, the treatment needs to be written in this section rather than in b455 Exercise Tolerance Functions.

One important issue with these functions is the level of oxygen in the blood. See "Oxygen" in the Techniques section for information on how to monitor oxygen saturation levels. Oxygen saturation levels are monitored when working with clients who have poor blood oxygen levels such as chronic obstructive pulmonary disease, as well as clients who are on oxygen therapy. Monitoring oxygen saturation levels provides immediate feedback about the client's activity tolerance, need or lack of need for further oxygen, and effectiveness of oxygen intake techniques when oxygen saturation levels fall below set parameters (e.g., taking slow and deep breaths through the nose to increase oxygen saturation levels).

Adaptations may need to be made so that the amount of effort and safety of the activity is appropriate for the client's condition.

b435 Immunological System Functions
Functions of the body related to protection against foreign substances, including infections, by specific and non-specific immune responses.
Inclusions: immune response (specific and non-specific); hypersensitivity reactions; functions of lymphatic vessels and nodes; functions of cell-mediated immunity, antibody-mediated immunity; response to immunization; impairments such as in autoimmunity, allergic reactions, lymphadenitis and lymphoedema
Exclusions: hematological system functions (b430)
- *b4350 Immune Response*
  Functions of the body's response to sensitization to foreign substances, including infections.
  - *b43500 Specific Immune Response*
    Functions of the body's response of sensitization to a specific foreign substance.
  - *b43501 Non-Specific Immune Response*
    Functions of the body's general response of sensitization to foreign substances, including infections.

o   *b43508 Immune Response, Other Specified*
o   *b43509 Immune Response, Unspecified*
- *b4351 Hypersensitivity Reactions*
  Functions of the body's response of increased sensitization to foreign substances, such as in sensitivities to different antigens.
- *b4352 Functions of the Lymphatic Vessels*
  Functions related to vascular channels that transport lymph.
- *b4353 Functions of Lymph Nodes*
  Functions related to glands along the course of lymphatic vessels.
- *b4358 Immunological System Functions, Other Specified*
- *b4359 Immunological System Functions, Unspecified*

Treatment for Immunological System Functions

These functions have to do with the immune system, both in the blood and in the lymph system. When it is working properly, the immune system is responsible for fighting infections. Problems with the immune system cause allergies and autoimmune diseases. Allergies, especially food allergies, can be life threatening. The therapist needs to know about any restrictions on the client's activities caused by deficits in these areas.

While recreational therapists do not evaluate these functions, they need to understand the limitations of clients who have deficits in any of these functions.

Treatment of underlying disorders is outside the therapist's scope of practice. However, discomfort caused by some of the deficits in this area (especially those caused by autoimmune diseases, such as the pain associated with fibromyalgia) may be alleviated by gentle exercise and/or passive and active stretching.

Adaptations need to be made so that the amount of effort and safety of the activity is appropriate for the client's condition. If there are deficits in the disease-fighting abilities of the client's immune system, the therapist needs to maintain careful control of the environment the client is exposed to. Strict isolation is a possibility. The therapist also needs to know about any allergies (including food allergies) so that s/he can make sure the client isn't exposed to dangerous allergens.

b439 Functions of the Hematological and Immunological Systems, Other Specified and Unspecified

Functions of the Respiratory System (b440-b449)

b440 Respiration Functions
Functions of inhaling air into the lungs, the exchange of gases between air and blood, and exhaling air.
Inclusions: functions of respiration rate, rhythm, and depth; impairments such as apnoea, hyperventilation, irregular respiration, paradoxical respiration, and bronchial spasm, and as in pulmonary emphysema
Exclusions: respiratory muscle functions (b445); additional respiratory functions (b450); exercise tolerance functions (b455)
- *b4400 Respiration Rate*
  Functions related to the number of breaths taken per minute.
  Inclusions: impairments such as rates that are too fast (tachypnea) or too slow (bradypnoea)
- *b4401 Respiratory Rhythm*
  Functions related to the periodicity and regularity of breathing.
  Inclusions: impairments such as irregular breathing
- *b4402 Depth of Respiration*
  Functions related to the volume and expansion of the lungs during breathing.
  Inclusions: impairments such as superficial or shallow respiration
- *b4408 Respiration Functions, Other Specified*
- *b4409 Respiration Functions, Unspecified*

Treatment for Respiration Functions

These functions have to do with the way air gets into the body, getting oxygen into the blood, and carbon dioxide out of the blood. Deficits in these functions may be life threatening. They certainly will have an effect on the client's ability to participate in activities, even ones with minimal physical demands.

While recreational therapists do not evaluate these functions, they need to understand the limitations of clients who have deficits. If one of these functions is the cause of deficits in exercise tolerance, the treatment needs to be written in this section rather than in b455 Exercise Tolerance Functions.

One important issue with these functions is the level of oxygen in the blood. See "Oxygen" in the Techniques section for information on how to monitor oxygen saturation levels. Recreational therapists may also need to monitor respirations within activity in particular client groups that are at risk for, or have, respiration impairments (e.g., chronic obstructive pulmonary disease, asthma, recovery stage after heart surgery). See "Vital Signs" in the Techniques section for information on how to monitor and document respiration.

Recreational therapists can work with the rest of the medical team to provide therapy under this section. See the treatment for exercise tolerance functions for more ideas on general programming. Some specific diagnoses that the therapist may treat that are covered in this section include asthma and bronchial spasms, hyperventilation (especially if it is caused by psychological issues), and expansion of the lungs. Some of these issues are covered in the Techniques section on "Relaxation and Stress Reduction." Working on expansion of the lungs involves finding ways to get the client to take deeper breaths. Simple activities, such as contests where the client is using a straw to blow a ping-pong ball across a table, can be used to increase lung function in a way that reduces the emphasis on "therapy" and is more likely to elicit the client's compliance.

Sometimes there is no effective treatment for the condition. Adaptations need to be made so that the required amount of effort is appropriate for the client's condition.

b445 Respiratory Muscle Functions

Functions of the muscles involved in breathing.
Inclusions: functions of thoracic respiratory muscles; functions of the diaphragm; functions of accessory respiratory muscles
Exclusions: respiration functions (b440); additional respiratory functions (b450); exercise tolerance functions (b455)

- *b4450 Functions of the Thoracic Respiratory Muscles*
  Functions of the thoracic muscles involved in breathing.
- *b4451 Functions of the Diaphragm*
  Functions of the diaphragm as involved in breathing.
- *b4452 Functions of Accessory Respiratory Muscles*
  Functions of the additional muscles involved in breathing.
- *b4458 Respiratory Muscle Functions, Other Specified*
- *b4459 Respiratory Muscle Functions, Unspecified*

Treatment for Respiratory Muscles Functions

These functions have to do with the muscles used to get air into and out of the body. Deficits in these functions are often the result of damage to the nerves that control the muscles (e.g., spinal cord injury, ALS). The problems will be written in two places: where the damage to the nerves is discussed and here where the deficits resulting from the nerve damage are described. Other deficits in the functions of the respiratory muscles may be caused by damage to the muscles themselves.

These problems may be life threatening. They certainly will have an effect on the client's ability to participate in activities, even ones with minimal physical demands.

Recreational therapists need to understand the limitations of clients who have these deficits. If one of these functions is the cause of deficits in exercise tolerance, the treatment needs to be written in this section rather than in b455 Exercise Tolerance Functions.

As with everything related to respiration and blood circulation, the level of oxygen in the blood is an important issue, as well as heart rate, blood pressure, and respiration. See "Oxygen" and "Vital Signs" in the Techniques section for information on how to monitor these issues.

Recreational therapists can work with the rest of the medical team to provide therapy under this section. See the treatment for exercise tolerance functions for more ideas on general programming.

Sometimes there is no effective treatment for the condition. Adaptations need to be made so that the required amount of effort is appropriate for the client's condition.

b449 Functions of the Respiratory System, Other Specified and Unspecified

Additional Functions and Sensations of the Cardiovascular and Respiratory Systems (b450-b469)

b450 Additional Respiratory Functions

Additional functions related to breathing, such as coughing, sneezing, and yawning.
Inclusions: functions of blowing, whistling, and mouth breathing

Treatment for Additional Respiratory Functions

These functions cover all of the leftover functions related to respiration.

There is one area where the recreational therapist may be involved with evaluation in this section. Abnormal patterns in one of these functions may be easier to note with the extended interactions recreational therapists often have with their clients. For example, a doctor taking a physical may not notice if the client yawns a time or two. A recreational therapist is much more likely to notice if the client yawns a hundred times during a group activity. It is important to report abnormal patterns to the rest of the medical team.

Recreational therapists can work with the rest of the treatment team to provide therapy under this section. Some of the therapy will be building skills.

Other parts will be extinguishing inappropriate behaviors.

b455 Exercise Tolerance Functions

Functions related to respiratory and cardiovascular capacity as required for enduring physical exertion.
Inclusions: functions of physical endurance, aerobic capacity, stamina, and fatigability
Exclusions: functions of the cardiovascular system (b410-b429); hematological system functions (b430); respiration functions (b440); respiratory muscle functions (b445); additional respiratory functions (b450)

- b4550 General Physical Endurance
  Functions related to the general level of tolerance of physical exercise or stamina.
- b4551 Aerobic Capacity
  Functions related to the extent to which a person can exercise without getting out of breath.
- b4552 Fatigability
  Functions related to susceptibility to fatigue, at any level of exertion.
- b4558 Exercise Tolerance Functions, Other Specified
- b4559 Exercise Tolerance Functions, Unspecified

Treatment for Exercise Tolerance Functions

Recreational therapists frequently address exercise tolerance functions for rehabilitation and health promotion. Healthy People 2010 recommends that healthy adults participate in 30 minutes of moderate physical activity five times a week to maintain health. Children and teenagers are recommended to engage in 60 minutes of moderate physical leisure activity five times a week to maintain health. The amount of time, intensity, and frequency of exercise for people who have health issues will vary depending on the person's limitations and abilities.

This section is used to document impairments in exercise tolerance that are not caused by other conditions. Many of the ideas presented here can be used for deficits documented in other parts of this chapter. The recreational therapist should check other sections to make sure they understand what is causing the deficit and only document in b455 if there is no other known cause for a lack of exercise tolerance. Given the average level of exercise for people in Western civilizations, this is likely to be a heavily used code.

Exercise functions are measured by frequency (how often the client engages in the specific activity), time (amount of time the client is able to engage in the specific activity), and intensity (mild, moderate, vigorous). Vital signs are used as a measure to assess and evaluate a client's functioning within each of the measures described. See "Vital Signs" in the Techniques section for more information.

See "Exercise Basics" in the Techniques section for information that must be obtained prior to a client's engagement in physical activity. Prior to establishing exercise tolerance goals, therapists are fully aware of (and document) any medical complications that could compromise optimal exercise tolerance functions.

The therapist makes the following notations during activities:

- Amount of time engaged in cardiovascular activity.
- The intensity of the cardiovascular activity.
- The client's ability to self-monitor vital signs and outward signs of fatigue.
- The client's ability to adapt exercises within the program to meet needs (e.g., range restrictions, intensity alterations).
- The client's ability to perform the exercises correctly and safely.
- The client's reaction to participation in the exercise program.
- Vital sign measurements (see "Vital Signs" in the Techniques section for information on how to document vital signs).

Treatment and adaptations for deficits in exercise tolerance are covered in the Techniques section under "Exercise Basics."

b460 Sensations Associated with Cardiovascular and Respiratory Functions

Sensations such as missing a heart beat, palpitation, and shortness of breath.
Inclusions: sensations of tightness of chest, feelings of irregular beat, dyspnoea, air hunger, choking, gagging, and wheezing
Exclusions: sensation of pain (b280)

Treatment for Sensations Associated with Cardiovascular and Respiratory Functions

These functions cover some of the other cardio-respiratory conditions that can affect a client. Many of them are serious sensations that should not be ignored. The therapist should be aware of these symptoms and plan any treatment in a way that takes them into account.

If these symptoms have been noted and precautions have been outlined for a client, the therapist must be careful not to exceed any recommended levels of activity or violate any of the other precautions. Sometimes the therapist will be the first to hear reports of these sensations. Most of them are serious enough that the therapist should stop any physical activity and call for appropriate medical assistance.

Adaptations can be made in activities to allow the client to monitor his/her own sensations and adjust the level of activity as required to maintain appropriate functioning. The therapist should watch for signs that self-monitoring is not being done appropriately, especially when a client thinks s/he needs to "tough it out." Monitoring by the therapist is appropriate when the client is unable to do it. Activities can be adapted to meet a client's needs.

b469 Additional Functions and Sensations of the Cardiovascular and Respiratory Systems, Other Specified and Unspecified

b498 Functions of the Cardiovascular, Hematological, Immunological, and Respiratory Systems, Other Specified

b499 Functions of the Cardiovascular, Hematological, Immunological, and Respiratory Systems, Unspecified

Chapter 5 Functions of the Digestive, Metabolic, and Endocrine Systems

This chapter is about the functions of ingestion, digestion, and elimination, as well as functions involved in metabolism and endocrine glands.

Functions Related to the Digestive System (b510-b539)

b510 Ingestion Functions

Functions related to taking in and manipulating solids or liquids through the mouth into the body.

Inclusions: functions of sucking, chewing and biting, manipulating food in the mouth, salvation, swallowing, burping, regurgitation, spitting, and vomiting; impairments such as dysphagia, aspiration of food, aerophagia, excessive salvation, drooling, and insufficient salivation

Exclusions: sensations associate with digestive system (b535)

- *b5100 Sucking*
  Functions of drawing into the mouth by a suction force produced by movements of the cheeks, lips, and tongue.
- *b5101 Biting*
  Functions of cutting into, piercing, or tearing off food with the front teeth.
- *b5102 Chewing*
  Functions of crushing, grinding, and masticating food with the back teeth.
- *b5103 Manipulation of Food in the Mouth*
  Functions of moving food around the mouth with the teeth and tongue.
- *b5104 Salivation*
  Function of the production of saliva within the mouth.
- *b5105 Swallowing*
  Functions of clearing the food and drink through the oral cavity, pharynx, and esophagus into the stomach at an appropriate rate and speed.
  Inclusions: oral, pharyngeal, or esophageal dysphagia; impairments in esophageal passage of food
  - ○ *b51050 Oral Swallowing*
    Function of clearing the food and drink through the oral cavity at an appropriate rate and speed.
  - ○ *b51051 Pharyngeal Swallowing*
    Function of clearing the food and drink through the pharynx at an appropriate rate and speed.
  - ○ *b51052 Esophageal Swallowing*
    Function of clearing the food and drink through the esophagus at an appropriate rate and speed.
  - ○ *b51058 Swallowing, Other Specified*
  - ○ *b51059 Swallowing, Unspecified*

- *b5106 Regurgitation and Vomiting*
  Functions of moving food or liquid in the reverse direction to ingestion, from stomach to esophagus to mouth and out.
- *b5108 Ingestion Functions, Other Specified*
- *b5109 Ingestion Functions, Unspecified*

Treatment for Ingestion Functions

It is not anticipated that recreational therapists will score ingestion functions. If a client has ingestion function impairments, it will most likely be the speech language pathologist or the ear, nose, and throat specialist who will score the extent of the client's impairment in these areas. Recreational therapists, however, need to be aware of ingestion impairments and address the impact that ingestion functions have on activity participation and the client's ability to follow correct swallowing techniques and adhere to diet levels in a real-life environment.

Ingestions functions can be impaired as a result of brain injury (e.g., cerebrovascular accident that impairs muscular functions related to swallowing), mouth impairments (e.g., missing teeth), damage to the esophagus (e.g., from burns), and surgery (e.g., wired jaw).

A common problem resulting from cerebrovascular accident or traumatic brain injury is dysphagia. Dysphagia is defined as difficulty swallowing due to impaired neurological functions that control ingestion functions or from some obstruction of the esophagus such as an esophageal tumor. Obstructions generally allow swallowing liquids; impaired neurological function may prevent swallowing both solids and liquids. If a client has difficulty swallowing, s/he could choke or aspirate food and liquids causing harm or injury.

The speech language pathologist evaluates the client's ingestion functions through a swallowing study that allows the therapist to see how the client bites, chews, manipulates, and swallows food. The results of the study will indicate to the therapist the type of diet the client should follow. There are four common food levels (pureed, mechanical soft, chopped, and regular) and three common liquid levels (thicks, nectars, and thins).

- *Pureed foods* are blenderized.

- *Mechanical soft* foods are those that require little or no chewing such as mashed potatoes, short flat noodles, and cooked carrots.
- *Chopped diet* consists of foods that require some, but not rigorous chewing, such as cubed chicken, chopped lasagna, and chopped string beans.
- *Regular diet* has no food texture restrictions.
- *Thin liquids* include water, ice tea, coffee, and lemonade.
- *Thick liquid* diet means that thin liquids need to be thickened. A product called "Thick It" is commonly used to thicken thin liquids. As per the product's label, a certain amount of the "Thick It" powder is stirred into the thin liquid to make it the desired consistency.
- *Nectars* are in the middle of thins and thicks. It is a thick fruit juice such as peach nectar.

In addition to determining the diet level, the speech language pathologist will recommend specific swallowing techniques to decrease risk of aspiration such as thorough chewing, tucking in the chin, and swallowing twice.

People who do not have dysphagia, but who do have other difficulties with chewing and swallowing (e.g., missing teeth, burned esophagus, wired jaw) will also have specific recommendations. Individuals who are missing moderate amounts of teeth may have difficulty chewing and manipulating food resulting in the recommendation of eating mechanical soft and chopped foods (e.g., soup, rice, boiled and chopped chicken). Certain foods may irritate a burned esophagus and, depending on the extent of damage to the esophagus, a feeding tube may be needed. A person who has a wired jaw will typically be allowed to eat small amounts of pureed foods and thin liquids through a straw.

Therapists document the type of diet the client is following (e.g., mechanical soft and thins), causes of swallowing impairments (e.g., client requires a mechanical soft diet secondary to missing teeth), ability of the client to adhere to special diet in real-life settings (e.g., client requires moderate cues to adhere to dietary restrictions in a community dining setting), ability of the client to follow swallowing techniques in real-life settings (e.g., client demonstrates modified independence secondary to increased time to integrate swallowing techniques into social dining), and any other restrictions or adaptations that are required by impairments in functioning (e.g., client needs additional liquid when eating because of minimal saliva production).

Treatment is aimed at restoring functions discussed in this section. Progression to a regular diet and thin liquids is possible in many cases with the aid of a speech language pathologist.

For treatment and adaptations, the recreational therapist needs to be aware of diet levels (both food and liquid) and recommended swallowing techniques for several reasons:

- To know what a client is allowed and not allowed to have during a therapy session (e.g., client asks for a glass of water; client wants to eat a cookie that was made in the therapy kitchen; when out in the community the client wants to order a specific food or liquid).
- To problem solve for the impact that diet levels have on activity participation (e.g., client refuses to engage in community socializing activities because food and drink are often available and the client does not want to use thickener in front of his peers).
- To reinforce proper food choice in a real-life community environment (e.g., what items on the menu are considered mechanical soft).
- To reinforce proper swallowing techniques in a real-life community environment (e.g., using swallowing techniques at a restaurant).

Adaptations seek to normalize to the greatest extent possible the client's experience of eating. Other adaptations include working with the client to deal with emotional issues resulting from difficulty in eating and working with family and friends to explain how they can help the client appropriately.

b515 Digestive Functions

Functions of transporting food through the gastrointestinal tract, breakdown of food and absorption of nutrients.

Inclusions: functions of transport of food through the stomach, peristalsis; breakdown of food, enzyme production, and action in stomach and intestines; absorption of nutrients and tolerance to food; impairments such as in hyperacidity of stomach, malabsorption, intolerance to food, hypermotility of intestines, intestinal paralysis, intestinal obstruction, and decreased bile production

Exclusions: ingestion functions (b510); assimilation functions (b520); defecation functions (b525); sensations associated with the digestive system (b535)

- *b5150 Transport of Food through Stomach and Intestines*
  Peristalsis and related functions that mechanically move food through stomach and intestines.
- *b5151 Breakdown of Food*
  Functions of mechanically reducing food to smaller particles in the gastrointestinal tract.
- *b5152 Absorption of Nutrients*
  Functions of passing food and drink nutrients into the bloodstream from along the intestines.
- *b5153 Tolerance to Food*
  Functions of accepting suitable food and drink for digestion and rejecting what is unsuitable.

Inclusions: impairments such as hypersensitivities, gluten intolerance
- *b5158 Digestive Functions, Other Specified*
- *b5159 Digestive Functions, Unspecified*

Treatment for Digestive Functions

It is not anticipated that recreational therapists will score digestive functions. If a person has difficulty digesting foods and liquids, the person would be referred to a gastroenterologist for further evaluation and documentation of the extent of digestive function impairments. Recommendations from the gastroenterologist are followed by the health care team such as avoidance of certain foods (e.g., people who have reflux disease should avoid high fat foods that soften the sphincter muscle allowing acid to rise into the esophagus) or total restriction of food types (e.g., a person who has colitis should not consume spicy foods).

Documentation for the recreational therapist is generally limited to noting how well the client follows dietary restrictions in the community.

Adaptations may be required or particular skills, such as assertiveness in refusing to eat harmful foods, may need to be taught to the client.

b520 Assimilation Functions
Functions by which nutrients are converted into components of the living body.
Inclusions: functions of storage of nutrients in the body
Exclusions: digestive functions (b515); defecation functions (b525); weight maintenance functions (b530); general metabolic functions (b540)

Treatment for Assimilation Functions

Scoring or addressing impairments of assimilation functions is not within the scope of recreational therapy practice.

As with other functions in this chapter, the recreational therapist may need to teach skills required for appropriate adaptations caused by deficits in assimilation of food.

b525 Defecation Functions
Functions of elimination of wastes and undigested food as feces and related functions.
Inclusions: functions of elimination, fecal consistency, frequency of defecation; fecal continence, flatulence; impairments such as constipation, diarrhea, watery stool and anal sphincter incompetence or incontinence
Exclusions: digestive functions (b515); assimilation functions (b520); sensations associated with the digestive system (b535)

- *b5250 Elimination of Feces*
  Functions of the elimination of waste from the rectum, including the functions of contraction of the abdominal muscles in doing so.
- *b5251 Fecal Consistency*
  Consistency of feces such as hard, firm, soft, or watery.
- *b5252 Frequency of Defecation*
  Functions involved in the frequency of defecation.
- *b5253 Fecal Continence*
  Functions involved in voluntary control over the elimination function.
- *b5254 Flatulence*
  Functions involved in the expulsion of excessive amounts of air or gases from the intestines.
- *b5258 Defecation Functions, Other Specified*
- *b5259 Defecation Functions, Unspecified*

Treatment for Defecation Functions

Defecation functions are traditionally monitored and scored by nursing staff, so it is not anticipated that recreational therapists will score defecation function codes. Recreational therapists may document defecation functions as they impact a client's ability to participate in activities (e.g., client had three episodes of fecal incontinence during one hour afternoon session; excessive flatulence is a severe hindrance to social activity participation). Recreational therapists need to be aware of defecation functions that pose a health threat and monitor the client appropriately (e.g., proper hydration for a client with diarrhea; checking with nursing staff prior to going out of the hospital for community integration training to make sure that a client at risk for autonomic dysreflexia isn't having any bowel issues, such as impacted bowels). Recreational therapists may also monitor defecation functions to assist with tracking the amount of food consumed (e.g., clients who report being on a hunger strike, have anorexia). If working with toddlers who are potty training, frequency of bowel movements are routinely tracked since holding bowel movements can become habitual (e.g., doesn't want to stop playing and come inside to use the bathroom, had a painful bowel movement at one time and holds bowels to avoid painful feeling).

Defecation functions are managed through medication (e.g., laxatives, binders), diet (elimination, addition, or change in foods consumed), behavior modification (e.g., rewards for a toddler who has a bowel movement in the potty), and adaptive devices (e.g., a client with a spinal cord injury who lacks motor function to push bowels uses a suppository inserter and digital bowel stimulator to release bowels). See the Equipment section for information about adaptive devices for defecation functions. Undergarments may be worn for fecal incontinence that is not yet controlled.

Recreational therapists who conduct community integration training need to be aware of the defecation impairments of their clients to adequately prepare for possible situations (e.g., change of clothes, wipes, plastic bag, room spray — especially for teenagers who are easily embarrassed, cell phone to call emergency services if client goes into autonomic dysreflexia). See "Community Problem Solving" in the Techniques section for more ideas.

Some impairments in defecation functions require an ostomy as a temporary or permanent solution to an intestinal or anus malformation or disease (e.g., cancer of the intestines or colon, inability to push waste through intestines, malformation of the anus/rectal structure). An ostomy is a surgical procedure that, in a sense, disconnects the intestinal tract at a place that is predetermined (e.g., severs the intestinal tract above the area that is cancerous) and pulls the end of the intestine to the surface of the abdomen. An artificial opening is created on the abdomen and the intestine is pulled through. The portion of the intestine that exits the abdomen is called the stoma. It is red to pink and looks raw, although it is not painful because intestinal tissue does not have pain receptors. A pouch-like bag is attached around the stoma to collect bowel waste. As fecal material passes through the intestines, the body absorbs much of the liquid from the digesting food and the fecal material becomes firmer as it travels through the tract. Consequently, the location of the ostomy will determine the consistency of the fecal material (firm, soft, pasty, liquid-like). If an ostomy is at the jejunum of the small intestine it is called a jejunostomy. If the ostomy is at the ileum of the small intestine it is called an ileostomy. If the ostomy is done to the large intestine, it is called a colostomy. Fecal material that is excreted in a liquid-like form creates a high risk for skin breakdown and subsequent infections. The pouch-like bag is changed and replaced routinely throughout the day.

Psychosocial adjustment to having an ostomy can be difficult. Tight clothing is contraindicated so that the pouch does not become constricted. Activities that cause rubbing or pressure against the pouch are also contraindicated so precautions must be taken (e.g., avoidance of particular sexual positions, contact sports). Odor and leaking can become a hindrance to socialization (embarrassment) and forming intimate relationships (fear of rejection, humiliation). Within the American culture defecation functions are often seen as dirty. It is something that is not talked about and is done in private. Having an ostomy confronts the individual with challenges through the day (leaks, odors, hindrances to activity, awareness of its position and guarding it against contact such as a child jumping on the lap, a person sliding over too closely on a bench seat). Consequently, some clients eventually hate the ostomy and either consciously or unconsciously begin to neglect its care. This exacerbates problems (e.g., pouch becomes over filled and leaks, increased fecal material results in stronger odor, infections) and often strengthens the client's neglect of its care (the more problems it creates the more the client hates it; the more the client hates it, the more problems it creates, and so on).

- Recreational therapy's role in caring for an ostomy focuses primarily on psychosocial adjustment and integrating its care into real-life settings.
- The recreational therapist and primary nurse often collaborate to problem solve for leaking issues related to specific activity movements.
- Self-esteem is promoted by providing activities and experiences that result in success and highlight the person's strengths. Identifying a person's strengths and developing ongoing opportunities that highlight the person's strengths will continually foster good self-esteem and minimize the effect of the ostomy. See "Self-Esteem" in the Techniques section for specific treatment suggestions.
- Recreational therapists reinforce needed care for the ostomy and educate the person as needed about the role that defecation functions play in health.

b530 Weight Management Functions
Functions of maintaining appropriate body weight, including weight gain in the developmental period.
Inclusions: functions of maintenance of acceptable Body Mass Index (BMI); and impairments such as underweight, cachexia, wasting, overweight, emaciation and such as in primary and secondary obesity
Exclusions: assimilation functions (b520); general metabolic functions (b540); endocrine gland functions (b555)

Treatment for Weight Management Functions

Recreational therapists play an important role in weight management functions. See "Obesity" and "Eating Disorders" in the Diagnosis section for information.

b535 Sensations Associated with the Digestive System
Sensations arising from eating, drinking, and related digestive functions.

Inclusions: sensations of nausea, feeling bloated, and the feeling of abdominal cramps; fullness of stomach, globus feeling, spasm of stomach, gas in stomach and heartburn

Exclusions: sensation of pain (b280); ingestion functions (b510); digestive functions (b515); defecation functions (b525)

- *b5350 Sensation of Nausea*
  Sensation of needing to vomit.
- *b5351 Feeling Bloated*
  Sensation of distension of the stomach or abdomen.
- *b5352 Sensational of Abdominal Cramp*
  Sensation of spasmodic or painful muscular contractions of the smooth muscles of the gastrointestinal tract.
- *b5358 Sensations Associated with the Digestive System, Other Specified*
- *b5359 Sensations Associate with the Digestive System, Unspecified*

Treatment for Sensations Associated with the Digestive System

Nursing is the health discipline that traditionally monitors sensations associated with digestive functions. However, recreational therapists may document sensations associated with digestive functions if they impede or affect a client's ability to participate in activities (e.g., client complained of severe heartburn/abdominal cramping after lunch affecting his ability to participate in therapy; client is three months pregnant and reports vomiting twice a day after meals). Other causes of nausea, bloating, and cramping after food ingestion include food poisoning, food intolerance (e.g., dairy intolerance), and excessive food intake.

Treatment interventions will vary depending on the cause of the problem (e.g., medication, surgery to reduce or eliminate heartburn, change in foods consumed).

Recreational therapists report impairments to appropriate health professionals (e.g., therapist tells client's primary nurse that she is complaining of feeling nauseous) and are prepared to handle vomiting in a community environment (e.g., spill kit to clean up vomit, bags for vomiting, wipes, pair of hospital scrubs or other clothes in case a change of clothes is needed).

b539 Functions Related to the Digestive System, Other Specified and Unspecified

Functions Related to Metabolism and the Endocrine System (b540-b559)

b540 General Metabolic Functions
Functions of regulation of essential components of the body such as carbohydrates, proteins, and fats, the conversion of one to another, and their breakdown into energy.

Inclusions: functions of metabolism, basal metabolic rate, metabolism of carbohydrate, protein, and fat, catabolism, anabolism, energy production in the body; increase or decrease in metabolic rate

Exclusions: assimilation functions (b520); weight maintenance functions (b530); water, mineral, and electrolyte balance functions (b545); thermoregulatory functions (b550); endocrine glands functions (b555)

- *b5400 Basal Metabolic Rate*
  Functions involved in oxygen consumption of the body at specified conditions of rest and temperature.
  Inclusions: increase or decrease in basic metabolic rate; impairments such as in hyperthyroidism and hypothyroidism
- *b5401 Carbohydrate Metabolism*
  Functions involved in the process by which carbohydrates in the diet are stored and broken down into glucose and subsequently into carbon dioxide and water.
- *b5402 Protein Metabolism*
  Functions involved in the process by which proteins in the diet are converted to amino acids and broken down further in the body.
- *b5403 Fat Metabolism*
  Functions involved in the process by which fat in the diet is stored and broken down in the body.
- *b5408 General Metabolic Functions, Other Specified*
- *b5409 General Metabolic Functions, Unspecified*

Treatment for General Metabolic Functions

Scoring general metabolic functions is not within the scope of recreational therapy practice. However, recreational therapists need to be aware of metabolic impairments and their impact on activity. For example, if it is known that the client has a problem metabolizing fat, specific recommendations may be prescribed by the client's physician (e.g., limit amount of fats in the client's diet, increase physical activity to assist with fat metabolism) that need to be incorporated into activity (e.g., address issues surrounding food choices in a real-life setting, look for physical leisure interests to assist with increasing physical activity).

Recreational therapists document the specific impairment (e.g., impairment with carbohydrate metabolism resulting from diabetes) and their association with activity (e.g., goal is to increase moderate physical leisure activity to five times a week for 30 minutes to assist with managing diabetes).

Treatment and adaptations involve the ongoing coordination of efforts with the rest of the treatment team to effect changes in the client's level of activity and recreational choices that are appropriate for the deficits the client has.

b545 Water, Mineral, and Electrolyte Balance Functions

Functions of the regulation of water, mineral, and electrolytes in the body.

Inclusions: functions of water balance; balance of minerals such as calcium, zinc, and iron, and balance of electrolytes such as sodium and potassium; impairments such as in water retention, dehydration, hypercalcaemia, hypocalcaemia, iron deficiency, hypernatraemia, hyponatraemia, hyperkalaemia and hypokalaemia

Exclusions: hematological system functions (b430); general metabolic functions (b540); endocrine gland functions (b555)

- *b5450 Water Balance*
  Functions involved in maintaining the level or amount of water in the body.
  Inclusions: impairments such as in dehydration and rehydration
    - *b54500 Water Retention*
      Functions involved in keeping water in the body.
    - *b54501 Maintenance of Water Balance*
      Functions involved in maintaining the optimal amount of water in the body.
    - *b54508 Water Balance Functions, Other Specified*
    - *b54509 Water Balance Functions, Unspecified*
- *b5451 Mineral Balance*
  Functions involved in maintaining equilibrium between intake, storage, utilization, and excretion of minerals in the body.
- *b5452 Electrolyte Balance*
  Functions involved in maintaining equilibrium between intake, storage, utilization, and excretion of electrolytes in the body.
- *b5458 Water, Mineral, and Electrolyte Balance Functions, Other Specified*
- *b5459 Water, Mineral, and Electrolyte Balance Functions, Unspecified*

Treatment for Water, Mineral, and Electrolyte Balance Functions

Scoring water, mineral, and electrolyte balance functions is not within the scope of recreational therapy practice. Recreational therapists however need to be familiar with signs of dehydration (e.g., pruned lips, reduced tears, dry mouth, reduced urination) and causes of dehydration (e.g., prolonged

vomiting, diarrhea, lack of fluid intake, intense exercise, hot conditions). Dehydration can be fatal, especially in infants and young children, who dehydrate faster than adults. If dehydration is left untreated, seizures, coma, and death may occur.

Therapists must know when to offer clients appropriate fluids when activity is increased causing loss of fluids (physical activity increases metabolic rate, increased metabolic rate increases fluid loss through sweat, the body sweats to reduce internal body heat that is generated through activity). Appropriate fluids must be available during activities and the therapist must make sure that the clients drink the fluids as appropriate and learn to monitor their own fluid needs. If serious dehydration is believed to be present, the therapist brings it to the immediate attention of the client's primary nurse for further evaluation and treatment.

Similarly, the therapist must be aware of electrolyte balance during strenuous activities. Working with the dietary and nursing staff, the recreational therapist can provide fluids, such as sports drinks, that will replace electrolytes during activities. For some clients, use of fluids with electrolytes will need to be monitored and charted.

The other area covered by this section is mineral balance. Mineral balance impairments can present as psychiatric conditions. Two common examples are

- *Hypercalcemia* (excessive calcium in the blood): causes apathy, muscle weakness, delirium, and personality and cognitive changes.
- *Hypocalcemia* (decreased calcium): causes delirium and personality changes, seizures, and intracranial pressure in the brain.

Therapists should not be quick to suggest a client has a psychiatric condition, especially one that has an unexpected onset, prior to a physician ruling out underlying conditions and seeking evaluation from a psychiatrist, psychologist, or neuropsychologist.

b550 Thermoregulatory Functions

Functions of the regulation of body temperature.
Inclusions: functions of maintenance of body temperature; impairment such as hypothermia, hyperthermia

Exclusions: general metabolic functions (b540); endocrine gland functions (b555)

- *b5500 Body Temperature*
  Functions involved in regulating the core temperature of the body.
  Inclusions: impairments such as hyperthermia or hypothermia
- *b5501 Maintenance of Body Temperature*
  Functions involved in maintaining optimal body temperature as environmental temperature changes.
  Inclusions: tolerance to heat or cold

- *b5508 Thermoregulatory Functions, Other Specified*
- *b5509 Thermoregulatory Functions, Unspecified*

Treatment for Thermoregulatory Functions

Recreational therapists are not expected to score thermoregulatory functions. However, recreational therapists may assess and monitor body temperature in some situations (e.g., client complains of feeling feverish when on a camping trip). See "Vital Signs" in the Techniques section for information on how to assess, monitor, and document body temperature.

On community outings the therapist is responsible for being sure that all clients are appropriately dressed for the prevailing conditions. Many of these issues are covered in Activities and Participation.

b555 Endocrine Gland Functions
Functions of production and regulation of hormonal levels in the body, including cyclical changes.
Inclusions: functions of hormonal balance; hyperpituitarism, hypopituitarism, hyperthyroidism, hypothyroidism, hyperadrenalism, hypoadrenalism, hyperparathyroidism, hypoparathyroidism, hypergonadism, hypogonadism
Exclusions: general metabolic functions (b540); water, mineral and electrolyte balance functions (b545); thermoregulatory functions (b550); sexual functions (b640); menstruation functions (b650)

Treatment for Endocrine Gland Functions

It is not within the scope of recreational therapy practice to score endocrine gland functions. Recreational therapists are aware that endocrine gland impairments can affect behavior (erratic, volatile), mood (depressed, manic, irritable), energy level (fatigue, apathy, excitability), sleep problems (insomnia, excessive sleeping), mental functions (poor concentration, memory, and orientation; slowed thinking), psychological stability (delusions,

hallucinations, paranoia), and growth (both height and weight). An example of how endocrine dysfunction affects multiple areas of health is provided through the descriptions of hyperthyroidism and hypothyroidism, two common endocrine gland impairments:

- *Hyperthyroidism*: Feelings of fatigue and general weakness, insomnia, unexplained weight loss, heart palpitations, increased perspiration, agitated behavior, feelings of anxiousness. In severe cases the client can present with memory impairments, orientation impairments, manic excitement, delusions, and hallucinations.
- *Hypothyroidism*: Feeling mentally slow, unexplained weight gain, thin and dry hair that comes out easily when combing and brushing, cold intolerance, reduced hearing, a deeper voice sound, loss of the lateral eyebrow. In severe cases the client can present with paranoia, hallucinations, and depression.

Clients who are suspected of having deficits in endocrine gland functions are evaluated for underlying endocrine function impairments as part of the process for ruling out underlying medical conditions. A referral to a psychologist, psychiatrist, or neuropsychologist may also be made to rule out psychiatric conditions. Endocrine function impairments are predominately treated with medication and monitored by an endocrinologist. Adaptations may be required to take into account the presenting symptoms.

b559 Functions Related to Metabolism and the Endocrine System, Other Specified and Unspecified

b598 Functions of the Digestive, Metabolic, and Endocrine Systems, Other Specified

b599 Functions of the Digestive, Metabolic, and Endocrine Systems, Unspecified

Chapter 6 Genitourinary and Reproductive Functions

This chapter is about the functions of urination and the reproductive functions, including sexual and procreative functions.

Urinary Functions (b610-b639)

b610 Urinary Excretory Functions
Functions of filtration and collection of the urine.
Inclusions: functions of urinary filtration, collection of urine; impairments such as in renal insufficiency, anuria, oliguria, hydronephrosis, hypotonic urinary bladder, and ureteric obstruction
Exclusions: urination functions (b620)
- b6100 Filtration of Urine
  Functions of filtration of urine by the kidneys.
- b6101 Collection of Urine
  Functions of collection and storage of urine by the ureters and bladder.
- b6108 Urinary Excretory Functions, Other Specified
- b6109 Urinary Excretory Functions, Unspecified

Treatment for Urinary Excretory Functions

It is not within the scope of recreational therapy practice to score urinary excretory functions. If a person has difficulty with filtration of urine or collection of urine, the person is referred to a urologist (a physician who specializes in the urinary system) and appropriate treatment is prescribed. Recreational therapists do treat urination functions, as seen in the next set of codes.

b620 Urination Functions
Functions of discharge of urine from the urinary bladder.
Inclusions: functions of urination, frequency of urination, urinary continence; impairments such as in stress, urge, reflex, overflow, continuous incontinence, dribbling, automatic bladder, polyuria, urinary retention, and urinary urgency
Exclusions: urinary excretory functions (b610); sensations associated with urinary functions (b630)
- b6200 Urination
  Functions of voiding the urinary bladder.
  Inclusions: impairments such as in urine retention
- b6201 Frequency of Urination
  Functions involved in the number of times urination occurs.
- b6203 Urinary Continence
  Functions of control over urination.
  Inclusions: impairments such as in stress, urge, reflex, continuous, and mixed incontinence
- b6208 Urination Functions, Other Specified
- b6209 Urination Functions, Unspecified

Treatment for Urinary Functions

Nursing staff are the primary health professionals who monitor and record urination functions. However, recreational therapists may also score these components. Difficulty with urination functions can be caused by:
- *Neurological damage* (e.g., cerebrovascular accident, traumatic brain injury, spinal cord injury, diabetes).
- *Congenital malformations.*
- *Urinary tract infections.*
- *Bladder cancer.*
- *Intoxication.*
- *Seizures.*
- *Extreme fear or anxiety.*
- *Medication*
  o "Psychotherapy drugs can lead to urinary hesitation, dribbling, urinary retention, and increased urinary tract infections" (Sadock & Sadock, 2003, p 982).
  o Medication that has the primary purpose, or secondary effect of, increasing or retaining urination.

Other conditions that affect frequency of urination and urinary continence outside of physiological processes include:
- *Cognitive impairments*: Inability to respond appropriately to the signal of a full bladder resulting in frequent episodes of urinary incontinence throughout the day (e.g., dementia).
- *Lack of mobility*: Inability to get to a commode/toilet/urinal, which may result in urinary incontinence or decreased frequency of urination due to limited assistance with urination.
- *Communication impairments*: Leading to difficulty in ascertaining the location of a bathroom.

In young children, urinary incontinence is frequent. Approximately 82% of two year olds, 49% of 3 year olds, 26% of 4 year olds, and 7% of five year olds have episodes of urinary incontinence (enuresis) on a regular basis (Sadock & Sadock, 2003). "Psychosocial issues [that] precipitate some cases of enuresis [include]… the birth of a sibling, hospitalization between the ages of two and four, the start of school, the breakup of a family because of divorce or death, and a move to a new domicile" (Sadock & Sadock, 2003, p 1257).

Recreational therapists teach clients how to manage urinary functions in real-life settings and assist clients in problem solving for specific life tasks that are common to their lifestyle (e.g., flying on a airplane, taking long road trips, self-catheterizing in a public bathroom, going to the beach, locating bathrooms at the mall). Recreational therapists may consult with nurses or occupational therapists when needed (e.g., problem solve for positioning in a wheelchair to self-catheterize in a public bathroom, problem solving to hold Texas catheter in place).

Recreational therapists document the specific urinary function impairment (e.g., impairment with urinary continence), frequency of impairment (e.g., client had two episodes of urinary incontinence during a one-hour community outing), specific life activities that are affected by urinary function impairment (e.g., client reports that she only leaves the house for doctor's appointments secondary to fear of urinary incontinence), specific adaptations and recommendations (e.g., therapist recommends that the client use the accessible bathroom at the airport prior to boarding the plane, monitor the amount of liquids consumed, and wear a urinary sanitary pad while in flight in case of urinary urgency without access to an accessible bathroom), treatment initiated and outcomes (e.g., Four-year-old client given a star on a chart for each day he was continent. Client has been continent for three consecutive days.), and level of assistance (e.g., client requires maximal verbal cues to toilet every hour when in a community environment).

Treatment for urinary functions includes medication, behavioral modification (e.g., positive rewards for young children), changes in toileting routine (e.g., try to use the bathroom every half hour to decrease periods of incontinence from urinary urgency), use of materials to increase a child's awareness of being wet (e.g., padded underwear instead of a diaper, a bell and bed pad alarm — the bell rings when the bed pad becomes wet), urinary collection devices (indwelling catheter, Texas catheter, urinal), and devices to assist with releasing the bladder (e.g., straight catheterizing).

Some specific adaptations that have been found to be helpful with urinary functions are provided below.

- If a client is having difficulty closing the bathroom stall door: When propelling a wheelchair into a bathroom stall, hook one end of a bungee cord to some place on the stall door (e.g., bottom, side, latch). Hook the other end to some other place in the bathroom (e.g., toilet paper holder, wheelchair, side bar on the stall). Another idea is to use a dressing stick (a stick with a hook on the end of it) to grab the bottom of the stall door to pull it closed. A small dressing stick could be kept in a backpack.
- If there is a possibility that a client may have a bladder accident in the community: Clients who have problems with urinary incontinence (e.g., sense of urgency, unaware of urine release), should pack an extra change of clothes, as well as cleanup supplies and a Ziploc bag, in a backpack just in case of a bladder accident.

Also see "Community Problem Solving" in the Techniques section for more ideas. Other adaptive devices are described below.

Indwelling Catheter

An indwelling catheter is a flexible plastic tube that is placed into the urethra. At the end of the tube is a urine collection bag. The bag must be placed below the client's knees for best drainage; otherwise, the urine may back up in the tube. Urine may also back up in the tube if the bag becomes full and is not emptied. Urine that backs up into the bladder can cause infection and damage to the elasticity of the bladder. The bag is strapped onto the lower leg or hooked onto the bottom of a wheelchair. Clients should not walk holding onto the collection bag or hang it on a walker (not low enough for good flow). Indwelling catheters are used for the short term. Long-term use of an indwelling catheter is not recommended due to high risk of infections since any foreign item that enters the body puts a person at risk for infection.

Straight Catheterizing

Straight catheterizing is the insertion of a thin plastic tube into the urethra to stimulate the bladder to release the urine being held in the bladder. The inability to release urine from the bladder is a common problem in spinal cord injuries. Clients are initially taught (if able) to do this independently from a slightly elevated supine position in bed. The tube is sterile (packaged in individually sealed wraps) and is opened only when the client is ready to use it. A gel is placed on the tip of the tube for ease of insertion. Once the bladder is stimulated, the urine will release through the tube. The collection device at the end of the tube can be varied (e.g., a bottle, a urinal, a bedpan). Once the client becomes more comfortable with the technique, it behooves the client to learn how to straight catheterize from a seated position (if possible). The ability to lie down to straight catheterize is unrealistic in many real-life situations (e.g., shopping, working, school, sports, visiting). The recreational therapist working in a rehabilitation setting is typically the person who initiates the conversation with nursing about the client's readiness to learn how to straight catheterize from a sitting position. This is done in preparation for community integration training. The therapist and nurse discuss the client's performance. When ready, the ability to straight catheterize in a public bathroom is set as a community integration goal (e.g., client to straight catheterize in a public bathroom at modified independence secondary to increased time and assistive devices). Below is a list of ideas to assist a client in straight catheterizing from a seated position in a bathroom:

- Make cathing packs. Put everything that is needed for one cathing session into a plastic grocery bag, fold it over, and put it into a backpack (backpack can be hung on the back of a wheelchair). It is good to take a few extra packs just in case the client intentionally or unintentionally stays out later than anticipated or the client consumes more fluids than usual and needs to catheterize more often within a period of time. The more fluids consumed, the more often the need to catheterize. With normal fluid intake, people self-catheterize every four to six hours.
- When straight catheterizing in a public bathroom, take out a cathing pack from the backpack and hook one of the plastic bag handles onto the wheelchair (e.g., brake handle, armrest) and let the other end of the bag hang open. Open pants or raise skirt (loose clothing makes it easier). Get into a slightly reclined sitting position and then reach into the bag to retrieve supplies. Use one hand to insert the tube and the other to guide the end of the tube over the toilet.
- If a client is having difficulty keeping his/her pants flap open wide enough (e.g., jeans) when self-catheterizing in a reclined sitting position, use a bungee cord with rubber tips on the hooks. Hook one end to the inside of the pants flap and hook the other end somewhere on the wheelchair to provide tension. Using a bungee cord will free up both hands for catheterizing.
- If a client is unable to catheterize from a reclined sitting position, discuss issues related to finding places to lie down and catheterize in his/her typical community settings.

Texas Catheter

A Texas catheter is an external urine collection system. A condom-like device is placed onto the penis and a special tape is wrapped around the top of the device. At the base of the device is a thin plastic flexible tube that feeds into a urine collection bag that it strapped to the lower leg. The use of a Texas catheter is less likely to cause infection since it is an external, rather than an internal, collection device. However, it does have limitations. At times the tape can become loose and leak and some people find the device bothersome and uncomfortable. Texas catheters are also used by people who lack access to bathrooms (e.g., truck drivers, a person who is on a long airplane flight and lacks mobility to get to the airplane bathroom or is limited in his ability to use the bathroom because of its small size).

Urinal

A urinal is an external plastic collection device that is held over the penis to collect urine. Males can use a variety of collection devices outside of the medical style urinal. For example, a plastic bottle with a good leak-proof lid can be kept in a backpack for urination. The use of a bottle can be helpful when the client is unable to access a bathroom (e.g., bathroom at a friend's home is on the second floor). Once the bottle is used, the urine can be disposed of immediately (e.g., friend takes the bottle upstairs to the bathroom and dumps it in the toilet) or the bottle can be put back into the backpack to be emptied at a later date (e.g., once returned home). If the person prefers to empty the bottle at a later date, a dark sock can be pulled over the bottle to mask the contents of the bottle.

Sanitary Pads for Urination

Sanitary pads for women that are specially designed to hold urine can be helpful for urinary incontinence. They may also be used for situations when the client is unable to access a bathroom (e.g., a long car ride where finding an accessible bathroom is difficult). Consciously allowing oneself to urinate using a pad can be uncomfortable. Clients may find it helpful to use the pad within a safe environment (e.g., "try it out" at home) to decrease anxiety and worry about its effectiveness.

Importance of Urinary Continence

Urinary continence is important for several reasons:
- Urinary incontinence causes odors that can impede socialization.
- Urinary incontinence can negatively affect self-esteem.
- Urinary incontinence can limit a person's community activities (fears going out of the home and having a bladder accident) contribut-

ing to secondary conditions (e.g., muscle atrophy, deconditioning of the cardiopulmonary system).

- Urinary incontinence increases risk for skin breakdown, especially when skin remains wet for prolonged periods of time. See Body Functions Chapter 8 for more information about skin breakdown.

b630 Sensations Associated with Urinary Functions
Sensations arising from voiding and related urinary functions.
Inclusions: sensations of incomplete voiding or urine, feeling of fullness of bladder
Exclusions: sensations of pain (b280); urination functions (b620)

Treatment for Sensations Associated with Urinary Functions

Recreational therapists are responsible for documenting sensations associated with urinary functions and reporting information to the treatment team. The sensations may be a symptom of some dysfunction in urination functions, which would be treated under code b620. Other possibilities include treatment for pain or stress that would be coordinated with other members of the treatment team.

b639 Urinary Functions, Other Specified and Unspecified

Genital and Reproductive Functions (b640-b679)

b640 Sexual Functions
Mental and physical functions related to the sexual act, including the arousal, preparatory, orgasmic, and resolution stages.
Inclusions: functions of the sexual arousal, preparatory, orgasmic, and resolution phase; functions related to sexual interest, performance, penile erection, clitoral erection, vaginal lubrication, ejaculation, orgasm; impairments such as impotence, frigidity, vaginismus, premature ejaculation, priapism and delayed ejaculation
Exclusions: procreation functions (b660); sensations associated with genital and reproductive functions (b670)

- *b6400 Functions of Sexual Arousal Phase*
  Functions of sexual interest and excitement.
- *b6401 Functions of Sexual Preparatory Phase*
  Functions of engaging in sexual intercourse.
- *b6402 Functions of Orgasmic Phase*
  Functions of reaching orgasm.
- *b6403 Functions of Sexual Resolution Phase*
  Functions of satisfaction after orgasm and accompanying relaxation.

- *b6408 Sexual Functions, Other Specified*
- *b6409 Sexual Functions, Unspecified*

Treatment for Sexual Functions

Talking about sexual functioning can be uncomfortable for many clients. Some may find it embarrassing or inappropriate, while others may have questions they are apprehensive to ask due to the sensitive nature of the topic. Consequently, clients may bring up issues related to sexuality in indirect ways (e.g., making sexual jokes, making statements such as, "No one is ever going to want to date me"). Indirect statements (including jokes) provide the therapist with an opportunity to approach the subject. It is important to understand which part of sexual function the client is concerned about. For clients with a condition that changes their appearance or functioning (e.g., burns, spinal cord injury), it may be the sexual arousal phase. They may be worried that no one will ever be interested in them sexually again. A man who has had an operation for prostate cancer may need information about achieving an erection. For others, such as a client who had a heart attack, the concern may be whether s/he will be able to perform sexually during the orgasmic phase. Note that the functional issues related to sexuality are documented here. Related relationship issues are documented using d770 intimate relationships or one of the other relationship codes. Concerns with sexuality will usually have both components.

The manner that the therapist approaches the subject will vary depending on the client. However, it is always done with respect and sincerity (e.g., "In addition to the goals that we set for your stay here I was wondering if you would like information on issues related to sexuality. It is common for people to have questions about sexuality after having heart surgery. Would you like to talk about it with me or someone else on your team?"). Notice in the example provided that the therapist "normalizes" sexuality by saying that "many people have questions." This helps to lessen client anxiety. Other comments that can help to lessen anxiety include those that validate how the client is feeling, such as, "I know this must be an awkward conversation that you probably didn't expect to have" or "I sense that this topic makes you uncomfortable. Would you like to change the subject? Just know that if you change your mind, we can talk about it or, if you prefer, I can give you some information in a sealed envelop that you can read on your own."

A transdisciplinary approach is commonly used when addressing issues of sexuality in a health care setting (e.g., a physician may need to clear the client for engagement in sexual activity or give him/her a prescription for medication; physical therapy may address issues related to positioning; occupational therapy may address issues related to dressing/undressing; nursing may address adaptive devices; recreational therapy may address issues related to dating and socializing; psychology may address issues related to self-esteem and confidence). Although attention to sexual health is gaining more recognition in health care, a clear protocol on how to address these issues is not always available. Consequently, many issues are addressed by the team member who initiates the conversation or the team member the client confides his/her concerns to. Due to the strong focus on participation in real-life activities and the unique therapeutic relationship that is built, recreational therapists are often key professionals in addressing sexual health. Recreational therapists should consistently seek out information related to specific disabilities and sexuality to maintain and update their knowledge base and consult other health disciplines when needed for further recommendations (e.g., discuss with the client's physical therapist how to work around a client's movement limitations for sexual positioning).

Due to the sensitivity of the topic, many clients want assurance that the discussion is not documented or spoken about with other people. The therapist should inform the client that s/he will not discuss the specifics of the conversation with others. However, if specific questions need to be answered (e.g., clearance from physician to engage in sexual activity), the therapist will need to divulge the client's name. If it is determined that further information is needed or that the client could benefit from additional conversations with other staff (e.g., talk with the nurse about sexual aids), the therapist will check with the client first prior to making these arrangements. The therapist also informs the client that documentation will reflect the specific information provided, but the details of the conversation will not be part of the medical chart.

The therapist documents the specific education provided and the client's ability to apply the information learned. For example, "Client educated about sexual positions that will not aggravate back pain at request of client. Client able to recall information independently." Documentation may also include referrals (e.g., "Client agreed to talk with nursing about sexual devices for impotence. Primary nurse scheduled to meet with client this evening."). Unlike other functional skills, sexual activity is not an observed behavior, so evaluation of techniques and equipment comes from the client and must be documented as such (e.g., "Client reports that sexual position recommendations did not aggravate back pain" or "Client reports that suction device was effective for achieving erection").

Some of the common problems and general adaptations for sexual functioning are provided below.

Male Issues

Concern: Unable to Initiate or Maintain Erection
Recommendations:
1. *Stuffing*: Manually placing the flaccid penis into the vagina to promote hardness/erection.
2. *External vacuum pumps with ring*: Placing a tubular suction device over the penis draws blood into the penis that promotes erection. Once erect, a ring is placed at the base of the penis to maintain the erection. The ring should not be worn for an extended period of time due to the risk of tissue death from lack of freshly oxygenated blood. Many health care settings have sample devices and can instruct the client on how to obtain the device.
3. *Penile injections*: This is the direct injection of a chemical substance into the penis for erection. Encourage the client to speak with a urologist for more information on substances available.
4. *Penile implants*: There are several different types of implants that are placed permanently into the penis for manual erection. There can be some complications with skin breakthrough with use. Encourage the client to speak with a urologist for more information.
5. *Medication*: including Viagra and Cialis.

Concern: Unable to Ejaculate
Recommendations: There are three ways to retrieve sperm.
1. *Electroejaculation*: Achieved through the use of a rectal probe. This is done at a medical facility.
2. *Vibro massage*: Use of an external vibrator on the penis. Can be done at home.
3. *Chemical stimulation*: Injection of a substance. This is done at a medical facility.

Female Issues

Concern: Decreased Lubrication
Recommendations:
1. Encourage the client to have her partner check her lubrication prior to intercourse.
2. Encourage the use of a water-based lubricant such as KY Jelly. Do not use oil or Vaseline. They will not dissolve and will increase risks for infections.

Concern: Pregnancy

Recommendations:

There are various issues to take into consideration when planning a child. Pregnancy can affect sensation, skin breakdown, dysreflexia, spasticity, balance, etc. It is important for the client to discuss these issues with her physician/OB-Gyn so as to fully understand the implications and precautions specific to the situation.

Concern: Birth Control

Recommendation:

1. Any type of devices inserted into the vagina for birth control should be thoroughly checked by both the client and his/her partner to ensure proper positioning for effectiveness. If the client has decreased sensation or physical limitations, there is a chance that it may be positioned incorrectly rendering the birth control product ineffective.
2. Oral contraceptives are to be approved by the physician, as well as the OB-Gyn.
3. Use a variety of birth control methods to decrease risks of pregnancy (e.g., condom and vaginal insert).

Both Male and Female Issues

Concern: Decreased Sensation

Recommendations:

1. Decreased sensation directly affects the ability to reach orgasm, lubricate, and/or erect. Refer to the section on each of the individual concerns for recommendations.
2. Other erogenous zones may be present after a neurological injury. They are known to "move." For example, prior an injury the genital may have been a sensitive area and now the neck may be a sensitive area.

Concern: Unable to Have or Reach Orgasm

Recommendations:

1. There are two basic types of orgasms:
   a. Reflexive: sensation to the body part.
   b. Psychogenic: through thoughts/fantasies.
2. If an orgasm cannot be had or reached, encourage the client to think about what "sex" truly means to him/her. Does it need to include an orgasm? Is intimacy itself the valued outcome? Encourage the client to talk about this with his/her partner.

Concern: Bowel and Bladder

Recommendations:

1. Bowel and bladder accidents may occur during sexual activity in clients who have neurological

impairments (e.g., spinal cord injury, multiple sclerosis) due to muscle contraction and relaxation. There are several ways to decrease the chances of this happening.
   a. Empty the bowel/bladder prior to sexual activity.
   b. Place towels on the bed to catch the urine/bowel so that it is easy to clean up and resume activity.
   c. Place a urinal next to the bed.

Concern: Physical Mobility

Recommendations:

1. Chose positions that are most comfortable for the individual and couple.
2. Chose positions that do not break specific precautions or parameters set by other health professionals (e.g., physician, physical therapist).
3. Be aware of the required balance and strength for each position and make safe decisions.
4. Experiment with various positions.

Concern: Communication

Recommendations:

1. Encourage the client to discuss needs with his/her partner prior to sexual activity to decrease anxiety, as well as the anxiety of the partner. Discuss what may happen and how you would like to deal with it.
2. Encourage both partners to discuss their views about sexual expression (intimacy versus intercourse/orgasm).

b650 Menstruation Functions

Functions associated with the menstrual cycle, including regularity of menstruation and discharge of menstrual fluids.

- *b6500 Regularity of Menstrual Cycle*
  Functions involved in the regularity of the menstrual cycle.
- *b6501 Interval between Menstruation*
  Functions relating to the length of time between two menstrual cycles.
- *b6502 Extent of Menstrual Bleeding*
  Functions involved in the quantity of menstrual flow.
- *b6508 Menstruation Functions, Other Specified*
- *b6509 Menstruation Functions, Unspecified*

Treatment for Menstruation Functions

Menstrual functions are addressed primarily by the client's gynecologist; however, various members of the treatment team play roles in managing menstruation issues. For example, the recreational therapist may help the client problem solve for menstrual care in a community setting (e.g., positioning, changing sanitary napkins or tampons, responding to needs in various community settings). If difficulty with menstrual care is due to physical impairments, the occupational therapist may make recommendations for adaptive equipment or techniques that can also be carried over into the community setting for recreational therapists to further assess. Recreational therapists are not expected to score the codes in this section, but discipline-specific documentation should reflect these functions, interventions provided, and an assessment of the client's functioning in menstrual care as appropriate.

b660 Procreation Functions

Functions associated with fertility, pregnancy, childbirth, and lactation.

- *b6600 Functions Related to Fertility*
  Functions related to the ability to produce gametes for procreation.
- *b6601 Functions Related to Pregnancy*
  Functions involved in becoming pregnant and being pregnant.
- *b6602 Functions Related to Childbirth*
  Functions involved during childbirth.
- *b6603 Lactation*
  Functions involved in producing milk and making it available to the child.
- *b6608 Procreation Functions, Other Specified*
- *b6609 Procreation Functions, Unspecified*

Treatment for
Procreation Functions

Functions related to childbirth are commonly addressed by obstetricians. It is not within the scope of recreational therapy to score the codes within this section. However, recreational therapists may, in some settings, address related issues and assist the client in problem solving for barriers (e.g., strategies for reducing stress, problem solving with a client who has a spinal cord injury on how to breastfeed a child in a community setting). Notations about the specific problems, interventions, and assessment of the client's skills are written, as appropriate, within discipline-specific documentation.

b670 Sensations Associated with Genital and Reproductive Functions

Sensations arising from sexual arousal, intercourse, menstruation, and related genital or reproductive functions.

- *b6700 Discomfort Associated with Sexual Intercourse*
  Sensations associated with sexual arousal, preparation, intercourse, orgasm, and resolution.
- *b6701 Discomfort Associated with the Menstrual Cycle*
  Sensations involved with menstruation, including pre- and post-menstrual phases.
- *b6702 Discomfort Associated with Menopause*
  Sensations associated with cessation of the menstrual cycle.
  Inclusions: hot flushes and night sweats during menopause.
- *b6708 Sensations Associated with Genital and Reproductive Functions, Other Specified*
- *b6709 Sensations Associated with Genital and Reproductive Functions, Unspecified*

Treatment for
Sensations Associated with
Genital and Reproductive Functions

Recreational therapists are responsible for documenting sensations associated with genital and reproductive functions and reporting information to the treatment team. The sensations may be a symptom of some dysfunction, which would be coded under the appropriate function. Other possibilities include treatment for pain or stress that would be coordinated with other members of the treatment team.

b679 Genital and Reproductive Functions, Other Specified and Unspecified

b698 Genitourinary and Reproductive Functions, Other Specified

b699 Genitourinary and Reproductive Functions, Unspecified

References

Sadock, B. & Sadock, V. (2003). *Kaplan & Sadock's synopsis of psychiatry, 9th edition*. Philadelphia, PA: Lippincott Williams & Wilkins.

Chapter 7 Neuromusculoskeletal and Movement-Related Functions

This chapter is about the functions of movement and mobility, including functions of joints, bones, reflexes, and muscles.

Functions of the Joints and Bones (b710-b729)

b710 Mobility of Joint Functions

Functions of the range and ease of movement of a joint.

Inclusions: functions of mobility of single or several joints, vertebral, shoulder, elbow, wrist, hip, knee, ankle, small joints of hands and feet; mobility of joints generalized; impairments such as in hypermobility of joints, frozen joints, frozen shoulder, arthritis.

Exclusions: stability of joints (b715); control of voluntary movement functions (b760)

- *b7100 Mobility of a Single Joint*
  Functions of the range and ease of movement of one joint.
- *b7101 Mobility of Several Joints*
  Functions of the range and ease of movement of more than one joint.
- *b7102 Mobility of Joints Generalized*
  Functions of the range and ease of movement of joints throughout the body.
- *b7108 Mobility of Joint Functions, Other Specified*
- *b7109 Mobility of Joint Functions, Unspecified*

Treatment for Mobility of Joint Functions[2]

Limited joint mobility affects the range of motion of a joint. There are two major types of range of motion, active range of motion (AROM) and passive range of motion (PROM). AROM refers to the client's ability to voluntarily move a joint by his/her own efforts (e.g., a client lifts his arm above his head). PROM refers to a joint that is moved by another person (e.g., a client lacks voluntary control over the mobility of a joint but it can be moved by the therapist — therapist stretches a client's paralyzed fingers after activity to prevent development of contractures).

There are several causes for deficits with mobility in joints. They may be caused by damage to the joint. Some examples of disease-caused damage are osteoarthritis, rheumatoid arthritis, and cancers. Trauma, such as fractures and sprains can also limit joint mobility. Surgery on a joint, such as in total hip replacement, may require the client to limit mobility of the joint. Contractures, a tightening or loss of the elasticity of skin, fascia (fibrous connective tissue), muscle, or joint capsule, also cause a loss of range of motion. Muscle tissue tightness that causes a noticeable change in ability is usually considered to be a mild contracture.

It is also important to note that when muscle tissue has little or no movement for a period of time the tissue shortens in length. A shortening of muscle tissue length causes an overall reduction in the client's ability to move the nearby joints through their normal range of motion. It is common for pain to accompany a reduction in muscle length, which, in turn, causes the client to "guard" the muscle, further reducing movement.

Muscles become less resilient with age. As one ages the length of time that it takes a muscle and its related joints to stiffen decreases. It is not unusual for someone in his or her fifties and beyond to be stiff after sleeping. By the time someone is in their seventies, a good night's sleep can cause the individual to be stiff to the point of causing mobility problems for the first ten to twenty minutes.

An impairment of a client's range of motion is a common secondary diagnosis for clients in treatment.

When assessing joint mobility, recreational therapists are concerned about how it impacts performance during life activities and recreation (e.g., ability to reach shelves in the grocery store or ability to play a sport). Precautions will vary depending on the cause of the joint mobility dysfunction (e.g., surgery, muscle contractions) and can be obtained from the treating physician. ROM parameters and restrictions can be found in the medical chart in an acute care or rehab setting or can be requested from the primary treating physician. Joint protection interventions may be indicated for clients with conditions that respond negatively to repetitive ROM tasks (e.g., rheumatoid arthritis).

If joint mobility is acutely restricted because of a medical condition (e.g., hip or knee replacement, rheumatoid arthritis), specific abilities or precautions will be written in the medical chart for the recreational therapist to follow and incorporate into treatment. For the recreational therapist working in a community setting, it is important to have a full awareness of a client's joint mobility impairments so that the client is not challenged above his/her level, resulting in injury.

---

[2] Much of the discussion here also applies to b720 Mobility of Bone Functions.

Traditionally recreational therapists measure joint mobility function in a broad fashion to reflect the effect that it has on activity. Once the recreational therapist is aware of all the client's joint mobility precautions and restrictions, the common recreational therapy assessment includes the therapist asking the client to appropriately move his/her joints independently through active ranges (e.g., can you raise your arms over your head, reach out to the side, make a fist, stretch out your fingers, stretch out your legs).

Documentation usually discusses the limitations the joint mobility impairment places on life activities. For example, if a client has limited shoulder joint mobility and it impairs his ability to do a 360° golf swing, the therapist may document, "Client able to perform a 180° back to front golf swing. Limited shoulder joint mobility impairs client's ability to achieve a full 360° golf swing." If a client has impaired knee flexion making it difficult to squat down to garden, the therapist may document, "Recommend client garden from a seated position rather than a squatting position due to impaired knee flexion, which hinders balance and safety."

In some cases recreational therapists may measure joint mobility using a goniometer, especially within a rehabilitation center where the recreational therapist has been cross-trained by other professionals. A goniometer is a two-armed instrument that is jointed in the center by a pin. The pin is placed over the center of the joint where the motion occurs (e.g., on the side of the knee). One instrument arm is held in line with the stationary body segment (e.g., outside thigh) and the other arm is moved (opened) along with the motion of the body segment (e.g., side of lower leg). When the joint is fully in extension or flexion (whichever is being measured) the indicator shows the number of degrees the segment has moved (e.g., knee flexion 90°). The documentation is made in a specific format, determined by the facility, to record the range of motion in the joints measured.

Treatment for joint mobility impairments will vary depending on the reason. For example, a client who has a total hip replacement will have hip range of motion restrictions for several months after surgery to allow the prosthetic joint to stabilize. Range of motion restrictions will also vary for people with rheumatoid arthritis depending on the stage of the disease (see the diagnosis of rheumatoid arthritis for more information). Therefore therapists must fully understand the nature of the joint mobility dysfunction, whether protective (e.g., to avoid joint instability or inflammation) or restrictive (e.g., contractures that prevent full joint mobility) as it relates to a client's specific diagnosis.

In general, however, therapists encourage AROM within parameters to increase available range while employing joint protection techniques as appropriate. Activities are redesigned within (and slightly above, if appropriate) available ranges. Adaptive equipment is prescribed as necessary to maximize independence and task performance.

Mild contractures can usually be reduced with moderate and frequent activity combined with relaxation (a reduction in stress and muscle guarding). Activities such as playing with a pet, fixing a meal, gardening, and other enjoyable activities help reduce muscle tightness

If a client has joint mobility restrictions, proper precautions and adaptations must be taken to reduce injury and ensure safety. People who need to protect their joints need to be educated about joint protection techniques. Joint protection refers to the use of larger joints to do the work of small joints to limit repetitive small joint range of motion and unnecessary work load (e.g., use of a universal cuff to hold a paint brush so that the wrist and arm are doing most of the work and finger movement in minimized; use of lightweight gardening equipment to minimize joint stress and encourage work of larger muscles and joints to perform the task). Joint protection does not mean that joints should not be ranged or bear weight. Secondary complications may arise if joints are not ranged (e.g., contractures). Key concepts of joint protection mean the client should:

1. Respect joint pain as a signal to stop an activity.
2. Avoid positions of deformity (e.g., press water from a sponge rather than squeezing, hold stirring spoons so that the bowl of the spoon is on the ulnar side of the hand and avoid turning the wrist inwards).
3. Avoid pressure that pushes the finger and wrist joints in an ulnar direction (e.g., turn handles or lids in the direction of the radius even if this means using the non-dominant hand).
4. Avoid external and internal deforming forces (e.g., the strong pinch and grasp that are typically required for knitting or hammering).
5. Use each joint in its most stable anatomical and functional plane (e.g., avoid twisting the knees when standing up by standing up first and then turning).
6. Use the strongest and largest joints available for the job because proximal joints are stronger than distal joints, and their use protects the weaker distal ones (e.g., carry a pocketbook over the forearm instead of in the hand, carry heavy items by putting a hand and forearm flat underneath and steadying the object with the other hand).

7. Use correct patterns of motion. See "Body Mechanics and Ergonomics" in the Techniques section.
8. Avoid holding one position for any undue length of time.
9. Avoid starting an activity that cannot be stopped if it proves to be beyond the client's capability.

Also see "Find Hand Use Ergonomics" in the Techniques section for more information.

b715 Stability of Joint Functions

Functions of the maintenance of structural integrity of the joints.
Inclusions: functions of the stability of a single joint, several joints, and joints generalized; impairments such as in unstable shoulder joint, dislocation of a joint, dislocation of shoulder and hip.
Exclusions: mobility of joint functions (b710)
* *b7150 Stability of a Single Joint*
  Functions of the maintenance of structural integrity of one joint.
* *b7151 Stability of Several Joints*
  Functions of the maintenance of structural integrity of more than one joint.
* *b7152 Stability of Joints Generalized*
  Functions of the maintenance of structural integrity of joints throughout the body.
* *b7158 Stability of Joint Functions, Other Specified*
* *b7159 Stability of Joint Functions, Unspecified*

Treatment for Stability of Joint Functions

Recreational therapists do not treat unstable joints. However they need to be aware of unstable joints and any precautions or parameters that must be followed to ensure that further injury does not occur.

The recreational therapist may need to adapt activities for the client when there are deficits in joint stability. For example, a client with a shoulder dislocation may be required to wear a protective harness to prevent the arm from being raised above the head. Activities that require raising the arms will need to be modified or adaptive equipment may be required, such as a grabber to reach objects on a high shelf.

Joint instability may be caused by activities run by a recreational therapist (e.g., playing a sport). If joint instability from an injury is suspected (e.g., the client is in pain or a joint appears to be out of correct alignment), medical attention should be sought immediately.

b720 Mobility of Bone Functions

Functions of the range and ease of movement of the scapula, pelvis, carpal, and tarsal bones.

Inclusions: impairments such as frozen scapula and frozen pelvis.
Exclusions: mobility of joints functions (b710)
* *b7200 Mobility of the Scapula*
  Functions of the range and ease of movement of the scapula.
  Inclusions: impairments such as protraction, retraction, laterorotation, and medial rotation of the scapula.
* *b7201 Mobility of the Pelvis*
  Functions of the range and ease of movement of the pelvis.
  Inclusion: rotation of the pelvis
* *b7202 Mobility of Carpal Bones*
  Functions of the range and ease of movement of the carpal bones.
* *b7203 Mobility of Tarsal Bones*
  Functions of the range and ease of movement of the tarsal bones.
* *b7208 Mobility of Bone Functions, Other Specified*
* *b7209 Mobility of Bone Functions, Unspecified*

Treatment for Mobility of Bone Functions

Recreational therapists do not treat mobility of bone functions, but they are aware of bone mobility impairments as communicated through medical documentation by other health professionals. If mobility of a bone function is impaired, recreational therapists follow specific precautions and parameters as established (e.g., mobility of pelvis is compromised limiting pelvis rotation). Many of the causes and treatments for deficits in mobility of bones are similar to the causes and treatments for deficits in mobility of joint functions (b710). Review that section for more information. Activity adaptations to accommodate bone mobility impairments are made as appropriate.

b729 Functions of the Joints and Bones, Other Specified and Unspecified

Muscle Functions (b730-b749)

b730 Muscle Power Functions

Functions related to the force generated by the contraction of a muscle or muscle groups.
Inclusions: functions associated with the power of specific muscles and muscle groups, muscles of one limb, one side of the body, the lower half of the body, all limbs, the trunk and the body as a whole; impairments such as weakness of small muscles in feet and hands, muscle paresis, muscle paralysis, monoplegia, hemiplegia, paraplegia, quadriplegia, and akinetic mutism.
Exclusions: functions of structures adjoining the eye (b215); muscle tone functions (b735); muscle endurance functions (b740).

- *b7300 Power of Isolated Muscles and Muscle Groups*
  Functions related to the force generated by the contraction of specific and isolated muscles and muscle groups.
  Inclusions: impairments such as weakness of small muscles of feet and hands.
- *b7301 Power of Muscles of One Limb*
  Functions related to the force generated by the contraction of the muscles and muscle groups of one arm or leg.
  Inclusions: impairments such as monoparesis and monoplegia
- *b7302 Power of Muscles of One Side of the Body*
  Functions related to the force generated by the contraction of the muscles and muscle groups found on the left or right side of the body.
  Inclusions: impairments such as hemiparesis and hemiplegia
- *b7303 Power of Muscles in Lower Half of the Body*
  Functions related to the force generated by the contraction of the muscle groups found in the lower half of the body.
  Inclusions: impairments such as paraparesis and paraplegia
- *b7304 Power of Muscles of All Limbs*
  Functions related to the force generated by the contraction of muscles and muscle groups of all four limbs.
  Inclusions: impairments such as tetraparesis and tetraplegia
- *b7305 Power of Muscles of the Trunk*
  Functions related to the force generated by the contraction of muscles and muscle groups in the trunk.
- *b7306 Power of All Muscles of the Body*
  Functions related to the force generated by the contraction of all muscles and muscle groups of the body.
  Inclusions: impairments such as akinetic mutism
- *b7308 Muscle Power Functions, Other Specified*
- *b7309 Muscle Power Functions, Unspecified*

Treatment for
Muscle Power Functions

Muscle power (commonly called muscle strength) can be affected by many things such as

neurological impairment (e.g., hemiplegia from a stroke), deconditioning (e.g., from inactivity or chronic disease), lack of sleep, lack of proper nutrition, and diseases that attack the muscles (e.g., fibromyalgia). Muscle power functions may also be restricted due to specific health conditions or injuries (e.g., weight lifting restrictions after having a heart attack or bone/muscle injury). Refer to the specific diagnoses for more information on how to address muscle power dysfunction as it relates to a specific diagnosis.

In general, muscle power refers to the degree of muscle power when movement is resisted with objects or gravity. Common ways to measure muscle power include:

- *Subjective strength test*: Ask the client to perform specific actions and observe the client's performance. For example, ask the client to hold your hand and then instruct the client to hold onto your hand tightly and not to let go when you try to pull your hand away.
- *Weights*: Ask the client to perform a familiar strength task that has a specific weight (e.g., picking up a one-pound hammer or lifting a three-pound weight). Record the amount of weight the client is able to manipulate and the number of repetitions s/he is able to perform prior to fatigue.
- *Manual muscle evaluation* (MME): The MME is a classification of strength that allows therapists to rate a client's strength along a scale. The specific techniques used by a therapist to arrive at the classification may vary. See Table 15 for a possible method of scoring.

Recreational therapists commonly document muscle power dysfunction by describing the specific impairment (e.g., right hemiparesis), clarifying muscle power abilities and limitations (e.g., able to lift a maximum of five pounds in right hand; documenting MME grade), and documenting the impact of muscle power dysfunction as it relates to specific activities (e.g., client able to swing one-pound hammer using right upper extremity for two minutes prior to muscle fatigue).

Table 15: Manual Muscle Evaluation — Strength

100%	5	N	Normal	Complete range of motion against gravity with full resistance
75%	4	G	Good	Complete range of motion against gravity with some resistance
50%	3	F	Fair	Complete range of motion against gravity
25%	2	P	Poor	Complete range of motion with gravity eliminated
10%	1	T	Trace	Evidence of contractility
0%	0	0	Zero	No evidence of contractility
S			Spasm	If spasm or contracture exists, place S or C after the grade of a move-
C			Contracture	ment incomplete for this reason.

From burlingame (2001), used with permission.

Therapeutic interventions to improve muscle power functions will vary depending on the cause of the impairment. Impairment related to neurological dysfunction such as that caused by a stroke, respond best to neuroplasticity interventions along with general strength training, whereas people with muscle power impairment from deconditioning respond best to general strength training alone. General strength training includes the use of graduated tasks of weight and repetition (e.g., gradually increasing the weight of the item used/lifted/manipulated, number of times the item is used/lifted/manipulated in a given period of time). Other interventions may include those that assist with sleep quality and quantity (see b134 Sleep Functions for common interventions), nutritional intake, and other interventions that are disease specific (e.g., teaching clients with multiple sclerosis how to manage fatigue that ultimately affects muscle power, teaching clients with fibromyalgia how to manage stress that ultimately affects level of fatigue and thus muscle power functions). Refer to specific diagnoses for more information.

Adaptations for muscle power impairments include the redesign of activity components to meet muscle power restrictions or abilities. Lightweight adaptive equipment may also be prescribed to meet the client's abilities (e.g., lightweight gardening equipment).

b735 Muscle Tone Functions

Functions related to the tension present in the resting muscles and the resistance offered when trying to move the muscles passively.
Inclusions: functions associated with the tension of isolated muscles and muscle groups, muscles of one limb, one side of the body and the lower half of the body, muscles of all limbs, muscles of the trunk, and all muscles of the body; impairments such as hypotonia, hypertonia, and muscle spasticity.
Exclusions: muscle power functions (b730); muscle endurance functions (b740)

*   *b7350 Tone of Isolated Muscles and Muscle Groups*
    Functions related to the tension present in the resting isolated muscles and muscle groups and the resistance offered when trying to move those muscles passively.
    Inclusions: impairments such as in focal dystonias, e.g., torticollis
*   *b7351 Tone of Muscles of One Limb*
    Functions related to the tension present in the resting muscles and muscle groups in one arm or leg and the resistance offered when trying to move those muscles passively.
    Inclusions: impairments associated with monoparesis and monoplegia
*   *b7352 Tone of Muscles of One Side of Body*
    Functions related to the tension present in the resting muscles and muscle groups of the right or

left side of the body and the resistance offered when trying to move those muscles passively.
Inclusions: impairments associated with hemiparesis and hemiplegia

*   *b7353 Tone of Muscles in Lower Half of Body*
    Functions related to the tension present in the resting muscles and muscle groups in the lower half of the body and the resistance offered when trying to move those muscles passively.
    Inclusions: impairments associated with paraparesis and paraplegia
*   *b7354 Tone of Muscles in All Limbs*
    Functions related to the tension present in the resting muscles and muscle groups in all four limbs and the resistance offered when trying to move those muscles passively.
    Inclusions: impairments associated with tetraparesis and tetraplegia
*   *b7355 Tone of Muscles of Trunk*
    Functions related to the tension present in the resting muscles and muscle groups of the trunk and the resistance offered when trying to move those muscles passively.
*   *b7356 Tone of All Muscles of the Body*
    Functions related to the tension present in the resting muscles and muscle groups of the whole body and the resistance offered when trying to move those muscles passively.
    Inclusions: impairments such as in generalized dystonias and Parkinson's disease or general paresis and paralysis
*   *b7358 Muscle Tone Functions, Other Specified*
*   *b7359 Muscle Tone Functions, Unspecified*

Treatment for Muscle Tone Functions

Muscle tone is the degree of tension or resistance in a muscle at rest and in response to stretch. Muscle tone dysfunction is typically divided into two problems

*   *Flaccidity (or hypotonia)*: a decrease in muscle tone. A diminished resistance to passive movement will be noted, and muscles may feel abnormally soft and flaccid. Diminished deep tendon reflexes also may be noted.
*   *Rigidity (or hypertonia)*: an increase in muscle tone causing greater resistance to passive movement. Two types of rigidity may be seen: *lead pipe* and *cogwheel*. Lead pipe rigidity is a uniform, constant resistance felt by the examiner as the extremity is moved through a range of motion. Cogwheel rigidity is considered a combination of the lead pipe type with tremor. It is characterized by a series of brief relaxations or "catches" as the extremity is passively moved.

Muscle tone problems result from brain injury (e.g., traumatic brain injury, stroke) or neurological impairment (e.g., spinal cord injury, Parkinson's disease). See separate diagnoses for more information.

Decreased or increased muscle tone can affect activity performance. Therapists begin by observing the state of the client's muscles at rest and when performing activities (e.g., increased muscle tone noted with physical activity).

Therapists document muscle tone impairments by diagnosis (hypotonic, hypertonic) and location (e.g., right upper extremity), as well as activities impaired by muscle tone dysfunction (e.g., increased tone in right upper extremity impairs client's ability to cast a fishing line resulting in the need for moderate assistance with this task).

If muscle tone impairments are noted, interventions to maximize function and decrease secondary problems (e.g., contractures) are introduced as noted here:

- *Flaccidity*: If muscles are hypotonic due to brain impairment (e.g., stroke, traumatic brain injury), tactile stimulation to the muscle can be helpful to improve tone. Hypotonic muscles due to nerve injury (e.g., spinal cord injury) may respond to tactile stimulation only if it is an incomplete injury. Flaccid or hypotonic limbs due to brain injury can be incorporated into functional activities to promote neuroplasticity (see "Neuroplasticity" in the Techniques section), whereas the incorporation of flaccid and hypotonic limbs due to nerve injury into functional activities is helpful to prevent muscle contractures.

- *Rigidity*: Stretching muscles (active and passive range of motion) prior to and after activity performance is important to reduce increased tone caused by activity and prevent contractures. In some instances, however, range of motion may be contraindicated (e.g., when working with a tenodesis splint in a client with a tetraplegia). Splints may be prescribed to stretch out rigid muscles for prevention or reduction of muscle contractures. Recreational therapists need to be aware of and assist the client as needed to don/doff splints. If rigidity is causing functional problems (e.g., hindering the ability to walk), pharmacological interventions may be used to decrease muscle rigidity (e.g., nerve block).

Sometimes flaccidity and rigidity occur together because flaccid muscles often experience contractures. Treatment in those cases aims to eliminate the contractures while also using the muscles in a way that increases their tone.

Should muscle tone functions remain unresolved, precautions are taken to ensure client safety (e.g., devices), prevent contractures (e.g., range of motion, splints), and improve functional abilities (e.g., adaptive equipment).

b740 Muscle Endurance Functions
Functions related to sustaining muscle contraction for the required period of time.
Inclusions: functions associated with sustaining muscle contraction for isolated muscles and muscle groups, and all muscles of the body; impairments such as in myasthenia gravis.
Exclusions: exercise tolerance functions (b455); muscle power functions (b730); muscle tone functions (b735)

- *b7400 Endurance of Isolated Muscles*
  Functions related to sustaining muscle contraction of isolated muscles for the required period of time.

- *b7401 Endurance of Muscle Groups*
  Functions related to sustaining muscle contraction of isolated muscle groups for the required period of time.
  Inclusions: impairments associated with mono-paresis, monoplegia, hemiparesis and hemiplegia, paraparesis and paraplegia

- *b7402 Endurance of All Muscles of the Body*
  Functions related to sustaining muscle contraction of all muscles of the body for the required period of time.
  Inclusions: impairments associated with tetraparesis, tetraplegia, general paresis, and paralysis

- *b7408 Muscle Endurance Functions, Other Specified*

- *b7409 Muscle Endurance Functions, Unspecified*

Treatment for Muscle Endurance Functions

Muscle endurance functions can be affected by neurological impairments (e.g., stroke) and muscular impairments (e.g., fibromyalgia, deconditioning as a secondary complication from another health problem).

To assess muscle endurance functions, the therapist presents the client with a muscle endurance task that is within appropriate parameters and precautions for the client. The therapist monitors vital signs as needed (e.g., heart rate, blood pressure, oxygen saturation level). The therapist measures muscle endurance functions in terms of time (e.g., client presents with standing tolerance of 15 minutes prior to muscle fatigue), weight (e.g., client able to perform 10 bicep curls with five-pound weight prior to muscle fatigue), and intensity (e.g., low intensity ball toss with eight-ounce ball results in upper extremity muscle endurance of six minutes whereas high intensity ball toss with same weight ball results in upper extremity muscle endurance of four minutes).

Therapists promote muscle endurance through the use of graduated muscle endurance tasks (e.g., increasing time, frequency, and intensity of the activity).

If muscle endurance does not recover to normal levels or if there are specific muscle endurance precautions (e.g., not allowed to sustain high intensity muscle activity for more than five minutes), activity adaptations are made. Some examples might be to decrease the weight of objects to decrease muscle workload, redesign an activity to meet compromised muscle endurance needs, decrease the task speed, decrease the task intensity, decrease the distance, decrease the task time, increase rest periods, explore energy saving techniques, and explore adaptive equipment to assist with managing muscle endurance (e.g., using an electric scooter at the grocery store, using a golf cart on the golf course).

b749 Muscle Functions, Other Specified and Unspecified

Movement Functions (b750-b789)

b750 Motor Reflex Functions
Functions of involuntary contraction of muscles automatically induced by specific stimuli.
Inclusions: functions of stretch motor reflex, automatic local joint reflex, reflexes generated by noxious stimuli and other exteroceptive stimuli; withdrawal reflex, biceps reflex, radius reflex, quadriceps reflex, patellar reflex, ankle reflex
- *b7500 Stretch Motor Reflex*
  Functions of involuntary contractions of muscles automatically induced by stretching.
- *b7501 Reflexes Generated by Noxious Stimuli*
  Functions of involuntary contractions of muscles automatically induced by painful or other noxious stimuli.
  Inclusion: withdrawal reflex
- *b7502 Reflexes Generated by Other Exteroceptive Stimuli*
  Functions of involuntary contractions of muscles automatically induced by external stimuli other than noxious stimuli.
- *b7508 Motor Reflex Functions, Other Specified*
- *b7509 Motor Reflex Functions, Unspecified*

Treatment for Motor Reflex Functions

A reflex is a reaction that occurs in response to a stimulus without conscious thought or will. Often the reflex is a result of nerve impulses that do not even reach the brain, such as the patellar ("knee jerk") reflex, which is one of the deep tendon reflexes included in b7502. Other reflexes occur as a result of the proprioceptors in muscles noticing a stretch, noxious stimuli, and other external stimuli.

The recreational therapist will usually not assess a reflex response unless it is being used to track some aspect of the client's state. For example, a pinprick may be used to distinguish between the lowest three levels on the Rancho Los Amigos Scale. The patellar reflex may be used with a client to assess some kinds of stress. See Table 16 for scoring a deep tendon reflex. Documentation involves the type of reflex and the numeric rating.

There is no specific treatment related to reflexes. Treatment should be directed at the underlying cause of the reflex deficit.

Some adaptations may be necessary. Clients who do not properly respond to noxious stimuli (e.g., potentially damaging heat) will need to be protected from dangerous situations and learn strategies to avoid injury. See b270 for some additional ideas.

b755 Involuntary Movement Reaction Functions
Functions of involuntary contractions of large muscles or the whole body induced by body position, balance, and threatening stimuli.
Inclusions: functions of postural reactions, righting reactions, body adjustment reactions, balance reactions, supporting reactions, defensive reactions
Exclusion: motor reflex functions (b750)

Treatment for Involuntary Movement Reaction Functions

Involuntary movement reaction functions are movements that the body makes in reaction to a position (e.g., leaning forward to stand or sit), balance challenge (e.g., moving arms during loss of balance in attempt to regain balance), and threatening

Table 16: Rating System for Deep Tendon Reflexes

Numeric Rating	Description of Function
4+	brisk, hyperactive, clonus
3+	is more brisk than normal, but does not necessarily indicate a pathologic process, gross functional ability not usually impaired
2+	Normal
1+	Low normal, with slight diminution in response, having minor impact on functional ability
0	no response

From burlingame (2001), p. 261. Used with permission.

stimuli (e.g., putting hands over face or head to protect it from injury). Reaction impairments are often a sign of central nervous system injury.

Therapists assess reaction impairments through observation during activity (e.g., walking, catching a ball). If the reaction movement is present, it is said to be positive. If it is not present, it is said to be negative. If the reaction movement is present but not at full intensity, the level of impairment is noted (e.g., mildly impaired) and explained as needed (e.g., slowed righting reactions).

For documentation, the specific activity used for observation and its conditions are documented (e.g., during dynamic standing activity of plant care client had moderately impaired righting reactions).

Recovery of movement reactions may occur in some cases depending on the cause of the problem (e.g., traumatic brain injury). Reaction impairments that are not recovered may cause significant impairments in life activities that may require the use of devices (e.g., walking devices, extra body protection gear during sporting activities).

Some of the most important involuntary movement reaction functions involve maintaining balance, posture, and stability in a variety of situations. Improving or maintaining balance, posture, and stability are underlying, basic functional skills required to participate in everyday activities. See the discussion of "Balance" in the Techniques section for more information on the relationship between balance and involuntary movement functions and techniques for improving balance.

b760 Control of Voluntary Movement Functions

Functions associated with control over and coordination of voluntary movements.
Inclusions: functions of control of simple voluntary movements and of complex voluntary movements, coordination of voluntary movements, supportive functions of arm or leg, right left motor coordination, eye hand coordination, eye foot coordination; impairments such as control and coordination problems, e.g., dysdiadochokinesia

- *b7600 Control of Simple Voluntary Movements*
  Functions associated with control over and coordination of simple or isolated voluntary movements.
- *b7601 Control of Complex Voluntary Movements*
  Functions associated with control over and coordination of complex voluntary movements.
- *b7602 Coordination of Voluntary Movements*
  Functions associated with coordination of simple and complex voluntary movements, performing movements in an orderly combination.
  Inclusions: right left coordination, coordination of visually directed movements, such as eye hand coordination and eye foot coordination; impairments such as dysdiadochokinesia

- *b7603 Supportive Functions of Arm or Leg*
  Functions associated with control over and coordination of voluntary movements by placing weight either on the arms (elbows or hands) or on the legs (knees or feet).
- *b7608 Control of Voluntary Movement Functions, Other Specified*
- *b7609 Control of Voluntary Movement Functions, Unspecified*

Treatment for Control of Voluntary Movement Functions

This section looks at the four aspects of controlling voluntary movement. The first two codes look at controlling simple and complex movements. The third code looks at coordination of movement, while the fourth code looks at the specific problem of using the arms or legs as supports for voluntary movement.

Control of Simple and Complex Voluntary Movement

Voluntary movement functions refer to the voluntary control of muscles. An example of a simple voluntary movement would be raising your hand to answer a question. An example of a complex voluntary movement would be positioning yourself into an advanced yoga posture. Voluntary movement functions can be hindered by damage to the brain or nervous system (e.g., brain injury, stroke, multiple sclerosis).

Therapists assess voluntary movement disorders by asking the client to perform specific voluntary movements and observing a client's performance of voluntary movements in an activity. Observation of performance within an activity is especially needed when cognitive impairments are present that could hinder the person's ability to understand the performance you are requesting (e.g., a person with a left cerebrovascular accident who has resultant receptive aphasia will have difficulty processing spoken language).

Voluntary movement disorders that are affected by underlying brain or nervous system problems that have the potential for recovery (e.g., incomplete spinal cord injury, brain injury, cerebrovascular accident, Guillain-Barré syndrome) are addressed through the use of neuroplasticity or other retraining interventions (see "Neuroplasticity" in the Techniques section and specific diagnoses). Voluntary movement disorders, although having a potential for recovery, are not always fully recovered, and some voluntary movement disorders are not able to be recovered (e.g., complete spinal cord injury). In this situation, the therapist aims to adapt activities so they match the client's abilities. When voluntary movement is restricted, secondary problems can occur such as muscle contractures (b710 Mobility of Joint Functions), joint instability (e.g., dislocated shoulder in a flaccid upper extremity caused by a stroke — b715 Stability of Joint Functions), muscle atrophy (affecting b730 Muscle Power Functions and b740 Muscle Endurance Functions), increased or decreased muscle tone (b735 Muscle Tone Functions), and pain (b280 Sensation of Pain).

Therapists document the specific impairment, the specific activity affected, the level of assistance, and any recommendations. Impairment of voluntary function is often documented by the amount of active range of motion. (e.g., "Voluntary movement of the right upper extremity is impaired resulting in moderately impaired finger/wrist/elbow flexion and extension. Consequently, client is able to perform only 50% of a simple repotting task. Client instructed on how to use right upper extremity as a functional assist for task and is able to incorporate techniques learned with minimal assistance.").

Coordination of Voluntary Movements

Coordination is the ability to execute smooth, accurate, controlled movements. The ability to produce these movements is a complex process, which is dependent on a fully intact neuromuscular system. Coordinated movements are characterized by appropriate speed, distance, direction, rhythm, and muscle tension. In addition, they involve appropriate synergist influences, easy reversal between opposing muscle groups, and proximal fixation to allow distal motion or maintenance of a posture. Incoordination and coordination deficit are general terms used to describe abnormal motor function characterized by awkward, extraneous, uneven, or inaccurate movements (O'Sullivan & Schmitz, 1988).

Some of the deficits that affect control of voluntary movement functions include:

- *Asthenia*: Characterized by generalized muscle weakness. Client may also have difficulty initiating voluntary movement, stopping a movement, or changing the force, speed, or direction of a movement.
- *Ataxia*: This is a general term that describes general difficulty with coordination of motor function of the muscles involved with walking. (Also see b770 Gait Pattern Function.)
- *Dysdiadochokinesia*: Impairment in ability to perform rapid alternating movements (e.g., rapid alternation between pronation and supination of the forearm). Movements are irregular, with a rapid loss of range and rhythm.

- *Dysmetria*: Impairment in the ability to accurately judge the distance or range of a movement needed to reach an item or goal (e.g., how far to reach forward to grab a hammer, proper height of the foot to put it on a step). If it is an overestimation, it is referred to as *hypermetria*. If it is an underestimation, it is referred to as *hypometria*.
- *Movement decomposition*: Impairment in ability to perform a smooth sequence of movements. Movements are performed in separate single sequential steps rather than as a smooth and integrated movement. For example, if a client is asked to touch her nose with her index finger, she may first extend her index finger, then extend her arm from the shoulder, and then flex her elbow so that her index finger touches her nose.
- *Nystagmus*: Impairment of the oscillatory movement of the eyes resulting in "jumpy" vision making it difficult to fixate. When trying to fixate on a peripheral object, an involuntary drift back to the midline position is observed. See b215 Functions of Structures Adjoining the Eye for more information or to code this impairment. Several deficits related to eye movements are associated with cerebellar lesions.

Recreational therapists do not typically use standardized tests for upper and lower extremity coordination. Clients are usually challenged with a coordination task that directly relates to functional tasks that are part of the client's lifestyle (e.g., typing on a computer keyboard, throwing a ball) and observations of impairments/abilities are made. However, the therapist must be familiar with the appropriate terminology that reflects coordination deficits and be aware of standardized tests that can provide further assessment of suspected problems. Some of these are discussed in "Coordination Tests" in the Assessment section. Therapists must also be aware of age-specific developmental changes (e.g., slower reaction time with aging) and disability restrictions (e.g., range of motion) that may influence test performance. Documentation of the deficits found is also described in "Coordination Tests" in the Assessment section.

Supportive Functions of the Arm or Leg

The voluntary movement of purposively placing weight through the arms (elbows or hands) or legs (knees or feet) is needed for mobility (d410 Changing Basic Body Positions, d415 Maintaining a Body Position, d420 Transferring Oneself, d430 Lifting and Carrying Objects, d435 Moving Objects with Lower Extremities, d445 Hand and Arm Use, d450 Walking, d455 Moving Around). Weight bearing through the arms and legs supports the body to perform specific movements (e.g., leaning one hand on a table to provide upper body support when reaching for a high object, lunging forward with one leg to support the upper body when throwing a baseball). Although these movements in some situations are performed quickly without much forethought, they are under voluntary control. Some clients may intentionally limit the amount of weight they place through the arms or legs due to specific precautions set by the physician (e.g., fracture), pain (e.g., tender spot on foot), impaired sensation (e.g., a client using a prosthetic leg has difficulty "feeling" the amount of weight being placed through the limb causing impairments with using the limb for supportive functions), and psychological issues (e.g., lacks confidence in his/her strength). This code refers to specific body functions that impair the ability to use arms or legs as supports. This is most commonly caused by brain and nervous system impairments (e.g., brain injury, multiple sclerosis, cerebrovascular accident, Parkinson's disease, pinched nerve in the back that causes legs to buckle at times, Guillain-Barré syndrome).

Therapists document the specific impairment, the specific activity affected, the level of assistance, and any recommendations (e.g., "Requires moderate assistance for throwing a baseball due to impaired supportive function of the left lower extremity").

Therapists address the supportive functions of arms and legs by assisting the client into a position that incorporates arm and leg support (e.g., have the client practice using the left arm as a support by placing the client's left hand on a table and having him reach and grasp high items; have the client practice using her right leg as a support by having her step forward with her right foot when throwing a dart). Continued use of the arm or leg as a support assists with re-teaching the client how to use the arms and legs as supports, as well as developing muscle strength and bone density that is needed for good support. In some cases, supportive functions of an arm or leg may not be possible (e.g., flaccid arm from a stroke). Therapists then aim to teach the client alternative ways to support the body within different tasks to maximize performance and safety (e.g., performing the task in a seated position instead of a standing position; using a walking device; using a piece of adaptive equipment to reduce the need for supportive functions, such as a fishing rod holder).

Therapists seek to resolve voluntary movement dysfunctions by using the methods described in "Motor Learning and Training Strategies" in the Techniques section. Other techniques that can be used to improve voluntary motor functions, especially the aspects of using the legs appropriately for support, can be found in "Balance" in the Techniques section. Some of these techniques are aimed at improving strength, but they also improve balance and coordination by repeated use of neural pathways related to movement and coordination. Whether the pathways are damaged from disease or trauma or not functioning because of lack of use, the therapeutic repetition of skills promotes neuroplasticity and restrengthening of functionality, thus assisting the return of previous levels of ability to perform voluntary movement (see "Neuroplasticity" in the Techniques section).

If impairments are not resolved or only resolved partially, the therapist re-designs activities to maximize independence, safety, and performance. Assistive devices such as walkers and canes may be used to help with balance.

b765 Involuntary Movement Functions
Functions of unintentional, non- or semi-purposive involuntary contractions of a muscle or group of muscles.
Inclusions: involuntary contractions of muscles; impairments such as tremors, tics, mannerisms, stereotypies, motor perseveration, chorea, athetosis, vocal tics, dystonic movements, and dyskinesia
Exclusions: control of voluntary movement functions (b760); gait pattern functions (b770)

- *b7650 Involuntary Contractions of Muscles*
  Functions of unintentional, non- or semi-purposive involuntary contractions of a muscle or group of muscles, such as those involved as part of a psychological dysfunction.
  Inclusions: impairments such as choreatic and athetotic movements; sleep-related movement disorders

- *b7651 Tremor*
  Functions of alternating contraction and relaxation of a group of muscles around a joint, resulting in shakiness.

- *b7652 Tics and Mannerisms*
  Functions of repetitive, quasi-purposive, involuntary contractions of a group of muscles.
  Inclusions: impairments such as vocal tics, coprolalia, and bruxism

- *b7653 Stereotypies and Motor Perseveration*
  Functions of spontaneous, non-purposive movements such as repetitively rocking back and forth and nodding the head or wiggling.

- *b7658 Involuntary Movement Functions, Other Specified*

- *b7659 Involuntary Movement Functions, Unspecified*

Treatment for
Involuntary Movement Functions

Involuntary movement functions are primarily caused by lesions in the basal ganglia. Basal ganglia lesions are common in Parkinson's disease, Wilson's disease, and Huntington's disease. Below is a list of common involuntary movement dysfunctions.

- *Athetosis*: Characterized by slow, involuntary, writhing, twisting, "wormlike" movements. Distal upper extremities are primarily affected (e.g., hyperextension of the wrist and fingers and then return to a flexed position) along with rotary movements of the extremity. Athetosis is a clinical feature of cerebral palsy.
- *Bradykinesia*: Characterized by slowed or decreased movements (e.g., decreased arm swing, slow shuffling gait, difficulty initiating or changing direction of movement, lack of facial expression, difficulty stopping a movement once begun).
- *Chorea*: Characterized by involuntary, rapid, irregular, and jerky movements; also referred to as choreiform movements. This is a clinical feature of Huntington's disease.
- *Choreoathetosis*: A movement disorder with features of both chorea and athetosis.
- *Dystonia*: Characterized by involuntary muscle contraction of the extremities resulting in bizarre twisting movements. A prolonged contraction at the end of a movement, it is called a *dystonic posture*.
- *Hemiballismus*: Characterized by a sudden, jerky, forceful, wild, flailing motions of the arm and leg of one side of the body.
- *Tremors*: An involuntary oscillatory movement resulting from alternating contractions of opposing muscle groups. Two types of tremors are associated with cerebellar lesions. An *intention, or kinetic, tremor* occurs during voluntary motion of a limb and tends to increase as the limb nears its extended goal (e.g., tremor begins when the arm begins to reach forward towards an item and increases as the arm reaches full extension). Intention tremors are diminished or absent at rest. *Postural, or static, tremors* may be evident by back-and-forth oscillatory movements of the body while the patient maintains a standing posture. They also may be observed as up-and-down oscillatory movements of a limb when it is held against gravity. There are many different types of tremors. burlingame (2001, p. 305) lists some of them:
  - *Action tremor*: Involuntary oscillating and rhythmic movements of the outstretched upper limb during activity.
  - *Coarse tremor*: Slow, rhythmic movements.
  - *Essential tremor*: Inherited tendency to develop a fine tremor, usually after the age of fifty. Also known as a familial tremor.
  - *Fine tremor*: Fast, rhythmic movements.
  - *Intension tremor*: Increase in intensity when the individual attempts a voluntary movement that requires coordination.
  - *Intermittent tremor*: Occurs when voluntary movement is attempted or occurs in hemiplegia.
  - *Motofacient tremor*: In muscle groups of the face.
  - *Passive tremor*: Only seen when the client is at rest.
  - *Persistent tremor*: Present whether the client is resting or attempting activity.
  - *Resting tremor*: Present when the limb is supported and the patient is at rest, as in Parkinsonism. Resting tremors typically disappear or reduce with voluntary movement and they may increase with emotional stress.
  - *Volitional tremor*: Seen through the entire body during voluntary movement, as in multiple sclerosis.

Additional tremors that are common to Parkinson's disease include a "pill-rolling" movement. It looks like the client is rolling a pill up and down the first two fingers with his/her thumb. Another tremor movement is the pronation and supination of the forearm, as well as tremor of the head.

Involuntary motor functions are assessed through observation during functional activity, at rest, and through equilibrium and non-equilibrium coordination tests (discussed in "Coordination Tests" in the Assessment section).

Involuntary motor functions are primarily controlled fully or partially through pharmacology. The therapist redesigns activities to minimize/eliminate interference with motor responses (e.g., remove unnecessary/unsafe items from the work area where poor motor responses could result in task interference) and minimizes chances of harm or injury.

b770 Gait Pattern Functions
Functions of movement patterns associated with walking, running, or other whole body movements.
Inclusions: walking patterns and running patterns; impairments such as spastic gait, hemiplegia gait, paraplegic gait, asymmetric gait, limping, and stiff gait pattern
Exclusions: muscle power functions (b730); muscle tone functions (b735); control of voluntary movement functions (b760); involuntary movement functions (b765)

Treatment for
Gait Pattern Functions

Although physical therapists are the primary health care professionals to evaluate and prescribe treatment interventions related to walking and moving, all health care professionals must be familiar with gait cycle terminology and approaches to treatment so that strategies and equipment can be carried over into everyday functional and/or leisure-based tasks. Gait patterns are important as part of d450-d469 Walking and Moving Around.

On the unit the physical therapist may measure the client's stride length and cadence through a simple text called the *Fifty-Foot Walk Test*. (See the Assessment section.) Because walking within the hospital setting is often less complex than walking in the community (less visual, auditory, and neuromusculoskeletal stimulation) a client's functional level could be different in the two settings. The recreational therapist may want to use the *Fifty-Foot Walk Test* with clients while in a community setting to determine if the client 1. has a significant difference in skill between the unit and the community, 2. is able to walk efficiently, 3. is at an increased risk of falling, or 4. has difficulty dividing attention well enough to walk and pay attention to other stimulation at the same time (d1402).

In addition to the stride length and cadence information from the *Fifty-Foot Walk Test* there are other methods to describe and measure a client's functional ability. Recreational therapists who are typically addressing walking and moving in a functional environment measure walking and moving by the following:

- *Distance*: How far did the client walk? Distance is easily measured in the community by re-walking the distance when the client is resting. Therapists should know the length of their stride so they can make good estimates of distances. If the therapist knows his/her stride length, all s/he needs to do is walk the same distance as the client and multiply the number of strides times the stride length. If the therapist took 100 normal stride steps and has a 2.5-foot stride, the client walked approximately 250'. With practice, the therapist will become adept at "eyeing" a distance and being able to approximate the number of feet walked by the client.
- *Surface*: What type of surface did the client move across? The therapist can provide broad descriptions (e.g., uneven community surfaces) or specific descriptions (grass, gravel, cobblestone, inclines, etc.) depending upon the situation. For example, if the client displayed different needs (e.g., amount of assistance, cueing) for

walking on grass as compared to cobblestone, then distinctions must be drawn in the documentation. If the client's performance was consistent throughout the evaluation, then the therapist may opt to broadly describe the surface. It is always a good idea to err on the side of over-description rather than under-description, especially if specific surfaces are deemed important to the client or rehab team (e.g., client will be required to walk 50' on an graded incline, 20' over grass, and 10' over gravel to move from his home to the train station each morning for work).

- *Amount of Assistance*: What type of assistance and how much assistance did the client require? This is typically measured by the FIM scale (see the Assessment section) or by the degree of assistance needed (e.g., minimum, moderate, or maximum assist). Also include detailed information on the amount of supervision required for safety, the type of device (if any) used by the client (e.g., small-based quad cane, platform crutches), and amount and type of cueing (e.g., minimal verbal cueing required for step length).

All of these descriptors are to be reflected in the documentation. Examples:

- Client walked approximately 150' on outdoor uneven surfaces with a rolling walker and minimal assistance for right knee buckling.
- Client walked approximately 50' over grassy surface with a single point cane and close supervision secondary to need for max verbal and tactile cues to decrease walking speed.
- Client walked approximately 45' on cobblestone, 25' on gravel, and 60' on slightly uneven concrete without an assistive device at modified independence secondary to increased time. Client independent in initiating rest break.

Treatment for functional problems with gait patterns has many aspects. They include strength, endurance, flexibility, and several balance issues. Most of these are covered in other sections of the ICF.

Adaptations for problems with gait patterns include making sure that the client has as many visual cues as possible, teaching the use of assistive devices such as canes, and using other mobility devices (e.g., wheelchairs and banana carts) when the client needs to move faster or through more obstacles than his/her abilities allow.

Please refer to Activities and Participation Chapter 4 Mobility for information on mobility treatment as well as the Techniques section for information on "Walking Techniques." The Concepts section has additional information about "Gait."

b780 Sensations Related to Muscles and Movement Functions

Sensations associated with the muscles or muscle groups of the body and their movement.

Inclusions: sensations of muscle stiffness and tightness of muscles, muscle spasm or constriction, and heaviness of muscles

Exclusion: sensation of pain (b280)

- *b7800 Sensation of Muscle Stiffness*
  Sensation of tightness or stiffness of muscles.
- *b7801 Sensation of Muscle Spasm*
  Sensation of involuntary contraction of a muscle or a group of muscles.
- *b7808 Sensations Related to Muscles and Movement Functions, Other Specified*
- *b7809 Sensations Related to Muscles and Movement Functions, Unspecified*

Treatment for Sensations Related to Muscles and Movement Functions

Muscle stiffness can be due to a variety of disorders (e.g., arthritis), muscle shortening when in prolonged rest, and general deconditioning (e.g., muscle stiffness from inactivity). Muscle spasms can be caused by a lack of potassium (e.g., charley horse leg spasm) or from a neurological injury that impairs muscle nerve innervation.

Muscle stiffness and spasm are assessed through observation (e.g., stiff walking, sighs with movement), assessing a limited range of motion, and direct questioning of the client. Muscle spasm, like muscle stiffness, is assessed through direct observation of involuntary muscle contractions within activity and at rest, as well as direct questioning of the client.

Therapists document the specific impairment noted and the related cause, if known, as well as the extent of impairment that it causes with specific activities (e.g., client reports that bilateral leg spasms severely limit his ability to transfer into a car).

Muscle stiffness and spasms are treated according to the origin of the problem. This may include the use of pharmacology and exercise.

Muscle stiffness and spasms that are not able to be controlled can result in increased chances of injury or harm to the client (e.g., increased risk for falls). Precautions should be taken to reduce falls (e.g., using a walking aid). The therapist should also provide adaptations for activities that are affected by impairments (e.g., adding extra time to the morning routine to reduce feelings of stiffness upon waking up).

b789 Movement Functions, Other Specified and Unspecified

b798 Neuromusculoskeletal and Movement-Related Functions, Other Specified

b799 Neuromusculoskeletal and Movement-Related Functions, Unspecified

References

burlingame, j. (2001). *Idyll Arbor's therapy dictionary*, 2nd ed. Ravensdale, WA: Idyll Arbor, Inc:

Rose, D. (2003). *Fallproof!: A comprehensive balance and mobility training program.* Champaign, IL: Human Kinetics.

O'Sullivan, S. & Schmitz, T. (1988). *Physical rehabilitation: Assessment and treatment.* Philadelphia, PA: F.A. Davis Company.

Patla, A. (1997). Understanding the roles of vision in the control of human locomotion. *Gait and Posture*, 5:54-69.

Chapter 8 Functions of the Skin and Related Structures

This chapter is about the functions of skin, nails, and hair.

Recreational therapists need to understand the protective and restorative functions of the skin and related sensations as they pertain to skin care within real-life activity. This is particularly important for:

1. Clients who have impaired sensation (e.g., a client with a complete spinal cord injury who loses sensation below the waist and must be diligent in performing weight shifts, keeping skin clean and dry, and performing routine skin inspections to prevent decubitus ulcers from forming; clients who have peripheral neuropathy from diabetes need to conduct daily inspections of the feet for development of ulcers).
2. Clients who are taking blood thinning medications that require careful protection of the skin from injury (medication thins blood to decrease clotting therefore skin openings will continue to bleed rather than clot).
3. Clients who are taking medication that affect the skin's sensitivity to light (e.g., some medications make the skin more sensitive to sunlight and require more protection from sunlight than is normally required).
4. Clients who have compromised immune systems (e.g., skin openings provide an opportunity for bacteria to enter the bloodstream).
5. Clients who have an infectious disease that can be spread via bodily fluids (e.g., a person with HIV or hepatitis who has a skin opening that bleeds may put others at risk if the blood is touched by another person who also has a skin opening for the infected blood to enter).
6. Clients who have skin damage and require special care in activities (e.g., a client with severe burns needs to be protected from activities that could cause physical contact and related pain; a client with an extremity amputation requires routine and diligent inspection of the skin on the stump during prosthetic training to assess the fit of the prosthetic, prosthetic toler-ance, and skin tolerance to friction).

Functions of the Skin (b810-b849)

b810 Protective Functions of the Skin
Functions of the skin for protecting the body from physical, chemical, and biological threats.
Inclusions: functions of protecting against the sun and other radiation, photosensitivity, pigmentation, quality of skin; insulting function of skin, callus formation, hardening; impairments such as broken skin, ulcers, bedsores, and thinning skin

Exclusions: repair functions of skin (b820); other functions of the skin (b830)

Treatment for Protective Functions of the Skin

Recreational therapists document the specific skin problem (e.g., decubitus ulcer on buttock), the specific care that is required within activity (e.g., weight shifts every 20 minutes), the client's ability to perform and problem solve for such care (e.g., client requires moderate verbal cues to perform weight shifts during activity; client able to independently problem solve for barriers that limit routine weight shifts), and special precautions taken by the therapist to ensure skin protection and optimal conditions for skin repair (e.g., client instructed on importance of thoroughly drying skin after swimming to prevent conditions that contribute to the development of decubitus ulcers; client able to verbally repeat information independently, however was only 75% effective in drying skin completely after swimming due to limited mobility; plan is to contact client's occupational therapist to problem solve for adaptive devices to maximize ability to dry skin thoroughly after swimming).

In addition to the issues discussed, therapists also document any noted skin changes and action taken (e.g., "When changing in the pool locker room, therapist noted a 1" by 2" reddened area on client's left hip. Primary nurse notified."; "When checking residual limb after walking, an abnormal reddened area was evident. For duration of community integration session, prosthetic was removed and wheelchair was utilized for mobility. Upon return, therapist notified nursing for skin care and physical therapy to reassess prosthetic fit and appropriateness of prosthetic adjustments.").

Refer to specific diagnoses (e.g., diabetes, spinal cord injury, burns) for diagnosis-specific skin care issues. Refer to "Skin Breakdown" in the Techniques section for information on prevention and treatment of skin breakdown.

b820 Repair Functions of the Skin
Functions of the skin for repairing breaks and other damage to the skin.
Inclusions: functions of scab formation, healing, scarring; bruising and keloid formation
Exclusions: protective functions of the skin (b810); other functions of the skin (b830)

Treatment for
Repair Functions of the Skin

Repair functions of the skin can be enhanced through therapeutic interventions when needed. Refer to the specific diagnoses for information for specific therapeutic interventions to promote skin repair (e.g., burns, skin breakdowns). Interventions may include:

- *Bandaging*: e.g., cover with gauze and medical tape.
- *Antibiotics*: topical, oral, or intravenous.
- *Protection*: Guard against agents that further injure the skin or diminish healing capacity (e.g., removal of pressure from the area of skin breakdown; avoidance of activities that could break fragile, healing skin).

Recreational therapists document the specific interventions they use to prevent further injury to compromised skin as well as promote the healing process. For example, if a client has an early stage decubitus ulcer on top of the left knee from crossing his legs, the therapist may document: Client required minimal verbal cues to protect ulcer on top of left knee during activity.

b830 Other Functions of the Skin

Functions of the skin other than protection and repair, such as cooling and sweat secretion.
Inclusions: functions of sweating, glandular functions of the skin, and resulting body odour
Exclusions: protective functions of the skin (b810); repair functions of skin (b820)

Treatment for
Other Functions of the Skin

The skin functions as a cooling agent by sweating to decrease internal heat. Internal heat, however, may not always be fully released through sweating and can cause additional problems (e.g., heat stroke). People who have complete spinal cord injuries often do not sweat below the level of injury, therefore decreasing the efficiency of the skin to cool down the body. Excessive sweating, on the other hand, can cause social problems and body odor. See "Vital Signs" for more information about body temperature.

Recreational therapists need to be aware of the environment and activity as it relates to body temperature (e.g., a physical sports activity on a hot day will cause people to become hot and sweaty). Therapists problem solve to reduce the chances of heat stroke (e.g., areas for shade, cool water, brimmed sport hats, times for rest) and closely monitor clients who are at a high risk for health issues related to heat (e.g., people who have spinal cord injuries). Depending on the intensity of the activity and the temperature of the day, the activity may be contraindicated for some (e.g., people with high level complete spinal cord injuries, elderly people with heart conditions, people with multiple sclerosis).

Sweating can also cause problems because it creates a moist area. Skin breakdowns become more likely, transfers can be more difficult because of increased friction, and infection risk is increased because bacteria have a more hospitable area in which to grow. Precautions need to be taken to keep sensitive areas dry.

Therapists document the specific actions taken to cool body temperature when appropriate to diagnosis (e.g., client demonstrated ability to independently plan for and use cooling agents when outdoors in the heat; therapist recommended that client carry a cool water bottle and washcloth in backpack to cool down body on hot days).

b840 Sensation Related to the Skin

Sensations related to the skin such as itching, burning sensation, and tingling.
Inclusions: impairments such as pins and needles sensation and crawling sensation
Exclusion: sensation of pain (b280)

Treatment for
Sensations Related to the Skin

Sensations of the skin such as pins and needles, crawling sensations, itching, burning, and tingling are caused by different things. For example, the feeling of pins and needles is commonly felt when there is lack of blood flow to the area. Crawling sensations may be induced by drugs that cause hallucinations. Itching and burning can be caused by an irritant (e.g., allergic reaction to a plant or chemical) and tingling may be the result of nerve damage (e.g., peripheral neuropathy from diabetes). The cause must first be identified to treat the problem. Refer to the specific diagnosis for more information.

In most cases, with the exception of nerve damage, odd sensations of the skin are short-lived and have simple cures. For example, the feeling of pins and needles can be halted by increasing blood flow to the area (e.g., repositioning and rubbing the affected area to promote blood flow). Itching and burning caused by an irritant can often be treated by using a topical medication to reduce the reaction and avoiding of the irritant. Crawling sensations that are drug induced will commonly cease once the drug is no longer taken.

Sometimes adaptations need to be made for clients who are not able to monitor and act on their own. For example, a client may complain about pins and needles but lack the cognitive ability to understand that moving the affected area will help the situation. The recreational therapist should document the concern about restricted blood flow and be sure to add monitoring the client's position on a routine basis to the treatment plan. In cases where medications cause uncomfortable sensations, the therapist can provide information on relaxation, mental imagery, or other techniques that help the client tolerate the sensations.

b849 Functions of the Skin, Other Specified and Unspecified

Functions of the Hair and Nails (b850-b869)

b850 Functions of the Hair
Functions of the hair, such as protection, coloration, and appearance.
Inclusions: functions of growth of hair, pigmentation of hair, location of hair; impairments such as loss of hair or alopecia

Treatment for
Functions of the Hair

It is not within the scope of recreational therapy practice to score functions of the hair, but recreational therapists need to be aware of the functions of hair within activities and report on issues as they impact activity performance and participation. For example, clients who have hair loss (e.g., from cancer treatments) may have lower self-esteem, confidence, and body image. Hair loss may require added head protection in sunny weather and in cold weather. Use of a wig may require the therapist to assist the client in problem solving for wig care in specific situations such as rain or physical activity.

Recreational therapists document the specific hair problem (e.g., hair loss), the specific care that is required within activity (e.g., use of a baseball cap when interacting with peers lessens client's anxiety as per client report), the client's ability to perform and problem solve for such care (e.g., client independently dons and doffs baseball cap; client able to independently problem solve for situations when baseball cap may not be available to reduce anxiety), and special precautions taken by the therapist to ensure protection and optimal conditions (e.g., client instructed on importance of keeping head warm in cold weather; client able to verbally repeat information independently and demonstrate ability to protect head in cold weather as observed during community integration training session).

In addition to the issues discussed, therapists also document any noted hair changes and action taken (e.g., "When brushing hair prior to therapy session, excessive hair loss in brush was noted. Client reports that this is a new occurrence and is concerned. Nursing notified and informed client that hair loss is a side effect of XYZ medication.").

b860 Functions of the Nails
Functions of the nails, such as protection, scratching, and appearance.
Inclusions: growth and pigmentation of nails, quality of nails

Treatment for
Functions of the Nails

Clients who have brittle nails (e.g., clients who are malnourished) may have changes in the structure of fingernails and toenails that lead to splitting. Other clients may have behaviors that impair the functions of the nails, such as biting the nails. Both may increase the risk of infection, so therapists need to be aware of thorough hand washing and protective measures, such as gloves, during activities. Irritating chemicals that could enter the skin should be avoided.

Nail funguses can cause concerns about appearance. They may also be somewhat contagious, so precautions may need to be taken. Systemic medicines used to treat nail fungus can have side effects that the therapist needs to be aware of.

Recreational therapists document the specific nail problem (e.g., client bites nails down to the quick), the specific care that is required within activity (e.g., gloves are to be worn to prevent nail biting), the client's ability to perform and problem solve for such care (e.g., client has other material that is appropriate for chewing on), and special precautions taken by the therapist to ensure protection and optimal conditions.

In addition to the issues discussed, therapists also document any noted nail changes and action taken (e.g., "Client's nails are now long enough to use for peeling an orange.").

b869 Functions of the Hair and Nails, Other Specified and Unspecified

b898 Functions of the Skin and Related Structures, Other Specified

b899 Functions of the Skin and Related Structures, Unspecified

Body Structures

Body Structures is a list of the anatomical parts of the body used to indicate the extent, nature, and location of an impairment.

Scoring

Recreational therapists usually will not score codes in this component. However, it is important for therapists to understand how to read the scoring of this component for interpretative purposes.

Body structures are anatomical parts of the body such as organs, limbs, and their components.

Impairments are problems in body functions or structures representing a significant deviation or loss.

To score a Body Structures impairment the therapist first identifies the appropriate code to score using the General Coding Guidelines shown to the right.

The code is written down in its entirety. This includes the letter and number (all Body Structures codes begin with the letter "s"). A decimal point is placed after the code. After the decimal point, the score for the first qualifier, second qualifier, and third qualifier are placed in this order.

The scoring scale for Body Structures is shown in Table 17. There are two recommended qualifiers and one suggested qualifier.

Body Structures Code	1st Qualifier (Extent of Impairment)	2nd Qualifier (Nature of Impairment)	3rd Qualifier (suggested) (Location of Impairment)
s7300.	1	6	1

General Coding Guidelines

1. Choose the appropriate codes that best reflect the client's functioning as it relates to the purpose of the encounter.
2. Only choose codes that are relevant to the context of the health condition. For example, if a person has impairments of the heart, but is being evaluated for neurological functioning, only neurological functioning should be coded.
3. Do not make inferences (assumptions) about a client's functioning in other areas based on a Body Structures impairment. Each function should be evaluated and then scored separately. For example, just because a person has a moderate structure impairment of the heart (s4100 Heart), it does not mean that the client will have difficulty with b4550 General Physical Endurance.
4. Only choose codes that reflect the specific predefined timeframe. Functions that relate to a timeframe outside of the predefined timeframe should not be coded.
5. Use the most specific code whenever possible. For example, if a client has an impairment of the knee joint score the specific code of s75011 Knee Joint rather than the broad code of d7501 Structure of Lower Leg.

Example: A client has a mild deviating position impairment of the right upper arm. The Body Structures code for upper arm is s7300. The code appropriately written would look like this: s7300.161

Table 17: Body Structures Qualifiers

First Qualifier Extent of Impairment	Second Qualifier Nature of Impairment	Third Qualifier (suggested) Location of Impairment
0 NO impairment 1 MILD impairment 2 MODERATE impairment 3 SEVERE impairment 4 COMPLETE impairment 8 not specified 9 not applicable	0 no change in structure 1 total absence 2 partial absence 3 additional part 4 aberrant dimensions 5 discontinuity 6 deviating position 7 qualitative changes in structure, including accumulation of fluid 8 not specified 9 not applicable	0 more than one region 1 right 2 left 3 both sides 4 front 5 back 6 proximal 7 distal 8 not specified 9 not applicable

Chapter 1 Structures of the Nervous System

s110 Structure of Brain
- *s1100 Structure of Cortical Lobes*
  - ○ *s11000 Frontal Lobe*
  - ○ *s11001 Temporal Lobe*
  - ○ *s11002 Parietal Lobe*
  - ○ *s11003 Occipital Lobe*
  - ○ *s11008 Structure of Cortical Lobes, Other Specified*
  - ○ *s11009 Structure of Cortical Lobes, Unspecified*
- *s1101 Structure of Midbrain*
- *s1102 Structure of Diencephalon*
- *s1103 Basal Ganglia and Related Structures*
- *s1104 Structure of Cerebellum*
- *s1105 Structure of Brain Stem*
  - ○ *s11050 Medulla Oblongata*
  - ○ *s11051 Pons*
  - ○ *s11058 Structure of Brain Stem, Other Specified*
  - ○ *s11059 Structure of Brain Stem, Unspecified*
- *s1106 Structure of Cranial Nerves*
- *s1108 Structure of Brain, Other Specified*
- *s1109 Structure of Brain, Unspecified*

s120 Spinal Cord and Related Structures
- *s1200 Structure of Spinal Cord*
  - ○ *s12000 Cervical Spinal Cord*
  - ○ *s12001 Thoracic Spinal Cord*
  - ○ *s12002 Lumbosacral Spinal Cord*
  - ○ *s12003 Cauda Equina*
  - ○ *s12008 Structure of Spinal Cord, Other Specified*
  - ○ *s12009 Structure of Spinal Cored, Unspecified*
- *s1201 Spinal Nerves*
- *s1208 Spinal Cord and Related Structures, Other Specified*
- *s1209 Spinal Cord and Related Structure, Unspecified*

s130 Structure of Meninges

s140 Structure of Sympathetic Nervous System

s150 Structure of Parasympathetic Nervous System

s198 Structure of the Nervous System, Other Specified

s199 Structure of the Nervous System, Unspecified

Chapter 2 The Eye, Ear, and Related Structures

s210 Structure of the Eye Socket

s220 Structure of Eyeball
- *s2200 Conjunctiva, Sclera, Choroid*
- *s2201 Cornea*
- *s2202 Iris*
- *s2203 Retina*
- *s2204 Lens of Eyeball*
- *s2205 Vitreous Body*
- *s2208 Structure of Eyeball, Other Specified*
- *s2209 Structure of Eyeball, Unspecified*

s230 Structures Around the Eye
- *s2300 Lachrymal Gland and Related Structures*
- *s2301 Eyelid*
- *s2302 Eyebrow*
- *s2303 External Ocular Muscles*
- *s2308 Structures Around Eye, Other Specified*
- *s2309 Structure Around Eye, Unspecified*

s240 Structure of External Ear

s250 Structure of Middle Ear
- *s2500 Tympanic Membrane*
- *s2501 Eustachian Canal*
- *s2502 Ossicles*
- *s2508 Structure of Middle Ear, Other Specified*
- *s2509 Structure of Middle Ear, Unspecified*

s260 Structure of Inner Ear
- *s2600 Cochlea*
- *s2601 Vestibular Labyrinth*
- *s2602 Semicircular Canals*
- *s2603 Internal Auditory Meatus*
- *s2608 Structure of Inner Ear, Other Specified*
- *s2609 Structure of Inner Ear, Unspecified*

s298 Eye, Ear, and Related Structures, Other Specified

s299 Eye, Ear, and Related Structure, Unspecified

Chapter 3 Structures Involved in Voice and Speech

s310 Structure of Nose
- *s3100 External Nose*
- *s3101 Nasal Septum*
- *s3102 Nasal Fossae*
- *s3108 Structure of Nose, Other Specified*
- *s3109 Structure of Nose, Unspecified*

s320 Structure of Mouth
- *s3200 Teeth*
- *s3201 Gums*
- *s3202 Structure of Palate*
  - *s32020 Hard Palate*
  - *s32021 Soft Palate*
- *s3203 Tongue*
- *s3204 Structure of Lips*
  - *s32040 Upper Lip*
  - *s32041 Lower Lip*
- *s3208 Structure of Mouth, Other Specified*
- *s3209 Structure of Mouth, Unspecified*

s330 Structure of Pharynx
- *s3300 Nasal Pharynx*
- *s3301 Oral Pharynx*
- *s3308 Structure of Pharynx, Other Specified*
- *s3309 Structure of Pharynx, Unspecified*

s340 Structure of Larynx
- *s3400 Vocal Folds*
- *s3408 Structure of Larynx, Other Specified*
- *s3409 Structure of Larynx, Unspecified*

s398 Structures Involved in Voice and Speech, Other Specified

s399 Structures Involved in Voice and Speech, Unspecified

Chapter 4 Structures of the Cardiovascular, Immunological, and Respiratory Systems

s410 Structure of Cardiovascular System
- s4100 Heart
  - s41000 Atria
  - s41001 Ventricles
  - s41008 Structure of Heart, Other Specified
  - s41009 Structure of Heart, Unspecified
- s4101 Arteries
- s4102 Veins
- s4103 Capillaries
- s4108 Structures of Cardiovascular System, Other Specified
- s4109 Structures of Cardiovascular System, Unspecified

s420 Structure of Immune System
- s4200 Lymphatic Vessels
- s4201 Lymphatic Nodes
- s4202 Thymus
- s4203 Spleen
- s4204 Bone Marrow
- s4208 Structures of Immune System, Other Specified
- s4209 Structures of Immune System, Unspecified

s430 Structure of Respiratory System
- s4300 Trachea
- s4301 Lungs
  - s43010 Bronchial Tree
  - s43011 Alveoli
  - s43018 Structure of Lungs, Other Specified
  - s43019 Structure of Lungs, Unspecified
- s4302 Thoracic Cage
- s4303 Muscles of Respiration
  - s43030 Intercostal Muscles
  - s43031 Diaphragm
  - s43038 Muscles of Respiration, Other Specified
  - s43039 Muscles of Respiration, Unspecified
- s4308 Structure of Respiratory System, Other Specified
- s4309 Structure of Respiratory System, Unspecified

s498 Structures of the Cardiovascular, Immunological, and Respiratory Systems, Other Specified

s499 Structures of the Cardiovascular, Immunological, and Respiratory Systems, Unspecified

Chapter 5 Structures Related to the Digestive, Metabolic, and Endocrine Systems

s510 Structure of Salivary Glands

s520 Structure of Oesophagus

s530 Structure of Stomach

s540 Structure of Intestine
- *s5400 Small Intestine*
- *s5401 Large Intestine*
- *s5408 Structure of Intestine, Other Specified*
- *s5409 Structure of Intestine, Unspecified*

s550 Structure of Pancreas

s560 Structure of Liver

s570 Structure of Gall Bladder and Ducts

s580 Structure of Endocrine Glands
- *s5800 Pituitary Gland*
- *s5801 Thyroid Gland*
- *s5802 Parathyroid Gland*
- *s5803 Adrenal Gland*
- *s5808 Structure of Endocrine Glands, Other Specified*
- *s5809 Structure of Endocrine Glands, Unspecified*

s598 Structures Related to the Digestive, Metabolic, and Endocrine Systems, Other Specified

s599 Structures Related to the Digestive, Metabolic, and Endocrine Systems, Unspecified

Chapter 6 Structures Related to the Genitourinary and Reproductive Systems

s610 Structure of Urinary System
- s6100 Kidney
- s6101 Ureters
- s6102 Urinary Bladder
- s6103 Urethra
- s6108 Structure of Urinary System, Other Specified
- s6109 Structure of Urinary System, Unspecified

s620 Structure of Pelvic Floor

s630 Structure of Reproductive System
- s6300 Ovaries
- s6301 Structure of Uterus
  - s63010 Body of Uterus
  - s63011 Cervix
  - s63012 Fallopian Tubes
  - s63018 Structure of Uterus, Other Specified
  - s63019 Structure of Uterus, Unspecified
- s6302 Breast and Nipple
- s6303 Structure of Vagina and External Genitalia
  - s63030 Clitoris
  - s63031 Labia Majora
  - s63032 Labia Minora
  - s63033 Vaginal Canal
- s6304 Testes
- s6305 Structure of the Penis
  - s63050 Glans Penis
  - s63051 Shaft of Penis
  - s63058 Structure of Penis, Other Specified
  - s63059 Structure of Penis, Unspecified
- s6306 Prostate
- s6308 Structures of Reproductive Systems, Other Specified
- s6309 Structures of Reproductive Systems, Unspecified

s698 Structures Related to the Genitourinary and Reproductive Systems, Other Specified

s699 Structures Related to the Genitourinary and Reproductive Systems, Unspecified

Chapter 7 Structures Related to Movement

s710 Structure of Head and Neck Region
- s7100 Bones of Cranium
- s7101 Bones of Face
- s7102 Bones of Neck Region
- s7103 Joints of Head and Neck Region
- s7104 Muscles of Head and Neck Region
- s7105 Ligaments and Fasciae of Head and Neck Region
- s7108 Structures of Head and Neck Region, Other Specified
- s7109 Structure of Head and Neck Region, Unspecified

s720 Structure of Shoulder Region
- s7200 Bones of Shoulder Region
- s7201 Joints of Shoulder Region
- s7202 Muscles of Shoulder Region
- s7203 Ligaments and Fasciae of Shoulder Region
- s7208 Structure of Shoulder Region, Other Specified
- s7209 Structure of Shoulder Region, Unspecified

s730 Structure of Upper Extremity
- s7300 Structure of Upper Arm
  - s73000 Bones of Upper Arm
  - s73001 Elbow Joint
  - s73002 Muscles of Upper Arm
  - s73003 Ligaments and Fasciae of Upper Arm
  - s73008 Structure of Upper Arm, Other Specified
  - s73009 Structure of Upper Arm, Unspecified
- s7301 Structure of Forearm
  - s73010 Bones of Forearm
  - s73011 Wrist Joint
  - s73012 Muscles of Forearm
  - s73013 Ligaments and Fasciae of Forearm
  - s73018 Structure of Forearm, Other Specified
  - s73019 Structure of Forearm, Unspecified
- s7302 Structure of Hand
  - s73020 Bones of Hand
  - s73021 Joints of Hand and Fingers
  - s73022 Muscles of Hand
  - s73023 Ligaments and Fasciae of Hand
  - s73028 Structure of Hand, Other Specified
  - s73029 Structure of Hand, Unspecified
- s7308 Structure of Upper Extremity, Other Specified
- s7309 Structure of Upper Extremity, Unspecified

s740 Structure of Pelvic Region
- s7400 Bones of Pelvic Region
- s7401 Joints of Pelvic Region
- s7402 Muscles of Pelvic Region
- s7403 Ligaments and Fasciae of Pelvic Region
- s7408 Structure of Pelvic Region, Other Specified
- s7409 Structure of Pelvic Region, Unspecified

s750 Structure of Lower Extremity
- s7500 Structure of Thigh
  - s75000 Bones of Thigh
  - s75001 Hip Joint
  - s75002 Muscles of Thigh
  - s75003 Ligaments and Fasciae of Thigh
  - s75008 Structure of Thigh, Other Specified
  - s75009 Structure of Thigh, Unspecified
- s7501 Structure of Lower Leg
  - s75010 Bones of Lower Leg
  - s75011 Knee Joint
  - s75012 Muscles of Lower Leg
  - s75013 Ligaments and Fasciae of Lower Leg
  - s75018 Structure of Lower Leg, Other Specified
  - s75019 Structure of Lower Leg, Unspecified
- s7502 Structure of Ankle and Foot
  - s75020 Bones of Ankle and Foot
  - s75021 Ankle Joint and Joints of Foot and Toes
  - s75022 Muscles of Ankle and Foot
  - s75023 Ligaments and Fascia of Ankle and Foot
  - s75028 Structure of Ankle and Foot, Other Specified
  - s75029 Structure of Ankle and Foot, Unspecified
- s7508 Structure of Lower Extremity, Other Specified
- s7509 Structure of Lower Extremity, Unspecified

s760 Structure of Trunk
- s7600 Structure of Vertebral Column
  - s76000 Cervical Vertebral Column
  - s76001 Thoracic Vertebral Column
  - s76002 Lumbar Vertebral Column
  - s76003 Sacral Vertebral Column
  - s76004 Coccyx
  - s76008 Structure of Vertebral Column, Other Specified
  - s76009 Structure of Vertebral Column, Unspecified
- s7601 Muscles of Trunk
- s7602 Ligaments and Fasciae of Trunk
- s7608 Structure of Trunk, Other Specified
- s7609 Structure of Trunk, Unspecified

s770 Additional Musculoskeletal Structures Related to Movement
- *s7700 Bones*
- *s7701 Joints*
- *s7702 Muscles*
- *s7703 Extra-articular Ligaments, Fasciae, Extramuscular Aponeuroses, Retinacula, Septa, Bursae, Unspecified*
- *s7708 Additional Musculoskeletal Structures Related to Movement, Other Specified*

- *s7709 Additional Musculoskeletal Structures Related to Movement, Unspecified*

s798 Structures Related to Movement, Other Specified

s799 Structures Related to Movement, Unspecified

Chapter 8 Skin and Related Structures

s810 Structure of Areas of Skin
- *s8100 Skin of Head and Neck Region*
- *s8101 Skin of the Shoulder Region*
- *s8102 Skin of Upper Extremity*
- *s8103 Skin of Pelvic Region*
- *s8104 Skin of Lower Extremity*
- *s8105 Skin of Trunk and Back*
- *s8108 Structure of Areas of Skin, Other Specified*
- *s8109 Structure of Areas of Skin, Unspecified*

s820 Structure of Skin Glands
- *s8200 Sweat Glands*
- *s8201 Sebaceous Glands*
- *s8208 Structure of Skin Glands, Other Specified*
- *s8209 Structure of Skin Glands, Unspecified*

s830 Structure of Nails
- *s8300 Finger Nails*
- *s8301 Toe Nails*
- *s8308 Structure of Nails, Other Specified*
- *s8309 Structure of Nails, Unspecified*

s840 Structure of Hair

s898 Skin and Related Structures, Other Specified

s899 Skin and Related Structures, Unspecified

Activities and Participation

Activities and Participation contain some of the most important codes for recreational therapy practice. Included in this section are the activities of learning, performing tasks, communication, mobility, self-care, interpersonal interactions, major life areas, and community and social life. Everything we *do* as humans is included here.

Relationship between Activities and Participation and Other ICF Sections

When problems are seen in a client's ability to do activities or participate in the community, the problems can usually be traced to an impaired body function or body structure deficit. Determining treatment requires understanding the underlying cause of the problem. What recreational therapists see in their practice is a deficit at the activity and participation level. What they need to do to treat the problem is to find the underlying problem in body function or body structure.

A body function is a skill or ability to carry out a defined task or action. In some cases the client will be able to consciously modify performance, while in other cases the client will be unable to do so. Some examples of the types of body functions listed by the World Health Organization include sustaining attention (b1400), regulating the rate of the heart's rhythm (b4101), and speed of speech (b3302).

Some tasks cannot be performed because the body structure required to perform the task is no longer functioning. Some of the structures include the spinal cord (s1200) and the pelvic region (s740).

To understand how the codes interact, let's consider a client who has a problem with balance while bowling. One body structure code to check is the vestibular labyrinth in the inner ear (s2601). The Body Functions code is b2351 Vestibular Function of Balance. If either of these codes shows a deficit, the client will probably have trouble with balance. Treatment in this case would most likely consist of finding adaptations that allow the client to continue bowling using codes in Environmental Factors Chapter 1 Products and Technology.

However, there are other possibilities. One of the most important is that the client may not be strong enough to handle the weight of a bowling ball. One of the Muscle Power functions (b750) may be the problem. (There are many other possibilities.) The therapist's responsibility is to document more than the problem with bowling. The therapist and the rest of the treatment team should find the appropriate codes to document the observation at the body function and/or body structure level. In this example, documenting the weakness of the client will allow the therapist to carry out appropriate treatment with the goal of making the client strong enough to bowl.

All the parts of the ICF tie together to create a picture of the whole person. It is important to code appropriately in all sections of the codes to be sure the picture is accurate.

Scoring

Recreational therapists score Activities and Participation (A&P) codes in many practice settings.

Activity is the execution of a task or action by a client.

Activity limitations are difficulties a client may have in executing activities.

Capacity is a client's ability to execute an activity in a standardized testing environment (e.g., the therapy gym or clinic).

Participation is involvement in a life situation.

Participation restrictions are problems a client may experience with involvement in life situations.

Performance is a client's ability to participate in a life situation (an activity within his/her real-life environment such as a client's neighborhood, church, grocery store, senior center, home).

Assistance is the use of assistive devices or personal assistance. Personal assistance includes both hands-on assistance (e.g., providing moderate assistance for a transfer) and non-hands-on assistance such as cueing and emotional support.

Environmental factors (EF) make up the physical, social, and attitudinal environment in which people live. Environmental factors are a separate component of the ICF (referred to as e-codes). The EF definition is provided in this section because e-codes will commonly be attached to A&P codes and you will see them in the A&P examples.

To score an A&P difficulty the therapist first identifies the appropriate code to score using the General Coding Guidelines shown on the next page.

General Coding Guidelines

1. Choose the appropriate codes that best reflect the client's functioning as it relates to the purpose of the encounter.
2. Only choose codes that are relevant to the context of the health condition. For example, if a person has difficulty with d6500 Making and Repairing Clothes, but is being evaluated for community mobility (d4600 Moving Around in Different Locations) only mobility functioning should be coded.
3. Do not make inferences about a client's functioning in other areas based on an A&P difficulty. Each function should be evaluated and then scored separately. For example, just because a person has a moderate difficulty with d450 Walking it does not mean that the client will have difficulty with d4600 Moving Around in Different Locations.
4. Only choose codes that reflect the specific predefined timeframe. Functions that relate to a timeframe outside of the predefined timeframe should not be coded.
5. Use the most specific code whenever possible. For example, if a client has difficulty with manipulating small game pieces, score the specific code of d4402 Manipulating rather than the broader code of d440 Fine Hand Use.

The code is written down in its entirety. This includes the letter and number (all A&P codes begin with the letter "d"). A decimal point is placed after the code. After the decimal point there are four qualifiers and an additional fifth qualifier that is still in development.

The scoring for A&P is shown in Table 18. There are four qualifiers. The first and second qualifiers are required. The third and fourth qualifiers are optional.

1st Qualifier (required)	2nd Qualifier (required)	3rd Qualifier (optional)	4th Qualifier (optional)
Performance	Capacity (without assistance)	Capacity (with assistance)	Performance (without assistance)

Table 18: Scoring for Activities and Participation

Scoring for Each Qualifier		
0 NO difficulty	(none, absent, negligible...)	0-4%
1 MILD difficulty	(slight, low...)	5-24%
2 MODERATE difficulty	(medium, fair...)	25-49%
3 SEVERE difficulty	(high, extreme...)	50-95%
4 COMPLETE difficulty	(total...)	96-100%
8 not specified		
9 not applicable		

Example: A 6-year-old client named Sarah is admitted to an inpatient physical rehabilitation center. Her shyness in peer group play in the hospital playroom causes her severe difficulty with engagement in play. When the therapist (e335 Health Professionals) provides encouraging words and gently guides her into group play activities, her level of difficulty with engagement decreases to mild difficulty. The therapist conducts a home visit and asks her mother to invite two of Sarah's friends to the home. While at home, Sarah requires minimal verbal cues from her mother (e310 Immediate Family) to engage in play with her friends. With this prompting Sarah initiates and engages in play without any difficulty. The A&P code for play is d9200 Play. The code appropriately written using all four qualifiers and related e-codes would look like this: d9200.0311, E-codes: e335+2, e310+1. Scoring A&P qualifiers can be complex. The rest of the introduction will continue this example to show how the values for these qualifiers were assigned.

A&P Code	
A&P code	d9200.
1st Qualifier (performance)	0
2nd Qualifier (capacity without assistance)	3
3rd Qualifier (capacity with assistance)	1
4th Qualifier (performance without assistance)	1

E-code	
E-code	Extent of barrier or facilitator
E335	+2
E310	+1

Qualifier Scoring Descriptions

This section describes how the scores were determined for each of the qualifiers in the example above.

First Qualifier (required)

The first qualifier (performance) indicates the client's level of difficulty participating in a life situation with all usual and realistic supports (facilitators) and constraints (barriers).

Example: The real-life setting is the client's home. The usual and realistic facilitator is the mother's prompting. Since Sarah plays with no problems when the mother's prompting is available, she scores a "0" for no difficulty. Although she requires some assistance from her mother, the mother's assistance is usual and realistic. When this assistance is provide, there is no residual difficulty. The score would be written out like this: d9200.0 _ _ _.

Meaning of the Score

Level of difficulty with participation in a life situation with usual and realistic assistance. This score tells us how much help the client needs to do this activity in real life with the usual and realistic supports in place.

Key points

Exclude any assistance offered by the therapist: Assistance provided by the therapist is not a usual and realistic facilitator in a client's life because the therapist will not be part of the client's life after discharge. Only facilitators and barriers that are in the client's usual real-life situation are considered. This does not mean that the therapist cannot offer assistance in a real-life setting if it is needed, but the therapist must exclude his/her assistance from the total picture to arrive at an appropriate score for the first qualifier. For example, if the therapist was providing the prompting for Sarah to engage in play instead of her mother, the first qualifier would be scored a 1 for mild difficulty because in a real-life setting (when the therapist is not there), Sarah would have mild difficulty engaging in play.

Only score residual difficulty: When assistance is provided, the therapist scores the amount of difficulty that is left over (residual, unattended). So, if a client has moderate difficulty participating in a life situation and the client's spouse provides assistance to the client so that no difficulty remains, the client would be scored as having no difficulty. If a spouse provides a client with assistance but the client still struggles with the task (continues to exhibit mild difficulty with the task despite the assistance), the client would be scored as having mild difficulty. This is a very different way of thinking for therapists. Basically, it challenges health professionals to say, "It doesn't matter if the client needs minimal assistance to engage in play, her mom provides the prompting that she needs. There is no difficulty here." As health professionals we have been trained to see any deviation from independence as a problem. The ICF design reflects the true disability movement. If there are things in our environments that make up for our limitations (and we all have limitations of one

kind or another), we should not be labeled as deficient.

Score the average: The first qualifier is supposed to represent the client's level of functioning in his/her real-life setting when an average number of barriers and facilitators are present. This level of functioning can be very difficult to obtain. Recreational therapists who work in rehabilitation settings may only have the opportunity to do integration training one or two times with a client before s/he is discharged, making it difficult to get a true gauge of the average number of barriers and facilitators present in a specific life situation (e.g., all of the barriers or facilitators may not be present or the average may be misrepresented leading the therapist to an invalid score). Another problem is that life situations are always changing. For example, in one moment a family can be very supportive and helpful and in another moment an argument can break out causing the family to withdraw from the client and refuse to offer assistance. Consequently, the score assigned should try to reflect the average based on the therapist's best clinical judgment.

When to score this qualifier: It is unlikely that a therapist will have enough information on admission to score this qualifier. Therapists usually do not use integration training until later in the client's stay after s/he is medically stable. While it is possible to use the available information and clinical judgment to estimate the client's anticipated level of difficulty with a specific life situation, it is usually better to leave the qualifier blank until a more accurate score can be given. Do not use the score 8 (not specified) or 9 (not applicable). A blank space indicates that the qualifier is not being used. If this is a readmission for the same diagnosis with no significant change in the client's condition, then the therapist will be able to score this qualifier fairly accurately using information from the client and other sources. When integration training is started or more real-life situations are encountered later in the client's stay, the therapist will be able to score this qualifier much more accurately.

Second Qualifier (required)

The second qualifier (capacity without assistance) indicates the client's level of difficulty with an activity in a standardized testing environment without any assistance (person or device).

Example: The standard environment is the hospital playroom where children play on their own. When assistance is not provided, Sarah has severe difficulty engaging in play. (She chooses to withdraw from the activity area more than 50% of the time.) Severe difficulty as shown in Table 18 is scored as a

"3." The score for d9200 Play, including the first two qualifiers, would be written out like this: d9200.03 _ _.

Meaning of the Score

Level of difficulty with an activity in a standard environment without assistance from a person or device. This score tells us the client's baseline of functioning in a standard environment (e.g., clinic) when no assistance is being given. Baseline data is used to set treatment goals and objectives and measure progress.

Key points

Provide assistance if unsafe or unethical: Clients are never asked to perform a task or action that has the potential to cause the client harm (e.g., asking a client to walk without assistance). If it was unethical or unsafe to withhold personal assistance or a device, the therapist would use professional judgment through informal and formal assessment tools to arrive at an anticipated level of difficulty if the assistance or device was not provided.

Score the average: As with the first qualifier, a client's level of difficulty with an activity can vary due to many variables (e.g., mood, motivation, time of day). Therapists choose the average difficulty level from all of those observed for the activity.

How to assess baseline functioning: Therapists assess this function by providing the client with a task or requesting an action in a standardized environment and assessing the client's response (e.g., "Can you please read this to me?", "Do you remember my name?", "Can you raise your arm over your head?"). It can be difficult to obtain a true baseline, even in a standardized testing environment. The culprits that affect the baseline are mostly related to the client (e.g., level of motivation, energy, interest). A client's level of functioning can vary from day to day, with the time of day, and because of who is around. Consequently, the score that the therapist assigns should try to best reflect the average.

Third Qualifier (optional)

The third qualifier (capacity with assistance) indicates the client's level of difficulty with a task or action in a standardized testing environment with the assistance of a person or device.

Example: The standard environment is the hospital playroom. When assistance is provided by the therapist, Sarah has mild difficulty engaging in play. With the therapist helping her get started in activities, she is able to continue playing more than three fourths of the time, but not all of the time, so she would score a "1" for mild difficulty. The score

for d9200 Play, including the first three qualifiers, would be written out like this: d9200.031 _.

Meaning of the Score

Level of difficulty with an activity in a standard environment with assistance from a person or device. This score tell us how much difficulty a client has with an activity in the place of treatment when help from a person or device is provided (the client's optimal level of functioning in the hospital).

Key points

Only score residual difficulty: When assistance is provided, the therapist scores the amount of difficulty that is left over (residual, unattended). So, if a client has moderate difficulty participating in a task and the therapist provides assistance to the client so that no difficulty remains, the client would be scored as having no difficulty. If a therapist provides a client with assistance but the client still struggles with the task (continues to exhibit mild difficulty with the task despite the assistance), the client would be scored as having mild difficulty. This is a very different way of thinking for therapists. Therapists usually score the level of assistance that the client requires. Here the therapist scores only the level of difficulty that remains outside of the assistance provided. As health professionals we have been trained to see any deviation from independence as a problem. The ICF design reflects the true disability movement. If there are things in our environments that make up for our limitations (and we all have limitations of one kind or another), we should not be labeled as deficient.

Score the average: Like the second qualifier, it can be difficult to get a true score due to the many variables that can affect a client's level of functioning within a standardized testing environment (e.g., level of motivation, energy, interest). Consequently, the score that the therapist assigns should try to best reflect the average.

Fourth Qualifier (optional but highly recommended by the authors)

The fourth qualifier (performance without assistance) indicates the client's level of difficulty participating in a life situation without assistance from another person or the use of a device with consideration of environmental factors (and personal factors although not recorded) that could influence his/her performance.

Example: The real-life setting is the client's home. The usual and realistic facilitator is the mother's prompting. If this assistance (the mother's prompting) is taken away, Sarah would have mild difficulty engaging in play in her real-life environment. The mother has observed that Sarah will leave her friends about 10% of the time because of frustration with not being able to do something, so she would have a score of "1" for mild difficulty. The score for d9200 Play, with all of the qualifiers, would be written out like this: d9200.0311

Meaning of the Score

Level of difficulty that a client has participating in a life situation without assistance. This score tells us the worst-case scenario: If the client was home (participating in this specific activity in his/her real-life environment) and s/he had no assistance from a person or a device (which is possible at any time, e.g., family is unavailable to help), this is how much difficulty the client would have with this activity.

When compared to the first qualifier (performance), it highlights the importance (or hindrance) of environmental factors on the client's level of difficulty in a life situation. The question is, what is it specifically, that causes this difference? If we can identify the causes, then there is a chance that we can manipulate in a positive direction by encouraging continuation of positive influences (facilitators) or eliminating or reducing negative influences (barriers). These are referred to as Environmental Factors. Although there are several ways to list Environmental Factors, we highly recommend that they are attached to A&P codes to highlight variables that are affecting a client's level of difficulty.

Within the ICF, this qualifier is identified as being optional. Only the first two qualifiers are required. We strongly suggest that therapists complete the fourth qualifier whenever possible for the following reasons:

Better reflection of true performance: The first qualifier (performance) reflects the norm and the fourth qualifier (performance without assistance) reflects the worst-case scenario. As therapists, we understand that situations can change quickly and the client needs to be prepared to deal with challenges. There will be times when things go better than the norm and when things go worse. For planning purposes, it is important to know how much worse the situation can get.

Performance without assistance is not clearly deduced: It can be unclear in some cases (when looking at just the first qualifier) how much difficulty the client would have participating in life situations if assistance was taken away, especially if e-codes are not attached to the A&P code. For example, the first qualifier may reflect that the client has no difficulty with d630 Preparing Meals in a life situation with usual and realistic supports and constraints. This is misleading to the reader because it does not tell you that the reason she has no difficulty in preparing meals is because her sister (e310 Immediate Family) helps her with 75% of the work. Now, if an e-code was attached to the A&P code to reflect the help from

the sister and it was rated a substantial facilitator (d630.0 _ _ _, E-code: e310+3), the reader could see that if the facilitator was taken away, the client would have severe difficulty with the task of Preparing Meals. The first qualifier "0" would become a "3" without the sister's help. So, e-codes help. But even if e-codes are attached to A&P codes, the reader may still not be able to get a clear picture of the worst-case scenario if the assistance is not provided. Health professionals may not attach all of the appropriate e-codes. There may be so many e-codes that the reader can't figure out what the client's level of difficulty would be if the assistance was not provided. A client's participation in real-life situations is a strong focus of recreational therapy practice. By scoring the fourth qualifier we can provide more accurate levels of community functioning.

Promotes attention to environmental factors: When we can easily see the difference in functioning between the first and fourth qualifier, it highlights the importance of environmental factors that are causing the difference. Disparities get attention. The more disparities that are reflected between the first and fourth qualifier, the more attention it can bring to reviewers of the importance of encouraging and promoting facilitators and eliminating or reducing barriers that are outside of the immediate person. Changes within the environment can play a large role in making changes in health.

Key points

Exclude assistance from all sources: When determining the score for this qualifier, the therapist uses clinical judgment (in most cases) to determine the level of difficulty that a client would have participating in a specific life situation without assistance from a person or device. This includes assistance not only from the therapist, but also from any other person who would help the client with participation in the specific life situation (e.g., other health care professionals, family, friends).

Provide assistance if unsafe or unethical: Like the second qualifier, clients are never asked to participate in a life situation that has the potential to cause the client harm (e.g., asking a client to walk around the neighborhood without assistance or a device that is needed for safety). In this case, the therapist would use professional judgment through informal and formal assessment tools to arrive at an anticipated level of difficulty if the assistance or device was not provided.

Score the average: Like the previous qualifiers, identifying a true score is almost impossible because of the constant fluctuation of internal and external variables that can affect a client's level of functioning. Consequently, the score that the therapist assigns should reflect the average. Like the first qualifier, it can be difficult for recreational therapists who work in a rehabilitation setting to identify an accurate score for this qualifier due to the often limited number of integration training sessions with clients.

Fifth Qualifier

The fifth qualifier is currently not shown or scored. It is unknown and is still in development. It is possible that it might be used to reflect the client's level of involvement in the activity or subjective satisfaction.

Blended Scores

Turn to the A&P section of this book and take a look at some of the A&P codes. You will find that they are all blended activities. What this means is that they are all activities that are comprised of multiple skill sets. For example, d4554 Swimming is defined as "propelling the whole body through water by means of limb and body movements without taking support from the ground underneath." This requires many skills including; mobility of joints (b710 Mobility of Joint Functions), upper body and lower body strength (b730 Muscle Power Functions), endurance (b740 Muscle Endurance Functions), and control and coordination of voluntary movements (b7601 Control of Complex Voluntary Movements, b7602 Coordination of Voluntary Movement).

It is important not to get caught up in the Body Functions skills and look at the A&P questions, how well does the client swim? Regardless of how it is done (as long as it's swimming of some kind), the therapist scores the amount of difficulty the client has with getting in and out of the pool and swimming from one point to another. We suggest scoring the level of difficulty for the part of the task the client needs the most help with. It really doesn't matter that the client can get in the water and swim with no difficulty. If s/he has moderate difficulty getting out

of the water, the activity of swimming is scored as moderate difficulty.

A&P codes that include a variety of activities can also pose a problem. For example, d9201 Sports is defined as "engaging in competitive and informal or formally organized games or athletic events, performed alone or in a group, such as bowling, gymnastics, or soccer." If a client participates in three different sports and has different average levels of difficulty for each sport, there can be a problem in scoring. Let's say the client had mild difficulty engaging in bowling, moderate difficulty with baseball, and severe difficulty with tennis. In this case, the therapist would need to choose the maximum level of difficulty the client has with sports (severe difficulty with tennis in this example). Another possibility that might be considered occurs if the client participates in tennis only because his best friend plays. The client might not consider it a sport at all. Then it might be better to score the activity of tennis as d7500 Informal Relationships with Friends and not d9301 Sports. In that case baseball would be the most difficult sport, so the overall score would be d9201 Sports, moderate difficulty. The appropriate way to blend scores is not settled yet, so therapists will need to score codes as they feel is appropriate and stay aware of the latest thinking in the field.

Addition of a Participation Score

When scoring codes in A&P Chapter 9 Community, Social, and Civic Life, we suggested that recreational therapists write in an additional Dehn code to the right of the scored ICF code. The Dehn code is not part of the ICF. It is an additional code that would help clarify a client's level of participation. See "Participation" in the Concepts section for more information on how this code can be helpful and how it can complement ICF scoring in this chapter.

Chapter 1 Learning and Applying Knowledge

This chapter is about learning, applying the knowledge that is learned, thinking, solving problems, and making decisions.

This section is the cousin to Body Functions Chapter 1 Mental Functions. The Body Functions reflects brain functions and Activities and Participation reflects brain activities. It is very difficult for the clinician to differentiate between the two because therapists use activities to determine the functioning of the brain. For example, a therapist presents the client with a problem solving activity to assess the brain function of problem solving. Examples of codes that are closely related include:

- b1646 Problem-Solving versus d175 Solving Problems.
- b1400 Sustaining Attention versus d160 Focusing Attention.
- b1720 Simple Calculation versus d150 Learning to Calculate.

Consequently, much of the description on how to assess, treat, document, and adapt for cognitive/mental tasks is in Body Functions Chapter 1 Mental Functions. Within this section the reader is directed to the appropriate Body Functions code for more information. For a review of the normal functioning of the brain, refer to "Nervous System" in the Concepts section.

Purposeful Sensory Experiences (d110-d129)

Purposeful Sensory Experiences comprises the activities of watching, listening, and other purposeful sensing. A description will follow each code directing the therapist to the appropriate codes that impact a person's ability to perform the activity. In general a person needs to be conscious, and have skills on some level of mental attention. Refer to b110 Consciousness and b140 Attention Functions for information on how to assess, treat, document, and adapt for these precursor skills of "Purposeful Sensory Experiences."

d110 Watching
Using the sense of seeing intentionally to experience visual stimuli, such as watching a sporting event or children playing.

Treatment for
Watching

To be able to use the sense of watching to intentionally experience visual stimuli a client needs to possess those skills mentioned at the beginning of the code set (b110 Consciousness and b140 Attention Functions) and have vision. Refer to b210 through

b229 Seeing and Related Functions for information on how to assess, treat, document, and adapt for consciousness and seeing functions that are needed for watching.

d115 Listening
Using the sense of hearing intentionally to experience auditory stimuli, such as listening to a radio, music, or a lecture.

Treatment for
Listening

To be able to use the sense of hearing to intentionally experience auditory stimuli the client needs to possess the skills mentioned at the beginning of the code set (b110 Consciousness and b140 Attention Functions) and have the sense of hearing. Refer to b230 Hearing Functions for information on how to assess, treat, document, and adapt for consciousness and hearing functions that are needed for listening.

d120 Other Purposeful Sensing
Using the body's other basic senses intentionally to experience stimuli, such as touching and feeling textures, tasting sweets, or smelling flowers.

Treatment for
Other Purposeful Sensing

To be able to use other basic senses to intentionally experience stimuli, such as touching and feeling textures, tasting sweets, or smelling flowers a client needs to have the skills mentioned at the beginning of the code set (b110 Consciousness and b140 Attention Functions) and have the sense of touch, taste, and smell. Refer to b265 Touch Function, b250 Taste Function, and b255 Smell Function for information on how to assess, treat, document, and adapt for consciousness, touch, taste, and smell functions that are needed for other purposeful sensing.

d129 Purposeful Sensory Experiences, Other Specified and Unspecified.

Basic Learning (d130-d159)
Basic learning comprises the activities of copying, rehearsing, learning to read, learning to write, learning to calculate, and acquiring skills. A description will follow each code directing the therapist to the appropriate Mental Functions codes that impact a person's ability to perform the activity.

In general a person needs to be conscious, and have skills on some level of mental attention, memory, and perception to perform the activities in this section. Refer to b110 Consciousness, b140 Attention Functions, b144 Memory Functions, and b156 Perceptual Functions for information on how to assess, treat, document, and adapt for these precursor skills of Basic Learning.

d130 Copying
Imitating or mimicking as a basic component of learning, such as copying a gesture, a sound, or the letters of an alphabet.

Treatment for
Copying

To be able to mimic a basic component of learning such as copying a gesture, sound, or letter of the alphabet a variety of mental and physical skills are needed (including those mentioned at the beginning of this code set). The specific skills will vary depending on the desired activity (e.g., mimicking a sound requires different skills than copying a gesture). The therapist will need to determine the components of the specific activity through task analysis. (See "Activity and Task Analysis" in the Techniques section.) Once the components are identified, specific areas of breakdown can be identified and then referred to in this book for information on how to assess, treat, document, and adapt for the specific skill. For example, if the client is having problems with joint mobility impacting her ability to mimic a hand gesture, then the therapist would refer to b710 Mobility of Joint Functions for information on how to assess, treat, document, and adapt for the problem.

d135 Rehearsing
Repeating a sequence of events or symbols as a basic component of learning, such as counting by tens or practicing the recitation of a poem.

Treatment for
Rehearsing

To be able to repeat a sequence of events or symbols such as counting by tens or practicing the recitation of a poem, the client requires a variety of mental and/or physically based skills (including those mentioned at the beginning of this code set). The specific skills will vary depending on the desired activity (e.g., repeating a dance sequence requires different skills than reciting a poem). The therapist will need to determine the components of the specific activity through task analysis. (See "Activity and Task Analysis" in the Techniques section.) Once the

components are identified, specific areas of breakdown can be identified and then referred to in this book for information on how to assess, treat, document, and adapt for the specific skill. For example, if the client is having problems with memory impacting his ability to recite a poem, then the therapist would refer to b144 Memory Functions for information on how to assess, treat, document, and adapt for the problem.

d140 Learning to Read
Developing the competence to read written material (including Braille) with fluency and accuracy, such as recognizing characters and alphabets, sounding out words with correct pronunciation, and understanding words and phrases.

Treatment for
Learning to Read

To be able to read written material (including Braille) with fluency and accuracy a variety of mental and/or physically based skills are needed (including those mentioned at the beginning of this code set). The specific skills will vary depending on the desired activity (e.g., sounding out letters requires different skills than recognizing Braille words), however the following additional basic precursor skills should be considered:

- *For sounding out letters/words*: b310 Voice Functions, b320 Articulation Functions, b330 Fluency and Rhythm of Speech Functions, b340 Alternative Vocalization Functions, and b230 Hearing Functions.
- *For reading written words*: b167 Mental Functions of Language, b210 Seeing Functions.
- *For reading Braille words*: b1564 Tactile Perception.

The therapist will need to determine the components of the specific activity through task analysis. (See "Activity and Task Analysis" in the Techniques section.) Once the components are identified, specific areas of breakdown can be identified and then referred to in this book for information on how to assess, treat, document, and adapt for the specific skill. For example, if the client is having problems with attention that are impacting her ability to read written words, then the therapist would refer to b140 Attention Functions for information on how to assess, treat, document, and adapt for the problem.

d145 Learning to Write
Developing the competence to produce symbols that represent sounds, words, or phrases in order to convey meaning (including Braille writing), such as spelling effectively and using correct grammar.

Treatment for
Learning to Write

To be able to produce symbols that represent sounds, words, or phrases to convey meaning a variety of mental and/or physically based skills are needed (including those mentioned at the beginning of this code set). The specific skills will vary depending on the desired activity (e.g., painting Chinese symbols requires different skills than writing a letter), however the following additional basic precursor skills should be considered:

- *Writing with sight*: b167 Mental Functions of Language, b210 Seeing Functions, d440 Fine Hand Use, d4463 Turning or Twisting the Hands or Arms.
- *Writing without sight*: All of above except b210 Seeing Functions. Additionally, b1564 Tactile Perception.

The therapist will need to determine the components of the specific activity through task analysis. (See "Activity and Task Analysis" in the Techniques section.) Once the components are identified, specific areas of breakdown can be identified and then referred to in this book for information on how to assess, treat, document, and adapt for the specific skill. For example, if the client is having a problem with grasping a pen and it is impacting his ability to write, then the therapist would refer to d4401 Grasping for information on how to assess, treat, document, and adapt for the problem.

d150 Learning to Calculate
Developing the competence to manipulate numbers and perform simple and complex mathematical operations, such as using mathematical signs for addition and subtraction and applying the correct mathematical operation to a problem.

Treatment for
Learning to Calculate

To be able to manipulate numbers and perform simple and complex mathematical operations, a client needs a variety of mental and/or physically based skills (including those mentioned at the beginning of this code set). The specific skills will vary depending on the desired activity (e.g., adding two single digit numbers requires different skills than balancing a checkbook), however the following additional basic precursor skills should be considered: b172 Calculation Functions and b210 Seeing Functions, as well as d440 Fine Hand Use and b710 Mobility of Joint Functions (for operation and manipulation of a pencil, calculator, etc.). The therapist will need to determine the components of the specific activity

through task analysis. (See "Activity and Task Analysis" in the Techniques section.) Once the components are identified, specific areas of breakdown can be identified and then referred to in this book for information on how to assess, treat, document, and adapt for the specific skill. For example, if the client is having problems with the mental skill of addition and they are impacting her ability to learn how to calculate, then the therapist would refer to b1720 Simple Calculation for information on how to assess, treat, document, and adapt for the problem.

d155 Acquiring Skills
Developing basic and complex competencies in integrated sets of actions or tasks so as to initiate and follow through with the acquisition of a skill, such as manipulating tools or playing games like chess.
Inclusions: acquiring basic and complex skills

- *d1550 Acquiring Basic Skills*
  Learning elementary, purposeful actions, such as learning to manipulate eating utensils, a pencil, or a simple tool.
- *d1551 Acquiring Complex Skills*
  Learning integrated sets of actions so as to follow rules, and to sequence and coordinate one's movements, such as learning to play games like football, or to use a building tool.
- *d1558 Acquiring Skills, Other Specified*
- *d1559 Acquiring Skills, Unspecified*

Treatment for
Acquiring Skills

There are two kinds of skills that are especially important for recreational therapists, leisure activity skills and skills related to advanced activities of daily living. Leisure activity skills are skills that allow an individual to "engage in any form of play, recreation, or leisure activity, such as informal or organized play and sports, programs of physical fitness, relaxation, amusement or diversion, going to art galleries, museums, cinemas, or theatres; engaging in crafts or hobbies, reading for enjoyment, playing musical instruments; sight seeing, tourism, and traveling for pleasure" (d920 Recreation and Leisure). Advanced activities of daily living include shopping, banking, related travel, and other complex activities required for daily life.

This code covers the process of teaching clients new activity skills such as learning a new game, hobby, or sport. It is not the process of restoring lost skills and advancing developmental skills (e.g., improving memory skills, direction following). Skills development assumes that the client possesses the underlying skills to learn a new activity and the therapist is the facilitator to teach the client the new activity.

Although recreational therapy uses the term leisure skills development, the ICF does not recognize this term. Because the ICF is client-centered rather than therapy-centered, it does not look at teaching; it looks at learning. Therefore, therapists determine a client's ability to acquire basic skills (d1550) and acquire complex skills (d1551) according to the extent of impairment. Activities that are taught to the client (e.g., tennis, fishing) are reflected by using these two codes. The specific activity (e.g., tennis) can be noted to the right of the scoring area. Many activity skills that are taught to a client can be scored under these two codes, although there are also many places in Activities and Participation that refer to specific leisure activity skills (e.g., d6505 Taking Care of Plants, d6500 Making and Repairing Clothes). Therapists should be careful not to use the d920 Recreation and Leisure code set (in the Activities and Participation Chapter 9 Community, Social, and Civic Life) for leisure skills development because the d920 Recreation and Leisure code set reflects *participation* in a specific activity (e.g., d9201 Sports) rather than *acquiring* activity skills (e.g., acquiring skills to play the game of football).

d159 Basic Learning Skills, Other Specified and Unspecified

Applying Knowledge (d160-d179)

Applying Knowledge comprises the activities of focusing attention, thinking, reading, writing, and calculating, solving problems, and making decisions. Note that there is a difference in this section of *applying knowledge* compared to the previous section of *acquiring skills*. For example, in the previous section d140 Learning to Read addressed *learning* the skill whereas in this section d166 Reading addresses the *application* of the skill (to read for the purpose of obtaining general knowledge or specific information). A description will follow each code directing the therapist to other appropriate codes that impact a person's ability to perform the activity. In general a person needs to be conscious, and have skills on some level of mental attention to perform the activities in this section. Refer to b110 Consciousness, b140 Attention Functions, and b160 Thought Functions for information on how to assess, treat, document, and adapt for these precursor skills of "Applying Knowledge."

d160 Focusing Attention
Intentionally focusing on specific stimuli, such as by filtering out distracting noises.

Treatment for Focusing Attention

To focus on specific stimuli and filter out distractions, a variety of mentally based skills are needed (including those mentioned at the beginning of this code set). More specifically one or more of the subcomponents of b140 Attention Functions are needed depending on the specific task that requires focused attention (b1400 Sustaining Attention, b1401 Shifting Attention, b1402 Dividing Attention, b1403 Sharing Attention). The therapist will need to determine the components of the specific activity through task analysis. (See "Activity and Task Analysis" in the Techniques section.) Once the components are identified, specific areas of breakdown can be identified and then referred to in this book for information on how to assess, treat, document, and adapt for the specific skill. For example, if the client's problem with focusing attention in a group activity is impacting his ability to complete the task at hand, the therapist may refer to b1402 Shifting Attention for information on how to assess, treat, document, and adapt for the problem.

d163 Thinking
Formulating and manipulating ideas, concepts, and images, whether goal-oriented or not, either alone or with others, such as creating fiction, proving a theorem, playing with ideas, brainstorming, meditating, pondering, speculating, or reflecting.
Exclusions: Solving Problems (d175), Making Decisions (d177)

Treatment for Thinking

To formulate and manipulate ideas, concepts, and images a variety of mentally based skills are needed (including those mentioned at the beginning of this code set). Additional skills that may be needed, depending on the complexity of the task, include subcomponents of b144 Memory Functions, b160 Thought Functions, b164 Higher-level Cognitive Functions (b1640 Abstraction, b1641 Organization and Planning, b1642 Time Management, b1643 Cognitive Flexibility, b1644 Insight, b1645 Judgment, b1646 Problem Solving). The therapist will need to determine the components of the specific activity through task analysis. (See "Activity and Task Analysis" in the Techniques section.) Once the components are identified, specific areas of breakdown can be identified and then referred to in this book for information on how to assess, treat, document, and adapt for the specific skill. For example, if client is having problems with abstraction that are impacting his ability to complete the thinking task at hand, the therapist may refer to b1640 Abstraction for information on how to assess, treat, document, and adapt for the problem.

d166 Reading

Performing activities involved in the comprehension and interpretation of written language (e.g., books, instructions, or newspapers in text or Braille), for the purpose of obtaining general knowledge or specific information.
Exclusions: Learning to Read (d140)

Treatment for Reading

To perform reading activities involved in the comprehension and interpretation of written language, the client needs a variety of mentally based skills (including those mentioned at the beginning of this code set). More specifically, subcomponents of b144 Memory Functions and those skills needed for code d140 Learning to Read (for reading written words: b167 Mental Functions of Language, b210 Seeing Functions; for reading Braille words: b1564 Tactile Perception). The therapist will need to determine the components of the specific activity through task analysis. (See "Activity and Task Analysis" in the Techniques section.) Once the components are identified, specific areas of breakdown can be identified and then referred to in this book for information on how to assess, treat, document, and adapt for the specific skill. For example, if the client is having a problem with feeling the raised Braille symbols and it is impacting her ability to comprehend and interpret the text, the therapist may refer to b1564 Tactile Perception for information on how to assess, treat, document, and adapt for the problem.

d170 Writing

Using or producing symbols or language to convey information, such as producing a written record of events or ideas or drafting a letter.
Exclusions: Learning to Write (d145)

Treatment for Writing

To perform writing activities involved in using or producing symbols or language to convey information, the client needs a variety of mentally and physically based skills (including those mentioned at the beginning of this code set). More specifically the skills that are needed for the code d145 Learning to Write (writing with sight: b167 Mental Functions of Language, b210 Seeing Functions, d440 Fine Hand Use, d4463 Turning or Twisting the Hands or Arms; writing without sight:

all of above except b210 Seeing Functions, additionally b1564 Tactile Perception). Depending on the complexity of the writing activity, subcomponents of b164 Higher Level Cognitive Functions may also be needed. The therapist will need to determine the components of the specific activity through task analysis. (See "Activity and Task Analysis" in the Techniques section.) Once the components are identified, specific areas of breakdown can be identified and then referred to in this book for information on how to assess, treat, document, and adapt for the specific skill. For example, if the client is having problems with organizing skills that are impacting his ability to organize a letter, the therapist may refer to b1641 Organization and Planning for information on how to assess, treat, document, and adapt for the problem.

d172 Calculating

Performing computations by applying mathematical principles to solve problems that are described in words and producing or displaying the results, such as computing the sum of three numbers or finding the result of dividing one number by another.
Exclusions: Learning to Calculate (d150)

Treatment for Calculating

To perform computations by applying mathematical principles to solve problems, the client needs a variety of mentally and physically based skills (including those mentioned at the beginning of this code set). Specific required skills include the ones that are needed for code d150 Learning to Calculate (b172 Calculation Functions, b210 Seeing Functions, d440 Fine Hand Use, b710 Mobility of Joint Functions). Depending on the complexity of the calculating activity, subcomponents of b164 Higher Level Cognitive Functions may also be needed. The therapist will need to determine the components of the specific activity through task analysis. (See "Activity and Task Analysis" in the Techniques section.) Once the components are identified, specific areas of breakdown can be identified and then referred to in this book for information on how to assess, treat, document, and adapt for the specific skill. For example, if the client is having difficulty with problem solving that is impacting her ability to perform computations, the therapist may refer to b1646 Problem Solving for information on how to assess, treat, document, and adapt for the problem.

d175 Solving Problems

Finding solutions to questions or situations by identifying and analyzing issues, developing options and solutions, evaluating potential effects of solutions,

and executing a chosen solution, such as in resolving a dispute between two people.
Inclusions: solving simple and complex problems
Exclusions: thinking (d163), making decisions (d177)

- *d1750 Solving Simple Problems*
  Finding solutions to a problem involving a single issue or question, by identifying and analyzing the issue, developing solutions, evaluating the potential effects of the solutions, and executing a chosen solution.
- *d1751 Solving Complex Problems*
  Finding solutions to a complex problem involving multiple and interrelated issues, or several related problems, by identifying and analyzing the issue, developing solutions, evaluating the potential effects of the solutions, and executing a chosen solution.
- *d1758 Solving Problems, Other Specified*
- *d1759 Solving Problems, Unspecified*

Treatment for
Solving Problems

Finding solutions to questions or situation by identifying and analyzing issues, developing options and solutions, evaluating potential effects of solutions, and executing a chosen solution requires a variety of mentally (and possibly physically) based skills (including those mentioned at the beginning of this code set). More specifically, b164 Higher Level Cognitive Functions and its subcomponents, b160 Thought Functions, and b144 Memory Functions may be required. The therapist will need to determine the components of the specific activity through task analysis. (See "Activity and Task Analysis" in the Techniques section.) Once the components are identified, specific areas of breakdown can be identified and then referred to in this book for information on how to assess, treat, document, and adapt for the specific skill. For example, if the client's difficulty with short-term memory is impacting her ability to solve problems, the therapist may refer to b1440 Short Term Memory for information on how to assess, treat, document, and adapt for the problem.

d177 Making Decisions
Making a choice among options, implementing the choice, and evaluating the effects of the choice, such as selecting and purchasing a specific item, or deciding to undertake and undertaking one task from among several tasks that need to be done.
Exclusions: thinking (d163), solving problems (b175)

Treatment for
Making Decisions

To make a choice among options, implement the choice, and evaluate the effects of the choice, the client needs a variety of mentally and possibly physically (e.g., writing options on paper to help make decisions) based skills (including those mentioned at the beginning of this code set). More specifically b164 Higher Level Cognitive Functions and its subcomponents, b160 Thought Functions, and b144 Memory Functions may be required. The therapist will need to determine the components of the specific activity through task analysis. (See "Activity and Task Analysis" in the Techniques section.) Once the components are identified, specific areas of breakdown can be identified and then referred to in this book for information on how to assess, treat, document, and adapt for the specific skill. For example, if the client has difficulty being optimistic (perhaps feeling that it doesn't matter what choice she makes because it will always result in a negative outcome), the therapist may refer to b1265 Optimism for information on how to assess, treat, document, and adapt for the problem.

d179 Applying Knowledge, Other Specified and Unspecified

d198 Learning and Applying Knowledge, Other Specified

d199 Learning and Applying Knowledge, Unspecified

Chapter 2 General Tasks and Demands

This chapter is about general aspects of carrying out single or multiple tasks, organizing routines, and handling stress. These items can be used in conjunction with more specific tasks or actions to identify the underlying features of the execution of tasks under different circumstances.

Introduction

This chapter is about *tasks*. A task is the direct effort of one person or a group to complete a goal. A task generally occurs in a sequential order and has a beginning point and a target outcome (Peabody, 2001). This chapter is also about *demands*. A demand is either an internal or an external motivation to take action to fulfill a need. The majority of work done with a client can be boiled down to helping clients master tasks to fulfill demands.

The World Health Organization recognizes the ability to complete many different tasks as the basis for taking care of oneself and fitting into one's community. Because of the importance of being able to undertake and complete all types of tasks, the World Health Organization made *tasks* its own, major chapter in its system of categorization. *General Tasks and Demands* is the second of nine Activities and Participation (A&P) categories, or chapters. Therapists are expected to assess the client's ability to perform these functions and provide interventions when appropriate. To be able to do this, it helps to understand what types of skills are included within each of the subcategories of General Tasks and Demands.

The category of General Tasks and Demands is divided into four subcategories: 1. undertaking a single task, 2. undertaking multiple tasks, 3. carrying out daily routine, and 4. handling stress and other psychological demands. The rest of this chapter will explain each of these subcategories and provide suggestions and guidelines for recreational therapy interventions. As discussed in the introduction to this section, the category of General Tasks and Demands requires the therapist to understand the other parts of the ICF because the tasks rely on physical, mental, social, or psychological body functions; body structures; and environmental factors.

Notice that the Tasks and Demands categories include Carrying Out Daily Routine and Handling Stress and Other Psychological Demands. At first it might seem like these two categories don't belong in this section. The reason that they are included is because the ability to carry out a daily routine is a general life task and handling stress and other psychological demands is part of our everyday lives. To help the therapist address client needs in these areas this chapter not only explains the subcategories,

but also provides references to numerous intervention techniques included in the Techniques section.

When problems are seen in a client's ability to perform a task, it is usually a result of an impaired body function, a body structure deficit, or an inappropriate environment. The one most amenable to treatment is a problem with a body function.

In some cases the client will be able to consciously modify body function performance while in other cases the client will be unable to do so. Some examples of the types of body functions listed by the World Health Organization include sustaining attention (b1400), regulating heart rate and heart rhythm (b4100 and b4101), and speed of speech (b3302). The therapist's job is to have an activity analysis of a task to compare the client's performance against the task analysis. (See the Techniques section for more information on "Activity and Task Analysis.") The client's ability (or inability) to perform each of the functions that are part of the task in the correct sequential order helps the therapist identify where functional breakdown occurs.

To address isolated skills the therapist has to understand the body functions required to carry out the skill. For example, a therapist must understand the basic anatomy of the brain and how it works. This understanding helps the therapist appreciate the theories of neuroplasticity (adaptability, flexibility, and malleability of brain cells) and cognitive retraining, which help enhance cognitive functioning. If the therapist doesn't understand the workings of the brain, then s/he will not be able to grasp the value of interventions. While this chapter covers many different tasks and the related interventions, the therapist will need to refer to other portions of this book for additional information.

As an example, let's look at a therapist working with a client who has difficulty undertaking a single task of repotting a plant. By watching the client try to pot the plant, the therapist finds that the client has difficulty because she 1. has tremors in both of her hands (problems with b765 Involuntary Movement because of tremors) and 2. is neglecting the tools and supplies on the left side of the table (problems with left neglect b2101 Visual Field Functions). After the recreational therapist reports these problems to the team, the occupational therapist searches her database for tasks that require visual field functions and together both therapists work on a unified approach to address this impairment. The physical therapist and physician work on a combined treatment and medication protocol to reduce problems with involuntary movement. The recreational therapist will be able to report on the success of the interventions by continued observation of the client in activities.

Therapeutic Interventions Used for Tasks

The therapist will use both educational techniques and counseling techniques when addressing client impairments related to general tasks and demands. See "Education and Counseling" in the Techniques section for more information.

The first three subcategories under General Tasks and Demands relate to the ability to *act*. The fourth subcategory relates to the client's ability to regulate his/her emotional *reaction* to demands. While the distinction between leisure education and leisure counseling is not well established in the field of recreational therapy, we believe it is best to apply leisure education (actions) interventions to the first three subcategories and apply leisure counseling techniques (related to feelings, attitudes, values, and beliefs that impact how a person reacts) to the fourth subcategory. This is not a perfect division because the therapist might use either technique in any of the categories. However, the therapist is likely to rely on leisure counseling techniques more heavily in self-regulation interventions.

d210 Undertaking a Single Task
Carrying out simple or complex and coordinated actions related to the mental and physical components of a single task, such as initiating a task, organizing time, space, and materials for a task, pacing task performance, and carrying out, completing, and sustaining a task.
Inclusions: undertaking a simple or complex task; undertaking a single task independently or in a group
Exclusions: acquiring skills (d155); solving problems (d175); making decisions (d177); undertaking multiple tasks (d220)
- *d2100 Undertaking a Simple Task*
  Preparing, initiating, and arranging the time and space required for a simple task; executing a simple task with a single major component, such as reading a book, writing a letter, or making one's bed.
- *d2101 Undertaking a Complex Task*
  Preparing, initiating, and arranging the time and space for a single complex task; executing a complex task with more than one component, which may be carried out in sequence or simultaneously, such as arranging the furniture in one's home or completing an assignment for school.

- *d2102 Undertaking a Single Task Independently*
  Preparing, initiating, and arranging the time and space for a simple or complex task; managing and executing a task on one's own and without the assistance of others.
- *d2103 Undertaking a Single Task in a Group*
  Preparing, initiating, and arranging the time and space for a single task, simple or complex; managing and executing a task with people who are involved in some or all steps of the task.
- *d2108 Undertaking Single Tasks, Other Specified.*
- *d2109 Undertaking Single Tasks, Unspecified*

Treatment for Undertaking a Single Task

A single task can be either a very simple action such as turning on a light or a very complex task such as determining the area of a pentagram. A single task usually involves both mental and physical components. For example, when a client walks into a dark room s/he realizes that the light needs to be turned on so that s/he can see and reaches out for the wall switch to turn on the light. The actions required for a single task would include initiating the action; organizing the time needed, the space needed, and materials required for completing the action; maintaining a reasonable pace of activity; and sustaining the mental and physical actions needed to carry out and complete the activity.

The skill of undertaking a single task requires the use of many skills. This is why it is referred to as an *application* skill. All Activities and Participation categories are application skills. Undertaking a single task is the application of isolated skills related to body functions (e.g., voluntary movement and visual field functions). Therapists evaluate a client's ability to perform application skills, but to address the problem, the isolated skills that make up the task must be evaluated, problems clearly identified, and methods to improve the client's performance developed. To identify the specific isolated skills of a task, the therapist conducts a task analysis. (See "Activity and Task Analysis" in the Techniques section.) Once specific deficits are identified, the therapist designs a treatment plan to restore, develop, or adapt for the problem. Consult the index of this book for information on a specific dysfunction.

Many clients need to have interventions directed at the level of undertaking a simple task. Clients with brain injuries, chronic mental illness, and mental retardation will be working on this level. At this level the recreational therapist is likely to be teaching the client skills related to specific activities such as playing bingo, swimming, making a clay pot, ordering from a restaurant menu, making a phone call, playing cards, and yoga.

As clients increase their skill levels they will begin to give their attention to more than one task at a time. If a client has been able to overlearn an activity skill, it will be easier for him/her to integrate more than one activity at a time. The therapist will help a client succeed if s/he does not push the client too fast into working on multiple tasks.

d220 Undertaking Multiple Tasks

Carrying out simple or complex and coordinated actions as components of multiple, integrated, and complex tasks in sequence or simultaneously.

Inclusions: undertaking multiple tasks; completing multiple tasks; undertaking multiple tasks independently or in a group

Exclusions: acquiring skills (d155); solving problems (d175); making decisions (d177); undertaking single tasks (d210)

- *d2200 Carrying Out Multiple Tasks*
  Preparing, initiating, and arranging the time and space needed for several tasks, and managing and executing several tasks, together or sequentially.
- *d2201 Completing Multiple Tasks*
  Completing several tasks, together or sequentially.
- *d2202 Undertaking Multiple Tasks Independently*
  Preparing, initiating, and arranging the time and space for multiple tasks, and managing and executing several tasks together or sequentially, on one's own and without the assistance of others.
- *d2203 Undertaking Multiple Tasks in a Group*
  Preparing, initiating, and arranging the time and space for multiple tasks, and managing and executing several tasks together or sequentially with others who are involved in some or all steps of the multiple tasks.
- *d2208 Undertaking Multiple Tasks, Other Specified*
- *d2209 Undertaking Multiple Tasks, Unspecified*

Treatment for Undertaking Multiple Tasks

In a clinical setting (either inpatient or outpatient) the types of challenges that a therapist presents to clients tend to be single task challenges. This is because it is easier to evaluate a client's actual skill level when the therapist has to look at one skill at a time. However, life in the community is seldom that simple and planned. The ability to juggle many different demands at the same time requires a complex set of skills that are hard to define and harder to measure. Often, when a client fails to complete multiple tasks, it is hard for the therapist to determine if the client failed because s/he was not

able to perform a specific skill (one of the many tasks being evaluated) or if s/he was not able to integrate the "higher level" skill of planning and coordinating multiple tasks at once.

As an example, the therapist sets up a situation in which a group of clients are in the kitchen to make a complete meal. One group of clients is responsible for preparing the chef salad, another group is responsible for making cornbread, and a third group is responsible for making chocolate chip cookies. One of the clients making the cookies, Barbara, is given the task of listening to Steve (another client) read the recipe out loud, measuring out the ingredients, and mixing the cookie dough. When the dinner is all done and the cookies baked, everyone takes one bite and spits the cookie out. It appears that Barbara put in two *tablespoons* of salt instead of one-eighth *teaspoon* of salt. Did Barbara fail to measure the salt correctly because she could not handle a set of tasks read to her step-by-step (d2103; Undertaking a Single Task in a Group) or did she get distracted because of others working on different tasks (d2203 Undertaking Multiple Tasks in a Group)? In the first case the impairment may be related to listening, reading, or a lack of basic kitchen skills. In the second case the impairment may be related to an inability to execute a sequential attention span (being able to pay attention to one task, move on to the next task, ignoring things she didn't need to pay attention to, and so forth), an inability to prioritize actions, or a lack of being able to observe someone else using a tablespoon to measure salt for the cornbread while she needed to use a quarter teaspoon to measure salt for the cookies.

Because many of the tasks related to recreation and leisure involve multiple tasks, the recreational therapist needs to become very skilled in observing clients engaged in multiple tasks and identifying the area(s) of impairment (e.g., impairment because of a lack of skill related to a simple task or because of a lack of skill related to juggling multiple tasks). This is especially true for the therapist working with clients in a community setting.

The ICF makes a distinction between carrying out multiple tasks and completing multiple tasks. A client can be good at preparing, initiating, arranging time and space, and managing and executing several tasks, but that does not necessarily equate to being able to complete the tasks. For example, a client may be able to manage and carry out the tasks needed to organize a family vacation (making phone calls for camping sites, evaluating the calendar and individual family members' schedules, looking at a map), but that does not mean that the vacation ever gets fully planned and carried out. The ability to complete several tasks together or sequentially often requires greater integration of cognitive and personality traits (e.g., persistence, confidence, problem solving).

The observation of failure in carrying out, undertaking, or completing multiple tasks will require the therapist to conduct a task analysis to further determine the specific dysfunction hindering capacity or performance. Once the specific dysfunction is identified, the therapist identifies and implements a treatment plan to optimize functioning.

This is the level where many recreational therapists address a client's ability to engage in leisure activities, including the steps needed to get to the movie theater, take a trip downtown to go shopping, or go to a baseball game. The *Community Integration Program* (Armstrong & Lauzen, 1994) is a set of twenty-two assessment and treatment protocol modules used by recreational therapists to address skills at the multiple task level. This is also an appropriate level to work on the concept of leisure balance: that the combined set of leisure activities the client engages in on a regular basis is balanced between physical, social, and emotional development opportunities.

Just as the progression from undertaking a simple task to undertaking multiple tasks represents the skills to take an action and execute it in a progressively more complex and stimulating situation, the move from undertaking multiple tasks to carrying out a daily routine represents another significant jump in ability.

d230 Carrying Out Daily Routine
Carrying out simple or complex and coordinated actions in order to plan, manage, and complete the requirements of day-to-day procedures or duties, such as budgeting time and making plans for separate activities throughout the day.
Inclusions: managing and completing the daily routine; managing one's own activity level
Exclusions: undertaking multiple tasks (d220)
- *d2301 Managing Daily Routine*
  Carrying out simple or complex and coordinated actions in order to plan and manage the require-ments of day-to-day procedures or duties.
- *d2302 Completing the Daily Routine*
  Carrying out simple or complex and coordinated actions in order to complete the requirements of day-to-day procedures or duties.
- *d2303 Managing One's Own Activity Level*
  Carrying out actions and behaviors to arrange the requirements in energy and time [for] day-to-day procedures or duties.
- *d2308 Carrying Out Daily Routine, Other Specified*
- *d2309 Carrying Out Daily Routine, Unspecified*

Treatment for
Carrying Out Daily Routine
Once a client has managed to learn an activity skill, the therapist challenges the client's skill so that s/he is able to complete the activity with other distractions and demands thrown into the mix. The progression to being able to carry out daily routine is another step in complexity and self-management.

While undertaking a simple task generally relates to having the skills necessary to carry out a specific activity (such as walking to the store), and undertaking multiple tasks generally relates to having the ability to sequentially pay attention to and carry out numerous activities at one time (such as talking to a friend who is walking with you to the store, creating a shopping list as you walk), carrying out a daily routine generally relates to how well you are able to get done what needs to get done (such as making sure that you schedule time to go to the store in time to fix dinner, arranging with your friend to walk with you, and ensuring that you have a means to pay for the food).

Just as with Undertaking Multiple Tasks, the ICF makes a distinction between managing (d2301 Managing Daily Routine) and completing (d2302 Completing the Daily Routine). Managing daily routine refers to the client's ability to carry out actions in order to plan and manage his/her daily responsibilities and duties (e.g., making a to do list, looking at all of the tasks of the day and arranging them in a manner that optimizes the best outcomes, considering transportation schedules that affect abilities to carry out tasks, considering the impact of tasks on other tasks that need to be done, actually carrying out multiple tasks). Managing daily routine does not equate to completing the daily routine. For example, a client with multiple sclerosis may be able to independently plan and manage a daily routine but finds herself often unable to complete the planned routine due to fatigue.

This leads into the next code of managing one's activity level. We only have so much energy and time to do what we want or need to do. It is not about managing the routine or completing the routine, but the client's ability to arrange actions and behaviors to allow for time and energy constraints. For example, a client with multiple sclerosis may be able to plan and manage a daily routine and even complete it, but at the end of the day she is so fatigued that come evening she is having multiple falls. Clients who have disorders that impact their energy level (such as multiple sclerosis, chronic fatigue syndrome, fibromyalgia, and bipolar disorder) will most often have to pay particular attention to the impact of their activity level on health. Clients with disorders that impact their ability to remember all that needs to be done, such as clients with early Alzheimer's disease, autism, or stroke, will be working on adaptations to keep track of all the tasks.

Therapists are also 1. aware of the secondary problems caused by poor management and execution of a daily routine and activity level, such as increased stress and inappropriate demand on the physical, mental, social, and emotional functions and 2. are careful to fully evaluate the dysfunction to find underlying daily routine and activity level causes that can be remediated (e.g., reducing or eliminating stressors related to management, execution, or completion of a daily routine rather than the sole intervention of teaching stress management techniques).

Therapists can evaluate the client's ability to manage his/her daily routine by
- Asking the client to fill out an activity pattern (see "Activity Pattern Development" in the Techniques section). This will also give the therapist an opportunity to evaluate the client's routine in relation to his/her energy and time constraints.
- Asking the client to fill out the "Pie of Life" (in the Techniques section). The purpose of the Pie of Life is to help the client understand how much time s/he spends at various activities and then evaluate whether changes can or should be made in his/her daily routine. There are multiple versions of this very popular activity. The therapist can use whichever ones work best for the client.

However, what a client says and what a client does are not always the same thing. Clients can be given the task of managing their daily routine in the current setting (whether capacity or performance) and be observed for their ability to complete the routine. Through observation and discussion, the therapist can also ascertain how well the daily routine meets the client's time and energy requirements. There can be many areas of difficulty (e.g., lack of knowledge of energy conservation techniques, pressure to perform at a higher level from others, lack of assistance, cognitive problems). Therefore the specific treatment interventions will vary depending on the individual needs of the client.

d240 Handling Stress and Other Psychological Demands
Carrying out simple or complex and coordinated actions to manage and control the psychological demands required to carry out tasks demanding significant responsibilities and involving stress, distraction, or crises, such as driving a vehicle during heavy traffic or taking care of many children.

Inclusions: handling responsibilities; handling stress and crisis
- *d2400 Handling Responsibilities*
  Carrying out simple or complex and coordinated actions to manage the duties of task performance and to assess the requirements of these duties.
- *d2401 Handling Stress*
  Carrying out simple or complex and coordinated actions to cope with pressure, emergencies, or stress associated with task performance.
- *d2402 Handling Crisis*
  Carrying out simple or complex and coordinated actions to cope with decisive turning points in a situation or times of acute danger or difficulty.
- *d2408 Handling Stress and Other Psychological Demands, Other Specified*
- *d2409 Handling Stress and Other Psychological Demands, Unspecified*

Treatment for Handling Stress and Other Psychological Demands

This section looks at how the client handles the psychological demands required to carry out tasks. While the previous sections of Chapter 2 looked at the actions and choices themselves, this section looks at the psychological issues associated with demands. While carrying out a daily routine revolves around the self-management of time, resources, and duties, the ability to handle stress and other psychological demands is the ability to self-regulate response to situations that tax the client's capabilities. The most common term for the response is stress.

Stress is a natural and healthy emotion, although it can turn into a big problem if it becomes excessive, unrelenting, or unmanaged. Unfortunately, people often don't give stress the attention it deserves. Stressful events and situations are typically viewed as things that one has little control over (e.g., "that's just the way life goes" — external locus of control) and when someone talks about managing stress the common reaction is, "yeah, right" (in conjunction with a laugh). The word "stress" is a part of our everyday vocabulary. It doesn't have a shock value like the word "cancer." People joke about it, put funny pictures on mugs about it, and depict daily stressors in the Sunday comics. Those things are funny because many of us can relate to them, but they may cause us to forget the potentially devastating effects that stress can have on our lives.

There are two kinds of stress, acute and chronic. Acute stress refers to stress that comes up in relation to current events in the client's life. Chronic stress is stress that seems as if it will never end. It can be there because the client has not dealt with a past event appropriately or because some kind of acute stress is ongoing.

Acute Stress

There are many sources of stress: environment, occupation, health, relationships, finances, etc. Whether they are positive or negative events does not matter. Changes of any kind can be sources of stress (e.g., moving to a new home, starting a new job, having a baby, graduating from school). Sources of stress are not universal either. What is stressful for one person may not be stressful for another. How the event is perceived has a lot to do with whether it is classified as stressful.

Here is a list of some of the stressors that may be addressed as part of recreational therapy treatment:

- *Emotional and psychological*: Feelings about oneself, the sources of emotional needs, and awareness about emotional needs.
- *Environment*: This may include work, neighborhood, school, or home and be caused by noise, crowding, lighting, signs, odors, colors, and litter, as well as interpersonal interactions.
- *Finances*: Money is one of the top stressors. Not making enough money and not having enough money are constant stressors in most lower and middle class families. It is also a stressor for many people who are experiencing a dramatic change in their income due to disability.
- *Health*: Including adjustment to disability and other health-related limitations.
- *Life crises*: Major life changes, whether good or bad, are sources of stress. This could include death of a loved one, change of job, disability, moving to a new home, or having a child.
- *Relationships*: Dynamics occurring within relationships can be sources of stress (spouse, partner, children, parents, co-workers, and friends).
- *Time*: Feeling crunched for time (more responsibilities than able to accomplish in a set amount of time) or lacking the ability to cope with time demands.
- *Work*: Including relationship with boss and coworkers, type of work, work conditions, or commute.

Obviously there is a great deal of overlap in the areas of stress described. In dealing with stress, it is important to see the problem from the client's perspective.

Chronic Stress

Some people experience chronic (long-term) stress. Chronic stress can be the result of ongoing unrelieved stressors, whether real or perceived (e.g., a physical illness or disability, financial problems, a mental illness such as generalized anxiety disorder,

many consecutive small stressors). With chronic stress, the outside portion (cortex) of the adrenal glands are stimulated and the chemical cortisol is released into the bloodstream. Cortisol slowly and steadily prepares the body to deal with a long-term stressor, rather than a short-term stressor. To maximize the amount of physical energy needed to deal with the stressor, the body suppresses other essential bodily functions (in addition to continuing the initial bodily reactions to stress) including the immune system, the reproductive system, the digestive system, tissue repair and growth, and the inflammatory system (Davis et al, 2000). In addition, cholesterol levels rise, a person's mood often becomes irritable, the person may become hyperalert, the heart beat slows down, the immune system is severely depressed, blood pressure rises slowly[3], metabolism drops, fats are stored instead of burned, and blood clots may form from the increased supply of platelets (Eliot, 1994).

Chronic stress can also cause a variety of other problems:

- Chronic stress is a risk factor for stroke (cerebrovascular accident) because sustained high blood pressure can result in a brain hemorrhage or it can loosen a blood clot from an artery wall and send it traveling to the brain where it can become lodged and cause a blockage (stroke caused by an embolism).
- Chronic stress depresses the body's immune system, thus allowing the start of an illness or disease that lay quietly within the body or leaving a vulnerable area of the body open to disease, illness, or complications (e.g., a specific organ that was operated on). Some people are more susceptible to certain diseases and illnesses given their genetic make-up, environment in which they live, diet, family history, etc. Stress is one of those variables that exacerbate the beginnings of a disease. A compromised immune system, in general, will make a person more susceptible to colds and flu. This can be very detrimental to someone whose health is fragile (e.g., recovering from major surgery, having AIDS or cancer).
- Chronic stress can contribute to an exacerbation of multiple sclerosis, hypertension (chronic high blood pressure), myocardial infarction (heart attack), fibromyalgia, ulcers, gastrointestinal problems (e.g., reflux disease, irritable bowel syndrome), migraine headaches, reproductive problems (lack of ovulation in women, impo-

---

[3] When blood pressure remains high over a period of time, the body adopts the new level as being normal rather than just a short-term reaction to a stressor. Pressure sensors in the blood vessels called baroreceptors become set at this new level

tence in men, loss of sex drive, premature labor), and mental illness (e.g., major depressive disorder, generalized anxiety disorder, schizophrenia).

- Chronic stress affects the body's ability to repair itself. If this compromises a person's ability to weight bear through the legs (stand up for a reasonable amount of time), bones will lose calcium, thus increasing the person's risk of fractures and osteoporosis. This in turn will limit the person's activity level, thus further increasing the person's risk of developing secondary complications from inactivity.
- Chronic stress can worsen certain conditions such as chronic pain (stress heightens sensitivity to pain), arthritis (can contribute to inflammation of joints), and diabetes (blood sugar levels rise).

Chronic stress can become a vicious cycle that continues to affect a person's physical, mental, social, and emotional functioning. It impacts life tasks (e.g., difficulty concentrating at school, missed workdays, short temper with children or disabled parent) and gives rise to further stressors. Stressors exacerbate problems and then problems heighten stressors. Ultimately a person can become emotionally and/or physically disabled from untreated chronic stress.

Reactions to Stress

People respond to stress in many different ways. Some responses are done consciously (e.g., go out for a run, go to the bar for a drink), some are emotional reactions (e.g., crying), while others are done unconsciously (e.g., defensive mechanisms). What is it that influences the coping mechanisms we choose? Many of our coping and defensive mechanisms are learned behavior from past experiences and observation of others (e.g., parents). People choose a coping style that works for them, whether healthy or unhealthy, and they are chosen based on many factors.

When stressors are experienced or perceived, the cerebral cortex sends a distress signal to the hypothalamus alerting it to the threat. In turn, the hypothalamus sends messages along the sympathetic nervous system to the inner part (medulla) of the small adrenal glands (located on top of each kidney). The adrenal glands release a family of chemicals called catecholamines (including adrenaline and noradrenaline). Adrenaline provides a surge of energy for strenuous physical tasks. Noradrenaline provides a fighting response. Both of these chemicals work "simultaneously with other physiologic reactions to create the complex network of survival"

(Eliot, 1994, p 23). This is often called the "fight or flight" response because it prepares the body to be as effective as possible at either fighting or escaping. It also significantly reduces the brain's ability to think about the situation.

When the "fight or flight" alarm system is activated, the body reacts in many ways. They include:

- The skeletal muscles require increased energy to respond to the stressors (to be able to run or fight). The body does this by 1. increasing the heart rate to deliver an increased volume of oxygenated blood to power major muscles, 2. diverting oxygenated blood from the digestive organs to the skeletal muscles to power major muscles, and 3. increasing blood sugar levels to supply increased energy to the muscles.
- The blood clots more rapidly to quickly heal wounds.
- The pupil of the eye dilates (widens) to increase visual acuity and awareness.
- Respiration rate increases to increase the amount of oxygen to the body.
- The body stimulates production of catecholamines, endorphins (body's natural painkillers), and hormones that increase visual and auditory acuity.

When the threat is gone, the body typically returns to a relaxed state. We say typically because research has shown that some peoples' bodies do not return to a normal relaxed state.

Other reactions to stress vary depending on the client. For a discussion of some of the views on coping and defense mechanisms see "Coping with Stress" in the Techniques section.

Assessment

During the assessment process, therapists help clients identify their specific stressors and strengths. Knowing the source of stress and the resources (strengths) of the client are essential to building a stress treatment plan. Therapists conduct a clinical interview with open-ended questions that encourage verbalizations of strengths and stressors (e.g., "What is different for you now?") and help the client to narrow down stressors and strengths into specific measurable objectives (e.g., poor communication skills do not allow the client to get his/her needs met; wheelchair mobility is required on a school campus that is not fully wheelchair accessible). The therapist also observes and evaluates indirect expressions of stress during activity through the client's defensive and coping mechanisms (e.g., putting self down, denial), behavioral responses to stressful situations (e.g., violence, yelling, withdrawn behavior), and physiological responses to stress (e.g., rise in blood pressure, dilation of eye pupils, excessive sweating). Of course, many of the signs of stress can also be attributed to other physiological changes in the body (e.g., side effect of medication, mental illness, chronic hypertension). It is the combination of observation, an understanding of the client's medical history and medications, and the context of the situation that helps the therapist differentiate among possible contributors to behavioral, physiological, and emotional states.

It may also be worthwhile for the therapist to look at self-awareness issues (discussed in "Education and Counseling" in the Techniques section). While these are not universal because some cultures do not have a bias toward individual expression, they are appropriate issues to look at in Western culture.

Areas of Stress

Some areas of life can be especially stressful. The cause of the stress can affect the type of treatment the therapist uses. Here are some considerations for particular areas of stress.

- *Emotional and psychological*: Feelings about oneself, the sources for meeting emotional needs, and awareness about emotional needs can all be sources of stress. For example, low self-esteem ("I am unworthy"), pessimism ("Nothing ever goes right"), and an external locus of control ("It doesn't matter what I do") promote poor coping strategies. Looking towards others to provide direction for one's life restricts a person from looking inward, identifying one's own values, and living one's "true" life (personal aspirations instead of aspirations of others). For the client facing a new disability or a health crisis, many of these issues surface, contributing to stress. For example, a client may not see self-esteem as a source of stress, but a therapist knows that self-esteem is an integral component of being able to respond to life's stressors in a healthy manner. The same is true for a client who has not "found himself." Meaning, that he isn't really clear on what he values in life, what he wants out of life, and where he fits in life. A client who is not self-assured and grounded will be influenced by others and searching for validation to define himself/herself. This is a common developmental stage for adolescents (trying on many roles to find the one that fits) and sometimes a person who was once self-assured becomes insecure when his/her life changes drastically.

- *Environment*: The environment has a huge impact on stress. This includes noise, crowding, lighting, signs, odors, colors, and litter. Clients who identify their environments (work, neighborhood, school, home) as stressful work with therapists to find ways to alter these environments (e.g., closing windows to shut out noise, repainting walls, cleaning out closets, burning scented candles, turning on classical music, wearing headphones). In some cases, clients opt to move from an urban to a rural environment in an attempt to escape these stressors. Clients must be careful to fully evaluate this move since a rural area may have inherent stressors that the client is unaware of (e.g., lack of transportation, loss of current social relationships, loss of close conveniences like a bank and grocery store). In the hospital setting, a clean and sterile environment often lacks the comfort and relaxing atmosphere of a home (e.g., nurses and carts going up and down the hall, people crying or screaming, a roommate that has the television on all night long, the odor of rubbing alcohol). Clients who find the hospital environment stressful should be encouraged to ask loved ones to bring in familiar items from home as appropriate (e.g., CD player, stuffed animals, a quilt and pillow sham from home).

- *Finances*: Money is one of the top stressors. Not making enough money and not having enough money are constant stressors in most lower and middle class families. It is also a stressor for many people who are experiencing a dramatic change in their income due to disability. Money issues can cause arguments, and an inability to pay the bills can cause tremendous stress. Therapists often avoid this topic believing that it is the personal business of the client, and some clients refuse to discuss it. We believe that therapists should not avoid this topic and approach the subject with the client in a caring and helpful manner. It is not possible for a therapist to know and understand the full context of a client's finances, nor is it appropriate to do so. However, asking the client if s/he is on a tight budget and expressing an understanding of the difficult situation encourages a client to share information (e.g., "I don't know what we are going to do now that I am out of work. My brother is helping us pay the bills right now."). Getting a sense of the client's finances helps to identify a need for assistance and points the client in the right direction to find help. Many people do not like to talk about money and therefore do not receive the support that they are entitled to. Second, having a sense of the client's finances helps the therapist identify activities that are within the client's budget. The identification of financial assistance and exploration of tasks that are within the client's budget can be helpful in reducing stress related to finances. Some clients also benefit from existential counseling (the meaning of one's life) because sometimes people get so caught up in keeping up with the Joneses that they don't really look at what they truly value and want in their life. Addressing money issues is not forbidden. Recreational therapists address money management issues when it is necessary for the client's independence or successful task engagement (e.g., a client with multiple sclerosis has trouble with her memory and vision and needs help designing a new system to manage her checkbook; a client who is blind needs help to design a system of identifying money in his wallet to be able to pay for groceries).

- *Health*: Good health does not precipitate stress unless the client is preoccupied with his/her health and fears health problems (e.g., cancerous tumor has been removed and client is now in remission, however client's fear of cancer growing back is a significant source of stress). People who have health problems, however, do not always perceive their health as a source of stress. If a problem is well managed and does not significantly impact functioning, quality of life, and independence, it may not be a source of stress. The same holds true for clients who have adapted well to limitations imposed by health conditions and have a strong internal locus of control. Even so, therapists who work with clients in a health care setting (e.g., rehabilitation, acute hospitalization) will often find that the clients report their current health condition as a source of high stress. Therapists help clients to adjust to disability (see "Adjustment to Disability" in the Techniques section) and address the client's primary concerns. Therapists focus on a variety of issues as they pertain to the client's unique situation to foster functioning, independence, and quality of life.
- *Life crises*: Major life changes, whether good or bad, are sources of stress. This could include death of a loved one, change of job, disability, moving to a new home, or having a child. Therapists ask the client to tell him/her about any changes that have occurred during the last year. The more changes, the more stress. Therapists cannot control change, but they can help clients adapt and cope with change. The interventions will vary depending on the changes (e.g., needs

referral for grief counseling for loss of spouse, needs to develop a circle of friends because of a move, client feels anxious about anticipated changes and could benefit from general relaxation training).

- *Relationships*: Dynamics occurring in relationships can be sources of stress (spouse, partner, children, parents, co-workers, friends). Issues that may cause stress include, but are not limited to, inadequate quality time with a spouse (too many other responsibilities), caring for an elderly parent, and lack of positive feelings from relationship (e.g., doesn't feel appreciated, listened to, respected). If a client is having trouble in a relationship (e.g., delinquent child, violence in the home) appropriate referrals are made. Issues related to quality of time and positive and healthy communication are commonly addressed by recreational therapists. Therapists identify activities and interactions that improve quality of time, as well as teach positive and healthy communication skills to promote growth and connectedness within relationships. Looking at another part of the issue, those who lack friendship, close relationships, and connectedness have higher mortality rates. Recreational therapists help clients to develop or enhance healthy relationships by identifying and integrating clients into social opportunities and addressing issues within the scope of recreational therapy practice that impact the ability to participate in social environments (e.g., communication skills, self-esteem, self-confidence, anxiety). In the hospital setting, therapists are aware of relationship changes regarding access to primary relationships for support (e.g., availability of spouse) and the need for continuing relationships in the hospital (especially prolonged hospitalization, such as waiting for a heart transplant). Therapists encourage family and friends to continue to provide support and provide them with methods to do so, as appropriate (e.g., making videos, sending e-mails, phone calls, cards, banners, quality time alone with a spouse). Therapists also identify alternative supports and facilitate them (e.g., introduce one client to another client who is also waiting for a heart transplant, provide a social environment for clients to meet, talk, and engage in activity).
- *Time*: Feeling crunched for time (client has more responsibilities than she can accomplish in a set amount of time) or lacking the ability to cope with time demands contributes to stress. A client may feel stressed because of lack of time, and the resultant feeling of being unable to control

his/her life can exacerbate certain behaviors and feelings that impact the ability to deal with stress (e.g., short fused, irritable, frustrated, anxious). These feelings can also be exacerbated within a hospital setting when therapies and care needs are scheduled without a break. Therapists evaluate responsibilities, demands, and desires of the client and compare them to the time available to decide if the client needs more skills related to time management (e.g., setting priorities, organizing skills, delegation, eliminating unnecessary double work, relevance of tasks). In the hospital setting, therapists try to alter the client's therapy and nursing care schedules so that the client and staff do not feel stressed about time.

- *Work*: Work can be a source of stress for many different reasons (relationship with boss, type of work, work conditions, commute, etc.). If work is a significant source of stress and the stress cannot be remedied, the client may want to explore a new worksite or change in career. People who have disabilities may need to make worksite or career changes depending on their abilities and limitations (e.g., was a carpenter and now has tetraplegia). People who anticipate problems returning to work because of a disability or who are unable to return to their career because they are now unable to perform the required skills are referred to the Office of Vocational Rehabilitation (OVR). OVR is a state program that assesses a client's ability to return to work and facilitates the client's ability to become part of the workforce. OVR will assist clients financially to return to school, obtain needed equipment related to return to work (e.g., hand controls for car, ramp to enter/exit home). Clients are referred to OVR by a social worker or case manager. Clients are put on a waiting list and are usually called within a few months. The goal is to find the client a career that matches his/her interests and abilities. Therapists also educate clients about their rights under the Americans with Disabilities Act as it pertains to employment. In some facilities, recreational therapists perform worksite evaluations and assist the client and employer in identifying needed changes. Recreational therapy is beginning to do more in this area (worksite evaluations, work skills, employer ADA training, worksite integration) because of the rising older adult population who are choosing to work for pleasure and enjoyment rather than as a necessary life task to pay the bills.

Contributors to Stress

There are some contributors to stress that the therapist may want to consider when designing a program.

- *Alcohol*: Alcohol is a CNS depressant. Short-term behavioral effects can include disinhibition, relaxation, or anger and violence. Alcohol affects physical coordination, memory, concentration, and insight. See Substance-Related Disorders for more information. Alcohol use can cause stress for an individual who feels pressured to drink or is trying to quit and is experiencing related frustration. Reactions of others in the home or at work to the amount of alcohol the client is drinking can also be a source of stress. Therapists address this issue by teaching the client assertiveness skills, relaxation training, and stress management skills, as well as addressing issues related to susceptibility to peer pressure (e.g., low self-esteem). Alcohol use can also impact the client's ability to deal with stress effectively (e.g., alcohol induced violent behavior impacts response to immediate stressor) and actions can continue to cause problems after alcohol is no longer in the system (e.g., behavior offended girlfriend and caused relationship stressors). Although alcohol is a legal drug, therapists discourage its use when cognitive and behavioral changes contribute to emotional and physical stress. Clients who wish to cease social alcohol consumption and find it difficult to do so explore the "pay offs" of social drinking (e.g., relaxation, stress reduction, enjoys social atmosphere, fitting in with peers) and address each issue with a therapist to find alterative ways to meet these needs. Treatment for abuse of alcohol or alcoholism is not the same as reducing social drinking. The therapist needs to apply different techniques and abstinence is generally considered to be a requirement for the client.
- *Body weight*: Clients who are overweight are putting a significant amount of stress on their body's systems (cardiovascular, muscular, pulmonary, and skeletal) putting themselves at increased risk for disease and illness (e.g., cardiac problems, diabetes, and stroke) and health-related problems related to inactivity (e.g., muscle atrophy, general deconditioning). A client who has a current health condition should be particularly concerned about his/her body weight because it often plays a large role in the development of secondary problems that affect functioning, independence, and quality of life. For example, excess body weight contributes to the pain level of a client with chronic back pain

because it adds to pressure on the back when the stomach accentuates the lumbar curve by pulling it forward. Pain causes the client to sit or lie down to reduce the pain. Prolonged periods of inactivity contribute to further problems causing the client to lose function. Loss of function may require the client to seek assistance from others thus impacting his/her level of independence. Needing assistance from others combined with decreased functioning can significantly impact the client's ability to perform desired life tasks that contribute to quality of life. Excess body weight can also be a source of emotional stress if the client is trying to lose weight and is experiencing frustration with the task or is the target of jokes and ridicule. Therapists help clients to meet their ideal body weight determined by the Body Mass Index and/or the recommendation of the physician. Therapists help clients reduce body weight by encouraging regular physical activity and a proper diet. Therapists must receive approval from the physician to begin an exercise program, as well as an order that describes additional information relevant to participation in an exercise program (e.g., precautions, parameters). Therapists identify activities that are enjoyed by the client that have the potential to be a form of physical exercise. For example, if a client enjoys talking and socializing, involvement in an exercise program that promotes talking and socializing might be well-received (e.g., a walking club) compared to a form of exercise that does not promote such interactions (e.g., walking on a treadmill). Of course, the therapist must fully evaluate how realistic the exercise choice is, the resources available to the client, the client's current health status as it relates to performance of the task, and the client's willingness and motivation to participate in the activity. The report, Healthy People 2010, recommends that people participate in moderate physical activity three to five times a week for a period of 20-30 minutes. This recommendation is for people who do not have a current health condition. People who have health conditions must seek medical clearance from their physician and guidelines for exercise participation to avoid further injury or harm. Therapists must also be aware of other problems that can cause an increase in body weight that may require assistance from other health professionals (e.g., psychotherapy for depression, metabolism problems). See "Obesity" in the Diagnosis section and "Exercise Basics" in the Techniques section for more information.

- *Caffeine*: Caffeine is a central nervous system stimulant. After it is ingested (coffee, tea, soda, chocolate), effects are experienced in about 30 minutes and maximum levels are reached within two hours (Julien, 2004). Caffeine increases mental alertness so quality and amount of sleep can be affected. Heavy consumption of caffeine (12+ cups per day) causes agitation, anxiety, tremors, rapid breathing, and insomnia (Julien, 2004). Behavioral responses of agitation and anxiety can affect a client's ability to implement healthy coping mechanisms (e.g., yells instead of talking out the problem). Lack of sleep affects concentration, attention, mental alertness, and stress tolerance compounding the problem when caffeine is no longer in the system. Clients may not view caffeine intake as a stressor, but it can significantly impact the client's ability to cope and deal with stress. Caffeine is not a nutritional requirement so it should be eliminated from diets unless it is prescribed by a physician (may be prescribed for migraine headaches). Withdrawal symptoms from caffeine can include headache, irritability, fatigue, dysphoric mood changes, muscle pain and stiffness, flu-like feelings, nausea, and craving for caffeine products. Clients should be encouraged to reduce caffeine intake in increments until it is fully eliminated from the diet to help minimize withdrawal symptoms. Therapists also assist clients to identify alternative contributors to mental alertness (e.g., physical exercise, quality and amount of sleep, proper diet, stress reduction, and relaxation training).

- *Diet*: Inadequate nutrition can lead to health and behavioral problems that can contribute to or affect the ability to manage stress. Lack of a proper diet can affect mental and physical energy levels possibly contributing to the level of effort that is needed to cope with stress (e.g., lacking physical strength to go for a long walk). Therapists need to understand the basic food pyramid and make recommendations consistent with the American Dietetic Association's balanced diet. Therapists should know the nutritional recommendations from the client's physician (e.g., low fat diet), dietician (sets specific guidelines, e.g., calories, food groups), and speech therapist (determines food consistency needs, e.g., chopped, pureed, soft). If a therapist believes that a client is not eating a well-balanced and healthy diet, a consult should be made to a nutritionist for a full evaluation. Recommendations from the nutritionist are incorporated into the client's lifestyle with the help of the recreational therapist (e.g., eating out, social eating, stress eating). Clients who present with an eating disorder require more intense treatment.

- *Lack of exercise*: Lack of exercise can contribute to secondary problems that cause stress, especially if there is a pre-existing health condition. Exercise is also a very effective intervention for managing stress because it induces a relaxation response, clears thinking, and expends energy.
- *Nicotine*: Nicotine increases blood pressure, increases heart rate, and stimulates the release of adrenaline that produces "fight or flight" response as discussed above. Smoking, or the use of any tobacco product that contains nicotine, may also be a source of stress if the person is trying to quit and is frustrated with this task (e.g., feeling irritable, pressure from loved ones). Therapists do not condone smoking and encourage clients to quit since it adversely affects health. If the physician recommends that the client stop smoking, it is helpful for both the therapist and the physician to have a meeting with the client. The physician explains to the client why s/he should quit smoking, prescribes something to assist the client with smoking cessation, if needed and appropriate (e.g., a nicotine patch), and explains to the client that nicotine withdrawal typically takes two to four weeks, although full withdrawal can take six months or longer (Julien, 2004). The client will also have to combat the psychological dependence and social components of smoking. The physician makes clear to the client that these two issues are just as important as nicotine withdrawal to successfully quit smoking and that s/he has ordered a recreational therapy consult to address these issues and integrate them into a post-discharge plan. Once the meeting is terminated, the recreational therapist schedules a separate session to evaluate when, where, and why the client smokes and identifies strategies for combating the desire. This could include making small changes in routine to decrease associations, increasing activity levels, learning healthy coping strategies for stress triggers, identifying non-prescription external aids that can help the client quit smoking (e.g., chewing gum), and education on the benefits of activity with particular attention to the power of relaxation and distraction for smoking cessation. Therapists also discuss the social consequences of not smoking that are concerns of the client (e.g., smoke breaks at work, bars). All of identified interventions are then reflected in the client's activity pattern (see "Activity Pattern Development" in the Techniques section).

- *Sleep*: Lack of sleep or impaired quality of sleep can lead to problems paying attention, concentrating, and tolerating stressful situations. Therapists help clients improve sleep by identifying and addressing causes of sleep problems (e.g., frequent urination in the middle of the night, stress, caffeine, depression). Further evaluation and sleep studies may also need to be conducted (e.g., sleep apnea). See b134 Sleep Functions for more information.
- *Telephone*: The telephone can be intrusive and demand attention. In the hospital setting, a ringing telephone can prompt a client to move too quickly to retrieve the call; it can be upsetting when the client receives yet another phone call having to explain the current situation; and it can be bothersome when trying to rest. Clients can request to have the telephone removed from their room and they have the right to turn off the ringer. Clients can also tell family and friends to only call between certain hours or designate a person or two to pass along information to others instead of each person calling the client. Once at home, the client can continue this by turning off the ringer and answering messages at his/her convenience and/or keeping a cordless or cell phone in a pant's pocket or apron pocket to use in case of an emergency (e.g., a fall) and to answer phone calls without having to rush to the phone.
- *Work ethic*: With the high work ethic in the American culture, the choice to play, relax, have fun, and laugh are often given second place to other responsibilities at the sacrifice of emotional, physical, social, and cognitive health. Recreational therapists heighten the client's awareness of the relationship between leisure and health and help to bring balance to the client's life. Engagement in tasks that offer relaxation and leisure experiences is imperative for good health. Recreational therapists need to have a full understanding of the benefits of leisure and help clients who are not leading a healthy leisure lifestyle to develop one. Engagement in activities that are enjoyable and relaxing opens the mind to new ideas and thoughts that help us cope with stress.

Clinical Treatment of Stress

There are five steps for the treatment of stress 1. Identify stressors and strengths, 2. Measure responses to stress, 3. Provide education, 4. Implement interventions, and 5. Reevaluate. Each are reviewed below.

1. Identify Stressors and Strengths

Therapists help clients identify their specific stressors and strengths. Knowing the source of stress and the resources (strengths) of the client is essential to building a stress treatment plan. An assessment tool developed by Eliot (1994) at the Institute of Stress Medicine is the *Quality of Life Index*. (The complete assessment is shown in the Assessment section). We like this tool because 1. it is quick to administer (10-15 minutes), 2. it is easy to score (15 minutes), 3. it indirectly educates the client to items that contribute to stress and the management of stress, 4. it evaluates a wide spectrum of items related to stress (including recreation and leisure) and provides the therapist with several scores that are easy to see and integrate, and 5. it looks at stress from the client's point of view. The last point is important because the most effective way to build a treatment plan for stress control "is to deal with the individual's perception of a stressful situation rather than with the actual situation or threat itself. We cannot control others; we can only control our reactions to them. There is much evidence that our unique perceptions and coping strategies are the primary catalyst for stress-linked disorders within our bodies" (Eliot, 1994, p. 87).

In addition to the QLI, therapists should conduct a clinical interview. Therapists should pose open-ended questions that encourage verbalizations of strengths and stressors (e.g., "What is different for you now?") and help the client to narrow down concerns about stressors and strengths so they can be turned into specific measurable objectives (e.g., poor communication skills do not allow the client to get his/her needs met; wheelchair accessibility on a school campus makes getting to class difficult). The therapist also observes and evaluates indirect expressions of stress during activities by watching the client's defensive and coping mechanisms (e.g., putting self down, denial), behavioral responses to stressful situations (e.g., violence, yelling, withdrawn behavior), and physiological responses to stress (e.g., rise in blood pressure, dilation of eye pupils, excessive sweating).

2. Measure Responses to Stress

Once stressors have been identified, the therapist measures the client's response to stress. Measuring the client's physiological, cognitive, and behavioral response to stress will provide a baseline of functioning to show if the interventions are effective. If possible, measure the client's reactions to stress in a real-life setting (e.g., overcoming physical barriers on a community outing). If this is not possible, monitor responses in simulated environments (e.g., overcoming physical barriers on hospital grounds) or during designed challenges that challenge the client's ability to deal with stress (e.g., count backwards from 300 by sevens without using paper, pencil, or calculator; play an increasingly challenging computer game).

Physiological response: The easiest ways to measure a client's physiological response to stress is through blood pressure monitoring and observation of physiological changes. Eliot (1994) recommends that blood pressure should be taken every other day over the course of ten days (five days of monitoring in all). Blood pressure should be taken several times each day, especially when entering, during, or exiting a stressful situation or when the client is believed to be in a relaxed state. Each blood pressure reading is calculated to determine the mean arterial blood pressure. To calculate the mean subtract the diastolic blood pressure from the systolic blood pressure, divide the answer by three, and then add back the diastolic blood pressure (e.g., if the blood pressure is 120/80, 120-80 = 40, 40 divided by 3 equals 13, 13 plus 80 equals 93. 93 is the mean arterial blood pressure of 120/80). Eliot (1994) divides blood pressure means into categories to determine to what extent a person is a hot reactor, as shown in Table 19. Therapists look for the highest mean over the course of the monitoring period. The highest peak is the best predictor of how the client will physiologically react to periods of high stress.

Cognitive response: Therapists ask the client to focus on internal and external cognition as they relate to dealing with stress and then write them in a daily journal for a set period of time (e.g., one week). Therapists look for patterns in the thought processes of the client (especially defensive mechanisms and coping mechanisms) and develop a plan to change distorted thinking patterns into healthy thinking patterns (e.g., changing "I can't do this" to "I can do this").

Behavioral response: Therapists look for

Table 19: Reactions to Stress

Reactor	Level	Classification	Mean Arterial Blood Pressure
Hot Reactor	Level 4	Severe	127 or greater
Hot Reactor	Level 3	Moderate	117-126
Hot Reactor	Level 2	Mild	107-125
Normal	Level 1	Normal	97-106
Cool Reactor	N/A	N/A	96 or below

behavioral manifestations of stress when the client is experiencing a stressful situation (e.g., punching walls, fidgeting, pulling hair). Behaviors are measured in terms of description (e.g., pulling one's hair, three small clumps of hair were pulled out by the client) and frequency (e.g., three times within a half hour session). Stress is not always revealed in verbalizations (e.g., client denies any stress, "I'm fine") and cognitions are not always apparent (e.g., client has internal dialogue rather than vocal dialogue). Stress, however, appears in other ways. If it is not verbally expressed, then it may manifest itself behaviorally, mentally (e.g., mental illness), or physically (e.g., physical illness).

3. Education

Clients are educated about the consequences of uncontrolled high levels of stress as it pertains to their specific situation (e.g., health, ability to perform life tasks, quality of life). Many people do not fully understand the detrimental effects of stress on their lives. Gaining insight can help clients to take control over their lifestyle and implement positive lifestyle changes.

4. Implement Interventions

The step reflects the coming together of many key components. Clients identify signs and symptoms of stress (steps 1 and 2), triggers of stress (steps 1 and 2), and managing/coping strategies for stress (step 3) so that they do not become barriers to health and therapeutic progress (step 4). Eliot (1994) comments on the relevance of managing stress through planned interventions and strategies. He says, "Life-threatening overreaction to stress is neither innate nor inevitable. We were not born with this trait. We have learned it. We can unlearn it" (p 92). Therapists convey this message to clients to highlight the control that they have in making positive lifestyle changes.

5. Reevaluate

When the program is running, it is important to check periodically to be sure that it is effective. The stressors may have changed, the client may have learned to deal with some of the stress and need new goals, the interventions may not feel comfortable any more. Depending on the particular situation it may be appropriate to do a brief reevaluation daily at the start of a program. Later there can be weekly or monthly checkups.

Program Ideas

There are many different ways to manage stress and to relax. Managing stress is very different from relaxation training, although one may affect the other.

Managing stress refers to the client's ability to take control over his/her stressors by making alterations or changes to promote positive change (e.g., time management skills, problem solving, accessing resources). Relaxation training, on the other hand, focuses on the use of specific techniques to induce a relaxation response when stress levels are high (e.g., deep breathing, progressive muscle relaxation). Relaxation training exercises are a stress management technique since they have long-term effects that enhance a person's ability to manage stress when it arises (e.g., daily meditation helps to relax the mind and body, yet it also trains the mind to stay calm and focused throughout the day).

Choosing stress management and/or relaxation training strategies requires the therapist to evaluate and integrate variables that are unique to each client. A common approach to this process is to start out by briefly reviewing several types of stress management and relaxation-training techniques that are initially thought to match the client's needs. This gives the therapist a general feel for what is appealing to or disliked by the client (e.g., a client may find yoga a very attractive intervention, yet adamantly refuse to participate in a visualization exercise because "I just don't like to do that."). Therapists must remember that although these techniques are labeled as stress management and relaxation training interventions, they do not have that effect on all people. Some people may find some of these techniques bothersome, frustrating, and annoying. We have found from experience that people who are highly stressed often have difficulty with relaxation training interventions that require a long period of time (e.g., guided imagery) and react better to beginning with simple techniques that offer an immediate physiological response (e.g., deep breathing). People who are highly stressed also seem to react better to interventions that challenge managerial skills such as problem solving, time management, and goal setting (all techniques that reflect a sense of control — an attribute that people who are highly stressed are often searching for). This is not always true, yet it does offer the therapist a viewpoint to consider when working with clients who are highly stressed.

Since therapists are aware that not all stress management and relaxation training strategies work with all people, provided below are guidelines to consider when identifying strategies:

- *Lifestyle*: Interventions must easily fit into the client's lifestyle (e.g., deep breathing is quick and discreet, while meditation requires a separate quiet space for a specific amount of time).
- *Interests*: They should align with the client's interests. Some clients do not like specific activities and will therefore balk at certain

suggestions from a therapist (e.g., doesn't like to sweat so doesn't like to go running, doesn't like to play singles tennis because reflexes are not quick enough to play both sides of the court).

- *Personality*: The interventions must fit with the personality of the client (e.g., quiet and reserved so doesn't like social activities).
- *Resources available* (e.g., would love to take up swimming but there isn't a community swimming pool in the area; the client doesn't drive and there is no paratransit service available in the community to take him to the next county to go swimming).
- *Finances* (e.g., client doesn't have enough money in her budget to participate in a community art program).
- *Level of support* (e.g., husband doesn't support his wife participating in a drama club).
- *Health abilities and limitations* (e.g., stress management technique of visualization would not be appropriate for someone who has schizophrenia; going out for a neighborhood walk might not be safe for a client who lives in a developing rural area with busy streets, no sidewalks, and a hilly terrain that surpasses the client's abilities).

Some strategies have proven to be effective for managing stress. Here is a list of some of the most popular stress management strategies to consider for clients:

- *Combating distorted thinking* and thought stopping (see "Education and Counseling" in the Techniques section).
- *Goal setting*.
- *Time management*.
- *Assertiveness training*.
- *Good nutrition*: eliminate stimulants such as caffeine, sugar, and nicotine (especially with psychosocial stresses).
- *Problem solving*: Problem solving for specific stressors with the goal of extinguishing or diminishing the stressor may be an appropriate stress management intervention (e.g., problem solve on how to identify accessibility issues prior to going to an unfamiliar place to decrease anxiety and stress associated with going to a new place). The therapist must be careful to focus on solving problems within the client's control. For example, a therapist would not help a client problem solve on how to change her sister's negative reaction to hearing "no" from the client. The therapist would help the client identify ways to deal with the sister's response.
- *Exercise*: Regular moderate exercise (three to five times a week for 20-30 minutes) decreases

stress-related symptoms and increases ability to cope with stressors.

- *Activity*: Engagement in activity, whether physically, socially, cognitively, or emotionally stimulating, can provide a relaxation response if it provides the client with a sense of enjoyment.
- *Specific skill enhancement*: The therapist focuses on impaired skills that affect the client's ability to handle stress (e.g., self-esteem, communication skills).

More ideas on dealing with stress will be found in the Techniques section: "Relaxation and Stress Reduction," "Adjustment to Disability," "Psychoneuroimmunology," and "Anger Management."

d298 General Tasks and Demands, Other Specified

d299 General Tasks and Demands, Unspecified

References

American Psychiatric Association. (1994). *Diagnostic and statistical manual of mental disorder, 4th edition.* Washington, DC: American Psychiatric Association.

Austin, D. (2004). *Therapeutic recreation processes and techniques, 5th edition.* Champaign, IL: Sagamore Publishing.

Boshes, L. & Gibbs, F. (1972). *Epilepsy handbook, 2nd ed.* Springfield, IL: Charles C. Thomas.

Brammer, L. (1988). *The helping relationship: Process and skills, 4th edition.* Englewood Cliffs, New Jersey: Prentice Hall.

burlingame, j. & Blaschko, T. (2002). *Assessment tools for recreational therapy and related fields, 3rd edition.* Ravensdale, WA: Idyll Arbor, Inc.

Corey, G. (1996). *Theory and practice of counseling and psychotherapy, 5th edition.* Pacific Grove, CA: Books/Cole Publishing Company.

Davis, M., Eshelman, E. R., & McKay, M. (2000). *The relaxation and stress reduction workbook, 5th edition.* Oakland, CA: New Harbinger Publications, Inc.

Dattilo, J., & Williams, R. (2000). Leisure education. In J. Dattilo (Ed.), *Facilitation techniques in therapeutic recreation.* State College, PA: Venture Publishing.

Edginton, C., Jordan, D., DeGraff, D. & Edginton, S. (1995). *Leisure and life satisfaction: Foundational perspectives.* Dubuque, IA: Brown & Benchmark Publishers.

Eliot, R. (1994). *From stress to strength.* New York, New York: Bantam Books.

Feldman, S. & Elliott, G. (1990). *At the threshold: The developing adolescent.* Cambridge, MA: Harvard University Press.

Griffiths, R., Evans, S., Heishman, S., Preston, K., Sannerud, C., Wolf, B., & Woodson, P. (1990). Low-dose caffeine physical dependence in humans. *Journal of Pharmacology and Experimental Therapeutics* 255:1123-1132.

Julien, R. (2004). *A Primer of Drug Action, 10th edition.* New York: Worth Publishers.

Luborsky, L. (1984). *Principles of psychoanalytic psychotherapy: A manual for supportive expressive treatment.* New York: Basic Books.

Mobily, K., Lemke, J., & Gisin, G. (1991). The idea of leisure repertoire. *Journal of Applied Gerontology, 10:*208-223.

Pary, R., Sikla, V., & Blaha, S. (1995). *Manual of clinical hospital psychiatry.* (Thienhaus, O., ed.). Washington, DC: American Psychiatric Press.

Peabody, L. (2001). *How to write policies, procedures, and task outlines: Sending clear signals in written directions.* Lacy, WA: Writing Services.

Purtilo, R., & Haddad, A. (2002). *Health professional and patient interaction (6th edition).* Philadelphia, PA: W.B. Saunders Company.

Sadock, B. & Sadock, V. (2003). *Kaplan and Sadock's synopsis of psychiatry, 9th edition.* Philadelphia, PA: Lippincott Williams & Wilkins.

St. Vincent Pallotti Center. (2004). The pie of life. www.pallotticenter.org/current/activityoftheweek/pie_of _life.

Stolov, W., & Clowers, M. (1981). *Handbook of severe disability.* Washington, DC: US Department of Education.

Stumbo, N. & Peterson, C. (2004). *Therapeutic recreation program design: Principles and procedures.* (4th Ed.) San Francisco, CA: Pearson Benjamin Cummings.

Trombly, C. (1989). *Occupational therapy for physical dysfunction, 3rd edition.* Baltimore, MD: Williams & Wilkins.

World Health Organization. *Panafrican emergency training centre,* Addis Ababa, July 1998.

Zuckerman, E (2000). *Clinician's thesaurus, 5th edition.* New York, New York: Guilford Press.

Chapter 3 Communication

This chapter is about general and specific features of communicating by language, signs, and symbols, including receiving and producing messages, carrying on conversations, and using communication devices and techniques.

Communication is one of the most important aspects of recreational therapy. When thinking about the skills a recreational therapist teaches a client, it is hard to think of any that don't require some form of communication. Physicians can treat illness without communicating with their clients (although treatment may not be optimal). Recreational therapists, on the other hand, are almost always working on activities that require explanation (receptive communication) or the client's interaction with others (expressive communication). Even the simple act of finding out what the client likes to do requires communication.

In the absence of specific known body function issues, assessing deficits in communication can be a complicated task. The therapist will note first that something is going wrong in the interaction, perhaps questions are answered inappropriately, instructions may be consistently misunderstood, or psychological issues may get in the way of conversation and discussion. Most of these problems will be the result of deficits in Body Functions (including Chapter 1 Mental Functions). Once the therapist notes the communication deficit in one of the areas in this chapter, s/he needs to look at the underlying code in Body Functions to determine the treatment required. In the sections of this chapter, there are suggested Body Functions areas to check, but others may be involved, too.

The results of communication problems will be seen in many other areas of functioning for Activities and Participation. Some of the possible areas are given in this chapter, but be sure to look for other possibilities when working with a client.

Communicating — Receiving (d310-d329)

d310 Communicating with — Receiving — Spoken Messages
Comprehending literal and implied meanings of messages in spoken language, such as understanding that a statement asserts a fact or is an idiomatic expression.

Treatment for Communicating with — Receiving — Spoken Messages

Comprehending literal and implied meanings of messages in spoken language requires the integration of many skills (e.g., b230 Hearing Functions, b1670 Reception of Language, b140 Attention Functions,

b1560 Auditory Perception). Additionally, deficits could affect functioning in other activities (e.g. d6200 Shopping, d660 Assisting Others, all skills listed in Activities and Participation Chapter 7 Interpersonal Interactions and Relationships).

If deficits are noted in this area, the therapist conducts a task analysis to determine the specific problem areas and then refers to the codes in this book for further information on how to assess, treat, document, and adapt for the dysfunction found (e.g., b16700 Reception of Spoken Language).

d315 Communicating with — Receiving — Nonverbal Messages
Comprehending the literal and implied meanings of messages conveyed by gestures, symbols, and drawings, such as realizing that a child is tired when she rubs her eyes or that a warning bell means that there is a fire.
Inclusions: communication with — receiving — body gestures, general signs and symbols, drawings, and photographs
- d3150 Communicating with — Receiving — Body Gestures
  Comprehending the meaning conveyed by facial expressions, hand movements or signs, body postures, and other forms of body language.
- d3151 Communicating with — Receiving — General Signs and Symbols
  Comprehending the meaning represented by public signs and symbols, such as traffic signs, warning symbols, musical or scientific notations, and icons.
- d3152 Communicating with — Receiving — Drawings and Photographs
  Comprehending the meaning represented by drawings (e.g., line drawings, graphic designs, paintings, three-dimensional representations), graphs, charts, and photographs, such as understanding that an upward line on a height chart indicates that a child is growing.
- d3158 Communicating with — Receiving — Nonverbal Messages, Other Specified
- d3159 Communicating with — Receiving — Nonverbal Messages, Unspecified

Treatment for Communicating with — Receiving — Nonverbal Messages

Comprehending the literal and implied meanings of messages conveyed by gestures, symbols, and drawings requires the integration of many skills (e.g., b1672 Integrative Language Functions, b210 Seeing

Functions, b140 Attention Functions, b1561 Visual Perception, b1640 Abstraction, b16702 Reception of Sign Language). Additionally, deficits could affect functioning in other activities (e.g., d350 Conversation, d860 Basic Economic Transactions, d9201 Sports, d475 Driving).

If deficits are noted in this area, the therapist conducts a task analysis to determine the specific problem areas and then refers to the codes in this book for further information on how to assess, treat, document, and adapt for the dysfunction found (e.g., b21023 Visual Picture Quality).

d320 Communicating with — Receiving — Formal Sign Language Messages
Receiving and comprehending messages in formal sign language with literal and implied meaning.

Treatment for
Communicating with — Receiving —
Formal Sign Language Messages

Receiving and comprehending messages in formal sign language with literal and implied meaning requires the integration of many skills (e.g., b140 Attention Functions, b144 Memory Functions, b16702 Reception of Sign Language). Additionally, deficits could affect functioning in other activities (e.g., d350 Conversation, d140 Learning to Read, d810-d839 Education, d920 Recreation and Leisure).

If deficits are noted in this area, the therapist conducts a task analysis to determine the specific problem areas and then refers to the codes in this book for further information on how to assess, treat, document, and adapt for the dysfunction found (e.g., b1440 Short Term Memory).

d325 Communicating with — Receiving — Written Messages
Comprehending the literal and implied meanings of messages that are conveyed through written language (including Braille), such as following political events in the daily newspaper or understanding the intent of religious scripture.

Treatment for
Communicating with — Receiving
— Written Messages

Comprehending the literal and implied meanings of messages that are conveyed through written language (including Braille) requires the integration of many skills (e.g., b140 Attention Functions, b144 Memory Functions, b16701 Reception of Written Language, b210 Seeing Functions). Additionally, deficits could affect functioning in other activities (e.g., d166 Reading, d6200 Shopping, d9203 Crafts

[if reading skills are needed to understand craft directions]).

If deficits are noted in this area, the therapist conducts a task analysis to determine the specific problem areas and then refers to the codes in this book for further information on how to assess, treat, document, and adapt for the dysfunction found (e.g., b1400 Sustaining Attention).

d329 Communicating — Receiving, Other Specified or Unspecified

Communicating — Producing (d330-d349)

d330 Speaking
Producing words, phrases, and longer passages in spoken messages with literal and implied meaning, such as expressing a fact or telling a story in oral language.

Treatment for
Speaking

Producing words, phrases, and longer passages in spoken messages with literal and implied meaning, requires the integration of many skills (e.g., b160 Thought Functions, b1641 Organization and Planning, b16710 Expression of Spoken Language). Additionally, "Speaking" could affect functioning in other activities (e.g., d355 Discussion, d620 Acquisition of Goods and Services, d7200 Forming Relationships, d845 Acquiring, Keeping, and Terminating a Job, d9205 Socializing, d910 Community Life).

If deficits are noted in this area, the therapist conducts a task analysis to determine the specific problem areas and then refers to the codes in this book for further information on how to assess, treat, document, and adapt for the dysfunction found (e.g., b1603 Control of Thought).

d335 Producing Nonverbal Messages
Using gestures, symbols, and drawings to convey messages, such as shaking one's head to indicate disagreement or drawing a picture or diagram to convey a fact or complex idea.
Inclusions: producing body gestures, signs, symbols, drawings, and photographs
- *d3350 Producing Body Language*
  Conveying meaning by movements of the body, such as facial gestures (e.g., smiling, frowning, wincing), arm and hand movements, and postures (e.g., such as embracing to indicate affection).
- *d3351 Producing Signs and Symbols*
  Conveying meaning by using signs and symbols (e.g., icons, Bliss board, scientific symbols) and symbolic notations systems, such as using musical notation to convey a melody.

- *d3352 Producing Drawings and Photographs*
  Conveying meaning by drawing, painting, sketching, and making diagrams, pictures, or photographs, such as drawing a map to give someone directions to a location.
- *d3358 Producing Nonverbal Messages, Other Specified*
- *d3359 Producing Nonverbal Messages, Unspecified*

Treatment for Producing Nonverbal Messages

Using gestures, symbols, and drawings to convey messages requires the integration of many skills (e.g., b160 Thought Functions, b1641 Organization and Planning, skills listed in Body Functions Chapter 7 Neuromusculoskeletal and Movement Related Functions [to make physical gestures], b1672 Integrative Language Functions). Additionally, deficits could affect functioning in other activities (e.g., d175 Solving Problems, d172 Calculating, d9201 Sports, d9203 Crafts, d7200 Forming Relationships).

If deficits are noted in this area, the therapist conducts a task analysis to determine the specific problem areas and then refers to the codes in this book for further information on how to assess, treat, document, and adapt for the dysfunction found (e.g., b710 Mobility of Joint Functions).

d340 Producing Messages in Formal Sign Language
Conveying, with formal sign language, literal and implied meaning.

Treatment for Producing Messages in Formal Sign Language

Conveying literal and implied meaning using formal sign language requires the integration of many skills (e.g., b710 Mobility of Joint Functions, b7202 Mobility of Carpal Bones, b735 Muscle Functions, b765 Involuntary Movement Functions, b160 Thought Functions, b16712 Expression of Sign Language, b1672 Integrative Language Functions). Additionally, deficits could affect functioning in other activities (e.g., d7200 Forming Relationships, d910 Community Life, d9200 Play, d810-d839 Education, d840-d859 Work and Employment).

If deficits are noted in this area, the therapist conducts a task analysis to determine the specific problem areas and then refers to the codes in this book for further information on how to assess, treat, document, and adapt for the dysfunction found (e.g., b7352 Tone of Muscles of One Side of Body).

d345 Writing Messages
Producing the literal and implied meanings of messages that are conveyed through written language, such as writing a letter to a friend.

Treatment for Writing Messages

Producing the literal and implied meanings of messages that are conveyed through written language requires the integration of many skills (e.g., skills listed in Body Functions Chapter 7 Neuromusculoskeletal and Movement Related Functions related to using the hand for writing such as b710 Mobility of Joint Functions and b735 Muscle Tone Functions; d440 Fine Hand Use for picking up, grasping, manipulating, and releasing a writing utensil; d170 Writing; b16711 Expression of Written Language). Additionally, deficits could affect functioning in other activities (e.g., d810-d839 Education, d840-d859 Work and Employment, d660 Assisting Others).

If deficits are noted in this area, the therapist conducts a task analysis to determine the specific problem areas and then refers to the codes in this book for further information on how to assess, treat, document, and adapt for the dysfunction found (e.g., d4401 Grasping).

d349 Communication — Producing, Other Specified and Unspecified

Conversation and Use of Communication Devices and Techniques (d350-d369)

d350 Conversation
Starting, sustaining, and ending an interchange of thoughts and ideas, carried out by means of spoken, written, sign, or other forms of language, with one or more people one knows or who are strangers, in formal or casual settings.
Inclusions: Starting, sustaining, and ending a conversation; conversing with one or many people
- *d3500 Starting a Conversation*
  Beginning a dialogue or interchange, such as by introducing oneself, expressing customary greetings, and introducing a topic or asking questions.
- *d3501 Sustaining a Conversation*
  Continuing and shaping a dialogue or interchange by adding ideas, introducing a new topic, or retrieving a topic that has been previously mentioned, as well as by taking turns in speaking or signing.
- *d3502 Ending a Conversation*
  Finishing a dialogue or interchange with customary termination statements or expressions and by bringing closure to the topic under discussion.

- *d3503 Conversing with One Person*
  Initiating, maintaining, shaping, and terminating a dialogue or interchange with one person, such as in discussing the weather with a friend.
- *d3504 Conversing with Many People*
  Initiating, maintaining, shaping, and terminating a dialogue or interchange with more than one individual, such as in starting and participating in a group interchange.
- *d3508 Conversation, Other Specified*
- *d3509 Conversation, Unspecified*

Treatment for
Conversation

Starting, sustaining, and ending an interchange of thoughts and ideas, carried out by means of spoken, written, sign, or other forms of language, with one or more people one knows or who are strangers, in formal or casual settings requires the integration of many skills (e.g., b110 Consciousness Functions, b122 Global Psychosocial Functions, b1260 Extraversion, b1304 Impulse Control, b140 Attention Functions, b144 Memory Functions, b1560 Auditory Perception, b1561 Visual Perception, b1603 Control of Thought, and many more). Additionally, deficits could affect functioning in other activities (e.g., d910 Community Life, d810-d839 Education, d840-d859 Work and Employment, d660 Assisting Others, d9205 Socializing, d9201 Sports, d9300 Organized Religion [if taking part in a religious conversation], d7200 Forming Relationships, d770 Intimate Relationships).

If deficits are noted in this area, the therapist conducts a task analysis to determine the specific problem areas and then refers to the codes in this book for further information on how to assess, treat, document, and adapt for the dysfunction found (e.g., b1304 Impulse Control).

d355 Discussion
Starting, sustaining, and ending an examination of a matter, with arguments for or against, or debate carried out by means of spoken, written, sign, or other forms of language, with one or more people one knows or who are strangers, in formal or casual settings.
Inclusions: discussion with one person or many people
- *d3550 Discussion with One Person*
  Initiating, maintaining, shaping, or terminating an argument or debate with one person.
- *d3551 Discussion with Many People*
  Initiating, maintaining, shaping, or terminating an argument or debate with more than one individual.
- *d3558 Discussion, Other Specified*
- *d3559 Discussion, Unspecified*

Treatment for
Discussion

Discussion requires the integration of many skills (e.g., b110 Consciousness Functions, b122 Global Psychosocial Functions, b1260 Extraversion, b1304 Impulse Control, b140 Attention Functions, b144 Memory Functions, b1560 Auditory Perception, b1561 Visual Perception, b1603 Control of Thought, and many more). Additionally, deficits could affect functioning in other activities (e.g., d910 Community Life, d810-d839 Education, d840-d859 Work and Employment, d9201 Sports, d9300 Organized Religion [if taking part in a Bible Study discussion group], d7200 Forming Relationships, d770 Intimate Relationships).

If deficits are noted in this area, the therapist conducts a task analysis to determine the specific problem areas and then refers to the codes in this book for further information on how to assess, treat, document, and adapt for the dysfunction found (e.g., b1266 Confidence).

d360 Using Communication Devices and Techniques
Using devices, techniques, and other means for the purposes of communicating, such as calling a friend on the telephone.
Inclusions: using telecommunication devices, using writing machines and communication techniques
- *d3600 Using Telecommunication Devices*
  Using telephones and other machines, such as facsimile or telex machines, as a means of communication.
- *d3601 Using Writing Machines*
  Using machines for writing, such as typewriters, computers, and Braille writers, as a means of communication.
- *d3602 Using Communication Techniques*
  Performing actions and tasks involved in techniques for communicating, such as reading lips.
- *d3608 Using Communication Devices and Techniques, Other Specified*
- *d3609 Using Communication Devices and Techniques, Unspecified*

Treatment for
Using Communication Devices
and Techniques

Using devices, techniques, and other means for the purposes of communicating requires the integration of many skills (e.g., b140 Attention Functions, b144 Memory Functions, b1564 Tactile Perception, b210 Seeing Functions, b230 Hearing Functions, b2702 Sensitivity to Pressure, skills in Body Functions Chapter 3 Voice and Speech Functions, skills in Body Functions Chapter 7

Neuromusculoskeletal and Movement Related Functions that are needed to operate the specific communication device such as b710 Mobility of Joint Functions, b730 Muscle Power Functions, b735 Muscle Tone Functions, b760 Control of Voluntary Movement Functions, and b765 Involuntary Muscle Functions). Additionally, deficits could affect functioning in other activities (e.g., d350 Conversation, d355 Discussion, d155 Acquiring Skills, d175 Solving Problems, d2402 Handling Crisis, d7200 Forming Relationships, d910 Community Life, d810-d839 Education, d840-d859 Work and Employment).

If deficits are noted in this area, the therapist conducts a task analysis to determine the specific problem areas and then refers to the codes in this book for further information on how to assess, treat, document, and adapt for the dysfunction found (e.g., b2300 Sound Detection).

d369 Conversation and Use of Communication Devices and Techniques, Other Specified and Unspecified

d398 Communication, Other Specified

d399 Communication, Unspecified

Chapter 4 Mobility

This chapter is about moving by changing body position or location or by transferring from one place to another, by carrying, moving, or manipulating objects, by walking running or climbing, and by using various forms of transportation.

Prior to 2001 the term mobility generally referred to the ability to move from one place to another. For example, the 2000 *Dorland's Illustrated Medical Dictionary* defined mobility as "capability of movement, or being moved." (p. 1122) Most aspects of mobility were assigned to the physical therapist, who worked with walking, mobility, and adapting equipment (such as wheelchairs, walkers, canes, splints) to help the client move from one place to another.

The scope of the term mobility has been greatly expanded by the World Health Organization. Mobility now encompasses walking and moving, use of transportation options, and participation in many different types of activities (e.g., catching, running).

The scope of practice for the recreational therapist includes many elements of mobility training and enhancement. While it is common for a physical therapist to determine the type of walking and moving appropriate for a client after a disabling condition, it is often the recreational therapist who helps the client problem solve barriers to mobility, especially related to moving around the community and using adaptive mobility equipment for sports and recreational activities. The occupational therapist often determines the techniques and adapted equipment to be used by the client for carrying, moving, and handling objects. The recreational therapist uses his/her specialized knowledge to help the client integrate the equipment and techniques into everyday life.

To illustrate that the definition of mobility has clearly moved into the scope of practice of the recreational therapist look at d465.

Changing and Maintaining Body Position (d410-d429)

d410 Changing Basic Body Position
Getting into and out of a body position and moving from one location to another, such as getting up out of a chair to lie down on a bed, and getting into and out of positions of kneeling and squatting.
Inclusion: Changing body position from lying down, from squatting or kneeling, from sitting or standing, bending and shifting the body's center of gravity
Exclusions: transferring oneself (d420)
* *d4100 Lying Down*
  Getting into and out of a lying down position or changing body position from horizontal to any

other position, such as standing up or sitting down.
Inclusion: getting into a prostrate position
* *d4101 Squatting*
  Getting into and out of the seated or crouched posture on one's haunches with knees closely drawn up or sitting on one's heels, such as may be necessary in toilets that are at floor level, or changing body position from squatting to any other position, such as standing up.
* *d4102 Kneeling*
  Getting into and out of a position where the body is supported by the knees with legs bent, such as during prayers, or changing body position from kneeling to any other position, such as standing up.
* *d4103 Sitting*
  Getting into and out of a seated position and changing body position from sitting down to any other position, such as standing up or lying down.
  Inclusions: Getting into a sitting position with bent legs or cross-legged; getting into a sitting position with feet supported or unsupported.
* *d4104 Standing*
  Getting into and out of a standing position or changing body position from standing to any other position, such as lying down or sitting down.
* *d4105 Bending*
  Tilting the back downwards or to the side, at the torso, such as in bowing or reaching down for an object.
* *d4106 Shifting the Body's Centre of Gravity*
  Adjusting or moving the weight of the body from one position to another while sitting, standing, or lying, such as moving from one foot to another while standing.
  Exclusions: transferring oneself (d420), walking (450)
* *d4108 Changing Basic Body Position, Other Specified*
* *d4109 Changing Basic Body Position, Unspecified*

Treatment for Changing Basic Body Position

For clients to be able to change or maintain body positions they need to work on the underlying functional skills associated with body position. There are four underlying principles associated with changing or maintaining body position. These are 1. functions of the joints and bones, 2. muscle functions,   3. movement   functions,   and

4. proprioceptive function. There are many reasons that clients may have problems with changing and maintaining body positions. The impairments may originate from a loss of muscle (being out of shape, muscle degeneration, or deconditioning), loss of muscle control (through neurological or brain damage), loss of tissue mobility, loss of the sensory feedback, or impairment in processes that allow balance. Because the causes of impairment vary, so will the approaches taken by the recreational therapist.

The primary body tissues that allow individuals to change or maintain position are soft-tissue (muscle, connective tissue, and skin) and boney tissue (bones and the associated joint structure). Conditions that cause a reduction in tissue mobility include "1. prolonged immobilization, 2. restricted mobility, 3. connective tissue or neuromuscular diseases, 4. tissue pathology due to trauma, and 5. congenital and acquired boney deformities." (Kisner & Colby, 1990, p. 109)

Refer to Body Functions Chapter 7 Neuromusculoskeletal and Movement Related Functions for information on how to assess, treat, document, and adapt for joint, bones, muscle, and movement functions.

Refer to Body Functions Chapter 2 Sensory Functions and Pain (specifically code b260 Proprioceptive Function) for information on how to assess, treat, document, and adapt for proprioceptive dysfunction.

Recreational therapists consult with the physical and occupational therapist for recommended techniques for changing body positions (e.g., technique used by the client to move from sitting to supine). Techniques are based on client's abilities, limitations, and precautions/parameters (e.g., weight-bearing restrictions). Techniques used by PTs and OTs may need to be adapted to meet the needs of the client in different settings (e.g., kneeling techniques for outdoor gardening may vary from how they are done indoors due to the lack of a sturdy support). Recreational therapists assist the client in problem solving for change of position and address the development of change of position skills in real-life environments. Below are common approaches to changing position.

- *Sit to stand*: Scoot to the edge of the seat, tuck the feet slightly behind the knees, place the hands on armrests, lean forward (nose over toes), push up using the leg muscles with the arms pushing up from the armrest for added support, fully stand to upright position.
- *Stand to sit*: Back up to the chair so that the back of the legs are touching the chair, reach back for the armrests while leaning slightly forward,

slowly lower bottom onto the chair using the leg muscles and arms on the armrest for added support, readjust into a comfortable sitting position.
- *Lying to sitting*: While on a bed, roll onto the side facing the edge of the bed, flex the elbow and wrist of the arm on the bottom. While pushing up with the arm to a sitting position, swing the legs off the side of bed. The final position is sitting on the edge of the bed with the legs dangling off the side.
- *Sitting to lying*: Sit down on the bed two thirds of the way up from the bottom, rotate the trunk and place the palms of both hands on the bed, swing the legs onto the bed one at a time, stretch out the legs and gently lower self onto the bed using the arms for support.
- *Stand to kneel*: Upper body support is helpful. Place the left hand on a sturdy support and step back one step with the left foot, place the right hand on the right knee, flex both knees until the left knee rests on ground and the right knee is at a 90° angle, slide the right foot backwards and gently lower the right knee onto the ground.
- *Kneel to stand*: Place the left hand on a sturdy support, slide the right foot forward to raise the right knee to a 90° angle, place the right hand on the right knee, push up into a standing position using the left hand on sturdy support and the right hand on the right knee.

d415 Maintaining a Body Position
Staying in the same body position as required, such as remaining seated or remaining standing for work or school.
Inclusions: maintaining a lying, squatting, kneeling, sitting, and standing position.
- *d4150 Maintaining a Lying Position*
  Staying in a lying position from some time as required, such as remaining in a prone position in bed.
  Inclusions: staying in a prone (face down or prostrate), supine (face upwards), or side-lying position
- *d4151 Maintaining a Squatting Position*
  Staying in a squatting position for some time as required, such as when sitting on the floor without a seat.
- *d4152 Maintaining a Kneeling Position*
  Staying in a kneeling position where the body is supported by the knees with legs bent for some time as required, such as during prayers in church.
- *d4153 Maintaining a Sitting Position*
  Staying in a seated position, on a seat or the floor, for some time as required, such as when sitting at a desk or table.

Inclusions: staying in a sitting position with straight legs or cross-legged, with feet supported or unsupported

- *d4154 Maintaining a Standing Position*
  Staying in a standing position for some time as required, such as when standing in a queue.
  Inclusions: staying in a standing position on a slope, on slippery or hard surfaces
- *d4158 Maintaining a Body Position, Other Specified*
- *d4159 Maintaining a Body Position, Unspecified*

Treatment for Maintaining a Body Position

Maintaining a body position requires the skills reviewed in the previous code set, Changing Body Position, although a greater degree of strength and control is needed to maintain the position in some instances (e.g., maintaining a squatting position requires more strength and control than maintaining a lying position).

The skill of maintaining a position means that there is no movement for a prolonged period of time, such as sitting still at a desk or standing during church. It does not encompass movement (e.g., shooting basketballs while standing). Therefore, therapists should be careful not to use this code for dynamic positions (movement within a position). Dynamic positions are not separately described in the ICF. Rather they are included in the various activities listed in the ICF. For example, throwing, catching, and reaching are in d445 Hand and Arm Use, jumping is in d455 Moving Around, and kicking is in d435 Moving Objects with Lower Extremities. These codes, although they indicate movement within a body position, do not require a specific body position for the function (e.g., the codes do not say that a person has to be standing in order to show full function with kicking — kicking can be from any position including sitting or lying down).

Maintaining a position is often documented by the length of time that a person can hold the position (e.g., client able to maintain a standing position for eight minutes prior to fatigue) and the level and/or type of assistance that is needed to maintain the position (e.g., client requires bilateral upper extremity support of table to maintain a standing position for four minutes; client able to maintain an unsupported sitting position for six minutes with moderate physical assistance from therapist).

If difficulty is noted in the person's ability to maintain a body position, the specific problem is identified through task analysis (see "Activity and Task Analysis" in the Techniques section) and/or direct observation to determine the area of breakdown. Once the dysfunction is isolated, the therapist consults the specific function in this book to learn how to assess, document, treat, and adapt for the problem.

d420 Transferring Oneself

Moving from one surface to another, such as sliding along a bench or moving from a bed to a chair, without changing body positions.
Inclusions: transferring oneself while sitting or lying
Exclusions: changing basic body position (d410)

- *d4200 Transferring Oneself While Sitting*
  Moving from a sitting position on a seat to another seat on the same or a different level, such as moving from one bed to another.
  Inclusions: moving from a chair to another seat, such as a toilet seat; moving from a wheelchair to a car seat
  Exclusions: changing basic body position (d410)
- *d4201 Transferring Oneself While Lying*
  Moving from one lying position to another on the same or a different level, such as moving from one bed to another.
  Exclusions: changing basic body position (d410)
- *d4208 Transferring Oneself, Other Specified*
- *d4209 Transferring Oneself, Unspecified*

Treatment for Transferring Oneself

The ability to transfer to or from various surfaces is a basic skill required for many leisure activities. Scooting into a booth at a restaurant, moving from one seat to another in a canoe, or moving over on the couch so that a friend may join you to watch a movie are all activities that involve transferring. Clients who use wheeled mobility devices or who are in a bed in a health care setting have an even greater need to transfer to engage in leisure activities. Many activities require specialized seating (snow mobiles, bicycles, cars, horseback riding) or take place using equipment that does not accommodate the size and structure of a wheelchair, but will allow a standard chair (for example, many picnic table designs, some restaurant seating). The recreational therapist working either in a clinical setting or in the community will need to know how to implement transfers and how to train clients to use transfers (called transfer training).

It is often the physical therapist or the occupational therapist who provides basic transfer training for clients. To help the client participate in activities the recreational therapist needs to know how to safely implement or modify transfers for two reasons:

1. The recreational therapist will be expected to help the client transfer during activities. For example, a client using a wheelchair comes to the pool for aquatic therapy. The client's orders from his physician specify that the client needs

to have moderate assistance to safely transfer from his wheelchair and the client needs to transfer to a bench to change his clothes. The recreational therapist needs to know how to implement the moderate assistance needed by the client so the client may change into swimming trunks.

2. Some leisure activities will require modifications or special problem solving so that clients can engage in the activity. For example, a client using a wheelchair has decided to try out the hand-peddled bicycle that the recreational therapist has in the gym. Transferring to a bicycle seat is different from transferring to a chair so the client may need instruction to transfer safely and efficiently.

To be able to transfer oneself (or for the therapist to help a client transfer), there are some basic guidelines to follow. See "Transfers" in the Techniques section for guidelines and types of transfers.

d429 Changing and Maintaining Body Position, Other Specified or Unspecified

Carrying, Moving, and Handling Objects (d430-d449)

d430 Lifting and Carrying Objects
Raising up an object or taking something from one place to another, such as when lifting a cup or carrying a child from one room to another.
Inclusions: lifting, carrying in the hands or arms, or on shoulders, hip, back, or head; putting down
- *d4300 Lifting*
  Raising up an object in order to move it from a lower to a higher level, such as when lifting a glass from the table.
- *d4301 Carrying in the Hands*
  Taking or transporting an object from one place to another using the hands, such as when carrying a drinking glass or a suitcase.
- *d4302 Carrying in the Arms*
  Taking or transporting an object from one place to another using the arms and hands, such as when carrying a child.
- *d4303 Carrying on Shoulders, Hip, and Back*
  Taking or transporting an object from one place to another using the shoulders, hip, or back, or some combination of these, such as when carrying a large parcel.
- *d4304 Carrying on the Head*
  Taking or transporting an object from one place to another using the head, such when as carrying a container of water on the head.
- *d4305 Putting Down Objects*
  Using hands, arms, or other parts of the body to place an object down on a surface or place, such

as when lowering a container of water to the ground.
- *d4308 Lifting and Carrying, Other Specified*
- *d4309 Lifting and Carrying, Unspecified*

Treatment for Lifting and Carrying Objects

Lifting and carrying objects is such a basic skill that dysfunction could greatly inhibit a person's ability to participate in life activities. Our arms are used routinely throughout the day to lift and carry objects to meet our needs for work, play, recreation, and self-care (e.g., lifting and carrying a briefcase, food items, craft supplies, children, laundry). Impairments that can affect someone's ability to lift, carry, and put down objects include upper extremity amputations, congenital arm deformities, severe rheumatoid arthritis, severe burns on the upper extremities, paralysis, weakness (e.g., hypotonia, severe deconditioning), involuntary motor impairments (e.g., tremors), muscle contractures, lifting restrictions (e.g., after a heart attack), cognitive problems (e.g., severe inattention to the task), and devices that hinder a person's ability to transport items in the hands (e.g., holding onto a walker with two hands does not allow the person to carry something in the hands while walking).

Therapists document the specific dysfunction (e.g., lifting restriction of five pounds), the level of dysfunction that it causes with the activity (e.g., restricts client from carrying his cello), the level of assistance that is needed (e.g., client is dependent for transport of cello due to lifting restrictions), and adaptations recommended (e.g., until lifting restrictions are removed, client's sister to transport cello).

Proper body mechanics are to be used for lifting, carrying, and putting down objects to prevent injury. Refer to "Body Mechanics and Ergonomics" in the Techniques section for more information.

If problems are anticipated, the therapist identifies the specific limitations (e.g., medical orders, clinical assessment) and consults other health care professionals as needed to problem solve for alternative techniques (e.g., one-handed lifting techniques for large items). Some adaptations for lifting and putting down objects include scooping using the forearms and using adaptive devices such as a "reacher." Adaptations for carrying objects are numerous including the use of backpacks (on the back or on the back of a wheelchair), baskets (on a bike, under a wheelchair), waist packs, pocketbooks, pockets, baby sling carriers, and bags (small lightweight bag to hang on side of a walker).

d435 Moving Objects with Lower Extremities
Performing, coordinated actions aimed at moving an object by using the legs and feet, such as kicking a ball or pushing pedals on a bicycle.
Inclusions: pushing with lower extremities; kicking
* *d4350 Pushing with Lower Extremities*
  Using the legs and feet to exert a force on an object to move it away, such as pushing a chair away with a foot.
* *d4351 Kicking*
  Using the legs and feet to propel something away, such as kicking a ball.
* *d4358 Moving Objects with Lower Extremities, Other Specified*
* *d4359 Moving Objects with Lower Extremities, Unspecified*

Treatment for
Moving Objects with Lower Extremities

Moving objects with the lower extremities (e.g., pushing, kicking, sliding) is common in sports and recreational activities (e.g., soccer, kickball). Impairments that can affect someone's ability to move objects with the lower extremities include lower extremity amputations; congenital leg deformities; severe rheumatoid arthritis or osteoarthritis in the hips, knees, and ankles; involuntary motor impairments (e.g., tremors, clonus); leg joint restrictions (e.g., limitations in knee flexion after knee replacement surgery); cognitive problems (e.g., severe inattention to the task); paralysis; extreme weakness; muscle contractures; and devices that hinder a person's ability to move objects with the lower extremities (e.g., a knee ankle foot orthosis or cast/splint).

Therapists document the specific dysfunction (e.g., knee flexion limited to 45°), the level of dysfunction that it causes with the activity (e.g., restricts client from kicking the soccer ball with his daughter), the level of assistance that is needed (e.g., client independent in stopping the rolled soccer ball with lower extremities but is dependent in kicking it back to his daughter), and adaptations recommended (e.g., until knee flexion/extension improves, client to play the part of goalie when practicing soccer with his daughter in the backyard).

If problems are anticipated, the therapist identifies the specific limitations (e.g., medical orders, clinical assessment) and consults with other health care professionals as needed to problem solve for alternative techniques (e.g., designing a push stick so the client can send a soccer ball back to his daughter when practicing in the back yard). Some adaptations for moving objects with the lower extremities include the use of devices (e.g., push stick, broom) or modification of the activity (e.g., instead of kicking a soccer

ball back and forth with his daughter the client plays the part of a goalie).

d440 Fine Hand Use
Performing the coordinated actions of handling objects, picking up, manipulating, and releasing them using one's hand, fingers, and thumb, such as required to lift coins off a table or turn a dial or knob.
Inclusions: picking up, grasping, manipulating, and releasing
Exclusions: lifting and carrying objects (d430)
* *d4400 Picking Up*
  Lifting or taking up a small object with hands and fingers, such as when picking up a pencil.
* *d4401 Grasping*
  Using one or both hands to seize and hold something, such as when grasping a tool or a door knob.
* *d4402 Manipulating*
  Using fingers and hands to exert control over, direct or guide something, such as when handling coins or other small objects.
* *d4403 Releasing*
  Using fingers and hands to let go or set free something so that it falls or changes position, such as when dropping an item of clothing.
* *d4408 Fine Hand Use, Other Specified*
* *d4409 Fine Hand Use, Unspecified*

Treatment for
Fine Hand Use

Fine hand use can be affected by a variety of conditions including rheumatoid arthritis, Parkinson's disease, multiple sclerosis, stroke, brain injury, peripheral neuropathy (e.g., from diabetes), upper extremity amputations, upper extremity congenital deformities, severe burns on the upper extremities, carpal tunnel syndrome, trigger finger, and muscle contractures.

Fine hand use (previously called fine motor skills, fine coordination, and/or dexterity) is a primary component of many activities. To help clients improve fine hand use the therapist should have a basic understanding of hand grasps (see Table 20) and of ways to improve client performance through modification of the environment.

Prior to addressing fine hand use functions, the therapist identifies any specific precautions or parameters (e.g., joint protection of the hands) and conducts an assessment of fine hand skills. Assessments that look at fine hand use include:
* *General Recreation Screening Tool* (GRST) for mental retardation/developmental disability and pediatric settings.
* *Comprehensive Evaluation in Recreational Therapy — Physical Disabilities* (CERT Phys/Dys) for people five years or older with loss of function

- *Recreation Early Development Screening Tool* (REDS) for individuals with severe or profound mental retardation or severe developmental disabilities who are adaptively under one year of age.
- *Therapeutic Recreation Activity Assessment* (TRAA) for people age four and older who have some obvious loss including clients with brain trauma, developmental disabilities, psychiatric disorders, and/or clients who are receiving some manner of supportive care such as residents in nursing homes, group homes, or assisted living.
- *Jebsen-Taylor Hand Function Test* to measure hand function with seven subtests covering the hand functions required for daily activities.

Fine hand use can also be assessed by asking the client to:
- Touch each finger to the thumb (finger thumb opposition).
- Make a fist and stretch out fingers (flexion and extension of fingers).
- Make a circle with the wrist (wrist rotation).
- Pinch the therapist's thumb or skin between thumb and index finger (pinch).
- Stretch out fingers straight (to observe any finger deformities or contractures).
- Fan fingers open and closed (abduction and adduction of fingers).
- Bend palms and fingers up and down (wrist flexion and extension).
- With hand in a gentle fist, stretch out one finger and then put it back into the fist (do this with each finger and thumb to evaluate digit isolation).
- Pick up items. Place different size items in front of the client and observe the client's grasp (see Table 20). Items might include a penny, a card, a pen, a paint bottle, a game board box, etc. Observe the type of grasp the client uses to pick up each item. Ask the client to pick up a specific item using a specific grasp if the typical grasp is not used (e.g., instead of picking up a penny using a pincer grasp the person slides it to the edge of the table and uses a scissor grasp. Use items that are common in the client's typical life activities when possible.

Therapists document the specific fine hand dysfunction and the specific problem it causes with fine hand use (e.g., intension tremors impacting ability to manipulate objects smaller than two-inch diameter), the level of assistance required (e.g., client able to pick up coins using a pincer grasp with minimal assistance), or the percentage or ratio of performance (e.g., client able to successfully and

Table 20: Developmental Levels of Hand Grasps

	Palmer Grasp: Adducted Thumb. Generally developed by age 5 months.
	Scissor Grasp: Object held between side of finger and thumb. Generally developed by age 8 months.
	Radial-Digital Grasp: Object held between the thumb and fingers so that it is not touching the palm. Generally developed by age 8 months.
	3-Jaw Chuck Grasp: Holding an object using the thumb and two fingers. Generally developed by age 10 months.
	Pincer Grasp: The use of the index finger and the thumb to pick up and hold an object. Usually developed by age 10 months.

From burlingame, j. and Blaschko, T. (2002). *Assessment Tools for Recreational Therapy and Related Fields, Third Edition.* Ravensdale, WA: Idyll Arbor. Used with permission.

independently pick up 10 out of 20 coins one at a time using a right pincer grasp).

Modalities used to improve fine hand use depend upon the underlying problems. Refer to the specific diagnosis for more information. In general:
- Conditions due to brain impairment (e.g., stroke, brain injury): focus on the use of graduated fine hand activities and repetition to develop neural connections to promote fine hand use. (See "Neuroplasticity" in the Techniques section.)
- Conditions due to joint impairments such as rheumatoid arthritis: focus on activity adaptation to protect joints (see b710 Mobility of Joint Functions for information on joint protection; also see "Body Mechanics and Ergonomics" and "Fine Hand Use Ergonomics," in the Techniques section) and encourage routine gentle range of motion of the hands.
- Conditions resulting in peripheral neuropathy: focus on teaching the client how to compensate for difficulty with fine hand use by greater reliance on his/her vision and adapting objects so they are easier to handle.
- Conditions due to chronic neurological conditions such as multiple sclerosis and Parkinson's disease: focus on routine range of motion exercises for the fingers and hands along with

activity adaptations to make it easier to handle objects.

- Conditions due to congenital deformities and overuse injury (e.g., carpal tunnel syndrome, trigger finger): focus on adaptation of activities to make it easier to handle objects.
- Conditions that result in muscle contractures (e.g., secondary complication of upper extremity paresis that is not routinely ranged or used in functional activities): focuses on release of contractures (if possible) through gentle passive range of motion and heat.

See "Grip Aids" in the Equipment section for common adaptations, such as:
- Increasing the size of the object.
- Using a universal cuff.
- Using stabilizing materials.

Also consider substituting for the activity (e.g., switching from embroidery to plastic canvas work because it requires less fine hand skills).

d445 Hand and Arm Use
Performing the coordinated actions required to move objects or to manipulate them by using hands and arms, such as when turning door handles or throwing or catching an object.
Inclusions: pulling or pushing objects; reaching; turning or twisting the hands or arms; throwing; catching
Exclusions: fine hand use (d440)
- *d4450 Pulling*
  Using fingers, hands, and arms to bring an object towards oneself, or to move it from place to place, such as when pulling a door closed.
- *d4451 Pushing*
  Using fingers, hands, and arms to move something from oneself, or to move it from place to place, such as when pushing an animal away.
- *d4452 Reaching*
  Using the fingers, hands, and arms to extend outwards and touch and grasp something, such as when reaching across a table or desk for a book.
- *d4453 Turning or Twisting the Hands or Arms*
  Using fingers, hands, and arms to rotate, turn, or bend an object, such as is required to use tools or utensils.
- *d4454 Throwing*
  Using fingers, hands, and arms to lift something and propel it with some force through the air, such as when tossing a ball.
- *d4455 Catching*
  Using fingers, hands, and arms to grasp a moving object in order to bring it to a stop and hold it, such as when catching a ball.
- *d4458 Hand and Arm Use, Other Specified*
- *d4459 Hand and Arm Use, Unspecified*

Treatment for Hand and Arm Use

Problems with hand and arm use can be affected by the conditions described in Fine Hand Use (the previous code set). Evaluation of hand use is the same as the evaluation discussed in Fine Hand Use. To evaluate arm use add additional components looking at joint and bone functions, muscle functions, and movement functions, all of which can be found in Body Functions Chapter 7 Neuromusculoskeletal and Movement Related Functions. That chapter also has information on assessment, documentation, treatment, and adaptation of dysfunction in areas affecting hand and arm use.

d449 Carrying, Moving, and Handling Objects, Other Specified and Unspecified

Walking and Moving (d450-d469)

d450 Walking
Moving along a surface on foot, step by step, so that one foot is always on the ground, such as when strolling, sauntering, walking forwards, backwards, or sideways.
Inclusions: walking short or long distances; walking on different surfaces; walking around obstacles
Exclusions: transferring oneself (d420); moving around (d455)
- *d4500 Walking Short Distances*
  Walking for less than a kilometer, such as walking around rooms or hallways, within a building or for short distances outside.
- *d4501 Walking Long Distances*
  Walking for more than a kilometer, such as across a village or town, between villages or across open areas.
- *d4502 Walking on Different Surfaces*
  Walking on sloping, uneven, or moving surfaces, such as on grass, gravel, or ice and snow, or walking aboard a ship, train, or other vehicle.
- *d4503 Walking around Obstacles*
  Walking in ways required to avoid moving and immobile objects, people, animals, and vehicles, such as walking around a marketplace or shop, around or through traffic or other crowded areas.
- *d4508 Walking, Other Specified*
- *d4509 Walking, Unspecified*

Treatment for Walking

In the past the term *ambulation* was used to mean *walking* (with or without adaptive equipment). While the term ambulation is frequently heard in treatment settings, the World Health Organization has moved away from using the term ambulation and instead uses the easier to understand term "walking."

When a client uses a method other than walking to get from one place to another the term now used is "moving." The simplification of this terminology makes translation of concepts easier (all languages have a word meaning walking) and helps demystify health care by using words clients are comfortable with.

Information on mobility devices, which can be used while walking, can be found in the Equipment section. For information on the types of gaits associated with the use of crutches and other mobility devices, see "Gait" in the Concepts section. Information on how to document walking can be found in b770 Gait Pattern Functions.

Prior to having a client walk who has experienced a condition, illness, or injury, medical orders are reviewed by the therapist. Medical orders provide information on any precautions or parameters that need to be followed (e.g., weight-bearing precautions, heart rate parameters, blood pressure parameters, restrictions to prolonged and direct sunlight, oxygen saturation levels, range restrictions). See "Vital Signs" and "Oxygen" for specific information, as well as consulting the specific diagnoses for information on diagnosis-specific precautions or parameters. Recreational therapists next consult with the primary physical therapist working with the client after reading the latest physical therapy clinical notes. The clinical notes will inform the recreational therapist of the current walking skills of the client (distance, device, level of assistance, specific gait deviations). Consulting with the physical therapist is helpful when further information is needed (e.g., specific cueing or guarding technique used by the physical therapist when walking with the client).

Recreational therapists address functional walking, meaning that walking is addressed within real-life activities (e.g., walking on outdoor surfaces, walking around obstacles, walking through manual doors, walking while performing a task such as watering the garden or walking a pet). Recreational therapists focus on using learned walking techniques in real-life settings and activities. Consequently, recreational therapists address the skill of walking after the client achieves functional walking skills. Functional skills are usually defined by distance and level of assistance. For distance, walking at least 50' for indoor activities, 250' for short community distances, and greater than 500' for general community activities is considered functional. Regarding level of assistance, the client must require minimal assistance or less by one person. Moderate assistance is typically more than a family member or caregiver can handle, making it an unrealistic mobility choice for home and community activities.

Although this is a general rule of thumb, it is important to note that there are exceptions to the rule that are made on an individual basis.

The best way to enhance community mobility skills is to "just do it." Practice and repetition will enhance the client's confidence and skills, and allow for increased opportunities to find solutions for barriers and attitudes. The therapist may find it helpful to start out by reviewing the techniques and then practicing outdoor walking and moving techniques on the facility's campus. Do not overwhelm the client by trying everything in one day. Provide positive feedback. Empathize with client's reservations and fears about walking and moving outdoors. The therapist will need to discuss issues related to outdoor and other community tasks and assist the client in problem solving outdoor walking and moving skills (e.g., how can the client safely use her walker and carry mail from the mail box? Is it appropriate for the client to walk with a cane while walking his pet poodle?). The therapist may also wish to write up guidelines and give them to the client for reference after discharge. Educate the client's family, friends, and caregivers who will be walking with the client outdoors so they are aware of how to best assist the client.

Clients with impairments often need to keep their hands free for balance or for using mobility aids such as canes and crutches. Adaptation of techniques or equipment can increase the client's walking and moving ability. Some common adaptations and equipment to assist with functional walking and moving include:

- *Baskets*: When the clients' hands need to be on the walker, it is hard to carry things. By attaching a basket to the front of a walker for carrying items, clients' hands remain free. Do not put too much weight in basket or the walker will become front heavy and tip over.
- *Waist packs*: Instead of using a pocket book, encourage clients to use a waist pack so that arms and hands are free to maintain balance and good posture.
- *Ice pick tip*: A retractable ice pick attachment is available for canes that can be very helpful for clients who want to hike on uneven dirt paths.
- *Backpacks*: A backpack is a good alternative for carrying items (laundry, groceries, crafts, etc.). Instruct clients in appropriate fitting and weight limits.
- *Cell phone or hand radio*: Cell phones are an important safety device. For example, if a client riding the bus gets off at the wrong stop, s/he can use the cell phone to get assistance. Hand radios (also called "walkie-talkies") are good for communication within short ranges (e.g., a

young child who wants to walk independently to a friend's home around the corner and needs to stay in contact with a parent for assistance or to ensure safety; a person who is gardening in the back yard and needs to contact his spouse who is indoors should he need assistance with walking back to the house from the garden).

Additional therapy interventions associated with walking and moving are "Energy Conservation Training" and "Community Accessibility Training" in the Techniques section. Information on the "Americans with Disabilities Act Education" in the Techniques section also applies to a client's legal rights for accessibility in walking and moving.

d455 Moving Around
Moving the whole body from one place to another by means other than walking, such as climbing over a rock or running down a street, skipping, scampering, jumping, somersaulting, or running around obstacles.
Inclusions: crawling, climbing, running, jogging, jumping, and swimming
Exclusions: transferring oneself (d420), walking (d450)
- *d4550 Crawling*
  Moving the whole body in a prone position from one place to another on hands, or hands and arms, and knees.
- *d4551 Climbing*
  Moving the whole body upwards or downwards, over surfaces or objects, such as climbing steps, rocks, ladders or stairs, curbs, or other objects.
- *d4552 Running*
  Moving with quick steps so that both feet may be simultaneously off the ground.
- *d4553 Jumping*
  Moving up off the ground by bending and extending the legs, such as jumping on one foot, hopping, skipping, and jumping, or diving into water.
- *d4554 Swimming*
  Propelling the whole body through water by means of limb and body movements without taking support from the ground underneath.
- *d4558 Moving Around, Other Specified*
- *d4559 Moving Around, Unspecified*

Treatment for Moving Around

Crawling, climbing, running, and jumping, with the exception of swimming, are all developmental skills. Crawling typically begins between six and nine months and is fully developed by nine to 12 months. Climbing stairs with assistance usually occurs around 15-18 months and children usually climb basic household objects (e.g., chair, bed) well by the age of two. Small hops are seen in toddlers

around 18-24 months and by two years of age a toddler can jump and run.

Alternative ways of "moving around" other than walking is an important consideration. For instance, a person who has both legs amputated at the hip may be able to use a swing-through gait or a modified crawl as an alternative to a wheelchair to get around within the home. Alternative forms of mobility are also evident in many sport and recreation activities (e.g., running, jogging, swimming, skating, sliding, skipping, hopping, rolling, climbing). These movements are areas of concern for the recreational therapist who is concerned with a person's involvement in recreation and sport activities.

Like walking, the therapist must first review precautions and parameters that the client may have related to mobility (e.g., physician notes in the medical record) and consult with the physical therapist to discuss issues related to "moving around" in a specific manner (e.g., sliding down a sliding board). The specific interventions used to work on problems associated with the form of mobility will vary depending on the diagnosis. Problems with the form of mobility (e.g., dynamic sitting balance) are noted through direct observation, task analysis (see "Activity and Task Analysis" in the Techniques section), and formal testing. Therapists document, at a minimum, the specific form of mobility, the specific problems noted, and the level of assistance required for the activity (e.g., client requires minimal assistance to maintain dynamic sitting balance in moderate ranges when sliding down a 40° sliding board). If the person requires or uses a piece of equipment for mobility (e.g., walker, wheelchair, skates) the code b465 Moving Around Using Equipment is used.

d460 Moving Around in Different Locations
Walking and moving around in various places and situations, such as walking between rooms in a house, within a building, or down the street of a town.
Inclusions: moving around within the home, crawling or climbing within the home; walking or moving within buildings other than the home, and outside the home and other buildings
- *d4600 Moving Around within the Home*
  Walking and moving around in one's home, within a room, between rooms, and around the whole residence or living area.
  Inclusions: moving from floor to floor, on an attached balcony, courtyard, porch, or garden
- *d4601 Moving Around within Buildings Other Than Home*
  Walking and moving around within buildings other than one's residence, such as moving around other people's homes, other private buildings, community and private or public buildings and enclosed areas.

Inclusions: moving throughout all parts of buildings and enclosed areas, between floors, inside, outside, and around buildings, both public and private

- *d4602 Moving Around outside the Home and Other Buildings*
  Walking and moving around close to or far from one's home and other buildings, without the use of transportation, public or private, such as walking for short or long distances around a town or village.
  Inclusions: walking or moving down streets in the neighborhood, town, village, or city; moving between cities and further distances, without using transportation
- *d4608 Moving Around in Different Locations, Other Specified*
- *d4609 Moving Around in Different Locations, Unspecified*

Treatment for
Moving Around in Different Locations

Moving around within the home, outdoors, and within other buildings requires different skills than moving around in a clinical setting. There are various environmental factors that have the potential to hinder or facilitate mobility (see Environmental Factors). These could be physical objects (e.g., furniture), the natural and man-made environment (e.g., weather, hills, broken sidewalk, curb cuts outs), or services, systems, and policies (e.g., non-compliance with accessibility laws). As reviewed in the walking code set, recreational therapists focus on moving around in real-life settings and activities such as the activities within the home, outdoors, and in other buildings outside of the home.

Note that the term "moving around" does not denote a specific way of moving around, although it is limited to moving around *without* equipment and it does not include the use of transportation. If the client uses a piece of equipment, use code d465 Moving Around Using Equipment. If the therapist wants to score the client's ability to move around using transportation, refer to the code set d470-d489 Moving Around Using Transportation.

Recreational therapists conduct a holistic assessment of the environment, as well as outlining variables that have the potential to hinder or facilitate moving around in different locations. Problems with barriers are solved for and facilitators are noted. Depending on the setting, therapists may opt to "practice" moving around in different locations by simulating the specific environment to build confidence, decrease anxiety, and provide opportunities for problem solving in a safe environment. Community integration training at the specific site (e.g., client's home, client's neighborhood) is ideal

whenever possible to fully assess, problem solve, and adapt for moving around in the alternative setting.

Refer to the following sections of the Techniques section for more information:

- "Community Problem Solving"
- "Emergency Response"
- "Integration"
- "Walking Techniques"

Refer to specific diagnoses for information on specific issues related to moving around and other sections as needed.

d465 Moving Around Using Equipment

Moving the whole body from place to place, on any surface or space, by using specific devices designed to facilitate moving or create other ways of moving around, such as with skates, skis, or scuba equipment, or moving down the street in a wheelchair or a walker.
Exclusions: transferring oneself (d420); walking (d450); moving around (d455); using transportation (d470); driving (d475)

Treatment for
Moving Around Using Equipment

Moving around using equipment includes moving around using any piece of mobility equipment (whether for assistance or sport) on any surface and in any space. This code is going to be challenging mainly for therapists who work in rehabilitation settings who assess, treat, document, and adapt for individual mobility skills with a piece of equipment. For example, therapists individually document a person's ability to go up and down stairs, up and down curbs, walk on uneven outdoor surfaces, walk on indoor level surfaces, up and down hills, in and out of manual doors, and in and out of elevators. Therapists document skills separately because a person's needs and abilities vary from activity to activity. It also allows the therapist a clear way of documenting progress with specific mobility activities. It is unclear at this time how therapists will go about using this code. A therapist might score this code by the average level of difficulty of all the mobility skills that use equipment or the therapist may opt to score a specific mobility skill and designate the specific skill scored to the right of the scored area in the additional notes section.

For information on how to assess, document, treat, and adapt for moving around using equipment, please refer to the following in the Techniques section:

- "Wheelchair Mobility"
- "Walking Techniques"

Also, refer to the Equipment section for information on specific pieces of common mobility equipment including canes, crutches, and walkers.

d469 Walking and Moving, Other Specified and Unspecified

Moving Around Using Transportation (d470-d489)

d470 Using Transportation
Using transportation to move around as a passenger, such as being driven in a car or on a bus, rickshaw, jitney, animal-powered vehicle, or private or public taxi, bus, train, tram, subway, boat, or aircraft.
Inclusions: using human-powered transportation; using private motorized or public transportation
Exclusions: moving around using equipment (d465); driving (d475)

- *d4700 Using Human-Powered Vehicles*
  Being transported as a passenger by a mode of transportation powered by one or more people, such as riding in a rickshaw or rowboat.
- *d4701 Using Private Motorized Transportation*
  Being transported as a passenger by private motorized vehicle over land, sea, or air, such as by a taxi or privately owned aircraft or boat.
- *d4702 Using Public Motorized Transportation*
  Being transported as a passenger by a motorized vehicle over land, sea, or air designed for public transportation, such as being a passenger on a bus, train, subway, or aircraft.
- *d4708 Using Transportation, Other Specified*
- *d4709 Using Transportation, Unspecified*

Treatment for Using Transportation

Community integration training is one of the primary focuses of recreational therapy practice, of which travel training is a major component. Travel training is a complex process that involves functional skills within all domains. While using private and public transportation is a complex task, the World Health Organization devotes only one category to getting from one place to another using transportation, which emphasizes the movement aspect of transportation.

Mobility in the community could be a relatively easy process in which the therapist needs to address dysfunction in only one area for successful integration. For example, a client with a left lower extremity amputation is admitted for prosthetic training. He uses the subway to go back and forth to work and desires to continue using this type of transportation. The client has no cognitive impairments and needs only to address functional skills related to mobility: the ability to climb stairs, board the subway train, get on and off the subway seat, use an escalator, and walk to and from the destination prior to and after boarding.

In other situations the therapist may need to address a variety of skills within many domains. For example, a client with a traumatic brain injury who exhibits moderate cognitive and social impairments may need to relearn a broad base of skills. Physically the client has mildly impaired walking and moving endurance. The client is to take a public bus three times a week to a community brain injury program. In this example, the therapist needs to address money management skills, using a bus map and schedule, problem solving skills, safety skills, social interaction skills, and time management skills. The therapist may need to adapt or modify the task to increase client safety and his functional ability to utilize the bus (e.g., designing a simplified bus map and time schedule, pre-making bus money envelopes, or the utilization of cue cards for dealing with common problems).

The therapist must be very adept at evaluating the deficits and needs of the client, as well as being creative with the adaptation or modification of thought processes to enhance function and safety. The therapist may also need to provide education and counseling related to the travel process (e.g., rights under the Americans with Disabilities Act, accessibility guidelines, community energy conservation techniques, travel resources and services) to further enhance traveling skills. See the *BUS* assessment for more ideas.

Transportation equals independence for many clients. It provides clients with the ability to leave their homes and access places in the community that contribute to health maintenance and promotion.

The recreational therapist establishes a baseline of functional travel skills (e.g., walking and moving endurance in terms of time or terrain, cues required to effectively interact with strangers in community, amount of assistance needed to transfer on and off the bus seat). The therapist should also document the purpose of travel training (e.g., source of transportation to go back and forth to work, the senior center, to another state to visit or live with family, for a planned vacation).

The *Community Integration Program* (Armstrong & Lauzen, 1994) is a good resource for more information on transportation training. Also refer to the specific diagnoses and other documents as needed to complement transportation training (e.g., "Americans with Disabilities Act Education," "Walking Techniques," and "Wheelchair Skills" in the Techniques section)

d475 Driving

Being in control of and moving a vehicle or the animal that draws it, traveling under one's own direction or having at one's disposal any form of transportation, such as a car, bicycle, boat, or animal-powered vehicle.

Inclusions: driving human-powered transportation, motorized vehicles, animal-powered vehicles

Exclusions: moving around using equipment (d465); using transportation (d470)

- *d4750 Driving Human-Powered Transportation*
  Driving a human-powered vehicle, such as a bicycle, tricycle, or rowboat.
- *d4751 Driving Motorized Vehicles*
  Driving a vehicle with a motor, such as an automobile, motorcycle, motorboat, or aircraft.
- *d4752 Driving Animal-Powered Vehicles*
  Driving a vehicle powered by an animal, such as a horse-drawn cart or carriage.
- *d4758 Driving, Other Specified*
- *d4759 Driving, Unspecified*

Treatment for Driving

Occupational therapists and recreational therapists may be part of an adaptive driving program at a rehabilitation facility. Generally, further specialized training in adaptive driving is needed by clinical professionals to participate in this type of program. Driving, as reviewed in the previous section, plays a vital role in independence and is a valued skill that people do not like to give up easily. There are many adaptations that allow people with disabilities to drive including:

- A steering wheel knob that allows a person to drive using one hand.
- A push/pull arm next to the steering wheel that allows a person to push for gas and pull for brake with one hand.
- Various switches that can be mounted in various places in a vehicle to operate a variety of vehicle functions (e.g., tap a switch with the left elbow to operate the windshield wipers).
- Converted mini vans that have a ramp that automatically folds out.
- Converted mini vans that have the driver seat removed so that a wheelchair can be manipulated into a driving position and strapped or snapped down to the floor.

In addition to driving an automobile, this code set includes driving human powered transportation (e.g., bicycle, rowboat), motorized vehicles besides automobiles (e.g., motorcycles, motorboats, aircraft, riding lawn mowers), and animal-powered vehicles (e.g., horse-drawn cart or carriage). Clearance is often necessary to operate a vehicle after an injury

(e.g., when neurological injury has occurred and the client desires to return to driving an automobile), however medical clearance is not always necessary (although highly recommended to ensure the safety of the person and others) to operate personal modes of transportation (e.g., bicycle, rowboat, riding lawn mower).

Recreational therapists conduct a task analysis and evaluate it against the person's skills for operating vehicles other than automobiles (unless specially certified and working within the capacity of that role).

Therapists document the specific vehicle that the client wants to operate, the level of assistance needed to perform the task, and any other issues that are relevant to the situation (e.g., Client requires minimal assistance to maintain dynamic sitting balance to pedal 16" bicycle while wearing right lower extremity prosthesis and using a right pedal clip).

Therapists assist clients in their desire to operate vehicles through treatment and adaptation. Treatment and adaptation will vary depending on the particular mode of transportation, diagnosis, and abilities and limitations of the client. For example, in one situation a therapist may work with a client to learn alternative ways for steering a powerboat with one hand, while in another case a therapist may work with a client who has had an amputation in teaching her how to ride a bicycle using a lower or upper extremity prosthesis.

d480 Riding Animals for Transportation

Traveling on the back of an animal, such as a horse, ox, camel, or elephant.

Exclusions: driving (d475); recreation and leisure (d920)

Treatment for Riding Animals for Transportation

Within the United States, the most common animal used for transportation is the horse (e.g., horseback riding through the park). However, riding a horse for leisure would not be scored under this code. It would be coded under d920 Recreation and Leisure (note the exclusion written within this code). This code refers to the riding of an animal for traveling. Therefore, if a client was riding an animal (e.g., a horse) to get from one place to another for the purpose of transportation (e.g., a client who lives in a rural environment and rides a horse to the local store) this code could be used. Recreational therapists who are unfamiliar with the skills involved in riding a particular animal will need to seek out qualified professionals to conduct an appropriate assessment of the client's abilities to ride the animal. Specific deficits identified are addressed as appropriate.

Dysfunctions that are identified can be referenced in this book for further guidance on assessment, documentation, treatment, and adaptation for the problem (e.g., balance).

Adaptations may include a modified saddle, a standing box to assist a person in mounting an animal, and modified steering systems.

d489 Moving Around Using Transportation, Other Specified and Unspecified

d498 Mobility, Other Specified

d499 Mobility, Unspecified

References

Armstrong, M. & Lauzen, S. (1994). *Community integration program, 2nd ed.*, Ravensdale, WA: Idyll Arbor.

burlingame, j. and Blaschko, T. (2002). *Assessment tools for recreational therapy and related fields, third edition.* Ravensdale, WA: Idyll Arbor.

Dorland's Illustrated Medical Dictionary, 29th Ed. (2000). Philadelphia: W. B. Saunders.

Kisner, C. & Colby, L. (1990). *Therapeutic exercise: Foundations and techniques*, 2nd ed. Philadelphia, PA: F. A. Davis.

Chapter 5 Self-Care

This chapter is about caring for oneself, washing, and drying oneself, caring for one's body and body parts, dressing, eating, and drinking, and looking after one's health.

d510 Washing Oneself

Washing and drying one's whole body, or body parts, using water and appropriate cleaning and drying materials or methods, such as bathing, showering, washing hands and feet, face and hair, and drying with a towel.

Inclusions: washing body parts, the whole body, and drying oneself

Exclusions: caring for body parts (d520), toileting (d530)

- *d5100 Washing Body Parts*
  Applying water, soap, and other substances to body parts, such as hands, face, feet, hair, or nails, in order to clean them.
- *d5101 Washing Whole Body*
  Applying water, soap, and other substances to the whole body in order to clean oneself, such as taking a bath or shower.
- *d5102 Drying Oneself*
  Using a towel or other means for drying some part or parts of one's body, or the whole body, such as after washing.
- *d5108 Washing Oneself, Other Specified*
- *d5109 Washing Oneself, Unspecified*

Treatment for Washing Oneself

Washing the whole body is an activity that occurs commonly within the home, (e.g., showering in the morning), although it may also occur in a community setting (e.g., showering in a locker room at a health club or school). Washing body parts on the other hand may occur more frequently in community settings (e.g., hand washing) for routine hygiene and health. Drying body parts or the whole body accompanies both of these tasks in most situations (with exception of showering before entering a pool). Recreational therapists holistically evaluate the skills and tasks required to participate in recreational and community activities of which washing and drying the whole body or parts of the body may be a part (e.g., washing hands before dining when eating out, showering before entering a pool, removing nail polish, washing and drying a residual amputated limb in a community setting when it becomes sweaty with odor, rinsing sand off of the feet at the beach shower). Washing and drying is much more than the typical morning or evening shower.

Washing and drying, although sounding quite simple, can require special techniques and equipment, as well as require the individual to follow special instructions including contraindications (e.g., unable to get a leg cast wet when bathing, use of a long-handled sponge or tub bench, not allowed to use oil-based products because it could breed bacteria in a wound, one-handed techniques for drying one's hair). Recommendations for washing and drying can come from a variety of health professionals (e.g., occupational therapist, nurse, physician, wound care specialist, prosthetist), including recreational therapists who identify washing and drying as components of a particular activity (e.g., swimming, dining out, going to the beach). Therapists evaluate the current recommendations for techniques and equipment, as well as contraindications from all sources, and teach a client how to integrate those recommendations into specific activities. In some cases, recommendations cannot easily be transferred into recreational and community activities (e.g., how to wash and dry residual limb when out in a community setting, how to operate a pull-cord shower at the beach and wash oneself while only having the use of one hand, how to shower in a health club locker room when a tub bench is not available). Recreational therapists assist clients in problem solving for these types of situations through the identification of modified techniques and equipment (e.g., at a beach shower, hook one end of a bungee cord to the pull shower cord and the other end to the top of a flip flop or water shoe to keep tension on the shower cord for continuous water flow), as well as address related issues that are foreseen as possible barriers to washing and drying during recreational and community activities.

In the ICF, recreational therapists document washing and drying skills by level of difficulty. Other ways to document performance include level of assistance required, equipment and techniques utilized, and contraindications followed.

Also see the Equipment section for information on "Bathing Aids" (e.g., long handled sponge, tub bench).

d520 Caring for Body Parts

Looking after those parts of the body, such as skin, face, teeth, scalp, nails, and genitals, that require more than washing and drying.

Inclusions: caring for skin, teeth, hair, finger and toe nails

Exclusions: washing oneself (d510), toileting (d530)

- *d5200 Caring for Skin*
  Looking after the texture and hydration of one's skin, such as by removing calluses or corns, and using lotions or cosmetics.
- *d5201 Caring for Teeth*
  Looking after dental hygiene, such as by brushing teeth, flossing, and taking care of a dental prosthesis or orthosis.
- *d5202 Caring for Hair*
  Looking after the hair on the head and face, such as by combing, styling, shaving, or trimming.
- *d5203 Caring for Fingernails*
  Cleaning, trimming, or polishing the nails of the fingers.
- *d5204 Caring for Toenails*
  Cleaning, trimming, or polishing the nails of the toes.
- *d5208 Caring for Body Parts, Other Specified*
- *d5209 Caring for Body Parts, Unspecified*

Treatment for
Caring for Body Parts

Caring for skin, teeth, hair, fingernails, and toenails is important for hygiene and prevention of health issues (e.g., losing teeth, skin cancer due to prolonged sun exposure without use of protective lotions, hair lice, finger or toenail infections). Some of these tasks are performed in the client's home (e.g., brushing teeth and shaving in the morning), and some are also performed in community and social settings (e.g., brushing hair during recess at school, applying sunscreen lotion when outdoors, polishing fingernails with friends). Therefore, performance of these activities and consequences of not following proper hygiene procedures can affect social relationships (e.g., bad breath, unkempt hair, and ragged fingernails influence perception of peers; difficulty caring for body parts may hinder participation in social activities such as going to a slumber party or camping trip).

Recreational therapists are concerned with caring for body parts as it impacts participation in life activities (e.g., forming social relationships, participation in activities that have a component of body part care such as putting on sunscreen at an outdoor pool). Therapists assist the client in problem solving for specific skills and situations and make recommendations for adaptive equipment, modifications, and techniques (e.g., A five-year-old boy uses a beige universal cuff to hold a hair comb. The boy is embarrassed to use the adaptive comb at school because his peers make fun of him, but they also make fun of him when his hair is unkempt. Either way, he is teased by his peers. The therapist learns that many of the boys in the class like dinosaurs, so she purchases a small stuffed dinosaur and hot glues it to the top of the universal cuff

making the dinosaur appear to be holding the comb. The adaptive comb is now perceived as being "cool" by the boy and his peers.).

In the ICF, recreational therapists document the level of difficulty that a client is having with the task. Other ways to document caring for body parts include the level of assistance required, specific adaptive equipment and techniques utilized, and impact on specific life activities.

d530 Toileting
Planning and carrying out the elimination of human waste (menstruation, urination, and defecation), and cleaning oneself afterwards.
Inclusions: regulating urination, defecation, and menstrual care
Exclusions: washing oneself (d510), caring for body parts (d520)

- *d5300 Regulating Urination*
  Coordinating and managing urination, such as by indicating need, getting into the proper position, choosing and getting to an appropriate place for urination, manipulating clothing before and after urination, and cleaning oneself after urination.
- *d5301 Regulating Defecation*
  Coordinating and managing defecation such as by indicating need, getting into the proper position, choosing and getting to an appropriate place for defecation, manipulating clothing before and after defecation, and cleaning oneself after defecation.
- *d5302 Menstrual Care*
  Coordinating, planning, and caring for menstruation, such as by anticipating menstruation, and using sanitary towels and napkins.
- *d5308 Toileting, Other Specified*
- *d5309 Toileting, Unspecified*

Treatment for
Toileting

Regulating urination, defecation, and menstrual care in recreational and community activities can be a complex process for some clients resulting in lack of activity engagement (e.g., client fears having an accident when in the community so s/he chooses to stay home rather than participate).

Managing urination, defecation, and menstrual care may seem like simple tasks, but for someone with a disability it can be a complex process requiring the integration of many components. Body structures and functions (including mental and psychological functions) must be free of deficits or alternatives will need to be sought. This may include the use of medications (e.g., stool softeners, medications to control bladder spasms), adaptive equipment (e.g., use of a digital stimulator, catheter, pads that hold urine), and/or special techniques (e.g., changes in body position, using a toileting time schedule). Urination, defecation, and menstrual care can also be very time consuming, especially if the client requires the use of extensive medications, equipment, and techniques. For example, a client with complete tetraplegia will need to devote about two and a half hours a day to bladder and bowel care (e.g., self-catheterize every four to six hours requiring about one and half hours a day, waiting one hour after taking a suppository for it to loosen the stools and then using other methods to assist in stool release such as a digital stimulator). This does not include the time needed to set-up, dress/undress, and transfer.

If urination, defecation, or menstrual care is not well controlled (e.g., sitting in urine or feces for prolonged periods of time; continuous bowel, bladder, or menstrual accidents that soak one's clothes) severe secondary complications can occur including skin breakdowns and infection (see "Skin Breakdown" in the Techniques section for more information). Skin breakdowns can be life threatening, especially for those who have compromised immune systems and severe mobility limitations. From a social perspective, the odor of urine, feces, and menstrual blood (as well as the observation of soiled clothes) deters initiation of social interaction from others, affecting social relationships and health.

The chance of accidents, the difficulty in trying to toilet in the community or other people's homes that do not meet the client's accessibility needs, the amount of time required to perform the task, and the level of assistance needed to perform the task are common obstacles to recreation and community activities. The recreational therapist assists the client in problem solving for the identified barriers in the specific real-life situations of the client, and addresses the development of new skills and techniques as appropriate. New skills and techniques are taught when previously learned skills do not transfer well into real-life situations:

Example: A client was taught how to use a transfer board to transfer from the wheelchair to the toilet. This works well for the client in his home bathroom, however it does not work well in a public bathroom because the size of the stall is too small to use the transfer board. The client's caregiver is not able to transfer the client onto the toilet because of back problems. The recreational therapist suggests the use of a Texas catheter for community activities, limiting the appropriate amount of liquids consumed prior to going out, and using the bathroom at home before leaving. See "Community Accessibility Training" and "Community Problem Solving" in the Techniques section, "Toileting" in the Equipment

section, and b6 Genitourinary and Reproductive Functions for more ideas.

In the ICF, therapists document the level of difficulty that a client has with each task. Therapists may also document the level of assistance needed, adaptive equipment and techniques, the setting, and activities that are impacted by difficulties in this area.

d540 Dressing
Carrying out the coordinated actions and tasks of putting on and taking off clothes and footwear in sequence and in keeping with climatic and social conditions, such as by putting on, adjusting, and removing shirts, skirts, blouses, pants, undergarments, saris, kimonos, tights, hats, gloves, coats, shoes, boots, sandals, and slippers.
Inclusions: putting on or taking off clothes and footwear and choosing appropriate clothing
- *d5400 Putting on Clothes*
  Carrying out the coordinated tasks of putting clothes on various parts of the body, such as putting clothes on over the head, over the arms and shoulders, and on the lower and upper halves of the body; putting on gloves and headgear.
- *d5401 Taking off Clothes*
  Carrying out the coordinated tasks of taking clothes off various part of the body, such as pulling clothes off and over the head, off the arms and shoulders, and off the lower and upper halves of the body; taking off gloves and head-gear.
- *d5402 Putting on Footwear*
  Carrying out the coordinated tasks of putting on socks, stockings, and footwear.
- *d5403 Taking off Footwear*
  Carrying out the coordinated tasks of taking off socks, stocking, and footwear.
- *d5404 Choosing Appropriate Clothing*
  Following implicit or explicit dress codes and conventions of one's society or culture and dressing in keeping with climatic conditions.
- *d5408 Dressing, Other Specified*
- *d5409 Dressing, Unspecified*

Treatment for Dressing

Dressing is commonly thought about as the domain of occupational therapy, but recreational therapists also play an important role in this code set. Dressing, as described in this ICF code set, is more than just putting on major clothing items such as shirts and pants, it also includes undergarments, gloves, hats, headgear (e.g., for wrestling), socks, footwear (e.g., roller skates, water shoes), and jackets (e.g., band jacket, ski jacket). This is much more than the dressing skills that are typically considered. This code set also includes the choice of appropriate clothing to follow a dress code (e.g., explicit dress codes for school or work, implicit dress codes such as those that are followed by peers), conventions of one's society or culture (e.g., Amish dress, proper dress for religious functions including wearing acceptable clothing items and specific religious garments such as a yarmulke), and dressing according to climatic conditions (e.g., wearing a jacket when it is cold outside — difficulty with this skill is often due to disabilities from sensory impairments, mental impairments such as schizophrenia and dementia, and lack of experience, such as young children who choose clothing based on likes or novice hikers who do not understand the danger of alpine weather).

Choosing appropriate clothing for dress codes and conventions of society or culture will also have an impact on other life areas including the development of social relationships, level of group acceptance, and attitudes of others towards the client (e.g., an adolescent client wears pre-teen clothing styles that are perceived by peers as being childish and odd). This can lead to impaired participation in life activities (e.g., client stops going to church because people tell her that she is dressed inappropriately). In most cases, people judge others by their appearance and clothing is a major factor (e.g., "She has no respect for God because she is wearing jeans in church." "She wears fancy clothes so she must be stuck up." "How can his parents allow him to go out of the house dressed like that? They must not be upstanding people.").

Recreational therapists evaluate the needs and requirements related to dressing for recreational and community activities that are part of the client's lifestyle, as well as explicit and implicit dress codes and standards for the client's culture and society. If difficulties are noted, therapists seek to reduce or eliminate the dysfunction through the identification of resources (e.g., money to buy appropriate clothing), adaptive equipment (e.g., dressing aids), and techniques (e.g., how to tie roller skate laces with impaired hand function). The current adaptive equipment and techniques utilized by the client are evaluated for appropriateness in other life situations and recommendations are then suggested (e.g., client was taught how to dress from a supine position but this will not work for trying on clothes at a store).

In the ICF, the recreational therapist documents the level of difficulty that the client has with each task. Therapists may also document on discipline-specific forms the level of assistance needed, the specific setting, adaptive equipment and techniques utilized, and activities impacted by difficulties in this area. Dressing, in some cases (although not currently coded this way in the ICF), may be a barrier to a particular life activity (e.g., difficulties is choosing

appropriate clothing for church results in difficulties in organized religion).

See the Equipment section for more information on "Dressing Aids."

d550 Eating

Carrying out the coordinated tasks and actions of eating food that has been served, bringing it to the mouth, and consuming it in culturally acceptable ways, cutting or breaking food into pieces, opening bottles and cans, using eating implements, having meals, feasting, or dining.
Exclusions: drinking (d560)

Treatment for Eating

Eating is more than the act of opening containers, using utensils, breaking or cutting food into pieces, bringing food to the mouth and swallowing the food. It includes the skill of consuming food in culturally acceptable ways, as well as having meals, feasting, and dining. Culturally acceptable ways of eating will vary depending upon the culture of the client, as well as the culture in which s/he is eating. For example, someone who is Chinese may be expected to use chopsticks and share bowls of food with others at the table when at home, but when out at a fancy restaurant, the client chooses to use utensils and food is not shared. During certain religious holidays or cultural events, manners for food consumption may also change (e.g., a higher standard of manners may be expected during Christmas dinner than during non-holiday family meals).

This leads into the differences between meals, feasting, and dining. Meals are commonly defined by food that is routinely eaten periodically during the day (e.g., eating a sandwich at lunchtime, having a dinner meal with the family). Feasting, on the other hand, often indicates a celebration (e.g., a holiday feast), while dining is often characterized as an elegant meal in a community setting (e.g., upscale restaurant). Food consumption behaviors for each of these differ. For example, during a meal in the home a client may sip the last bit of soup from the bowl and use his sleeve to wipe his mouth without any negative remarks or looks from his family because it is normal eating behavior in his home. However, if the client behaved in the same manner while dining out, it would most likely be perceived as inappropriate. The client realizes that this manner of food consumption is not appropriate for dining out and instead tips the soup bowl and uses a spoon to get the last bit of broth and uses a napkin to blot his mouth clean. Feast behavior can be a bit harder to categorize, but during most celebratory feasts people tend to eat more and socialize more. Food consumption manners may be reduced (e.g., people handing other people food, sharing plates of food with children, people sitting in different location such as at the table or while walking around). Therapists are aware that food consumption behaviors are influenced by culture, religion, society, setting, and purpose and address the expected behaviors. If food consumption behaviors are not appropriate, secondary problems can result (e.g., rejected by peers, negative judgments of others towards the client, decreased invitations to events) affecting other health areas. Although the ICF does not currently code in this manner, eating impairments can be a barrier to other life activities.

Despite the focus of this discussion on food consumption, recreational therapists are also concerned with the client's ability to perform basic eating skills such as opening containers, using utensils, breaking or cutting food, bringing food to the mouth, and swallowing. The therapist evaluates the current techniques used by the client and evaluates the functionality of those skills in real-life settings. For example, a client may use a special plate that has raised sides like a bowl so that she is able to scoop food easily onto the spoon by sliding it up the side of the plate. This type of bowl is not available at restaurants and the client does not feel comfortable bringing her own bowl (having to move food from the restaurant plate onto her special plate would be difficult for her and she does not feel comfortable asking the waiter or the chef to use the plate). In this situation, the therapist may recommend the use of a plate guard (a piece of plastic that hooks around the outside of standard plate) or the therapist may work with the client to help her be more assertive. What is important is finding a way to allow the client to eat out because it is part of normal social life.

In the ICF the therapist documents the level of difficulty the client has with each task. Therapists may also document within discipline-specific documentation the level of assistance needed, specific adaptive equipment and techniques utilized, the specific setting, and other activities that are affected by any dysfunction.

See the Equipment section for more information on "Eating and Drinking Equipment."

d560 Drinking

Taking hold of a drink, bringing it to the mouth, and consuming the drink in culturally acceptable ways, mixing, stirring, and pouring liquids for drinking, opening bottles and cans, drinking through a straw or drinking running water such as from a tap or a spring; feeding from the breast.
Exclusions: eating (d550)

Treatment for Drinking

To be able to drink something, a container is opened; the drink is poured, stirred, or mixed and brought to the mouth and drunk in a culturally acceptable manner. This also includes the use of drinking fountains, breast-feeding, straws, and running water (e.g., cupping hands under a faucet). There are a variety of adaptive drinking devices such as weighted drinking glasses, cups with specially designed handles and lids, and drinking aids such as cups with special spouts or specially designed straws (long, bendable). Therapists evaluate the use of the client's current devices for drinking and determine if they are appropriate to meet the needs of the client in recreational and community activities that are part of the client's lifestyle. In some instances, they will not meet the client's needs and further recommendations will be needed (e.g., specialized drinking bottle doesn't fit in a standard bike water bottle holder; the client has a specialized cup at home but encounters difficulty when she goes out to eat because she is unable to hold onto a standard drinking glass at a restaurant).

Drinking also includes the consumption of liquids in a culturally acceptable manner. For example, at home you may drink water from a water bottle, but at a restaurant it is expected that you pour the water from the bottle into a glass. Another example may be that at a restaurant you do not share a drinking glass, but at church everyone takes a sip of wine from the chalice. Recreational therapists are aware of the differences in liquid consumption behaviors that are influenced by culture, religion, society, setting, and purpose and address the related behaviors. If behaviors are not appropriate (e.g., refused to drink from the chalice at church, puts mouth on the water fountain), secondary problems can result (e.g., rejection by peers, negative judgments from others about the client) that can impair health (e.g., social health declines, possibly mental health could decline if social supports decline). Although the ICF does not currently code in this manner, drinking impairments can be a barrier to other life activities.

In the ICF, recreational therapists document the level of difficulty that a client has with each task. Therapists may also document in discipline-specific documentation the level of assistance needed, adaptive equipment or techniques utilized, the setting, and other life activities that are affected by dysfunction in this area.

See the Equipment section for more information on "Eating and Drinking Equipment."

d570 Looking After One's Health

Ensuring physical comfort, health, and physical and mental well-being, such as by maintaining a balanced diet, and an appropriate level of physical activity, keeping warm or cool, avoiding harms to health, following safe sex practices, including using condoms, getting immunizations and regular physical exams.

Inclusions: ensuring one's physical comfort; managing diet and fitness; maintaining one's health

- *d5700 Ensuring One's Physical Comfort*
  Caring for oneself by being aware that one needs to ensure, and ensuring, that one's body is in a comfortable position, that one is not feeling too hot or cold, and that one has adequate lighting.
- *d5701 Managing Diet and Fitness*
  Caring for oneself by being aware of the need and by selecting and consuming nutritious foods and maintaining physical fitness.
- *d5702 Maintaining One's Health*
  Caring for oneself by being aware of the need and doing what is required to look after one's health, both to respond to risks to health and to prevent ill-health, such as by seeking professional assistance; following medical and other health advice; and avoiding risks to heath such as physical injury, communicable diseases, drug-taking, and sexually transmitted diseases.
- *d5708 Looking After One's Health, Other Specified*
- *d5709 Looking After One's Health, Unspecified*

Treatment for Looking After One's Health

Looking After One's Health (d570) and its components d5700 Ensuring One's Physical Comfort, d5701 Managing Diet and Fitness, and d5702 Maintaining One's Health are important codes for the recreational therapist. They are broad codes that encompass a variety of issues under the scope of recreational therapy practice. Therapists can use the broad code of d570 Looking After One's Health or can be more specific by choosing the descriptive codes underneath this heading.

Ensuring One's Physical Comfort

Common issues addressed by recreational therapy that fall under this code include:

1. Education and client utilization of joint protection techniques (e.g., for rheumatoid arthritis). See b710 Mobility of Joint Functions for information on joint protection techniques.
2. Awareness of and making changes for temperatures that affect one's functioning (e.g., heat exacerbates multiple sclerosis symptoms, temperature changes may not be noticed by someone who has sensory deficits such as a complete spinal cord injury). See b270 Sensory Functions Related to Temperature and Other

Stimuli for more information on how to assess, treat, document, and adapt for dysfunction in this area.

3. Awareness and proper positioning of the body including ergonomics and body mechanics (e.g., a client who lacks awareness of a limb such as a possible result of a stroke, a client who is responsible for positioning her body correctly in a device such as a wheelchair or a splint, comfortable use of a computer workstation, proper body mechanics in an activity). See "Body Mechanics and Ergonomics" and "Fine Hand Use Ergonomics" in the Techniques section, and Activities & Participation Chapter 4 Mobility for information on how to assess, treat, document, and adapt for dysfunction in these areas.
4. Education and problem solving to ensure proper lighting (e.g., a client who has low vision may benefit from direct white light on a subject to increase visibility of the subject — where to purchase such a light, how to set it up correctly at the working area, etc.).

Managing Diet and Fitness

Common interventions addressed by recreational therapy that fall under this code include issues related to nutrition and physical fitness. Recreational therapists address nutritional needs as they relate to choosing and consuming nutritious foods in real-life situations (e.g., restaurants, eating-on-the-go). The therapist obtains recommendations from the client's nutritionist, physician, and/or speech therapist (e.g., dietary restrictions related to swallowing, such as food and liquid consistencies) and evaluates the possible barriers that could hinder the client's ability to follow through with their recommendations (e.g., choosing healthy foods at a restaurant, portable snacks to maintain good glucose levels, healthy cooking techniques, reading food labels in the grocery store). Integration training in settings that pose difficulty for the client can be helpful to reinforce newly learned nutrition behaviors.

Recreational therapists put a strong emphasis on client engagement in healthy forms of physical leisure that are safe and appropriate based on the client's abilities and limitations. Engagement in regular physical leisure activity is one of the Healthy People 2010 initiatives that recreational therapists strive to instill in their clients. Engagement in regular physical leisure activity at moderate intensity can decrease risks for illness and disease, promote recovery, prevent secondary complications from inactivity, aid in better sleep, contribute to psychological health (e.g., reduce feelings of depression and anxiety), and promote the development of muscle strength, coordination, balance, and range of motion. Recreational therapists explore the client's interests to identify forms of physical leisure activity that have inherent characteristics that are attractive to the client (e.g., social, outdoor, competitive, reflective — see "Activity Pattern Development" in the Techniques section for information on interest exploration).

Once a safe, appropriate, and realistic form of physical leisure is identified and clearance for participation in the activity is given by the client's physician, the therapist addresses the development of functional skills that are necessary for participation (e.g., how to monitor pulse, how to move around in the water with an amputation, how to safely change exercise intensity within an exercise session should vital signs exceed parameters). (See "Exercise Basics" and "Vital Signs" in the Techniques section for more information.) The therapist helps the client to identify resources for participation (e.g., location of the client's local walking club, financial assistance available to join the local health club[4]) and problem solves for anticipated barriers (e.g., client becomes tired at the 5th golf hole when friends want to play 18 holes, lack of adaptive bathroom equipment at the YMCA. See d175 Solving Problems and "Community Problem Solving" and other relevant topics in the Techniques section as applicable to identified barriers (e.g., "Community Accessibility Training"). Lastly, integration training provides the therapist with the opportunity to assess the client's performance in his/her real-life setting, address unforeseen issues, and provide emotional and professional support. Score the findings under the specific community activity, e.g., d4702 Using Public Motorized Transportation, d4602 Moving Around Outside the Home and Other Buildings, d9201 Sports, d4601 Moving Around within Buildings Other Than Home. See "Integration" in the Techniques section for more information.

Maintaining One's Health

This code relates to a client's activities and behaviors needed to maintain his/her health. The specific activities and behaviors are determined by each client's needs and will therefore vary from

client to client (e.g., implementation of fall-prevention techniques, joint protection techniques, proper body mechanics, ergonomics, a healthy nutrition plan, a regular exercise program, smoking cessation, healthy coping strategies, adaptations and techniques for activities, pain management strategies, precautions and parameters, recommendations by health professionals, social circles, leisure activities, community involvement). This code is different from other codes in this A&P chapter because it focuses on "awareness" and "action." It challenges the therapist to ask the questions: "Is the client aware of activities and behavior that impact his/her health? and, "Is the client able to follow through on what is required for maintaining his/her health by implementing recommendations, carrying over learned skills, and making healthy choices that impact health, level of functioning, independence, and quality of life?" In essence, can the client pull it all together and integrate what s/he needs to do to stay healthy?

Therapists in a rehabilitation setting are able to assess a client's "awareness" through verbalizations and discussions about what needs to be done to stay healthy. A healthy activity pattern for after discharge can be developed.

Evaluating the client's ability to act on a plan can be harder, though. Sometimes the initial phases of the activity plan can be started while the client is still working with the recreational therapist to evaluate how well the client will be able to fulfill the plan. Another way to assess the client's ability to perform required actions is to give out homework assignments and see how well they are carried out (e.g., assigning the client homework such as exercising for 30 minutes each evening, talking with other clients on the floor to work on making friends, listening to a visualization CD when lying in bed to aid in sleep). Even if this kind of assessment isn't possible, therapists are typically aware of the client's activities and behaviors during structured and unstructured time through their observations and reports from other health care professionals (e.g., talking with the night nurse assigned to the client). Using the available information, the therapist can evaluate the client's ability to follow through with health activities and behaviors and make a guess as to how well the client will be able to maintain his/her health. Ideally, the client will be seen for follow-up evaluations after discharge to get a more accurate picture of health maintenance if there is a concern in this area.

The code does not allow the therapist to delineate between "awareness" and "action," therefore the therapist needs to ask both of these questions:

1. To what extent is the client aware of the health activities and behaviors that affect his/her health? (knowledge, measured as a fraction).

---

[4] Resource awareness does not have a specific code. The code used will reflect the specific resource given, e.g., if you were talking with a client about adaptive recreation resources, the code to use would be e1401 Assistive Products and Technology for Culture, Recreation, and Sport and, if you were talking about places in the community that provide opportunities to engage in physical leisure, you might use the code d9201 Sports. See "Community Leisure Resource Awareness" and "Personal Leisure Resource Awareness" in the Techniques section for more on this topic.

2. To what extent is the client able to carry over healthy activities and behaviors into his/her daily life? (action, measured as a fraction).

A suggestion on how to score this code is to look at both components that are required for maintaining one's health, awareness and action. To find out how many of the actions a client will actually do to maintain his/her health multiply the awareness fraction times the action fraction. For example, if a client has 50% of the knowledge required to maintain his health and acts on it every time, he still is able to do only 50% of the things required to maintain his health. Similarly, if a client knows everything that she needs to do to maintain her health, but acts on it only 50% of the time, she will also be doing 50% of the things required to maintain her health. The multiplication is required when a client does not know everything and does not act on everything s/he knows. For example, a client who knows 50% of what is required and acts on it 50% of the time will be doing only 25% of what is required to maintain health (.5 times .5). From a treatment perspective it is usually best to work on the component (awareness or action) that is lower.

See "Lifestyle Alteration Education" in the Techniques section as a sample guide for treatment to promote positive health maintenance and ways to increase a client's awareness of health issues as they relate to maintaining health.

d598 Self-Care, Other Specified

d599 Self-Care, Unspecified

Chapter 6 Domestic Life

This chapter is about carrying out domestic and everyday actions and tasks. Areas of domestic life include acquiring a place to live, food, clothing and other necessities, household cleaning and repairing, caring for personal and other household objects, and assisting others.

Acquisition of Necessities (d610-d629)

d610 Acquiring a Place to Live

Buying, renting, furnishing, and arranging a house, apartment, or other dwelling.

Inclusions: buying or renting a place to live and furnishing a place to live

Exclusions: acquisition of goods and services (d620); caring for household objects (d650)

- *d6100 Buying a Place to Live*
  Acquiring ownership of a house, apartment, or other dwelling.
- *d6101 Renting a Place to Live*
  Acquiring the use of a house, apartment, or other dwelling belonging to another in exchange for payment.
- *d6102 Furnishing a Place to Live*
  Equipping and arranging a living space with furniture, fixtures and other fittings and decorating rooms.
- *d6108 Acquiring a Place to Live, Other Specified*
- *d6109 Acquiring a Place to Live, Unspecified*

Treatment for Acquiring a Place to Live

Situations that arise to necessitate the need of acquiring a place to live include 1. no available pre-established home for the client to return to or move into, 2. desire by the client or client's guardian to live someplace different, 3. a current living situation that is no longer appropriate for the client (e.g., a home that doesn't meet accessibility needs), or 4. discharge from a residential program. The most common situation for a recreational therapist is assisting a client who is being discharged from a residential treatment setting.

Recreational therapists assist clients in identifying their specific living needs such as how much money is available to purchase/rent and maintain a home, proximity to important destinations (e.g., close to family, work, bus line, accessible train station, shopping areas), type of home (e.g., needs one floor living, needs living quarters without maintenance), accessibility of the home (e.g., steps, size of rooms, hallways, and doorways; accessibility of appliances), the surrounding environment (e.g., needs to live in a neighborhood that has sidewalks and no hills), and available resources (e.g., needs to live in an particular county that provides special assistance or services that other counties do not provide).

Therapists also assist clients in identifying appropriate furnishings (e.g., choosing furniture that provides adequate support for the client so that s/he can safely transfer onto and off of the furniture) and amount of space needed around furnishings for safe mobility. Common adaptations to standard furnishings will depend upon the needs of the client (e.g., touch lights, lever door handles). See "Americans with Disabilities Act Education" in the Techniques section for more information about accessibility space planning.

Integration training will further facilitate the process to allow the therapist to determine the actual level of accessibility and the ability of the surrounding environment to meet the client's needs. See "Integration" in the Techniques section for information on conducting a home assessment.

In the ICF, therapists document the level of difficulty that the client has with each task, as well as listing any environmental factors that hinder or facilitate the task. Therapists may also document more specific skills in discipline-specific documentation such as level of assistance, barriers and facilitators to the activity, issues related to acquiring a place to live, client needs related to a living place, and the impact that it has on other life activities (e.g., impact on participation in current recreational and community activities).

d620 Acquisition of Goods and Services

Selecting, procuring, and transporting all goods and services required for daily living, such as selecting, procuring, transporting, and storing food, drink, clothing, cleaning materials, fuel, household items, utensils, cooking ware, domestic appliance, and tools; procuring utilities and other household services.

Inclusions: shopping and gathering daily necessities

Exclusions: acquiring a place to live (d610)

- *d6200 Shopping*
  Obtaining, in exchange for money, goods and services required for daily living (including instructing and supervising an intermediary to do the shopping), such as selecting food, drink, cleaning materials, household items, or clothing in a shop or market; comparing quality and price of the items required, negotiating and paying for selected goods or services, and transporting goods.
- *d6201 Gathering Daily Necessities*
  Obtaining, without exchange of money, goods and services required for daily living (including instructing and supervising an intermediary to

gather daily necessities), such as by harvesting vegetables and fruits, and getting water and fuel.

- *d6208 Acquisition of Goods and Services, Other Specified*
- *d6209 Acquisition of Good and Services, Unspecified*

Treatment for Acquisition of Goods and Services

Recreational therapists, particularly those who work in the independent living movement and rehabilitation settings, address the skills related to acquisition of goods and services (shopping, gathering necessities). Shopping and gathering daily necessities, although commonly considered things that one has to do, are also things from which one can derive pleasure, satisfaction, and health. The act of shopping, for instance, is more than just buying groceries. It is also an opportunity to get out of the house for exercise (walking up and down the aisles, carrying heavy grocery bags), socialization (talking with the cashier, seeing and talking with neighbors and friends who are also shopping, conversing with strangers in aisles and grocery lines), and cognitive stimulation (comparing prices, staying within a grocery budget).

Likewise, the skills required for shopping and gathering daily necessities are also complex, including mobility skills (walking on outdoor and indoor surfaces, car transfers, electric store scooter transfers, toilet transfers, changing body positions to reach items), cognitive skills (basic and complex math, attention, memory, problem solving, direction following, reading and comprehending aisle signs), vision (to read signage, avoid obstacles), social skills (interacting with familiar and unfamiliar people; assertion of needs/requesting assistance from others), physical skills (e.g., strength to lift items, push a store cart, carry bags; balance; endurance functions).

Due to the number and complexity of the skills required to shop and gather daily necessities, it is recommended that the therapist identify and score all of the codes that lie outside of this code set that are relevant to the client's ability to shop or gather daily necessities. For example, if the client needs to perform car transfers to be able to go shopping, the therapist would score d4200 Transferring Oneself While Sitting. If a client needs to lift grocery items, the therapist would score d4300 Lifting. If a client needs short-term memory skills to recall a shopping list, then b1440 Short Term Memory would be scored. The number of skills that are involved in performing any community activity are numerous and it would be a daunting task for the therapist to identify and code every related code, therefore the best approach is to identify the skills within the

community task that are difficult for the client and identify and score only those codes (see "Activity and Task Analysis" in the Techniques section). So if a client does not have difficulty with short-term memory, then there is no need to identify and score the code of short-term memory even though it is a skill that occurs with the task of shopping and gathering daily necessities.

Outside of functional skill development, common educational interventions related to shopping and gathering daily necessities may include education about community energy conservation techniques (ways to conserve the amount of energy that a client expends during community activities to maximize safety and productivity as discussed in "Energy Conservation Training" in the Techniques section), community accessibility training (education about what a community facility has to have in order to meet the accessibility needs of the client so that s/he does not get "stuck" as discussed in "Community Accessibility Training" in the Techniques section), outdoor mobility techniques (techniques for walking or using a wheelchair in a community setting as discussed in "Walking Techniques" and "Wheelchair Mobility" in the Techniques section), problem solving for community barriers (see "Community Problem Solving" in the Techniques section), social skills training (see "Social Skills Development" in the Concepts section and "Social Skills Training" in the Techniques section), and the Americans with Disabilities Act (to know what services clients are entitled to and the level of accessibility to be provided as discussed in "Americans with Disabilities Act Education" in the Techniques section). Family/caregiver training may also need to be a component of training if their assistance is required for task performance.

Recreational therapists will typically begin with functional skill development and education related to the tasks of shopping and gathering daily necessities, followed by community integration training to the specific stores and other locations that the client frequents. Common sites for integration training related to acquiring goods and services include grocery stores, hardware stores, department stores, drug stores, and clothing stores (see "Integration" in the Techniques section for more information). For example, the therapist may begin with teaching the client outdoor wheelchair mobility techniques, problem solve for community barriers, and then take the client to the client's local grocery store to assess his ability to carry over learned skills into a real-life setting, as well as provide therapeutic learning interventions (e.g., posing the client with "what if" questions, assisting the client to problem solve through an unexpected situation).

In the ICF, therapists document the level of difficulty that the client has with the task of shopping and/or gathering daily necessities. In discipline-specific documentation, therapists will also document the level of assistance required for each specific skill within the task (e.g., transfers, walking, assertion), recommendations (e.g., level of assistance or supervision needed after discharge to perform the task), adaptive equipment or techniques utilized, and the problems that the difficulty with shopping imposes on other life activities and needs (e.g., nutrition as covered in d5701 Managing Diet and Fitness).

d629 Acquisition of Necessities, Other Specified and Unspecified

Household Tasks (d630-d649)

d630 Preparing Meals
Planning, organizing, cooking, and serving simple and complex meals for oneself and others, such as by making a menu, selecting edible food and drink, getting together ingredients for preparing meals, cooking with heat and preparing cold foods and drinks, and serving the food.
Inclusions: preparing simple and complex meals
Exclusions: eating (d550); drinking (d560); acquisition of goods and services (d620); doing housework (d640); caring for household objects (d650); caring for others (d660)
- *d6300 Preparing Simple Meals*
  Organizing, cooking, and serving meals with a small number of ingredients that require easy methods of preparation and serving, such as making a snack or small meal, and transforming food ingredients by cutting and stirring, boiling, and heating food such as rice or potatoes.
- *d6301 Preparing Complex Meals*
  Planning, organizing, cooking, and serving meals with a large number of ingredients that require complex methods of preparation and serving, such as planning a meal with several dishes, and transforming food ingredients by combined actions of peeling, slicing, mixing, kneading, stirring, presenting, and serving food in a manner appropriate to the occasion and culture.
  Exclusions: using household appliances (d6403)
- *d6308 Preparing Meals, Other Specified*
- *d6309 Preparing Meals, Unspecified*

Treatment for Preparing Meals

Preparing simple and complex meals is a basic need to sustain life, unless there is another person or service that prepares meals for us (e.g., a parent, guardian, home delivery program). Preparing meals is often thought of something that is done within the home, although preparation of simple and complex meals is also performed in many other settings (e.g., during recreational activities such as camping and hiking; work; school; volunteer work at a soup kitchen; recreational cooking groups). The skill of preparing meals can also be a precursor skill to involvement in other life activities (e.g., need to prepare simple meals to give a birthday party over the lunch hour; need to prepare a complex dish to take to a "celebration of life" of a deceased loved one; need to prepare simple meals for an elderly neighbor to fulfill the provider's emotional need for helping others). The key point is to recognize that, if a client has difficulty preparing simple or complex meals, it could impact involvement in other life activities that provide many benefits.

A client may acquire knowledge and skills of simple meal preparation from other health professionals (usually occupational therapists), however it is the recreational therapist who evaluates and addresses 1. the impact of meal preparation skills on participation in life activities, 2. the skills required to prepare simple and complex meals in various community and recreational settings, 3. adaptive equipment and techniques in addition to those provided by other health care professionals to minimize difficulty with meal preparation in real-life settings, and 4. integration training to the specific area where the client performs meal preparation activities (e.g., home kitchen, cooking group center, soup kitchen). Recreational therapists who work in independent living and assisted living may additionally address meal preparation in the home setting for the purpose of teaching and promoting independence with basic life tasks.

In the ICF, therapists document the level of difficulty that a client has with each of the tasks in this code set. In discipline-specific documentation, therapists will additionally document the level of assistance required for each specific skill in the task of meal preparation, recommendations (e.g., level of assistance or supervision needed), adaptive equipment or techniques utilized, and the problems that the difficulties with meal preparation impose on other life activities and needs (e.g., d7200 Forming Relationships).

d640 Doing Housework
Managing a household by cleaning the house, washing clothes, using household appliances, storing food, and disposing of garbage, such as by sweeping, mopping, washing counters, walls, and other surfaces; collecting and disposing of household garbage; tidying rooms, closets, and drawers; collecting, washing, drying, and ironing clothes; cleaning footwear; using brooms, brushes, and

vacuum cleaners; using washing machines, driers, and irons.

Inclusions: washing and drying clothes and garments; cleaning cooking area and utensils; cleaning living area; using household appliances, storing daily necessities, and disposing of garbage

Exclusions: acquiring a place to live (d610); acquisition of goods and services (d620); preparing meals (d630); caring for household objects (d650); caring for others (d660)

- *d6400 Washing and Drying Clothes and Garments*
  Washing clothes and garments by hand and hanging them out to dry in the air.
- *d6401 Cleaning Cooking Area and Utensils*
  Cleaning up after cooking, such as by washing dishes, pans, pots, and cooking utensils, and cleaning tables and floors around cooking and eating area.
- *d6402 Cleaning Living Area*
  Cleaning the living areas of the household, such as by tidying and dusting, sweeping, swabbing, mopping floors, cleaning windows and walls, cleaning bathrooms and toilets, and cleaning household furnishings.
- *d6403 Using Household Appliances*
  Using all kinds of household appliances, such as washing machines, driers, irons, vacuum cleaners, and dishwashers.
- *d6404 Storing Daily Necessities*
  Storing food, drinks, clothes, and other household goods required for daily living; preparing food for conservation by canning, salting, or refrigerating, keeping food fresh and out of the reach of animals.
- *d6405 Disposing of Garbage*
  Disposing of household garbage such as by collecting trash and rubbish around the house, preparing garbage for disposal, using garbage disposal appliances, burning garbage.
- *d6408 Doing Housework, Other Specified*
- *d6409 Doing Housework, Unspecified*

Treatment for Doing Housework

Housework includes washing and drying clothes, cleaning cooking area and utensils, cleaning living area, using household appliances, storing daily necessities, and disposing of garbage. Housework, although commonly thought of as being performed solely within the client's primary home, occurs in many different settings (e.g., camping, vacationing, visiting others at their residences for an extended period of time). For example, washing and drying clothes may need to be performed at a campsite, cleaning a cooking area and utensils may need to be performed at a picnic, using household appliances such as a travel iron when vacationing, storing daily necessities in coolers and suitcases for travel, and

disposing of garbage while hiking through a park. If difficulty with housework imposes a barrier to involvement in other life activities further dysfunction can result (e.g., doesn't go on camping trips with daughter's Girl Scout troop impacting d7601 Child-Parent Relationships; limits hike so does not have to pack necessities or worry about disposing of garbage impacting d5701 Managing Diet and Fitness).

A client may acquire knowledge and skills of housework from other health professionals (usually occupational therapy), however it is the recreational therapist who evaluates and addresses 1. the impact of housework on participation in other life activities, 2. the skills required of housework in various community and recreational settings, 3. adaptive equipment and techniques in addition to those provided by other health professionals to minimize difficulty with housework in real-life settings, and 4. integration training to the specific area where the client performs housework activities (e.g., camping trailer). Recreational therapists who work in independent living and assisted living may additionally address housework with clients in the residential setting for the purpose of teaching and promoting independence with basic life tasks.

In the ICF, therapists document the level of difficulty that a client has with each of the tasks in this code set. In discipline-specific documentation, therapists will additionally document the level of assistance required for each specific skill in the task of housework, recommendations (e.g., level of assistance or supervision needed), adaptive equipment or techniques utilized, and the problems that the difficulty of housework imposes on other life activities and needs (e.g., d7601 Child-Parent Relationships).

d649 Household Tasks, Other Specified and Unspecified

Caring for Household Objects and Assisting Others (d650-d669)

d650 Caring for Household Objects
Maintaining household and other personal objects, including house and contents, clothes, vehicles, and assistive devices, and caring for plants and animals, such as painting or wallpapering rooms, fixing furniture, repairing plumbing, ensuring the proper working order of vehicles, watering plants, grooming and feeding pets and domestic animals.

Inclusions: making and repairing clothes; maintaining dwelling, furnishings, and domestic appliances; maintaining vehicles; maintaining assistive devices; taking care of plants (indoor and outdoor) and animals

Exclusions: acquiring a place to live (d610); acquisition of goods and services (d620); doing housework (d640); caring for others (d660); remunerative employment (d850)

- *d6500 Making and Repairing Clothes*
  Making and repairing clothes, such as by sewing, producing, or mending clothes; reattaching buttons and fasteners; ironing clothes, fixing, and polishing footwear.
  Exclusions: using household appliances (d6403)
- *d6501 Maintaining Dwelling and Furnishings*
  Repairing and taking care of dwelling, its exterior, interior, and contents, such as by painting, repairing fixtures and furniture, and using required tools for repair work.
- *d6502 Maintaining Domestic Appliances*
  Repairing and taking care of all domestic appliances for cooking, cleaning, and repairing, such as by oiling and repairing tools and maintaining the washing machine.
- *d6503 Maintaining Vehicles*
  Repairing and taking care of motorized and non-motorized vehicles for personal use, including bicycles, carts, automobiles, and boats.
- *d6504 Maintaining Assistive Devices*
  Repairing and taking care of assistive devices, such as prostheses, orthoses, and specialized tools and aids for housekeeping and personal care; maintaining and repairing aids for personal mobility such as canes, walkers, wheelchairs, and scooters; and maintaining communication and recreational aids.
- *d6505 Taking Care of Plants, Indoors and Outdoors*
  Taking care of plants inside and outside the house, such as by planting, watering, and fertilizing plants; gardening and growing foods for personal use.
- *d6506 Taking Care of Animals*
  Taking care of domestic animals and pets; watching over the health of animals or pets, planning for the care of animals or pets in one's absence.
- *d6508 Caring for Household Objects, Specified*
- *d6509 Caring for Household Objects, Unspecified*

Treatment for Caring for Household Objects

Recreational therapists address many of the skills in this section because they are not only necessities; they are also forms of leisure. Sewing, home remodeling, fixing household appliances, working on cars, maintaining recreation equipment (e.g., waxing skis), indoor and outdoor gardening, and caring for pets are all listed under this section and participation in these tasks, for the most part, is the choice of the individual. For example, one client may choose to buy clothes at the department store rather than making them due to lack of sewing skills or lack of time or interest in the activity, while another client may have the money and means to buy clothing but

chooses to make her own clothes because it is enjoyable. The same goes for fixing cars and home remodeling and so on. Many Americans are fortunate to have this choice; however, some do not. For those whom these activities are necessities (e.g., the client has to make his/her own clothes because s/he cannot afford to buy clothes; religious clothing is difficult to find at a local retailer, therefore it is easier to make one's clothing; client lives in a rural environment where there aren't local clothing retailers) they are often given priority in the occupational therapy treatment plan. For those whom these activities are primarily leisure driven, they are incorporated into the recreational therapy treatment plan. An exception to this is those recreational therapists who work in settings where part of their role is to assist clients with the development of necessary daily living skills that may not necessarily be leisure driven (e.g., independent living movement, assisted care program).

Caring for household objects, although commonly thought of as being performed solely within the client's primary home, occurs in many different settings (e.g., mending a button when out in the community, repairing a piece of furniture at a friend's home because he has the proper tools, taking a household appliance to the repair shop, fixing a boat that is docked, repairing a skateboard at the skateboard park, growing food at a neighborhood garden, exercising a pet by going for walks in the park). Consequently, recreational therapists identify and address issues related to caring for household objects in community settings (e.g., handling the dog to go the veterinarian, transporting furniture and appliances, communicating repair needs). Impaired ability to care for household objects, especially those that involve community settings, can have an impact on other life activities, thus impacting other areas of health (e.g., difficulty exercising the dog by walking through the park affects d5701 Managing Diet and Fitness).

A client may acquire knowledge and skills of caring for household objects from other health professionals (often occupational therapists), however, it is the recreational therapist who evaluates and addresses 1. the impact of caring for household objects on participation in other life activities, 2. the skills required to care for household objects in various community and recreational settings, 3. adaptive equipment and techniques in addition to those provided by other health professionals to minimize difficulty with caring for household objects in real-life settings, and 4. integration training to the specific area where the client cares for household objects (e.g., the park where the client walks the dog, the neighborhood garden). Recreational therapists who work in independent living and assisted living may additionally address caring for household objects with clients in the residential setting for the purpose of teaching and promoting independence with basic life tasks.

In the ICF, therapists document the level of difficulty that a client has with each of the tasks in this code set. In discipline-specific documentation, therapists will additionally document the level of assistance required for each specific skill within the task of caring for household objects, recommendations (e.g., level of assistance or supervision needed), adaptive equipment or techniques utilized, and the problems that the difficulty of caring for household objects imposes on other life activities and needs (e.g., d5701 Managing Diet and Fitness).

Some of the common adaptations for tasks in this code set are provided below.

Making and repairing clothes: There are a variety of adaptations for making and repairing clothes including the repositioning of the sewing machine foot pedal (e.g., mounting the foot pedal to a side wall to be operated with the outside of the knee), using needle threaders, direct lighting, hemming clips instead of pins to hold a hem, use of a rotary cutter instead of scissors, adaptive scissors (table mounted scissors that are pressed down with a wrist or forearm, spring scissors that spring back open after release), and using strips of Dycem wrapped around the thumb and index finger to help grip the needle. Also see "Sewing" in the Equipment section. When doing an evaluation of this code, be sure to also check e115 Products and Technology for Personal Use in Daily Living or e140 Products and Technology for Culture, Recreation, and Sport. If one of these is relevant for making and repairing clothes, include it in the documentation along with d6500 Making and Repairing Clothes.

Maintaining dwellings and furnishings: Adaptive tools and techniques for maintaining the interior and exterior of a home include adaptive cuffs, pole extenders, and adaptive tools (e.g., tools with ergonomic design, limited impact, light weight, automatic start, automatic function). Examples include pole extenders for paintbrush rollers, the use of a clamp to stabilize a piece of broken furniture, putting a piece of putty on a piece of wood and then placing the nail into the putty so that it holds it steady when a client who only has use of one hand is getting the nail started, a lightweight, self-coiling hose to wash the exterior of the home, or a long-handled sponge to wash windows. Adaptive equipment and techniques for dusting, sweeping, swabbing, mopping, cleaning windows and walls, cleaning bathrooms and toilets, and cleaning household furniture include the use of adaptive tools (e.g., long-

handled, lightweight, cuffed, pole extenders, ergonomic) that are either specially designed or on the general market. Some examples include the use of a long-handled duster, an automatic floor vacuum that does not require a human to push it, disposable floor cleaning systems that do not require wringing a mop, a lightweight automatic sweeper instead of a broom, sitting on a chair outside of the tub and cleaning the bathtub with a long-handled scrubby, and the use of spray-on products that do not require scrubbing (spray on and then wipe off).

Maintaining domestic appliances: Repairing and taking care of domestic appliances (including maintenance of appliances) may include the use of adapted tools that are specially designed or are on the general market and techniques that are standard modifications or individualized. Examples include the use of automatic and power tools (e.g., an automatic screwdriver, cordless drill), homemade items (e.g., magnet on the end of a stick to retrieve fallen nails), and individualized techniques (e.g., using a long-handled mirror to see places on appliances the client couldn't otherwise see because of limitations in body positioning).

Maintaining vehicles: Repairing and taking care of motorized and non-motorized vehicles for personal use, including bicycles, carts, automobiles, and boats, may require the use of adaptive tools that are specially designed or are on the general market and techniques that are standardized modifications or individualized. Examples include the use automatic and power tools (e.g., an air gun to take off lug nuts instead of using a wrench), a bicycle lift that raises the bike up into the air so that it is easier to work on, placing small parts on a tray or a piece of Dycem so they do not roll away, and built-up tool handles using foam tubing for people who have impaired hand grasp.

Maintaining assistive devices: Repairing and taking care of assistive devices may require the use of adaptive tools that are specially designed or on the general market and techniques that are standardized modifications or individualized. Examples include the use of soft cloth that sticks to a Velcro mitt, the use of electric tools (e.g., electric screwdriver), the use of a palm sander to hold a buffing cloth for skis, or using built-up handles on pliers to tighten a butterfly nut on a pair of skates.

Taking care of plants: Taking care of indoor and outdoor plants may require the use of assistive tools that are specially designed or on the general market and techniques that are standardized modifications or individualized. Examples include the use of long-handled, lightweight tools (e.g., made of fiberglass instead of wood), use of raised garden beds and flower boxes, a "hi-low" (a device that allows a person to raise or lower a hanging flower basket with an automatic release pulley system), a lightweight, self-coiling hose, the use of a wrapping paper tube to slide seeds down to a specific area on the ground, use of a post hole digger instead of a shovel, specially designed gardening tools to maximize joint protection and use larger muscle groups, garden kneelers, and gardening chairs.

Taking care of animals: Taking care of domestic animals and pets may require the use of assistive tools that are specially designed or on the general market and techniques that are standardized modifications or individualized. For example, using a long-handled pooper scooper to clean out a kitty litter box, using a basket with a stiff handle to raise and lower animal food to the ground, kitty litter boxes with an automatic cleaning grid, a clothesline to hook a long leash onto so that the dog can get out for exercise in an unfenced yard, modifying a bird cage with a larger door opening to be able to easily access the pet, and adapted pet brushes.

The skills needed to participate in the activities of this code set are many. If deficits are suspected in this area, the therapist conducts a task analysis to determine the specific areas of difficulty. Refer to the code that reflects the area of difficulty (e.g., b455 Exercise Tolerance Functions) for information on assessment, document, treatment, and adaptation.

d660 Assisting Others
Assisting household members and others with their learning, communicating, self-care, movement, within the house or outside; being concerned about the well-being of household members and others.
Inclusions: assisting others with self-care, movement, communication, interpersonal relations, nutrition, and health maintenance
Exclusion: remunerative employment (d850)
- *d6600 Assisting Others with Self-Care*
  Assisting household members and others in performing self-care, including helping others with eating, bathing, and dressing; taking care of children or members of the household who are sick or have difficulties with basic self-care; helping other with their toileting.
- *d6601 Assisting Others in Movement*
  Assisting household members and others in movements and in moving outside the home, such as in the neighborhood or city, to or from school, place of employment, or other destination.
- *d6602 Assisting Others in Communication*
  Assisting household members and others with their communication, such as by helping with speaking, writing, or reading.
- *d6603 Assisting Others in Interpersonal Relations*
  Assisting household members and others with their interpersonal interactions, such as by

helping them to initiate, maintain, or terminate relationships.
- *d6604 Assisting Others in Nutrition*
  Assisting household members and others with their nutrition, such as by helping them to prepare and eat meals.
- *d6605 Assisting Others in Health Maintenance*
  Assisting household members and others with formal and informal health care, such as by ensuring that a child gets regular medical check-ups, or that an elderly relative takes required medication.
- *d6608 Assisting Others, Other Specified*
- *d6609 Assisting Others, Unspecified*

Treatment for Assisting Others

Assisting others, like caring for household objects, can be a necessity or a choice. For example, it is necessary for an adult to assist a child with self-care (e.g., washing, dressing), but it may not be necessary for a person to assist others with transportation (e.g., a client volunteers to help older people who belong to the church get to and from doctor appointments). Like the other codes within this chapter, assisting others occurs in many different contexts and environments, including community settings (e.g., assisting an elderly parent with routine exercise by going for daily walks around the neighborhood, assisting a child in making friends at the playground, helping an adult family member who has trouble reading to read directions for putting together a piece of recreational equipment). Consequently, recreational therapists identify and address issues related to assisting others in community settings. Impaired ability to care for others can have an impact on other life activities, thus impacting other areas of health (e.g., difficulty caring for an elderly parent requires the client to hire private assistance impacting the client's finances and thus other life activities that require money).

A client may acquire knowledge and skills of assisting others from other health professionals, however, it is the recreational therapist who evaluates and addresses 1. the impact of assisting others on other life activities (e.g., caring for others is negatively affecting self-care), 2. the skills required to assist others in various community and recreational settings (e.g., assisting a disabled child with wheelchair mobility in the home is different than in an outdoor environment), 3. adaptive equipment and technique recommendations in addition to those provided by other health professionals to minimize difficulty with assisting others in real-life settings, and 4. integration training to the specific area where the client assists others (e.g., the playground, the recreation center).

In the ICF, therapists document the level of difficulty that a client has with each of the tasks in this code set. In discipline-specific documentation, therapists will additionally document the level of assistance required for each specific skill in the task of assisting others, recommendations (e.g., level of assistance needed), adaptive equipment or techniques utilized, and the problems that the difficulty of assisting others imposes on other life activities and needs (e.g., d240 Handling Stress and Other Psychological Demands).

d669 Caring for Household Objects and Assisting Others, Other Specified and Unspecified

d698 Domestic Life, Other Specified

d699 Domestic Life, Unspecified

Chapter 7 Interpersonal Interactions and Relationships

This chapter is about carrying out the actions and tasks required for basic and complex interactions with people (strangers, friends, relatives, family members, and lovers) in a contextually and socially appropriate manner.

This chapter is about how people interact with others. The skills needed to interact with others are complex and often difficult to learn, even without any type of impairment. Recreational therapists, in the past, have covered these skills under the heading of social skills. The ICF does not use the same skill divisions, so this chapter will suggest ways to use the techniques that are already available to recreational therapists and adapt them for the ICF context.

Many different members of the treatment team address the development of social skills and relationship skills. The recreational therapist is one of the primary team members who help a client with interpersonal interactions and relationships. Because these skills can be practiced more easily in leisure and recreational situations than in other interactions in health care settings, this chapter places a heavy emphasis on the use of games, groups, and leisure activities as the modality to teach the skills. Refer to "Social Skills Training" and "Interpersonal Relationship Activities" in the Techniques section for specific techniques and activities related to the development of interpersonal interactions and relationships. Therapists should also refer to "Basic Awareness of Self" in the Concepts section for information about precursor social skills.

Some interaction deficits, especially when they are part of psychological problems related to family and intimacy, are outside the scope of practice of recreational therapists and should be left to psychologists or psychiatrists. When dealing with relationship issues, it is especially important for the recreational therapist to maintain an appropriate relationship with the client.

General Interpersonal Interactions (d710-d729)

d710 Basic Interpersonal Interactions
Interacting with people in a contextually and socially appropriate manner, such as by showing consideration and esteem when appropriate, or responding to the feelings of others.
Inclusions: showing respect, warmth, appreciation, and tolerance in relationships; responding to criticism and social cues in relationships; and using appropriate physical contact in relationships.
- *d7100 Respect and Warmth in Relationships*
  Showing and responding to consideration and esteem, in a contextually and socially appropriate manner.

- *d7101 Appreciation in Relationships*
  Showing and responding to satisfaction and gratitude, in a contextually and socially appropriate manner.
- *d7102 Tolerance in Relationships*
  Showing and responding to understanding and acceptance of behavior, in a contextually and socially appropriate manner.
- *d7103 Criticism in Relationships*
  Providing and responding to implicit and explicit differences of opinion or disagreement, in a contextually and socially appropriate manner.
- *d7104 Social Cues in Relationships*
  Giving and reacting appropriately to signs and hints that occur in social interactions.
- *d7105 Physical Contact in Relationships*
  Making and responding to bodily contact with others, in a contextually and socially appropriate manner.
- *d7108 Basic Interpersonal Interactions, Other Specified*
- *d7109 Basic Interpersonal Interactions, Unspecified*

Treatment for Basic Interpersonal Interactions

There are a set of basic interpersonal skills that are required before a person is able to develop meaningful relationships with others. These skills are normally developed while growing up, but some conditions, such as autism and mental retardation, limit a person's ability to develop appropriate skills. Psychological disorders, such as obsessive-compulsive disorder and schizophrenia, are often accompanied by deficits in the ability to interact with others appropriately (refer to specific diagnosis). These skills can also be lost as a result of brain injuries. (Even mild brain injuries may result in some loss of ability to handle interpersonal interactions.) For a discussion of the development of skills related to interpersonal interactions, see "Social Skills Development" in the Concepts section. Many of the clients that we serve will be working on these prerequisite skills to improve their ability to interact with others.

Some of the underlying skills will be found in Body Functions. The most important ones are b152 Emotional Functions, b1800 Experience of Self, and b126 Temperament and Personality Functions. Without these basic building blocks, it is hard to have interpersonal interactions. Other parts of b1 Mental Functions, such as b1142 Orientation to Person, are important to maintaining interpersonal interactions, but they are not required at this basic level. It is not uncommon to hear stories of clients with dementia who still act appropriately with other people even when they have forgotten most of their own lives and can't remember who the other person is. Clients with dementia do need a basic sense of themselves, though, as described in "Basic Awareness of Self as Part of Socialization" in the Concepts section.

Assessment of basic interpersonal interaction skills is not a simple process. It requires a multifaceted approach characterized by pre-assessment, on-going evaluation, and post-assessment. Consistent with behavioral and learning theories, this model assesses interpersonal interactions within a behavioral framework.

There are many ways that behaviors can be assessed within a behavioral framework. Because a client's interpersonal interactions may differ in various situations, assessment in more than one setting is warranted. At this level direct observation of the client's behavior and behavioral checklists or rating scales that record information on social strengths and weaknesses are the most appropriate tools. Some of the assessment tools that can be used are the *Leisure Social/Sexual Assessment* (*LS/SA*), the *CERT-Psych/R*, the *FOX*, the *School Social Behavior Scales*, the *Home and Community Social Behavior Scales*, and the *Social Attributes Checklist*. Summaries of these assessments may be found in the Assessment section. Each of these tools is discussed in detail in *Assessment Tools for Recreational Therapy and Related Fields, Third Edition* by burlingame and Blaschko (2002).

The therapist documents the deficits found and plans the appropriate interventions. Teaching skills in this area requires that assessment and intervention are integrally related. Assessment is ongoing, so that the training changes as an individual's performance changes. The pre-assessment techniques can also be used to evaluate how well the objectives have been met. Progress is measured only in relationship to stated objectives about specific problem areas that have been identified in the ongoing assessments.

Treatment involves an ongoing process where the client learns skills or relearns previously understood skills in a developmentally appropriate order. See "Social Skills Training" in the Techniques section for an appropriate sequence of skill development and techniques to use when teaching the skills. Some activities that teach these skills can be found in "Interpersonal Relationship Activities" in the Techniques section.

Adaptations are often required for clients with deficits in interpersonal interaction. Generally it involves working with the caregivers of the client to explain what the client's deficits are and why they happen. This is especially important when the deficits occur to a person who previously had appropriate social skills, such as the result of a brain injury or a stroke. It is often hard for caregivers to understand and accept an interpersonal skill deficit when no or minimal physical deficits are present. Consequently, caregivers are educated on how to best respond to inappropriate social behaviors. The two primary issues are making sure the behaviors of the client do not harm him/her (physically, emotionally, or in relationships) and re-educating the client in interpersonal skills.

The response of the caregiver to inappropriate social behaviors often comes from a place of love and caring (e.g., "I told him not to talk to his daughter like that because he was not picking up on her feelings of sadness and was reacting inappropriately to her behavior. I love my daughter and my husband and I do not want their relationship to be harmed."), feelings of upset or fear ("I have to be careful about what I say because sometimes he takes it the wrong way, becomes infuriated, and starts throwing things. I'm afraid he is going to hurt himself or one of us."), or feelings of protection (e.g., "He is so vulnerable that whenever someone criticizes him he does what the other person wants him to do without any thought as to the consequences. One day, a guy at work told him he was an arrogant person and no one at the shop liked him. My husband now takes donuts into the shop every morning trying to win back some friendship with his co-workers, but now they just make fun of him. It pains me and I want to protect him, so that's why I say the things I do.")

Caregivers also need to learn about the issues involved in continued interpersonal skill recovery. If inappropriate behavior is allowed to continue, it will become a more ingrained response, making it even more difficult to change down the line. Also, when considering theories related to neuroplasticity (see "Neuroplasticity" in the Techniques section), if faulty connections are allowed to continue, the caregiver is actually fostering the development of the faulty connections and telling the brain that the correct connections are not needed and can therefore be discarded.

The response of the caregiver to inappropriate social behaviors will vary depending on the response it elicits in the client, the situation at hand, and feelings provoked in the caregiver. Teaching the caregiver to respond in an even-toned voice that is non-judgmental is often the best course of action. For example, instead of saying, "Why did you say that to him?" which automatically puts a person on the defensive, the caregiver should say, "Mike is clearly upset after your talk with him. He is crying. What do you think we should do?" or "I know it is hard. We have to remind ourselves that yelling at him does not help him and that what he really needs is for us just to sit and listen to him sometimes." Other approaches may include cueing (e.g., touch the client's arm and make eye contact when s/he is being inappropriate as a cue to change the current behavior) and, although difficult and not always possible, manipulate the interactions (e.g., teaching children how to best talk to and respond to dad; inviting one friend over instead of two friends because the client is better at responding to social cues when interacting with one person at a time). See "Social Skills Training" in the Techniques section for more information.

The role of the caregiver as a teacher can take a major toll on the relationship. For example, the wife of a client may begin to feel more like a parent to her husband than a wife, which can affect other life areas such as emotional closeness, sexual life, and family roles and responsibilities (e.g., wife now helps the children more with emotionally charged issues rather than the husband; wife becomes the primary person to deal with situations of conflict). It is also important for therapists to remember that caregivers have needs as well. They need to feel loved, appreciated, and cared for. If they are not getting this from their loved one, even if they understand the reasons, it can leave the caregiver feeling unfulfilled, lonely, and stressed. Therefore, attention to the needs of the caregiver should also be a priority (e.g., information on relaxation training, importance of forming social networks, support for the caregiver's own self care, permission to feel angry, and healthy ways to release feelings of anger).

d720 Complex Interpersonal Interactions

Maintaining and managing interactions with other people, in a contextually and socially appropriate manner, such as by regulating emotions and impulses, controlling verbal and physical aggression, acting independently in social interactions, and acting in accordance with social rules and conventions.
Inclusions: forming and terminating relationships; regulating behaviours within interactions; interacting according to social rules; and maintaining social space

- *d7200 Forming Relationships*
  Beginning and maintaining interactions with others for a short or long period of time, in a contextually and socially appropriate manner, such as by introducing oneself, finding and establishing friendships and professional relationships, starting a relationship that may become permanent, romantic, or intimate.
- *d7201 Terminating Relationships*
  Bringing interactions to a close in a contextually and socially appropriate manner, such as by ending temporary relationships at the end of a

visit, ending long-term relationships with friends when moving to a new town or ending relationships with work colleagues, professional colleagues, and service providers, and ending romantic or intimate relationships.
- *d7202 Regulating Behaviors within Interactions*
  Regulating emotions and impulses, verbal aggression and physical aggression in interactions with others, in a contextually and socially appropriate manner.
- *d7203 Interacting According to Social Rules*
  Acting independently in social interactions and complying with social conventions governing one's role, position, or other social status in interactions with others.
- *d7204 Maintaining Social Space*
  Being aware of and maintaining a distance between oneself and others that is contextually, socially, and culturally appropriate.
- *d7208 Complex Interpersonal Interactions, Other Specified*
- *d7209 Complex Interpersonal Interactions, Unspecified*

Treatment for Complex Interpersonal Interactions

The second part of this chapter (d720 Complex Interpersonal Interactions) explores the development of basic social skills related to general interpersonal interactions. The majority of clients who require this level of training will have cognitive impairments that greatly reduce their ability to understand and interpret social rules and interactions. For clients in this category "overlearning" social skills will be needed so that the actions are executed without much thought; they are so well learned that they are implemented naturally.

As with the previous section, underlying skills will be found in the body functions chapter, including b152 Emotional Functions, b1800 Experience of Self, and b126 Temperament and Personality Functions. The client will also need b1 Mental Functions, such as b1142 Orientation to Person, to maintain interpersonal interactions. Assessment of basic interpersonal interaction skills is not a simple process. It requires a multifaceted approach characterized by pre-assessment, on-going evaluation, and post-assessment. Consistent with behavioral and learning theories, this model assesses interpersonal interactions in a behavioral framework.

There are many ways that behaviors can be assessed in a behavioral framework. Because a client's interpersonal interactions may differ in various situations, assessment in more than one setting is warranted. Each assessment should include an interview to obtain information about the client's social behavior, direct observation of the client's behavior, and behavioral checklists or rating scales that record information on social strengths and weaknesses. The best tool for evaluation of interpersonal interactions at this level is the *Leisure Social/Sexual Assessment* (*LS/SA*). It is especially appropriate for clients with life-long cognitive or psychosocial impairments. Some other assessment tools that can be used are the *CERT-Psych/R*, the *FOX*, the *School Social Behavior Scales*, the *Home and Community Social Behavior Scales*, and the *Social Attributes Checklist*. Summaries of these assessments may be found in the Assessment section. Each of these tools is discussed in detail in *Assessment Tools for Recreational Therapy and Related Fields, Third Edition* by burlingame and Blaschko (2002).

Other methods of assessment include further behavioral observations in a variety of settings. The recreational therapist is especially appropriate for conducting these assessments because s/he is responsible for taking the client into the community where a variety of settings may be found. Teaching a client with a brain injury how to ride the bus can be done with verbal instruction in a medical setting. Some limited role-playing can also help to make sure that the client understands all of the steps required. However, only an actual ride on the bus will demonstrate that the client has the necessary *social* skills to ride the bus successfully. The failure to have appropriate interactions with other riders and the bus driver cause more problems than cognitive deficits (burlingame, 1989). Similar kinds of problems can be assessed and documented in other community settings.

The therapist documents the deficits found and plans the appropriate interventions. Teaching skills in this area requires that assessment and intervention are integrally related. Assessment is ongoing, so that the training changes as an individual's performance changes. The pre-assessment techniques can also be used to evaluate how well the objectives have been met. Progress is only measured in relationship to stated objectives and specific problems areas identified in the ongoing assessments.

Treatment involves an ongoing process where the client learns skills or relearns previously understood skills in a developmentally appropriate order. See "Social Skills Training" and "Interpersonal Relationship Activities" in the Techniques section for an appropriate sequence of skill development, techniques to use when teaching the skills, and activities that teach these skills. Participating in activities in the community is strongly tied to appropriate social interactions. Two books that provide structured activities in the community are the *Community Integration Program* by Armstrong and

Lauzen (1994) and *Out in the World* by Johnson and Orichowskyj (1999). Managing emotions can be extremely difficult for someone with a brain injury (including stroke). It is important to explain to clients and caregivers the need to be in calm surroundings as much as possible, that it is all right to take a time out when things become too stressful, and that the emotional overload may be easier to handle as the brain heals. See b152 Emotional Functions for more thoughts on handling emotional issues.

As with the basic interpersonal interaction skills, adaptations are often required for clients with deficits. Adaptations usually involve working with the caregivers of the client to explain what the client's deficits are and why they happen. This is especially important when the deficits occur to a person who previously had appropriate social skills, such as the result of a brain injury or a stroke. It is hard to see from the outside that there have been changes. The inside is very different, though, and caregivers and others who come in contact with the client need to understand how to handle situations so that the client can be successful.

Some specific requirements are

1. accepting the social deficits of the client (e.g., realizing the client will not pick up on social cues as well and that humor may not be understood);
2. giving very specific, concrete statements about inappropriate behavior when it is displayed to halt the behavior, minimize adverse consequences of the behavior, and encourage awareness of social deficits; and
3. making it clear to the client that loved ones understand and accept his/her social deficits and are willing and able to provide needed assistance.

d729 General Interpersonal Interactions, Other Specified and Unspecified

Particular Interpersonal Relationships (d730-d779)

d730 Relating with Strangers
Engaging in temporary contacts and links with strangers for specific purposes, such as when asking for directions or making a purchase.

Treatment for
Relating with Strangers

Relating to strangers, for most clients, involves the application of basic and complex interpersonal skills already described. Sometimes there are psychosocial issues, such as shyness, or psychological issues, including autism, anxiety disorders, and psychoses, that make it difficult to make contact with any other person. These will show up in most interpersonal interactions and can be handled using the techniques in d710 and d720.

There is one set of clients who need to have special consideration when dealing with strangers, clients with MR/DD. Clients who have MR/DD often do not have a good understanding of what a stranger is and will follow the instructions of anyone who appears friendly. They may not be able to distinguish between helpers, such as clerks in stores, and people who wish to do them harm. Recreational therapists need to assess the client's ability to recognize helpers and other strangers, as described in "Social Skills Development" in the Concepts section. Then they need to teach the clients appropriate ways to interact with strangers as discussed in "Social Skills Training" in the Techniques section.

d740 Formal Relationships
Creating and maintaining specific relationships in formal settings, such as with employers, professionals, or service providers.
Inclusions: relating with persons in authority, with subordinates, and with equals
- *d7400 Relating with Persons in Authority*
  Creating and maintaining formal relations with people in positions of power or of a higher rank or prestige relative to one's own social position, such as an employer.
- *d7401 Relating to Subordinates*
  Creating and maintaining formal relations with people in positions of lower rank or prestige relative to one's own social position, such as an employee or servant.
- *d7402 Relating to Equals*
  Creating and maintaining formal relations with people in the same position of authority, rank, or prestige relative to one's own social position.
- *d7408 Formal Relationships, Other Specified*
- *d7409 Formal Relationships, Other Unspecified*

Treatment for Formal Relationships

Formal relationships add a layer of complexity to the relationship skills covered in d710 and d720. These relationships require the client to follow the special rules of his/her society in the way s/he treats other people in structured situations. In North America formal relationships are most likely to be seen in the workplace (including the military, which probably has the most formal structure found in Western society). Prisons are also highly formalized. For teenagers and children, these relationships will occur at school and when playing team sports. In a medical setting, problems with the relationship between the medical personnel, clients, and people

associated with clients would probably be scored with this code.

Deficits in this area can be caused by many diagnoses. Clients with MR/DD may not have learned the relationships yet. Inability to function in formal relationships is a defining characteristic of some psychological diagnoses, and is present in many others. Clients with brain injuries may have lost the understanding of how to act in formal situations or they may not be able to tolerate having to follow authority figures. Some clients may be in denial or simply fed up with a frustrating medical condition and are, therefore, unwilling to follow medical prescriptions.

Measuring deficits in formal relationships is usually done through observation. There are some formal tools used to record the observations including the *CERT-Psych/R*, the *School Social Behavior Scales*, and the *Home and Community Social Behavior Scales*. Often the behavior will be recorded just as a chart note.

Treatment depends on the cause of the deficit. For clients with MR/DD the information in "Social Skills Development" in the Concepts section can be used to teach these relationships. Other clients will usually fail in these relationships because of cognitive issues, such as not being able to accomplish the task required, and/or emotional issues, such as anger. Many of the aspects of b1 Mental Functions or other parts of the A&P chapters may come into play. Some possible areas to look at in the Techniques section are "Anger Management," "Adjusting to Disability," and "Coping with Stress."

d750 Informal Social Relationships
Entering into relationships with others, such as casual relationships with people living in the same community or residence, or with co-workers, students, playmates, or people with similar backgrounds or professions.
Inclusions: informal relationships with friends, neighbours, acquaintances, co-inhabitants, and peers
- *d7500 Informal Relationships with Friends*
  Creating and maintaining friendship relationships that are characterized by mutual esteem and common interests.
- *d7501 Informal Relationships with Neighbours*
  Creating and maintain informal relationship with people who live in nearby dwellings or living areas.
- *d7502 Informal Relationships with Acquaintances*
  Creating and maintaining informal relationships with people whom one knows but who are not close friends.
- *d7503 Informal Relationships with Co-inhabitants*
  Creating and maintaining informal relationships with people who are co-inhabitants of a house or

other dwelling, privately or publicly run, for any purpose.

- *d7504 Informal Relationships with Peers*
  Creating and maintaining informal relationships with people who share the same age, interest, or other common feature.
- *d7508 Informal Social Relationships, Other Specified*
- *d7509 Informal Social Relationships, Unspecified*

Treatment for Informal Social Relationships

Informal social relationships are based on the relationship skills covered in d710 and d720. These relationships require the client to maintain appropriate interactions with people the client knows.

Deficits in this area can be caused by many diagnoses. Clients with MR/DD may not have learned the relationships yet. Inability to function in casual relationships can be part of many psychological diagnoses. Clients with brain injuries may have lost the understanding of how to act in these situations. They may be unable to function in these situations because they can no longer process the subtle social cues that are required to act appropriately or they may not be able to tolerate dealing with the frustrations that interacting with other people often brings.

Measuring deficits in informal relationships is usually done through observation. There are some formal tools used to record the observations including the *CERT-Psych/R*, the *School Social Behavior Scales*, and the *Home and Community Social Behavior Scales*. Often the behavior will be recorded just as a chart note. It is important to document the type of deficit and the particular situation where the deficit occurs, so that treatment can be planned appropriately and progress can be measured.

Measurement can be difficult in some situations. For example, a client in a long-term care facility may not interact with other clients because s/he can't hear what they are saying. This would be a deficit in b230 Hearing Functions, not in relationships. Other clients may be in situations where there are few opportunities for informal social relationships, even if the client is able to participate in them. Clients in psych facilities and clients in medical isolation are in two possible situations where it might be difficult to create and maintain informal social relationships.

Treatment depends on the cause of the deficit. For clients with MR/DD the information in "Social Skills Development" in the Concepts section can be used to teach these relationships. Other clients will usually fail in these relationships because of cognitive issues, such as not being able to accomplish the task required, and/or emotional issues, such as

fear or anger. Many of the aspects of b1 Mental Functions or other parts of the A&P chapters may come into play. Some possible areas to look at in the Techniques section are "Anger Management," "Integration," and "Coping with Stress."

d760 Family Relationships

Creating and maintaining kinship relations, such as with members of the nuclear family, extended family, foster and adopted family, and step-relationships, more distant relationships such as second cousins, or legal guardians.

Inclusions: parent-child and child-parent relationships, sibling and extended family relationships

- *d7600 Parent-Child Relationships*
  Becoming and being a parent, both natural and adoptive, such as by having a child and relating to it as a parent or creating and maintaining a parental relationship with an adoptive child, and providing physical, intellectual, and emotional nurture to one's natural or adoptive child.
- *d7601 Child-Parent Relationships*
  Creating and maintaining relationships with one's parent, such as a young child obeying his or her parents or an adult child taking care of his or her elderly parents.
- *d7602 Sibling Relationships*
  Creating and maintaining a brotherly or sisterly relationship with a person who shares one or both parents by birth, adoption, or marriage.
- *d7603 Extended Family Relationships*
  Creating and maintaining a family relationship with members of one's extended family, such as with cousins, aunts and uncles, and grandparents.
- *d7608 Family Relationships, Other Specified*
- *d7609 Family Relationships, Unspecified*

Treatment for Family Relationships

Family relationships are based on the relationship skills covered in d710 and d720. These relationships require the client to maintain appropriate interactions with people the client knows well. Sorting out and modifying family relationships can be one of the most difficult tasks for any medical professional. If significant changes are required, the deficits should usually be handled by a psychologist or other professional trained to deal with family dynamics. Recreational therapists may be involved when the basic family relationship is sound, but some change in the client's condition requires the family to change how they relate to the client. Serious illnesses, significant physical disabilities, and brain injuries are areas where the recreational therapist may be able to provide services.

Measuring deficits in family relationships is usually done through observation in both hospital and community settings. There are some formal tools used to record the observations including the *Home and Community Social Behavior Scales*. Often the behavior will be recorded just as a chart note. It is important to document the type of deficit and the particular situation where the deficit occurs, so that treatment can be planned appropriately and progress can be measured. Note that the deficits recorded may be deficits that the client has or they may be deficits with members of the family. Sometimes the most significant problem is that the family has not figured out how to deal with the new condition of the client and/or the client has not adjusted to his/her role change in the family. For example, a client is a single parent of a fifteen-year-old daughter. Due to a physical disability, the client now requires physical assistance from the daughter who willingly provides the needed assistance. The client is now struggling with maintaining a parent-child relationship with her daughter because the family roles have changed. She reports that it is difficult to reprimand her daughter for poor behavior because she fears that the daughter may not provide her with the physical assistance that she needs.

Treatment depends on the cause of the deficit. For clients with MR/DD the information in "Social Skills Development" in the Concepts section and "Social Skills Training" in the Techniques section can be used to teach these relationships. Many of the aspects of b1 Mental Functions or other parts of the A&P chapters may come into play for other clients. Family issues are often treated by providing accurate information about how the client's abilities have changed. For both clients and their families look at "Anger Management," "Integration," "Adjusting to Disability," and "Coping with Stress" in the Techniques section.

d770 Intimate Relationships

Creating and maintaining close or romantic relationships between individuals, such as husband and wife, lovers, or sexual partners.

Inclusions: romantic, spousal, and sexual relationships

- *d7700 Romantic Relationships*
  Creating and maintaining a relationship based on emotional and physical attraction, potentially leading to long-term intimate relationships.
- *d7701 Spousal Relationships*
  Creating and maintaining an intimate relationship of a legal nature with another person, such as in a legal marriage, including becoming and being a legally married wife or husband or an unmarried spouse.
- *d7702 Sexual Relationships*
  Creating and maintaining a relationship of a sexual nature, with a spouse or other partner.

- *d7708 Intimate Relationships, Other Specified*
- *d7709 Intimate Relationships, Unspecified*

Treatment for Intimate Relationships

The fourth section of this chapter looks at skills related to intimacy and its appropriate expression, regulation, and range. Intimate relationships are based on the relationship skills covered in d710 and d720. These relationships require the client to maintain appropriate interactions with people the client is extremely close to. Sorting out and modifying intimate relationships can be almost as difficult as sorting out family relationships. If significant changes are required, the deficits should usually be handled by a psychologist or other professional trained to deal with these dynamics.

Recreational therapists may be involved when the basic relationship is sound, but some change in the client's condition requires a change in the relationship. Serious illnesses, significant physical disabilities, and brain injuries are areas where the recreational therapist may be able to provide services. The recreational therapist will also be involved in teaching the skills required for intimate relationships to clients with MR/DD.

The client's expression of sexuality is often uncomfortable for staff. In too many settings the client's sexuality is avoided or discouraged. Since, in most situations, an individual's development and expression of intimate relationships (including his/her expression of sexuality) is most appropriate in non-work settings, the recreational therapist should be prepared to work with a client on his/her appropriate expression of social skills, including ones related to intimate relationships and sexuality. See b640 Sexual Functions for specific information on how recreational therapists address sexuality with clients.

Assessment of deficits in intimate relationships is almost always the result of the client or someone who knows the client presenting the information to the treatment team. The one major exception to this is with clients who have MR/DD where the therapist uses a tool such as the *Leisure Social/Sexual Assessment* (described in the Assessment section) to measure the client's knowledge about intimate relationships. The interview part of that assessment is a useful tool for gathering information about the client's social behavior, which will aid in selection, grouping, and development of objectives. In order to develop an appropriate individualized program for gaining leisure and social/sexual knowledge and skills it is necessary to obtain information about the client's present use of time, knowledge, skills, and interests. If conducted by a professional trained in assessment techniques, the interview has a high degree of validity and reliability for broad assessment.

For a discussion of the development of skills related to intimate relationships for clients with MR/DD, see "Social Skills Development" in the Concepts section and "Social Skills Training" in the Techniques section.

For all clients, the development of a client's social skills, especially related to his/her expression of intimate relationship skills, is a difficult area of treatment. The therapist needs to help the client develop intimate skills without creating a sexually charged atmosphere during treatment and without the client developing intimate feelings for the therapist. This is especially challenging when working with clients who have cognitive impairments.

Treatment for other clients depends on the underlying cause of the deficit. See b640 Sexual Functions for a discussion of how to treat physical and emotional issues related to sexuality. Psychological issues, with their intricate interactions with family relationships, are probably best handled by a psychologist specifically trained to deal with sexual and relationship issues.

d779 Particular Interpersonal Relationships, Other Specified and Unspecified

d798 Interpersonal Interactions and Relationships, Other Specified

d799 Interpersonal Interactions and Relationships, Unspecified

Reference

Armstrong, M. & Lauzen, S. (1994). *Community integration program, 2ⁿᵈ ed.* Ravensdale, WA: Idyll Arbor.

burlingame, j. (1989). *Bus utilization skills assessment.* Ravensdale, WA: Idyll Arbor.

burlingame, j. & Blaschko, T. M. (2002). *Assessment tools for recreational therapy and related fields, third edition.* Ravensdale, WA: Idyll Arbor.

Johnson, R. P. & Orichowskyj, R. M. (1999). *Out in the world: A community living skills manual, 2nd ed.* Bisbee, AZ: Imaginart.

Chapter 8 Major Life Areas

This chapter is about carrying out the tasks and actions required to engage in education, work, and employment and to conduct economic transactions.

Education (d810-d839)

d810 Informal Education
Learning at home or in some other non-institutional settings, such as learning crafts and other skills from parents or family members, or home schooling.

d815 Preschool Education
Learning at an initial level of organized instruction, designed primarily to introduce a child to the school-type environment and prepare it for compulsory education, such as by acquiring skills in a day-care or similar setting as preparation for advancement to school.

d820 School Education
Gaining admission to school, engaging in all school-related responsibilities and privileges, and learning the course material, subjects, and other curriculum requirements in a primary or secondary education programme, including attending school regularly, working cooperatively with other students, taking direction from teachers, organizing, studying, and completing assigned tasks and projects, and advancing to other stages of education.

d825 Vocational Training
Engaging in all activities of a vocational programme and learning the curriculum material in preparation for employment in a trade, job, or profession.

d830 Higher Education
Engaging in the activities of advanced educational programmes in universities, colleges, and professional schools and learning all aspects of the curriculum required for degrees, diplomas, certificates, and other accreditations, such as completing a university bachelor's or master's course of study, medical school, or other professional school.

d839 Education, Other Specified and Unspecified

Treatment for Education

Carrying out tasks and actions required to engage in informal or formal education (e.g., learning, gaining admission, engaging in school-related responsibilities and privileges, attending, working cooperatively with others, organizing, studying, completing tasks and projects, advancing to other stages of education) encompasses many different skill sets (e.g., d7202 Regulating Behaviors within Interactions, d140 Learning to Read, b144 Memory Functions).

Recreational therapists who work in school settings regularly address barriers to education. Recreational therapists who work in rehabilitation settings also address barriers to education (e.g., problem solving for architectural barriers, developing peer social skills, assertiveness training) and integrate the client into the specific educational setting (e.g., client's home, recreation center, elementary school). It is important for therapists to note that informal education can occur in a variety of settings (e.g., home, recreation center, discussions at church) and that informal, as well as formal, education can be related to recreation and leisure (e.g., pursuing a new hobby, advancing education for personal pleasure versus career gain). Additionally, engaging in school-related privileges includes school activities such as sport rallies, plays, and other social and recreational activities outside of the standard formal curriculum. If a recreation or sport activity takes place in an educational setting, the therapist would score one of these codes rather than the recreation and leisure codes in Activities and Participation Chapter 9.

Therapists assist clients in evaluating school activities, barriers, and facilitators. Active problem solving and functional skill development are implemented to minimize barriers, identify further facilitators, and maintain/improve participation and functioning in school activities. Outside of basic academic work, involvement in structured school activities (e.g., sports, clubs, groups) and unstructured school activities (e.g., socializing in the lunchroom, engaging in activity with others at recess) are integral parts of health.

Therapists then provide integration training in the school and continue to evaluate the client's functioning in his/her real-life setting (performance qualifier). Outside of client evaluation, the therapist talks with relevant school staff and makes recommendations as needed (e.g., request a key for the client to use the school elevator, talk with the school nurse about the need for the client to have a private area to self-cath in a supine position, get clearance for the client to arrive five minutes late to class if required because of mobility issues, take out a chair in the auditorium to create a space for the client to sit in his/her wheelchair, install an automatic door). See "Integration" in the Techniques section for more information on conducting a school evaluation.

In the ICF the therapist documents the client's level of difficulty. In discipline-specific documentation, the therapist makes additional notes about the level of assistance required with the subtasks of school participation (e.g., wheelchair propulsion, interaction with others, coping style), recommendations (e.g., level of assistance needed, recommendations given to the school), and adaptive equipment or techniques utilized (e.g., changing the club meeting to a first floor classroom), and the problems that the difficulty of education imposes on other life activities and needs (e.g., going to school put an increased financial strain on the family because the client used to work and contribute to the household finances).

Work and Employment (d840-d859)

d840 Apprenticeship (Work Preparation)
Engaging in programmes related to preparation for employment, such as performing the tasks required of an apprenticeship, internship, articling, and in-service training.
Exclusions: vocational training (d825)

d845 Acquiring, Keeping, and Terminating a Job
Seeking, finding, and choosing employment, being hired, and accepting employment, maintaining, and advancing through a job, trade, occupation, or profession, and leaving a job in an appropriate manner.
Inclusions: seeking employment; preparing a resume or curriculum vitae; contacting employers and preparing interviews; maintaining a job; maintaining one's own work performance; giving notice; and terminating a job

- *d8450 Seeking Employment*
  Locating and choosing a job, in a trade, profession, or other form of employment, and performing the required tasks to get hired, such as showing up at the place of employment or participating in a job interview.
- *d8451 Maintaining a Job*
  Performing job-related tasks to keep an occupation, trade, profession, or other form of employment, and obtaining promotion and other advancements in employment.
- *d8452 Terminating a Job*
  Leaving or quitting a job in the appropriate manner.
- *d8458 Acquiring, Keeping, and Terminating a Job, Other Specified*
- *d8459 Acquiring, Keeping, and Terminating a Job, Unspecified*

d850 Remunerative Employment
Engaging in all aspects of work, as an occupation, trade, profession, or other form of employment, for payment, as an employee, full or part time, or self-employed, such as seeking employment and getting a job, doing the required tasks of the job, attending work on time as required, supervising other workers or being supervised, and performing required tasks alone or in groups.
Inclusions: self-employment, part-time and full-time employment

- *d8500 Self-Employment*
  Engaging in remunerative work sought or generated by the individual, or contracted from others without a formal employment relationship, such as migratory agricultural work, working as a free-lance writer or consultant, short-term contract work, working as an artist or crafts person, owning and running a shop or other business.
  Exclusions: part-time and full-time employment (d8501, d8502)
- *d8501 Part-Time Employment*
  Engaging in all aspects of work for payment on a part-time basis, as an employee, such as seeking employment and getting a job, doing the tasks required of the job, attending work on time as required, supervising other workers or being supervised, and performing required tasks alone or in groups.
- *d8502 Full-Time Employment*
  Engaging in all aspects of work for payment on a full-time basis, as an employee, such as seeking employment and getting a job, doing the required tasks of the job, attending work on time as required, supervising other workers or being supervised, and performing required tasks alone or in groups.
- *d8508 Remunerative Employment, Other Specified*
- *d8509 Remunerative Employment, Unspecified*

d855 Non-Remunerative Employment
Engaging in all aspects of work in which pay is not provided, full-time or part-time, including organized work activities, doing the required tasks of the job, attending work on time as required, supervising other workers or being supervised, and performing required tasks alone or in groups, such as volunteer work, charity work, working for a community or religious group without remuneration, working around the home without remuneration.
Exclusions: Chapter 6 Domestic Life

d859 Work and Employment, Other Specified and Unspecified

Treatment for Work and Employment

Treatment for employment includes apprenticeship; acquiring, keeping, and terminating a job; remunerative employment; and non-remunerative employment. Employment is actively addressed by a variety of health disciplines and programs including the profession of recreational therapy (e.g., office of vocational rehabilitation, work readiness programs, trade teachers, therapists, job facilitators).

Examples of recreational therapists addressing employment include:

- Recreational therapists who work with troubled youth may assist them in developing life skills including the skills needed to acquire, keep, and terminate a job (e.g., interviewing skills, developing a resume, choosing appropriate clothing, communicating with superiors, time management skills).
- Recreational therapists who work in a developmentally disabled job program assist clients during job performance to facilitate use of job skills (e.g., task performance, utilizing adaptive techniques, asking for assistance when needed, managing time, working in a group).
- Recreational therapists who work in long-term care may assist residents in identifying volunteer opportunities inside or outside of the residential setting (non-remunerative employment).
- Recreational therapists who work in physical rehabilitation may incorporate worksite evaluations and job analysis into integration training sessions.
- Recreational therapists who work in psychiatric care may assist clients with the development of coping mechanisms for stressful situations (including situations that occur at work).

Employment, whether paid or unpaid, provides many health benefits outside of monetary compensation or required obligations. The primary health benefits of employment for an individual are evaluated on an individual basis. For example, a 65-year-old client who works part time at the local hardware store (remunerative employment) states that he doesn't work for the money but rather for the socialization that it provides (talking with all the "guys" who come in for supplies). Another example is a 35-year-old woman whose mother died of breast cancer. She finds that raising money for breast cancer campaigns makes her feel like she is "doing something" to help other people who are going through what her mom went through, ultimately working as a coping strategy for this woman. A final example is an adolescent who writes articles and poems and submits them to a teen magazine. She is paid for the pieces that are accepted and the money is appreciated, but the adolescent states that acknowledgement of her ideas and thoughts is more rewarding. Therapists understand that work is not just work, but it can have a deeper meaning and purpose, that, if not pursued, could cause dysfunction in other life areas (e.g., social health, emotional health).

It is important for therapists to note that employment can occur in a variety of settings (e.g., work from home, office, on the road), each with their own individual characteristics (e.g., quiet and alone in the home, noisy and crowded in an office) and that employment can be related to recreation and leisure (e.g., volunteering at a local nursing home for one's own pleasure rather than fulfilling a duty; working part time at the ice cream shop for the purpose of socialization rather than for monetary gain). Additionally, engaging in employment tasks and projects may also be recreation or sport related (e.g., entertaining clients by taking them to the Super Bowl, participating in the mandatory office basketball team). If a recreation or sports activity takes place in an employment setting (e.g., pro tennis player), the therapist would score one of these codes rather than the recreation and leisure codes in Activities and Participation Chapter 9.

Once the therapist identifies that work and employment are areas that need to be addressed in treatment, therapists assist clients in:

1. Developing needed skills (e.g., social skills, direction following, relating to superiors).
2. Minimizing barriers (e.g., changing attitudes of others, educating the client about his/her rights to employment under the Americans with Disabilities Act, educating other people as appropriate to the client's needs and abilities).
3. Identifying and promoting facilitators (e.g., attitudes of people in positions of authority, products and technology).
4. Evaluating the environment of the work or employment setting and making recommendations.

In the ICF therapists score the level of difficulty that client has with work and employment. In discipline-specific documentation, therapists will additionally document the level of assistance required with each subtask of the work/employment activity, adaptive equipment and techniques, recommendations given, education provided, and the impact that dysfunction in work/employment has on other life tasks (e.g., d9205 Socializing, d610 Acquiring a Place to Live).

See "Integration" in the Techniques section for information on work evaluations. Also see "Americans with Disabilities Act Education" in the Techniques section for further information about work accommodations.

Economic Life (d860-d879)

d860 Basic Economic Transactions

Engaging in any form of simple economic transaction, such as using money to purchase food or bartering, exchanging goods or services; or saving money.

d865 Complex Economic Transactions

Engaging in any form of complex economic transaction that involves the exchange of capital or property, and the creation of profit or economic value, such as buying a business, factory, or equipment, maintaining a bank account, or trading in commodities.

d870 Economic Self-Sufficiency

Having command over economic resources, from private or public sources, in order to ensure economic security for present and future needs.

Inclusions: personal economic resources and public economic entitlements

- *d8700 Personal Economic Resources*
  Having command over personal or private economic resources, in order to ensure economic security for present and future needs.
- *d8701 Public Economic Entitlements*
  Having command over public economic resources, in order to ensure economic security for present and future needs.
- *d8708 Economic Self-Sufficiency, Other Specified*
- *d8709 Economic Self-Sufficiency, Unspecified*

d879 Economic Life, Other Specified and Unspecified

Treatment for Economic Life

Economic skills of basic and complex economic transactions and economic self-sufficiency are skills required for independent living, unless another person carries the responsibility for the individual (e.g., as a guardian).

Recreational therapists who work in rehabilitation and residential programs regularly address barriers to economic life and promote facilitators, especially with clients who are cognitively impaired or are striving to reach developmental milestones (e.g., teaching a seven-year-old how to perform basic economic transactions at the toy store with her birthday gift card). Economic transactions are needed for many recreation and leisure activities (e.g., buying movie tickets, buying flowers for a date, buying recreation equipment) and are therefore commonly addressed. Integration of economic skills into the client's real-life community is also an intervention (e.g., withdrawing money from the ATM machine, purchasing tickets at the movie theater). Addressing economic self-sufficiency (e.g., saving money) is not commonly included in inpatient rehabilitation programs, however it is often a component of the recreational therapy treatment plan when working with clients in an independent living program as part of learning basic life skills.

Economic issues have the potential to affect the basic human needs of shelter and food in either a positive or negative way, as well as participation in other life activities (e.g., recreational pursuits).

If a problem is suspected with economic life, the therapist conducts a task analysis to identify the specific areas of dysfunction (e.g., d172 Calculating, d177 Making Decisions, d4402 Manipulating). Deficits are then addressed. Please refer to the specific problem in this book for information on how to assess, document, treat, and adapt for the identified problem.

In the ICF therapists document the client's level of difficulty. In discipline-specific documentation, therapists document the level of assistance required with each of the subtasks of the skill, adaptive equipment and techniques, recommendations, and impact of the dysfunction on other life tasks (e.g., relationship with spouse, participation in activities, nutrition).

d898 Major Life Areas, Other Specified

d899 Major Life Areas, Unspecified

Chapter 9 Community, Social, and Civic Life

This chapter is about the actions and tasks required to engage in organized social life outside the family, in community, social, and civic areas of life.

These are very difficult sections for the recreational therapist to score. It is difficult because the categories are broad and few, not allowing for a true reflection of the client's performance in a specific task (see the introduction to the Activities and Participation section). Additionally, the term "engaging" is not fully defined and the score given does not allow the therapist to delineate participation patterns. We will review these issues in detail below and suggest ways to increase the reliability of scores in this section.

Defining the Term "Engaging"

When you look at the definition of each of the categories in this section, the word "engaging" is used in their definitions (e.g., engaging in pastimes, engaging in needlecrafts). The problem is that "engaging" is not a therapeutic term commonly used in our practice and could therefore cause some difficulties in scoring if it is not interpreted the same way by all therapists. Since the ICF is based on health rather than on disability (all definitions are functionality or ability definitions, not problem definitions), we feel comfortable making the assumption that the term "engaging" means "healthy participation" in the activity. In that case, engaging in a social activity means initiating and sustaining conversation, participating in healthy group activities, and exhibiting appropriate social skills such as eye contact, ability to read social situations, and good social decisions.

With this in mind, let's look at one of the recreation and leisure codes

d9202 Arts and Culture: Engaging in, or appreciating, fine arts or cultural events, such as going to the theatre, cinema, museum, or art gallery, or acting in a play, reading for enjoyment, or playing a musical instrument.

Notice that the code includes a range of participation. For example, the skill of appreciating fine art such as looking through a museum catalog is very different from the more physically active task of playing a cello. This causes a problem for the field of recreational therapy because the skill sets for these tasks are quite different and a client may participate in a variety of "Arts and Culture" activities. This means that one therapist may score the client as having no difficulty with "Arts and Culture" (aware of only the client's ability to look through a collection of museum catalogs) while another therapist may score the client has having moderate difficulty (thinking only about the client's ability to play the cello).

Another aspect of the problem recreational therapists have is that there are two ways to look at healthy participation. The first looks at the ability of the client to perform the actions required in the activity. The second looks at whether the client is participating in a healthy way or merely going through the motions (whether the client is truly "engaging" in the activity). Both need to be scored to give an accurate picture of the client's ability to engage in organized social life.

To score the ICF code hold the mental picture of "healthy participation" in your mind, measure how much difficulty the client has in performing the tasks required for this level of "healthy participation" and choose the appropriate score. If the client's level of difficulty ranges tremendously with the activity (e.g., client has maximal difficulty throwing a bowling ball, no difficulty in keeping score, minimal difficulty taking turns, and moderate difficulty putting on the bowling shoes), the therapist should take the lowest score (i.e., maximal difficulty).

The additional recommendation of the authors is for the therapist to write the name of the specific activity (e.g., bowling), along with a description of the participation level (e.g., Dehn's level 3: Active Participation) to the left of the scored code. Another example would be "Playing the cello, Dehn's level 4: Creative Participation." For an explanation of levels of participation see "Participation" in the Concepts section.

Scoring the ability of the client to engage in activities from two perspectives will provide a better description of what is being observed, as well as communicate more accurately to the other readers the specific activity and participation level found. In discipline-specific documentation, therapists are encouraged to use the Dehn level to further describe the level of activity participation.

d910 Community Life
Engaging in all aspects of community social life, such as engaging in charitable organizations, service clubs, or professional social organizations.
Inclusions: informal and formal associations; ceremonies

Exclusions: non-remunerative employment (d855); recreation and leisure (d920); religion and spirituality (d930); political life and citizenship (d950)

- *d9100 Informal Associations*
  Engaging in social or community associations organized by people with common interests, such as local social clubs or ethnic groups.
- *d9101 Formal Associations*
  Engaging in professional or other exclusive social groups, such as associations of lawyers, physicians, or academics.
- *d9102 Ceremonies*
  Engaging in non-religious or social ceremonies, such as marriages, funerals, or initiation ceremonies.
- *d9108 Community Life, Other Specified*
- *d9109 Community Life, Unspecified*

Treatment for Community Life

Community life can best be described as engaging in community groups and clubs with specific people joining together for a specific interest. Notice that this code excludes recreation and leisure, religion and spirituality, and political life. However the groups and clubs can be related to recreation, leisure, religion, spirituality, or politics (e.g., engaging in a social club, ceremony within a church). There is a distinction, although it is subtle. The community life code set is about engaging in community groups and clubs, whereas recreation, leisure, religion, spirituality, and political code sets are about engaging in the specific activity (in the home or the community). For example, if a client belonged to a senior citizen social club, the therapist would score "informal associations" related to the level of difficulty that he has engaging in the construct of a club (group membership skill such as calling people to action, voting, following group rules, expressing opinions within a group, following unstated social rules). This same client, while at the social club, engages in card playing. Card playing is a specific recreation activity, so the therapist would score his level of difficulty with card playing under the Recreation and Leisure code set (d9200 Play).

Engaging in community groups and clubs is one of the major areas of recreational therapy practice. The result of engaging in community life can directly affect a person's health in a positive or negative way. For example, a client who participates in a community group that raises money for children in need may reap the positive benefits of having a social network, getting exercise through physical challenges that raise money, and raising her sense of self-esteem in being part of an organization that gives to the community. On the other hand, another client may belong to a neighborhood gang (d9100 Informal Associations) that is involved with illegal activities (e.g., selling illegal drugs, destroying other's property). The client may state the same benefits as our previous client such as the benefits of having a social network, getting physical exercise by fighting with other gangs, and raising his sense of pride in being a part of a gang that accepts only a select few.

This is a perfect example of the need to use Dehn's levels. (See "Participation" in the Concepts section.) Let's say that this client has no difficulty in engaging within the gang, yet the gang activities themselves are dangerous to him and others. The therapist could score d9100 Informal Associations within all qualifiers a "0" for no difficulty and write to the left of the code "Neighborhood Gang: Dehn's level –2 Harm to Others." If this information was not provided after the code, any other person reading the score of "0" would think that the person is fully independent in the activity, which he is, but it does not alert the reader to the further issue of how engaging in this "informal association" might harm the client's health or the health of others.

From these examples it is evident that the level of difficulty that a client has with an activity or task does not relate to the level of health brought about by the activity. The ICF also does not currently allow the therapist to code Body Functions or Activities and Participation as barriers or facilitators of other activities (e.g., how engagement in d9100 Informal Associations facilitates b1266 Confidence). If the International Classification of Functioning, Disability, and Health is to accurately reflect a client's "health" we cannot overlook the facts that 1. the level of difficulty does not equate with the level of health in all situations and 2. the inability to link Body Structures, Body Functions, and Activities and Participation codes as facilitators and barriers to other Body Structures, Body Functions, and Activities and Participation codes poses a problem in being able to look at the holistic interaction of variables affecting a client's level of heath. The ICF is a wonderful classification system, but it is not perfect yet. With further use and recommendations, changes to the ICF will surely be made along these lines.

Recreational therapists evaluate the health of a client's lifestyle, which includes evaluation of community life. The difficulties that a client may have with engagement in community life can range considerably. It may be that the client is unaware of:

1. *Resources* (see "Community Leisure Resource Awareness" in the Techniques section).
2. *Human rights* (see d940 Human Rights, "Americans with Disabilities Act Education" in the Techniques section).

3. *Community barriers* (see "Community Problem Solving" and "Community Accessibility Training" in the Techniques section).
4. *Energy conservation* (see "Energy Conservation Training" in the Techniques section).
5. *Adaptations for engagement* (e.g., how to assert needs within a community group when unable to speak).

The client may also have difficulty with specific skills that are inherent in the specific club or group, such as:
1. *Social skills* (see Activities and Participation Chapter 7, see "Social Skills Development" in the Techniques section).
2. *Time management* (see d230 Carrying Out Daily Routine).
3. *Mobility* (see Activities and Participation Chapter 4, "Wheelchair Mobility" and "Walking Techniques" in the Techniques section).
4. *Anger management* (see "Anger Management" in the Techniques section).
5. *Adjustment to disability* (see "Adjustment to Disability" in the Techniques section).

Therapists are to refer to the specific code (e.g., d7202 Regulating Behaviors in Interactions) and/or specific chapters (e.g., "Activities and Participation" in the Techniques section and Chapter 4 Mobility) for information on how to assess, document, treat, and adapt for dysfunction in any of these areas.

Therapists will also want to consult "Integration" in the Techniques section for specific techniques on how to integrate clients into various community life activities.

d920 Recreation and Leisure
Engaging in any form of play, recreational, or leisure activity, such as informal or organized play and sports, programmes of physical fitness, relaxation, amusement, or diversion, going to art galleries, museums, cinemas, or theatres; engaging in crafts or hobbies, reading for enjoyment, playing musical instruments; sightseeing, tourism, and traveling for pleasure.
Inclusions: play, sports, arts and culture, crafts, hobbies, and socializing
Exclusions: riding animals for transportation (d480); remunerative and non-remunerative work (d850 and d855); religion and spirituality (d930); political life and citizenship (d950)
- *d9200 Play*
  Engaging in games with rules or unstructured or unorganized games and spontaneous recreation, such as playing chess or cards or children's play.
- *d9201 Sports*
  Engaging in competitive and informal or formally organized games or athletic events, performed alone or in a group, such as bowling, gymnastics, or soccer.
- *d9202 Arts and Culture*
  Engaging in, or appreciating, fine arts or cultural events, such as going to the theatre, cinema, museum, or art gallery, or acting in a play, reading for enjoyment, or playing a musical instrument.
- *d9203 Crafts*
  Engaging in handicrafts, such as pottery or knitting.
- *d9204 Hobbies*
  Engaging in pastimes such as collecting stamps, coins, or antiques.
- *d9205 Socializing*
  Engaging in informal or casual gatherings with others, such as visiting friends or relatives or meeting informally in public places.
- *d9208 Recreation and Leisure, Other Specified*
- *d9209 Recreation and Leisure, Unspecified*

Treatment for Recreation and Leisure

Engaging in recreation and leisure is an integral component of health and it is exciting to see it recognized by the World Health Organization. Recreation and leisure in the ICF are related to specific categories of activities that are commonly performed for pleasure and enjoyment. For example, playing an instrument falls under d9202 Arts and Culture. If a client plays an instrument for pleasure and enjoyment, the therapist would use this code. If the client plays an instrument for any other reason (e.g., work), the therapist would code the appropriate code instead (e.g., d850 Remunerative Employment).

The terms recreation and leisure are often used synonymously. The field of recreational therapy, however, often divides the terms. Recreation is commonly defined as activity, compared to leisure that is defined as a state of mind. Looking at this code set, it is obvious that it is activity focused. Leisure, however, as a state of mind, can be reflected in many of the ICF codes (e.g., d9100 Informal Associations, d6200 Shopping, d630 Preparing Meals, d6500 Making and Repairing Clothes, d6501 Maintaining Dwelling and Furnishings, d6503 Maintaining Vehicles, d6506 Taking Care of Animals). It could be argued that the other codes in the ICF, as mentioned above, are related to tasks that *need* to be done rather than tasks that are done for pleasure and enjoyment. However, to say that would mean that pleasure and enjoyment are absent from all activities outside of those categorized in the recreation and leisure code set. This is simply not true. Consequently, recreational therapists must decide if it is more appropriate to score an activity done for pleasure as a recreation and leisure code or to use a code that more specifically reflects the specific activity (e.g., if a client has the hobby of gardening, the therapist can use the code d6505 Taking Care of Plants or d9204 Hobbies; if a client builds hot rod cars for fun, the therapist can use the code d6504 Maintaining Vehicles or d9204 Hobbies). Therapists must also be careful when choosing codes for physical activities. For example, in Activities and Participation Chapter 4 Mobility there are a variety of codes that reflect a type of movement that is also a sport (e.g., d4551 Climbing, d4552 Running, d4553 Jumping, d4554 Swimming). If the therapist desires to score a type of movement, the mobility codes would be used (e.g., d4554 Swimming). However, if the therapist wants to score swimming as a sport, the recreation and leisure code would be used (d9201 Sports).

When scoring the codes in this area, there will be times when a client will be active in more than one activity that needs to be scored under this code. He may be better at one activity than another. The only way to provide an accurate assessment is to list all of the activities with a separate score for each. Unfortunately the ICF requires a single score for the item. We suggest the therapist analyze all that the client needs to do to have a healthy level of participation in recreation and leisure and score this item according to the level of difficulty that the client has in reaching this level of participation. As discussed at the beginning of the chapter, include the name of the activity, the maximum level of difficulty, and Dehn's level of participation for each activity.

Not all clients will have a healthy recreation and leisure lifestyle, so very often a therapist will need to begin with education about the consequences of an inappropriate leisure lifestyle and the benefits of recreation and leisure participation as it pertains to the current needs of the client whether it is a lack of physical exercise, mental stimulation, or emotional engagement. (See "Consequences of Inactivity" and "Maslow's Hierarchy of Needs" in the Concepts section. See "Lifestyle Alteration Education" in the Techniques section.)

The client may require leisure interest testing and exploration (see "Activity Pattern Development" in the Techniques section). Inaccurate information may need to be corrected (e.g., educating a client about adaptive equipment, techniques, and resources to engage in an activity that the client thought was only for able-bodied people) and counseling interventions may be employed (see "Education and Counseling" in the Techniques section.) Functional skill development related to activity participation commonly follows. The specific functional skills addressed will depend on the activity and the needs of the client. An activity analysis is conducted to determine areas of difficulty (see "Activity and Task Analysis" in the Techniques section). Therapists can refer to the specific skill in this book for information on how to assess, document, treat, and adapt for any deficits (e.g., if a client is having trouble with fine motor skills, refer to code d440 Fine Hand Use). Integration training typically follows, allowing the therapist to address issues that arise in a real-life setting and further assess the client's ability to integrate skills into his life (see "Integration" in the Techniques section).

d930 Religion and Spirituality

Engaging in religious or spiritual activities, organizations, and practices for self-fulfillment, finding meaning, religious or spiritual value, and establishing connection with a divine power, such as is involved in attending a church, temple, mosque, or synagogue, praying or chanting for a religious purpose, and spiritual contemplation.

Inclusions: organized religion and spirituality

- *d9300 Organized Religion*
  Engaging in organized religious ceremonies, activities, and events.
- *d9301 Spirituality*
  Engaging in spiritual activities or events, outside of organized religion.
- *d9308 Religion and Spirituality, Other Specified*
- *d9309 Religion and Spirituality, Unspecified*

Treatment for Religion and Spirituality

Ninety to 95% of people in the United States say that they believe in God or a higher being (Miller & Thoresen, 2003), yet religion and spirituality are rarely addressed in the health care setting. This is mostly due to fears of invading a person's privacy and overstepping the client-therapist boundary. Spirituality, however, whether obtained through religious or non-religious activities, is becoming increasingly recognized as being a benefit for health that needs to be addressed in the healthcare setting. (It is already a requirement in facilities operated under OBRA regulations, Tag 248: Activities.)

The terms religion and spirituality are often used interchangeably, however there are distinct differences between the two. Religion is an external expression of faith in God or a higher being. There are specific beliefs, values, and practices that unite a person with a religious community (e.g., Roman Catholic, Jewish, Hindu). Spirituality, on the other hand, is an intrinsic quality (e.g., "She is a spiritual person."). It is a feeling of connectedness with oneself, nature, the world, and/or a higher spirit. The ability to "stand outside of his/her immediate sense of time and place and to view life from a larger, more detached perspective" describes a common component of spirituality called spiritual transcendence (Rowe & Allen, 2004, p. 1). Spirituality can arise from the practice of religion, but the practice of a religion is not necessary to be spiritual.

Components of Spiritual Growth

Seaward (1997) theorizes that there are four specific internal processes that nurture spiritual health — centering, emptying, grounding, and connecting.

- *Centering*: Centering is a process of turning inwards and exploring personal thoughts, feelings, attitudes, and perceptions to gain a greater sense of the self. Activities such a meditation and yoga and rhythmic exercises such as running, walking, and swimming are common interventions to facilitate centering.
- *Emptying*: Emptying is a process of letting go of destructive thoughts, feelings, and actions that inhibit spiritual growth. Journaling can be helpful to increase awareness of thoughts, feelings, attitudes, values, and perceptions that inhibit a person from reaching his/her full life potential and satisfaction. Destructive traits that inhibit this growth often come to light and can then be released (emptied). Once the consciousness is cleared, the spirit (soul, core) is ready to receive new insights and move on to grounding.
- *Grounding*: In grounding a person 1. reflects inward to find inner resources to face the challenges that lie before him/her and 2. sharpens coping skills to manage stressful encounters in a healthy and self-fulfilling way. Meditation or prayer can be helpful to find inner strength and peace. Stress management and relaxation training strengthen coping skills. Problem solving and communication skills can also prove helpful in the development and tuning of healthy coping skills. Seaward recommends the additional modalities of paying attention to nature, participating in rituals, reading, discussing ideas and values with others, and simply paying attention to life as ways that help with grounding the spirit.
- *Connecting*: In the first three processes (centering, empting, grounding), the person focuses on connecting with the self. In the final process, the person focuses on connecting with others, nature, and with a higher power or spirit. Seaward states, "Those people who engage fully in the connecting process, without the influence of judgment, greed or fear, show an undeniable enthusiasm for life" (Seaward, 1997, p. 153).

Much of the literature about spirituality reports that meaning in one's life, connecting with a higher power, feeling connected to the world (as a system), having a nurturing relationship with oneself, having a strong personal value system, and having a meaningful purpose in the world affect health in a positive way.

Benefits and Interventions

"Spirituality is one of several known psychosocial variables that influence the course of health over an individual's lifetime...[and] it may play an independent role in helping individuals attend to positive elements in their life" (Bartlett et al, 2003, p. 780). It has been linked with happiness and positive health perceptions (Daaleman, Perera, & Studenski, 2004), positive affect and outlook (Myers, 2000; Diener, 2000; Rowe & Allen, 2004), decreased vulnerability to depression (even in the face of grief and loss) (Ellison & Levin, 1998; McIntosh, Silver, & Wortman, 1993), enhanced immune functioning, enhanced ability to adapt and cope with illness or disability (Bartlett et al, 2003; Rowe & Allen, 2004), and an increased ability to look at things from different perspectives along with creative problem solving (Ashby, Isen, & Turken, 1999).

Interestingly, a significant positive correlation between spirituality and age has been reported (Rowe & Allen, 2004), perhaps because increased spirituality is required to cope with the realization of mortality (Reed, 1991).

Although spirituality may have a significant correlation with age, health care professionals must not forget about the spiritual needs of a child. Elkins & Cavendish (2004) remind health professionals that attitudes and values expressed by a child are often influenced by the family's spiritual ideas and beliefs. Children have spiritual lives and they deserve to be continued and fostered in a health care setting. Spirituality is a growth process and, although people's development of spirituality varies, basic building blocks of spirituality often begin in childhood. Therapists should interview the parents, as discussed below, to determine any specific spiritual or religious needs that should be implemented in the hospital setting (e.g., prayers before bed, reminding the child that her special spirit is with her) and pay attention to signs of spiritual needs in the child. Elkins & Cavendish (2004) report that "children may use humor, poetry, stories, spiritual readings, religious artifacts, pictures, and art to send cues related to spiritual needs" (p. 181).

Health care professionals who provide education and counseling, teach disease management, or conduct client/family support groups should incorporate the development of spirituality whenever possible (Rowe & Allen, 2004). Although religion and spirituality are not totally neglected in clinical practice, Hathaway, Scott, & Garver (2004) found that they do not receive an adequate level of clinical attention in everyday practice. They recommend that professionals incorporate an assessment of religious and spiritual health into everyday clinical practice. Clinicians can begin by asking simple preliminary questions that probe the faith and spirituality of a client and expand exploration of the issues as relevant and appropriate. Therapists should also educate the client on the health benefits of spirituality and explain that it is an element of health that is routinely addressed in practice in order to provide the best services possible, as well as to respect the client's beliefs. A common line of questioning might look like this:

1. Ask the client if s/he is affiliated with a specific religion. If yes, what religion? Does the client consider himself/herself to be a spiritual person? What does being spiritual mean to the client? Has this helped the client navigate through life's challenges? The client may be wondering why you are asking these questions and possibly feeling a little uncomfortable because religion and spirituality have typically been kept private. Explain to the client why you are asking these questions and ask if it is okay to continue with a few more questions (explain that spirituality is an area of health that is gaining more attention because of the health benefits it can bring and that spirituality has an effect on the client's condition).

2. Ask the client if s/he participates regularly in specific rituals to meet his/her spiritual needs (e.g., church, meditation) and if there are specific restrictions that staff should be aware of (e.g., no meat on Fridays during Lent, no one is allowed to see the client's hair except her husband).

3. Develop a spiritual health treatment plan that meets the needs of the client and fosters spiritual growth (e.g., opportunities to participate in religious services, quiet area for meditation or prayer, a book and pen for journaling).

If the client is not affiliated with a specific religion and s/he states no spirituality in his/her life, the client should be briefly educated on why spirituality is assessed in therapy and that there is no intention to offend. However, because spirituality is recognized as an aspect of health, it should not be disregarded due to the client's verbalizations of lack of spirituality. Clients should be given experiences to grow and the word "spirituality" does not necessarily have to be used (especially if the client isn't able to

grasp the difference between religion and spirituality and feels that the therapist is pushing religion). For example, a client can be encouraged to sit outside in the fresh air before therapy begins or be given a journal. These techniques are not modalities only for spiritual growth. They are also aids to help decrease stress, open the mind to new ideas, and induce relaxation.

Summary

"Spiritual health is a dynamic and flexible dimension of health, one that can be enhanced as a result of prolonged and conscientious effort" (McGee, Nagel, & Moore, 2003). Interventions that foster centering, emptying, grounding, and connecting can deepen spirituality. Therapists should keep an open mind, ask open-ended questions and validate the importance of the individual's spirituality (e.g., "What would you like to pray about this evening?", "I understand that attending the morning religious service is important to you so how about I schedule your therapy sessions in the afternoon?"). Additionally, therapists who work with terminally ill children or adults may find that "spiritual care may be the only source of comfort when a cure is not possible" (Elkins & Cavendish, 2004, p. 184).

d940 Human Rights
Enjoying all nationally and internationally recognized rights that are accorded to people by virtue of their humanity alone, such as human rights as recognized by the United Nations Universal Declaration of Human Rights (1948) and the United Nations Standard Rules for the Equalization of Opportunities for Persons with Disabilities (1993); the right to self-determination or autonomy; and the right to control over one's destiny. Exclusions: political life and citizenship (d950)

Treatment for Human Rights

The term "enjoying" is different from "engaging" which is used for the other parts of this chapter's code set. Enjoying means that a client benefits fully from, profits from, and takes advantage of his/her human rights. Difficulty with enjoying human rights can be due to a number of things:

1. The client is unaware of his/her rights.
2. The client does not know how to achieve his/her rights.
3. The client lacks the appropriate skills to achieve his/her rights (e.g., lacks assertiveness skills).
4. The client has been overpowered and stripped of his/her rights (e.g., held a prisoner by someone who does not recognize the client's rights).
5. The client is being denied his/her human rights (e.g., public facility refusing to build a wheel-

chair ramp although is legislated to do so under the Americans with Disabilities Act, a woman is forced to wear a religious garb by her caretaker when she is afforded the right within her country not to wear it if she so chooses, a child is kept in a basement without food or clothing).

6. Organization/facilities/other people are unaware of human rights they are to be providing (e.g., company is unaware that they are to make accommodations for someone who has a disability).

Recreational therapists are knowledgeable about basic disability law and general human rights, teach client's about their rights and how to access those rights, assist clients in developing skills to achieve their rights, and educate others that are affecting the client's ability to fully enjoy his/her human rights.

Common environmental factors affecting human rights include products and technology (e.g., a facility lacks the resources to build a ramp), support and relationships (e.g., emotional support and assistance from others to take advantage of human rights, such as emotionally encouraging the client to fight for his/her rights or helping the client write a letter or use a communication device), attitudes (e.g., societal attitudes and attitudes of people in authority that make it difficult for a client to access human rights), and services, systems, and policies (e.g., services, systems, and policies that are identified as a need and have not yet been developed to protect a particular human right).

In the ICF, therapists document the level of difficulty that a client has with enjoying his/her human rights. It is recommended that along with documenting specific rights that are not available, therapists compare the percent of rights enjoyed to the total afforded to determine the level of difficulty. In discipline-specific documentation, therapists make additional notations about the specific human rights that are not being enjoyed, barriers that hinder enjoyment, recommendations for change, related skill development, and level of assistance required from another person to enjoy human rights. If a client is being denied his/her basic human rights and it poses a danger to the client (e.g., abused elder), it is the responsibility of the therapist to report it immediately to appropriate authorities (e.g., police, social worker, child welfare office).

See "Americans with Disabilities Act Education" in the Techniques section for more detailed information about the rights that people with disabilities are afforded under the Act.

d950 Political Life and Citizenship

Engaging in the social, political, and governmental life of a citizen, having legal status as a citizen and enjoying the rights, protections, privileges, and duties associated with that role, such as the right to vote and run for political office, to form political associations; enjoying the rights and freedoms associated with citizenship (e.g., the rights of freedom of speech, association, religion, protection against unreasonable search and seizure, the right to counsel, to a trial, and other legal rights and protection against discrimination); having legal standing as a citizen.

Exclusion: human rights (d940)

Treatment for Political Life and Citizenship

The code measures the degree to which the client engages in life as a citizen and how fully the client enjoys the rights, protections, privileges, and duties associated with citizenship. In the United States people have freedom to vote, run for office, form political associations, and enjoy freedom of speech, freedom of religion, freedom of association, protection against unreasonable search and seizure, the right to counsel and to a fair trial, and protection from discrimination. However, despite having these rights and freedoms there are instances when these rights and freedoms are not fully afforded (e.g., clients are not provided with ways to vote).

Recreational therapists are knowledgeable about basic rights, protections, and privileges that correlate with citizenship, teach clients about their rights as appropriate (e.g., recent immigrant to the United States does not realize that he has freedom to practice religion), and educate others that are affecting the client's ability to enjoy the rights and privileges of citizenship (e.g., having a discussion with the activity leader about non-discrimination law).

Common environmental factors affecting a client's ability to enjoy rights, privileges, and freedoms of citizenship include attitudes (e.g., societal attitudes and attitudes of people in authority that make it difficult for a client to access citizenship rights) and the lack of appropriate services, systems, and policies (e.g., absentee ballots requests are not available).

In the ICF, therapists document the level of difficulty that a client has with enjoying his/her political life and citizenship. It is recommended that therapists, along with documenting specific rights that are not available, compare the percent of rights enjoyed to the total that should be available. In discipline-specific documentation, therapists make additional notations about the specific rights of citizenship that are not being enjoyed, barriers that hinder enjoyment, recommendations for change, related skill development, and level of assistance required for enjoying citizenship rights. If a client is being denied his/her basic political or citizenship rights and danger to the client is possible (e.g., client is being harassed because of her religion), it is the responsibility of the therapist to encourage the client to make a police report. If the client refuses, and danger is believed to be imminent, the therapist may need to report it to appropriate authorities (e.g., police, social worker).

d998 Community, Social, and Civic Life, Other Specified

d999 Community, Social, and Civic Life, Unspecified

References

Ashby, F. G., Isen, A.M., & Turken, A. U. (1999). A neuropsychological theory of positive affect and its influence on cognition. *Psychol Rev, 106*(3), 529-550.

Bartlett, S. J., Piedmont, R., Bilderback, A., Matsumoto, A. K., & Bathon, J. M. (2003). Spirituality, well-being and quality of life in people with rheumatoid arthritis. *Arthritis Rheum 49*(6):778-783.

Daaleman, T., Perera, S., & Studenski, S. (2004). Religion, spirituality, and health status in geriatric outpatients. *Annuals of Family Medicine, 2*(1).

Dattilo, J. (1994). *Inclusive leisure services: Responding to the rights of people with disabilities.* State College, PA: Venture Publishing.

Dehn, D. (1995). *Leisure Step Up.* Ravensdale, WA: Idyll Arbor.

Diener, E. (2000). Subjective well-being: The science of happiness and a proposal for a national index. *American Psychology; 55*:34-43.

Elkins, M. & Cavendish, R. (2004). Developing a plan for pediatric spiritual care. *Holistic Nurse Practitioner, 18*(4):179-184.

Ellison, C. & Levin, J. (1998). The religion-health connection: Evidence, theory, and future directions. *Health Education Behavior; 25*:700-20.

Hathaway, W., Scott, S., & Garver, S. (2004). Assessing religious/spiritual functioning: A neglected domain in clinical practice? *Professional Psychology: Research and Practice, 35*(1).

Koenig, H., George, L., & Titus, P. (2004). Religion, spirituality, and health in medically ill hospitalized older patients. *Journal of American Geriatrics Society, 52*(4):554-562.

McGee, M., Nagel, L., Moore, M. (2003). A study of university classroom strategies aimed at increasing spiritual health. *College Student Journal, 37*(4).

McIntosh, D., Silver, R., & Wortman, C. (1993). Religion's role in adjustment to a negative life event: Coping with the loss of a child. *Journal of Personal Social Psychology; 65*:812-21.

Miller, W. R. & Thoresen, C. E. (2003). Spirituality, religion, and health: An emerging research field. *American Psychologist, 58*:24-35.

Myers, D. (2000). The funds, friends, and faith of happy people. *American Psychology; 55*:56-67.

Reed, P. G. (1991). Self-transcendence and mental health in oldest-old adults. *Nursing Research, 40*(1):5-11.

Rowe, M., & Allen, R. (2004). Spirituality as a means of coping with chronic illness. *American Journal of Health Studies, 19*(1).

Seaward, B. (1997). *Stand like mountain, flow like water: Reflections on stress and human spirituality.* Deerfield Beach, FL: Health Communications, Inc.

Turner, L. (2001). Medical facilities as moral worlds. http://mh.bmjjournals.com on 4/26/2004

Environmental Factors

Environmental Factors are things in the environment that facilitate or present barriers for the client.

Scoring

Recreational therapists score environmental factors codes (e-codes) in many practice settings.

Environmental factors make up the physical, social, and attitudinal environment in which people live and conduct their lives.

The ICF lists over 66 environmental factors that have the potential to influence a client's level of impairment and difficulty. They are referred to as e-codes. E-codes are on a positive-negative Likert scale. The therapist can use a negative score (with only the decimal point) to show that an environmental factor is a barrier (e.g., e1650 Financial Assets is a barrier to paying for involvement in d920 Recreation and Leisure) or a positive score to show that an environmental code is a facilitator (e.g., e350 Domesticated Animals is a facilitator to d2401 Handling Stress). The scoring scale for environmental factors is shown in Table 21. The "e___" is the specific environmental code and the number after the decimal point or + sign denotes the extent the code acts as a barrier or facilitator.

To score environmental factors the therapist first identifies the appropriate code to score as described in General Coding Guidelines on the next page. The code is written down in its entirety. This includes the letter and number (all environmental factor codes begin with an "e"). If the environmental factor is a barrier, a decimal point is placed after the code. After the decimal point the extent of the barrier is recorded. If the environmental code is a facilitator, a + sign is placed after the code. After the + sign the extent of the facilitator is recorded.

There are a variety of options to document e-codes. E-codes can be written:

- *After each ICF component*: Therapists can make a list of e-codes that affect one ICF component. For example, the therapist may identify six e-codes as barriers and four e-codes as facilitators for Body Functions as a whole.
- *After each code*: Therapists can attach e-codes after each code for which a barrier or facilitator is identified (e.g., a client's pet dog is a moderate facilitator for handling stress: d2401 Handling Stress, E-code: e350+2)
- *As a separate entry*: Therapists can list e-codes as a separate group unrelated to a specific ICF component or specific ICF code (e.g., E-codes: e350+2, e1650.3).

The recreational therapist will most likely find it helpful to note e-codes after each specific ICF code. This reflects the recreational therapy clinical process and provides the reader with a better understanding of the barriers and facilitators as they relate to a specific impairment or difficulty.

Table 21: Scoring for Environmental Factors

Scoring for Each Qualifier		
e____ .0 NO barrier	(none, absent, negligible…)	0-4%
e____ .1 MILD barrier	(slight, low…)	5-24%
e____ .2 MODERATE barrier	(medium, fair…)	25-49%
e____ .3 SEVERE barrier	(high, extreme…)	50-95%
e____ .4 COMPLETE barrier	(total…)	96-100%
e____ +0 NO facilitator	(none, absent, negligible…)	0-4%
e____ +1 MILD facilitator	(slight, low…)	5-24%
e____ +2 MODERATE facilitator	(medium, fair…)	25-49%
e____ +3 SEVERE facilitator	(high, extreme…)	50-95%
e____ +4 COMPLETE facilitator	(total…)	96-100%
e____ .8 barrier, not specified		
e____ +8 facilitator, not specified		
e____ .9 not applicable		

How to determine extent of barrier/facilitator

A major question in using e-codes is how to decide if an environmental factor is mild, moderate, severe, or complete? The ICF does not tell us clearly how to delineate among the levels, so it appears that it is left to the judgment of the clinician to determine the level of barrier or facilitator. To reduce the subjectivity of the scores, we propose that recreational therapists use the following formula.

E-codes as facilitators: If the environmental factor is taken away, how many levels of impairment or difficulty does the client drop down? If the client's level of impairment or difficulty does not change when the facilitator is removed, then it is a +0 (no facilitator). If the client's level of impairment or difficulty drops by one level when the facilitator is removed (e.g., mild difficulty to moderate difficulty), then it is a +1 (mild facilitator). If the client's level of impairment or difficulty drops by two levels when the facilitator is removed, then it is a +2 (moderate facilitator). If the client's level of impairment or difficulty drops by three levels when the facilitator is removed, then it is a +3 (substantial facilitator). If the client's level of impairment or difficulty drops by four levels, then it is a +4 (complete facilitator).

E-codes as barriers: If the environmental factor is taken away (the barrier is removed), how many levels of impairment or difficulty does the client improve? If the client's level of impairment or difficulty does not change when the barrier is removed, then it is a .0 (no barrier). If the client's performance improves by one level when the barrier is removed (e.g., complete difficulty to severe difficulty), then it is a .1 (mild barrier). If the client's performance improves by two levels when the barrier is removed, then it is a .2 (moderate barrier). If the client's performance improves by three levels when the barrier is removed, then it is a .3 (severe barrier). If the client's performance improves by four levels (complete difficulty to no difficulty), then it is a .4 (complete barrier).

Of course there will be times when using the formula will be difficult, especially when the e-code is just one of several environmental variables. If this is the case, best clinical judgment will need to be used.

Issues with e-codes

E-code as Barrier and Facilitator

In some situations, an e-code can be scored as both a facilitator and a barrier. *Example from EF 1 Products and Technology:* A client who lives in a long-term care facility only attends entertainment

---

General Coding Guidelines

1. Choose the appropriate codes that best reflect the client's functioning as it relates to the purpose of the encounter.

2. Only choose codes that are relevant to the context of the health condition. It is unrealistic to think that a health professional has the time to assess the extent that each environmental factor is a barrier or facilitator for every client. Health professionals should evaluate and assess environmental factors as barriers or facilitators for the specific impairment, activity, or life situation that is being addressed in the encounter.

3. Do not make inferences about other environmental factors based on ones that have already been identified. Meaning, 1. just because an e-code is a barrier or facilitator for one activity does not mean that it is a barrier for other activities and 2. just because an e-code has been identified as a barrier or facilitator does not mean that environmental codes that are typically related are barriers or facilitators as well (e.g., although e1650 Financial Assets may be a barrier for participation in an activity, it cannot be assumed that lack of money results in lack of needed assistive devices).

4. Only choose codes that reflect the specific predefined timeframe. Environmental factors that relate to a timeframe outside of the predefined timeframe should not be coded.

5. Use the most specific code whenever possible. For example, if light intensity is identified as a facilitator for d9203 Crafts, score the specific code of e2400 Light Intensity rather than the broader code of e240 Light.

---

events when food is provided. When food is not provided, the client does not attend. This is an example of how e1100 Food can be a facilitator to d9202 Arts and Culture. The scoring of d9202 Arts and Culture that reflects the impact of e1100 Food could look like this: d9202.0 _ _ 4, E-code: e1100+4 OR like this d9202.0 _ _ 4, E-code: e1100.4. The first d-code qualifier reflects the level of difficulty that the client has in a real-life setting with assistance (performance) and the fourth qualifier reflects his level of difficulty in a real-life setting when assistance is not provided (performance without assistance). The e-code could be rated a +4 or a .4 because when food is provided the client's level of difficulty reduces (engaging in Arts and Culture) by four levels, but in the same sense when food is not provided the client's level of difficulty increases by four levels. The ICF does not provide the therapist with direction on how to resolve this problem. The authors recommend that therapists score the e-code as a facilitator rather than a barrier in this type of situation. Barriers are often thought of as being constant (always or most always present) and facilitators are often thought of as something that can be introduced to increase or improve action or task performance. This helps the therapist in teaching others (e.g., activity director, family) about the use of facilitators to decrease the level of difficulty a client has with a specific action, task, or activity. The identified facilitator is also already in the client's environment. It is usually easier to keep something in an environment that is already present than to try to remove something or add something.

E-code is Qualifier Specific

In some situations, the e-code is qualifier specific. *Example taken from EF 4 Attitudes*: A 23-year-old client with tetraplegia attends college (lives off campus). He has a personal care attendant with him at all times to assist with overcoming barriers (e.g., pushing elevator buttons), self-care (e.g., catheterizing), and schoolwork (e.g., note taking). When the client tries to strike up a conversation with other students outside of class, the attendant rushes him along and says, "We don't have time for this." When the attendant is not present (e.g., takes a break to use the bathroom), the client has no difficulty with d9205 Socializing. When the attendant is present, the client has total difficulty socializing. The scoring of d9205 Socializing that reflects the impact of e440 Individual Attitudes of Personal Care Providers and Personal Assistants would look like this: d9205.4 _ _ 0, E-code: e440.4. The first qualifier reflects the level of difficulty that the client has in a real-life setting with assistance (performance) and the fourth qualifier reflects his level of difficulty in a real-life setting when assistance is not provided (performance without assistance). The e-code was rated a .4 because it increased his level of difficulty with the task by four levels. The same attendant, however, facilitates the client's socialization in therapy sessions (cues the client to strike up conversations). The dilemma for the therapist attempting to score the level of barrier or facilitator of the attendant for socialization is now difficult. The therapist has two choices for scoring. First, the therapist can score the average. Is the attendant, on average, more of a facilitator or barrier to socialization for the client? If the attendant is more of a barrier than a facilitator, the therapist would score the average negative impact that s/he has on the client's engagement in socialization (vice versa if the attendant is more of a facilitator). Second, if there is no average (the attendant just has different attitudes that are reflected differently in capacity versus performance environments), then the therapist should designate this after the e-code. For example, d9205.4040, E-code: e440.4 (performance), e440+4 (capacity).

The Use of .0 and +0

In some situations, the .0 or +0 should be used. The therapist may identify a specific barrier or facilitator to engagement in an activity or life situation with a very small overall impact. In this situation, the therapist should still score the e-code rather than delete it because it puts the e-code on the "radar screen" of the people who will be evaluating the data. If barriers (even if they are slight) do not gain attention, they can easily become larger, making them more difficult to eliminate or reduce. Likewise, if facilitators (even if they are slight) are brought to the attention of data reviewers, they may be able to be encouraged within our society. *Example from EF 1 Products and Technology*: A client has moderate difficulty walking on uneven surfaces. He would like to go for walks at the local park but the paths are unpaved, hilly, and full of tree roots making it dangerous and unrealistic. This is an example of how e1603 Products and Technology of Parks, Conservation, and Wildlife Areas can be a barrier to d4602 Moving Around Outside the Home and Other Buildings. The scoring of d4602 that reflects the impact of e1603 as a barrier would look like this: d4602.2 _ _ 2, E-code: e1603.0. The fourth qualifier reflects the client's average level of difficulty moving around outside the home in his current life situation given supports and constraints as a whole (not just in the park). The e-code is rated a .0 because it was determined by the therapist that the park trails (if paved) would not change (or negligibly change) the overall level of difficulty that the client has with all of the aspects of Moving Around Outside the Home and Other Buildings.

Chapter 1 Products and Technology

This chapter is about the natural or human-made products or systems of products, equipment, and technology in an individual's immediate environment that are gathered, created, produced, or manufactured. The ISO 9999 classification of technical aids defines these as "any product, instrument, equipment, or technical system used by a disabled person, especially produced or generally available, preventing, compensating, monitoring, relieving, or neutralizing" disability. It is recognized that any product or technology can be assistive. (See ISO 9999: Technical aids for disabled persons — Classification (second version); ISO/TC 173/SC 2, ISO/IDS 9999 (rev.)) For the purposes of this classification of environmental factors, however, assistive products and technology are defined more narrowly as any product, instrument, equipment, or technology adapted or specially designed for improving functioning of a disabled person.

e110 Products or Substances for Personal Consumption
Any natural or human-made object or substance gathered, processed, or manufactured for ingestion.
Inclusions: food, drink, and drugs
- *e1100 Food*
  Any natural or human-made object or substance gathered, processed, or manufactured to be eaten, such as raw, processed, and prepared food and liquids of different consistencies, herbs, and minerals (vitamin and other supplements).
- *e1101 Drugs*
  Any natural or human-made object or substance gathered, processed, or manufactured for medicinal purposes, such as allopathic and naturopathic medication.
- *e1108 Products or Substances for Personal Consumption, Other Specified*
- *e1109 Products or Substances for Personal Consumption, Unspecified*

Considerations for Products or Substances for Personal Consumption

Food

Food is a basic human need. Without a healthy, balanced diet of enough food and proper kinds of food, body structures and functions are harmed, ultimately affecting life activities. Severe nutritional deficiencies, whether caused by the environment (e.g., famine) or from personal choice (e.g., anorexia), can also result in death. Lack of proper nutrition can be caused by lack of food availability, impaired access to healthy foods, behavioral issues (e.g., child refusing to eat certain foods), or from a mental illness. Consequently, food can be a barrier to the health of a specific body structure or function, as well as a barrier to life activities (e.g., d5701 Managing Diet and Fitness, d630 Preparing Meals). Lack of food, caused by any means, may also affect other life activities, specifically activities that are closely tied to food. Within the Western culture, food has become more than just a basic human need. It has

also become closely linked with social activities, thus making food (in some situations) a barrier or facilitator of social and recreational activities (e.g., lack of food in the home may be a barrier for a client to invite someone over to his home to visit thus impacting d7200 Forming Relationships; the need to have pureed food at a restaurant is embarrassing for a client, who then chooses to limit her engagement in d9100 Informal Associations; the lack of availability of healthy food options at school is hindering a child with diabetes from maintaining proper glucose levels). Food as a facilitator can be described in much the same way. For example, food can contribute to the health of a specific body structure or function, as well as facilitate involvement in social, community, and recreational activities. Interestingly, the pairing of food with recreational activities often yields higher attendance rates in residential facilities (e.g., the availability of free food on a college campus increases a client's participation in d9205 Socializing; the offering of healthy snacks at an exercise class in a long-term care setting increases a client's participation in exercise — d5701 Managing Diet and Fitness).

Recreational therapists consider the role of food in hindering or facilitating engagement in life activities and design appropriate interventions to either:
1. Reduce or eliminate the negative effect of food on a particular life activity (e.g., problem solving for d6201 Gathering Daily Necessities because it is a barrier for the client to inviting people over to socialize, identifying pureed foods offered by the restaurant that will not draw attention to the client so that she continues to engage in dining out with friends for maintaining relationships — d7200 Forming Relationships).
2. Maintain or further facilitate the positive impact of food on life activities (e.g., ensure that healthy snacks continue to be offered at exercise class to increase engagement in d5701 Managing Diet and Fitness; talk with the client's social worker to make sure that the client is still eligible for food stamps so that he feels comfortable in his

availability of food to invite others over for d9205 Socializing).

Example (Food as a Facilitator and Barrier)

A client who lives in a long-term care facility only attends art and culture events when food is provided (in this example, food is an expected part of entertainment activities). When food is not provided, the client does not attend. This is an example of how e1100 Food can be a facilitator to d9202 Arts and Culture. The scoring of d9202 Arts and Culture that reflects the impact of e1100 Food would look like this "d9202.0 _ _ 4, E-code: e1100+4" or like this "d9202.0 _ _ 4, E-code: e1100.4." The first qualifier reflects no difficulty in his current life situation with arts and culture with all available supports and constraints (performance). The fourth qualifier reflects complete difficulty in his current life situation when assistance is not provided (performance without assistance). The e-code could be rated a +4 or a .4 because when food is provided the client's level of difficulty with engaging in Arts and Culture reduces by four levels, but in the same sense when food is not provided it increases the client's level of difficulty by four levels. In this situation, the therapist yields to the positive and scores food as a facilitator (see Issues with E-Codes in Scoring the ICF for reasoning).

Drugs

The use of prescription and non-prescription drugs in Western culture is quite common and often relied on as a primary means of treating illness or disease. Medication, therefore, can be a major facilitator in the health of a body structure or function, supporting greater performance in life activities. However, side effects of medications can have devastating effects on life activities as well (e.g., medication that causes severe drowsiness impacting the ability to engage in d910 Community Life). There are also drugs that are manufactured and sold illegally. Use of illegal substances can lead to substance dependence, impacting not only specific body structures and functions, but significantly impairing life activities (e.g., d845 Acquiring, Keeping, and Terminating a Job; d760 Family Relationships). Outside of ingesting drugs, whether legal or illegal, the presence of drugs in a neighborhood can also impact activity levels (e.g., a child not being allowed outside to play due to fear of drug peddlers impacting d9200 Play; a client refusing to walk to the local store due to fear of drug peddlers impacting d5701 Managing Diet and Fitness).

Recreational therapists consider the role of drugs in hindering or facilitating engagement in life activities and design appropriate interventions to either:
1. Reduce or eliminate the negative effect of drugs on a particular life activity (e.g., identify safe places to exercise where the client does not feel threatened by neighborhood drugs; discuss with the client's physician the negative effect that a drug is having on a client's participation in community activities to problem solve for other approaches/medications).
2. Maintain or further facilitate the positive impact of drugs on life activities (e.g., the recreational therapist, as a clinical team member, reinforces the importance of taking needed medication that positively effects engagement in healthy life activities).

Example (Drugs as a Barrier)

A client is addicted to cocaine. In the treatment facility, he exhibits severe difficulty maintaining relationships with family members when they come to visit. The family reports that he had no problem with this skill before he started using drugs. This is an example of how e1101 Drugs can be a barrier to d7503 Informal Relationships with Co-Inhabitants. The scoring of d7503 that reflects the impact of e1101 as a barrier would look like this: "d7503._ 4 _ _, E-code: e1101.4." The second qualifier (capacity without assistance) reflects complete difficulty with creating and maintaining relationships with people who live in the home while in the standardized environment of a treatment facility. The e-code is rated a .4 because drugs increase the client's level of difficulty with maintaining relationships by four levels (no difficulty to complete difficulty).

Example (Drugs as a Facilitator)

A client has a mood disorder that causes a moderate impairment in emotional regulation. A prescription medication helps her to regulate her emotions but she still has a residual, mild impairment. This is an example of how e1101 Drugs can be a facilitator for b1521 Regulation of Emotion. The scoring of b1521 that reflects the impact of e1101 as a facilitator would look like this: "b1521.1, E-code: e1101+1." The qualifier reflects the client's current level of impairment (mild impairment) with regulation of emotion. The e-code is rated a +1 because the prescription medication improves her level of impairment by one level (moderate impairment to mild impairment).

e115 Products and Technology for Personal Use in Daily Living

Equipment, products, and technologies used by people in daily activities, including those adapted or specially designed, located in, on, or near the person using them.

- *e1150 General Products and Technology for Personal Use in Daily Living*
  Equipment, products, and technologies used by people in daily activities, such as clothes, textiles, furniture, appliances, cleaning products, and tools, not adapted or specially designed.
- *e1151 Assistive Products and Technology for Personal Use in Daily Living*
  Adapted or specially designed equipment, products, and technologies that assist people in daily living, such as prosthetic and orthotic devices, neural prostheses (e.g., functional stimulation devices that control bowels, bladder, breathing, and heart rate), and environmental control units aimed at facilitating individuals' control over their indoor setting (scanners, remote control systems, voice-controlled systems, timer switches).
- *e1158 Products and Technology for Personal Use in Daily Living, Other Specified*
- *e1159 Products and Technology for Personal Use in Daily Living, Unspecified*

Considerations for Products and Technology for Personal Use in Daily Living

Products and technology for daily activities whether general or adapted can a barrier or a facilitator to body structures, body functions, and life activities. It is quite easy for therapists to understand how products and technology can be a facilitator (e.g., ventilator as a facilitator for b440 Respiration Functions; adaptive gardening tools as a facilitator for d6505 Taking Care of Plants, Indoors and Outdoors). It is through continued exploration of products and technology by reading catalogs, researching on the internet, talking with other professionals, designing and trying out devices, and attending professional conferences and workshops that the therapist's awareness (and skills related to making devices) grows and flourishes.

Technology however, is not always a good thing. In some situations, extensive adaptations may inhibit health maintenance or promotion (e.g., a client using extensive switches and timers to perform tasks that he could perform otherwise). Also, common everyday items, such as the clothes we wear and the furniture in our homes can pose a barrier, especially if it impedes our abilities (e.g., clothes with small buttons can be a barrier to d540 Dressing for a client who has use of only one hand; furniture that is too low can be a barrier to 4103 Sitting for a client that

does not have the strength to push up into a standing position from a low surface).

Recreational therapists consider the role products and technology for personal use in daily living play in hindering or facilitating engagement in life activities and design appropriate interventions to either:

1. Reduce or eliminate the negative effect of technology for daily living on a particular life activity (e.g., identify bathing suit style options that are easier to put on and take off to increase engagement in a water exercise class; identify an environmental control that opens the door to the craft room).
2. Maintain or further facilitate the positive impact of technology for daily living on life activities (e.g., assess current technology to determine if newer technology would even further benefit the client; encourage continued use of technology for daily living).

Example (Products and Technology for Personal Use in Daily Living as a Barrier)

At home, a client has complete difficulty putting on clothes due to poor hand and arm function. This is an example of how e1150 General Products and Technology for Personal Use in Daily Living (clothing) can be a barrier for d5400 Putting On Clothes. The scoring for d5400 that reflects the impact of e1150 as a barrier would look like this: "d5400._ _ _ 4, E-code: e1150.4." The fourth qualifier reflects complete difficulty in his current life situation with putting on clothing without assistance (performance without assistance). In the therapist's clinical judgment, the client would have no difficulty putting on clothes if adaptive clothing were provided, thus the Products and Technology for Personal Use in Daily Living (specifically clothing) is believed to be increasing his level of difficulty by four levels (no difficulty to complete difficulty). Thus, the e-code is rated a .4.

Example (Products and Technology for Personal Use in Daily Living as a Facilitator)

In a clinic setting, a client with multiple sclerosis has severe difficulty holding a hairbrush. However, when using a cuff to hold the brush, she has no difficulty brushing her hair. This is an example of how e1151 Assistive Products and Technology for Personal Use in Daily Living can be a facilitator for d5202 Caring for Hair. The scoring for d5202 that reflects the impact of e1151 as a facilitator would look like this: "d5202._ 3 0 _, E-code: e1151+3." The second qualifier reflects severe difficulty caring for hair in a clinic setting without assistance of the cuff (capacity without assistance). The third qualifier reflects her ability to brush her hair in a clinic setting with assistance of the cuff (capacity with assistance). The e-code was rated a +3 because it improved her level of difficulty by three levels (severe difficulty to no difficulty).

e120 Products and Technology for Personal Indoor and Outdoor Mobility and Transportation
Equipment, products, and technologies used by people in activities of moving inside and outside buildings, including those adapted or specially designed, located in, on, or near the person using them.

- *e1200 General Products and Technologies for Personal Indoor and Outdoor Mobility and Transportation*
Equipment, products, and technologies used by people in activities of moving inside and outside buildings, such as motorized and non-motorized vehicles used for the transportation of people over ground, water, and air (e.g., buses, cars, vans, other motor-powered vehicles and animal-powered transporters), not adapted or specially designed.

- *e1201 Assistive Products and Technology for Personal Indoor and Outdoor Mobility and Transportation*
Adapted or specially designed equipment, products, and technologies that assist people to move inside and outside buildings, such as walking devices, special cars and vans, adaptations to vehicles, wheelchairs, scooters, and transfer devices.

- *e1208 Products and Technology for Personal Indoor and Outdoor Mobility and Transportation, Other Specified*

- *e1209 Products and Technology for Personal Indoor and Outdoor Mobility and Transportation, Unspecified*

Considerations for Products and Technology for Personal Mobility and Transportation

Products and technology, whether general or assistive, for personal indoor and outdoor mobility and transportation can be barriers or facilitators to body structures, body functions, and life activities. To determine if it is a barrier or a facilitator, the therapist must first identify the products and technology for mobility and transportation that are pertinent to the client (e.g., what is currently being used, what is desired, what problems are identified, what is needed). Although products for personal indoor and outdoor mobility and transportation can be numerous (e.g., plane, train, wheelchair, cane), therapists must also be aware of non-traditional forms of mobility and transportation used by a client (e.g.,

roller skates, bicycles, skateboards). See e140 Products and Technology for Culture, Recreation, and Sport if mobility devices are used for recreation or sport.

Products and technology for mobility and transportation can be facilitators or barriers to engagement in life activities such as d6200 Shopping, d9202 Arts and Culture, d450 Walking (e.g., client needs a rolling walker for outdoor mobility but her insurance does not cover the full cost of the walker so she does not have one — not having a walker is a barrier under e1201 Assistive Products and Technology for Personal Indoor and Outdoor Mobility and Transportation, and lacking proper equipment coverage identifies e5802 Health Policies as an additional barrier). Impaired engagement or lack of engagement in life activities as a result of a barrier to Personal Indoor and Outdoor Mobility and Transportation can directly or indirectly affect body functions, body structures, and life activities (e.g., lack of transportation requires the client to walk to the store, facilitating b455 Exercise Tolerance Functions and b730 Muscle Power Functions; lack of transportation in a rural environment limits the client's d9205 Socializing that negatively impacts d2401 Handing Stress and b1265 Optimism). Improperly prescribed or unprescribed use of adaptive mobility or transportation equipment can hinder health maintenance and promotion (e.g., a client is using an electric scooter for community activities when she could walk without injury or harm). The currently used form of general or assistive transportation may not meet the needs of the client (e.g., a client has been using a public bus for transportation, even though the first step into the bus is rather high. Several times the client has lost her balance and a stranger has kept her from falling).

Recreational therapists consider the role of products and technology for outdoor mobility and transportation in hindering or facilitating engagement in life activities and design appropriate interventions to either:
1. Reduce or eliminate the negative effect of outdoor mobility and transportation on a particular life activity (e.g., A client with a lower extremity prosthetic is having difficulty riding a bicycle for transportation because the prosthetic foot keeps sliding off the pedal. The recreational therapist prescribes a toe clip to hold the prosthetic foot on the pedal.).
2. Maintain or further facilitate the positive impact of outdoor mobility and transportation on life activities (e.g., assess current mobility and transportation to determine if newer products or technology would even further benefit the client;

encourage continued use of products and technology for mobility and transportation).

Example (Products and Technology for Personal Mobility and Transportation as a Barrier)

A client uses the public bus system for transportation. She has advanced rheumatoid arthritis that causes her to have severe difficulty lifting her foot onto the first step of the bus (it is about an 18-inch high step). The client is able to step up and down an eight-inch step with a rail with no difficulty. This is an example of how e1200 General Products and Technology for Personal Indoor and Outdoor Mobility and Transportation can be a barrier for d4702 Using Public Motorized Transportation. The scoring of d4702 that reflects the impact of e1200 as a barrier would look like this: "d4702._ _ _ 3, E-code: e1200.3." The fourth qualifier reflects severe difficulty with using public motorized transportation in a life situation without assistance (performance without assistance). This score was determined by identifying the average level of difficulty the client had with the whole task, not just her ability to step up the bus step. (The information to arrive at this level is not shown in this example.) The e-code was rated a .3 because the height of the bus step increases the client's level of difficulty to board the bus by three levels (no difficulty stepping up an eight-inch step with a rail to severe difficulty stepping up an 18" bus step).

Example (Products and Technology for Personal Mobility and Transportation as a Facilitator)

The same client in the previous example finds out that there are "kneeling buses" available along the local bus routes. The kneeling bus is able to lower the first bus step to 10". The client has mild difficulty stepping up and down the 10-inch bus step but a stranger is usually kind enough to provide her with assistance. This is an example of how e1201 Assistive Products and Technologies for Personal Indoor and Outdoor Mobility and Transportation can be a facilitator for d4702 Using Public Motorized Transportation. The scoring of d4702 that reflects the impact of e1201 as a facilitator would look like this: "d4702. 0 _ _ 3, E-code: e1201+2." The first qualifier reflects no difficulty in her ability to board the bus in her current life situation with all available supports and constraints, including the kneeling bus and the assistance of a stranger (performance). The fourth qualifier reflects a severe difficulty in her ability to board the bus in her current life situation without assistance of the kneeling bus or a stranger

(performance without assistance). The e-code was rated a +2 because the kneeling bus improved her level of difficulty from severe difficulty (the level of difficulty to step up and down a standard bus step as reviewed in the first example) to mild difficulty due to the assistance of a kneeling bus. The assistance of a stranger further improves her level of difficulty with boarding the bus by one level from mild difficulty to no difficulty. The new scoring string incorporating e345 Strangers would look like this: "d4702. 0 _ _ 3, E-codes: e1201+2, e345+1."

e125   Products   and   Technology   for Communication
Equipment, products, and technologies used by people in activities of sending and receiving information, including those adapted or specially designed, located in, on, or near the person using them.
- *e1250 General Products and Technology for Communication*
  Equipment products and technology used by people in activities of sending and receiving information, such as optical and auditory devices, audio recorders and receivers, television and video equipment, telephone devices, sound transmission systems, and face-to-face communication devices, not adapted or specially designed.
- *e1251 Assistive Products and Technology for Communication*
  Adapted or specially designed equipment, products, and technologies that assist people to send and receive information, such as specialized vision devices, electro-optical devices, specialized writing devices, drawing or hand writing devices, signaling systems and special computer software and hardware, cochlear implants, hearing aids, FM auditory trainers, voice prostheses, communication boards, glasses, and contact lenses.
- *e1258 Products and Technology for Communication, Other Specified*
- *e1259 Products and Technology for Communication, Unspecified*

Considerations for Products and Technology for Communication

Products and technology for communication can be a barrier or facilitator. For example, a television, radio, instant messaging on the computer, and video conference calls can be a facilitator for many life activities (e.g., d6200 Shopping, d7200 Forming Relationships, d8451 Maintaining a Job). The same technology can also be a barrier when the client uses it in an addictive or escapist way by watching too much television, playing too many computer games, or becoming addicted to gambling or pornography on the Internet. Products and technology for communication can also be a barrier when they hinder participation in life activities (e.g., client is unable to operate a computer, telephone, fax machine).

Adaptive communication products and technology are usually facilitators when general products and technology are not sufficient (e.g., a telephone that has a flashing light when it rings as a facilitator for d3600 Using Telecommunication Devices). Assistive products and technology that are misprescribed or unprescribed (client uses a piece of adaptive equipment that is not prescribed by a qualified professional) can prove to be a barrier in situations where the piece of equipment does not perform in the manner expected or desired (e.g., a mouthstick a client ordered through a catalog does not have the correct bend on it to easily access computer keyboard keys resulting in neck pain and ineffective communication).

Recreational therapists consider the role of products and technology for communication in hindering or facilitating engagement in life activities and design appropriate interventions to either:
1. Reduce or eliminate the negative effect of products and technology for communication on a particular life activity (e.g., A client with a hearing impairment does not hear the high pitch of a telephone ring. The therapist prescribes a special light for the telephone that flashes when it rings.).
2. Maintain or further facilitate the positive impact of products and technology for communication on life activities (e.g., assess current products and technology for communication to determine if newer products or technology would further benefit the client; encourage continued use of products and technology for communication).

Example (Products and Technology for Communication as a Barrier)

A client who is deaf has complete difficulty using a standard telephone in the clinic. This is an example of how e1250 General Products and Technology for Communication can be a barrier to d3600 Using Telecommunication Devices. The scoring of d3600 that reflects the impact of e1250 as a barrier would look like this: "d3600._ 4 _ _, E-code: e1250.4." The second qualifier reflects complete difficulty in ability to use a standard telephone in a clinic setting without assistance (capacity without assistance). It is the clinical judgment of the therapist that the use of an adaptive telephone (TTY) would result in the client having no difficulty in using the telephone. The e-code is rated

a .4 because the standard telephone (when compared to a TTY) increases the client's level of difficulty by four levels (no difficulty to complete difficulty).

Example (Products and Technology for Communication as a Facilitator)

The same client in the previous example is given and shown how to use an adaptive telephone (TTY). She has mild difficulty using the TTY, but with assistance from the therapist, there is no residual difficulty. This is an example of how e1251 Assistive Products and Technology for Communication can be a facilitator for d3600 Using Telecommunication Devices. The scoring of d3600 that reflects the impact of e1251 as a facilitator would look like this: "d3600. _ 4 0 _, E-code: e1251+4." The second qualifier reflects complete difficulty using a standard telephone without assistance in the clinic (capacity without assistance). The third qualifier reflects no difficulty using a TTY with assistance of the therapist in the clinic (capacity with assistance). The e-code was rated a +4 because the communication product/technology improved her level of difficulty by four levels (complete difficulty to no difficulty).

e130 Products and Technology for Education
Equipment, products, processes, methods, and technology used for acquisition of knowledge, expertise, or skill, including those adapted or specially designed.
- *e1300 General Products and Technology for Education*
  Equipment, products, processes, methods, and technology used for acquisition of knowledge, expertise, or skill at any level, such as books, manuals, educational toys, computer hardware or software, not adapted or specially designed.
- *e1301 Assistive Products and Technology for Education*
  Adapted and specially designed equipment, products, processes, methods, and technology used for acquisition of knowledge, expertise, or skill, such as specialized computer technology.
- *e1308 Products and Technology for Education, Other Specified*
- *e1309 Products and Technology for Education, Unspecified*

Considerations for Products and Technology for Education

Products and technology for education can be a barrier or facilitator. General products such as books, educational toys, and computer programs can assist with learning (a facilitator). Likewise, adaptive products and technology such as adaptive learning toys, Braille books, or voice activated computer programs also can facilitate education. Products and technology, whether general or adapted, can be a barrier for education when it is not affordable, accessible, acceptable, and appropriate to promote the acquisition of knowledge, expertise, or skill. This may include products and technology that are inappropriate for the specific age, learning style, educational level, or knowledge/skill desired.

Recreational therapists consider the role of products and technology for education in hindering or facilitating engagement in life activities and design appropriate interventions to either:

1. Reduce or eliminate the negative effect of products and technology for education on a particular life activity (e.g., A client with low vision is unable to see textbook materials. Therapist prescribes a specialized magnification device to allow the client to see textbook print.).

2. Maintain or further facilitate the positive impact of products and technology for education on life activities (e.g., assess current products and technology for education to determine if newer products or technology would further benefit the client; encourage continued use of products and technology for education).

Example (Products and Technology for Education as a Barrier)

A 4-year-old girl with mild mental retardation attends a mainstream pre-school. The school does not have adaptive learning toys (e.g., switch toys) and the teaching methods are not geared for children who have disabilities. The parents and teacher agree that the child is not progressing in this type of environment and is only engaging in about 40% of the learning activities. This is an example of how e1300 General Products and Technology for Education can be a barrier to d815 Preschool Education. The scoring of d815 that reflects the impact of e1300 as a barrier would look like this: "d815.3 _ _ _, E-code: e1300.3." The first qualifier reflects severe difficulty with engaging in preschool learning activities in the client's current life situation. This is calculated by the level of difficulty determined through amount of non-engagement in learning activities even with the assistance of the teachers and current devices (performance). The therapist anticipates that the child would have no difficulty engaging in learning activities if placed in a pre-school program specially designed for children with mild retardation. Consequently, the e-code is rated a .3 because the current teaching toys and methods are believed to be increasing her level of difficulty with engagement in learning activities by three levels (no difficulty to severe difficulty).

Example (Products and Technology for Education as a Facilitator)

The same child in the previous example now attends a pre-school program that is specially designed for children who have mild retardation. She exhibits no difficulty in engaging in learning activities. This is an example of how e1301 Assistive Products and Technology for Education can be a facilitator for d815 Preschool Education. The scoring of d815 that reflects the impact of e1301 as a facilitator would look like this: "d815.0 _ _ 3, E-code: e1301+3." The first qualifier reflects no difficulty with preschool in her current life situation with all available supports and constraints, which includes the assistive products and technology available in her new classroom (performance). The fourth qualifier reflects severe difficulty with preschool if assistance is removed as shown in the previous example (performance without assistance). The e-code is rated a +3 because the assistive products and technology for education improve her level of difficulty by three levels (severe difficulty to no difficulty).

e135 Products and Technology for Employment
Equipment, products, and technology used for employment to facilitate work activities.

- *e1350 General Products and Technology for Employment*
  Equipment, products, and technology used for employment to facilitate work activities, such as tools, machines, and office equipment, not adapted or specially designed.

- *e1351 Assistive Products and Technology for Employment*
  Adapted or specially designed equipment, products, and technology used for employment to facilitate work activities, such as adjustable tables, desks, and filing cabinets; remote control entry and exit of office doors; computer hardware, software, accessories, and environmental control units aimed at facilitating an individual's conduct of work-related tasks and aimed at control of the work environment (e.g., scanners, remote control systems, voice-controlled systems, and timer switches).

- *e1358 Products and Technology for Employment, Other Specified*

- *e1359 Products and Technology for Employment, Unspecified*

Considerations for Products and Technology for Employment

Products and technology, whether general or assistive, for employment can be a barrier or a facilitator to body structures, body functions, and activities and participation. For example, if a client operates a computer at work and has carpal tunnel syndrome, lack of an ergonomically correct computer station could be a barrier for pain management in the hands (e.g., b28016 Pain in Joints) as well as impair specific body structures of the hand muscles. Consequently, the lack of a proper computer system could impact her ability to maintain her job (d8451 Maintaining a Job) and also affect her financial security (e.g., d870 Economic Self-Sufficiency). On the other hand, if an ergonomic computer station was provided for this person, it could act as a facilitator for b28016 Pain in Joints, d8451 Maintaining a Job, and d870 Economic Self-Sufficiency.

Products and technology for employment may also be a barrier if they are improperly prescribed, resulting in dysfunction, or if they do not meet the needs of the client (e.g., client provided with a screwdriver when he really needs a cordless drill). Any product or technology must also be available, affordable, acceptable, and accessible in order to be a facilitator. In some instances, this is not the case and further environmental factors may need to be identified as the underlying causes of difficulty (e.g., e430 Individual Attitudes of People in Positions of Authority, e590 Labor and Employment Services, Systems, and Policies).

Recreational therapists consider the role of products and technology for employment in hindering or facilitating engagement in life activities and design appropriate interventions to either:

1. Reduce or eliminate the negative effect of products and technology for employment on a particular life activity (e.g., A client works part time at the local hardware store. He has multiple herniated discs and needs to change his body position often throughout the day to alleviate sensations of pain. The therapist prescribes a stool for periodic sitting and floor blocks to periodically place one foot to shift body weight.).

2. Maintain or further facilitate the positive impact of products and technology for employment on life activities (e.g., assess current products and technology for employment to determine if newer products or technology would even further benefit the client; encourage continued use of products and technology for employment).

Example (Products and Technology for Employment as a Barrier)

A client has carpal tunnel syndrome in both hands. She is a typist. Using a standard keyboard she is able to perform only 55% of her typing responsibilities due to wrist pain. Her boss told her that if she does not increase her productivity to at least 80% she will be terminated. This is an example of how e1350 General Products and Technology for Employment can be a barrier for d8451 Maintaining a Job. The scoring of d8451 that reflects the impact of e1350 as a barrier would look like this: "d8451.2 _ _ _ , E-code: e1350.2." The first qualifier reflects moderate difficulty in her current real-life work situation with maintaining a job given all available supports and constraints (performance). This score was determined by figuring out the percent of her job that she is not currently performing (45% equals moderate difficulty). The client has no other difficulties at work affecting her ability to maintain her job. In the clinical judgment of the therapist, the client would have no difficulty with maintaining her job if adaptive computer equipment was provided and utilized. The e-code is rated a .2 because her current computer equipment is believed to be increasing her level of difficulty in maintaining her job by two levels (no difficulty with assistive equipment to moderate difficulty without equipment).

Example (Products and Technology for Employment as a Facilitator)

The client in the previous example is prescribed mobile wrist supports and an ergonomic keyboard. The use of the adaptive devices raises her productivity to 80% (20% difficulty remaining) and she is able to keep her job. This is an example of how e1351 Assistive Products and Technology for Employment can be a facilitator for d8451 Maintaining a Job. The scoring of d8451 that reflects the impact of e1351 as a facilitator would look like this: "d8451.0 _ _ 2, E-code: e1351+2." The first qualifier reflects no difficulty maintaining her job in her current life situation with all available supports and constraints that now includes adaptive computer equipment (performance). The score of no difficulty was chosen because her boss asked her to reach a level of 80% to keep her job. The fourth qualifier reflects moderate difficulty with maintaining her job without the use of the adaptive equipment as explained in the previous example (performance without assistance). The e-code is rated a +2 because the adaptive computer equipment improved her level of difficulty by two levels (moderate difficulty to no difficulty).

e140 Products and Technology for Culture, Recreation, and Sport
Equipment, products, and technology used for the conduct and enhancement of cultural, recreational, and sporting activities, including those adapted or specially designed.

- *e1400 General Products and Technology for Culture, Recreation, and Sport*
  Equipment, products, and technology used for the conduct and enhancement of cultural, recreational, and sporting activities, such as toys, skis, tennis balls, and musical instruments, not adapted or specially designed.
- *e1401 Assistive Products and Technology for Culture, Recreation, and Sport*
  Adapted or specially designed equipment, products, and technology used for the conduct and enhancement of cultural, recreational, and sporting activities, such as modified mobility devices for sports, adaptations for musical and other artistic performance.
- *e1408 Products and Technology for Culture, Recreation, and Sport, Other Specified*
- *e1409 Products and Technology for Culture, Recreation, and Sport, Unspecified*

Considerations for Products and Technology for Culture, Recreation, and Sport

Products and technology, whether general or assistive, for culture, recreation, and sport can be a barrier or a facilitator to body structures, body functions, and activities and participation. For example, if a client engages in the sport of skiing and owns his own skis, then general products for culture, recreation, and sport would be a facilitator for d9201 Sports. Likewise, if a client has a spinal cord injury and uses an adaptive sit-ski to engage in skiing, then e1401 Assistive Products and Technology for Culture, Recreation, and Sport would be a facilitator for d9201 Sports.

Products and technology for culture, recreation, and sport can also be a barrier to participation if they are not available, accessible, affordable, or acceptable. Also, if it is improperly prescribed, dysfunction can occur or it may not meet the needs of the client (e.g., child given an adult size guitar instead of a junior size guitar). In some instances, further environmental factors may need to be identified as the underlying causes of difficulty (e.g., policy issues at the school for giving out instruments — e585 Education and Training Services, Systems, and Policies).

Recreational therapists consider the role of products and technology for culture, recreation, and sport in hindering or facilitating engagement in life activities and design appropriate interventions to either:

1. Reduce or eliminate the negative effect of products and technology for culture, recreation, and sport on a particular life activity (e.g., A client wants to participate in wheelchair racing but lacks the appropriate equipment of a racing wheelchair. The therapist assists the client in problem solving and identifying available resources to obtain a racing wheelchair.).
2. Maintain or further facilitate the positive impact of products and technology for culture, recreation, and sport on life activities (e.g., assess current products and technology for culture, recreation, and sport to determine if newer products or technology would even further benefit the client; encourage continued use of products and technology for culture, recreation, and sport).

Example (Products and Technology for Culture, Recreation, and Sport as a Barrier)

A 15-year-old boy had a traumatic lower extremity amputation. Prior to the amputation he was on the school track team. He desires to run track again but does not have a sport prosthetic. He has a standard non-sport prosthetic that severely inhibits his ability to run (severe difficulty). This is an example of how of e1400 General Products and Technology for Culture, Recreation, and Sport is a barrier for d4552 Running. The scoring of d4552 that reflects the impact of e1400 as a barrier would look like this: "d4552.3 _ _ _, E-code: e1400.3." The first qualifier reflects severe difficulty with running in his current life situation including all currently available supports and constraints (performance). In the clinical judgment of the therapist, the client would have no difficulty running if he had a sport prosthetic. The e-code is rated a .3 because it is believed that the current prosthetic causes him to have an increased level of difficulty with running by three levels when compared to the foreseen level of difficulty when using a sport prosthetic (no difficulty to severe difficulty).

Example (Products and Technology for Culture, Recreation, and Sport as a Facilitator)

The same client in the previous example now has a specially designed prosthetic for running. He is able to run using the new prosthetic without difficulty. Engaging in the sport of track, however, he has mild difficulty. Although the sport prosthetic allows him to compete, he feels insecure in his abilities. This is an example of how e1401 Assistive Products and Technology for Culture, Recreation, and Sport can be a facilitator for d4552 Running and d9201 Sports. The scoring of d4552 and d9201 that reflects the impact of e1401 as a facilitator would look like this: "d4552. 0 _ _ 3, E-code: e1401+3, d9201.1 _ _ 4, E-code: e1401+3." The first qualifier of d4552 reflects no difficulty with the skill of running in his current life situation given all available supports and constraints including the sport prosthetic (performance). The fourth qualifier reflects severe difficulty with the skill of running in his current environment if all available supports were removed including the sport prosthetic (performance without assistance). The first qualifier of d9201 reflects mild difficulty engaging in sports in his current life situation given all available supports and constraints including the sport prosthetic (performance). The fourth qualifier reflects complete difficulty engaging in sports in his current life situation if all available supports were removed (performance without assistance). The e-code for both A&P codes are rated a +3 (moderate facilitator) because the product and technology (sport prosthetic) improved the client's level of difficulty by three levels.

e145 Products and Technology for the Practice of Religion or Spirituality

Products and technology, unique or mass-produced, that are given or take on a symbolic meaning in the context of the practice of religion or spirituality, including those adapted or specially designed.

- *e1450 General Products and Technology for the Practice of Religion or Spirituality*
  Products and technology, unique or mass-produced, that are given or take on a symbolic meaning in the context of the practice of religion or spirituality, such as spirit houses, maypoles, headdresses, masks, crucifixes, menorahs, and prayer mats, not adapted or specially designed.
- *e1451 Assistive Products and Technology for the Practice of Religion or Spirituality*
  Adapted or specially designed products and technology that are given, or take on a symbolic meaning in the context of the practice of religion or spirituality, such as Braille religious books, Braille tarot cards, and special protection for wheelchair wheels when entering temples.
- *e1458 Products and Technology for the Practice of Religion or Spirituality, Other Specified*
- *e1459 Products and Technology for the Practice of Religion or Spirituality, Unspecified*

Considerations for Products and Technology for the Practice of Religion or Spirituality

Products and technology, whether general or assistive, for the practice of religion or spirituality can be a barrier or a facilitator to body structures, body functions, and activities and participation. For example, wearing a cross necklace that makes her feel protected helps a client manage stressful situations, then e1450 General Products and Technology for the Practice of Religion or Spirituality would be a facilitator for d2401 Handling Stress. Likewise, if a client has a special prayer written for him by his pastor that he finds helpful in

managing feelings of anxiety in stressful situations, then e1451 Assistive Products and Technology for the Practice of Religion and Spirituality would be a facilitator for d2401 Handling Stress.

Products and technology for the Practice of Religion and Spirituality can also be barriers to participation in such activities if they are not available, accessible, affordable, or acceptable. Also, if it is improperly prescribed, dysfunction can occur or it may not meet the needs of the client (e.g., spiritual bracelet is too big and cannot be worn). Products and technology for religion or spirituality may also impact life activities in a negative way if they cause the client or others harm. For example, a negative impact might be a belief in a product or technology that affects a client's judgment, such as "I can jump off this six-story building and I will not be injured because I am wearing a special religious medal that keeps me from harm." In this example, if the medal was not adapted or specially designed, e1450 General Products and Technology for the Practice of Religion or Spirituality would be a barrier to b1645 Judgment.

Recreational therapists consider the role of products and technology for the practice of religion and spirituality in hindering or facilitating engagement in life activities and design appropriate interventions to either:

1. Reduce or eliminate the negative effect of products and technology for the practice of religion and spirituality on a particular life activity (e.g., A client wants to participate in a specific spiritual dance but lack of hair due to chemotherapy means that the headdress will not stay on his head. The therapist researches and identifies a product to hold the headdress onto the head.).
2. Maintain or further facilitate the positive impact of products and technology for the practice of religion and spirituality on life activities (e.g., assess current products and technology for the practice of religion and spirituality to determine if newer products or technology would further benefit the client; encourage continued use of products and technology for the practice of religion and spirituality).

Example (Products and Technology for the Practice of Religion and Spirituality as a Barrier)

A client believes that a religious medal that she wears on a necklace keeps her from harm. She has attempted several times (an average of 25%) while at the clinic to engage in unsafe activities (e.g., walking without needed assistance), stating that the religious medal will keep her from falling. This is an example of how e1450 General Products and Technology for the Practice of Religion can be a barrier to b1645 Judgment. The scoring of b1645 that reflects the impact of e1450 as a barrier would look like this: "b1645.3, E-code: e1450.2." The qualifier reflects severe judgment impairment. The level of judgment impairment was determined through testing and observation including the observation of the unsafe incidents. The e-code was rated a .2 (moderate barrier) because the therapist determined through testing that the client's belief in the religious medal appears to account for 25% of her judgment impairment while the other 75% appears to be related to other cognitive impairments.

Example (Products and Technology for the Practice of Religion and Spirituality as a Facilitator)

A client is currently experiencing many life changes and unfortunate situations causing a high level of stress. In the hospital, the client finds comfort in her spiritual beliefs (a higher power guiding and helping her). She carries a small carved stone dove in her pocket as a physical reminder. With the emotional comfort of staff, her spiritual beliefs, and the stone dove, she is able to handle stress with minimal difficulty. This is an example of how e1450 General Products and Technology for the Practice of Spirituality can be a facilitator for d2401 Handling Stress. The scoring of d2401 that reflects the impact of e1450 as a facilitator would look like this: "d2401.__1_, E-code: e1450+1." The third qualifier reflects mild difficulty in handling stress with assistance in the hospital (capacity with assistance). It would not be appropriate to take away the stone dove to determine the extent of its facilitation. The extent could be estimated by the frequency the client reaches into her pocket and grasps the dove, talks about the dove, and carries the dove. In this situation, the therapist rated the e-code a +1 because it was her clinical judgment that the dove is a mild facilitator in the multitude of coping mechanisms used by the client (spiritual faith, emotional comfort of others).

e150 Design, Construction, and Building Products and Technology of Buildings for Public Use

Products and technology that constitute an individual's indoor and outdoor human-made environment that is planned, designed, and constructed for public use, including those adapted or specially designed.

- *e1500 Design, Construction, and Building Products and Technology for Entering and Exiting Buildings for Public Use*
  Products and technology of entry and exit from the human-made environment that is planned, designed, and constructed for public use, such as design, building, and construction of entries and exits to buildings for public use (e.g., workplaces, shops, and theater), public buildings, portable and stationary ramps, power-assisted doors, lever doors handles, and level door thresholds.
- *e1501 Design, Construction, and Building Products and Technology for Gaining Access to Facilities inside Buildings for Pubic Use*
  Products and technology of indoor facilities in design, building, and construction for public use, such as washroom facilities, telephones, audio loops, lifts or elevators, escalators, thermostats (for temperature regulation), and dispersed accessible seating in auditoriums or stadiums.
- *e1502 Design, Construction, and Building Products and Technology for Way Finding, Path Routing, and Designation of Locations in Buildings for Public Use*
  Indoor and outdoor products and technology in design, building, and construction for public use to assist people to find their way inside and immediately outside buildings and locate the places they want to go to, such as signage, in Braille or writing, size of corridors, floor surfaces, accessible kiosks, and other forms of directories.
- *e1508 Design, Construction, and Building Products and Technology of Buildings for Public Use, Other Specified*
- *e1509 Design, Construction, and Building Products and Technology of Buildings for Public Use, Unspecified*

Considerations for Design, Construction, and Building Products and Technology of Buildings for Public Use

Design, construction, and building products and technology of buildings for public use can be a barrier or a facilitator to body structures, body functions, and life activities. For example, the construction of a ramp to enter a public building (e1500 Design, Construction, and Building Products and Technology for Entering and Exiting Buildings for Public Use) could be a facilitator for d9300 Organized Religion (entering a church). In another example, wheelchair accessible seating in a theatre could be a facilitator for d9202 Arts and Culture. A final example would be large print signage in a building as a facilitator for d6200 Shopping (reading grocery aisle signs) for someone with a vision impairment.

Design, construction, and building products and technology of buildings for public use can also be a barrier to participation in activities if it is not available, accessible, affordable, or acceptable. Also, if it is improperly prescribed, dysfunction can occur (e.g., ramp is too steep causing the client to lose control of her wheelchair) or it may not meet the needs of the client (e.g., wheelchair accessible bathroom on the second floor but no elevator to get to the second floor).

Recreational therapists consider the role of design, construction, and building products and technology of buildings for public use in hindering or facilitating engagement in life activities and design appropriate interventions to either:

1. Reduce or eliminate the negative effect of products and technology of buildings for public use on a particular life activity (e.g., A client wants to attend his granddaughter's dance recital in a school auditorium. He requires the use of a wheelchair. Wheelchair accessible seating is at the back of the auditorium. However it is not feasible for him to sit there because he also has a vision impairment that hinders his ability to see the stage from a distance. So, although wheelchair accessible seating is provided, it does not meet his needs. The therapist educates the client about the Americans with Disabilities Act and the school's requirement to accommodate his needs in a way that is reasonable. The client calls the school and discusses his situation. The school identifies a safe area in front of the stage for the client to sit in his wheelchair for the recital.).

2. Maintain or further facilitate the positive impact of products and technology of buildings for public use on life activities (e.g., assess current products and technology of buildings for public use to determine if newer products or technology would even further benefit the client; encourage continued use of products and technology of buildings for public use).

See "Americans with Disabilities Act Education" in the Techniques section for information on how to obtain a copy of the current ADA accessibility guidelines for public buildings.

Example (Design, Construction, and Building Products and Technology of Buildings for Public Use as a Barrier)

A client who uses a manual wheelchair reports having difficulty getting into buildings that provide opportunities for social and community associations because there are steps at the entrances (no ramps). This is an example of how e1500 Design,

Construction, and Building Products and Technology for Entering and Exiting Buildings for Public Use can be a barrier for d9100 Informal Associations. The scoring of d9100 that reflects the impact of e1500 as a barrier would look like this: "d9100. 2 _ _ _, E-code: e1500.1." The first qualifier reflects moderate difficulty with overall engagement in informal associations in his current life situation given all currently available supports and constraints (performance). This qualifier was scored a 2 from testing and observation that showed difficulty with 40% of the task due to multiple issues (e.g., poor communication skills, lack of self-confidence in abilities). As determined by the therapist, the inaccessible entrances account, on average, for one level of the difficulty with engagement in informal associations. If the barrier were removed by installing ramps, the client would still have a residual mild difficulty with engagement in informal associations. This is why the e-code was rated a .1 (accounts for one level of difficulty with engagement in informal associations).

Example (Design, Construction, and Building Products and Technology of Buildings for Public Use as a Facilitator)

The same client in the previous example learns about portable ramps. He educates the workers at the places he likes to go (e.g., recreation center) about where they can be purchased. Some of the places purchase a portable ramp and now place them over the steps when he visits. He also keeps one in his car trunk and requests assistance from the workers at the site to help him set it up if they do not have one. This is an example of how e1500 Design, Construction, and Building Products and Technology for Entering and Exiting Buildings for Public Use can be a facilitator for d9100 Informal Associations. The scoring of d9100 that reflects the impact of e1500 as a facilitator would look like this: "d9100.1 _ _ 2, E-code: e1500+1." The first qualifier reflects mild difficulty engaging in informal associations in his current life situation given all available supports and constraints (performance). This score reflects the one level positive change due to the use of portable ramps as discussed in the previous example. The fourth qualifier reflects moderate difficulty engaging in informal associations in his current life situation when supports are removed (performance without assistance). See the previous example for an explanation of this score. The e-code was rated a +1 because the portable ramps improved his level of difficulty with engagement in informal associations by one level.

e155 Design, Construction, and Building Products and Technology of Buildings for Private Use
Products and technology that constitute an individual's indoor and outdoor human-made environment that is planned, designed, and constructed for private use, including those adapted or specially designed.
- *e1550 Design, Construction, and Building Products and Technology for Entering and Exiting of Buildings for Private Use*
  Products and technology of entry and exit from the human-made environment that is planned, designed, and constructed for private use, such as entries and exits to private homes, portable and stationary ramps, power-assisted doors, lever door handles, and level door thresholds.
- *e1551 Design, Construction, and Building Products and Technology for Gaining Access to Facilities inside Buildings for Private Use*
  Products and technology of indoor facilities in design, building, and construction for private use, such as washroom facilities, telephones, audio loops, kitchen cabinets, appliances, and electronic controls in private homes.
- *e1552 Design, Construction, and Building Products and Technology for Way Finding, Path Routing, and Designation of Locations in Buildings for Private Use*
  Indoor and outdoor products and technology in design, building, and construction of path routing, for private use, to assist people to find their way inside and immediately outside buildings and locate the places they want to go to, such as signage, in Braille or writing, size of corridors, and floor surfaces
- *e1558 Design, Construction, and Building Products and Technology of Buildings for Private Use, Other Specified*
- *e1559 Design, Construction, and Building Products and Technology of Buildings for Private Use, Unspecified*

Considerations for Design, Construction, and Building Products and Technology of Buildings for Private Use

See e1500 Design, Construction, and Building Products and Technology for Buildings for Public Use. The only difference is that this code set refers to buildings for private use. See "Americans with Disabilities Act Education" in the Techniques section for information about accessibility requirements for public and private buildings.

e160 Products and Technology of Land Development
Products and technology of land areas, as they affect an individual's outdoor environment through the implementation of land use policies, design, planning,

and development of space, including those adapted or specially designed.
- *e1600 Products and Technology of Rural Land Development*
  Products and technology in rural land areas, as they affect an individual's outdoor environment through the implementation of rural land use policies, design, planning, and development of space, such as farm lands, pathways, and signposting.
- *e1601 Products and Technology of Suburban Land Development*
  Products and technology in suburban land areas, as they affect an individual's outdoor environment through the implementation of suburban land use policies, design, planning, and development of space, such as curb cuts, pathways, signposting, and street lighting.
- *e1602 Products and Technology of Urban Land Development*
  Products and technology in urban land areas as they affect an individual's outdoor environment through the implementation of urban land use policies, design, planning, and development of space, such as curb cuts, ramps, signposting, and street lighting.
- *e1603 Products and Technology of Parks, Conservation, and Wildlife Areas*
  Products and technology in land areas making up parks, conservation, and wildlife areas, as they affect an individual's outdoor environment through the implementation of land use policies and design, planning, and development of space, such as park signage and wildlife trails.
- *e1608 Products and Technology of Land Development, Other Specified*
- *e1609 Products and Technology of Land Development, Unspecified*

Considerations for Products and Technology of Land Development

Products and technology of land development can be a barrier or a facilitator to body structures, body functions, and life activities. For example, changes in street lighting could be a facilitator to evening activities in an area that has been previous unlit (d1601 Products and Technology of Suburban Land Development as a facilitator to d9205 Socializing in the evening). Another example would be the development of land in rural areas for a shopping center (d1600 Products and Technology of Rural Land Development as a facilitator to d6200 Shopping).

Products and technology of land development can also be a barrier to activity participation if it is improperly designed (e.g., does not meet ADA accessibility guidelines) or doesn't meet the needs of the client (e.g., pathways are developed but they do not have curb cuts or they have a gravel surface making them inaccessible for people who use manual wheelchairs).

Recreational therapists consider the role of products and technology of land development in life activities and design appropriate interventions to either:

1. Reduce or eliminate the negative effect of products and technology of land development on a particular life activity (e.g., A client wants to walk a three-mile path in a park. The paths in the park are paved, but they are not marked, making it difficult for the client to find her way back. The client and therapist call their local representative and identify the process to install appropriate park path markers.).
2. Maintain or further facilitate the positive impact of products and technology of land development on life activities (e.g., assess current products and technology of land development to determine if newer products or technology would further benefit the client; encourage continued use of products and technology of land development).

See "Americans with Disabilities Act Education" in the Techniques section for information on how to obtain a copy of the current ADA accessibility guidelines for land development.

Example (Products and Technology of Land Development as a Barrier)

A client has moderate difficulty walking on uneven surfaces. He would like to go for walks at the local park but the paths are unpaved, hilly, and full of tree roots making is dangerous and unrealistic. This is an example of how e1603 Products and Technology of Parks, Conservation, and Wildlife Areas can be a barrier to d4602 Moving Around Outside the Home and Other Buildings. The scoring of d4602 that reflects the impact of e1603 as a barrier would look like this: "d4602.2 _ _ 2, E-code: e1603.0." The fourth qualifier reflects the client's average level of difficulty moving around outside the home in his current life situation given supports and constraints as a whole (not just within the park). The e-code is rated a .0 because it was determined by the therapist that the park trails (if paved) would not change (or negligibly change) the level of overall difficulty that the client has with d4602 Moving Around Outside the Home and Other Buildings.

Example (Products and Technology of Land Development as a Facilitator)

A client recently moved from the city to a rural farm area. There is no street signage. His friends, who live in the city, do not come to visit him because they get lost easily. This affects his ability to socialize with his city friends (d9205 Socializing). The client has mild difficulty socializing with peers in his new neighborhood for various reasons. He petitioned the county to put up street signs. Once the street signs were posted, his friends from the city visit about two times a month since they do not fear getting lost. This is an example of how e1600 Products and Technology of Rural Land Development can be a facilitator for d9205 Socializing. The scoring of d9205 Socializing that reflects the impact of e1600 would look like this: "d9205.1 _ _ 2, E-code: e1600+0." The first qualifier reflects mild difficulty socializing in his current life situation given supports and constraints (performance). The mild difficulty with socializing is due to a variety of issues related to the move (e.g., feels uncomfortable around new peers). The fourth qualifier reflects moderate difficulty socializing when assistance is not provided (performance without assistance). The support is the encouragement of his parents to socialize with new neighborhood peers. The facilitator that is paired with this A&P code only affects socialization with a small group of peers on an infrequent basis. The therapist determines that, although the installation of street signs was a good thing, it did not have a profound enough effect on the client's engagement in socialization to show a level change in difficulty. Consequently, the e-code is scored a +0.

e165 Assets

Products or objects of economic exchange such as money, goods, property and other valuables that an individual owns or of which he or she has rights of use.

Inclusions: tangible and intangible products and goods, financial assets

*   *e1650 Financial Assets*
    Products, such as money and other financial instruments, which serve as a medium of exchange for labor, capital goods, and services.
*   *e1651 Tangible Assets*
    Products or objects, such as houses and land, clothing, food, and technical goods, which serve as a medium of exchange for labor, capital goods, and services.
*   *e1652 Intangible Assets*
    Products, such as intellectual property, knowledge, and skills, which serve as a medium of exchange for labor, capital good, and services.
*   *e1658 Assets, Other Specified*
*   *e1659 Assets, Unspecified*

Considerations for
Assets

Assets can be a barrier or a facilitator to body structures, body functions, and life activities. For example, financial assets could be a facilitator to participate in d9204 Hobbies. It could also be a barrier to participation in d9204 Hobbies if the client lacks the financial assets to pay for needed hobby materials. The exchange of tangible assets (e.g., clothing or food) for labor, goods, and services, as well as the exchange of intangible assets such as knowledge and skills for labor, goods, and services is also part of Western culture. It is commonly used for informal trade instead of a formalized exchange (often called bartering in Western culture). For example, your elderly neighbor does not like to cook, so you agree to make her a casserole each week in exchange for teaching your son how to play the piano. Another example would be helping your brother-in-law to build a shed in the backyard in exchange for him helping you to hang a new front door (intangible asset).

Recreational therapists consider the role of assets in life activities and design appropriate interventions to either:

1. Reduce or eliminate the negative effect of assets on a particular life activity (e.g., a client wants to exercise at the local YMCA but does not have the financial assets to pay for the membership. The client and therapist contact the YMCA to see if there are scholarship funds available or the availability and appropriateness of the client providing other assets in exchange for the membership, such as helping at the front desk.).
2. Maintain or further facilitate the positive impact of assets on life activities (e.g., assess current assets to determine if other assets would further benefit the client; encourage continued use of current assets).

Example (Assets as a Barrier)

A client desires to learn how to play the guitar. She does not have enough money to pay for lessons. This is an example of how e1650 Financial Assets can be a barrier to d155 Acquiring Skills. (Note that the code d155 Acquiring Skills is used instead of code d9202 Arts and Culture because d9202 reflects playing the guitar, while d155 reflects learning how to play the guitar). The scoring of d155 that reflects the impact of e1650 as a barrier would look like this: "d155.2 _ _ 3, E-code: e1650.3." The first qualifier

reflects the level of difficulty that the client has with acquiring skills in her current life situation with available supports and constraints (her grandmother gives her money to help her pay for acquiring new skills through classes and programs) showing that overall she has moderate difficulty acquiring new skills (performance). The fourth qualifier is the level of difficulty that she has acquiring new skills when no money is received from her grandmother (performance without assistance). The e-code is rated a .3 because when the therapist looks at the client's overall life situation, financial assets appear to account for 80% of the barrier related to acquiring skills.

Example (Assets as a Facilitator)

The same client in the previous example spoke with a neighbor who knows how to play the guitar. The neighbor agreed to give her free guitar lessons if she would take the neighbor's dog for a walk two times a week. The client agreed. This is an example of how e1652 Intangible Assets can be a facilitator for d155 Acquiring Skills. The scoring of d155 that reflects the impact of e1652 as a facilitator would look like this: "d155.2 _ _ 3, E-code: e1652+0." The first and fourth qualifiers are the same as the previous example. There has been no change in the A&P code of d155 despite the introduction of a new facilitator (the neighbor who is willing to barter for guitar lessons). Remember that d155 encompasses the average level of difficulty that a client has with acquiring skills. In this example, learning to play the guitar is only one of many skills that the client is trying to acquire. Therefore, it did not have enough impact to reduce her level of difficulty in acquiring skills in life situations with assistance or without assistance. The e-code was rated a +0 because it had a negligible impact (not enough to decrease her level of difficulty) on her ability to acquire skills. If there is no change in level of difficulty, then why even acknowledge the facilitator? Facilitators should always be acknowledged and scored. It tells the therapist to encourage continuation of the facilitator and suggests areas where more facilitators may be found. It also brings awareness to the people analyzing the incoming data to support continuation (or further implementation) of facilitators to enhance health and quality of life.

e198 Products and Technology, Other Specified

e199 Products and Technology, Unspecified

Chapter 2 Natural Environmental and Human Made Changes to Environment

This chapter is about animate and inanimate elements of the natural or physical environment, and components of that environment that have been modified by people, as well as characteristics of human populations within that environment.

e210 Physical Geography
Features of land forms and bodies of water.
Inclusions: features of geography included within orography (relief, quality, and expanse of land and land forms, including altitude) and hydrography (bodies of water such as lakes, rivers, sea)
- *e2100 Land Forms*
  Features of land forms, such as mountains, hills, valleys, and plains.
- *e2101 Bodies of Water*
  Features of bodies of water, such as lakes, dams, rivers, and streams.
- *e2108 Physical Geography, Other Specified*
- *e2109 Physical Geography, Unspecified*

Considerations for Physical Geography

Physical geography can be a barrier or facilitator to life activities and functions. Recreational therapists consider the role of physical geography in life activities and design appropriate interventions to either:

1. Reduce or eliminate the negative effect of physical geography on a particular life activity. In some cases, changing the physical geography of the client's home may be possible (e.g., leveling out the driveway and paving it to make it easier to walk), however, in most cases the client will need to be taught how to compensate for the barriers. Examples include putting a specialized ice pick end on the bottom of a standard cane to help with walking on uneven surfaces or changing the type of food being grown to one that will thrive in poor soil. In some situations, it might be best for the client to consider moving to a new location that is more geographically favorable (e.g., if drinking water source is contaminated and affecting health).

2. Maintain or further facilitate the positive impact of physical geography on life activities: If the physical geography of the client's area is a facilitator for life activities and functioning, therapists bring this to the attention of the client and encourage the client to consider physical geography when making any life changes.

Example (Bodies of Water as a Barrier)

A client desires to grow a crop. He finds that the local water supply is contaminated and cannot be used for irrigation. This is an example of how e2101 can be a barrier to d6505 Taking Care of Plants. The scoring of d6505 that reflects the impact of e2101 as a barrier would look like this: "d6505.4 _ _ _, E-code: e2101.4." The first qualifier reflects complete difficulty in being able to care for plants in his current life situation given supports and constraints (performance). If the water was not contaminated, it is the clinical judgment of the therapist that the client would have no difficulty caring for plants. The e-code is rated a .4 because the water contamination increases the client's level of difficulty by four levels (no difficulty to complete difficulty).

Example (Bodies of Water as a Facilitator)

A client engages in fishing during the summer months. He lives in an area where lakes are prevalent. This is an example of how e2101 Bodies of Water can be a facilitator for d9201 Sports. The scoring of d9201 that reflects the impact of e2101 would look like this: "d9201. 0 _ _ 0, E-code: e2101+0." The first qualifier reflects no difficulty overall with engagement in sports (this includes fishing but is not limited to fishing) in his current life situation given supports and constraints (performance). The fourth qualifier reflects the client's level of difficulty with fishing in his current life situation if supports were removed (performance without assistance). Since the client is independent with engaging in sports (requires no assistance), the fourth qualifier is the same as the first qualifier. The e-code is rated a +0 because although it has an impact on the sport of fishing (wouldn't be able to fish if there wasn't any water), his level of difficulty with engaging in sports would not change overall.

Example (Land Forms as a Barrier)

A client lives in a hilly neighborhood. He sustained an injury that now requires him to use a manual wheelchair. He does not drive. He used to walk to the stores to do his shopping. Now he lacks the strength and mobility to propel the wheelchair and carry supplies up and down steep hills. This is an example of how e2100 Land Forms can be a barrier to d6200 Shopping. The scoring of d6200 that reflects the impact of e2100 would look like this: "d6200. 0 _ _ 4, E-code: e2100.1." The first qualifier reflects no difficulty shopping in his current life situation if assistance is provided by someone who pushes him in the wheelchair or if he orders supplies by internet or telephone (performance). The fourth qualifier reflects complete difficulty if assistance is not provided (performance without assistance). The e-code is rated a .1 because it only slightly hinders the client's ability to shop (because he can still shop by phone/internet). The land forms, using this example, might be better coded as a barrier to d5701 Maintaining Diet and Fitness or to b4550 General Physical Endurance if outdoor mobility is hindered to the point where it is affecting his ability to maintain fitness, health, and endurance functions.

e215 Population
Groups of people living in a given environment who share the same pattern of environmental adaptation.
Inclusions: demographic change; population density
- *e2150 Demographic Change*
  Changes occurring within groups of people, such as the composition and variation in the total number of individuals in an area caused by births, deaths, ageing of a population, and migration.
- *e2151 Population Density*
  Number of people per unit of land area, including features such as high and low density.
- *e2158 Population, Other Specified*
- *e2159 Population, Unspecified*

Considerations for Population

The population that a client is part of can be a facilitator or barrier to life activities and functioning. Recreational therapists consider the role of population in life activities and design appropriate interventions to either:

1. Reduce or eliminate the negative effect of population on a particular life activity: In some cases, changing the population of the client's living area may be possible (e.g., moving into a larger apartment), however, in most cases the client will need to be taught how to compensate for the barriers. For example, if a client is having difficulty adapting to the change of population in the neighborhood, therapists assist clients in identifying new sources of social support that meet the client's needs (e.g., instead of conversing so much with neighbors, the client may benefit from participation in a private club that caters to a group that is similar to the client).

2. Maintain or further facilitate the positive impact of population on life activities: If the population of the client's area is a facilitator for life activities and functioning of the client, the therapist brings this to the attention of the client and encourages the client to consider population when making any life changes.

Example (Population as a Barrier and Facilitator)

An 85-year-old client reports that many of his neighborhood friends have passed away. Young families are purchasing the homes and there aren't many older people left in his neighborhood to socialize with. He finds it difficult to relate to the younger generation and has difficulty forming relationships with them. This is an example of how e2150 Demographic Change can be a barrier to d7200 Forming Relationships. The scoring of d7200 to reflect the impact of e2150 as a barrier would look like this: "d7200. 3 _ _ _, E-code: e2150.3." The first qualifier reflects severe difficulty in forming relationships in his current life situation given available supports and constraints (performance). This score was determined through conversation and observation by the therapist. In the clinical opinion of the therapist, if the demographic change in his neighborhood has added more people similar to the client, his level of difficulty with forming relationships would improve to no difficulty (improvement by three levels). Given this premise, the e-code is rated a .3 because demographic change is believed to be the cause of increasing his level of difficulty with socializing by three levels. (Note: If the neighborhood was changing so that new people moving in were more similar to the client, then e2150 Demographic Change could be a facilitator to d7200 Forming Relationships. Having other people to talk with might also be a facilitator for d2401 Handing Stress).

e220 Flora and Fauna
Plants and animals.
Exclusions: domesticated animals (e350); population (e215)
- *e2200 Plants*
  Any of various photosynthetic, eukaryotic, multicellular organisms of the kingdom Plantae characteristically producing embryos, containing chloroplasts, having cellulose cell walls, and lacking the power of locomotion, such as trees, flowers, shrubs, and vines.
- *e2201 Animals*
  Multicellular organisms of the kingdom Animalia, differing from plants in certain typical characteristics such as capacity for locomotion, non-photosynthetic metabolism, pronounced response to

stimuli, restricted growth, and fixed bodily structure, such as wild or farm animals, reptiles, birds, fish, and mammals.
Exclusions: assets (3165); domesticated animals (e350)

- *e2208 Fauna and Flora, Other Specified*
- *e2209 Fauna and Flora, Unspecified*

Considerations for Flora and Fauna

Plants and animals can be facilitators or barriers to life activities and functions. Recreational therapists consider the role of plants and animals in life activities and design appropriate interventions to either:

1. Reduce or eliminate the negative effect of plants and animals on a particular life activity: In some cases, changing the flora and fauna of the client's areas of functioning may be possible (e.g., planting or cutting down trees, taking out plants that cause allergies). In most cases the client will need to be taught how to compensate for the barriers. For example, if a client is having allergic reactions to plants when outdoors, allergy medications may need to be explored. If a client benefits from shaded areas, then it would be beneficial to explore the possibility of planting shade trees in the client's environment.
2. Maintain or further facilitate the positive impact of plants and animals on life activities: If flora and fauna within the client's areas of living are facilitators to life activities and functioning, the therapist brings this to the attention of the client and encourages the client to consider flora and fauna when making any life changes.

Example (Plants as a Barrier)

An 8-year-old girl has severe allergic reactions to pollen. Consequently her outdoor play activities are restricted during the spring. This is an example of how e2200 Plants (as well as e2255 Seasonal Variation) can be a barrier to d9200 Play. The scoring of d9200 to reflect the impact of e2200 and e2255 as barriers would look like this: "d9200. 1 _ _ 3, E-code: e2200.1, e2255.1." The first qualifier reflects mild difficulty engaging in play in the client's current life situation given available supports and constraints (performance). This score was determined through client observation not shared in this example. The fourth qualifier reflects severe difficulty engaging in play in her current life situation should assistance be removed (performance without assistance). This would include removal of allergy medication and assistance from her caregivers. This is not safe or ethical, so this score reflects the clinical

judgment of the therapist. Both e-codes are rated a .1 because plants and seasonal variation affect her engagement in play only during one season and, when looking at all of the difficulties that the client has engaging in play (which are not shared in this example), the therapist determined that the plants and seasonal variation only account for one level of change in difficulty.

Example (Plants as a Facilitator)

A 34-year-old female with multiple sclerosis needs to stay out of the sun to avoid fatigue. Her backyard is shaded by trees and this allows her to participate in activities with her children outdoors without experiencing extreme fatigue. This is an example of how e2200 Plants can be a facilitator for d920 Recreation and Leisure. The scoring of d920 to reflect the impact of e2200 as a facilitator would look like this: "d920.1 _ _ 3, E-code: e2200+1." The first qualifier reflects mild difficulty engaging in recreation and leisure in her current life situation given available supports and constraints (performance). The fourth qualifier reflects severe difficulty engaging in recreation and leisure in her current life situation without assistance (performance without assistance). The scores chosen were based on the average level of difficulty within a broad range of recreational activities (not just summer activities) not shared in this example. The e-code was rated a +1. This was determined through clinical judgment by evaluating the impact of shade on the client's engagement in recreational activity as a whole. The percent of recreational activities affected by shade was limited since it was only a benefit during the hot summer months. Consequently, it is only a minimal facilitator to engagement in recreational activities.

Example (Animals as a Barrier)

A client with osteoporosis has a history of falls. Many of her falls (80%) are related to tripping over her pet cat within her home. This is an example of how e2201 Animals can be a barrier to d4600 Moving Around Within the Home. The scoring of d4600 to reflect the impact of e2201 as a barrier would look like this: "d4600. 3 _ _ _, E-code: e2201.3." The first qualifier reflects severe difficulty moving around the house in her current life situation given available supports and constraints (performance). The e-code is rated a .3 because it is the pet cat that is causing 80% of her falls (severe barrier).

Example (Animals as a Facilitator)

A client had her right knee replaced. She is able to walk short community distances without a device and exhibits good balance. She has a pet dog that requires walking every day. She reports that her pet dog is a motivator for her to go outside for a walk every day. This is an example of how e2201 Animals can be facilitator to d4500 Walking Short Distances. The scoring of d4500 to reflect the impact of e2201 as a facilitator would look like this: "d4500.0 _ _ 0, E-code: e2201+0." The first qualifier reflects that she has no difficulty walking short distances in her current life situation given supports and constraints (performance). The fourth qualifier reflects that she has no difficulty walking short distance in her current life situation without assistance (performance without assistance). The client does not use a device or require assistance from another person, therefore her score for the fourth qualifier remains the same as the first qualifier. Although the dog is a primary motivator, it does not change her level of difficulty walking short distances, therefore the e-code is rated a +0. If the client reported that she wouldn't walk as much as necessary without the dog, it might be correct to score the performance at 1 or more and rate the e-code +1 or better, accordingly. If the client had a large unruly dog that could not be left at home alone, it is possible that the dog would hinder her ability to walk. In this example, e2201 Animals could be a barrier to d4500 Walking Short Distances.

e225 Climate
Meteorological features and events, such as the weather.
Inclusions: temperature, humidity, atmospheric pressure, precipitation, wind, and seasonal variations
- *e2250 Temperature*
  Degree of heat or cold, such as high and low temperature, normal or extreme temperature.
- *e2251 Humidity*
  Level of moisture in the air, such as high or low humidity.
- *e2252 Atmospheric Pressure*
  Pressure of the surrounding air, such as pressure related to height above sea level or meteorological conditions.
- *e2253 Precipitation*
  Falling of moisture, such as rain, dew, snow, sleet, and hail.
- *e2254 Wind*
  Air in more or less rapid natural motion, such as a breeze, gale, or gust.
- *e2255 Seasonal Variation*
  Natural, regular, and predictable changes from one season to the next, such as summer, autumn, winter, and spring.
- *e2258 Climate, Other Specified*
- *e2259 Climate, Unspecified*

Considerations for Climate

Climate can be a barrier or facilitator to life activities and functions. Recreational therapists consider the role of climate on life activities and design appropriate interventions to either:
1. Reduce or eliminate the negative effect of climate on a particular life activity: It is not possible to change the climate of the client's areas of living, so the client will need to be taught how to compensate for the barriers. For example, if a client with multiple sclerosis fatigues easily with heat, then she would be encouraged to keep her core body temperature as low as possible by drinking cold water, wearing a brimmed hat, wearing breathable clothing such as cotton, and using a portable battery-operated fan. Another example would be for the client who is unable to go to church during the winter months to consider other acceptable ways to engage in religious activities (e.g., having a Eucharistic minister come to the house, watching a Mass on television, inviting people over to the house for Bible study).
2. Maintain or further facilitate the positive impact of climate on life activities: If the climate in the client's areas of living is a facilitator to life activities and functioning, the therapist brings this to the attention of the client and encourages the client to consider the climate when making any life changes.

Example (Temperature and Humidity as a Barrier)

A client has multiple sclerosis. On average she is able to engage in the task of shopping with moderate difficulty. When the humidity and/or temperature are high, it affects her level of functioning. She experiences greater fatigue and weakness and this affects her ability to go shopping in the community resulting in severe difficulty. This is an example of how e2250 Temperature and e2251 Humidity can be a barrier to d6200 Shopping. The scoring of d6200 Shopping that reflects the impact of e2250 and e2251 would look like this: "d6200.2 _ _ 4, E-code: e2250.2, e2251.2." The first qualifier reflects her average level of difficulty (moderate difficulty) with shopping in her current life situation given support and constraints (performance). The fourth qualifier reflects complete difficulty to engage in the task of shopping in her current life situation when assistance is not provided (performance without assistance). This score was chosen based on clinical observation and testing by the therapist that is not shared in this example. Both e-codes are rated a .2 because the change in temperature and humidity causes a 2 level change in her ability to engage in shopping. (Note: If the temperature and humidity were low, e2250 Temperature and e2251 Humidity could be facilitators to d6200 Shopping. As reviewed in Issues Related to E-Codes in ICF Scoring, it may be better to score e-codes as a facilitator rather than as a barrier when they can be both a barrier and a facilitator).

Example (Temperature as a Facilitator)

A 10-year-old boy with mental retardation loves to swim in his backyard outdoor pool. He lives in California where it is often hot enough to swim outdoors. This is an example of how e2250 Temperature can be a facilitator for d4554 Swimming. The scoring of d4554 to reflect the impact of e2250 as a facilitator would look like this: "d4554.0 _ _ 4, E-code: e2250+4." The first qualifier reflects the client's level of difficulty with swimming in his current life situation given supports and constraints (performance). The fourth qualifier reflects his level of difficulty with swimming if assistance is removed (e.g., life vest). The e-code was rated a +4 because if the temperature is not hot enough it would completely limit his ability to swim (if indoor swimming was not available).

Example (Seasonal Variation as a Barrier)

A client has a complete spinal cord injury and requires the use of a manual wheelchair for mobility. He lives in an area where it snows and sleets heavily for three months out of the year. During these months, he does not attend church because it is too dangerous to go outside. This is an example of how e2253 Seasonal Variation can be a barrier to d9300 Organized Religion. The scoring of d9300 to reflect the impact of e2253 as a barrier would look like this: "d9300.1 _ _ 0, E-code: e2253.1." The first qualifier reflects that on average he has mild difficulty engaging in organized religion in his current life situation given usual supports and constraints (performance). This score reflects the average amount of difficulty (no difficulty nine months out of the year and complete difficulty three months out of the year). The e-code is rated a .1 because it causes a one level change in a negative direction (no difficulty to mild difficulty).

e230 Natural Events
Geographic and atmospheric changes that cause disruption in an individual's physical environment, occurring regularly or irregularly, such as earthquakes and severe or violent weather conditions, e.g., tornadoes, hurricanes, typhoons, floods, forest fires, and ice-storms.

Considerations for Natural Events

Natural events will most likely be only coded as barriers to activities. Except for people such as firefighters who are employed (d8451 Maintaining a Job) because of natural events, it is hard to think of a situation when an earthquake, flood, forest fire, or ice storm could be a facilitator to life activities or functions. These codes will most likely be barriers to codes in Activities and Participation Chapter 2 General Tasks and Demands, Chapter 4 Mobility, Chapter 6 Domestic Life, Chapter 8 Major Life Areas, and Chapter 9 Community, Social, and Civic Life.

Recreational therapists consider the role of natural events on life activities and design appropriate interventions to reduce or eliminate the negative effect of natural events on a particular life activity. Therapists working with clients who have experienced a natural event recognize that further counseling and assistance may be needed. Therapists assist clients in identifying appropriate resources to initiate needed support (e.g., referring the client to the social worker). If the client lives in an area where natural events are common and lives are regularly disrupted, the client may need to consider relocation to a more stable area, especially if recovery from the natural event requires more skills and abilities than the client has available (e.g., client is not able to go up on the roof and make repairs each storm season like he did before he was injured).

Example (Natural Events as a Barrier)

A client's home was destroyed in a tornado. She is now having trouble finding a new place to live in the area because many of the homes were destroyed. This is an example of how e230 Natural Events can be a barrier to d610 Acquiring a Place to Live. The scoring of d610 to reflect the impact of e230 as a barrier would look like this: "d610.4 _ _ _ , E-code: e230.4." The first qualifier reflects the client's complete difficulty in acquiring a place to live in her current life situation given usual supports and constraints (performance). The e-code is rated a .4 because it causes a four level change in a negative direction (no difficulty to complete difficulty).

e235 Human-Caused Events
Alterations or disturbances in the natural environment, caused by humans, that may result in the disruption of people's day-to-day lives, including events or conditions linked to conflict and wars, such as the displacement of people, destruction of social infrastructure, homes and lands, environmental disasters, and land, water, or air pollution (e.g., toxic spills).

Considerations for Human-Caused Events

Human-caused events will most likely be coded as barriers to life activities and functions. It is hard to imagine how a human-caused event such as displacement of people, wars, destruction of social infrastructure, and environmental disasters could be a facilitator to life activities, except for the few employed because of the event.

Therapists working with clients who have experienced a human-caused event recognize that further counseling and assistance may be needed. Therapists assist clients in identifying appropriate resources to initiate needed support (e.g., referring the client to the social worker). If the client lives in an area where human-caused events are common and lives are regularly disrupted, the client may need to consider relocation to a more stable area, especially if recovery from the human-caused event requires more skills and abilities than the client has available (e.g., client is not able to quickly hide within the home when fighting breaks out in the street).

Example (Human-Caused Events as a Barrier)

A 23-year-old male is sent to war. He returns home two years later. He has recurrent night terrors and is unable to successfully cope with daily stressors. This is an example of how e235 Human Caused Events can be a barrier to d2401 Handling Stress. The scoring of d2401 to reflect the impact of e235 as a barrier would look like this: "d2401.3 _ _ 4, E-code: e235.4." The first qualifier reflects the client's severe difficulty in coping with stress in his current life situation given usual supports and constraints (performance). The fourth qualifier reflects the client's complete difficulty in coping with stress when assistance is not provided (e.g., support of others). The e-code is rated a .4 because it is anticipated based upon testing, discussion, and observation that if the human-caused event of war did not occur, the client's ability to cope with stress would rise by four levels.

e240 Light
Electromagnetic radiation by which things are made visible by either sunlight or artificial lighting (e.g., candles, oil, or paraffin lamps, fires, and electricity), and which may provide useful or distracting information about the world.
Inclusions: light intensity; light quality; colour contrasts
- *e2400 Light Intensity*
  Level or amount of energy being emitted by either a natural (e.g., sun) or an artificial source of light.

- *e2401 Light Quality*
  The nature of the light being provided and related colour contrasts created in the visual surroundings, and which may provide useful information about the world (e.g., visual information on the presence of stairs or a door) or distractions (e.g., too many visual images).
- *e2408 Light, Other Specified*
- *e2409 Light, Unspecified*

Considerations for Light

Light can be a barrier or facilitator to life activities and functioning. Recreational therapists consider the role of light on life activities and design appropriate interventions to either:
1. Reduce or eliminate the negative effect of light on a particular life activity: In most cases, changes in light in the client's areas of living may be possible (e.g., use of artificial light, shading sunlight), however in some cases the client will need to be taught how to compensate for the barriers. For example, if a client is having difficulty seeing a task clearly due to problems with light intensity or quality, adaptations need to be sought. Such adaptations include the use of direct light and high intensity light, increased time (e.g., walking slowly and carefully when walking up a flight of stairs when the edge of the steps are difficult to see due to limited light), and use of items with high contrast (e.g., black on white or white on black).
2. Maintain or further facilitate the positive impact of light on life activities: If the light in the client's areas of living is a facilitator to life activities and functioning, the therapist brings this to the attention of the client and encourages the client to consider light when making any life or activity changes.

Example (Light Intensity and Light Quality as Facilitator and Barrier)

A client has impaired vision. She reports that she has not engaged in making dried flower crafts for several years because she is unable to see the items and craft clearly. Using a high intensity, artificial white light the client is able to see the items and craft clearly. This is an example of how e2400 Light Intensity and e2401 Light Quality can be facilitators for d9203 Crafts. The scoring of d9203 to reflect the impact of e2400 and e2401 as facilitators would look like this: "d9203. 0 _ _ 4, E-code: e2400+4, e2401+4." The first qualifier reflects no difficulty with crafts in her current life situation given usual supports and constraints, including the adaptive light (performance). The fourth qualifier reflects complete difficulty in her current life situation when assistance (the light) is not provided (performance without assistance). Both e-codes are rated a +4 because without them the client's level of difficulty would fall 4 levels. Prior to the adaptation, e2400 Light Intensity and e2401 Light Quality would have been a barrier to d9203 Crafts.

e245 Time-Related Changes
Natural, regular, or predictable temporal change.
Inclusions: day/night and lunar cycles
- *e2450 Day/Night Cycles*
  Natural, regular, and predictable changes from day through to night and back to day, such as day, night, dawn, and dusk.
- *e2451 Lunar Cycles*
  Natural, regular, and predictable changes of the moon's position in relation to the earth.
- *e2458 Time-Related Changes, Other Specified*
- *e2459 Time-Related Changes, Unspecified*

Considerations for Time-Related Changes

Time-related changes can be a barrier or facilitator to life activities and functions. Some suggest lunar cycles are correlated with behavior, even if it is just because the client believes it.

Day/night and lunar cycles cannot be changed. If they present a barrier for life activities and functioning, the client will need to learn to compensate and adapt for the barriers.

Example (Day/Night Cycles as a Barrier and Facilitator)

A 5-year-old girl has a rare condition of extreme photosensitivity. Sunlight, whether direct or indirect, may not touch her skin. If it does, severe burns occur. She plays outside after the sun goes down and if she needs to go outside during the day, she has to wear a special protective hat, gown, and gloves that cover her entire body. This is an example of how e2450 Day/Night Cycles can be both a barrier and facilitator to d9200 Play. The scoring of d9200 to reflect the impact of e2450 as a barrier would look like this: "d9200. 0 _ _ 4, E-code: e2450.4." The first qualifier reflects no difficulty with play in her current life situation with current supports and constraints (e.g., gown, playing outdoors after sunset, playing indoors with shades drawn during the day) (performance). The fourth qualifier reflects complete difficulty when assistance is not provided (performance without assistance). The e-code is rated a .4 because day/night cycles can result in a change of four levels if adaptations and assistance is not provided. In this same example, the inability of the child to attend a normal public school and participate in daytime peer

activities is another example of how e2450 Day/Night Cycles could be a barrier to d9205 Socializing and d7200 Forming Relationships).

e250 Sound
A phenomenon that is or may be heard, such as banging, ringing, thumping, singing, whistling, yelling, or buzzing, in any volume, timbre, or tone, and that may provide useful or distracting information about the world.
Inclusions: sound intensity; sound quality
- *e2500 Sound Intensity*
  Level or volume of auditory phenomenon determined by the amount of energy being generated, where high energy levels are perceived as loud sounds and low energy levels as soft sounds.
- *e2501 Sound Quality*
  Nature of a sound as determined by the wavelength and wave pattern of the sound and perceived as the timbre and tone, such as harshness or melodiousness, and which may provide useful information about the world (e.g., sound of dog barking versus a cat meowing) or distractions (e.g., background noise).
- *e2508 Sound, Other Specified*
- *e2509 Sound, Unspecified*

Considerations for Sound

Sound can be a barrier or facilitator to life activities and functions. Recreational therapists consider the role of sound on life activities and design appropriate interventions to either:
1. Reduce or eliminate the negative effect of sound on a particular life activity: In many cases, changes in sound in the client's areas of living may be possible (e.g., change the sound intensity and quality of things in the environment such as alarm clocks). In some cases the client will need to be taught how to compensate for the barriers. For example, if a client is very sensitive to loud noises, then it might be helpful to explore wearing earplugs when others are using loud equipment nearby. If the client is having difficulty hearing because of the sound intensity or quality, then auditory devices may be explored.
2. Maintain or further facilitate the positive impact of sound on life activities: If sounds in the client's living environment are facilitators to life activities and functioning, the therapist brings this to the attention of the client and encourages the client to consider sound when making any life or activity changes.

Example (Sound as a Facilitator and Barrier)

A client is legally blind. She has learned how to use her sense of hearing to identify sounds that give her information she used to get from vision (e.g., listening for the clicking noise that denotes traffic light changes) when walking in the community. This is an example of how e250 Sound can be a facilitator for d4602 Moving Around Outside the Home and Other Buildings. The scoring of d4602 that reflects the impact of e250 as a facilitator would look like this: "d4602.0 _ _ 4, E-code: e250+4." The first qualifier reflects that she has no difficulty moving around outside the home and other buildings in her current life situation with all available supports and constraints (performance). The fourth qualifier reflects that she would have complete difficulty with this task if assistance were removed (performance without assistance). The e-code was rated a .4 because without sound, it is anticipated through clinical judgment that her ability to move around outside would reduce by four levels.

Example (Sound Intensity as a Barrier and Facilitator)

A client who had a traumatic brain injury is very sensitive to noise. Loud noises easily cause him to become agitated. This is an example of how e2500 Sound Intensity can be a barrier to b1263 Psychic Stability. The scoring of the ICF to reflect the impact of e2500 as a barrier would look like this: "b1263.2, E-code: e2500.2." The qualifier reflects the client's moderate impairment with psychic stability as determined through testing and observation. The e-code was rated a .2 because, when loud noises are present, they increase the client's level of difficulty by two levels. If soft sounds surrounded the client's living areas, then e2500 Sound Intensity could be a facilitator to b1263 Psychic Stability.

e255 Vibration

Regular or irregular to and fro motion of an object or an individual caused by a physical disturbance, such as shaking, quivering, quick jerky movements of things, buildings, or people caused by small or large equipment, aircraft, and explosions.
Exclusions: natural events (e230), such as vibrations or shaking of the earth caused by earthquake

Considerations for Vibration

Vibration can be a barrier or facilitator to life activities and functions. Recreational therapists consider the role of vibration on life activities and design appropriate interventions to either:

1. Reduce or eliminate the negative effect of vibration on a particular life activity: In some cases, changes in vibration in the client's areas of living may be possible (such as in the example below), however in many cases the client will need to be taught how to compensate for the barriers. For example, if a client's spasms are heightened by vibration and there is a lot of vibration in the client's environment, anti-spasm medications may be an area to explore or the client may benefit from moving to another location, such as sleeping in another room farther from the source of vibration.
2. Maintain or further facilitate the positive impact of vibration on life activities: If vibrations in the client's living environment are facilitators to life activities and functioning, the therapist brings this to the attention of the client and encourages the client to consider vibrations when making any life or activity changes.

Example (Vibration as a Barrier)

For a 37-year-old-male with a developmental disability, vibrations cause increased leg spasms with pain and discomfort. The path through the local park is full of tree roots making it a very bumpy ride in a wheelchair. This is an example of how e255 Vibration can be a barrier to d920 Recreation and Leisure. The scoring of d920 to reflect the impact of e255 as a barrier would look like this: "d920.2 _ _ 4, E-code: e255.1." The first qualifier reflects the client's moderate difficulty with all recreational activities in his current life setting with all available supports and constraints (performance). The fourth qualifier reflects the client's level of difficulty with recreational activities if assistance was not provided (e.g., no wheelchair, medications). The qualifier scores are an average of all skills in the blended activity of recreation and leisure as determined by the therapist through testing and observation. The e-code is rated a .1 because, although it completely limits his ability to go through the park, vibration affects only a minimal percentage of his overall recreational activities, therefore it only changes his overall difficulty with recreational activities by one level.

Example (Vibration as a Facilitator)

An 8-week-old infant is very colicky at night. She cries through most of the night. The mother found a device that attaches to the crib and vibrates the mattress. The vibration relaxes the infant and lets her sleep for longer periods of time during the night. This is an example of how e255 Vibration can be a facilitator to b134 Sleep Functions. The scoring of b134 to reflect the impact of e255 as a facilitator would look like this: "b134.0, E-code: e255+4." The qualifier reflects that the client has no difficulty with sleep functions and that the e-code is a complete facilitator in achieving this level of difficulty. If the vibration was removed it is anticipated that her level of impairment would increase by four levels, thus reflecting the change of four levels. If the infant cried because of vibrations, for example because she sleeps above a vibrating generator, then e255 Vibration would be a barrier to b134 Sleep Functions.

e260 Air Quality
Characteristics of the atmosphere (outside buildings) or enclosed areas of air (inside buildings), and which may provide useful or distracting information about the world.
Inclusions: indoor and outdoor air quality
* e2600 Indoor Air Quality
  Nature of the air inside buildings or enclosed areas, as determined by odour, smoke, humidity, air conditioning (controlled air quality), or uncontrolled air quality, and which may provide useful information about the world (e.g., smell of leaking gas) or distractions (e.g., overpowering smell of perfume).
* e2601 Outdoor Air Quality
  Nature of the air outside buildings or enclosed areas, as determined by odour, smoke, humidity, ozone levels, and other features of the atmosphere, and which may provide useful information about the world (e.g., smell of rain) or distractions (e.g., toxic smells).
* e2608 Air Quality, Other Specified
* e2609 Air Quality, Unspecified

Considerations for Air Quality

Air quality can be a barrier or facilitator to life activities and functions. Recreational therapists consider the role of air quality on life activities and design appropriate interventions to either:
1. Reduce or eliminate the negative effect of air quality on a particular life activity: In some cases, changes in air quality in the client's areas of living may be possible (e.g., using an air purifier system in the home), however in most cases the client will need to be taught how to compensate for the barriers. For example, if a client has difficulty breathing outdoors due to poor air quality, then the client may need to limit the amount of time spent outdoors, use an inhaler when breathing difficulty occurs, or avoid certain activities that contribute to poor air quality (e.g., smoking).
2. Maintain or further facilitate the positive impact of air quality on life activities: If air quality in the client's living environments is a facilitator to

life activities and functioning, the therapist brings this to the attention of the client and encourages the client to consider air quality when making any life or activity changes.

Example (Outdoor Air Quality as a Barrier and Facilitator)

An 11-year-old girl with severe asthma lives in an urban city. The outdoor air quality is poor making it difficult for her to breathe outdoors. This limits the amount of time she can play outdoors with peers. This is an example of how e2601 Outdoor Air Quality can be a barrier to d9205 Socializing, d9200 Play, d7200 Forming Relationships, and b440 Respiration Functions. Let's look at how to score one of these codes. The scoring of b440 to reflect the impact of e2601 as a barrier would look like this: "b440.2, E-code: e2601.2." The qualifier reflects her current level of respiration function impairment. The e-code was rated a .2 because outdoor air quality can increase her level of difficulty with respiration functions by two levels to complete impairment. If the outdoor air quality was good, then e2601 Outdoor Air Quality would be a facilitator to all of the activities and functions listed above.

Example (Indoor Air Quality as a Barrier)

A client lives in a retirement community. She becomes ill and is transferred to the skilled nursing unit in the retirement community. The skilled care center has a strong odor of urine. The woman's friend is very sensitive to smells and cannot tolerate the odor, so she does not visit her best friend while she is there and the relationship deteriorates. This is an example of how e2600 Indoor Air Quality can be a barrier to maintaining a friendship (d7200 Forming Relationships). The scoring of d7200 to reflect the impact of e2600 as a barrier would look like this: "d7200.3 _ _ 4, E-code: e2600.3." The first qualifier reflects her severe difficulty in forming relationships in her current living environment (the skilled care unit). This is due to a variety of reasons, not just related to the issue going on with her best friend (performance). Remember, this is an overall score, not just a score related to this particular situation. The fourth qualifier reflects that there would be a complete difficulty with forming relationships without assistance if there was no initiation of conversation by staff and no encouragement by staff to come out of her room (performance without assistance). The e-code was rated a .3 because the indoor air quality is severely limiting her ability to maintain her previous friendships. It is anticipated that if the indoor air quality was good, her friends would visit and she would have no difficulty in maintaining her friendships, thus reflecting a change in three levels.

e298 Natural Environment and Human-Made Changes to Environment, Other Specified

e299 Natural Environment and Human-Made Changes to Environment, Unspecified

Chapter 3 Support and Relationships

This chapter is about people or animals that provide practical physical or emotional support, nurturing, protection, assistance, and relationships to other persons, in their home, place of work, school, or at play or in other aspects of their daily activities. The chapter does not encompass the attitudes of the person or people that are providing the support. The environmental factor being described is not the person or animal, but the amount of physical and emotional support the person or animal provides.

e310 Immediate Family
Individuals related by birth, marriage, and other relationship recognized by the culture as immediate family, such as spouses, partners, siblings, children, foster parents, adoptive parents, and grandparents.
Exclusions: extended family (e315); personal care providers and personal assistants (e340)

e315 Extended Family
Individuals related through family or marriage or other relationships recognized by the culture as extended family, such as aunts, uncles, nephew, and nieces.
Exclusions: immediate family (e310)

e320 Friends
Individuals who are close and ongoing participants in relationships characterized by trust and mutual support.

e325 Acquaintances, Peers, Colleagues, Neighbours, and Community Members
Individuals who are familiar to each other as acquaintances, peers, colleagues, neighbours, and community members, in situations of work, school, recreation, or other aspects of life, and who share demographic features such as age, gender, religious creed, or ethnicity or pursue common interests.
Exclusions: associations and organizational services (e5550)

e330 People in Positions of Authority
Individuals who have decision-making responsibilities for others and who have socially defined influence or power based on their social, economic, cultural, or religious roles in society, such as teachers, employers, supervisors, religious leaders, substitute decision-makers, guardians, or trustees.

e335 People in Subordinate Positions
Individuals whose day-to-day life is influenced by people in positions of authority in work, school, or other settings, such as students, workers, and members of a religious group.
Exclusions: immediate family (e310)

e340 Personal Care Providers and Personal Assistants
Individuals who provide services as required to support individuals in their daily activities and maintenance of performance at work, education, or other life situation, provided either through public or private funds, or else on a voluntary basis, such as providers of support for home-making and maintenance, personal assistants, transport assistants, paid help, nannies, and others who function as primary caregivers.
Exclusions: immediate family (e310); extended family (e315); friends (3320); general support services (e5750); health professionals (e355)

e345 Strangers
Individuals who are unfamiliar and unrelated, or those who have not yet established a relationship or association, including persons unknown to the individual but who are sharing a life situation with them, such as substitute teachers, co-workers, or care providers.

e350 Domesticated Animals
Animals that provide physical, emotional, or psychological support, such as pets (dogs, cats, birds, fish, etc.) and animals for personal mobility and transportation.
Exclusions: animals (e2201); assets (e165)

e355 Health Professionals
All service providers working within the context of the health system, such as doctors, nurses, physiotherapists, occupational therapists, speech therapists, audiologists, orthotist-prosthetists, and medical social workers.
Exclusions: other professionals (e360)

e360 Other Professionals
All service providers working outside the health system, including lawyers, social workers, teachers, architects, and designers.
Exclusions: health professionals (e355)

e398 Support and Relationships, Other Specified

e399 Support and Relationships, Unspecified

Considerations for Support and Relationships

Therapists use the codes in this chapter to reflect the amount of physical and emotional support that a person or animal provides to the client. Recreational therapists consider the role of support and relationships on life activities and design appropriate interventions to either reduce or eliminate the negative effect of support and relationships on a particular life activity or maintain or further facilitate the positive impact of support and relationships on life activities. Being aware of supports and relationships that facilitate or hinder the level of difficulty with a function, task, or activity is necessary to improve client functioning. It highlights the possible need for training (e.g., training caregiver on how to best provide appropriate physical or emotional support). It also cues the therapist to remind clients that appropriate support increases functioning and health, making it worthwhile to seek out or change support to optimize functioning.

Physical Support

Physical support refers to hands on assistance provided to the client such as helping the client to walk, transfer, dress, or bathe. It also refers to physical support that does not require physical contact with the client (physical support not physical assistance) such as help with carrying shopping bags, providing transportation, picking up tennis balls after play, putting down the kneeler at church, or running errands. Hands on and non-hands on physical support can greatly affect a client's ability to engage in activities. In some cases, physical support can be a facilitator (contributes in a positive manner to the level of difficulty that a client has with an activity) while in other cases it can be a barrier (contributes in a negative manner to the level of difficulty that a client has with an activity). Examples are provided below.

Example (Physical Support as a Facilitator):

A client has moderate difficulty with d7200 Forming Relationships. When in social situations her friend gives her non-verbal cues when she begins to say something that is not appropriate. This support decreases the level of difficulty that the client has with d7200 Forming Relationships to mild difficulty. The scoring of d7200 Forming Relationships that reflects the impact of e320 Friends would look like this: "d7200.1 _ _ 2, E-code: e320+1." The first qualifier of d7200 is the level of difficulty that the client has in her current life situation with all available supports and constraints (performance). The fourth qualifier reflects her level of difficulty in a real-life setting when support is not provided (performance without assistance). The e-code was rated a +1 because it lowered her level of difficulty by one level.

Example (Physical Support as a Barrier):

A client has minimal difficulty with walking outdoors (d465 Moving Around Using Equipment).

His wife is very anxious about him walking outdoors because she is afraid that he will fall. Consequently, she holds tightly onto his arm when they walk outside. This gets in the way of him being able to correctly hold onto the walker and actually increases the level of difficulty that he has with d465 Moving Around Using Equipment to moderate difficulty. The scoring of d465 Moving Around Using Equipment that reflects the impact of e310 Immediate Family would look like this: "d465.2 _ _ 1, E-code: e310.1." The first qualifier of d465 is the level of difficulty that the client has in his current life situation with all available supports and constraints (performance). The fourth qualifier reflects his level of difficulty in his current life situation when support is not provided (performance without assistance). The e-code was rated a .1 because it increased his level of difficulty with the task by one level.

Emotional and Psychological Support

Emotional and psychological support can contribute just as much as physical support to level of difficulty. This includes verbal support such as encouraging words, motivational speeches, and guidance without judgment, as well as non-verbal support such as listening, a smile, a pat on the shoulder, sitting with someone, holding hands, and embracing. Animals (e350) provide emotional and psychological support through unconditional love, physical contact (e.g., petting), and dependency (positive feelings about oneself can occur from being needed and being able to provide needed care).

Example (Emotional and Psychological Support as a Facilitator)

A client is shy in peer group play in the hospital, which limits her level of engagement to severe difficulty. When the therapist provides encouraging words and gently guides her into group play, her level of difficulty with engagement decreases to mild difficulty. The scoring of d9200 Play that reflects the impact e335 Health Professionals would look like this: "d9200. _ 3 1 _, E-code: e355+2." The second qualifier is the level of difficulty that a client has in a standard clinic environment without support from the therapist (capacity without assistance). The third qualifier reflects the client's level of difficulty in a standard clinic environment when support is provided by the therapist (capacity with assistance). The e-code was rated a +2 because it decreased her level of difficulty by two levels.

Example (Emotional and Psychological Support as a Barrier)

A client with a progressive chronic illness is struggling to cope with the rapid changes in her life. Her aunt, although believing that she is being helpful, forces the client to problem solve and account for all of her activities (e.g., How are you going to care for your children? Why are you doing so much?). When her aunt is not at the hospital, her level of difficulty with coping is mild. When her aunt comes to the hospital and offers unwanted input, her level of difficulty with coping becomes severe. The scoring of d2401 Handling Stress that reflects the impact of e315 Extended Family would look like this: "d2401. _ 1 3 _, E-code: e315.2." The second qualifier is the client's current level of difficulty handling stress in a standard clinic environment without support (capacity without assistance). The third qualifier reflects her level of difficulty in a standard clinic environment when support is provided (capacity with assistance). The e-code is rated a .2 because it increases the client's level of difficulty by two levels.

Chapter 4 Attitudes

This chapter is about the attitudes that are the observable consequences of customs, practices, ideologies, values, norms, factual beliefs, and religious beliefs. These attitudes influence individual behavior and social life at all levels, from interpersonal relationships and community associations to political, economic, and legal structures; for example, individual or societal attitudes about a person's trustworthiness and value as a human being that may motivate positive, honorific practices or negative and discriminatory practices (e.g., stigmatizing, stereotyping, and marginalizing or neglect of the person). The attitudes classified are those of people external to the person whose situation is being described. They are not those of the person themselves. The individual attitudes are categorized according to the kinds of relationships listed in Environmental Factors Chapter 3. Values and beliefs are not coded separately from attitudes as they are assumed to be the driving forces behind the attitudes.

e410 Individual Attitudes of Immediate Family Members
General or specific opinions and beliefs of immediate family members about the person or about other matters (e.g., social, political, and economic issues), that influence individual behavior and actions.

e415 Individual Attitudes of Extended Family Members
General or specific opinions and beliefs of extended family members about the person or about other matters (e.g., social, political, and economic issues), that influence individual behavior and actions.

e420 Individual Attitudes of Friends
General or specific opinions and beliefs of friends about the person or about other matters (e.g., social, political, and economic issues), that influence individual behavior and actions.

e425 Individual Attitudes of Acquaintances, Peers, Colleagues, Neighbours, and Community Members
General or specific opinions and beliefs of acquaintances, peers, colleagues, neighbours, and community members about the person or about other matters (e.g., social, political, and economic issues), that influence individual behavior and actions.

e430 Individual Attitudes of People in Positions of Authority
General or specific opinions and beliefs of people in positions of authority about the person or about other matters (e.g., social, political, and economic issues), that influence individual behavior and actions.

e435 Individual Attitudes of People in Subordinate Positions
General or specific opinions and beliefs of people in subordinate positions about the person or about other matters (e.g., social, political, and economic issues), that influence individual behavior and actions.

e440 Individual Attitudes of Personal Care Providers and Personal Assistants
General or specific opinions and beliefs of personal care providers and personal assistants about the person or about other matters (e.g., social, political, and economic issues), that influence individual behavior and actions.

e445 Individual Attitudes of Strangers
General or specific opinions and beliefs of strangers about the person or about other matters (e.g., social, political, and economic issues), that influence individual behavior and actions.

e450 Individual Attitudes of Health Professionals
General or specific opinions and beliefs of health professionals about the person or about other matters (e.g., social, political, and economic issues), that influence individual behavior and actions.

e455 Individual Attitudes of Other Professionals
General or specific opinions and beliefs of other professionals about the person or about other matters (e.g., social, political, and economic issues), that influence individual behavior and actions. [modified from ICF to match group described in e360]

e460 Societal Attitudes
General or specific opinions and beliefs generally held by people of a culture, society, subcultural or other social group about other individuals or about other social, political, and economic issues, that influence group or individual behavior and actions.

e465 Social Norms, Practices, and Ideologies
Customs, practices, rules, and abstract systems of values and normative beliefs (e.g., ideologies, normative world views, and moral philosophies) that arise within social contexts and that affect or create societal and individual practices and behaviors, such as social norms of moral and religious behavior or etiquette; religious doctrine and resulting norms and practices, norms governing rituals or social gathering.

e498 Attitudes, Other Specified

e499 Attitudes, Unspecified

Considerations for
Attitudes

This chapter is about the attitudes of others as they impact the level of impairment or difficulty that a client has with a particular function or activity. It is not about the attitudes of the client. In the code descriptions, the term "attitude" appears to be described as an opinion, belief, or value. However, the chapter description notes that beliefs and values are the driving force of attitudes. Consequently, although titled as "attitudes," this chapter incorporates a broad spectrum of beliefs, values, and opinions from individuals and groups, including customs, practices, rules, abstract systems of values and normative beliefs, moral philosophies, moral and religious behavior or etiquette, religious doctrine and resulting norms and practices, and norms governing rituals or social gatherings. Although it is not reflected in the ICF, there are differences in the meaning of attitudes, beliefs, and values. To understand the differences in the terms, see "Education and Counseling" in the Techniques section.

Looking at the number of individuals and groups listed in this chapter, as well as the descriptions of each code, brings an awareness of the number of people and groups that can facilitate or hinder impairment and task difficulty. Addressing attitudinal barriers has been a long-standing component of recreational therapy practice in both community and treatment settings.

Basic information related to possible sources of attitudinal influence is obtained during the intake and initial assessment. Knowing and synthesizing this information provides the therapist with a springboard for identifying attitudinal influences. This includes the client's:

- *Religion*: Knowing a client's religion and the extent to which the client practices religious beliefs helps the therapist understand the actions and behaviors of the client. It also helps the therapist to identify possible sources of influence (e.g., the Koran, priest, members of fellowship).
- *Culture*: Knowing the culture that the client lives in helps the therapist understand the actions and behaviors of the client. A therapist cannot assume that a client of a particular cultural descent practices that culture. For example, a client may be of Chinese descent, but live an Americanized life. Identifying the client's culture of practice will help the therapist to identify possible sources of influence.
- *Living situation*: Knowing who lives with the client tells the therapist possible people of influence (e.g., spouse).

- *Age*: Knowing the client's age helps the therapist identify who is likely to have the most influence over the client. For children, parental attitudes are more influential than peers. For adolescents, attitudes of classmates are more influential than parents although parental attitudes still weigh in heavily. And in the college years, peers far outweigh parental attitudes.

Health care facilities, although non-discriminatory, often serve a predominant group of people because of their locations (e.g., a high population of African-Americans). Through hands-on experience and their own research, therapists become aware of particular norms related to the population they serve (e.g., religion, culture, and age). For example, African-American women typically have a strong spirituality. Since they are adults, self-esteem theories say that their likely group of influence is similar peers (e.g., other members of the church). Consequently, a therapist who is assigned to work with an African-American adult woman should plan to explore the effect of religion (e465 Social Norms, Practices, and Ideologies) and friends (e420 Individual Attitudes of Friends) on impairments and difficulties.

Therapists additionally explore attitudinal influences by listening closely to verbalizations, observing behavior, and asking exploratory questions to better understand sources of influence. If a source of influence can be identified, then there is a chance that it can be used. For example, a client is out at a mall for integration training with his therapist. He is normally a very talkative and assertive person. The therapist notices that he is avoiding asking questions of people in the community (e.g., "I'll just figure it out myself.", "She looks too busy.", "No, I really just don't want to.") and seems withdrawn. The therapist brings this change in behavior to the attention of the client and prompts the client to analyze the variables influencing his behavior (e.g., "Joe, it seems that you are trying to avoid talking to the people in the stores? This isn't like you. You are usually very talkative and outgoing. Do you notice this? What do you think is causing this change?"). The therapist finds out that the client has had several recent bad experiences with store employees talking down to him. The client says that he would rather just avoid the interactions altogether than feel like a "little kid." This is an example of how e445 Individual Attitudes of Strangers can be a barrier to using assertion and social interactions for getting needs met.

To continue with this example, now that the attitude of influence has been identified, the therapist can seek to decrease the extent of the barrier and/or increase the client's coping skills for the barrier to positively increase functioning. For example, if this had occurred at a particular place frequented by the client, such as the client's health club, it may be helpful for the therapist to educate the employees on proper etiquette when talking to a client who uses a wheelchair. In the mall scenario, education for all employees in the mall is not realistic. Teaching the client coping skills for dealing with the actions of others would provide a better outcome. Possibilities include teaching the client to view behaviors of others from different viewpoints or to use simple, non-aggressive remarks to change the behavior of others (or at least increase their awareness of their behavior).

On the other hand, if attitudes of specific individuals or groups are facilitators, the therapist may find it helpful to incorporate the specific people in the client's treatment to further facilitate progress. For example, if the positive attitude of the client's sister is a facilitator for motivation, then asking her to attend therapy sessions could prove to be beneficial. Highlighting the positive influences of a person or group to the client can also be helpful so that the client and therapist can discuss how to maintain involvement with the person or group for continued benefits. Finally, clients are encouraged to consider the impact of life changes on these resources (e.g., the client may lose the positive influences of neighbors if moves to another neighborhood).

Scoring attitudes as barriers or facilitators to impairment and life activities can be done as shown in these examples.

Example (Attitudes as a Barrier)

In the example also discussed at the beginning of the Environmental Factors section, a 23-year-old client with tetraplegia attends college. When attending classes, he has a personal care attendant with him at all times to assist with overcoming barriers, self-care, and schoolwork. When the client tries to strike up a conversation with other students outside of class, the attendant rushes him along and says, "We don't have time for this." When the attendant is not present (e.g., takes a break to use the bathroom), the client has no difficulty d9205 Socializing. When the attendant is present, the client has complete difficulty socializing. The scoring of d9205 Socializing that reflects the impact of e440 Individual Attitudes of Personal Care Providers and Personal Assistants as a barrier would look like this: "d9205.4 _ _ 0, E-code: e440.4." The first qualifier reflects the level of difficulty that the client has in his current life situations given all available supports and constraints (performance). The fourth qualifier reflects his level of difficulty in his current life situation when assistance is not provided (performance without assistance). The e-code was rated a .4 because it increased his level of difficulty with socializing by four levels.

Example (Attitudes as a Facilitator)

A client's motivation for engagement in therapy is poor (severe impairment). When her sister attends therapy sessions, the client's motivation improves to mild impairment. The scoring of b1301 Motivation to reflect the impact of e410 Individual Attitudes of Immediate Family Members as a facilitator would look like this: "b1301.3, E-code: e410+2." The qualifier reflects the client's average level of impairment for motivation. The e-code is rated a +2 because the positive attitude of the client's sister improves the client's motivation impairment by two levels.

Chapter 5 Services, Systems, and Policies

This chapter is about:
1. Services that provide benefits, structured programmes and operations, in various sectors of society, designed to meet the needs of individuals. (Included in services are the people who provide them). Services may be public, private, or voluntary, and may be established at a local, community, regional, state, provincial, national, or international level by individuals, associations, organizations, agencies, or governments. The goods provided by these services may be general or adapted and specially designed.
2. Systems that are administrative control and organizational mechanisms, and are established by governments at the local, regional, national, and international levels, or by other recognized authorities. These systems are designed to organize, control, and monitor services that provide benefits, structured programmes and operations in various sectors of society.
3. Policies constituted by rules, regulations, conventions, and standards established by governments at the local, regional, national, and international levels, or by other recognized authorities. Policies govern and regulate the systems that organize, control, and monitor services, structured programmes, and operations in various sectors of society.

e510 Services, Systems, and Policies for the Production of Consumer Goods
Services, systems, and policies that govern and provide for the production of objects and products consumed or used by people.
- *e5100 Services for the Production of Consumer Goods*
  Services and programmes for the collection, creation, production, and manufacturing of consumer goods and products, such as for products and technology used for mobility, communication, education, transportation, employment, and housework, including those who provide these services.
  Exclusions: education and training services (e5850); communication services (e5350); Chapter 1: Products and Technology
- *e5101 Systems for the Production of Consumer Goods*
  Administrative control and monitoring mechanisms, such as regional, national, or international organizations that set standards (e.g., International Organization for Standardization) and consumer bodies, that govern the collection, creation, production, and manufacturing of consumer goods and products.
- *e5102 Policies for the Production of Consumer Goods*
  Legislation, regulations, and standards for the collection, creation, production, and manufacturing of consumer goods and products, such as food and drug regulations.
- *e5108 Services, Systems, and Policies for the Production of Consumer Goods, Other Specified*
- *e5109 Services, Systems, and Policies for the Production of Consumer Goods, Unspecified*

Considerations for Production of Consumer Goods

Recreational therapists advocate for services, systems, and policies related to the production of consumer goods (e.g., production of adaptive equipment) mostly from a professional level through support and involvement in professional organizations. If a service, system, or policy is identified as a barrier to engagement in a life activity, recreational therapists provide the client with relevant information (e.g., information on the Americans with Disabilities Act) and then seek out appropriate health professionals who are best to intervene and provide further guidance, such as a social worker or case manager. Consequently, other health professionals will most often use these e-codes as descriptors. If the service barrier is on a local level and pertains directly to engagement in a specific activity, the recreational therapist will commonly intervene (e.g., talking to the paratransit driver to clarify a scheduling policy that is troubling a client).

e515 Architecture and Construction Services, Systems, and Policies
Services, systems, and policies for the design and construction of buildings, public and private.
Exclusions: open space planning services, systems, and policies (e520)
- *e5150 Architecture and Construction Services*
  Services and programmes for design, construction, and maintenance of residential, commercial, industrial, and public buildings, such as house-building, the operationalization of design principles, building codes, regulations, and standards, including those who provide these services.
- *e5151 Architecture and Construction Systems*
  Administrative control and monitoring mechanisms that govern the planning, design, construction, and maintenance of residential, commercial, industrial, and public buildings, such as for implementing and monitoring building codes, construction standards, and fire and life safety standards.
- *e5152 Architecture and Construction Policies*
  Legislation, regulation, and standards that govern the planning, design, construction, and mainte-

nance of residential, commercial, industrial, and public buildings, such as policies on building codes, construction standards, and fire and life safety standards.

- *e5158 Architecture and Construction Services, Systems, and Policies, Other Specified*
- *e5159 Architecture and Construction Services, Systems, and Policies, Unspecified*

Considerations for Architecture and Construction

Recreational therapists advocate for services, systems, and policies related to architecture and construction (e.g., accessibility issues) mostly from a professional level through support and involvement in professional organizations. If a service, system, or policy is identified as a barrier to engagement in a life activity, recreational therapists provide the client with relevant information (e.g., information on the Americans with Disabilities Act) and then seek out appropriate health professionals who are best to intervene and provide further guidance such as social workers and case managers. Consequently, other health professionals will most often use these e-codes as descriptors. If the service barrier is on a local level and pertains directly to engagement in a specific activity, the recreational therapist will commonly intervene (e.g., educating the supervisor at the recreation center about reasonable accommodations under the Americans with Disabilities Act to reduce or eliminate barriers at the center for the client).

e520 Open Space Planning Services, Systems, and Policies
Services, systems, and policies for the planning, design, development, and maintenance of public lands (e.g., parks, forests, shorelines, wetlands) and private lands in the rural, suburban, and urban context.
Exclusions: architecture and construction services, systems, and policies (e515)
- *e5200 Open Space Planning Services*
  Service and programmes aimed at planning, creating, and maintaining urban, suburban, rural, recreational, conservation, and environmental space, meeting and commercial open spaces (plazas, open-air markets), and pedestrian and vehicular transportation routes for intended uses, including those who provide these services.
  Exclusions: products for design, building, and construction for public (e150) and private (e155) use; products of land development (e160)
- *e5201 Open Space Planning Systems*
  Administrative control and monitoring mechanisms, such as for the implementation of local, regional, or national planning acts, design codes, heritage or conservation policies, and environmental planning policy, that govern the planning, design, development, and maintenance of open

space, including rural, suburban, and urban land, parks, conservation areas, and wildlife reserves.
- *e5202 Open Space Planning Policies*
  Legislation, regulations, and standards that govern the planning, design, development, and maintenance of open space, including rural land, suburban land, urban land, parks, conservation areas, and wildlife reserves, such as local, regional, or national planning acts, design codes, heritage or conservation policies, and environmental planning policies.
- *e5208 Open Space Planning Services, Systems, and Policies, Other Specified*
- *e5209 Open Space Planning Services, Systems, and Policies, Unspecified*

Considerations for Open Space Planning

Recreational therapists advocate for services, systems, and policies related to open space planning (e.g., park trails) mostly from a professional level through support and involvement in professional organizations. If a service, system, or policy is identified as a barrier to engagement in a life activity, recreational therapists provide the client with relevant information (e.g., information on the Americans with Disabilities Act) and then seek out appropriate health professionals who are best to intervene and provide the client with further guidance, such as a social worker or case manager. Consequently, other health professionals will most often use these e-codes as descriptors. If the service barrier is on a local level and pertains directly to engagement in a specific activity, the recreational therapist will commonly intervene (e.g., educating the park supervisor about reasonable accommodations under the Americans with Disabilities Act to reduce or eliminate barriers at the park for the client).

e525 Housing Services, Systems, and Policies
Services, systems, and policies for the provision of shelters, dwellings, or lodging for people.
- *e5250 Housing Services*
  Services and programmes aimed at locating, providing, and maintaining houses or shelters for persons to live in, such as estate agencies, housing organizations, shelters for homeless people, including those who provide these services.
- *e5251 Housing Systems*
  Administrative control and monitoring mechanisms that govern housing or sheltering of people, such as systems for implementing and monitoring housing policies.
- *e5252 Housing Policies*
  Legislation, regulations, and standards that govern housing or sheltering of people, such as legislation and policies for determination of eligibility for housing or shelter, policies concern-

ing government involvement in developing and maintaining housing, and policies concerning how and where housing is developed.

- *e5258 Housing Services, Systems, and Policies, Other Specified*
- *e5259 Housing Services, Systems, and Policies, Unspecified*

Considerations for Housing

Recreational therapists do not typically advocate for services, systems, and policies related to housing. However, there may be times when certain groups of recreational therapists are a part of housing advocacy (e.g., recreational therapists who work in the independent living movement). If a service, system, or policy is identified as a barrier to engagement in a life activity, recreational therapists provide the client with relevant information (e.g., information on the Americans with Disabilities Act) and then seek out appropriate health professionals who are best to intervene and provide the client with further guidance (e.g., social worker, case manager). Consequently, other health professionals will most often use these e-codes as descriptors. If the service barrier is on a local level and pertains directly to engagement in a specific activity, the recreational therapist will commonly intervene (e.g., a recreational therapist working in the independent living movement advocates for a handicap parking space in front of the client's apartment by educating the apartment manager about the Americans with Disabilities Act).

e530 Utilities Services, Systems, and Policies
Services, systems, and policies for publicly provided utilities, such as water, fuel, electricity, sanitation, public transportation, and essential services.
Exclusion: civil protection services, systems and policies (e545)

- *e5300 Utilities Services*
  Services and programmes supplying the population as a whole with essential energy (e.g., fuel and electricity), sanitation, water, and other essential services (e.g., emergency repair services) for residential and commercial consumers, including those who provide these services.
- *e5301 Utilities Systems*
  Administrative control and monitoring mechanisms that govern the provision of utilities services, such as health and safety boards and consumer councils.
- *e5302 Utilities Policies*
  Legislation, regulations, and standards that govern the provision of utilities services, such as health and safety standards governing delivery and supply of water and fuel, sanitation practices in communities, and policies for other essential

services and supply during shortages or natural disasters.

- *e5308 Utilities Services, Systems, and Policies, Other Specified*
- *e5309 Utilities Services, Systems, and Policies, Unspecified*

Considerations for Utilities

Recreational therapists do not typically advocate for services, systems, and policies related to utilities. However, there may be times when certain groups of recreational therapists are a part of utility advocacy (e.g., recreational therapists working with a mission program who advocate as a mission group for better drinking water). If a service, system, or policy is identified as a barrier to engagement in a life activity, recreational therapists provide the client with relevant information and then seek out appropriate health professionals who are best to intervene and provide the client with further guidance (e.g., social worker, case manager). Consequently, other health professionals will use these e-codes as descriptors.

e535 Communication Services, Systems, and Policies
Services, systems, and policies for the transmission and exchange of information.

- *e5350 Communication Services*
  Services and programmes aimed at transmitting information by a variety of methods such as telephone, fax, surface and air mail, electronic mail, and other computer-based systems (e.g., telephone relay, teletype, teletext, and internet services), including those who provide these services.
  Exclusion: media services (e5600)
- *e5351 Communication Systems*
  Administrative control and monitoring mechanisms, such as telecommunication regulation authorities and other such bodies, that govern the transmission of information by a variety of methods, including telephone, fax, surface and air mail, electronic mail, and computer-based systems.
- *e5352 Communication Policies*
  Legislation, regulations, and standards that govern the transmission of information by a variety of methods including telephone, fax, post office, electronic mail, and computer-based systems, such as eligibility for access, requirements for a postal address, and standards for provision of telecommunications.
- *e5358 Communication Services, Systems, and Policies, Other Specified*
- *e5359 Communication Services, Systems, and Policies, Unspecified*

Considerations for Communication

Recreational therapists do not typically advocate for services, systems, and policies related to communication. If a service, system, or policy is identified as a barrier to engagement in a life activity, recreational therapists provide the client with relevant information (e.g., information on the Americans with Disabilities Act) and then seek out appropriate health professionals who are best to intervene and provide the client with further guidance, such as a social worker or case manager. Consequently, other health professionals will most often use these e-codes as descriptors. If the service barrier is on a local level and pertains directly to engagement in a specific activity, the recreational therapist will commonly intervene (e.g., a recreational therapist working with a client who is deaf may place a call to the phone company to find out information on policies for setting up a TTY service for the client).

e540 Transportation Services, Systems, and Policies

Services, systems, and policies for enabling people or goods to move or be moved from one location to another.

- *e5400 Transportation Services*
  Services and programmes aimed at moving persons or goods by road, paths, rail, air, or water, by public or private transport, including those who provide these services.
  Exclusion: products for personal mobility and transportation (e115)
- *e5401 Transportation Systems*
  Administrative control and monitoring mechanisms that govern the moving of persons or goods by road, paths, rail, air, or water, such as systems for determining eligibility for operating vehicles and implementation and monitoring of health and safety standards related to use of different types of transportation.
  Exclusion: social security services, systems, and policies (e570)
- *e5402 Transportation Policies*
  Legislation, regulations, and standards that govern the moving of persons or goods by road, paths, rail, air, or water, such as transportation planning acts and policies, policies for the provision and access to public transportation.
- *e5408 Transportation Services, Systems, and Policies, Other Specified*
- *e5409 Transportation Services, Systems, and Policies, Unspecified*

Considerations for Transportation

Recreational therapists do not typically advocate for services, systems, and policies related to transportation. However, there may be times when certain groups of recreational therapists are a part of transportation advocacy (e.g., recreational therapists who work within the independent living movement). If a service, system, or policy is identified as a barrier to engagement in a life activity, recreational therapists provide the client with relevant information (e.g., information on the Americans with Disabilities Act) and then seek out appropriate health professionals who are best to intervene and provide the client with further guidance, such as a social worker or case manager. Consequently, other health professionals will most often use these e-codes as descriptors. If the service barrier is on a local level and pertains directly to engagement in a specific activity, the recreational therapist will commonly intervene (e.g., a recreational therapist working in the independent living movement helps a client make a call to the local paratransit company to find out about its policies for scheduling rides).

e545 Civil Protection Services, Systems, and Policies

Services, systems, and policies aimed at safeguarding people and property.
Exclusion: utilities services, systems, and policies (e530)

- *e5450 Civil Protection Services*
  Services and programmes organized by the community and aimed at safeguarding people and property, such as fire, police, emergency, and ambulance services, including those who provide these services.
- *e5451 Civil Protection Systems*
  Administrative control and monitoring mechanisms that govern the safeguarding of people and property, such as systems by which provision of police, fire, emergency, and ambulance services are organized.
- *e5452 Civil Protection Policies*
  Legislation, regulations, and standards that govern the safeguarding of people and property, such as policies governing provision of police, fire, emergency, and ambulance services.
- *e5458 Civil Protection Services, Systems, and Policies, Other Specified*
- *e5459 Civil Protection Services, Systems, and Policies, Unspecified*

Considerations for Civil Protection

Recreational therapists do not typically advocate for services, systems, and policies related to civil protection. However, there may be times when certain groups of recreational therapists are a part of civil protection advocacy (e.g., recreational therapists who work in the independent living movement). If a service, system, or policy is identified as a barrier to engagement in a life activity, recreational therapists provide the client with relevant information and then seek out appropriate health professionals who are best to intervene and provide the client with further guidance, such as a social worker or case manager. Consequently, other health professionals will most often use these e-codes as descriptors. If the service barrier is on a local level and pertains directly to engagement in a specific activity, the recreational therapist will commonly intervene (e.g., a recreational therapist working in the independent living movement helps a client make a call to the local firehouse to alert the fire company that a person with a disability lives in the house so they can respond appropriately should there ever be a fire in the home).

e550 Legal Services, Systems, and Policies
Services, systems, and policies concerning the legislation and other law of a country.
*   *e5500 Legal Services*
    Services and programmes aimed at providing the authority of the state as defined in law, such as courts, tribunals, and other agencies for hearing and settling civil litigation and criminal trials, attorney representation, services of notaries, mediation, arbitration, and correctional or penal facilities, including those who provide these services.
*   *e5501 Legal Systems*
    Administrative control and monitoring mechanisms that govern the administration of justice, such as systems for implementing and monitoring formal rules (e.g., laws, regulations, customary law, religious law, international laws, and conventions).
*   *e5502 Legal Policies*
    Legislation, regulations, and standards, such as laws, customary law, religious law, international laws and conventions, that govern the administration of justice.
*   *e5508 Legal Services, Systems, and Policies, Other Specified*
*   *e5509 Legal Services, Systems, and Policies, Unspecified*

Considerations for Legal

Recreational therapists do not typically advocate for services, systems, and policies related to legal services. If a service, system, or policy is identified as a barrier to engagement in a life activity, recreational therapists provide the client with relevant information (e.g., information on the Americans with Disabilities Act) and then seek out appropriate health professionals who are best to intervene and provide the client with further guidance, such as a social worker or case manager. Consequently, other health

professionals will most often use these e-codes as descriptors. If the service barrier is on a local level and pertains directly to engagement in a specific activity, the recreational therapist will commonly intervene (e.g., a recreational therapist helps a client to process a parking placard application and then takes the client to the hospital notary to get it notarized).

e555 Associations and Organizational Services, Systems, and Policies
Services, systems, and policies relating to groups of people who have joined together in the pursuit of common, noncommercial interests, often with an associated membership structure.
*   *e5550 Associations and Organizational Services*
    Services and programmes provided by people who have jointed together in the pursuit of common, noncommercial interests with people who have the same interests, where the provision of such services may be tied to membership, such as associations and organizations providing recreation and leisure, sporting, cultural, religious, and mutual aid services.
*   *e5551 Associations and Organizational Systems*
    Administrative control and monitoring mechanisms that govern the relationships and activities of people coming together with common noncommercial interests and the establishment and conduct of associations and organizations such as mutual aid organizations, recreational and leisure organizations, cultural and religious associations, and not-for-profit organizations.
*   *e5552 Associations and Organizational Policies*
    Legislations, regulations, and standards that govern the relationships and activities of people coming together with common noncommercial interests, such as policies that govern the establishment and conduct of associations and organizations, including mutual aid organizations, recreational and leisure organizations, cultural and religious associations, and not-for-profit organizations.
*   *e5558 Associations and Organizational Services, Systems, and Policies, Other Specified*
*   *e5559 Associations and Organizational Services, Systems, and Policies, Unspecified*

Considerations for Associations and Organizations

Recreational therapists advocate for services, systems, and policies related to associations and organizational services (e.g., inclusion of people with disabilities into mainstream recreation associations) mostly from a professional level through support and involvement in professional organizations. If a service, system, or policy is identified as a barrier to engagement in a life activity, recreational therapists provide the client with relevant information (e.g., information on the Americans with Disabilities Act) and then seek out appropriate health professionals who are best to intervene and provide the client with further guidance, such as a social worker or case manager. Consequently, other health professionals will most often use these e-codes as descriptors. If the service barrier is on a local level and pertains directly to engagement in a specific activity, the recreational therapist will commonly intervene (e.g., educating the priest at the church about reasonable accommodations for a client to be able to participate at Mass).

e560 Media Services, Systems, and Policies

Services, systems, and policies for the provision of mass communication through radio, television, newspapers, and internet.

- *e5600 Media Services*
  Services and programmes aimed at providing mass communication, such as radio, television, closed captioning services, press reporting services, newspapers, Braille services, and computer-based mass communication (world wide web, internet), including those who provide these services.
  Exclusion: communication services (e5350)

- *e5601 Media Systems*
  Administrative control and monitoring mechanisms that govern the provision of news and information to the general public, such as standards that govern the content, distribution, dissemination, access to, and methods of communicating via radio, television, press reporting services, newspapers, and computer-based mass communication (world wide web, internet).
  Inclusions: requirements to provide closed captions on television, Braille versions of newspapers or other publications, and teletext radio transmissions.
  Exclusion: communication systems (e5351)

- *e5602 Media Policies*
  Legislation, regulations, and standards that govern the provision of news and information to the general public, such as policies that govern the content, distribution, dissemination, access to, and methods of communicating via radio, television, press reporting services, newspapers, and computer-based mass communication (world wide web, internet).
  Exclusion: communication policies (e5352)

- *e5608 Media Services, Systems, and Policies, Other Specified*

- *e5609 Media Services, Systems, and Policies, Unspecified*

Considerations for Media

Recreational therapists do not typically advocate for services, systems, and policies related to media. If a service, system, or policy is identified as a barrier to engagement in a life activity, recreational therapists provide the client with relevant information and then seek out appropriate health professionals who are best to intervene and provide the client with further guidance, such as a social worker or case manager. Consequently, other health professionals will most often use these e-codes as descriptors. If the service barrier is on a local level and pertains directly to engagement in a specific activity, the recreational therapist will commonly intervene (e.g., a recreational therapist working in the independent living movement helps a client make a call to the local newspaper to find out if a Braille copy is available).

e565 Economic Services, Systems, and Policies

Services, systems, and policies related to the overall system of production, distribution, consumption, and use of good and services.
Exclusion: social security services, systems, and policies (e570)

- *e5650 Economic Services*
  Services and programmes aimed at the overall production, distribution, consumption, and use of goods and services, such as the private commercial sector (e.g., businesses, corporations, private for-profit ventures), the public sector (e.g., public, commercial services such as cooperatives and corporations), financial organizations (e.g., banks and insurance services), including those who provide these services.
  Exclusions: utilities services (e5300); labour and employment services (e5900)

- *e5651 Economic Systems*
  Administrative control and monitoring mechanisms that govern the production, distribution, consumption, and use of goods and services, such as systems for implementing and monitoring economic policies.
  Exclusions: utilities systems (e5301); labour and employment systems (e5901)

- *e5652 Economic Policies*
  Legislation, regulations, and standards that govern the production, distribution, consumption, and use of goods and services, such as economic doctrines adopted and implemented by governments.
  Exclusions: utilities policies (e5302); labour and employment policies (e5902)

- *e5658 Economic Services, Systems, and Policies, Other Specified*

- *e5659 Economic Services, Systems, and Policies, Unspecified*

Considerations for
Economics

Recreational therapists do not typically advocate for services, systems, and policies related to economic services. If a service, system, or policy is identified as a barrier to engagement in a life activity, recreational therapists provide the client with relevant information (e.g., information on the Americans with Disabilities Act) and then seek out appropriate health professionals who are best to intervene and provide the client with further guidance, such as a social worker or case manager. Consequently, other health professionals will most often use these e-codes as descriptors. If the service barrier is on a local level and pertains directly to engagement in a specific activity, the recreational therapist will commonly intervene (e.g., A client who is out with a recreational therapist for integration training has his money access card eaten by the ATM machine. The recreational therapist assists the client in going to the bank and finding out what happened to the card and what procedures need to be followed to have it returned.).

e570 Social Security Services, Systems, and Policies
Services, systems, and policies aimed at providing income support to people who, because of age, poverty, unemployment, health condition, or disability, require public assistance that is funded either by general tax revenues or contributory schemes.
Exclusion: economic services, systems, and policies (e565)
- *e5700 Social Security Services*
  Services and programmes aimed at providing income support to people who, because of age, poverty, unemployment, heath condition, or disability, require public assistance that is funded either by general tax revenues or contributory schemes, such as services for determining eligibility, delivering or distributing assistance payments for the following types of programmes: social assistance programmes (e.g., non-contributory welfare, poverty, or other needs-based compensation), social insurance programmes (e.g., contributory accident or unemployment insurance), and disability and related pension schemes (e.g., income replacement), including those who provide these services.
  Exclusions: health services (e5800)
- *e5701 Social Security Systems*
  Administrative control and monitoring mechanisms that govern the programmes and schemes that provide income support to people who, because of age, poverty, unemployment, health condition, or disability, require public assistance, such as systems for implementation of rules and regulations governing the eligibility for social assistance, welfare, unemployment insurance payments, pensions, and disability benefits.

- *e5702 Social Security Policies*
  Legislation, regulations, and standards that govern the programmes and schemes that provide income support to people who, because of age, poverty, unemployment, health condition, or disability, require public assistance, such as legislation and regulations governing the eligibility for social assistance, welfare, unemployment insurance payments, disability, and related pensions and disability benefits.
- *e5708 Social Security Services, Systems, and Policies, Other Specified*
- *e5709 Social Security Services, Systems, and Policies, Unspecified*

Considerations for
Social Security

Recreational therapists do not typically advocate for services, systems, and policies related to social security. If a service, system, or policy is identified as a barrier to engagement in a life activity, recreational therapists provide the client with relevant information and then seek out appropriate health professionals who are best to intervene and provide the client with further guidance, such as a social worker or case manager. Consequently, other health professionals will most often use these e-codes as descriptors.

e575 General Social Support Services, Systems, and Policies
Services, systems, and policies aimed at providing support to those requiring assistance in areas such as shopping, housework, transport, self-care, and care for others, in order to function more fully in society.
Exclusions: personal care providers and personal care assistants (e340); social security services, systems, and policies (e570); health services, systems, and policies (e580)
- *e5750 General Social Support Services*
  Services and programmes aimed at providing social support to people who, because of age, poverty, unemployment, health condition, or disability, require public assistance in the areas of shopping, housework, transport, self-care, and care of others, in order to function more fully in society.
- *e5751 General Social Support Systems*
  Administrative control and monitoring mechanisms that govern the programmes and schemes that provide social support to people who, because of age, poverty, unemployment, health condition, or disability, require such support, including systems for the implementation of rules and regulations governing eligibility for social support services and the provision of these services.
- *e5752 General Social Support Policies*
  Legislation, regulations, and standards that govern the programmes and schemes that provide social support to people who, because of

age, poverty, unemployment, health condition, or disability, require such support, including legislation and regulations governing eligibility for social support.

- *e5758 General Social Support Services, Systems, and Policies, Other Specified*
- *e5759 General Social Support Services, Systems, and Policies, Unspecified*

Considerations for General Social Support

Recreational therapists advocate for services, systems, and policies related to general social support (e.g., support services for recreational activities) mostly from a professional level (e.g., through support and involvement in professional organizations). If a service, system, or policy is identified as a barrier to engagement in a life activity, recreational therapists provide the client with relevant information (e.g., information on the Americans with Disabilities Act) and then seek out appropriate health professionals who are best to intervene and provide the client with further guidance, such as a social worker or case manager. Consequently, other health professionals will most often use these e-codes as descriptors. If the service barrier is on a local level and pertains directly to engagement in a specific activity, the recreational therapist will commonly intervene (e.g., educating the supervisor at the supermarket about reasonable accommodations under the Americans with Disabilities Act to reduce or eliminate barriers at the supermarket for the client).

e580 Health Services, Systems, and Policies
Services, systems, and policies for preventing and treating health problems, providing medical rehabilitation, and promoting a healthy lifestyle.
Exclusion: general social support services, systems, and policies (e575)
- *e5800 Health Services*
  Services and programmes at a local, community, regional, state, or national level, aimed at delivering interventions to individuals for their physical, psychological, and social well-being, such as health promotion and disease prevention services, primary care services, acute care, rehabilitation, and long-term care services; services that are publicly or privately funded, delivered on a short-term, long-term, periodic, or one time basis, in a variety of service settings such as community, home-based, school, and work settings, general hospitals, specialty hospitals, clinics, and residential and non-residential care facilities, including those who provide these services.
- *e5801 Health Systems*
  Administrative control and monitoring mechanisms that govern the range of services provided to individuals for their physical, psychological,

and social well-being, in a variety of settings including community, home-based, school, and work settings, general hospitals, specialty hospitals, clinics, and residential and non-residential care facilities, such as systems for implementing regulations and standards that determine eligibility for services, provision of devices, assistive technology, or other adapted equipment, and legislation such as health acts that govern features of a health system such as accessibility, universality, portability, public funding, and comprehensiveness.
- *e5802 Health Policies*
  Legislation, regulations, and standards that govern the range of services provided to individuals for their physical, psychological, and social well-being, in a variety of settings including community, home-based, school, and work settings, general hospitals, specialty hospitals, clinics, and residential and non-residential care facilities, such as policies and standards that determine eligibility for services, provision of devices, assistive technology, or other adapted equipment, and legislation such as health acts that govern features of a health systems such as accessibility, universality, portability, public funding, and comprehensiveness.
- *e5808 Health Services, Systems, and Policies, Other Specified*
- *e5809 Health Services, Systems, and Policies, Unspecified*

Considerations for Health

Recreational therapists advocate for services, systems, and policies related to health (e.g., provision of recreational therapy services and programs) at their worksite and through professional organizations (e.g., American Therapeutic Recreation Association, National Therapeutic Recreation Society). If a service, system, or policy is identified as a barrier to engagement in a life activity, recreational therapists provide the client with relevant information (e.g., information on the Americans with Disabilities Act) and then seek out appropriate health professionals who are best to intervene and provide the client with further guidance (e.g., health insurance company). This code poses an interesting situation for therapists who identify residual needs for a client that are not addressed because of a health service, system, or policy (e.g., client would benefit from outpatient transportation training but the funding source does not cover the service). In our current health system, there is a danger of using the codes in this category too liberally because all health care professionals usually want more for their clients than is available. Therapists must be careful to not use this code routinely as a way to advocate for their profession by

1. judiciously choosing these codes as barriers only when well-informed about the service, policy, or system and 2. evaluating the total health care services being received by the client (e.g., recreational therapy may not be covered by the health care insurance company for outpatient transportation training while occupational therapy is covered for outpatient transportation training). In this example, the client is receiving the training (the codes are not profession-specific but rather holistic).

If the therapist is well informed about the specific service, policy, or system that is a barrier and the client is not able to receive the service from any other health care professional, the therapist can use the codes in this category to reflect the specific barrier. For example, a client with a stroke desires to return to playing golf. He used to play golf five times a week as a primary source of exercise for health promotion. He currently has moderate difficulty overall with the game. At this level of difficulty, the client refuses to return to the game of golf. He has no other forms of physical activity in his current lifestyle. In the clinical judgment of the therapist, the client can progress to no difficulty with individual outpatient therapy on the golf course along with support from his fellow players. The client states that he would return to the game of golf if he could achieve this level of playing. The therapist petitions for outpatient recreational therapy services and it is denied by the health insurance company. The therapist speaks with the occupational and physical therapists to review whether their outpatient therapy recommendations might include the recreational therapy objectives for golf. It is determined that it is unrealistic for the other therapies to absorb the golf objectives. In this case, the therapist could score e5801 Health Systems as a barrier to d9201 Sports and possibly d5701 Maintaining Diet and Fitness.

e585 Education and Training Services, Systems, and Policies

Services, systems, and policies for the acquisition, maintenance, and improvement of knowledge, expertise, and vocational or artistic skills. See UNESCO's International Standards Classification of Education (ISCED-1997).

- **e5850 Education and Training Services**
  Services and programmes concerned with education and the acquisition, maintenance, and improvement of knowledge, expertise, and vocational or artistic skills, such as those provided for different levels of education (e.g., preschool, primary school, secondary school, post-secondary institutions, professional programmes, training and skills programmes, apprenticeships, and continuing education), including those who provide these services.

- **e5851 Education and Training Systems**
  Administrative control and monitoring mechanisms that govern the delivery of education programmes, such as systems for the implementation of policies and standards that determine eligibility for public or private education and special needs-based programmes; local, regional, or national boards of education or other authoritative bodies that govern features of the education systems, including curricula, size of classes, numbers of schools in a region, fees and subsidies, special meal programmes, and after-school care services.

- **e5852 Education and Training Policies**
  Legislation, regulations, and standards that govern the delivery of education programmes, such as policies and standards that determine eligibility for public or private education and special needs-based programmes, and dictate the structure of local, regional, or national boards of education or other authoritative bodies that govern features of the education system, including curricula, size of classes, numbers of schools in a region, fees and subsidies, special meal programmes, and after school care services.

- **e5858 Education and Training Services, Systems, and Policies, Other Specified**

- **e5859 Education and Training Services, Systems, and Policies, Unspecified**

Considerations for Education and Training

Recreational therapists do not typically advocate for services, systems, and policies related to education. However, there may be times when certain groups of recreational therapists are a part of education advocacy, such as recreational therapists who work in the school system. If a service, system, or policy is identified as a barrier to engagement in a life activity, recreational therapists provide the client with relevant information (e.g., information on the Individualized Education Plans) and then seek out appropriate professionals who are best to intervene and provide the client with further guidance (e.g., teacher, social worker, case manager). Consequently, other professionals will most often use these e-codes as descriptors. If the service barrier is on a local level and pertains directly to engagement in a specific activity, the recreational therapist will commonly intervene (e.g., a recreational therapist working in the school system advocates for a student to receive recreational therapy services).

e590 Labour and Employment Services, Systems, and Policies

Services, systems, and policies related to finding suitable work for persons who are unemployed or looking for different work, or to support individuals already employed who are seeking promotion.

Exclusion: economic services, systems, and policies (e565)

- *e5900 Labour and Employment Services*
  Services and programmes provide by local, regional, or national governments, or private organizations to find suitable work for persons who are unemployed or looking for different work, or to support individuals already employed, such as services of employment search and preparation, reemployment, job placement, outplacement, vocational follow-up, occupational health and safety services, and work environment services (e.g., ergonomics, human resources and personnel management services, labour relations services, professional association services), including those who provide these services.

- *e5901 Labour and Employment Systems*
  Administrative control and monitoring mechanisms that govern the distribution of occupations and other forms of remunerative work in the economy, such as systems for implementing policies and standards for employment creation, employment security, designated and competitive employment, labour standards and law, and trade unions.

- *e5902 Labour and Employment Policies*
  Legislation, regulations, and standards that govern the distribution of occupations and other forms of remunerative work in the economy, such as standards and policies for employment creation, employment security, designated and competitive employment, labour standards and law, and trade unions.

- *e5908 Labour and Employment Services, Systems, and Policies, Other Specified*

- *e5909 Labour and Employment Services, Systems, and Policies, Unspecified*

Considerations for Labor and Employment

Recreational therapists do not typically advocate for services, systems, and policies related to labor and employment. However, there may be times when certain groups of recreational therapists are a part of education advocacy (e.g., recreational therapists who work in the independent living movement). If a service, system, or policy is identified as a barrier to engagement in a life activity, recreational therapists provide the client with relevant information (e.g., information on the Americans with Disabilities Act) and then seek out appropriate health professionals who are best to intervene and provide the client with further guidance, such as a social worker or case manager. Consequently, it will be other health professionals who will usually use these e-codes as descriptors. If the service barrier is on a local level and pertains directly to engagement in a specific activity, the recreational therapist will commonly intervene (e.g., a recreational therapist working in the

independent living movement assists the client in talking with an employer about job responsibilities and abilities).

e595 Political Services, Systems, and Policies
Services, systems, and policies related to voting, elections, and governance of countries, regions, and communities, as well as international political organizations.

- *e5950 Political Services*
  Services and structures such as local, regional, and national governments, international organizations, and the people who are elected or nominated to positions within these structures, such as the United Nations, European Union, governments, regional authorities, local village authorities, traditional leaders.

- *e5951 Political Systems*
  Structures and related operations that organize political and economic power in a society, such as executive and legislative branches of government, and the constitutional or other legal sources from which they derive their authority, such as political organizational doctrine, constitutions, agencies of executive and legislative branches of government, the military.

- *e5952 Political Policies*
  Laws and policies formulated and enforced through political systems that govern the operation of the political system, such as policies governing election campaigns, registration of political parties, voting, and members in international political organizations, including treaties, constitutional and other law governing legislation and regulation.

- *e5958 Political Services, Systems, and Policies, Other Specified*

- *e5959 Political Services, Systems, and Policies, Unspecified*

Considerations for Politics

Recreational therapists do not typically advocate for services, systems, and policies related to political policy. If a service, system, or policy is identified as a barrier to engagement in a life activity, recreational therapists provide the client with relevant information (e.g., information on voting rights for a person in a long-term care facility) and then seek out appropriate health professionals who are best to intervene and provide the client with further guidance, such as a social worker or case manager. Consequently, it will be other health professionals who will usually use these e-codes as descriptors.

e598 Services, Systems, and Policies, Other Specified

e599 Services, Systems, and Policies, Unspecified

Section 4: Recreational Therapy Treatment Issues

This section describes recreational therapy equipment, concepts, techniques, and assessments discussed in earlier parts of the book.

Equipment

This section looks at the equipment used by recreational therapists and their clients. Each piece of equipment used by recreational therapists includes a description, weight, fitting, authorization requirements, use, benefits, design challenges, cost, and primary treatment direction. Other equipment is described so that recreational therapists can understand some of the issues involved with its use. Places to buy some of this equipment are given in the "Equipment Resources" topic in this section.

Many of the devices included in this section are adaptive devices. Recreational therapists are eligible to become Assistive Technology Practitioners (ATP). Go to www.resna.org for a listing of each state's initiative project, information on how to become a certified ATP, and schedules of workshops discussing adaptive equipment.

There are other places in the Handbook that have more information on equipment. They include:

- *Sexuality*: b640 Sexual Functions.
- *Urinary devices*: b620 Urination Functions
- *Low vision and hearing impairment*: b2 Sensory Functions and Pain. Information on magnifiers and lighting can be found in the Equipment section.
- *Communication*: b3 Voice and Speech Functions and e125 Products and Technology for Communication.
- *Mouthstick*: "Computer" and "Card Playing" in this section.
- *Headpointer*: "Computer" in this section.
- *Typing aid*: "Computer" in this section.
- *Driving*: d470-d489 Moving Around Using Transportation.

Bathing Aids

Equipment commonly used for bathing includes a handheld shower hose, a long-handled sponge, a tub chair or bench, tub grab bars, a wash mitt, and a wheeled shower chair.

Handheld shower hose: A handheld shower hose is a five-foot long hose that connects from the shower arm to the shower sprayer. The shower sprayer at the end of the hose can be clipped to the shower arm so that it can be placed in the usual shower sprayer position or it can be unclipped and held by hand. Separate mounting brackets can be purchased and attached to different places on the wall giving the client choices on where to stabilize and position the shower sprayer for bathing.

Long-handled sponge: A long-handled sponge has a plastic or wooden handle that is eight inches to 27" long with a sponge on the end. Plastic handles can be heated with a heat gun and reshaped.

Tub chair and bench: A tub chair or tub bench is a non-slip seat that is set inside a tub or stall shower. Some have a back support (a tub chair looks like a chair) and others do not (a tub bench has a single bench seat without a back). Both tub chairs and tub benches come in extended models. Extended tub chairs and benches have a longer bench seat that goes over the side of the tub. Instead of all four legs being inside the tub, two legs are inside the tub and two legs are outside the tub. Tub chairs and benches are height adjustable and some have molded accessories (e.g., places for soap, a handheld shower hose, or a bottle of shampoo).

Tub grab bars: Tub grab bars are typically made out of steel and are chrome plated or nylon coated. They attach onto the tub wall or the outside edge of the tub.

Wash mitt: A wash mitt looks like a mitten. It is made out of terrycloth with a Velcro strap that goes around the wrist to hold it on the hand.

Wheeled shower chair: A wheeled shower chair looks like a standard chair (four legs, a seat, armrest, back). It is usually made out of tubular PVC and has small caster wheels on the base of each chair leg. Wheels are lockable. Some chairs have a seatbelt.

Weight

A handheld shower hose weighs about three pounds. A long-handled sponge and wash mitt weigh a few ounces. Tub benches weigh an average of 12 pounds. Tub grab bars vary depending on the length of the bar. They usually weigh less than three pounds. A wheeled shower chair is about 20 pounds.

Fitting

Handheld shower hose: NA

Long-handled sponge: Long-handled sponges are reshaped using a heat gun to obtain the best bend or curve so the client can access hard-to-reach body areas (e.g., back, feet).

Tub chair and bench: A tub chair or bench is used for clients when there are bathing safety concerns. These concerns include the inability to stand for the required amount of time to properly shower (poor standing endurance) and instability on a wet surface (poor balance or coordination). A client who has good unsupported sitting endurance, strength, and balance may need only a tub bench (no back support). A client who is not able to maintain unsupported sitting because of endurance, strength, or balance will need a tub chair with back support. Therapists prescribing a tub bench or chair must consider the client's lowest level of functioning on any given day to help choose the right piece of equipment (e.g., in the morning the client may have good unsupported sitting endurance but in the evening she does not). To use a standard tub bench or chair the client must be able to step into and out of the tub. Clients who have difficulty stepping over the edge of the tub and who need assistance transferring to and from the tub chair or bench would benefit from an extended tub bench. The extended tub bench allows the client to sit on the extension and lift one leg at a time into the tub while in a seated position.

Tub grab bars: Tub grab bars that attach onto the edge of the tub are not adjustable in height, but therapists determine where to place the bar along the edge of the tub. The placement of the bar depends on how the client is going to use it. If the client is going to stand in the tub for a shower and is going to use the bar to help step in and out of the tub, then it would be best placed towards the front of the tub to allow enough room to swing the legs over the edge of the tub. If the client plans on sitting in the tub and needs assistance lowering and standing up from the tub, then the bar is best placed slightly past the middle of the tub toward the back. This will align with the placement of the client's hands when in a seated position in the tub so that the bar can provide effective support for standing and lowering. Tub bars that attach to the tub wall are used for standing support (hold onto when standing in the shower) and/or help to sit in and stand up out of the tub or to sit or stand from the tub bench. Depending on the planned use of the grab bars, they are placed differently. If the client plans to use the bar for support when standing in the shower, the bar is best placed at the wrist level of the client in a horizontal position. If the client plans to use the bar for support to lower and stand up from a seated position in the tub the bar is best centered and placed at the base of the wall right above the edge of the tub. An additional vertical bar may also prove to be helpful for pulling up to a standing position. If the client plans on using the bar for assistance to sit and stand from a seated position in the tub, as well as support for standing, it is best placed on an angle (about 45°) with it pointing upward towards the showerhead. This will allow the client a variety of hand placements.

Wheeled Shower Chair: NA
Wash Mitt: NA

Authorization

This equipment is commonly prescribed by occupational therapists. Recreational therapists who perceive a need for such equipment discuss it with the client's primary occupational therapist.

Use

Handheld shower hose: One end of the hose screws onto the shower arm and the other end of the hose screws onto the shower sprayer. The shower sprayer can be clipped back up to the shower arm or it can be left hanging down from the shower arm. A client holds the shower sprayer when it is unclipped from the shower arm to rinse body areas. This is done from a standing or seated position. If additional mounting clips are attached to the tub wall (other than the clip on the shower arm), the shower sprayer can be hung (clipped) at additional places. This is particularly helpful for the client who is using a tub chair or bench. An additional mounting clip attached to the front or side wall of the tub will provide the client with an easy place to clip the shower sprayer when not in use (e.g., washing with a washcloth, shampooing hair). It can also be an additional mounting location to hold and angle the water spray for effective bathing. For example, if a client has paralysis of one arm, the client could clip the shower sprayer to a mount on the front wall so that it sprays the client's midsection. This would allow the client to lift the paralyzed arm with the non-affected arm to rinse under the paralyzed arm.

Long-handled sponge: The sponge is used to wash parts of the body that the client cannot reach without assistance or adaptive devices.

Tub bench and chair: If it is a standard tub bench or chair, all four legs are placed inside the tub. If it is an extended tub bench or chair, two legs are placed inside the tub and two legs are placed outside of the

tub. The tub bench faces the front of the tub so the client can access the faucets, drain, and shower sprayer. It should be slightly back from center to allow sufficient room to safely transfer on and off the seat. To use a standard tub bench or chair, the client steps into the tub and sits down on it. To use an extended tub bench, the client transfers onto the extended area of the tub bench that extends over the tub edge. The client then lifts one leg at a time into the tub and slides all the way over to the other side of the seat. It can be difficult to "slide" across a tub bench when undressed. Clients are instructed to do small buttock lifts to slide across the seat. It can also be helpful to place a towel on the seat.

Tub grab bars: See Fitting

Wheeled shower chair: A wheeled shower chair is used for clients who do not have good enough trunk control to sit on a tub bench (e.g., tetraplegia). The chair is placed inside a stall shower. It is not something that comes in and out of the shower stall easily unless the shower stall doesn't have a pan (no edges around it). The wheels are locked prior to transferring onto it. Once seated in the shower chair, the client can begin bathing. If there isn't a pan, the client can be wheeled out of the shower area to another area in the bathroom or adjoining room to dress or perform further tasks (e.g., toileting). Some shower chairs have a commode built into the bottom of the seat so that the client can do his/her bowel program while seated in the shower chair. For example, clients with a high-level spinal cord injury often find it helpful to do their bowel routine in conjunction with their shower. The suppository is inserted prior or during the shower. While showering the suppository begins to work and bowels are released. Being in the shower allows the client to fully bathe the perineal area after the bowels are released, often allowing this process to be accomplished independently rather than needing extended clean up assistance.

Wash mitt: See Description.

Benefits

Equipment for bathing increases safety and independence with the task of bathing.

Design Challenges

There are a variety of designs to meet the individual needs of clients. In some cases, therapists specially fabricate a piece of equipment or modify an existing piece of equipment.

Costs

A handheld shower hose costs about $15.00-$20.00. A long-handled sponge costs about $3.00-$7.00. The average cost of a tub bench or chair is $60.00. Tub grab bars that attach to the tub edge typically range from $50.00 to $75.00. A wheeled shower chair ranges from $200.00 to $300.00. A wash mitt costs about $6.00.

Treatment Direction

Recreational therapists contribute to discussions about bathing equipment needs of the client, especially as it pertains to transferring bathing skills into a community environment (e.g., showering at the pool or gym). Recreational therapists also teach clients how to use bathing equipment in a community setting (e.g., YMCA) and make bathing equipment recommendations as they relate to participation in community activities (e.g., being able to rinse off before entering a pool).

Canes

Canes as walking sticks are the most commonly used mobility device (School of Public Health, 2004). Canes have four common components: 1. the handle, 2. the shaft, 3. the base, and 4. the tip.

Cane Handles

There are many options for cane handles. The handle is the interface between the client and the walking aid so it needs to meet the needs of the client based on his/her abilities and impairments and the activities selected. To increase comfort, cane handles may be covered with foam or other materials that pad the handle. All handles should be evaluated for ease of cleaning. The primary types of handles are

- *Ball-topped handle*: a sphere located on top of the shaft of the cane. This type of cane places too much pressure on the palm of the hand and forces the wrist into a dorsiflexion position. This cane is not a good choice to use when the client must support a lot of weight on the cane or use the cane for extended periods.
- *Crooked handle*: A semicircular top formation of the cane. This type of cane is the one that is typically pictured in older movies and books. Because of the shape of the curved handle, the little finger and index finger must help grasp the cane in a partially flexed position while the two center fingers are flexed more. This is an unnatural position for the hand and can increase fine motor fatigue.
- *Pistol handle*: A pistol handle is a cane grip that extends from the cane shaft at approximately a 90° angle. This type of handle is especially good for clients with weak grasps. Research has found that 85% of cane users find pistol handles to be more comfortable than crook-handles (Wylde, 2004). Pistol handles are also called "T" handles. Ergonomically this type of handle puts most of the pressure on the centerline of the palm, increasing pain, callusing, and nerve compression.

Cane Shaft

- A number of types of materials are used for the shaft of a cane. In most cases, the material used in the shaft decides the weight of the cane. (The exception is with quad bases.)
- Aluminum shafts are usually the lightest with wood shafts being heavier. One of the added benefits of aluminum shafts is that many of them have height adjustment buttons to raise and lower the height of the cane. This not only allows a cane purchased at a local drug store to be fitted to a client, but it also allows the length of the cane to be adjusted based on the type of activity or the height of shoe heels.
- Some cane shafts are foldable. Folding canes are made of many different types of material including wood.
- There are two common accessories applied to cane shafts: wrist straps and cane holders. Wrist straps are straps clipped onto the shaft just below the handle. With the wrist strap around the wrist a person may "drop" the cane to use two hands for an activity and always have the cane close by. A cane holder is not actually a holder but a short 90° extension on the shaft (located below the handle) that can be used to lean the cane against a table or wall without the cane falling over.

Bases

Canes have one-point or four-point bases of support that are located at the bottom of the cane shaft. Four-point bases provide more stability than single base canes. Some clients may use single point bases for many activities and choose to use quad bases for activities that challenge the client's balance. Standard aluminum canes with adjustable buttons allow the client to interchange a one-point base with a quad (four-point) base.

- *Single bases*: Single base canes are also referred to as single point canes (SPC). Single point canes are effective in resolving minor instability and balance difficulties, as well as preventing falls. Minor instability and balance difficulties are common in the aging process.
- *Four-point bases*: Four-point bases are referred to as quad canes. They provide increased stability compared to a single base cane. There are two types of quad canes, small-base quad canes (SBQC), also called narrow-base quad canes (NBQC), and wide-base quad canes (WBQC), also called large-base quad canes (LBQC). A SBQC has a smaller base, thus challenging the client's balance more than a LBQC. The shaft of the cane is to the side of the base (it is not centered on the base). Therefore, the bases on the quad cane are right and left sensitive. The base must jut out away from the client. The base of a quad cane is adjustable. It can rotate to the left or the right so that it can be properly adjusted for the client.

Cane Tips

Cane tips are the unit that makes contact with the ground. They are selected based on the type of traction needed. There are many choices and the selection centers on the client's abilities and the activity.

- Most cane tips are removable allowing replacement of worn tips or the placement of specialized tips. An easy way to remove an old cane tip is to place it in a slightly closed door and twist and pull the cane.
- Icy conditions often cause clients to be homebound. Canes with rubber tips do not provide a good base of support on icy or snow-covered surfaces. Specialized ice attachments are available, most having retractable spikes so that the cane may be used in an icy parking lot and (with the spikes retracted) inside also.
- A tripod base is available that fits most canes. A tripod tip is a rubber tip with three "toes" extending two inches from the bottom of the tip with rubber "webs" between the toes. The toes are usually located at four, eight and twelve o'clock (if placed on a clock face). Tripod tips are helpful for walking on soft surfaces, such as dirt trails or lawns. Canes can stand upright without being held or propped against something with a tripod base.
- Clients should have extra tips available, especially while traveling, as smaller towns may not have places to purchase new tips.
- Cane tips must be replaced when they are worn because they will not grip the surface well, thus increasing the risk of falling. Worn cane tips will also make the cane shorter, therefore being a less effective support.

While canes increase independence, they also can make fashion statements offering clients the opportunity to express personal flair. Canes are offered in a variety of woods, metal, and modern materials. Some are made of multiple elements. For example, the handle may be made of brass, while the shaft is made of plastic designed to look like a plaid fabric. Wooden canes can easily be painted and shellacked to meet the individual's style (sand off the original shellac first so that new paint sticks).

Weight

Varies. The rule of thumb is to ensure that the cane selected for use is light enough that the client will not have difficulty lifting the device even when s/he is experiencing mild fatigue and that it is strong enough to support the weight of the client. Therapists also consider the weight of the cane in relation to its

use. For example, a client who was living in a tough neighborhood feared being attacked by local gangs. He was a young, strong client who had a below-knee amputation. The physical therapist prescribed a heavy-duty black metal cane (500-pound weight capacity weighing approximately two pounds). That was above the weight normally prescribed since a standard aluminum cane has a 250-350 pound weight capacity and weighs approximately 1 pound. The client possessed the strength to easily tolerate and manipulate the increased weight of the cane. Recreational therapy then taught the client self-defense techniques using the cane.

Fitting the Device

- Unless the client uses the cane for a limited time during recovery, the expectation should be that the client will have two or more canes or multiple interchangeable parts for use during different types of activities.
- The handle of the cane should be level with the client's hip joint. Some prescribing guidelines suggest that having the top of the cane reach the client's wrist when the arm is at his/her side is a better measurement. To know where to cut a wooden cane for proper length, turn it upside down so that the rounded cane handle rests on the floor and make a mark on the cane where it reaches the client's wrist and then cut it at that mark. Depending on the type of activity, the cane may need to be longer. For instance, if the client is hiking over hilly ground, the height of the cane handle may need to be six inches above the client's elbow to provide support going down-hill. Canes that are adjustable for length may be good choices in this situation. If the client hikes above the tree line, aluminum canes (usually the type of cane that is adjustable) may not be the safest choice, as the cane may become a light-ning rod during a thunderstorm.
- Clients who are over seventy years old may want to select a cane length two to three inches longer than described above.
- Canes that are too long increase stress on the shoulder and arm causing pain and decreasing endurance. Canes that are too short increase strain on the wrist and the back.
- Properly fitted canes for basic walking place the client's elbow at a 20-30° angle.
- When selecting the handle type, it is important that the handle fits the contour of the client's hand.
- A larger handle grip may be more comfortable for clients with arthritis.

Authorization

A prescription is not required for canes, but clients are encouraged to get assistance from a therapist or physician when selecting canes.

Use

The cane is placed on the opposite side of an injury or weakened side. See "Walking Techniques" in the Techniques section for information on how to walk and go up and down steps and curbs with a cane.

Benefits

Canes increase a client's options and independence by augmenting balance. Because canes are relatively inexpensive and interchangeable, using a cane provides a client with the ability to "custom fit" the cane to the activity.

Design Challenges

Almost all canes used today lack design components based on solid ergonomic principles (Diez, 1997). Cane handles using ergonomic principles would have handles that:

- Allow the wrist to remain in a near neutral position (straight wrist with minimal flexion, extension, or deviation). There are two benefits to using a cane with the wrist in a near neutral position: 1. grip strength is greater in a neutral position versus a flexed position, and 2. risk of developing carpal tunnel syndrome is reduced.
- Are cylindrical in shape and large enough in size to allow the surface pressure exerted on the hand and fingers to be more widely distributed.

Two other ergonomic challenges posed by most of the canes available today are related to repetition and vibration. Repetitive damage may occur as the wrist and fingers repetitively bend to move the cane forward during walking. Vibration and jarring occur each time the client places the tip on the ground during the gait cycle. With instruction clients can minimize these actions to reduce long-term damage to tissue and joints.

Costs

Most canes range between $5.00 and $75.00. Specialty canes may be well over $150.00. The rubber tips that are on the bottom of most canes wear out in less than a year. Replacement tips are not expensive, costing less than $3.00 apiece. Retractable ice attachments usually are available for under $15.00.

Treatment Direction

- Teach clients how to use a cane when walking over different surfaces (e.g., uneven outdoor surfaces).
- Contribute to the selection of an appropriate cane length based on activity or heel size.
- Assist clients in identifying appropriate cane tips to maximize safety in specific tasks.
- Help clients problem solve for proper cane placement when it is not in use. For example, where and how to place a cane when sitting at a table at a restaurant or on a city bus.

References

Diez, M. (1997). *Ergonomic projects.* http://ergo.human. cornell,edu/ErogPROJECTS/97/diez.htm.

School of Public Health. (2004). Take a step towards independence: Canes. University of Buffalo, New York. http://cat.buffalo.edu/newsletters/canes.php.

Wylde, M. (2004). Referenced in product catalog. The House of Canes and Walking Sticks. www.houseofcanes.com.

Card Playing Equipment

Card holders, shufflers, and adaptive cards are common adaptations for card playing. Card holders are devices that hold cards. Commercial card holders come in racks, narrow slots, and discs. A card shuffler is a device that shuffles the cards automatically. Adaptive cards include low vision cards and Braille cards.

- *Card racks*: Card racks are made out of wood. They have four grooves cuts into the holder (one behind another). The holder has a peg on the bottom in the back so that the holder sits on a slant making the cards easier to see (tiered). It sits on a flat surface like a table, an over-the-bed table, or the floor.
- *Narrow slots*: Some card holders have one long narrow slot to hold the cards. It is typically made out of a thin plastic. They sit on a flat surface like a table, an over-the-bed table, or the floor.
- *Discs*: Two small plastic discs are held together with a spring. The cards are placed into the disc fanned out. The disc is held in the hand and the cards are placed between the discs.
- *Card shuffler*: A card shuffler is a machine that automatically shuffles cards. It can shuffle up to two full decks of cards at one time. It is battery operated. Half of the cards at put on one side of the machine and half on the other. With a push of a button, the cards are shuffled into a box in the center of the machine. The client pulls out the box to retrieve the shuffled cards.
- *Adaptive cards*: Low vision cards are cards with extra large corner marks ("A," "9," "♦"). Braille cards are cards that have Braille letters and numbers. Adaptive cards are available for standard card decks, as well as Uno and Skip-Bo.

Weight

A card rack weighs about a pound. Narrow slot card holders and discs weigh only a few ounces. A card shuffler weighs about one and a half pounds. Adaptive cards are a few ounces when held together in a full deck.

Fitting

NA

Authorization

NA

Use

Card racks and narrow slots: Card racks and narrow slots are used for clients who have limited hand function, especially pinch, grasp, and strength. Clients who are unable to put cards into or take cards out of the holder can request another player to remove or retrieve a particular card (e.g., "Can you please take out the second card on your right and place it in the pile?"). Clients can also use a vertical pincher mouth stick (a tongue controlled pincher on the end of the mouth stick) to grab an upright card in a holder. The vertical pincher mouth stick will not be able to pick up a card that is lying flat on the table or in a stack. Card racks are used for card games that require the player to hold more than seven cards. Card holders with one narrow slot are used for card games that require seven cards or less.

Card discs: Card discs are best for clients who have minimal or moderate hand grasp but lack enough strength to hold onto the cards. Some clients can remove or retrieve their own cards from the holder. If the client lacks a strong enough pinch to hold the card, s/he can request another player to remove or place a card for him/her. Card discs are a popular choice because they hold the cards in a small area and resemble the normal way cards are held. If a client prefers the disc to a rack or narrow slot but is unable to hold onto it, the therapist can make an adaptation. Put a piece of self-adhesive Velcro on the bottom of the disc and another piece of Velcro on a block of wood. Stick the disc to the block of wood to stabilize it. Now it is a hands-free card holder like the card rack and narrow slot.

Adaptive cards: Although adaptive cards may be larger in size, or have larger corner marks or Braille markings, the use of the cards is the same as standard cards.

Benefits

Enables clients to increase their independence with card games.

Design Challenges

Card holders are very simple in design and therapists are often very creative in creating them for clients based on their individual needs. Here are some examples:

- Cut a telephone book clear through about two inches from the spine. Wrap the outside perimeter with duck tape to hold it upright so it doesn't flap open. Place cards into the pages.

- Use the bristles of a flat scrub brush to hold the cards.
- Put two round plastic lids back to back. Staple or tape the lids together from the middle down. Slide cards into the top round of the two lids.

Cost

A card rack costs about $16.00. A plastic card holder with a narrow slot costs about $5.00. A card disc costs about $7.00 for a pack of three. An automatic card shuffler costs about $20.00. Adaptive card playing equipment is not covered by health insurance because it is not viewed as being medically necessary. Adaptive cards range from $3.00 to $20.00 a deck.

Treatment Direction

Recreational therapists recommend card playing adaptive equipment, provide training in its use, and educate clients about places that recommended equipment can be purchased.

Computers

The use of computers for home, work, and recreational tasks is commonplace in our society. They are used to manage finances, personal or business files, communication (e-mail, instant messaging, chat rooms, written correspondence), graphic design, research, purchasing goods, and controlling the environment through environmental control units. Computers, which have a variety of adaptations for use, are very helpful as a functional tool for achieving independence for people who have physical or mental disabilities, and are a desired skill in our society.

Interfaces

There are many adaptations to the standard interfaces that make it easier for a client to use a computer.

Keyboards

- *Standard keyboards*: Standard keyboards are good for people who have full upper hand and arm function and for people who have tremors or spasticity (small keyboards make hitting specific keys difficult).
- *Small keyboards*: Small keyboards are about two thirds to one-half the size of standard keyboards. Some are even cordless. Small keyboards are good for people who use a mouthstick or headpointer since they require less head and neck range to hit the keys. Small keyboards are also good for mounting (e.g., place one on a goose-neck mount so that it can be positioned for clients who have restricted range).
- *On screen keyboards*: There are keyboard software programs that allow the client to see a keyboard on the screen and use a mouse or mouse adaptation to click on the keyboard character that s/he wishes to have appear in the application. A hardware keyboard is not required. Windows XP has an on-screen keyboard under "accessibility options."
- *Filter keys*: Settings on the way the keys on a keyboard work that ignore brief or repeated keystrokes. The timing can be modified.
- *Sticky keys*: Settings on the way keys work that require the client to depress a key for a set period of time for it to register. The timing can be modified.

Typing Adaptations

There are many different ways to type on the computer. These are the most common.

Typing aid: This is a plastic half moon cuff that slips around the palm of the client's hand. Extending from the cuff is a short plastic pointer with a rubber tip. The client can use a typing aid on one hand or on both hands. The rubber tip is used to hit the keys on the keyboard. The rubber tip helps keep the pointer from slipping off the key that is being pressed and hitting other keys accidentally. Typing aids are good to use with clients who have no or minimal finger function, but who posses enough shoulder and elbow flexion and strength to move across the keyboard and depress keys. A typing aid can be paired with a small keyboard if range is restricted. It can also be paired with filter keys and/or sticky keys for clients who might otherwise have trouble using a small keyboard because of tremors or spasticity.

Mouthstick: A mouthstick is a device that a client holds in his/her mouth. It consists of a bitewing (looks like a "V") that the client places in the mouth and a stick that extends from the bitewing. Some sticks are pliable and can be formed into different shapes to get a good angle for using the keyboard (slightly bent at the bottom). Some mouthsticks have a tongue button in the bitewing (a small spring loaded button that causes a pincher to open up on the bottom of the mouthstick when the button is pushed by the tongue). This is good for retrieving paper. Other mouthsticks have a solid stick. Personally, we have found the bendable mouthstick to be best for typing. However clients who do extensive computer work often find it difficult to use a mouthstick for a prolonged period of time because it takes a lot of facial and mouth muscles to hold and manipulate the mouthstick. Mouthsticks also need a "docking station," a place to put the mouthstick so that it can be easily released and then retrieved by the client. Docking stations vary and they can even be made. The most common docking station is a cylinder that is placed at an angle on the desk (looks like an angled pencil holder). Another docking system looks like a tray that extends off of the computer to allow the client to set down the mouthstick. The therapist can also attach a piece of heavy duty Velcro to the side of the computer monitor and wrap another piece around the stick of the mouthstick so that the client can stick it to the side of the computer.

Dragon Dictate: This is the most common voice controlled computer program. It types what the client says verbally and it also has a command mode that allows the user to tell the computer actions that s/he wants to make (e.g., click on a program, open a file). The program has to learn the client's voice (takes about three hours). It is supposed to be 100%

accurate after voice training, but it can become very frustrating at times when the program does not respond appropriately. Clients who want to learn Dragon Dictate should also be taught other ways to operate the computer (e.g., mouthstick, use of a universal cuff and pencil). Dragon Dictate is used with clients who have a high level spinal cord injury and do not have (or have very minimal) use of the upper extremities. If some function does exist, use of the function should be encouraged whenever possible to maintain strength, range, and functionality of the limb.

Headpointer: A headpointer looks like a helmet that goes on the client's head. A long pointer extends from the front of the helmet. The client uses neck muscles to manipulate the device. This is commonly used with clients who have no or minimal hand and arm use. Clients who use this device will often require assistance to put it on and take it off. It is a large device and it is very noticeable, causing some clients to dislike it from the start.

Universal cuff and pencil: A universal cuff is a loop of material that slips onto the client's hand over the four fingers. It has a pocket built into it. Pencils, hairbrushes, paintbrushes, etc. can be placed in the pocket. It helps the client hold onto a device. It is used for clients who do not have a good hand grasp. See d440 Fine Hand Use for more information. To type on the computer, a pencil can be put into the pocket (upside down so that the rubber tip is used). The client hits the keyboard keys with the rubber tip of the pencil. To use the universal cuff and an upside down pencil, the client must have wrist rotation because the pocket is on the underside of the palm so the pencil will jut out to the side. The client must turn his/her wrist to point the pencil down to hit the keys. This adaptation is usually well received by the client because it is inexpensive and simple. It is good for clients who have limited hand use, clients who have tremors, or clients who have spasms, especially when paired with filter keys and/or sticky keys.

Large print keyboard stickers: Large print stickers (black on white or white on black) can be purchased and put onto the keyboard keys. This allows people who have minimal vision impairments to easily identify the keys on the keyboard.

Mouse

There are many different kinds of computer mice. These are the most common.

- *Standard mouse*: This is the standard mouse that comes with a computer. It is a small oval shaped device that fits in the cup of a client's hand and has a right and left button. This is a good option for clients who are able to single out fingers to

press the buttons and have good hand-eye coordination.

- *Tracking ball*: Tracking balls come in many different sizes. They can be small or very large. We have found the large tracking balls to be an excellent adaptive device (e.g., Microsoft Easy Ball). They can be purchased at most computer stores. A large ball sits inside a cradle. The client can use his/her fingers, heel of the hand, forearm, typing aid, pencil in a universal cuff, or mouthstick to move the ball. The cradle holds the ball still and it rolls in the cradle. When the ball is pushed in a certain direction, the cursor moves on the screen. Since the ball stays in the cradle, the client does not have to have full range of motion to manipulate the ball. It also has a large right and left button that can be depressed easily and a third button that holds the right or left button depressed so that the client can let go of the button and then operate the mouse to be able to do a "click and drag."

- *Keyboard controlled*: Under "accessibility options" in Windows the arrows on the keyboard can be changed to operate the mouse (called mouse keys). The up arrow makes the curser on the screen move up; the down arrow makes the curser on the screen move down; and so on. This allows the client who is proficient with the keyboard to integrate the mouse functions into the keyboard.

Monitor

The monitor can be modified in magnification and contrast. Larger screen monitors are easier to see.

- *High contrast and screen magnification*: For clients who have low vision, an accessibility option in Windows allows the client to increase the high contrast and magnify a portion of the screen. High contrast allows the client to choose various contrasts that make the words and icons on the screen easier to see (e.g., black on white, white on black and yellow). The screen magnifier enlarges the toolbars, mouse, side slides, and screen space so that clients who have vision impairments are able to see the screen better.

- *Setting a larger font as the default*: If the client is having difficulty seeing the default font, teach the client how to change the size of the font and set it as a default font. To assess the font size that is best for the client, start with a basic font (e.g., Times New Roman) and gradually increase the size of the font until the client is able to see it clearly without squinting or moving closer to the screen. Ask the client to read a paragraph or two using the font to determine if it is comfortable for the client to read for a prolonged period of time. If it isn't, increase the font by another size. The identified font can be set as the default so that it comes up every time the client uses an application.

- *Scan and read software*: There are various software programs that allow the client to scan information into the computer (e.g., a book page) and the computer will read it to the client. This is good for clients who have visual impairments or reading problems (e.g., dyslexia, illiteracy).

Applications

Accessibility options: In Windows accessibility options can be found in the control panel. Click on the accessibility icon. Tabs will appear for the keyboard, mouse, display, sound, and general where changes can be made. Windows XP has a program that also walks the client through all of the available options.

Weight

The weight of each device varies. Therapists need to consider whether the weight of an item will be helpful (e.g., for tremors) or contraindicated (e.g., joint protection for rheumatoid arthritis).

Fitting

Devices are chosen, they are not fitted like a cane or a walker. Many of these devices can be adjusted for optimal position and placement. For example, a keyboard can be placed further to the right or to the left. It can be raised (e.g., on a book) or lowered (e.g., onto a beanbag lap tray on the client's lap). It can also be mounted on a stand that clamps onto a table and can be positioned as needed. The placement and position of a device is determined by the client's physical capabilities and the desired outcomes. For example, if a client has only head control, a switch may be mounted next to the client's head so that with a side tilt of the head the computer could be turned on or off. In addition, a mouthstick may be Velcroed to the side of the computer monitor (a makeshift docking station) so that the client can reach forward with his/her neck to retrieve and dock the mouthstick. In another example, a therapist may put the mouse on the right side of the keyboard (even though the client is left handed) to facilitate coordination or digit isolation in a hand that has been injured. The therapist might also switch the mouse to the client's non-dominant side to develop skills related to dominance switching. Switching dominance (e.g., right-handedness to left-

handedness) is common when functional restoration of skills in the dominant hand is not expected.

Authorization

NA

Use

There are many different pieces of equipment and techniques that can be used for the computer. New therapists should find out about their state's Initiative on Assistive Technology (e.g., Pennsylvania's Initiate on Assistive Technology). The initiatives offer low-cost computer technology workshops that not only teach you about the pieces of equipment, but also give you the opportunity to try out each piece of equipment and learn where it can be purchased. The average price for these workshops is about $40.00. Recreational therapists are also eligible to become Assistive Technology Practitioners (ATP). Go to www.resna.org for a listing of each state's initiative project and how to become a certified ATP.

Benefits

Assistive technology for computers can increase independence and improve function (e.g., use an adaptive mouse to play a game of Breakout on the computer to work on attention).

Design Challenges

There are a variety of designs to meet the individualized needs of clients. In some cases, therapists specially fabricate a piece of equipment or modify an existing piece of equipment.

Costs

Costs can vary greatly depending on the type of equipment.

Treatment Direction

- Recreational therapists evaluate, train, and prescribe adaptive computer equipment. Insurance companies typically do not reimburse the cost of a computer or adaptive computer equipment. The office of vocational rehabilitation (OVR) would reimburse a client for these expenses if they are necessary for the client to return to work and the funds are available. OVR is a state program that receives a certain amount of funding each year and, when it is gone, it is gone until next year's budget is received.
- Recreational therapists fabricate or modify computer equipment.

Crutches

There are three types of crutches: axillary crutches, forearm crutches, and platform crutches. Axillary crutches are the most common crutch. People who have a minimal injury and are required to maintain weight-bearing precautions (e.g., cast on one leg or sprained ankle) are typically prescribed axillary crutches. The crutches tuck underneath the arms and there is a bar for each hand to hold. The overall height and the hand bar height are both adjustable. Forearm crutches (also called Lofstrand crutches) have a cuff that slips onto the top of the forearm and horizontal handles for the client to hold. Forearm crutches are best for clients who have moderate problems with stability and generalized weakness throughout the lower extremities. Platform crutches (also known as triceps crutches) are similar to forearm crutches while providing more support because they have an additional upper cuff.

Weight

Axillary crutches weigh about 3 pounds a pair. Forearm crutches weigh about 5 pounds a pair. Platform crutches weigh about 6 pounds.

Fitting

Axillary crutches: Ask the client to stand normally (feet shoulder width apart) and lift his/her arms out to the side. Adjust the crutch so that it sits about two inches below the client's armpit (axilla) when the base of the crutch is six to eight inches out from the client's foot. The hand bar is then adjusted so that the elbow is bent 30° when the crutches are in line with the client's feet. An easy way to set this angle is to adjust the hand bar so that it is at the height of the client's wrist.

Forearm crutches: This crutch should allow the client to flex his/her elbow 15-30°. The increased flexion allows the arm to bear greater weight. Ask the client to stand in a normal position (feet shoulder-width apart). Place the base of the crutch two to four inches outside the foot and six inches forward of the foot. Adjust the cuff so that it sits 1-1½" below the back of the elbow.

Platform crutches: Ask the client to stand normally (feet shoulder-width apart). Place the base of the crutch two to four inches outside the foot and six inches forward of the foot. Adjust the upper cuff so that it sits about 2" below the skin fold of the armpit. Adjust the lower cuff so that it sits 1-1½" below the back of the elbow.

Authorization

Simple axillary crutches may be purchased from local stores. A prescription is needed for forearm or platform crutches.

Use

There are various ways to walk with crutches (crutch gaits). There are also specific techniques for standing and sitting with crutches and going up and down steps and curbs. See "Walking Techniques" in the Techniques section for detailed information.

Benefits

Crutches provide support for movement.

Design Challenges

NA

Costs

Axillary crutches cost about $20.00 to $45.00. Forearm crutches cost about $150.00. Platform crutches cost about $180.00.

Treatment Direction

Recreational therapists assess the client's ability to use crutches in a community setting and in functional tasks. They provide necessary training and recommendations (e.g., in a crowded community environment the crutches do not offer the client enough support to maintain balance, so a walker is recommended). Recreational therapists also make recommendations for crutch accessories (e.g., crutch bag).

Dressing Aids

There are six pieces of equipment commonly used as dressing aids: a buttonhook, a dressing stick, elastic shoelaces, a long-handled shoehorn, a sock donner, and a zip grip.

Buttonhook: A small loop of wire attached to a small built up handle.

Dressing stick: Dressing sticks have a lacquered dowel-like wood shaft that is about 5/8" in diameter and comes in lengths that vary from 24" to 34". At one end of the shaft is a C-hook and at the other end is a large plastic coated push/pull hook.

Elastic shoelaces: Shoelaces made out of elastic rather than cotton or nylon.

Long-handled shoehorn: Just like a standard shoehorn, but much longer (18-30").

Sock donner: A piece of plastic about nine inches long and six inches wide with the sides rounded up a bit. Attached to this piece of plastic is a long loop of material or cord.

Zip grip: A plastic ring that attaches onto a zipper pull.

Weight

All of these items weigh less than a few ounces.

Fitting

Dressing stick and long-handled shoehorn: Longer dressing sticks and shoehorns are chosen for clients who have bending or twisting precautions (e.g., total hip replacement, laminectomy) or who have very limited range of motion.

Sock donners: The sock donner chosen is based on whether or not the client has use of one or both hands. Sock donners that have one continuous loop of material or cord can be pulled using one hand. Sock donners that have two separate cords require the use of two hands (each hand pulls one cord).

Elastic shoelaces, buttonhooks, and zip grips: no special fitting requirements.

Authorization

Dressing aids are typically prescribed by occupational therapists. Recreational therapists who notice that a client needs dressing aids that have not already been prescribed should discuss it with the client's primary occupational therapist.

Use

Buttonhook: The metal loop of the buttonhook is put through the buttonhole and then over the button that goes into the buttonhole. The client then pulls the button through the hole by holding the handle of the buttonhook and pulling it through the buttonhole. Buttonhooks are good for clients who have poor fine hand coordination or strength or only have functional use of one arm.

Dressing stick: Dressing sticks have different hooks on each end. The stick provides the client with a way to reach clothing items that are out of reach (too low, too high, too far away) and the hooks provide the means for grabbing the items. Dressing hooks are also helpful to put clothes on or take clothes off (e.g., grab a belt loop with a hook to help pull up pants, reach stick over the opposite shoulder to reach the other sleeve of a button-down shirt). Dressing sticks are helpful for clients who have limited range of motion to retrieve, put on, or take off clothing (e.g., traumatic brain injury, stroke, total joint replacement, back surgery).

Elastic shoelaces: Elastic shoelaces are laced through a shoe just like regular shoelaces. Some of them tie like regular shoelaces and others form a knot at the last shoelace hole so tying is not required. Elastic shoelaces allow the shoe to stretch open and closed without having to tie and untie the shoelaces. (The elastic shoelaces that tie are for appearance, they do not have to be tied and untied.) This is good for people who are unable to bend down to tie or untie shoes (e.g., total hip replacement) or for clients who have difficulty tying and untying shoes (e.g., problems with fine hand coordination and strength). A long-handled shoehorn is often used in conjunction with elastic shoelaces to help slide the foot into the shoe.

Long-handled shoehorn: A long-handled shoehorn is used the same way as a regular shoehorn. It is just longer. The client opens up the shoelaces and tongue of the shoe and puts it on the floor. The client slides his/her foot into the shoe as far as it can go. When the foot is not able to slide all the way into the shoe, the long-handled shoehorn is inserted into the back heel of the shoe. The client lifts his/her heel so that it rests on the shoehorn. The shoehorn helps the foot slide into the shoe because it gives the foot a surface to push against (much like your fingers when you put them in the back of your shoe to help slide your foot into the shoe). Long-handled shoehorns are good for clients who are unable to bend down and use their hand to help slide the shoe onto the foot (e.g., total hip replacement, poor sitting balance) or a client who does not have good finger, hand, or wrist strength to provide a good amount of resistance to slide the foot into the shoe.

Sock donner: A sock is slid onto the base of the sock donner (the plastic part) so that the entire sock is scrunched onto it and the toe of the sock is tight at the end. The base is then lowered to the floor and the client wiggles his/her foot into the sock (the curved plastic base keeps the sock open so the foot can slide inside). Once the foot is fully into the base, the client pulls up on the loop of material. This pulls the base out of the sock and slides the sock onto the foot at the same time. Sock donners are good for people who are unable to bend down to put on their socks (e.g., total hip precautions), clients who have poor hand coordination or strength, and clients with sitting balance problems.

Zip grip: A zip grip is a plastic or metal ring that snaps through the small hole at the base of a zipper. The large ring is easier to grasp, making it easier to zip and unzip jackets, pants, sweaters, backpacks, fanny packs, etc. This is good for people who need to protect finger joints (e.g., rheumatoid arthritis) or for clients who have trouble with fine hand coordination or strength. Therapists can also make zip grips out of a variety of material. For example, the therapist can thread a piece of flower wire or pipe cleaner through the zipper hole, twist it together, and cover the sharp ends with tape. Another idea is to use a twist tie from a bag of bread (again making sure there are no sharp points).

Benefits

Dressing aids increase a client's independence with dressing.

Design Challenges

There are a variety of designs to meet the individual needs of clients. In some cases, therapists specially fabricate a piece of equipment or modify an existing piece of equipment.

Costs

A buttonhook ranges from $4.00 to $6.00. A dressing stick ranges from $5.00 to $12.00. Elastic shoelaces cost about $3.00 a pair. A long-handled shoehorn ranges from $5.00 to $10.00. A sock donner averages around $12.00. Zip grips cost about $2.00 for a pack of six.

Treatment Direction

- Recreational therapists are familiar with dressing equipment and how to use it because they teach clients how to use dressing aids in a community setting (e.g., trying on clothes in a store dressing room, donning and doffing pants in a bathroom, changing clothes in a locker room).
- Recreational therapists make suggestions to the client's primary occupational therapist for dressing aids when needs are noted for which equipment has not been prescribed.

Dycem

Dycem is a non-slip rubbery plastic that is used to stabilize and grasp items. It is non-toxic, latex free, colorfast, odorless, washable with soap and water, and can be affixed permanently with Super Glue. It can be purchased in many different sizes. It comes on a roll that is 8-16" wide and 2-10 yards long. The Dycem on the roll is 1/32" thick. It also comes in the form of 1/8" thick pads in various shapes (circles, squares, rectangles) and sizes (5-14" in diameter or length).

Weight

The roll Dycem is so thin that it doesn't add any measurable weight to an item. The Dycem pads weigh a pound or less.

Fitting

NA

Authorization

NA

Use

Dycem keeps things from sliding away. Roll Dycem can easily be cut with standard scissors to any size. Items can be placed on top of it to help with item stabilization (e.g., place a bowl on top of a piece of Dycem to keep it from sliding away while stirring, place a piece of Dycem on the table where a client with hemiparesis rests his/her arm so that the arm does not slip off the table). It can also be wrapped around items (e.g., cut strips and wrap them around a hammer to help keep the hammer from slipping out of the client's hand). Dycem is one of those products that every therapist needs to have in his/her cabinet. It can be wrapped around pencils, pens, markers, hairbrushes, toothbrushes, fishing pole handles, baseball bats, gardening shovels, and basically anything else that has a handle.

Benefits

It helps to solve many problems related to stabilization and grasping.

Design Challenges

NA

Costs

A two-yard roll of 16-inch Dycem costs about $35.00 and a 10-yard roll costs about $120.00. Dycem mats range from about $10.00 to $20.00.

Treatment Direction

Recreational therapists experiment with Dycem when the client has grasping problems or needs stabilization of an item and make recommendations for its use. Another non-slip product, although not usually as effective as Dycem, can be found in any store that sells drawer liners (e.g., Wal-Mart). It goes by different names but it looks like an open weave and it feels rubbery. This, too, can be cut with scissors and placed under objects. It does not stick to itself well enough, though, to be used for wrapping around items (e.g., a pen).

Eating and Drinking Equipment

There is a variety of adaptive equipment on the market specific to eating including cups, plates, straws, and utensils.

Cups: Therapists can prescribe a variety of adaptive cups and cup devices that allow clients increased independence and function when drinking liquids. There are adaptive aids that clip onto standard cups such as a Sure Grip Glass Holder and a Bilateral Glass Holder. A Sure Grip Glass Holder is tightened around a standard drinking glass and has a large flexible handle that can be bent to fit the client's hand. The Bilateral Glass Holder, like the Sure Grip Glass Holder slides onto a standard glass and can be tightened, however it has two "D" shaped handles (one on each side) for a client who requires the use of two hands to lift and tilt a glass. Therapists also prescribe fully formed adaptive drinking cups. There are "Nosey Cups" that have a pitcher-like spout, weighted cups, cups with leak-proof lids, cups that require suction to release the liquid (like pediatric sippy cups), and cups that will not leak when the client is lying on his/her back in bed).

Plates: Therapists may prescribe pieces of equipment that can be added to standard plates such as plate guards. A plate guard looks like a horseshoe that clips onto the outside rim of a plate. They are typically made out of plastic or stainless steel. They help with scooping and keeping food on the plate. Therapists may also prescribe fully formed adaptive plates that can help to increase a client's independence with eating. For example, a Hi-Lo Scoop Plate has a low front rim and a high back rim. Some molded plates have a high rim all the way around (resembling a bowl) and others have suction cups on the bottom or are divided into sections.

Straws: Therapists may prescribe the use of long drinking straws (18" tall). Rigid Plexiglas straws have a ¼" diameter and can be heated and shaped. Flexible polyethylene straws have a 3/16" diameter and are not able to be re-shaped. There are also drinking straw holders that attach onto the rim of the cup to keep the straw in place. One-way straws are also available that allow fluid to come up but do not allow it go back down, thus eliminating air in the straw at all times.

Utensils: Therapists can use adaptive materials and equipment to transform eating utensils so that they meet the needs of the client. For example, utensils can be built up with foam tubing (see Foam Tubing) or a utensil holder can be used (see Grip Aids). Therapists may also prescribe the use of specially made adaptive utensils. For example, flexible utensils have a 14" long flexible handle that can be manipulated into a variety of positions (e.g., wrapped around the client's wrist). There are also lightweight utensils (weighing only an ounce), weighted utensils (weighing anywhere from two to eight ounces and some have adjustable weights), rubber utensils, unbreakable plastic utensils, adjustable angle utensils, and utensils that have permanent built up handles that are dishwasher safe.

Weight

Adaptive cups, plates, and utensils typically range from one to eight ounces. Long straws weigh only an ounce or so.

Fitting

Eating aids are mostly devices that are chosen rather than fitted with the exception of a few devices.

Straws: Rigid Plexiglas straws can be heated and re-shaped (e.g., angled, curved) to meet the needs of the client. The therapist evaluates the placement and location of the cup in relation to the client's mouth and bends the straw to maximize access. For example, a client with tetraplegia has a water bottle in a cup holder on the side of his wheelchair. A rigid straw is used so that the client is able to turn his head to the side to reach the straw. If the straw is too high, it may need to be bent or curved so that the client can retrieve it.

Utensils: Flexible handle utensils can be bent or wrapped around a client's wrist and or forearm to provide appropriate support and position of the utensil.

Authorization

Eating and drinking equipment is commonly prescribed by occupational therapists. Recreational therapists who perceive a need for such equipment beyond what is already prescribed discuss it with the client's primary occupational therapist.

Use

Cups: Adaptive cups and glass holders all have the same purpose. They are designed to allow a client to hold, lift, tilt, drink from, lower, and release a cup. Glass holders (Sure Grip and Bilateral Grip) are good for clients who have trouble holding a cup due to weakness, tremors, or finger/wrist dysfunction. They are also good for clients who need to protect their hand and wrist joints (e.g., rheumatoid arthritis) since it transfers stress on the fingers to the larger joints and muscles of the wrist, forearm, and upper arm.

Nosey cups are good for clients who are unable to lift their chin to empty the contents of a cup (e.g., client using a wheelchair headrest, neck fusion, on a prone cart) or who should not lift their chin (e.g., people with swallowing disorders that are encouraged to lower and tuck their chin to swallow). Weighted cups are good for clients who have tremors. Cups with leak-proof lids are good for clients who have upper extremity tremors, poor coordination, spasms, or increased tone that might result in the cup toppling over. Cups that require suction to release the liquid are good for clients who typically take in too much liquid, clients who need a device to limit the amount of fluid (e.g., swallowing problems), or clients who are lying down in bed. There are also special cups like the Kennedy Cup that is leak-proof and has a straw (not a suction) that can be used in a lying down position.

Plates: Plate guards and adaptive plates have the same purpose: to keep food on the plate and to help with scooping. Other purposes may be the prescription of an adaptive plate so that it stays put on the table (e.g., suction cups or increased weight) or keeps food divided. Plate guards and adaptive plates are used by clients who have hand and upper arm impairments (e.g., tremors, spasms, restricted range of motion, lack of coordination).

Straws: Long straws are used for clients who have limited range of motion to reach a standard straw in a cup and who are unable to take hold of the cup and bring it to their lips (e.g., tetraplegia, full arm casts). Rigid straws, because of their larger diameter (1/4") can be used for drinking soups in addition to drinking liquids from a cup. One-way straws are good for clients who are using the Kennedy Cup since it keeps liquid in the straw and eliminates air.

Utensils: See "Grip Aids" and "Foam Tubing" for information on fitting these materials onto utensils. Flexible utensils are good for clients who have a poor grasp and benefit from minimal support of the wrist (wrap around the wrist) and forearm (wrap around forearm). Lightweight utensils are good for clients who have limited hand strength or who need to protect finger joints (e.g., rheumatoid arthritis). Weighted utensils are good for clients who have tremors because the added weight typically lessens the tremor although it fatigues the muscle

more quickly. Rubber utensils are good for clients who need to protect their teeth, but they are not appropriate for clients who are biters. Unbreakable utensils are good for clients who typically drop or throw utensils. Adjustable angle utensils are good for clients who have limited range of motion and require angled utensils to achieve a correct feeding position. Permanent built-up handles are good for clients who require a permanent built-up handle that is dishwasher safe. Built-up handles are good for clients who have a poor grasp.

Benefits

Eating aids increase a client's independence with the necessary life task of eating. They also have a direct impact on the client's safety (e.g., limits risk of spilling hot liquids or foods, dropping food, or spilling liquid on the floor).

Design Challenges

There are a variety of designs to meet the individual needs of clients. In some cases, therapists specially fabricate a piece of equipment or modify an existing piece of equipment.

Costs

See "Grip Aids." Glass holders typically range from $7.00 to $15.00 and adaptive cups range from $4.00 to $13.00. Plate guards cost about $5.00 and molded plates cost from $6.00 to $20.00. Long straws and one-way straws cost about $2.00 each. Adapted utensils can cost anywhere from $6.00 to $50.00 per utensil.

Treatment Direction

- Occupational therapists typically prescribe feeding equipment, however recreational therapists make suggestions to the treating OT when needs or problems are observed.
- Recreational therapists are familiar with feeding equipment and its use to assist the client in carrying over the use of feeding equipment into a community environment (e.g., restaurants, work, school, home, picnics).

Equipment Resources

Although this list is not exhaustive, here is a list of catalogs and contacts for adaptive equipment that we have found to be helpful. Some of the equipment ideas in the catalogs may give you ideas for designing your own equipment, especially if the client is not able to afford the equipment. Health insurance does not reimburse expenses for adaptive equipment if it is not viewed as being medically necessary (e.g., adaptive gardening equipment). Recreational therapists should have a workshop available for making equipment that contains various adaptation materials and tools. Therapists can also ask clients to bring in things that they already have at home that can be altered to make a piece of adaptive equipment (e.g., flat wooden scrub brush turned upside down can be used to hold cards). Recreational therapists should also seek out the assistance of other health professionals to design and make equipment. For example, I worked with an occupational therapist to make custom mouthsticks. She made a custom bite plate for the client with splinting materials and then wrapped the bite plate around a rigid straw and put a rubber tip on the end. The rigid straw could be reshaped with heat to form the bend or curve the client needed.

We encourage you to call each of the companies below and request a free catalog. Place them on your bookshelf for reference and ask the companies to keep you on their mailing list for updated catalogs.

Catalogs

These are the most frequently used catalogs in a rehabilitation setting for general adaptive equipment:

Access to Recreation and After-Therapy Catalog
2509 E. Thousand Oaks Blvd., Suite 430
Thousand Oaks, CA 91362
1-800-634-4351
(Adaptive equipment for recreation and daily activities)

Enrichments
145 Tower Drive, Dept. #D65
Burr Ridge, IL 60521
1-800-323-5547
(Adaptive equipment for everyday tasks)

Maxi Aids
42 Executive Blvd.
Farmingdale, NY 11735
1-800-522-6294
(Products for low vision, blind, deaf, hearing impaired, and other special needs)

Sammons Preston
PO Box 5071
Bolingbrook, IL 60440-5071
1-800-323-5547
(Rehabilitation equipment and supplies)

S & S Worldwide and Adapt Ability
PO Box 513
Colchester, CT 06415-0513
1-800-566-6678
(Crafts and adaptive equipment)

Other favorite catalogs, booklets, and resources:

ABLEDATA and NARIC (National Rehabilitation Information Center)
8455 Colesville Road, Suite 935
Silver Spring, MD 10910-3319
1-800-227-1216
(Electronically maintained database of information on assistive technology, rehabilitation and health-related problems)

Able-Net
1081 Tenth Ave. SE
Minneapolis, MN 55414-1312
1-800-322-0956
(Adaptive switches)

Access With Ease, Inc.
PO Box 1150
Chino Valley, AZ 86323
1-800-531-9479
("Nifty little gadgets" for people with disabilities)

Ann Morris Enterprises, Inc.
551 Hosner Mountain Rd
Stormville, NY 12582-5329
1-800-454-3175
(Low vision products)

Home Automation Systems, Inc.
151 Kalmus Drive, Suite L4
Costa Mesa, CA 92626
1-800-949-6255
(Home automation supplies — doors, locks, drapes, pet doors, lights, heating, etc.)

IBM Special Needs Systems
PO Box 1328
Boca Raton, FL 33431
1-800-426-4832
(Free fact sheets on how computers can help people with disabilities)

JC Penney Company
PO Box 100001
Dallas, TX 75301-4318
1-800-222-6161
("Easy Dressing Fashions" catalog)

National Easter Seal Society
70 East Lake Street
Chicago, IL 60601
312-726-6200
(Offers written materials and resources related to independence for people with disabilities)

National Lekotek Center
2100 Ridge Ave.
Evanston, IL 60201
708-328-0001
(Information on toys and play for children with disabilities)

National Handicapped Sports
451 Hungerford Drive, Suite 100
Rockville, MD 20850
1-800-966-4NHS (4647)
(Adaptive sports)

National Information Center for Children and Youths with Disabilities (NICHCY)
PO Box 1492
Washington, DC 20013
1-800-999-5599
(Free information, brochures, and booklets to assist parents, educators, caregivers, and advocates in helping children with disabilities to become participating members of the community)

National Stroke Association
8480 East Orchard Road, Suite 1000
Englewood, CO 80111-5015
1-800-STROKES (787-6537)
(Free booklet on "Adaptive Resources: A Guide to Manufacturers and Products")

Paralyzed Veterans of America
801 Eighteenth St. NW
Washington, DC 20006
1-800-424-8200
(Booklet on a variety of disabled sports and contact organizations)

Prentke Romich Company
1022 Heyl Road
Wooster, OH 44691
1-800-848-8008 or 1-800-262-1984/1990
(High-tech communication, computer-access, and environmental control devices)

RESNA
Rehabilitation Engineering and Assistive Technology Society of North America
1700 N. Moore St, Suite 1540
Arlington, VA 22209-1903
Phone 703-524-6686
Fax 703-524-6630

Technical Aids and Systems for the Handicapped, Inc. (TASH)
Unit 1-91 Station Street
Ontario, Canada L1S 3H2
1-800-463-5685
(Adaptive switches and mounting devices)

The Safety Zone
340 Poplar Street, Building 20
Hanover, PA 17333-0019
1-800-338-1635
(Variety of adaptive equipment for people with disabilities)

Toy Guide for Differently Abled Kids
Toys R Us
PO Box 8501
Nevada, IA 50201-9968
(Free booklet from any Toys R Us store)

Toys for Special Children
385 Warburton Ave.
Hastings-on-Hudson, NY 10706
1-800-TEC-TOYS (832-8697)
(Adaptive toys)

Walt Nicke Co
36 McLeod Lane
PO Box 433
Topsfield, MA 01983
978-887-3388
(Adaptive gardening equipment)

Foam Tubing

Foam tubing looks like a hose with a hole through the middle. Foam tubing comes in outer diameters ranging from ¾"-1 3/8" and inner diameters ranging from 3/8"-¼" (the size of the hole down the center of the tubing, referred to as the "bore"). Foam tubing comes in various lengths (4-24") and it can easily be cut to any length with standard scissors.

Weight

A few ounces.

Fitting

Hold up the handle of an item (e.g., a paintbrush). While holding onto the item, ask the client to grasp the item. Measure the gap between the item and the client's grasp to determine the outer diameter of the foam tubing needed. If the gap is larger than 1 3/8", then the therapist should use a universal cuff (see "Universal Cuff" in the Equipment section). Next, measure the diameter of the handle to determine what size bore is needed. The outer diameter of the foam tubing determines the bore that it comes with. There isn't a lot of choice. The larger the outer diameter, the larger the bore. Therapists can always adapt the foam tubing (see Use) to make the bore fit the handle of the item. In many cases, the therapist can chose a larger outer diameter (without affecting function) to have a bigger bore, but should not choose a smaller diameter because, if it is too small, the client will not be able to hold onto it. Therapists should have a piece of each size of foam tubing to be able to try out diameters during the evaluation. As for the length of the tubing, it should be long enough to fit the grasping patterns used to manipulate the tool.

Authorization

NA

Use

Foam tubing is used for clients who have a poor hand grasp. They need to be able to close their hand at least half way. Foam tubing is slipped onto cylindrical items (e.g., utensils, pens, paintbrushes, fishing pole handles, gardening tools). This makes the handles larger so they are easier to grasp. Foam tubing has a slip resistant outer surface making it easier for clients to hold. Foam tubing is also used for clients who have arthritis in the hands and need to follow joint protection precautions. Using a built up handle puts less stress on the finger joints and muscles (see "Joint Protection" in b710 Mobility of Joint Functions).

If the bore (inner hole) is too big for the device, fill up the gap by wrapping tape around the device (e.g., wrap medical tape a few times around a pen to increase the diameter of the pen so that it is held snugly inside the bore of the foam tubing). If the bore is too small for the device, cut a slit in the foam tubing lengthwise from top to bottom with a pair of scissors. The foam tubing can be pried open and stretched around the larger handle. It will not make it all the way around the handle, but it will still be effective. If it pops off the larger handle, wrap a thin layer of tape around the foam tubing.

Benefits

Foam tubing increases the width of a handle, making items easier to hold for clients who have decreased hand grasp. Larger and softer handles also lessen stress on hand joints and muscles. This promotes the use of larger muscle groups (wrist, arm) that aids in joint protection (see "Joint Protection" in b710 Mobility of Joint Functions).

Design Challenges

NA

Costs

One yard of foam tubing ranges from $5.00 to $12.00.

Treatment Direction

Recreational therapists prescribe and fit foam tubing for items used in activities.

Gardening Equipment

There are many different pieces of adaptive gardening equipment. This topic looks at kneelers, self-coiling hoses, lightweight tools, long-handled tools, Hi-Lo's, and cut and holds. There are other types of gardening equipment, not covered here, that may be appropriate for clients.

Kneeler: A kneeler is a U-shaped device made out of metal or plastic. It is placed on the ground in front of the area that the client wishes to garden. The kneeler gives the client a soft place to kneel (a cushion is placed at the bottom of the "U") and handles on each side give support to get into and out of a kneeling position. If you turn it over, it can be used as a seat.

Self-coiling hose: A self-coiling hose is made of plastic that sort of resembles a large slinky. When the client walks with the hose, it does not drag on the ground like a standard hose and it is lightweight. When the client lets go of the hose, it gently springs back to the hose bib and is easily gathered and lifted back onto a hose hook.

Lightweight, long-handled tools: Long-handled tools make gardening easier from a seated position. Choose long handled tools that are made of lightweight materials (e.g., fiberglass instead of solid wood) for less stress on joints and ease of movement.

Hi-Lo: The Hi-Lo is a pulley for raising and lowering hanging baskets. Attach the Hi-Lo onto a porch hook and then attach the hanging basket to the bottom of the Hi-Lo. Gently lift up on the bottom of the hanging basket to disengage the pulley and then raise or lower it to the desired height. Once at the desired height, gently push up to lock the pulley. This is a fantastic device for watering and cleaning out hanging baskets instead of standing on chairs or ladders.

Cut and hold: There are many different models of cut and holds. It basically cuts a stem or thin branch and then continues to hold the stem or branch in the jaws of the cutter instead of letting it fall to the ground.

Weight

The weight of gardening equipment varies depending on the model and manufacturer. Lightweight options are usually preferable

Fitting

Choose equipment that is appropriately sized for each client.

Authorization

NA

Use

Kneeler: Place the kneeler in front of the area to be gardened. Hold onto the handles for support and kneel down on the kneeler. To stand, hold the handles for support and stand up.

Self-coiling hose: If a client is not using a mobility device or is using a unilateral device (e.g., one cane), the client can hold the hose with one hand. Although not ideal, if the client is using a bilateral upper extremity device (e.g., walker), the client may be able to wrap his/her hand around both the walker handle and the hose. This type of hose is best for clients who have good balance, require no mobility device or use a unilateral device, and have the strength and function to hold onto the hose for extended periods of time so that it does not spring back to the hose bib when in use.

Lightweight, long-handled tools: Clients who are unable to kneel or sit on the ground to garden will need to garden from a seated position. Clients can sit on a gardening seat or a sturdy chair by the garden bed and use long-handled tools to reach the ground. Lightweight tools are ideal because they require less energy and strength. Short tools require the client to bend over to reach the ground. In some cases this may not be safe (e.g., falling forward out of the chair, breaking hip precautions). Clients who are unable to drag a chair to the gardening site are encouraged to keep a chair outside by the garden permanently. It may also be helpful to keep a plastic tote next to the garden bed and keep frequently used gardening tools in it so that the client does not have to carry tools from the shed to the garden bed. For some clients, carrying gardening tools across uneven terrain while using an assistive device is not safe.

Hi-Lo: See the description.

Cut and holds: This device is helpful for clients who do not have functional use of one upper extremity (e.g., stroke) or for clients who do not have good balance for reaching into garden beds (e.g., multiple sclerosis). Since the device cuts and then holds a thin branch or stem, it can be brought back to the client and placed into a trash bag for trimmings or into a basket for cut flowers.

Other tips: Here is a list of other tips that can promote gardening independence, functionality, and safety.

- Use a backpack to carry small tools and items to the gardening site.
- Explore the use of alternative ways to transport equipment (e.g., baby coach).
- Have the client take a cordless phone outside in case of an emergency.
- Consider the use of walkie-talkies for the client and another person in the house. This will allow the client and the other person to talk when needed. For example, if the client falls when outside in the garden, she can use the walkie-talkie to tell her husband who is inside the house that she needs help.
- Use sun block.
- Take a bottle of cold water outside to keep hydrated.
- Take frequent rest breaks. Avoid becoming over-fatigued because tired muscles make it difficult to walk back to the house, especially on uneven surfaces.
- Do not stand up quickly from a kneeling position because the quick change in blood pressure can cause dizziness.

Benefits

Gardening is a good form of exercise. Adaptive gardening equipment can increase the client's independence and enjoyment with the task.

Design Challenges

There are a variety of designs to meet the individual needs of clients. In some cases, therapists specially fabricate a piece of equipment or modify an existing piece of equipment.

Costs

Garden kneelers cost $20.00 to $40.00. Light-weight, long-handled gardening tools will vary depending in the tool chosen and material. A Hi-Lo is about $15.00. Cut and Holds vary in price from about $20.00 to $60.00. Gardening equipment is not viewed as being medically necessary, so it is not covered under health insurance. Clients must pay out of pocket for gardening equipment. Clients should check their local garden and home centers, order it through a catalog, or find a reliable on-line resource.

Treatment Direction

- Recreational therapists evaluate a client's abilities to engage in the activity of gardening and prescribe adaptive equipment and techniques, as needed, to ensure safety and maximize independence and enjoyment.
- Recreational therapists train clients on use of adaptive gardening equipment and techniques and give clients resources on where to purchase recommended equipment.

Grip Aids (Palmar Clip, Utensil Holder, and Universal Cuff)

The basic design of all three pieces of equipment is a loop of nylon, elastic, cotton, leather, or plastic that slides over the four fingers and down onto the palm. A tight pocket is built into the palm side of the strap so that the handle of an item can be put into it and held in place. With the palm facing down the item would extend out from the palm horizontally. This is a good angle for using eating utensils, but it is not a good angle for writing. If a more vertical pocket is desired, an accessory called a "right-angle pocket" can be placed into the existing cuff pocket. The equipment can be used for right or left hands.

There are three different designs: 1. a piece of elastic in a leather loop that can stretch and conform to the palm (referred to as a universal cuff), 2. a D-ring and Velcro closure so that it can be loosened to slide onto the palm and then tightened to fit the palm (referred to as a utensil holder; the pocket is thin to allow a tight grip on a flat utensil), or 3. a piece of plastic in the shape of a crescent moon (referred to as a palmar clip) attaches to the pocket so that clients who do not have the ability to stretch or tighten a cuff can just slide their hands into it (most often used for clients who have tetraplegia). The plastic can be heated with a heat gun and shaped to fit the client's palm. For clients who have a floppy wrist (unable to maintain hand and forearm alignment), a "wrist support with palmar clip" is helpful. It is a splint that wraps around the client's forearm, wrist, and palm. It has Velcro closures and a palmar clip with a pocket.

Weight

A few ounces.

Fitting

To determine the correct cuff size, the therapist measures the width of the client's palm in inches from the outside of the pinky finger to the outside of the index finger. The elastic universal cuffs usually come in small (fits 2½" width), medium (fits 3" width), and large (fits 3½ inch width). Utensil holders fit a range (e.g., 3¼"-4¼"). Palmar clips are adjusted to fit with a heat gun. Right-angled pockets can be heated and bent to achieve a desired bend.

Authorization

Occupational therapists commonly prescribe utensil holders. Both occupational therapists and recreational therapists prescribe palmar clips and universal cuffs.

Use

The palmar clip, utensil holder, and universal cuff are good for clients who do not have a functional hand grasp and for whom built up handles using foam tubing do not work because the diameter of the foam tubing is not sufficient. If a client is unable to actively pronate (palm facing down) and supinate (palm facing up) the palm, a standard clip, holder, or cuff will result in the client being able to hold items in a horizontal position only. This isolated position is effective for feeding, but it is not effective for more complex tasks like operating a computer keyboard or painting (see "Computers" for alternative typing devices for clients who are unable to pronate and supinate the palm). If a vertical hold is needed, a right-angle pocket will need to be added (it fits into the existing pocket).

Individuals who can pronate and supinate the palm or who are using a right-angled pocket will find a variety of uses for these devices. For example, an upside down pencil can be placed in the pocket (the rubber eraser is sticking out). Upside down pencils are good for pushing and sliding things (e.g., elevator buttons, a board game piece, computer keys). Placing the pencil in the pocket so that it sticks out is best to avoid excessive wrist rotation, extension, and flexion (e.g., place the universal cuff on the right hand so that the pocket opening is on the pinky side of the palm rather than the thumb side; when the upside down pencil is inserted, the pencil end will jut out to the right).

Benefits

Allows a client to "hold onto" items without having a functional grasp. These aids can help with eating and typing, as well as pushing buttons or sliding small items.

Design Challenges

There are a variety of designs to meet the individual needs of clients. In some cases, therapists specially fabricate a piece of equipment or modify an existing piece of equipment.

Costs

A palmar clip with a pocket costs about $16.00. A utensil holder costs about $7.00 to $10.00. A universal cuff costs about $8.00. A right-angle pocket costs about $16.00. A wrist support with palmar clip costs about $35.00. The devices are typically covered by insurance if they are documented as being medically necessary (e.g., tool for eating).

Treatment Direction

- Recreational therapists should have a variety of palmar clips, utensil holders, universal cuffs, right-angle pockets, and wrist supports with palmar clips to try out with the client to evaluate the best equipment choice. The choice of device is determined by the client's functional abilities (as described under "use") and the preferences of the client. The occupational therapist may have already ordered one of these devices for the client, so find out what piece is currently prescribed and try to use that specific piece of equipment for other functional tasks (e.g., typing, sliding game pieces). If another device is more suitable for these needs, the recreational therapist recommends the purchase of the device. If the health insurance company will not cover the cost of a second similar device, the client will have to pay for it out of pocket.

- The recreational therapist evaluates, educates, and trains the client on the use of the device as it pertains to completion of specific tasks (e.g., typing on a computer keyboard, playing checkers, pushing elevator buttons in the community).

Needlecrafts

Needlecrafts include embroidery, cross-stitch, plastic canvas, crochet, and knitting. All of these use needle threaders, magnifiers and lighting, and adaptive scissors, which are discussed in "Sewing" in the Equipment section. Clients may also use Dycem, which has its own entry in the Equipment section.

Embroidery: Embroidery uses colored thread to create various designs on material (cotton, linen). Embroidery includes a variety of stitches (e.g., backstitch, satin stitch, French knots). It can be done with or without a pattern depending on the abilities of the person. Materials can be purchased separately or a project package can be chosen. If an embroidery package is chosen, the material, thread, and needle are provided in addition to an illustration of the project, which is used as a guide to complete the project. The pattern is inked onto the fabric and the artist fills in the space with the designated color and stitch.

Cross-stitch: Like embroidery, cross-stitch uses colored thread to create various designs on material (mostly cotton). Cross-stitch uses primarily one stitch called, what else, the cross-stitch, which looks like an "X". There are two types of cross-stitch: counted cross-stitch and stamped cross-stitch. Counted cross-stitch is done on aida cloth. Aida cloth is a tightly woven cotton cloth that looks like a very small basket weave. The artist counts the basket squares to determine where to stitch. Stamped cross-stitch is done on flat cotton. The "Xs" are stamped on the cotton showing the person exactly where to place the cross-stitch

- *Equipment for embroidery and cross-stitch*: Embroidery holders can be used for both embroidery and cross-stitch. They come in various forms: a hoop on a stand that sits on a tabletop, a hoop placed on a gooseneck clamp that clamps onto a tabletop or a wheelchair arm, a scroll-like device that rolls the fabric from one side of the scroll to the other, and another hoop that attaches to a curved piece of wood that is held in place by the client's leg. Embroidery holders can be purchased through health care catalogs, but they are also available in craft stores. Many people who embroider or cross-stitch use these devices to decrease the stress of holding the piece for long periods of time.

Plastic canvas: Plastic canvas looks like a thick plastic mesh or screen. It has holes in it and it comes in sheets. A thick plastic or metal needle is used to run diagonal stitches through the mesh to make a design. Plastic canvas can be cut into shapes before it is filled in with yarn. It can also be stitched together (e.g., to make a tissue box, a Christmas ornament).

- *Equipment for plastic canvas*: If the client needs to stabilize the plastic canvas (e.g., only has use of one hand), a large piece of plastic canvas (e.g., 12" x 8") can be set on a wire book holder. It can rest in the book holder or be Velcroed or tied to the book holder. Smaller pieces can be taped or Velcroed onto the side of a tabletop in front of the client.

Crochet: Crochet uses one needle with a small hook on the end. Crochet needles come in various sizes. The smaller the needle, the smaller the stitch. The type of material used in crochet can vary from very thick yarns to make blankets to very thin threads to make doilies.

Knitting: Knitting is different from crochet. It uses two needles that have tapered ends. One is held in each hand.

- *Equipment for crochet and knitting*: A device called a "clamp-it" has suction cups on the bottom so it can stick to a tabletop or side wall (can be positioned horizontally or vertically) and a clamp that can be adjusted to hold items at any angle (available through Maxi Aids, in "Equipment Resources"). It can be used to hold knitting or crochet needles. It can also hold a magnifier and a variety of other items. This is a good device for one-handed knitting or crocheting.

Weight

Embroidery holders vary in weight depending on the style and material from which they are made. The "clamp-it" weighs approximately one pound.

Fitting

NA

Authorization

NA

Use

Embroidery holders: Embroidery holders sit on a table, clamp onto a table, slide under the leg, or roll on scrolls. In a hoop design, the outer hoop is removed. The fabric is laid on top of the inner hoop and the outer hoop is pushed down over top of the fabric to hold it taut. This is typically done before the device is set-up (e.g., clamped onto the table, put under the leg). The scroll design has two pieces of fabric, each attached down one side of a scroll. The project is sewn onto the fabric that is attached to each scroll. Once this is done, the project will be attached to the scrolls (scroll, fabric, project, fabric, scroll). The scrolls are tightened until the fabric is taut.

Book holder (wire): Open the book holder and set it on the table. The front legs of the book holder can open wide or close in tight to support the project. The project is placed on the book holder, which helps to stabilize it.

Clamp-it: Wet the suction cups on the bottom of the device and stick it to the tabletop. It should be positioned where the client would typically hold the needle. For example, if a client needed to use the "clamp-it" to hold a crochet needle, which she normally held in her left hand, then the clamp-it, would be placed on the table in front of the left hand and slightly to the center (or dead center, whichever is more comfortable for the client). The clamp is opened and the needle is placed into the clamp and tightened. The needle can be positioned at various angles and the therapist will adjust the angle of the needle to find the best functional position for the client. While knitting or crocheting, the chain of loops will begin to lower towards the floor. When the project is just being started sometimes the chain will flip around the needle because the hand is not being used to hold the chain down. To keep this from happening, clip a clothespin onto the bottom of the chain to give it some weight so that it will not flip around the needle. Once a few rows have been knitted or crocheted, the weight of the piece should keep it from flipping around the needle.

Benefits

Adaptive equipment for needlecrafts may allow a client to engage in needlecraft activities despite a functional loss.

Design Challenges

There are a variety of designs to meet the individual needs of clients. In some cases, therapists specially fabricate a piece of equipment or modify an existing piece of equipment.

Costs

Embroidery hoop holders can range from $40.00 to $100.00. They can be purchased through adaptive equipment catalogs and through local arts and crafts stores. A wire book holder costs a few dollars and a "clamp-it" costs about $10.00.

Treatment Direction

- Recreational therapists assess a client's functional abilities to engage in needlecrafts if it is an interest of the client or it will be used as a therapeutic modality to increase function.
- Adaptive equipment is tested and prescribed for needlecrafts as needed.
- Recreational therapists educate the client about each piece of adaptive equipment: its set-up, use, and maintenance.
- Adaptive needlecraft devices are not covered by health insurance because they are not viewed as being medically necessary. Recreational therapists tell clients where recommended devices can be purchased.
- If the client requires assistance in the use of a device (e.g., help to set up the device), the recreational therapist educates the client's caregivers, as appropriate.

Prosthesis

Healthcare professionals who prescribe and manufacture prostheses consider comfort, ease of donning (putting on) and doffing (taking off), weight (the lighter the better), durability, required maintenance (e.g., cleaning), visual cosmetic appeal, and functionality of the unit when choosing an appropriate prosthesis for a client. The average life of a prosthesis for an adult is two years with daily use. Teenagers and children may require more frequent prostheses due to growth. The weight of the prosthesis usually is about half the weight of the body segment it replaces, from 3-7 lbs for a below-knee prosthesis, and from 7-12 lbs for an above-knee prosthesis. Lightweight and sport prosthetics however, may also be considered (Kottke & Lehmann, 1990).

Lower Extremity Prosthesis

Lower extremity prosthesis components:
- *Socket*: The socket is a "bucket-like" component that slides onto the residual limb. It is designed to protect the residual limb, as well as to disperse the forces associated with standing and walking. The client's residual limb is measured by making a plaster mold from the limb or through computer-assisted technology. The socket should be wiped out daily with a damp cloth and mild soap. When not wearing the prosthetic, it should be laid down on its side on the floor so that it does not fall over and crack.
- *Sock or gel liner*: Socks of various plies are worn on the stump to make up for the gap between the limb and the prosthesis to ensure a good fit. See "Prosthetic Socks" in the Equipment section for more information.
- *Suspension system*: This is how the prosthesis stays on the limb without falling off. It may consist of a variety of belts and straps that bolt onto the socket and connect to a waist strap or it may be a suction suspension. The most common type of suction suspension is silicon suction. A silicon-based sock is worn over the residual limb and then is inserted into the socket. It forms an airtight seal that stabilizes the prosthesis.
- *Articulating joint* (if needed): This is the knee joint. The prosthetic knee must provide support during the swing phase and maintain unrestricted motion for sitting and kneeling. The prosthetic knee can have a single axis with a simple hinge and a single pivot point, or it may have a polycentric axis with multiple centers of rotation (Bodeau & Mipro, 2002b).

- *Pylon*: This is the metal shaft that attaches to the socket and the terminal device. It is the replacement for the femur and/or the tibia/fibula. Once all of the adjustments are made to the prosthesis as a whole so that it fits the client correctly, the pylon is covered in soft foam contoured to match the other limb with a hard laminated shell (exoskeleton) or covered with a cosmetic soft covering (endoskeleton).
- *Terminal device*: This is the foot, but it may take other forms for athletic activities (e.g., running). The ankle joint is typically part of the terminal device. However, like the foot, separate ankle joints can be fitted for demanding physical work or physically demanding recreational pursuits (e.g., rock climbing) that incorporate more complex motion and strength.

Upper Extremity Prosthesis

There are two types of upper extremity prostheses referred to as body-powered prostheses and myoelectric prostheses. Bodeau & Mipro (2002a) explain the difference between the two units:
- The body-powered prostheses are manipulated using cables/straps. They are the most durable prostheses and have higher sensory feedback. However, body powered prostheses are less cosmetically pleasing than a myoelectric unit, and they require more gross limb movement.
- Myoelectric prostheses, operated by myoelectricity, may give more proximal function and increased cosmetic appeal, but they can be heavy and expensive. They have less sensory feedback and require more maintenance. They function by sensing electrical activity on the residual limb muscles and transmitting the information to electric motors that operate the prosthetic.

Components depend on the amputation site.

Below Elbow Amputation (BEA)
- Voluntary opening (VO) split hook.
- Friction wrist.
- Double-walled plastic laminate socket.
- Flexible elbow hinge.
- Single-control cable system.
- Biceps or triceps cuff.
- Figure-of-eight harness.

Above Elbow Amputation (AEA)
Same as below elbow amputation except:

- Substitutes an internal-locking elbow for the flexible elbow hinge.
- Uses a dual control cable instead of a single control.
- Does not have a biceps or triceps cuff.

The upper extremity prosthesis tries to replicate hand functions of the missing hand. The five relevant grips are
- *Precision grip* (e.g., pincher grip): The pad of the thumb and index finger are in opposition to pick up or pinch a small object (e.g., small bead, grain of rice).
- *Tripod grip* (e.g., palmar grip, 3-jaw chuck pinch): The pad of the thumb is against pads of the index and middle finger.
- *Lateral grip*: The pad of the thumb is in opposition to the lateral aspect of the index finger to manipulate a small object (e.g., turning a key in a lock).
- *Hook power grip*: The distal interphalangeal (DIP) joint and proximal interphalangeal (PIP) joint are flexed with the thumb extended (e.g., carrying a briefcase by the handle).
- *Spherical grip*: Tips of fingers and thumb are flexed (e.g., screwing in a light bulb or opening a doorknob).

References

Bodeau, V. & Mipro, R. (2002a). Upper limb prosthetics. http://www.emedicine.com/pmr/ topic174.htm on 1/19/04.

Bodeau, V. & Mipro, R. (2002b). Lower limb prosthetics. http://www.emedicine.com/pmr/ topic175.htm on 1/19/04.

Kottke, F. & Lehmann, J. (1990). *Krusen's handbook of physical medicine and rehabilitation, 4th edition.* W.B. Saunders Company: Philadelphia, PA.

Prosthetic Socks

Prosthetic socks are made from nylon, cotton, wool, or synthetic material and are placed over an amputated limb to fill up the gap and ensure a good fit between the residual limb and the prosthetic. Prosthetic socks come in various lengths, widths, and plies. The length and width of socks are prescribed by the prosthetist (a professional who designs, makes, and fits prosthetics). The number of plies is determined by the therapist. A ply refers to the number of threads knitted together to make the sock. Some prosthetic socks have a gel insert to provide added cushioning. Prosthetic socks come in four plies.

- Nylon stocking (0 ply/thickness)
- White trim (1 ply/thickness)
- Yellow trim (3 ply/thickness)
- Green trim (5 ply/thickness)

A client's sock ply is determined by adding up all of the sock plies that the client needs to wear to fill the gap (e.g., one green sock (5 ply) + one yellow sock (3-ply) = 8 ply). Generally, more than 10 plies are too much. If more than 10 plies are needed, the socket may need to be redesigned or modified. A poor fit can cause secondary skin problems.

Weight

A few ounces.

Fitting

Prior to applying socks, the stump shrinker or ace wrap must be removed. The stump should always be clean and dry prior to applying socks. The skin should be inspected for signs of ulceration or infection every time socks are put on and every time the prosthetic and socks are removed. Any change in skin color that lasts more than 30 minutes deserves medical attention prior to further use of the prosthetic.

The nylon sock is put on first (0 ply), followed by the prosthetic socks initially recommended by the physical therapist and prosthetist. Each sock should fit smoothly without any wrinkles. The seams along the bottom of the sock are worn on the outside (not against the skin). The stump will continue to shrink as a result of atrophied muscles, pressure from the prosthesis, and wrapping. As a result, the client will need to have readjustments to the sock plies and, less often, the prosthesis. Residual limbs also change in volume throughout a day, so the client must always have extra socks readily available and make needed changes.

If the residual limb fits snugly (not too tight or loose), then no pain is felt, no ulceration or bruising is evident after wearing the prosthesis, and the pressure mark from wearing the prosthesis is not on a bony area (e.g., knee cap, elbow). For the below knee amputee, if the pressure mark is located below the kneecap and above the top of the shinbone then the number of sock plies is correct. If the pressure mark is on the kneecap, add one sock ply. If the pressure mark is on the shinbone, take off one sock ply. Continue modifying the number of plies until the pressure mark is in the correct location.

Skin checks are done before donning the prosthesis (putting it on) and after doffing the prosthesis (taking it off). The client will be put on a wearing schedule by the physical therapist. (See the "Amputation" diagnosis for more information on the wearing schedule.)

When the client is walking (lower extremity prosthesis) or using the prosthesis (upper extremity prosthesis), the therapist should be attentive to the fit of the prosthesis. Socks should be worn thick enough so that they do not slide up or down when in the socket of the prosthesis.

Authorization for use

NA

Use

See Fitting.

Benefits

Fills up the gap between the residual limb and the prosthesis. This ensures a good fit. A good fit is essential for proper functioning of the prosthesis, the client's safety, and maintaining the integrity of the skin.

Design Challenges

Cotton socks absorb moisture. This is a good thing because it takes moisture away from the skin. Prolonged moisture on the skin along with friction promotes skin breakdown. Because they absorb moisture, socks must be changed frequently throughout the day. The frequency of this will vary depending on the client's activity level, the weather, and perspiration. Socks must be washed by hand or on the gentle cycle daily in lukewarm water and mild soap. To dry the socks, wrap them in a towel (do not twist socks) and then lay them flat to air-dry. Socks should not be placed on a radiator, in a dryer, or in direct sunlight because that can shrink the sock. If a hole or run develops, the sock needs to be replaced. It should not be sewn or repaired. Sewing a sock may decrease the sock's dimensions or add seams that could result in a poor fit or skin irritation.

Costs

A standard cotton prosthetic sock costs about $25.00 per sock. Socks with gel liners typically range from $60.00 to $80.00 a sock.

Treatment Direction

- Recreational therapists perform skin checks, document findings, and talk with the primary physical therapist about observations to further assess the need for sock ply changes.
- Recreational therapists assist client with donning and doffing sock plies.
- Recreational therapists teach clients about the need to change socks in a community setting and identify comfortable places for the client to change his/her socks (e.g., dressing rooms).
- Recreational therapists help clients to identify ways to carry extra socks (and other prosthetic supplies) in a community setting (e.g., use of a lightweight backpack).
- See "Amputation" in the Diagnoses section for more specific information related to recreational therapy's role with prosthetic wear and monitoring.

Reachers

A reacher is an adaptive device for retrieving high, low, or out of reach items. They come in a variety of lengths ranging from 18-33". Reachers have three common components. Each has a jaw that holds the item, an aluminum or stainless steel shaft, and a trigger handle that is squeezed to engage the jaws.

Jaws: The jaws hold the item. Some are rubber tipped, some have suction cups, some can be rotated, and some are just ribbed plastic. Ribbed plastic is good for picking up clothing but it is not good for holding cans because the jaws slip off. Suction cups and rubber tips are good to hold round items and boxes. Some reachers have self-closing jaws, meaning that the client doesn't have to maintain a tight squeeze on the trigger handle to continue the hold on the item. Other jaws stay closed all the time and squeezing the trigger handle opens the jaws instead of closing the jaws. Most jaws have magnetic ends for retrieving small metal objects (e.g., safety pins, paper clips). Jaws typically open three to four inches.

Shaft: The shaft is the metal bar between the trigger handle and the jaws. The longer the shaft, the heavier the reacher. Some shafts are foldable making the reacher easy to transport (e.g., in a backpack).

Trigger handle: Squeezing the trigger handle with the hand closes the jaws. Some reachers maintain this closure until a lock is released so that the client does not have to maintain a tight squeeze on the trigger handle. If a client does not have finger movement but does have wrist movement, a reacher called a "quad reacher" may be helpful. The trigger handle is operated through wrist movements.

Accessories: Various holders can be purchased and placed on a wheelchair or walker to hold the reacher. It can also be placed in a pouch or bag on the back of a wheelchair. A wrist support is an available option with some models. It supports the forearm and wrist if muscle weakness is present.

Weight

Reachers have weight capacities, meaning that they can only pick up a certain amount of weight. Some reachers can only grasp and lift items that weigh less than a pound while others can grasp and lift items that weigh up to four pounds. The weight of a reacher also varies. Reachers can weigh anywhere from three to twelve ounces.

Fitting

Jaws: Therapists evaluate the purpose of the reacher. What are the most common items that the client needs to retrieve? Are they less than one pound? Are they greater than two pounds? What shape are they? How far does the jaw have to open to hold the item? Therapists choose a reacher that is able to grasp and lift these items (e.g., suction cup jaws because he client needs to retrieve a lot of round items; plastic ribbed jaws because the client needs to retrieve only clothing items that are less than one pound).

Length: Therapists choose a reacher length that best suits the needs of the client. Longer reachers are good for clients who have bending precautions (e.g., a total hip replacement, laminectomy) or who find it difficult to lean forward (e.g., a person with poor trunk control). The advantages of extra length are balanced against the added weight and difficulty of using a longer tool.

Trigger handle: Trigger handles that open the jaws when squeezed do not require the client to maintain a squeeze on the trigger handle to hold the item. The tension pulls the jaws together once the client opens the jaws. This type of jaw is good for clients who need to protect hand and wrist joints (e.g., rheumatoid arthritis, frail hands). Trigger handles that close the jaws when squeezed require the client to maintain the squeeze to hold the item. Some reachers have a lock that holds the squeeze. These are good for clients who have good hand, wrist, and arm strength.

Weight: Therapists consider the weight of the reacher as it affects the client's performance. Reachers that are shorter typically weigh less. Lightweight reachers are best for clients who must protect their joints (e.g., rheumatoid arthritis) or have limited arm, wrist, and finger strength.

Authorization

Occupational therapists commonly prescribe reachers for home use. Recreational therapists who identify the need for a specific type of reacher discuss their concerns with the occupational therapist. Health insurance will typically cover only one reacher. If one reacher has already been submitted for reimbursement, the recreational therapist will recommend that the client purchase the additional reacher out of pocket.

Use

Reachers are used for retrieving items that are out of reach for the client (too high, too low, too far away).

Benefits

Allows clients to retrieve items without assistance from another person.

Design Challenges

There are a variety of designs to meet the individual needs of clients. In some cases, therapists specially fabricate a piece of equipment or modify an existing piece of equipment.

Cost

The price for a reacher ranges from $15.00 to $45.00. The quad reacher costs about $140.00.

Treatment Direction

- Clients are taught how to operate the reacher and the limitations of the reacher (e.g., weight capacity).

- Clients practice using the reacher in a real-life or simulated real-life environment to learn how to 1. align themselves with the item to be retrieved, 2. slide or move other items out of the way to retrieve the desired item, 3. transport items over a long distance (grab item, place item on an accessible surface like a countertop, clip the reacher onto the holder mounted on the walker, walk a few more feet towards the destination, turn around to re-approach the item on the counter, grab the item, move it further down the counter, clip the reacher onto the holder mounted on the walker, and so on until the item is placed at the desired location). Clients are to avoid excessive twisting when retrieving, transporting, or releasing an item because it challenges the client's balance more than if the client faced the item forward.

- Therapists help clients to problem solve for transporting the reacher and prescribe clips and holders as needed. Therapists can also try using Velcro. Place a piece of loop Velcro on the shaft of the reacher and a piece of hook Velcro on the side of the walker or back of the wheelchair.

Sewing (machine and hand)

Sewing is the process of joining fabric together using a needle and thread. This is done for the purpose of making clothes and household items (curtains, table covers, quilts, costumes, pillows, dolls). There are 12 pieces of adaptive equipment or adaptations commonly used for this activity: needle threader; magnifier; lighting; adaptive scissors; hem clips; tape; cushioned board and pins; rotary cutters, mats, and rulers; pedal changes; and Dycem.

Needle threader: There are many different types of needle threaders, but they all have one thing in common: an easier way to thread a needle. Threading a needle, whether handheld or on a sewing machine, can be difficult for clients who have poor vision (decreased clarity, double vision, field cuts) or who have diminished fine motor skills (e.g., finger-thumb opposition, pinch, spasms, tremors).

Magnifier: A small magnifier can be attached to the sewing machine that magnifies the needle and sewing area by 2 times. There are also a variety of other magnifiers that can be used for cutting, seeing patterns, and piecing material.

Lighting: Direct lighting improves the client's ability to see the task. Table and floor lamps that provide bright white light (not fluorescent) are most helpful.

Adaptive scissors: Fiskars makes several brands of scissors that have soft grips and a spring-loaded handle. The soft handles make it easier to grasp and protect finger and wrist joints. These can be purchased at many local craft and sewing stores. PETA scissors are also spring activated. They have five different models, two of which are for people who have use of only one hand. These two models each have a base that rests on the table allowing the client to cut by pressing on a rectangular plastic piece that is mounted on top of the top blade. PETA scissors can be purchased from rehab catalogs (see Equipment Resources). An alternative to scissors is a rotary cutter (see rotary cutters and mats below).

Hem clips: Hem clips are four-inch long clips that hold a hem in place. A hem is created by folding in the bottom edge of the material (twice) to make a finished edge. The hem is then sewn in place. Hems are usually pinned in place. Hem clips are an alternative to pinning.

Tape use: Tape, especially medical tape, seems to work well for stabilizing fabric to a tabletop. The corners of a piece of fabric can be taped down to the table to hold it in place. Medical tape seems to pull fabric threads the least.

Cushioned board and pins: This is a fabricated piece of equipment. Purchase a large piece of Styrofoam (e.g., 24" x 24" x 2"). Cut a piece of cotton fabric so that it covers the top and sides of the Styrofoam with an additional three-inch allowance to wrap around the back and glue (use fabric glue). Purchase pins with large pinheads so they can be picked up easily. If you can't find them, glue a wooden bead or button to the top of a pinhead (Super Glue works well). To stabilize a piece of fabric, lay it down on top of the covered Styrofoam and push the large-headed pins through the fabric and into the Styrofoam board. This is good for small projects (e.g., making a pillow).

Rotary cutters, mats, and rulers: These are common supplies used for quilting but they can also be helpful for other types of sewing, especially for clients who have limited hand function. A rotary cutter looks like a small pizza cutter that is operated with one hand to cut through fabric. The fabric is laid on top of a quilter's mat (a special mat that protects the table from the rotary cutter). The rotary cutter will not cut through the mat. People who quilt are also familiar with quilting rulers. They come in various widths, lengths, and shapes. For making straight or angled cuts, the quilting ruler is laid on the fabric, held in place by putting pressure on top of the ruler, and cutting the fabric by running the rotary cutter along the edge of the ruler.

Pedal changes: Sewing machines have a pedal that sits on the floor. Applying pressure to the pedal with the foot makes the sewing machine sew. When pressure is gradually released, the sewing machine slows down, and when the pressure is fully removed, the sewing machine stops. Clients who do not have a foot that can operate a sewing machine pedal can change the location of the pedal. It can be mounted on a table leg so the client can operate it with the knee. Depending of the weight of the pedal, the therapist can use Velcro to hold the pedal to the table leg or the therapist can use an "Instant 'D' Ring Velstrap" (a Velcro product available in rehab catalogs). It is attached to either side of the pedal and then tightened down around the table leg. Another option is to place the pedal on top of the table so the client can operate it by using a hand or a combination of the forearm and elbow.

Dycem: Cut two small strips of Dycem about one inch wide and two inches long (see "Dycem" in the Equipment section). Wrap one around the client's thumb and the other around the index finger. A small piece of medical tape can hold the wrap closed if needed. This helps the client get a better grip (pinch) on the needle when pushing or pulling it through a piece of fabric while hand sewing.

Weight

Needle threaders, adaptive scissors, hem clips, tape, cushioned board and pins, and rotary scissors, mats, and rulers weigh very little. Magnifiers and lighting equipment will vary in weight depending on the model chosen. Therapists who anticipate the weight of an item will affect the client's ability to use the item should research the weight before suggesting its use to the client.

Fitting

Needle threaders, hem clips, tape, cushioned board and pins, rotary scissors, mats, and rulers, and Dycem do not require fitting. Some adaptive scissors are right or left handed. Magnifiers come in different magnifications (2x to 15x is typical). Therapists should have various types of magnifiers to determine the type of magnifier and magnification that works best for a desired task (e.g., a magnifier that stands independently on the table is helpful for tasks that require the use of two hands). Lighting that provides direct light on the item is desirable. Possible lights include a small reading lamp that sits on the table, a tall gooseneck lamp that sits on the floor next to a chair and can be adjusted to shine directly on the task (e.g., book, cross-stitch), or a combination device that provides both light and magnification. The therapist should have at least one tabletop lighting device that can be used to determine if direct light on the project provides the client with increased clarity and task performance.

Authorization

NA

Use

Needle threaders: The use of a needle threader varies depending on the model. The wire loop needle threader has a large diamond shaped wire loop that is easily seen. The tip of the diamond is pushed through the eye of the needle. Once it is through, the client puts the thread through the large diamond wire loop and then pulls it back through the eye to thread the needle. Another model, called the "infila automatic", requires the client to put the needle eye down into a small cylinder, place the thread through a small valley, and push a button to send the thread through the needle eye.

Magnifiers: The magnifier is held at least 12" from the subject to achieve full magnification. The closer it is held to the subject, the smaller the magnification.

Lighting: Lighting should be direct, 18-24" from the item.

Adaptive scissors: The use of adaptive scissors varies depending on the model chosen. Fiskar scissors have one loop for the thumb and a straight handle on the other blade to wrap all four fingers around. The scissors are then squeezed to close the blades (to cut). One-handed scissors from PETA rest on the table and are depressed using one finger, multiple fingers, the wrist, or the forearm.

Hem clips: To open hem clips, the end is pinched between the thumb and index finger. They are slid onto the fabric and then released.

Tape use: See "description."

Cushioned board and pins: See "description."

Rotary cutter, mats, and rulers: Place the mat on a table, put the fabric on top of the mat, place the ruler in position, and run the rotary cutter along the edge of the ruler to make the cut. The rotary cutter requires a good grip and gross motor arm movement compared to scissors that require more fine hand movement such as flexion and extension of fingers and more complex hand-eye coordination. The handle of the rotary cutter can also be built up with foam tubing for clients who have a limited grasp (see "Foam Tubing" in the Equipment section). The use of a quilting ruler will guide the rotary cutter. Rotary cutters are good for straight cuts. They are not good for making intricate or curved cuts.

Pedal changes: See "description."

Dycem: See "description."

Benefits

Adaptive sewing equipment and techniques can increase a client's independence and ability to sew. For some the skill of sewing is a necessary skill of daily living for making clothes and home materials, while other sew for leisure.

Design Challenges

There are a variety of designs to meet the individual needs of clients. In some cases, therapists specially fabricate a piece of equipment or modify an existing piece of equipment.

Costs

Needle threaders range from $.50 (wire loop needle threader) to $3.00 (infila automatic). Magnifiers cost anywhere from $9.00 to $90.00 depending on the magnification and size. Adaptive scissors can range from $15.00 to $30.00. Hem clips cost a few dollars at the most. Medical tape is also inexpensive. Making a cushioned board and pins costs about $15.00. Rotary cutters cost about $10.00. Rotary cutter mats range from $8.00 to $40.00 depending on the size. The cost of quilting rulers also varies depending on the size and shape, between $7.00 and $25.00. Refer to "Velcro" and "Dycem" in the Equipment section for cost information.

Treatment Direction

Recreational therapists perform a task analysis of the sewing skills desired by the client and identify areas of breakdown. Areas of breakdown are further assessed to determine the exact skill or skills that are causing the breakdown. Adaptive equipment needs are evaluated and modified techniques are tried with the goal of increasing the client's independence and level of engagement with the task. Recommendations are given to the client, as well as the client's caregivers, as appropriate (e.g., client requires supervision at all times when operating the sewing machine).

Switches

A switch is an electromechanical device that is used to activate or deactivate an electrical signal. There are thousands of switches that range from very tiny finger switches to large machinery switches. Some of the most common switches used in a therapy setting include: mechanical (push button, joystick, sip and puff, rockers, touch sensitive, etc.), infrared (e.g., light beam), and proximity (senses proximity of body part to switch to activate the switch without having to touch the switch).

A switch (input method) is a modality that allows the operation of electrical devices. Switches are commonly used for computers, powered mobility, augmentative communication devices, toys, and home automation (e.g., lights, doors, small appliances, stereo). Access to these applications, that may not be otherwise accessible, provides opportunities for engagement in life tasks at home, work, play, recreation, and leisure.

Switches can be single, dual, or multiple. Single switches are used to operate a simple on-off object (e.g., toy, radio, light). Dual switches are used for objects that require two operations (e.g., scanning and selecting as needed to operate a computer program). Multiple switches are used to operate objects that require three or more operations (e.g., a joystick to control the movement of a power wheelchair).

Switches operate in either momentary or latching mode. In momentary mode, the switch performs the action only as long as the switch is engaged (e.g., when pressure is applied to a switch button the toy moves, when pressure is released the toy stops). In latching mode, once the switch is activated, the response continues until the switch is reactivated to stop the response (e.g., when pressure is applied to a switch button the toy jumps, the toy continues to jump even though the pressure has been removed, when pressure is reapplied to the switch the toy stops jumping).

Switches can be placed on a flat surface (e.g., tabletop) or they can be attached to a mounting system.

Weight

Varies

Fitting

Switches are fitted to the individual needs of the client. To determine the type of switch, the placement of the switch, and the position of the switch, therapists evaluate the functioning of the client, the specific item, and the desired action. Type of switch and placement of the switch are also based on client preferences, outcomes of trial placements, data collection, observation, and professional opinion. The smallest movement is preferred (e.g., finger movement over forearm movement) because it means less fatigue. Switch hits should be accurate and reliable. Therapists consider using switches that use the hand or forearm first because the hand or forearm is the most natural. Following the hand or forearm is the full arm or shoulder. The full arm or shoulder typically requires the hand to be stabilized to ensure an accurate switch hit. Next, the foot or ankle is considered followed by the head or neck. The head and neck can interfere with visual attention and induce feelings of vertigo. Lastly, the use of the large joints such as the knee or hip is considered because the larger the joint, the more energy required, often resulting in quick fatigue.

Authorization

Switches may or may not be covered by health insurance. If seeking health insurance reimbursement, medical necessity must be proven.

Use

Will vary depending on the type of switch and the placement of the switch. Successful switch use requires practice.

Benefits

The ability to use a computer, communicate, play with a toy, operate a power wheelchair, and control electronics in the home are common life tasks that provide opportunities for physical, emotional, social, and cognitive health that improve independence, functioning, and quality of life.

Design Challenges

There are a variety of designs to meet the individual needs of clients. In some cases, therapists specially fabricate a piece of equipment or modify an existing piece of equipment.

Costs

Will vary depending on the switch and mounting system.

Treatment Direction

- Recreational therapists evaluate, prescribe, and train clients on the use of switches.
- Recreational therapists keep abreast of assistive technology through professional workshops orchestrated through the profession, assistive technology organizations (see RESNA in the resource section), consultation with assistive technology practitioners and suppliers, and individual research. See "Equipment Resources" for switch catalogs.

Therapy Putty

Therapy putty feels like a smooth clay. It is nontoxic, it doesn't dry out, and it doesn't stick under fingernails. Some forms of putty are also latex-free. It can be squeezed, stretched, twisted, or pinched. Putty typically comes in soft, medium-soft, medium, and firm and is color-coded for easy identification of consistency (e.g., yellow is soft, firm is blue). Therapy putty is used mostly to improve hand strength. In addition to a therapeutic medium to improve hand strength, recreational therapists have found therapy putty to be helpful for stabilizing hard to stabilize items (see Use).

Weight

Therapy putty can be purchased in small or large containers. A client is typically given two ounces of therapy putty to work with.

Fitting

NA

Authorization

NA

Use

Recreational therapists often use therapy putty as a substitute for playdough when working with children who need to improve hand strength because of its therapeutic property of resistance. Therapy putty, although not advertised to be used in this manner, is also a wonderful stabilizer for hard-to-stabilize, odd-shaped items. For example, a client went fly-fishing before he had a stroke. As a result of the stroke, he does not have a functional left-hand grasp. Prior to the stroke, he would spend several hours each week tying fishing flies, which consisted of many different complex knots. Therapy putty turned out to be an excellent way to stabilize the hook so he could learn to tie knots with one hand.

Firm therapy putty was used by pressing the bottom of the hook down into the putty while leaving the top of the hook exposed for tying knots. Using a combination of medical tape to hold one end of the line on the table, the client's right hand to go under and over with the other end of the line, and his teeth to help the hand pull knots tight, the client was able to tie a fishing knot. Once the fly was completed, he pulled the hook out of the putty and it came out clean without any putty sticking to it.

Benefits

Therapy putty is a medium to improve and challenge hand strength. It should also be considered as a stabilization material.

Design Challenges

NA

Costs

A two-ounce container of therapy putty costs about $4.00.

Treatment Directions

- Recreational therapists consider the use of therapy putty as a substitute for playdough when development of hand strength is needed. Squeezing therapy putty can also be a mechanism for stress reduction.
- Recreational therapists evaluate the use of therapy putty as a stabilization material for odd shaped items that are difficult to stabilize.

Toileting

There are many types of equipment that are used in toileting. Six common pieces of toileting equipment are discussed here: bidet, commode, raised toilet seat, suppository inserter and digital bowel stimulator, toilet grab bar, and urinal. See Body Functions Chapter 6 for information on other types of equipment including indwelling catheters, straight catheters, Texas catheters, urinals, and sanitary pads for urination.

Bidet: A bidet is a piece of equipment that releases an upward spray of water that cleans the perirectal area. Some bidets also release warm air to dry the area. They can be placed on top of or underneath the seat of a standard toilet.

Commode: A commode is a freestanding piece of equipment. It looks like a chair with a round or oval cutout in the seat. The arms and legs may be adjustable and some have a swing away arm to make it easier to transfer. Under the seat is a pail (also referred to as a bucket). The client sits on the commode to urinate or defecate. The pail is removed and emptied. Some commodes are able to fit over a standard toilet if the pail is removed, allowing the client to benefit from the added support of the commode chair while being able to use the toilet.

Raised toilet seat: A raised toilet seat is plastic ring that attaches onto the toilet bowl (underneath the toilet seat). It raises the height of the toilet seat an additional three to six inches. Some models allow the toilet seat to lower down on top of the raised toilet seat but many do not. The client sits directly on the raised toilet seat.

Suppository inserter and digital bowel stimulator: A client who is unable to put in a suppository by hand may be able to use a suppository inserter. It is a handled device that has a spring-loaded holder on the end. The suppository is inserted into the holder and, when adequate pressure is applied, the suppository is released. The digital bowel stimulator is also a handheld device. It has a tip on the end that is inserted into the rectum to stimulate the bowels to release. Both the inserter and the stimulator have a cuff on the handle so they are easy to hold. Some models are also adjustable in length or angle.

Toilet grab bars: Toilet grab bars are attached to the wall or walls that surround the toilet to provide the client with support to sit or stand. They are typically made out of steel.

Urinal: A urinal is a plastic container that is used for urination in a reclined or seated position. There are both male and female urinals. Some are clear with imprinted ounces and cubic centimeters for easy measuring.

Weight

Depending on the model, a bidet that attaches to a standard toilet can weigh from a few ounces to several pounds. A commode weighs from eight to fifteen pounds. A raised toilet seat weighs from three to six pounds. A suppository inserter, digital bowel stimulator, and urinal are a few ounces. The weight of toilet grab bars will vary depending on the length of the bar chosen. They typically do not weigh more than three pounds.

Fitting

NA for all devices except toilet grab bars. Toilet grab bars are attached to the wall in strategic places to provide the client with support to sit or stand. They are typically placed horizontally on the wall about a foot higher than a toilet seat or they are placed at an angle. If placed at an angle, they are typically angled down towards the toilet so that they provide a lower bar when sitting and higher bar when standing.

Authorization

Occupational therapists commonly prescribe toileting equipment. Recreational therapists who perceive a need for such equipment discuss it with the client's primary occupational therapist.

Use

Bidet: After relieving bowel and bladder, a button is commonly pushed for the bidet to release the spray of water and another button for warm air. This is best used by clients who are unable to attend to hygiene needs related to toileting due to arthritic hands, impaired arm and hand function, or spinal problems that limit flexion and extension of the trunk.

Commode: See "Description." Commodes are used in the hospital, rehab, residential living, and home setting. A commode may be placed over the toilet to provide support for standing or sitting or next to the client's bed if the client experiences a sense of bowel or bladder urgency, if the bathroom is too far away, or if the bathroom is occupied. A commode may be prescribed for home use for these same reasons or if the bathroom is on another floor that the client can't access.

Raised toilet seat: Once it is attached to the toilet bowl, there are no special instructions for its use. Raised toilet seats are used for clients who have total hip precautions (unable to bend more than 90°) or clients who have difficulty getting up and down from a regular height toilet (e.g., weak lower extremities).

Suppository inserter and digital bowel stimulator: See Description. Clients are typically taught how to use these devices by a nurse rather than a therapist. They are used by clients who need to use a suppository and are unable to use their hand to insert it. The stimulator is then used to empty the bowels if the bowels do not move on their own. These devices are commonly used by clients who have tetraplegia.

Toilet grab bars: Clients hold the bar when lowering themselves down onto the toilet and/or to push up from the toilet.

Urinal: Urinals can be used in a seated or standing position. Males have an easier time using a urinal than females because of anatomy. Urinals are used for a variety of reasons. They are used by clients who are unable to get out of bed, make it to the bathroom in time (urgency), or are unable to access a bathroom (e.g., bathroom is on a non-accessible floor or the bathroom itself does not meet the accessibility needs of the client). In general, urinals are good for hospital and home use but are not the best choice for community activities. If a client needs to take a urinal in the community, it is because the bathroom is not accessible (on another floor), the bathroom doesn't meet the accessibility needs of the client, or there is no bathroom available (e.g., on a boat, in a park). In these instances, the client may need to hold onto the urine until it can be properly disposed of or the client may prefer to hold onto the urine so as not to cause embarrassment (e.g., doesn't want to ask someone to run upstairs to the bathroom and empty the urinal for him/her). A male client should use a plastic bottle with a tight screw on lid. A dark sock can be pulled over the bottle to keep it covered for privacy (e.g., the full bottle is placed into the backpack and someone else goes into the backpack or takes it to the bathroom for the client). Female clients who have these same issues but have difficulty using the female urinal can choose different urine collection options such as wearing a sanitary pad that is designed to hold urine or watch fluid intake with careful attention not to dehydrate.

Benefits

Toileting equipment and devices allow a client to achieve greater independence and safety with this task. Proper care of bowel and bladder needs is necessary to prevent secondary complications (e.g., skin breakdown from sitting in wet clothes, impacted bowels, odor).

Design Challenges

There are a variety of designs to meet the individual needs of clients. In some cases, therapists specially fabricate a piece of equipment or modify an existing piece of equipment.

Costs

A bidet that attaches to a standard toilet ranges from $35.00 to $450.00. A commode ranges from $70.00 to $200.00. A raised toilet seat ranges from $15.00 to $100.00. A suppository inserter and digital bowel stimulator cost about $50.00 to $60.00 each. The cost of a toilet grab bars varies depending on the size. They range from $20.00 to $55.00 a bar. Urinals cost about $12.00.

Treatment Directions

- Recreational therapists assist clients to the bathroom, whether in the hospital or community setting, therefore they need to be familiar with toileting equipment.
- Recreational therapists need to be familiar with toileting equipment and its use to ensure the safety of the client.
- Recreational therapists help clients to use toileting skills in a community environment. Public bathrooms do not always meet the accessibility needs of the client nor is there always a bathroom when needed. Therapists help clients problem solve for these issues and recommend equipment and techniques to overcome identified barriers (e.g., using a plastic bottle with a screw on lid, wearing a pad made to collect urine, wearing a Texas Catheter, watching fluid intake, using the bathroom before going out, scheduling community tasks around bowel schedules, self-cathing in a public bathroom).

Transfer Aids

Transfer aids are devices that help the client transfer from one surface to another (e.g., move from the wheelchair to the car). Not all clients require the use of a device to transfer. Clients who do not use a device for walking or who use a cane or walker will not require a device for transferring. Clients who use a wheelchair may or may not need a device for transferring depending on their lower and upper body strength and general balance. Several types of transfer aids are discussed in this section.

Transfer boards: Transfer boards are typically made out of wood. They look like a wooden plank and they come in several different lengths from a short board that is 18" long to a long board that is 32" long. Each end of the board is rounded so there are no sharp corners. Some transfer boards have cutouts in the board for the client to grab the board with his/her hand to help with positioning it.

Disc board: A disc transfer board looks like a standard transfer board but it has a groove that runs along the length of the board. At one end of the groove is a disc. The disc slides from one end to the other through the groove.

Transfer disc: A transfer disc is like a flat lazy Susan with a non-skid surface that sits on the floor.

Leg or thigh lifter: The leg lifter looks like the "walking the invisible dog" toy. It is a length of material (about 42") with a loop on the end. It has aluminum inside to give it rigidity. A client who has difficulty moving a lower extremity can swing the loop around the end of his/her foot and use the device to manually move the leg (e.g., lift the leg onto the bed). A thigh lifter looks like a belt that straps around the thigh above the knee and has an added loop on the top. The client grabs the loop to lift up the leg and reposition it. This is a common device for people who have paraplegia or tetraplegia to position lower extremities for tasks (e.g., transfers, legs that have fallen off of wheelchair footplates). People who have paraplegia often readjust their legs using their arms without a thigh lifter but some find thigh lifters helpful.

Seat lifts: Seat lifts are cushions that are placed on a chair that either makes the seat higher (e.g., a four inch high portable cushion) or helps the client go from a seated to a standing position (e.g., a cushion that looks like this shape ">" is placed on a chair). It has springs or an electronic component that gives the client a boost to stand up.

Sit to and from stand aids: There are various devices for a bed, sofa, or chair that give the client extra support to sit or stand from these surfaces. Some are portable and some attach to the structure. A metal bar extends from the floor up to the seating area where a handle like grab bar is attached. Having a handle to hold can be helpful for surfaces that do not provide support (e.g., a bed, an armless chair, a sofa with too high, too low, or non-existent side arms).

Hoyer lift: A Hoyer lift is a large metal device that measures about 45" long, 26" wide, and five feet tall. A sling is cradled around the client and a cranking system lifts the client up in the air. The Hoyer lift pivots and lowers the client onto another surface. Two people are needed to ensure the safety of the client when using this device.

Transfer belt: This is a heavy-duty, wide belt that is strapped around a client's waist. It has generous loops around the belt for the therapist to hold. This is helpful for transferring clients who require maximal assistance because it gives the therapist better control over the transfer. It is also a helpful device that therapists use for gait training. Transfer belts are helpful when clients wear dresses instead of pants with belt loops because there isn't a good place for a therapist to get a good hold on the client to provide support for transferring or walking.

Weight

A transfer board weighs about two and a half pounds. A transfer disc weighs about five pounds. A leg lifter weighs a few ounces. A plain raised cushion is about one pound and a non-motorized seat lifter is about eight pounds. Sit to and from stand aids weigh about five pounds. A Hoyer lift weighs about 100 pounds. Transfer belts weigh a pound or less depending on the material used to make the belt.

Fitting

Transfer board: A short board is used when transferring to another close surface (e.g., wheelchair to chair). When a longer distance needs to be covered, a longer board is used (e.g., wheelchair to car).

Transfer disc, leg lifter, seat lifts, transfer belts: NA

Sit to and from stand aids: Most are adjustable. Attach or place the device in the desired area. Ask the client to sit on the surface and hold the support bar. Adjust the bar so that the elbow flexes at a 90° angle.

Hoyer lifts: The therapist is responsible for choosing the appropriate size sling to use on the Hoyer lift (e.g., small, medium, large, extra large). Not every Hoyer lift and sling system is the same. Therapists must receive training on how to operate each Hoyer lift prior to attempting its use. Therapists should ask the client's primary nurse what sling is recommended.

Authorization

Transfer boards, transfer discs, and leg lifters are commonly reimbursed by health insurance when it is medically necessary. Seat lifts and sit to and from stand aids are not typically reimbursed by health insurance and must be paid for by the client. Transfer belts are used in the clinic environment and they may also be helpful for caregivers. This is not typically reimbursed by health insurance but it is worth a try if you can argue that it is medically necessary for the safety of the client. Clients who require a Hoyer lift do not typically return to a home environment. Very often people who require this level of care are discharged to a skilled nursing facility. If a client is returning home and requires the use of a Hoyer lift, it is either rented or purchased by the health insurance company.

Use

Transfer boards: See "Transfers" in the Techniques section.

Hoyer lift: Hoyer lifts can be a bit complex to operate. Although they all operate the basically same way, it is important to receive training on the specific model being used. The Hoyer lift is on wheels. It is positioned next to the client so that the strapping system can be easily wrapped and hooked around the client. Once the client is properly strapped, a crank slowly lifts the client up into the air. The Hoyer lift is then wheeled to the transfer location. The client is lowered onto the transfer surface using the crank and then the straps are removed.

Transfer disc: The client is seated and instructed to place both feet on the transfer disc. The therapist lines up the transfer destination at a 90° angle from the surface that the client is currently sitting. The therapist assists the client into a sit pivot or stand pivot position and then rotates the client to the right or the left to line up with the transfer destination. This can be a helpful device for clients who require maximal assistance to transfer. The rotation motion can scare clients, however, and cause them to counteract the rotation, thus impeding its benefit.

Other aids: See "Description" above.

Benefits

Transfer aids increase independence.

Design Challenges

There are many different designs for transfer aids to meet the individual needs of clients.

Costs

A transfer board costs about $35.00 to $70.00. A transfer disc costs about $100.00. A Hoyer lift costs about $2,000.00. A transfer belt costs about $10.00 to $50.00. A sit to and from stand aid costs about $50.00 to $250.00. A seat lifter cushion is about $40.00 and the more complex spring or electric seat lifters range from $200.00 to $350.00. A leg or thigh lifter costs about $10.00 to $20.00.

Treatment Direction

- Recreational therapists assist clients in developing transfer skills and problem solve for transfer techniques in unfamiliar settings (e.g., transferring in a tight public bathroom stall).
- Recreational therapists make suggestions to the treatment team from client observations (e.g., needs a longer transfer board for car transfers).

Velcro

Velcro is one of those fabulous materials that can be found in every therapist's cabinet. Velcro is a material that grabs onto itself. It consists of hook and loop. Hook is the rough Velcro and loop is the soft Velcro. When hook and loop are pressed together, the fibers grab onto each other forming a closure. Velcro comes in many forms. The most common types of Velcro used by recreational therapists are self-adhesive Velcro, non-adhesive Velcro, and instant D-ring Velstrap. Self-adhesive Velcro has a peel off, sticky backing and the non-adhesive Velcro does not (it must be glued or sewn). Instant D-ring Velstrap is a ready-made strap with a D-ring and a Velcro closure.

Weight

Velcro is very light and only adds an ounce or so to an item.

Fitting

Velcro can be used for many different things therefore the process for fitting will vary depending on how it is used.

Authorization

NA

Use

Self-adhesive Velcro: Whenever you want to make something stick somewhere, consider Velcro. Examples: Apply loop Velcro to the squares on a board game and hook Velcro to the bottom of the game board pieces so that they are not easily knocked over by a client who has upper extremity tremors or spasms. Apply a piece of hook Velcro to the arm of a folding chair used for fishing and loop Velcro to the bottom of a small lure box to keep the lure box from toppling over onto the ground. Apply a piece of hook Velcro to the palm of a mitten or winter glove and play catch with a fuzzy tennis ball (the ball will stick to the hook Velcro making it easier to catch and hold). Wrap a small piece of loop Velcro around a mouthstick about an inch from the bottom and stick a piece of hook Velcro onto the side of the computer monitor. The client can independently "dock" the mouthstick by touching it to the hook Velcro. The mouthstick stays in an easily accessible spot so the client can grab it again when it is needed.

Non-adhesive Velcro: Non-adhesive Velcro is used when it is not appropriate to use self-adhesive Velcro (won't stick to the desired surface, won't maintain stick). This is mostly used for clothing or cloth items. Example: On a sweater, sew pieces of hook Velcro opposite the buttons and loop Velcro on top of the buttonholes to stick the sweater together rather than having to button.

Instant D-Ring Velstrap: This is used to make a cuff for an item with a handle (e.g., brush, small gardening tool, sanding block for woodworking). If a client is unable to hold an item because of decreased hand grasp and built up handles made out of foam tubing don't work (client unable to attain a functional grasp with a built up handle) or a utensil holder or universal cuff pocket is too small, consider using a Velstrap. Velstraps look and work like a utensil holder minus the pocket. They slide over the four fingers down onto the palm and an adjustable Velcro strap fits the cuff to the hand. Velstraps have a self-adhesive backing that makes applying the strap simple. If the adhesive is not adequate, small nails may be used to further anchor the strap, depending on the surface (e.g., wooden handle). If nailing is needed, it is recommended to pre-drill the holes to minimize the risk of the handle splitting. Examples: Attach a Velstrap to the handle of a small 12-inch gardening shovel, a hairbrush, a pool cue, or a sanding block for woodworking.

Benefits

Velcro is inexpensive. It is an easy material to use. Velcro is a commonly used material for everyday items (shoes, backpacks) so clients are familiar with it. Velcro is helpful for stabilization and positioning (keeps things from slipping away, holds things in their correct place). It grabs onto itself, making it easy to create closures.

Design Challenges

NA

Costs

- *Self-adhesive Velcro*: Ten yards of one-inch-wide hook or loop Velcro costs about $20.00. Ten yards of two-inch-wide hook or loop Velcro costs about $36.00.
- *Non-adhesive Velcro*: Ten yards of one-inch-wide hook or loop Velcro costs about $15.00. Ten yards of two-inch-wide hook or loop Velcro costs about $25.00.
- *Instant D-ring Velstrap*: Self-adhesive Velstraps that are one inch wide cost about $16.00.

Treatment Directions

- Recreational therapists use Velcro to adapt and modify equipment and items to meet the specific needs of a client.

- Recreational therapists teach clients how to use Velcro products and how to order Velcro products so that they are able to adapt materials on their own once therapy has ended.

Walkers

There are two types of walkers: standard walkers and rolling walkers. Walkers also have several attachments that make them easier for the client to use.

Standard Walkers

Standard walkers have four legs and feet. On the bottom of each foot is a rubber tip that keeps the walker from slipping when the client puts weight on it. Most standard walkers fold but some do not (each side folds into the center so that the walker becomes flat). There are handgrips on each side of the walker to help the client grip the walker. They are usually made out of foam, rubber, or plastic. Standard walkers are used when a client needs bilateral upper extremity support to advance a lower extremity (e.g., a client who has weight-bearing parameters, a client who has had a lower extremity amputation using the walker to hop on one leg, a client learning to walk with a lower extremity prosthesis where there is difficulty bearing weight through the prosthetic limb).

The hemi-walker is a variant on a standard walker. It is a small, four-legged device that is held with one hand to the side of the body. It is different from a quad cane because all four legs originate from the top of the device rather than just four small feet on a bottom platform. It provides more support than a quad cane and less support than a standard walker. Hemi-walkers are commonly used by clients who have paralysis of one upper extremity and require an assistive device that provides more support than a cane to walk.

Rolling Walkers

Rolling walkers are different from standard walkers because they have small wheels on the front or the front and back of the walker. Rolling walkers are used with clients who do not have weight-bearing precautions or impairments. They are commonly used with clients who have endurance and strength issues (e.g., cardiopulmonary issues) because they do not require the client to lift the walker to advance it like a standard walker. There are some variations that may be used in special cases.

- *Reverse walkers*: Reverse walkers are used for pediatrics. It looks like the child is using the walker backwards (it goes around the child's back). They typically have upright handles and automatic brakes that engage when the child puts pressure on the handgrips. The weight of the

device is to the back of the child therefore it encourages the child to stand upright.

- *Eva walkers*: Eva walkers provide maximum walking support. They are much larger than a typical walker and they are used only in a rehabilitation setting as a device for gait training. They are not sent home with the client. They have a large pad that wraps around the front and sides of the walker for the client to rest his/her forearms. There are also two upright handles for the client to grasp. The Eva walker has a wider and stronger base than a traditional walker.

- *Seated walkers*: There is a type of rolling walker that is geared towards the active adult. It is modern and sleek and comes in various colors. The usual features include a basket on the front, swivel wheels for increased agility, larger wheels than a typical walker with pneumatic or solid rubber tires to help transverse uneven community surfaces, hand brakes, and a built-in seat that flips down when the client needs to take a rest. It is commonly prescribed for clients who are able to walk consecutive short community distances (walk 150', rest for 10 minutes, walk another 150', and so on), need the security of having an immediate place to sit and rest, have the cognitive ability to operate and manipulate the device safely (put brakes on before sitting), and engage in community tasks requiring longer distances.

Walker Attachments

- *Glides*: Glides are small ski-like attachments that hook onto the bottom of the back feet of a rolling walker, only when the back feet do not have wheels. It keeps the back feet from catching on the floor (rubber feet on tile floors sometimes stick and catch) and keeps the walker from squeaking when the back feet rub against the floor. If the walker does not have glides and it is squeaking and catching, get two small Dixie cups from the water fountain and set each back walker foot inside a cup. It will stop squeaking and glide across a tiled floor. This is not a substitute for glides, but it works in a pinch. Another idea is to put a slit into a standard tennis ball and set each of the back feet of the walker inside a ball.

- *Platform*: A platform attachment is a metal rod that attaches to the side of a walker. On top of the rod is a forearm rest with an upright handle to the front of it for the client to hold. A Velcro strap wraps around the forearm to hold it on the forearm rest. These are commonly used for gait training with rolling walkers. They are also used for clients who have enough lower extremity strength to walk, have limited mobility or strength in one or both upper extremities, and require bilateral upper extremity support for balance.

- *Swing seat or foldaway seat*: Plastic or canvas seats are available for walkers. The hook to the four legs so that the client can sit "inside" the walker. Therapists must be careful when making this recommendation because the seat is not very stable (especially on rolling walkers) and it can be a tight squeeze to get into and out of the seat, possibly putting the client at an increased risk of falling. It is a good thing to have one in the equipment closet and to evaluate the client's ability to safely use this product before recommending it. If a client is fearful about not being able to find a place to sit and rest, consider the seated rolling walker or teach the client how to plan for and recognize resting areas in the community (see "Energy Conservation Training" in the Techniques section).
- *Baskets and pouches*: There are a variety of baskets and pouches that can be attached to the front or side of a walker. These are very important attachments so that the client does not attempt to carry items while also trying to hold onto the walker. They are not covered by insurance companies because they are not seen as medically necessary. Many clients are on a tight budget and find it difficult to spend $25.00 for a basket. Some hospitals have volunteers who make pouches out of cotton fabric and give them to the clients for free. Clients can also use a wicker bike basket and tie it to the front of the walker with heavy string. Clients who are going to use baskets or pouches must be warned that putting too much weight in the pouches or basket will affect the client's safety and performance. Too much weight in the front basket can cause the walker to tip forward and, if it is a standard walker, advancing the walker can become difficult because of the extra weight. Transporting extra weight using a standard walker increases energy demands. This could result in decreased walking distance (e.g., was able to walk 150' but with five pounds of items in pouches is able to walk only 100'). If clients need to carry bulky items (e.g., transport laundry from one room to another, carry several grocery items from the car into the house), the therapist may consider the use of a backpack. Like the swing seat, the client's ability to use a backpack and to determine an appropriate weight limit must be assessed. Other ideas for transporting

items include the use of a fanny pack (instead of a pocket book) and an apron with pockets.

Weight

A standard or rolling walker weighs approximately six pounds. A hemi-walker weighs about four pounds. An Eva walker weighs about 40 pounds. A seated rolling walker weighs about 17 pounds.

Fitting

Most walkers are height adjustable in one-inch increments. The height of the walker, just like the cane, should allow a 20-30° elbow flexion. A simple way to achieve this it to have the client place his/her hands down by his/her side and then adjust the walker height so that the walker handle comes up to the client's wrist. The width of the walker varies depending on the size of the person. A common width for an adult walker is 20" and a youth walker is 16". With hands down by the side, each walker handle should meet the client's hands. It should not adduct or abduct the shoulder.

Authorization

Walkers can be purchased from local stores. A letter of medical necessity is needed for insurance reimbursement.

Use

There are different techniques for walking with a standard walker, a hemi-walker, and a rolling walker. There are also specific techniques for going up and down curbs and stairs. See "Walking Techniques" in the Techniques section for detailed information.

Benefits

Walkers offer bilateral upper extremity support for people who have trouble with their balance. The variety of walkers offers the therapist flexibility in choosing an appropriate device to best suit the client's needs in real-life tasks.

Design Challenges

Walkers are pretty basic pieces of equipment and there aren't many fancy components to confuse the client. Simple is sometimes a good thing, especially for people who have cognitive impairments. The equipment companies have answered the call to develop walkers that are more functional in life activities (e.g., folding seats, baskets, pouches, brakes). They are lightweight and relatively inexpensive.

Costs

A standard walker costs about $75.00. A hemi-walker costs about $65.00. An Eva walker costs about $800.00. A rolling walker costs about $90.00. A seated rolling walker costs about $375.00. A reverse walker costs about $350.00.

Treatment Direction

- Recreational therapists evaluate a client's ability to use a walker in a community setting, on uneven outdoor and indoor surfaces, and while doing functional tasks (e.g., carrying items, transferring). They make recommendations for types of walkers, walker accessories, changes in technique, and ways to overcome physical barriers. For example, if a client lives alone on the second floor of a duplex and lacks the ability to carry the walker up and down the steps, how is he going to be able to take it out with him to go shopping? Is it possible for the client to get two walkers, one for inside the apartment and one to keep by the front door? Is it safe to keep it at the front door? Just because a device is functional in a clinic it does not mean that it fully meets the needs of the client in real life.

- If the recreational therapist is working with a client who is very active in the community, has a long-term or progressive disability, and is anxious about his/her ability to use a basic rolling walker in a community setting (afraid of not being able to find a seat, concerns about transporting items), the recreational therapist should consult with the physical therapist and explore the possibility of prescribing a seated rolling walker.

Wheelchairs, Scooters, and Wheelchair Accessories

There are three main types of seated mobility devices: manual wheelchairs, power wheelchairs, and scooters. The type of seated mobility chosen reflects the needs of the client. If a client is going to need the wheelchair for only a short period of time (e.g., total joint replacement), the client will probably rent a standard manual wheelchair. For a client who is ordering a custom wheelchair for long-term use, choosing a wheelchair can be difficult because it must match the client's physical needs, cognitive abilities, living environment, and activity patterns. Clients are presented with many different options and at times it can become a very confusing and frustrating process for the client, especially when the wheelchair chosen will not be replaced by the insurance company for several years. Some therapists prefer to order a custom wheelchair while the client is in inpatient rehab because it takes six to eight weeks for the wheelchair to be made. This may not always be ideal because it doesn't afford the client the opportunity to test-drive the wheelchair. What sounds good and looks good may not always feel right to the client. A developing trend is to send the client home with a trial wheelchair that is closely related to the wheelchair in consideration. This gives the client an opportunity to try out several different wheelchairs over a short period of time in his/her real-life environment in order to make a more informed choice.

Manual Wheelchairs

Advantages: Manual wheelchairs are lightweight. They do not require a battery and they have fewer parts than a power wheelchair thus requiring less maintenance. When compared to power wheelchairs and scooters, manual wheelchairs are less expensive to repair (no electric components), quieter (no motor), and more discreet (you see more of the person and less of the chair). Manual wheelchairs are easily transportable and foldable and provide more flexibility than power wheelchairs or scooters for overcoming obstacles (able to pop a wheelie, negotiate curbs and steps). Manual wheelchairs also help to maintain and improve muscle and cardiopulmonary strength and endurance and provide secondary health benefits related to the physical activity of pushing.

Disadvantages: Manual wheelchairs require upper body strength and endurance. Years of wheelchair propulsion can cause shoulder problems. A high degree of strength is required to overcome community barriers (e.g., hills) and the speed of the wheelchair varies depending on the client's physical ability, as well as endurance level (which can fluctuate throughout the day).

Types: There are two types of manual wheelchair frames, rigid and cross-brace.
- *Rigid frame*: The rigid frame is one tubular piece. It has a modern or sport-like appearance and is lighter than a cross-brace wheelchair. A rigid frame is stronger and more energy efficient than a cross-brace chair because it does not have a jointed frame piece (an advantage for the active person). A solid frame, however, is more sensitive to body movement and can be a challenge to manipulate on uneven surfaces. Rigid chairs have a tighter turning radius and offer a variety of options that cannot be ordered on a cross-brace wheelchair (e.g., seat bucket options; special sport designs for tennis, rugby, basketball, racing). To fold a rigid frame chair the wheels pop off and the back folds down making it look like a box. A folded rigid wheelchair does not fit easily into a standard car trunk. The client will need a van, pickup truck, or sport utility vehicle with a hatchback or the client can sit in the driver seat, fold the chair, and then pull it across his body and place it on the passenger seat. This is the most common because most clients who purchase a rigid frame wheelchair have paraplegia and are unable to load a wheelchair into a trunk independently. Rigid frame wheelchairs are custom ordered. They are not a standard rental wheelchair.
- *Cross-brace frame*: The cross-brace frame wheelchair has a cross-frame. The frame looks like an "X" under the wheelchair seat. This design allows the wheelchair to fold flat (take off leg rests and armrests, remove seat cushion, grab the front and the back of the wheelchair seat and pull up, the wheelchair will then collapse flat). When folded, the wheelchair can be placed flat in a trunk or put into a rooftop carrier. A button in the car opens the rooftop carrier and lowers a metal contraption down next to the driver's side door, the driver loads the wheelchair onto the contraption and then pushes the button to raise it up and slide it into the rooftop carrier. Roof top carriers are not available for rigid frame wheelchairs. The roof top carrier is an excellent choice for a client who does not have the strength to pull in or load the wheelchair without assistance. The cross-brace wheelchair has a traditional appearance and is stable on uneven surfaces. However, active clients often complain that the wheelchair has too much "shake" because the

center joint in the cross-brace can become loose with active use. It also requires more energy to push than a rigid frame wheelchair. Cross-brace chairs do not have as many options as rigid frame wheelchairs. Clients who have a short-term need for a wheelchair (e.g., a client who has a total hip replacement may require the use of a wheelchair for a month or two for long-distance mobility) are typically given a standard cross-brace rental wheelchair. A client who has a long-term need for a manual wheelchair can opt for a cross-brace wheelchair and it will be custom tailored (like the rigid frame wheelchair) to meet the specific needs of the client (e.g., width, height, options). Clients who opt for a cross-brace framed wheelchair are usually those with progressive muscular disabilities (e.g., multiple sclerosis) who would benefit from a wheelchair with greater stability.

Power Wheelchairs

Advantages: Powered wheelchairs conserve cardiopulmonary and muscular energy. When compared to a manual wheelchair, they provide greater ease overcoming uneven terrain (e.g., grass, ramps) and require the use of only one body part to control the wheelchair (e.g., hand, elbow, head) leaving the other limbs available for other tasks. Power wheelchairs are custom fitted and designed for the client with the goal of independent operation. Assistance from others may be required to change or charge the battery and perform routine maintenance. Power wheelchairs can also be designed with power tilt and recline to aid in pressure relief and comfort.

Disadvantages: Power wheelchairs can be difficult to transport. Some power wheelchairs can be dismantled and placed into a car trunk (the typical pieces weighing about 30 pounds), however the client would need to be able to transfer into a car and have another person who could dismantle and reassemble the wheelchair as well as provide assistance to transfer into the car. Another option is a wheelchair trailer that hooks onto a tow ball on the back of a car. The client transfers into the car and another person drives the wheelchair around to the back of the car and loads it on the trailer. Most clients who purchase a power wheelchair have significant motor loss making car transfers almost impossible. Therefore, most clients choose to purchase a custom van with a ramp or lift. Clients who desire to drive and have the ability to drive using adaptive equipment can also have a van tailored so that the power wheelchair locks down as the driver seat. When compared to the manual wheelchair, power wheelchairs require higher maintenance because there are more parts. They are

more expensive. They do not provide cardiovascular or muscular exercise (possibly promoting further deterioration). And they are bigger pieces of equipment (see more of the chair than the person). Some power wheelchairs can go up small curbs (two to four inches) although they do not have the flexibility of a manual wheelchair, which can be folded and carried up a flight of steps and can bump up high curbs.

Types: Power wheelchairs are described as being front wheel drive, rear wheel drive, or mid-wheel drive.

* *Front wheel drive*: The front wheel drive wheelchair gives the person the sensation that s/he is pulling the chair behind him/her. They are very agile (makes a full rotation in a tight space). They take skill to operate and may be difficult for those with cognitive deficits. The wheels in the front are larger and help to overcome small obstacles. A tilt option may make the chair unstable (weight transferred to the back may raise the front wheels making it difficult to operate).
* *Rear wheel drive*: The rear wheel drive gives the person the sensation that s/he is being pushed forward. The larger wheels are in the back. There is a greater sense of control at the sacrifice of agility (needs more room to make a full rotation). Anti-tippers may be needed because the wheelchair may have a tendency to tip with acceleration and inclines.
* *Mid-wheel drive*: The mid-wheel drive has a tight turning radius and it requires good upper body balance to operate. It doesn't perform well on rough terrain and it is best for hard flat surfaces.

Scooters

Advantages: Scooters are less expensive than power wheelchairs and some believe that they are more "socially acceptable" than a power wheelchair in the American culture. Like the power wheelchair, they conserve cardiovascular and muscular energy. However, when compared to the power wheelchair, the scooter is not able to meet complex positioning needs (e.g., tilt, recline, custom headrests and backrests). It is a good option for older adults who would not otherwise be able to engage in community tasks due to limited mobility and those who may be in the early stages of a disease such as multiple sclerosis. Scooters can be dismantled and put into a car trunk but they are heavy. There is a chain hoist that can be attached to the inside of a car trunk to lift, swing, and lower the scooter into the trunk. The scooter does have some unique extras that the manual wheelchair and power wheelchair do not have such as a basket on the front or back to transport items and the ability to place items on the running board.

Disadvantages: In contrast with the power wheelchair, the client requires good arm strength and adequate hand use to steer the scooter and operate buttons. The client also has to have good trunk control due to limited seat support. Although different seating options are available, they are not as extensive or adaptable to meet complex trunk and upper extremity needs. Scooters don't work well at tables and desks because the front steering system gets in the way. Like the power wheelchair, the scooter requires the use of a battery and does not provide cardiopulmonary or muscular exercise, possibly leading to deconditioning. Scooters cannot be tipped backwards to climb curbs and other physical obstacles, therefore the environment must be fully accessible.

Components of the Seat

Cushions: The primary function of a cushion is to prevent pressure ulcers and maintain postural stability. There are four main types of cushions:
* *Foam*: Foam cushions are inexpensive. The therapist can easily carve out areas in the cushion to decrease pressure on sensitive areas that are at a high risk for skin breakdown or that currently have skin breakdown. Foam cushions, however, wear out quickly (become flat). When the cushion becomes flat, it will not meet the comfort needs of the client and can result in secondary problems, such as skin breakdowns. Foam cushions come in a range of densities.
* *Gel*: Gel cushions have gel fluids placed in pouches inside of the cushion. They easily adapt to pressure distribution needs and clients say they are comfortable. Gel cushions are heavier than foam cushions and they do not absorb impact well (bouncing up and down). Some gel cushions can bottom out, so look for cushions that have separate compartments in the cushion if weight makes this an issue. Gel cushions can leak.
* *Air/dry floatation*: Support is maintained by air (e.g., Roho cushion: small, interconnected rubber balloons arranged in rows). They are waterproof, but they are less stable than other cushions. Air leaks can occur so air pressure should be checked frequently. They are lightweight.
* *Honeycomb*: Honeycomb cushions have individual "beehive" like cells. The skin is kept cooler. The cushions are lightweight, shock absorbent, and washable. There is no risk of leakage, and they provide good support. They

have a low profile appearance. They are relatively new, and no weaknesses have been noted so far.

Seat width (also referred to as chair width): This is the width of the wheelchair seat. If it is too wide, it can be difficult to manipulate the handrims (wheels) on a manual wheelchair. It also promotes poor posture and adds more weight to the wheelchair.

Seat depth: This is the length of the seat (front to back). If it is too shallow (short) it places increased pressure on the buttocks and lessens stability. If it is too deep, the client will not be able to rest effectively against the back of the seat. It will also add more weight to the chair.

Seat height: This is how high the seat is off the ground. The correct seat height depends on the length of the client's legs, clearance needed for footrests or running board, the integration of the seat height in standard environment (e.g., desk and table height), personal preferences of the client, and any restrictions due to the build of the chair.

Seat angle (manual wheelchairs): The seat does not have to be parallel to the floor; it can be angled forward or backward ("seat dump," "squeeze"). Clients with higher-level spinal cord injuries who lack good trunk and upper body control may benefit from a seat that is angled back because it keeps them back in the chair for added safety. However it can also make transferring in and out of the chair more difficult, as well as possibly promote secondary problems (back problems, ulcers).

Back support: There are many types of chair backs including rigid, cloth, and vinyl. Cloth and vinyl backs fold down on a rigid chair or fold in half vertically on a cross-brace chair. Rigid backs are removable and come in a variety of heights, widths, lateral supports, and curves to meet the needs of the client. Scooters do not have separate back supports because the seat is a one-piece unit.

Back angle: Some seat backs are adjustable. Although upright is usually desirable, the person's disability and positioning needs may make an angled back or tilt/recline back optimal.

Components of Propulsion

Push handles (wheelchairs only): If the back of the chair is low so that it only comes up to the middle of the client's back (a common feature of rigid chairs) push handles interfere when the client propels the wheelchair because they are hit by the back of the upper arm. Push handles are helpful in case the client needs assistance (e.g., needs someone to help bump up a high curb or down a flight of stairs). Push handles also provide support for the client who has poor trunk control and needs to lean forward (e.g., hook one arm around a push handle and lean forward with the other arm to retrieve an item).

Tires: Tires that are air-filled are called pneumatic tires. They provide a comfortable ride. However they puncture easily and often need to be replaced. Clients with pneumatic tires must be able to independently fix a flat tire and need to keep a patch kit, inner tube, and tools on the chair in case of an emergency. Solid rubber tires have a rougher ride but they never go flat. They are heavier than pneumatic tires. Rubber or foam filled inserts are available for tires instead of having a solid rubber tire. These tires won't go flat since no air is required and they have a softer ride than a solid rubber tire.

Wheels (manual wheelchair): Wheels for manual wheelchairs come in different diameters. They must be ergonomically correct in relation to the seat height (too high a tire can overstrain arms and be difficult to start propulsion, too low a tire can result in decreased force to propel the wheelchair). Spoked wheels are heavier than molded wheels and require adjustment for wheel balance. Molded wheels take more of an impact than spoked wheels and do not require adjustments.

- *Wheel placement*: The back wheels (also called the power wheels) can be moved more forward or backwards (axle adjustment). The more forward the back wheels, the tippier the wheelchair. The more backward the wheels, the more stable the wheelchair. If the client is to learn how to do wheelies and/or slight caster tips, then the wheels will need to be placed slightly forward. Start out with wheels in a more stable position and move them forward to the optimal position. You don't want the wheelchair to be too tippy for safety reasons. Weight and height of the person also determine how to position wheels to best achieve optimal stability and tip. In addition, the therapist considers the placement of wheels in relation to stress on the upper body to propel the wheelchair (if they are too far back it will be difficult for the client to push the wheels).
- *Camber*: Camber is the angle of the wheels. The wheels tilt in at the top and out at the bottom. The more camber a wheel has, the wider the total width of the wheelchair, which can make it difficult to maneuver through doorways and tight spaces. Camber provides the chair with a greater wheelbase and therefore gives the chair greater turning and lateral stability (e.g., leaning). Some wheelchairs have a fixed camber while others are adjustable. Sport chairs can have extreme camber so that the person does not fall out of the wheelchair easily. Everyday chairs may have a slight

camber to accommodate normal living movements. Camber adjustments can also cause the wheels to toe-in or toe-out making the chair more difficult to steer and propel.

Handrims (manual wheelchair): Like wheels, handrims come in different diameters. Handrims are usually made out of metal and are attached to the outside of the wheel. The client uses the handrims to propel the wheelchair. The smaller the diameter, the more force the client needs to apply to propel the chair. Most people who use wheelchairs push the wheelchair using the palms and heels of the hand on both the handrim and the tire. This technique requires less force to propel the chair and puts less stress on the hands. The problem with this technique is that clients can injury their hands because tires can pick up glass and other debris that could cut the skin. Clients who find this technique helpful must wear fingerless gloves (see "push gloves" later in this article) to protect their hands. For clients who have hand limitations, knobs can be placed on the handrims (short nubs that stick out from the handrim that allows the client to use the hand to push the chair without the use of fingers). Therapists can also wrap handrims in therabands, which make the handrim easier to grip. There are also devices that allow the user to push with only one hand.

Casters: Casters are the small wheels on the front of manual wheelchairs. They come in a variety of sizes and materials. Smaller casters are usually made of solid plastic. They have good agility and turn easily, but they have a bumpy ride and don't roll over obstacles easily, which means that the client will have to do a mini-wheelie to get over door thresholds and small cracks and may get stuck on sidewalk cracks or street grates. Sudden and unexpected stops from a caster that gets stuck can cause injury if the person is thrown from the chair. Pneumatic casters are air filled. They give a soft ride, overcome small obstacles easily, and are not as hard on the wheelchair frame, therefore adding extra years to the life of the chair. However, they can puncture easily. Solid rubber casters are another option. They come in a variety of sizes. They are a softer ride than the small plastic casters and will not go flat like pneumatic casters.

Control systems (power wheelchair and scooter): Power wheelchairs can be controlled by a joystick, sip and puff (breath controlled), chin control, or head control. Scooters are controlled by a two handed front steering system.

Batteries (power wheelchair and scooter): There are two types of wheelchair and scooter batteries (gel cell and wet cell). How long and far the chair will go depends on many other factors along with battery size: weight of chair, wheel size, surfaces negotiated, amount of equipment on the chair, extra weight carried on chair (e.g., heavy school backpack), driving style (stop and go really fast, slow and steady pace). Both types of battery must be charged and well maintained at all times.

- *Gel cell*: Gel cell batteries require less maintenance than wet cell batteries, but they don't last as long as a wet cell battery and they are slightly less powerful.
- *Lead cell/wet cell*: Wet cell batteries can be charged more times than a gel cell battery so they have a longer life span. They are popular among active users who would otherwise have to replace expensive batteries more often. They generally have about 10% more power (amp hours) than gel cell batteries.

Components for Safety

Wheel locks (manual and power wheelchair, scooter): Wheel locks or brakes are used to keep the wheelchair from moving. They are especially important when getting in or out of the wheelchair and when parked on an incline. There are a variety of wheelchair brakes. The most typical are mounted to the front of the wheel. However, for the person using a manual wheelchair, they can get in the way when propelling the wheelchair and hurt the thumb. The client may want to consider "scissor" brakes that disappear under the wheelchair when disengaged so they do not get in the way when propelling the chair. Brakes can also be mounted to the back of the wheel. Brakes will need adjustment from time to time because they can become loose or misaligned. If the wheelchair has pneumatic tires, brakes should be adjusted when the tires are at their correct tire pressure. If brakes become less effective, tires may need to be filled. The client can also request two different types of brakes (e.g., remove standard front locking brakes and use the scissor brakes when playing a sport). Some wheelchair locks come on automatically when there is no weight on the seat of the wheelchair. This feature prevents clients from falling when they transfer into or out of a wheelchair without setting the brakes. It is especially useful for clients with cognitive deficits. Power wheelchairs have a locking mechanism that is usually found in the middle of the back wheels. A small round metal plate sits inside the wheel and when turned in a certain direction will put the chair in manual or power mode. Manual mode allows the wheelchair to be pushed by another person. Power wheelchairs and scooters do not have manual locks. The wheels lock when the chair is turned off. The seat can be locked on a scooter (e.g., client swivels the scooter seat to the

right and then locks it in place so that it does not move when standing or transferring).

Anti-tippers (manual and power wheelchairs): Anti-tippers are downward-sloped attachments that click into the lever bars. The lever bars are the two bars that extend out the back of the wheelchair between the two wheels. They are easily removable or can be flipped up out of the way. Depending on the person's agility and skill, some clients can do this themselves while others require the assistance of another to remove or flip the anti-tippers. They resemble the shape of a half moon, round part down towards the ground. They prevent the chair from tipping backwards. This is a good safety precaution for clients who have a tendency to tip backwards. They can also be an obstacle and annoyance for the independent person who needs to tip the chair back to overcome obstacles (e.g., bump up a curb). If the client typically has a helper with him/her and would require the assistance of another to overcome such obstacles, it is better to err on the side of safety and opt for the anti-tipper bars. Anti-tippers can be designed to be one inch or more from the ground so different clearances can be achieved. This way a client who feels safer with anti-tippers but needs to tip the chair back a maximum of three inches to overcome obstacles in his/her community can have anti-tippers with a four-inch clearance.

Grade aids (manual wheelchair): A device that resembles the shape of a half moon that attaches below the wheel lock. They are easily locked and unlocked in the same manner as wheel locks. When locked, it prevents the wheel from rolling backwards. This is especially helpful for individuals who lack the strength or hand function to overcome inclines (e.g., multiple sclerosis, high-level spinal cord injury with minimum hand and arm involvement).

Seatbelt (manual and power wheelchairs): Although every wheelchair should have a seatbelt some of them do not or the client chooses not to wear it or opts to remove it from the chair. Seatbelts are a vital component of the wheelchair. Should the wheelchair come to an abrupt stop, the client can be thrown from the wheelchair resulting in serious injury. The seatbelt also provides additional trunk support.

Components for Arms and Legs

Armrests (manual and power wheelchairs, scooter): Armrests are helpful for many reasons. They help hold the seat cushion in place, offer support (e.g., when transferring) and stability (e.g., trunk stability), help with changing position in the chair and performing weight shifts, and provides an extra "handle" to maintain balance when reaching for an item with one arm. Armrests can also get in the way. If they are too long the client may have difficulty propelling the wheelchair or using a desk or table because the armrests bump up against the table edge preventing the client from getting close enough to the table. There are many different types of armrests: standard upholstered armrests in various lengths, flip-up armrests that swing up and behind the chair so there is no need to manually remove the armrests when transferring or using a table, tubular armrests that look sleek and modern (although they aren't as comfortable as standard armrests), and molded or sculpted armrests that are specially designed to provide arm support for clients who lack full upper body function (e.g., high level spinal cord injury). Armrests should not be too high or too low. Too high can cause pain in the neck and shoulders and too low can encourage a slumping posture resulting in back problems.

Footrests (manual and power wheelchairs; scooter has a running board): There are two different kinds of footrests.

- *Fixed legrests*: Fixed legrests (also referred to as roll bars) are part of the wheelchair frame and do not swing out of the way. They can be found on some pediatric power wheelchairs, but are most common on manual rigid frame wheelchairs. Fixed legrests are sleek and modern. They tuck the feet right below or slightly behind the knees, thus shortening the length of the chair. They also act as a "roller bar" that aids in keeping the chair from tipping forward. Transferring can be a bit cumbersome at first due to the added obstacle, but can be overcome. Feet and legs are kept from sliding off the roller bar with a calf strap that wraps behind and in front of the legs (usually with a Velcro closure). Roller bars, like swing away legrests, can be angled to help keep the feet from sliding off.
- *Swing away legrests*: Swing away legrests are two single footrests (one for each foot) and swing out to the side of the chair. They are used on manual and power wheelchairs. They are removable. Swing away legrests can be moved out of the client's way, therefore they can be advantageous for transferring (able to place feet flat on the floor unobstructed) or lowering the client's knees so s/he can fit under a table (place feet flat on the floor instead of on the legrests). Swing away legrests lengthen the chair due to the space needed for the footplates.

Both legrests can also be narrowed (depending of the style of the chair), thus keeping the legs closer together and giving the client a tighter turning radius. Footrests must be high enough to accommodate uneven surfaces and small obstacles (e.g., raised sidewalk block) but not so high that they create inappropriate knee and hip flexion.

Miscellaneous Components and Accessories

Suspensions (manual wheelchair): Some rigid and cross-brace manual chairs have suspension systems (springs) that allow better wheel contact with the ground when going over uneven surfaces, as well as a more comfortable/softer ride.

Clothing guards (manual and power wheelchairs): Clothing guards are typically a flat plastic piece that partially covers the side of the armrest. This prevents clothing from coming into contact with the wheels.

Cup holders: There are various types of cup holders that attach onto the wheelchair armrest or frame. A bottle of water could also be easily kept in a backpack on the back of the wheelchair. Water is important for hydration and taking medication.

Pouches: Backpack-like pouches for the back, side, or underside of a wheelchair or scooter.

Crutch holders (manual wheelchair, but could be put on a power wheelchair or scooter): This is a small metal tray that attaches to one of the tipper bars and a Velcro strap that wraps around the push handle. The crutches sit on the tray and the Velcro strap goes through the crutch handles to hold them in place.

Toolkits (manual and power wheelchair, scooter): Small toolkits can be purchased that have the tools and equipment needed to perform light repairs on a wheelchair or scooter. Clients can also ask the wheelchair vender for a list of recommended tools and supplies to be purchased independently.

Push gloves or cuffs (manual wheelchair): These are gloves that the client wears when pushing a wheelchair. They are often fingerless. Some have a thumb protector. The palm of the glove usually has a patch of leather, suede, or rubber that gives extra fiction for pushing the chair. Weight training gloves from a local sporting goods store are commonly preferred.

Backpacks: Backpacks can be purchased at a local store. The arm straps on the backpack can be hooked around the push handles of the wheelchair so that it hangs on the back of the wheelchair. Choose a backpack that is waterproof, won't show a lot of dirt (a dark color), and one that has zippers and pockets that match the client's needs and abilities. For example, if a client has limited hand function, choose a backpack with large pockets and zippers. Small pockets may be difficult for this client to get his/her hand inside and a backpack with a drawstring may be difficult to operate. Look at the number of pockets in the backpack. How many pockets does the client need (e.g., one for cathing supplies, one for change of clothes, one for a cell phone)? Consider the weight of the backpack and the fashion statement that it makes (e.g., a brown leather backpack versus a Spiderman backpack).

Weight

The weight of a wheelchair varies greatly depending on the type and extent of materials used, the weight of the cushion, and the type of wheels chosen (spoked wheels are heavier than molded wheels, solid rubber tires are heavier than pneumatic tires).

- *Power wheelchair*: 100-180 pounds (250-500 pound capacity). This excludes the batteries, which typically weigh about 75 pounds.
- *Scooter*: approximately 150 pounds (300 pound capacity).
- *Standard cross-brace aluminum wheelchair*: approximately 41-50 pounds (250 pound capacity) and 46 pounds (350 pound capacity).
- *Standard cross-brace lightweight wheelchair*: 28-36 pounds (250 pound capacity).
- *Standard rigid frame wheelchair*: 19-27 pounds (250 pound capacity).
- *Titanium rigid frame wheelchair*: approximately 18 pounds (250 pound capacity).
- *Sport wheelchairs*: 15-27 pounds (250 pound capacity).

General Maintenance

Manual Wheelchair

- *Chair*: At least once a week clean the chair with a mild detergent and soft cloth.
- *Cushion*: If washable, wash the cushion or cushion cover at least once a week. Wash more frequently if required due to soiling.
- *Frame*: Look for any cracks, scratches, sharp edges, loosened bolts, thin material (cloth seat/back, foam tubing on handgrips, etc.).
- *Tires*: Are they worn? Do they need to be replaced? If pneumatic, check tire pressure.
- *Casters and wheels*: Remove any debris that may be caught around caster/power wheels.
- *Axles/joints*: Do they need lubricating?
- *Wheels*: Do they spin freely? Do bearings need to be replaced?
- *Spoke tension*: Check at least monthly.
- *Casters and forks*: Should not shake with propulsion.
- *Alignment*: Do all four wheels touch the ground? Does the chair need to be aligned?
- *Wheel locks*: Do they lock tightly? Do they need adjustment?

Power Wheelchairs and Scooters

Become familiar with the "sound" of the chair. Should anything sound "off," a full inspection of the chair should be performed. This includes checking all the components listed for the manual wheelchair, as well as additional components special to the power wheelchair and scooter including electrical connections, belts, batteries, and tilt/recline mechanisms.

Fitting

Clients are fitted for a wheelchair or scooter by the vendor and the physical therapist.

Authorization

Wheelchairs and scooters: A physician's order, a certificate of medical necessity (CMN), and supporting documentation that justify prescription of a wheelchair.

Use

See "Wheelchair Mobility" in the Techniques section for detailed information.

Benefits

Using a wheelchair or scooter provides an opportunity for mobility. Mobility enables people to engage in life tasks for health. However, inappropriate use of a wheelchair or scooter can cause physical health deterioration (e.g., using a wheelchair more than recommended, using a scooter or wheelchair that provides more assistance than needed).

Design Challenges

The wheelchair and scooter have many parts and every part has many different kinds of designs. It is impossible to discuss all of the design challenges of the wheelchair and scooter, however the primary challenges revolve around material weight, strength, and durability; usability; cost; reliability; power and speed; and flexibility and adjustability of parts and accessories to meet the individual needs of the client.

Costs

- Power wheelchair: approximately $6,000.00
- Scooter: average cost is around $2,000.00
- Standard cross-brace aluminum wheelchair (includes pediatric): $450.00 to $1,700.00
- Standard cross-brace lightweight wheelchair (includes pediatric): $1,200.00 to $2,500.00
- Rigid frame wheelchair: $1,400.00-$2,500.00
- Sport wheelchairs: $2,000.00-$8,000.00
- Power wheelchair battery: $100.00-$200.00

Treatment Direction

- Traditionally, in the rehabilitation setting, the physical and occupational therapists, along with the wheelchair vendor identify and choose appropriate wheelchair options to present to the client. Recreational therapists are increasingly becoming more involved in the wheelchair selection process. The recreational therapist offers a view of the client's lifestyle that other therapists do not have. By having a holistic understanding of the client's current and desired recreational and community activities, along with the knowledge of the application of wheelchair components, recreational therapists can offer quality input.
- Recreational therapists assist clients in test-driving wheelchairs by scheduling community integration sessions that allow the client an opportunity to test one or more wheelchairs in a real-life environment.
- Recreational therapists teach clients how to manipulate mobility devices and overcome obstacles in a community environment. See "Wheelchair Mobility" in the Techniques section for directions on how to teach each specific wheelchair skills. See "Community Accessibility Training" in the Techniques section for information on how to educate clients about community accessibility issues.
- Recreational therapists teach clients how to problem solve for barriers that may occur with their wheelchair/scooter in a community setting (e.g., battery dies, flat tire). See "Community Problem Solving" in the Techniques section.
- Recreational therapists are part of the wheelchair prescription team to voice concerns and ideas about wheelchair and scooter prescriptions.

Concepts

This section looks at the concepts that were discussed in Sections 2 and 3. Understanding these concepts is important in the practice of recreational therapy.

Basic Awareness of Self as Part of Socialization

Until an individual is able to conceptualize that s/he is separate from the things around him/her and that s/he is able to influence others, it is hard to begin developing the skills to interact. Self-awareness involves being able to identify and express your own individual characteristics and understanding how those characteristics are similar to, or different from, others in your community. Many of these skills are relevant to mental functions, such as orientation to person (b1142) and experience of self (b1800), and participation functions, such as communicating with and receiving spoken messages (d310) and communicating with and receiving non-verbal messages (d315). The emphasis on awareness of self deals with the client's ability to better understand who s/he is so that expression of his/her characteristics to others is made easier. The key is interaction.

The therapist will find that it is not just clients with cognitive impairments who have a lack of skill and understanding in this area. Clients who have experienced emotional trauma, such as sexual abuse as a child, may not have established what are known as "boundaries." If a client does not have established boundaries, the therapist's efforts for emotional healing through therapy may actually cause additional harm. (Hislop, 2001)

From an early age people learn how to view themselves and how to fit into their world through play. Rogers (1986) described the process of learning about boundaries through play at a young age:

> Babies are, in fact, learning a lot through these games (peek-a-boo, clapping the baby's hands together, etc.), but it certainly is play. They are learning where parts of their bodies are located and what it feels like when people touch them. They are learning how to give pleasure by smiling and moving in certain ways that make Mother laugh and continue hugging and playing. Although the thoughts and words certainly aren't there, there is *experience* occurring that tells the baby, "I can make someone happy." Doesn't that experience have to be a cornerstone in the development of healthy self-esteem?

> In these games, babies play with their mothers' bodies almost as much as the other way around. In doing so, they learn what happens when they pull Mother's hair too hard or squeeze her nose too fiercely. They learn, from the "map" of their mothers' faces, how to read displeasure as well as pleasure. They learn to curb their more aggressive actions in favor of the things that clearly evoke delight. Doesn't that have to be the cornerstone in the development of healthy self-control (p. 5)?

Awareness of where "mine" (and my possessions) stop and where "yours" start is usually learned between the ages of 18 and 24 months. Without this awareness, the development of healthy relationships is difficult at best. Some therapists will work with clients who have celebrated many more birthdays than just two, who may also have knowledge and skills in many areas, and yet still lack the basic understanding of "mine/yours." The therapist's challenge will be to create a playful learning environment that is both age-appropriate and skill-level appropriate.

Playful leisure activities are a natural and appropriate place to learn about healthy boundaries. Just as babies don't learn about boundaries solely through lectures from mom or dad, our clients will develop a deeper understanding through the multi-sensory approach of learning through play. Some suggestions of how to set up a playful atmosphere that allows a client to learn about healthy boundaries include:

- Clients (especially clients with cognitive impairments) tend to develop a sense that the objects s/he uses during leisure and recreation are "his/hers" as the pleasurable experience of play is woven into the client's defining himself/herself by the activities in which s/he engages. Sharing these objects with others may be emotionally and mentally hard. The therapist can facilitate appropriate understanding of "mine" and "others" by identifying one or two objects that belongs to individual clients and gently enforcing the exclusive use. Clients at this level of understanding of "mine" and "yours" are not ready to learn about sharing; their first step is to learn about holding onto their own and leaving others' things alone. The experience of having others enforce the client's exclusive ownership of items helps him/her develop a sense of power and a sense of control of things. The feeling of power and control are critical underlying concepts for establishing appropriate boundaries and reducing the chance of the client becoming a victim of abuse.

- Once a client has developed a fundamental understanding of the concept of "mine" and "yours," the therapist can begin introducing leisure activities in which the clients share group items for short periods of time. The therapist uses verbal and gestured praise to reward sharing behavior. As soon as the therapist senses that the cooperative sharing is about to disintegrate, s/he should begin transitioning the activity into individual activity within the group sharing structure. For example, the group's task is to create a group collage that will display pictures of activities that at least one person in the group enjoys. Start the activity by having each client look through a few magazines in a pile in front of him/her. Place half as many bottles of glue on the table as there are clients. After each client has a few pictures torn out of the magazines, instruct the group to work with one other person to begin gluing the pictures onto the poster board. Before the activity degrades to grabbing, pushing, or other inappropriate expressions, the therapist may ask members of the group to look through their own pile of magazines again to see if they might find just one or two additional pictures. This helps create a smooth transition from a group activity to an individual activity (parallel play). When the group's individual behaviors seem ready to move back into a short period of sharing again, instruct the group to do so. Having the clients rotate their pile of magazines one person to the right (or left) may also help transition the client into the concept of sharing.

For clients to develop a clear understanding of "me" versus "you" some simple concepts need to be developed. Flemming, Hamilton, and Hicks (1977) developed a list of basic understandings that are the underlying concepts needed to develop an awareness of self. An awareness of self is an important first step to developing an awareness of boundaries. Their list of basic understandings includes:

- I'm me. I'm special. There is no one else just like me.
- I have a special name given to me when I was born. It is on my birth certificate.
- No one has a voice just like mine; no one has fingerprints just like mine.
- I am like others in some ways; I am different from others in some ways.

- I can do some things easily; I can do some things well.
- Some things are hard to do; some things I cannot do well yet.
- I can do many things now that I couldn't do when I was a baby.
- As I get older, I will be able to do more things than I can do now.
- I do not have to be good at everything; I can make mistakes.
- I have feelings; at different times I may be glad, sad, and angry, tired, or have other feelings.
- I can learn some good ways to show my feelings.
- If I know I am special, I know others can be special in their way, too.
- Others need to know that I think they are special; sometimes I need to know them better to know how special they are (in what ways they are special).
- No one can know what I think or how I feel unless I tell them or show them.
- When I share my own ideas or do things in my own way, I am being creative.
- My thoughts and ideas are important. Other people have good ideas, too.
- I am likeable (loveable) to someone. I can learn to like (love) others.
- I have a right to share the materials, equipment, and the attention of the therapist and to be safe and protected (p.87).

References

Flemming, M., Hamilton, S., & Hicks, D. (1977). *Resources for creative teaching in early childhood education*. New York, NY: Harcourt Brace Jovanovich.

Hislop, J. (2001). *Female sex offenders: What therapists, law enforcement and child protective services need to know*. Ravensdale, WA: Issues Press.

Rogers, F. (1986). *Mister Roger's playbook: Insights and activities for parents and children*. New York, NY: The Berkley Publishing Group.

Consequences of Inactivity

Staying in bed or being inactive for long periods of time can be dangerous to a client's health. Recreational therapists need to have a full understanding of the secondary complications from inactivity and educate clients and caregivers about them. Although knowledge does not always equal action, it is still a viable component in formulating lifestyle change. In some situations, educating the client first about the consequences of inactivity can be helpful for clients to understand the benefits of recreational therapy (e.g., "Recreational activities can help me to reduce my risks of developing these secondary conditions and I really don't want these problems because it will impact my ability to do [something that is meaningful to the client].").

Linking problems to their effect on activities that are meaningful to a client can make a profound impact (e.g., "If I don't become more active, I am at risk of losing more functioning and then I will need more help and possibly not be able to live alone anymore...and I don't want that because I value my independence.", "I love to do things with my grandchildren so I need to stay active to be a part of their activities."). Taking this approach means that the recreational therapist:

1. begins by talking with clients about their lifestyle,
2. finds out what is meaningful to the client (e.g., ability to take care of oneself independently, spend time with friends, go back to school, play with other children),
3. and then ties together the effect of how a sedentary/inactive lifestyle could negatively impact the ability to participate in activities that are meaningful to the client.

Complications Related to Inactivity and Bed Rest

There are many complications associated with inactivity and bed rest. Here are some of the important ones that recreational therapists address.

Contractures

As the old saying goes, "Use it or lose it." Muscles need to be stretched and joints ranged so that they do not contract. If muscles are not stretched, they shorten and tighten affecting the mobility (range of motion) of the joint. Prolonged inactivity of muscles can cause contractures (shortening of muscles that severely restrict range of motion). Once they occur, contractures are difficult to undo. Typical treatment is serial casting. The joint/limb is stretched

as much as possible and then a cast is applied to hold the stretch for a period of time to lengthen the muscle. The cast is then removed and the process is repeated until full range or optimal range is obtained. Contractures are common problems for people who spend a great amount of time in a fixed position (e.g., hip and knee contractures for someone who spends too much time in a sitting position; wrist and elbow contractures in a paralyzed limb that is not routinely ranged). Contractures can cause problems with self-care (e.g., unable to put on a shirt independently because of upper extremity contractures; difficulty standing upright due to hip and knee contractures; contractures in a paralyzed upper extremity prevent the client from using the limb as an assist during activities) and life activities (e.g., hip and knee contractures can make walking difficult).

Prevention
- Move each joint through its full range of motion at least once every eight hours.
- Intermittent lying on the abdomen will help prevent hip flexion contractures.
- Changing positions often (e.g., lying to sitting to standing).
- Involvement in physically active self-care, vocational, recreational, and community activities that hold meaning for the client to encourage movement.

Atrophy

Muscle fibers deteriorate from inactivity resulting in decreased strength. Total disuse of a muscle (as after paralysis, tendon tear, plaster casting, or severe pain on motion) will lead to the loss of about one-eighth of its strength each week. If paralysis exists, external electrical stimulation of the muscles is sometimes used to help prevent atrophy. If that is not the treatment of choice, the client must at least do range of motion exercises to prevent contractures. Clients who have had prolonged illness or inactivity will all have some degree of disuse atrophy of their muscles. Backache and fatigue during periods of inactivity may be caused by atrophied muscles. The heart is also a muscle, and it undergoes disuse atrophy like other muscles do when a person is inactive. If the heart muscle atrophies, it must work harder to do the same job as before. As a result, the client may experience shortness of breath, easy fatigability, palpitations, and/or lightheadedness with exertion. Trying to perform vigorous activities that are above current strength level can cause strains, pains, accidents, falls, and injury. This can limit independence, functioning, and quality of life.

Prevention
- Strengthen muscles regularly through therapeutic exercise, self-care activities, and recreational and community activities (see "Exercise Basics" in the Techniques section).

Osteoporosis and Kidney Stones

When weight bearing through the arms and legs (and when muscles pull and stretch at their connections) the body deposits and absorbs calcium in the bones. Bed rest and inactivity eliminate most of these stresses. Within three days of bed rest there are measurable increases in the amount of calcium in the urine because the bones are losing it. The bones then soften and weaken (osteoporosis), and even ordinary forces such as those encountered during transfers, therapy activities, or minor falls may cause bone fractures. Fractured vertebras are the most common result of osteoporosis in older persons. Ordinary x-rays do not show evidence of osteoporosis until more than 50% of the bone mineral has been lost.

Along with the loss of bone mass, there is the danger of kidney stones resulting from the increased calcium in the urinary system.

Prevention
- Weight bear through the arms and legs. For example, standing at a table and performing an activity that requires the client to use the upper extremities for support (e.g., weight bearing through the left arm to provide support to be able to reach with the right hand).
- Weight bearing can be promoted through therapeutic exercise, self-care activities, vocational activities, and recreation and community activities.
- Drink lots of fluids to yield 1.5-2 liters of urine output a day to decrease risk of kidney stones. Increased activity level increases thirst encouraging the client to drink more fluids. Increased fluid intake causes increased urination, helping to reduce stagnant urine in the bladder.

Urinary Tract Infection (UTI)

Emptying the bladder while lying down can prevent the bladder from fully emptying. The urine left over in the bladder can become stagnant, grow bacteria, and cause infection.

Prevention
- Drink urine acidifiers such as cranberry juice or vitamin C to decrease bacteria growth in the urine.
- Empty bladder in a standing or sitting position whenever possible.
- Increased activity level increases thirst, encouraging the client to drink more fluids. Increased fluid intake causes increased urination, helping to reduce stagnant urine in the bladder.

Deep Vein Thrombosis (DVT)

A DVT is a blood clot. It usually forms in the legs in people who are inactive for periods of time, sometimes as little as a few hours. Due to poor blood circulation, blood tends to pool in the lower extremities and blood clots form. The danger is that the blood clot could break loose and lead to an embolism (a blood clot blocking an artery) in the heart, lungs, or brain causing a heart attack, death, or stroke.

Prevention
- Move around frequently and vary positions to promote blood circulation (e.g., sit, stand, lie down, raise legs). Raising the legs can help to decrease edema (swelling due to fluid pooling in the legs from inactivity) and promote blood flow toward the heart.
- Use compression stockings (thick elastic stockings) that are worn on the legs to help push fluid and blood toward the heart and keep it from pooling in the legs.
- Perform leg exercises when sitting or lying for long periods of time (e.g., ankle flexion and extension, knee raises, knee flexion and extension, marching, abduction and adduction of the hips).

Orthostatic Hypotension

Bed rest and inactivity (even after one to two weeks) can cause blood pressure to drop when moving from one position to another position after having been in one position for an extended period of time (e.g., a client who has been lying down in bed stands up). Blood pressure that drops with a change in body position is called orthostatic hypotension. When a person has been in one position for an extended period of time and the body position is changed, blood pools to the legs and abdomen. The circulatory system needs to respond quickly to the change in body position to make sure the blood is available to the brain. If it does not respond quickly enough, because of inactivity, the blood pressure drops causing the client to feel dizzy, weak, or faint.

Orthostatic hypotension is rarely a chronic problem. With increased movement and changes in body positioning, the body learns to adjust the blood pressure quickly. However, for clients who stay in bed at home or sit for prolonged periods of time, orthostatic hypotension can be the cause of falls and injuries that could impact the client's ability to function and be independent (e.g., falls and fractures the hip).

Prevention
- Change body positions frequently throughout the day. This can be promoted through self-care, vocational, recreational, and community activities.

Pneumonia

Prolonged bed rest increases the risk for pneumonia. Lying down and poor posture result in a poor cough reflex (e.g., rounded shoulders with chin tucked when sitting in a wheelchair; propped up in bed). It also makes it difficult to take deep breaths. Air passages start to shut down and harmful bacteria begin to grow. Bacterial infections can affect other body functions and, in clients whose health is already compromised, death can result.

Prevention
- Change body positions frequently throughout the day. This can be promoted through self-care, vocational, recreational, and community activities.
- Sit upright.
- Breathe deeply at regular intervals.
- Use activities to stimulate coughing, breathing, and movement of secretions.

Malnutrition

Inactivity and prolonged bed rest can take a toll on a client's nutrition. It can be difficult to eat in a reclined position in bed or eat a proper meal when propped on up on the sofa. Consequently, clients tend to eat too much "junk food" and improperly balanced meals. Sedentary behavior can also increase food intake because there are less distractions and typically the television is on, which may cause the client not to realize how much food s/he is consuming. For some clients, decreased activity causes lack of appetite, also resulting in poor nutritional intake. Proper nutrition is necessary for the body to heal, repair, and maintain functioning.

Prevention
- Plan healthy meals and eat with other people.
- Do not eat in bed or sitting in front of the television. Eat sitting up at the table to increase awareness of what is being eaten.
- Seek help from a nutritionist if needed.
- Exercise stimulates appetite. This can be promoted through self-care, vocational, recreational, and community activities.

Constipation

Inactivity and bed rest can cause constipation. Whole body movements interact with the digestive system to stimulate the intestines. Food choices, as discussed earlier, may be less healthful when a client is on bed rest. Lack of proper hydration, which can also lead to constipation, may also occur during bed rest and inactivity.

Prevention
- Change body positions frequently throughout the day.
- Engage in physical activity.
- Both of the above can be promoted through self-care, vocational, recreational, and community activities.
- Eat a healthy diet with foods that have sufficient fiber.
- Drink sufficient amounts of fluids.

Skin Breakdown

Prolonged pressure on the skin over boney processes can result in the development of decubitus ulcers. When pressure over a boney process (e.g., hip bones, elbows, heels) is not relieved, blood circulation to the skin and underlying body tissue is impaired. Lack of oxygenated blood to the area causes damage to the cells and a skin breakdown. In some cases, a client may feel the discomfort but be unable to move into another position to relieve the pressure due to impaired mobility skills. In other cases, such as complete spinal cord injury, clients lack the sensation to feel the discomfort and must compensate by performing weight shifts every 20-30 minutes. See "Skin Breakdown" in the Techniques section for more information.

Prevention
- Use of special wheelchair cushions and bed mattresses designed to relieve pressure over boney processes.
- Frequent change of body position. This can be promoted through self-care, vocational, recreational, and community activities.

- Keeping the skin dry at all times. Moisture increases fragility of the skin, quickening skin breakdown.

Emotional and Social Health

Inactivity and bed rest can take a toll on more than just the physical functioning of the body. Anxiety, depression, hostility, social isolation, and learned helplessness can occur. This could be because fewer activities allow an increased focus on negative thoughts. The client may have: concerns about self-care or activities that need to be done by other people because the client is unable to perform them (e.g., worry about whether or not a sibling will follow through and go to the bank for him/her today), hostility and anger that could be due to poor coping strategies and heightened stress, social isolation due to decreased community activities and friends and family who tend to visit less often after the immediate health crisis is over, and learned helplessness due to over-helpful caregivers who induce helplessness behavior or fear on the part of the client related to the client's ability to perform certain tasks.

Prevention
- Emotional and social health can be affected by many other variables in addition to inactivity and bed rest. However, social networks and support can be helpful in offering advice, comfort, motivation, and coping skills. This can be promoted through social activities inside and outside the home, including recreational and vocational activities.
- Keep a healthy routine (e.g., regular sleep pattern, meaningful activities, regular exercise, healthy eating). See "Activity Pattern Development" in the Techniques section.
- Express feelings in a healthy manner. Seek counseling if needed. See "Coping with Stress" in the Techniques section.
- Explore healthy coping strategies (e.g., spirituality, exercise, meditation, talking with a trusted friend).
- Encourage self-reliance and independence with appropriate tasks.

Gait

Gait refers to the body mechanics used to walk. It includes the elements of rhythm, cadence, and speed. It includes walking using a device (e.g., crutches, cane, walker) but does not include moving around in a wheelchair.

Moving our bodies from point A to point B is a complex task that involves many different body functions and structures. For example, most of us rely on our vision to make sure we don't run into anything. Our bones help us remain upright against the pull of gravity and our muscles help us stay balanced while allowing movement. We use visual cues, vestibular information about balance, and proprioceptor nerves to let us know where our body parts are. Coordinating all of these is required for safe walking. By looking at a client's gait we can assess many aspects of a client's overall abilities.

This section will discuss the gait cycle, normal gait, some of the common abnormal gait patterns, and gaits using crutches.

Gait Cycle

A gait cycle is the time and actions required for one foot to touch the ground twice. This cycle typically takes about one second and has both a stance phase and a swing phase. The stance phase is the time that the foot is in contact with the ground and the swing phase is the time that the foot is in the air. Typically 60% of the cycle is spent in the stance phase and 40% is spent in the swing phase. Both feet are on the ground at the same time for approximately 20% of the cycle. The term used to describe the time that both feet are on the ground is called *double-support time.*

During each cycle there are three functional tasks that the body must accomplish: 1. weight acceptance, 2. single-limb support, and 3. limb advancement. Weight acceptance is the most challenging because it requires the integration of many tasks including establishing an initial contact with the ground in a smooth manner, anticipating the required knee flexion to absorb the shock of the body's weight (around 15° on level surfaces), coordinating muscle actions to accept the weight of the body and provide stability, and proprioceptor feedback to help keep the body's center of gravity moving forward to accomplish the next step. The primary muscles used in the weight acceptance are hip extensors, quadriceps, and dorsiflexors.

- Hip extensors provide limb stability.
- Quadriceps control knee flexion during weight acceptance.

- Dorsiflexors control the heel strike, place the foot on the ground, and prepare it for accepting the body's weight.

During the single-limb support phase, the two primary tasks are to support the body's total weight and simultaneously get ready to advance the leg. The primary muscles used in the single-limb support phase are hip abductors, trunk muscles, quadriceps, and plantar flexors.

- Hip abductors stabilize the hip during the weight-bearing phase.
- Trunk muscles help maintain an upright position.
- Quadriceps help prepare for the forward motion of the body's center of gravity.
- Plantar flexors control the tibia, which controls the forward movement during the weight-bearing phase.

The last phase of the cycle is the limb advancement phase where the body prepares for the swing of the leg and then executes the action. To facilitate the swing action the knee must be bent to around 35° (on level ground) in the pre-swing phase advancing to a 60° bend to keep the toes above the ground during the swing phase. The primary muscles used during this phase are the dorsiflexors, hamstrings, hip flexors, knee flexors, and quadriceps.

- Dorsiflexors keep the toes from touching the ground.
- Hamstrings cause the bend at the knee.
- Hip flexors move the leg forward.
- Knee flexors also control the position of the knee.
- Quadriceps extends the leg at the end of the advancement phase.

Normal Gait

A normal gait is called a heel-toe gait. In the heel-toe gait the heel strikes the ground first with the rest of the foot rolling down to the ground after the heel strike during the weight acceptance phase. Rose (2003) lists four attributes associated with normal gaits: "1. an adequate range of joint mobility; 2. appropriate timing of muscle activation across the gait cycle; 3. sufficient muscle strength to meet the demands involved in each phase of the gait cycle; and 4. unimpaired sensory input from the visual, somatosensory [skin and deep tissue sensations], and vestibular [sense of balance] systems" (p. 179).

While mobility is the general category associated with the process of movement from point A to point B, moving by using the legs (perhaps with the help of devices) requires functional skills that are found under b7 Neuromusculoskeletal and Movement Related Functions and b1 Mental Functions. To better understand what constitutes a normal gait the therapist should be familiar with the concepts of stride length, cadence, central pattern generators, avoidance strategies, and accommodation strategies.

There are two characteristics, *stride length* and *cadence*, that influence how fast the client walks. Stride length is the distance covered between the time one heel touches the ground (heel strike) and the next time that same heel touches the ground. Cadence is the number of steps a client takes within a specified length of time, often measured over a distance of 50'. Not only do stride length and cadence help the therapist determine if a client is able to move through the community at a reasonable speed, but it can also indicate if the client is at an increased risk of falling. A slow cadence and short stride length are signs of an increased risk of falling (Rose, 2003). One way to measure stride and cadence is described in the *Fifty-Foot Walk Test* in the Assessment section.

The spinal cord has groupings of nerves, often referred to as *central pattern generators*, that allow us to maintain a rhythm during movement that we often are not aware of. Central pattern generators are nerves that produce patterns of actions that are independent of sensory input. For individuals to be functionally independent in the community they must be able to use mental functions to neurologically override or modify the rhythm of movement created by their central pattern generators. For example, if a client is walking through a shopping mall and comes to a set of steps leading to the next level of the mall, he must be able to adjust his walking pattern by stepping higher to place his feet on the step. Clients with global mental function impairments, such as Alzheimer's, have difficulty with this process.

Patla (1997) describes two critical strategies for community mobility that are frequently impaired by disease, trauma, or old age. The first is *avoidance strategy* — the ability to momentarily modify one's movement patterns to avoid a barrier. The ability to change direction to walk around a mud puddle is an example of avoidance strategy. Clients with Parkinson's disease have difficulty stopping the gait cycle and are therefore at a greater risk of falling or otherwise hurting themselves. Clients with damage to the cerebellum area of the brain also have difficulty using avoidance strategies.

The second critical strategy for safe mobility is *accommodation strategy*. Clients accommodate the rhythm pattern associated with movement to adjust to a change in the environment. Slowing down, picking the foot up, and stepping over the dog's bone left in the center of the living room floor is an example of

using an accommodation strategy. Clients with peripheral neuropathies (damage to the nerves in the arms and legs) will have more difficulty adjusting to changes in the walking surface because they will not be able to perceive them. Clients with visual impairments will have significantly more problems avoiding obstacles.

Abnormal Gaits

There are impairments (diseases and disorders) that affect the gait cycle and clients' abilities to function in their community. The list below contains some of the more common gait patterns (burlingame, 2001).

- *Antalgic gait*: A gait that has a shortened limb support phase because the client is avoiding putting weight on a leg that hurts. A limp.
- *Arthogenic gait*: Also referred to as hip-hiking. A gait noted by the elevation of one hip and the swinging out of the leg (instead of a straight through swing). This gait is often caused by a deformity or stiffness of the hip or the knee.
- *Ataxic gait*: A gait characterized by an unsteady, wide gait that has two different forms:
  - *Spinal ataxia* is caused by a disruption of sensory pathways in the central nervous system. This gait is frequently seen in clients with tabes dorsalis (slow wasting away of the nerve roots in the spine due to syphilis), multiple sclerosis, or other disease processes that affect the central nervous system. The ataxic gait tends to become worse when the client closes his/her eyes. In addition to the broad-based gait, spinal ataxia is also identified by "double tapping" when the heel comes down first followed by the toes making a double slapping sound.
  - *Cerebellar ataxia* is caused by lesions in the cerebellum of the brain. Cerebellar ataxia is characterized by an inability to walk in a straight line but does not worsen when the client's eyes are closed.
- *Dystrophic gait*: Movement is achieved by rolling the hips from side to side producing a pronounced waddling or penguin gait. Because of the nature of this gait, the client's ability to run or to climb stairs or to hike up inclines is impaired. The most common reason for this gait is muscular dystrophy, but it is also seen in a variety of myopathies (diseases of the muscles that cause weakness or wasting that are not the result of nerve dysfunction). This gait is also referred to as a myopathic gait.
- *Festinating gait*: A gait in which the individual takes small steps while leaning forward. It is

common for the client to strike the ground with only the toes and ball of the foot (tiptoeing) during the limb support phase. Due to the forward position of the client's center of gravity, the gait becomes steadily faster as the client tries not to fall forward. Other abnormal characteristics of this gait include a loss of reciprocal arm swing and difficulty initiating movement during the limb advancement stage of the gait cycle. This gait is frequently seen in individuals with Parkinson's disease.

- *Footdrop gait*: A gait where the client slaps the foot to the ground after lifting the knee high on the affected side only (the client is unable to pull the toes up to get a heel strike, therefore the toes hit first or the whole foot slaps down flat). This gait causes increased jarring to the body. It limits, to some degree, the client's ability to achieve a high skill level in physical activities requiring highly coordinated foot and leg movements. The footdrop gait is frequently due to weak or paralyzed dorsiflexor muscles.
- *Gastrocnemius-soleus gait*: An abnormal gait where the affected side is dragged along due to the lack of heel lift on push off (limb advancement phase). Activities that involve going up inclines are affected most. Since this gait is usually due to weakened gastrocnemius and/or soleus muscles, a strengthening program involving activities that mildly stress those muscles may lead to increased function.
- *Hemiplegic gait*: also known as a *flaccid gait* This gait has two primary elements:
  - a swinging (circumduction) or pushing of the affected leg forward.
  - forefoot strike with a missing heel strike on the affected leg (also referred to as "footdrop").

Other problems with gait include dorsal (posterior) column deficits. The dorsal columns are responsible for mediating proprioceptive input from muscles and joint receptors. Proprioceptive input includes both position sense (awareness of the position of a joint at rest) and kinesthetic sense (awareness of movement). Problems observed may include a wide-based and swaying gait pattern, uneven step lengths, excessive lateral displacement, advancing leg lifted too high and then dropped abruptly, and dysmetria. Visual feedback helps compensate for proprioceptive deficits, therefore the client will perform better in well-lit areas compared to poorly lit areas.

Gaits Using Crutches

Clients who use crutches generally employ one or more of the following gaits depending on the walking surface and other conditions (burlingame, 2001).

- *Drag-to gait*: This gait is used when the client has very limited control or weight-bearing ability in the lower extremity and good to strong strength in the upper extremity. The client begins the modified gait cycle by placing both crutches in front of the body. The crutches are slightly wider than shoulder width and placed between one and two feet in front of the client. The client leans into the crutches, placing most of his/her body weight on the crutches. The client then drags his/her feet forward until they are between the crutches.
- *Four-point gait*: A gait where the client uses two crutches in addition to the use of two weight-bearing legs in walking. By alternating the movement of the crutches and the legs the patient is able to move while always having at least three points of support. This gait provides maximal support with stability but causes significant limitations to activities. This type of gait is usually slower than other types of gaits and requires the use of the hands, providing limited or no use of the hands while walking.
- *Swing-through gait*: This gait involves the movement of the crutches toward the direction that the patient is moving. The crutches are placed and then the patient swings his/her lower body to the point where the crutches are anchored and continues through beyond that point. The swing-through gait is most often used by patients who have difficulty with alternate leg movements either due to balance difficulties or due to paralysis.
- *Swing-to gait*: This gait involves the patient placing both crutches in front of him/her and swinging the legs to the position directly between the two crutches.
- *Three-point gait*: When the patient is unable to walk due to intolerance of weight bearing on one of the legs, two crutches are used to bear the weight instead of the unusable limb.
- *Two-point gait*: With this gait the client simultaneously advances the right foot and left crutch. Once both strike the ground, the left foot and right crutch are advanced.

See "Walking Techniques" in the Techniques section for more specific information on how to walk using a cane, crutches, or a walker.

References

burlingame, j. (2001). *Idyll Arbor's therapy dictionary*, (2nd ed.). Ravensdale, WA: Idyll Arbor, Inc.

Patla, A. E. (1997). Understanding the roles of vision in the control of human locomotion. *Gait and Posture, 5*:54-69.

Rose, D. (2003). *Fallproof! A comprehensive balance and mobility training program*. Champaign, IL: Human Kinetics.

Maslow's Hierarchy of Needs

Maslow's Hierarchy of Needs is a construct that helps the therapist identify a client's motivation for action based on human needs. It can be very helpful in guiding the therapist's approach.

The basic idea of the model is that some needs are more important than others. If a person is starving, they are going to try to find food before they try to paint a picture of the sunset. If a person is fed, sheltered, and psychologically safe, he might try to satisfy his need to create something beautiful. Maslow has defined five levels of needs as shown in Table 22 below.

Identifying a motivational level is important to effectively match the client's willingness and desire to address therapy issues. For example, a client who is fully immersed in needing to achieve physiological needs (Level One) will not be receptive to exploring leisure values and attitudes. Addressing inappropriate needs may damage the client-therapist relationship and impede client progress. Note that there is nothing in this model that requires the client to progress between levels in any pattern. A client who is meeting self-esteem needs by going on a community integration outing (Level Four) may suddenly become so tired that nothing matters more than getting back to bed and getting some sleep (Level One). Everyone moves between the various levels during the day. The important thing to remember is that the lower levels needs must be met first. Then we can go on to meet the higher level needs. Let's take a look at the levels.

Level One (Physiological Needs): The physiological needs include food, drink, air, sleep, freedom from pain, and an appropriate temperature. If a client has any of these needs, they will be of primary importance. In fact, nothing else will probably matter if the need is severe enough. Because we live in a rich country, hunger and thirst need to be put in perspective. Maslow is not talking about someone who is thinking a snack would be nice. He really isn't thinking about a person who is thirsty after a long walk. While those needs are real, they can be put off for a while. The serious Level One needs that can't be put off, such as severe dehydration, choking, or intolerable pain, are the ones the therapist must be aware of. These needs must be met immediately before any other therapy is attempted. However, the therapist may still ask the client to postpone satisfying a Level One need that hasn't become critical yet as part of the therapy process, as long as it is appropriate and safe. For example, the therapist may ask the client to finish a set of moderately uncomfortable exercises before taking pain medication if that is part of the treatment plan.

Level Two (Safety): Safety needs include establishing a stable and consistent environment. Some of the issues include knowing that we will have a home, that food will be available, that no one will attack us. It isn't an immediate need like the needs in Level One. It is knowing that the things we need will be available in the future. Therapists can help meet these needs by talking with the client about hospital services (e.g., role of the case manager) that will help him/her sort out issues related to finances, care for loved ones, and disposition after discharge. Therapists validate that concerns of safety and security are of utmost importance. Therapists emphasize recreational therapy's role in the restoration and adaptation of skills and tasks that help the client feel like his/her world will be a safe place.

Clients with Level Two needs are typically open to problem solving to facilitate security and predictability. Problem solving for basic tasks requires the therapist to analyze and discuss the task in a step-by-step fashion to assure the client that the therapist is trying to address and look at every aspect of the problem. This helps to calm fears and promote feelings of security. Examples of basic activities include walking on outdoor surfaces, toileting in a public restroom, grocery shopping, getting the mail, making sure the children are cared for, and finding transportation. Whenever these needs are met, the client can work on satisfying Level Three needs.

Level Three (Love and Belonging): Clients at Level Three are motivated by tasks that focus on feelings of acceptance, love, being wanted, and being respected. When clients perceive that basic survival needs are met (Level One) or feel confident that they are being addressed effectively (e.g., through therapy) and they feel a sense of security (Level Two) in

Table 22: Maslow's Hierarchy of Needs

Level	Category	Description
1	Physiological Needs	Food, drink, air, shelter, sleep, freedom from pain, comfortable temperature
2	Safety	Security, predictability, certainty, a place where one feels safe from harm
3	Love and belonging	Accepted, wanted, loved, respected
4	Self-esteem	Believe in self-competence and worth
5	Self-actualization	Self-development, autonomy, challenge

their life (they can predict what is most likely to happen after discharge; have more of a sense of how things are going to be), the client typically begins to search for connectedness. Does anyone care about me, love me, need me, or want me in their life? Am I respected? Where do I belong? Feeling connected is a basic and universal psychological need.

The therapist helps the client identify sources that can meet this need. Remember that other people are required to fulfill this need for the client so the therapist should focus on who is most likely to help meet this need. Therapists first look at the people who were actively involved in the client's life prior to the current situation (e.g., family, friends, neighbors, church, senior group, ballroom dancing partner). Ask the client if the people in his/her life made him/her feel loved, wanted, and accepted. If yes, address the issues and skills that are related to returning to the activities that s/he did with those people that promoted those feelings. Is it through conversations on the front porch? Is it ballroom dancing on Friday nights? Is it quiet and intimate time alone with one's spouse? Is it praising a higher spirit as part of a supportive group (e.g., a church)? Is it contributing to the upkeep of the home? Is it tucking the children in at night?

An important thing for the therapist to consider is that the current setting or the discharge location may isolate the client from prior sources of emotional love and support (e.g., neighbor, spouse). Clients may not have a system that continues to meet their needs for love and belonging. If a client reports that s/he feels disconnected or disconnection is suspected (e.g., sits alone, low level of socialization with others, symptoms of depression), the therapist identifies and facilitates connections and provides leisure activities that hold value and meaning to the client. In the long term, the therapist needs to look at what kind of connections the client will be able to keep after discharge and work to facilitate them. In the short term the therapist may be able to facilitate meeting Level Three needs by assisting the client in organizing a small event (e.g., inviting a few friends to the hospital to eat chips and watch the Super Bowl game) or other hospital service (e.g., allowing a spouse to stay overnight at the hospital) that promotes a renewed feeling of connectedness.

If a client reports that s/he felt disconnected prior to this situation and there are no connections to return to, the therapist needs to create and facilitate those connections. One way to do that is to find activities that the person likes. A benefit of participating in activities that one enjoys is meeting other people who also share the same interests. With common interest there is a purpose for conversation and with conversation there is connectedness. Relationships form and opportunities exist for support, encouragement, caring, and acceptance.

Up to this point, Maslow is discussing very basic needs of body, safety, and interconnectedness. Levels Four and Five are less clearly defined, as we will see.

Level Four (Self-Esteem): The fourth level of Maslow's Hierarchy of Needs is the motivation for self-esteem through feelings of competence and self-worth. It includes the need to feel good about oneself and to be respected by others. These are clearly human needs, but different cultures satisfy the need in different ways. The basic idea is to participate in activities that help us feel good about what we are doing and earn us the respect of those around us. In a health care setting, feeling good about oneself includes being competent in performing tasks and performing enough tasks to feel like a whole person. The therapist can help by structuring activities so the client is successful and increasing the difficulty and range of the activities until the client masters all of the activities that are required. If that is not possible, the therapist will need to work with the client so that the client accepts the fact that s/he has some limitations that were not there before. The client may no longer be able to perform all the tasks s/he feels s/he should perform. Self-esteem can be hard to feel when a person has lost functional abilities. The second part of self-esteem, the respect of others, can have a huge effect in these cases. If the client can see that others still respect and care for her, it can go a long way toward reducing the negative feelings that go along with a loss of competencies. For more on self-esteem, see "Self-Esteem" in the Techniques section.

Level Five (Self-Actualization): The fifth (and highest) level of Maslow's Hierarchy of Needs is self-actualization. People at this level "are no longer in a state of becoming, but, instead, are in a state of being. They are no longer attempting to remove deficiencies (the lower level of needs)... [but are in search of] truth, beauty, aliveness, uniqueness, justice, order, simplicity, meaningfulness, and playfulness" (Austin, 2004, p 248).

Clients at this level are seeking expanded growth. It may be looking at things from a different perspective (e.g., seeing beauty in something one didn't see beauty in before), incorporating or removing things in one's life (e.g., living a simpler life, pursuing new activities that hold meaning in one's life), and changing behaviors (e.g., joining into play instead of being reserved, speaking more plainly, searching for truth in a conflict). Much of this is an evolved way of thinking and acting.

Clients who were at this level prior to an injury or illness will need to satisfy the needs at the lower levels before they are concerned with self-actualization again. If the therapist has clients who are looking for self-actualization, the therapist can help identify and provide access to opportunities that will help the client reach the goal (e.g., finding a place or way to express uniqueness, overcoming barriers that hinder engagement in activities that make the person feel "alive").

All in all, Maslow provides a framework that helps the therapist understand what the client needs and why it is important to meet basic needs before trying to go on to needs on higher levels.

References

Austin, D. (2004). *Therapeutic recreation processes and techniques, 5th edition*. Champaign, IL: Sagamore Publishing.

Metabolic Equivalents

Metabolic equivalents are used to provide a standardized measure of the amount of energy used to do common tasks. A metabolic equivalent (MET) is the ratio of the work metabolic rate to the resting metabolic rate. One MET is defined as 1 kcal/kg/hour and is roughly equivalent to the energy cost of sitting quietly. A MET is also defined as a level of oxygen uptake of 3.5 ml/kg/min. As with the energy definition, one MET equals the oxygen cost of sitting quietly.

There is a Compendium of Physical Activities that lists the MET values for many common activities. It was developed for use in epidemiologic studies to standardize the assignment of MET intensities in physical activity questionnaires. Dr. Bill Haskell from Stanford University conceptualized the Compendium and developed a prototype for the document. The Compendium was first used in the Survey of Activity, Fitness, and Exercise (SAFE study — 1987 to 1989) to code and score physical activity records. Since then, the Compendium has been used in studies worldwide to assign intensity units to physical activity questionnaires and to develop innovative ways to assess energy expenditure in physical activity studies. Version 1 of the Compendium was published in 1993. An updated version was published in 2000.

Activities are classified by a 5-digit code that identifies the category (heading) as the first two digits and type (description) of activity as the last three digits. An example is shown in Table 23.

Recreational therapists can use the Compendium as a way to determine the relative intensity of activities. Recreational therapists, especially those who work on an inpatient cardiac unit, may have physician orders that require the therapist to use only activities that fall within a specific MET range (e.g., 1.0-2.5). Therefore, it is necessary for therapists to be familiar with the relative MET levels of certain activities.

There are some significant limitations on the MET numbers that the therapist needs to keep in mind. The Compendium was not developed to determine the precise energy cost of physical activity for a particular individual. Even the ratios of the activities will be different depending on characteristics such as body mass, adiposity, age, sex, efficiency of movement, geography, and environmental

conditions in which the activities are performed. Individual differences in energy expenditure for the same activity can be large and the true energy cost for an individual may or may not be close to the stated mean MET level as presented in the Compendium. Consequently, therapists use the Compendium of Physical Activities to identify, in a general sense, activities that tend to correlate with a specific MET level, knowing that clients with health conditions will use more METs than the number listed in the Compendium. Vital signs (such as blood pressure, pulse, and oxygen saturation levels) and observation are more important in evaluating a client's response to activity than MET numbers.

Example: A physician's order for a client with a cardiac condition states the MET range (e.g., 1.0-2.5), blood pressure parameters (no change in systolic or diastolic blood pressure greater than 20), oxygen saturation level (if oxygen levels drop below 94%, stop activity, if levels do not rise with cessation of activity and application of breathing techniques, client is to be put on two liters of oxygen and re-assessed), and pulse parameters (stop activity if change from resting heart rate is greater than 20). The therapist refers to the Compendium of Physical Activities to identify activities with a MET level of 1.0-2.5 (because a client with health conditions will expend more energy for activities than reflected in the Compendium, higher MET level activities outside of the MET level range orders are never attempted without physician clearance). The client is asked to perform an activity with the lowest MET first (e.g., standing activity with minimal movements at 1.0 MET). The therapist monitors the client's vital signs to see if the client can participate in the activity while maintaining precautions and parameters. If the client is unable to maintain precautions and parameters, the activity is stopped and the therapist follows the orders of the physician. Depending on the severity of the client's reaction to activity, immediate assistance may be warranted (e.g., page physician or primary nurse). If the client is able to participate and stay within precautions and parameters, the activity is upgraded to one with a higher MET level (e.g., standing activity with moderate movement). Again, vital signs are monitored along with observation to assess the client's physiological response to activity.

The Compendium can be found at

Table 23: MET code example

Code	Heading	Description	MET
01010	01 - bicycling	010 - Bicycling, < 10 mph, leisure, to work or for pleasure (Taylor Code 115)	4.0

http://prevention.sph.sc.edu/tools/compendium.htm. Researchers may download the compendium for use in their research. Users do not have permission to extract parts of it to use in commercial products, free products, or any other use without the author's permission as well as permission of Lippencott, Williams and Wilkins, who hold the copyright on the Compendium published in *Medicine and Science in Sports and Exercise.*

References

Ainsworth, B. E., Haskell, W. L., Leon, A. S., Jacobs, D. R. Jr., Montoye, H. J., Sallis, J. F., & Paffenbarger, R. S. Jr. (1993). Compendium of physical activities: Classification of energy costs of human physical activities. *Medicine and Science in Sports and Exercise, 25*:71-80.

Ainsworth, B. E., Haskell, W. L., Whitt, M. C., Irwin, M. L., Swartz, A. M., Strath, S. J., O'Brien, W. L., Bassett, D. R. Jr., Schmitz, K. H., Emplaincourt, P. O., Jacobs, D. R. Jr., & Leon, A. S. (2000). Compendium of physical activities: An update of activity codes and MET intensities. *Medicine and Science in Sports and Exercise, 32*(Suppl):S498-S516.

University of South Carolina Prevention Research Center. (2002). Info about the MET table. http://prevention.sph.sc.edu/tools/compendium.htm.

Nervous System

The nervous system is the extensive, complicated network of structures that sense the condition of the body and control all of its functions. There are two parts to the nervous system: the *central nervous system* (CNS) and the *peripheral nervous system* (PNS). The CNS is comprised of the brain and the spinal cord. The PNS is comprised of the nerves that enter/exit the spine (often referred to as spinal nerves), the cranial nerves, and the nerves in the body that connect to muscles and organs. The system sends and receives messages throughout the body. For example, if you want to move your right hand, the brain sends a message to the spinal cord. The message then travels down the spinal cord to the appropriate spinal nerves that hook up with the nerves that make the muscles of your right hand move. The neural path that sends a message from the brain is referred to as the *efferent system*. This contrasts with the *afferent system*. If you put your right hand in a pile of snow, the nerves in the skin of your right hand will send a message through the nerves in the body back to the spinal nerves that lead to the spinal cord and up to the brain to register the sensation of cold. This is the afferent system, which sends information from the environment and the organs to the brain.

The nervous system (including the brain) controls and directs every activity in the body, including thought processes like memory and attention, voluntary movement (e.g., raising one's arm), involuntary bodily functions (e.g., breathing, blood pressure, heart rate), the senses, emotions, behavior, language, and sexual function. Many bodily functions are controlled by the brain, but some are not. Reflexes, for example, travel only to the spinal cord and back. The nervous system concerned with digestion has a large number of nerves associated with it and the nerves seem to be connected in a structure that allows processing similar to the brain. The idea of acting on a "gut feeling" may have some basis in physiology. The extent to which this system and the brain interact is not clear at this time, but it is a good idea to be aware that decisions may not be controlled exclusively by the brain.

The nervous system is a very complex network that synthesizes and responds to multifaceted internal and external stimuli. It is this integrative process that allows us to achieve higher-level skills (e.g., understand nonverbal social cues, view things from a different perspective, analyze, and project consequences). The response of the nervous system to stimuli is just as complex. The nervous system primarily responds to stimuli through the release of chemicals (e.g., endorphins), the execution of an action (e.g., open hand to catch a ball, motor reflex act such as jerking your hand away when it touches a hot stove), and/or a change in an internal process (e.g., quickened heart rate, sweating, increased blood pressure). It is a marvelous system that is not yet fully understood.

Neurons

There are billions of neurons (nerve cells) in the nervous system that are responsible for sending, receiving, and processing information. Neurons typically look like young skinny trees (although they can be a variety of shapes and sizes). (See Figure 2.) The "roots" of the tree are called axon terminals, shown here as motor nerve endings. They connect to the "trunk of the tree" called an axon. The axon is coated in a myelin sheath (a fatty slippery substance that helps signals travel quickly).[5] At the top of the "tree trunk" there is a cell body (like an irregular blob) that contains a "nest" called the nucleus. Off of the cell body are "tree branches" called dendrites.

Messages, whether they are sent through the efferent system (from the brain) or the afferent system (to the brain), travel from one neuron to another in the same manner. Electric impulses (messages) are received by the "top of the tree" (the dendrites) and then travel towards the axon. Once the message is received by the axon's terminals, the axon releases a chemical (called a neurotransmitter) in the form of molecules into the space between the two neurons. (The space is called a synapse.) Neurons are very close to each other, but they do not touch each other. The neurotransmitter allows the message to "jump" (this is called a transmission) to the next neuron, where it again is received by the dendrites, travels down the axon, and then jumps to another neuron. The neurotransmitters that are released by the axon into the synapse bind with special molecules that are located on the cell membrane of the dendrites of the receiving neuron. These special molecules are called receptors. When enough receptors are activated, they stimulate an electrical response in the dendrites, triggering a message down the axon, and onto the next neuron, and so on.

---

[5] The rate of conduction of a nerve impulse along a heavily myelinated axon can be as fast as 394 feet a second (or 120 meters a second). In contrast, a nerve impulse can travel no faster than about 6.5 feet a second (or 2 meters a second) along an axon without myelin. The thickness of the myelin covering on an axon is closely linked to the function of the axon. For example, axons that travel a long distance, such as those that extend from the spinal cord to the foot, generally contain a thick myelin covering to facilitate faster transmission of the nerve impulse.

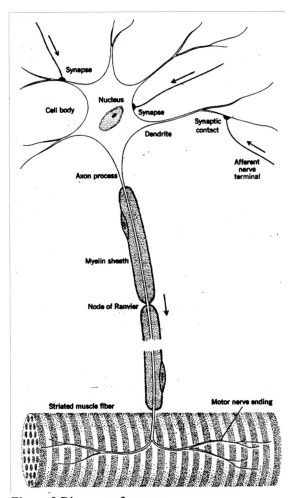

Figure 2 Diagram of a nerve

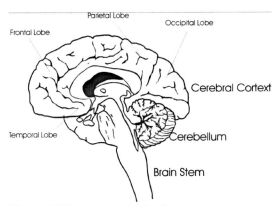

Figure 3 Diagram of the brain

Brain

The total weight of an adult brain is about three pounds and it is about the size of a cantaloupe. There are three major components of the brain: the brain stem, the cerebellum, and the cerebral cortex, as shown in Figure 3.

The brainstem connects the brain to the spinal cord. It is responsible for transmitting and integrating information that passes between the other parts of the brain and the body. Most of the cranial nerves arise from the brainstem.

The cerebellum sits behind the brain stem. It is relatively small and makes up only about an eighth of the total weight of the adult brain. The cerebellum is responsible for coordinating voluntary muscular activity.

Then there is the largest part of the brain. This is called the cerebral cortex. It appears very wrinkly and bumpy because the cerebral cortex is folded and scrunched together so that it is able to fit in the skull. Amazingly, if the cerebral cortex is laid out flat, it would be about 324 square inches (about the size of a full page of newspaper).

The cerebral cortex is made up of two hemispheres. Imagine a large baked potato cut lengthwise as if to put toppings on it. Each half of the potato would be called a hemisphere. Like the baked potato, the cerebral cortex has two sides, a right hemisphere and a left hemisphere. The right and left hemispheres are in constant communication with each other through a thick band of 200-250 million nerve fibers called the corpus callosum. The right hemisphere controls muscles on the left side of the body and seems to be responsible for creativity and abstract thought. The left hemisphere controls muscles on the right side of the body and seems to be responsible for logical thought, language, and math. However, the two hemispheres are in constant communication and signals interplay so that it is difficult to ascertain whether or not these characteristic hemispheric traits are truly segregated. The current belief is that they are more likely to occur on the expected side, but are not there exclusively. Clients with normal brain functioning that lack the ease of thinking abstractly or creatively, may benefit from therapeutic modalities (e.g., art) that encourage and stimulate right brain processing. Similarly, clients who have trouble following instructions may benefit from modalities that emphasize logic and linear processing.

The cerebral cortex is also divided into four lobes: the frontal lobe, the parietal lobe, the temporal lobe, and the occipital lobe. Each lobe occurs on both cerebral hemispheres, therefore there are a right frontal lobe and a left frontal lobe, a right parietal lobe and a left parietal lobe, and so on. Although all the lobes of the brain interact to form a very complex network, certain functions have been found to exist within each lobe. For specific information see the website http://www.headinjury.com/brainmap.htm.

Clinicians must be careful when assuming that damage to a particular lobe will result in the dysfunction of the skills associated with that lobe (e.g., all clients with a frontal lobe injury will have attention problems). Certain functions have been found consistently in certain lobes, but other lobes may also control some of that same function. For example, the ability to attend to an object or task (to pay attention) is found not only in the frontal lobe, but also in the parietal lobe. Therefore, if damage to the frontal lobe occurs, the parietal lobe might pick up more of the work in "paying attention." So, although the function of "paying attention" may have been damaged in the frontal lobe, the client may not present with problems in the area of attention because the parietal lobe is now doing the work. Another variable to consider is the severity and extent of the damage to the lobe. The severity of the brain damage (mild, moderate, severe), the extent of the brain damage (the amount of area affected), and the nature of the damage (focal or diffuse) will affect the presentation of the client. Consequently, the client may have problems with some or all skills associated with damage to a particular lobe and the extent of dysfunction with those skills may range from mild to severe.

So now the question is, if the clinician cannot assume that damage to a particular lobe will consistently result in the same presentation, what is the use in knowing this information? Knowing the possible problems that the client may have before you see him/her is vital to the assessment process. The clinician who knows what s/he might "see" has an idea what to look for (observe) and what to test for (evaluate). For example, if a client has a frontal lobe injury, the clinician knows to check for difficulties with problem solving (e.g., client is having difficulty operating the nurse call bell). Further testing (e.g., 1. asking the client a few questions that require problem solving — if someone was driving close to your car bumper what would you do? 2. presenting the client with a problem-solving task, such as a puzzle) will uncover specific problems. There are close, but not complete, ties between brain physiology and function. Understanding the functions of areas of the brain helps the clinician provide appropriate treatment for different brain injuries.

Spinal Cord

The spinal cord is the specialized component of the nervous system that connects the brain with the rest of the body. A lot of research has been done to identify the various components of the spinal cord and the types of deficits damage to the spinal cord causes.

Damage to a particular location along the length of the spinal cord will cause deficits in parts of the body below the damage. For example, damage in the lower back will affect the legs but not the arms. The severity of a spinal cord injury is usually measured by the American Spinal Injury Association Impairment Scale (AIS), which is a modification of the *Frankel Neurological Assessment for Spinal Injury*. This classification system has five levels of completeness (A through E) and describes the degree of motor and sensory function lost. The test for completeness is made in the sacral segments (S4-S5) because it provides a consistent measure of completeness during the healing process, which is not possible by measuring the completeness at higher levels on the spine. Spinal cord injuries impact more than just motor and sensory function. Patients with spinal cord injuries also frequently experience neurogenic symptoms (hypotension, bradycardia, and impairment of reflexes), bowel and bladder disorders (urinary retention and paralysis of the bowel), and loss of perspiration below the level of a complete spinal injury.

The "anatomical portion" of the spinal cord body injured also determines functional loss. The body of the spinal cord is divided into three columns (funiculi): the anterior (primary functions include motor function, posture reflexes, light touch, and pressure), the lateral (primary functions include subconscious proprioception for control of locomotion, temperature, and motor function), and the posterior (primary functions include proprioception, two-point discrimination, deep pressure, touch, and vibration). When the sensory testing for spinal cord injury is done, both pinprick and light touch are used to help determine which of the three columns are affected. (burlingame, 2001) See the Spinal Cord Injury diagnosis for more information.

References

burlingame, j. (2001). *Idyll Arbor's Therapy Dictionary, 2nd Edition.* Ravensdale, WA: Idyll Arbor.

Participation

Recreational therapists do not view participation in an activity as an either/or scenario (either the client participated or s/he did not). Recreational therapists study participation patterns (also called levels). Evaluation of a client's participation level helps to clarify the client's quality of participation in an activity. This is important to form a baseline of the client's participation pattern, to note changes (progress, regression), and to formulate and measure the attainment of goals. The quality of participation in an activity deserves special attention since the quality of participation in an activity brings with it specific health benefits (the health benefits of being a spectator are very different from the benefits of actively participating in a physical activity).

Many recreational therapists are familiar with Dehn's Leisure Step Up model (Dehn, 1995) that provides a hierarchy of healthy leisure participation levels; and burlingame (2001) clarification of the differences between attendance and participation, which can be seen by looking at the involvement of the client. These definitions were developed to help therapists and researchers clarify client participation levels and patterns in a way that leads to a better understanding of how activities affect the client's life.

Attendance: Attendance is defined as how many times or how often a client shows up for an activity. Attendance does not measure effort, quality of participation, emotional involvement, behavior, or attitude. It only measures if the client is there or not. Attendance is a good measure for monitoring use of an activity, facility, or equipment to help with determining staffing needs, budget needs, and maintenance needs. Attendance is also used to measure the very basic skill of showing up at an activity. This may be a good way to measure progress in a client who has trouble initiating this basic skill due to compliance or follow through issues. For clients with these issues, just showing up at an activity can be progress. The ICF is not concerned with "attendance," though. The ICF goal is to measure the level of the client's abilities, therefore the term "attendance" is not used in the ICF code. The definition of attendance is provided in this section to give the therapist a clear understanding of its difference from participation.

Participation: Participation measures the quality of the client's actions and the amount of effort that the clients puts into the activity. The ICF is concerned with participation. A whole section of the ICF is called "Activities and Participation." Participation, unlike attendance, can be measured on a spectrum of healthy (beneficial to self and others) to unhealthy (harmful to self or others). Dehn (1995) describes nine levels of leisure participation along this spectrum as part of his Leisure Step Up program, as described below. Therapists will find that adding Dehn's levels is helpful when scoring codes in Activities and Participation Chapter 9 (see the chapter for detailed suggestions). Clients are encouraged to achieve a healthy balance among the positive levels while avoiding participation on the negative levels.

Positive Levels

There are five positive levels in the model ranging from uninvolved spectator up to cathartic. Clients may participate in an activity on any of these levels. In deciding on the level of the client's participation it is appropriate to ask the client and to make independent observations based on the client's attitude and demeanor.

- *Level 1 (Uninvolved Spectator)*: This level is described as being an uninvolved spectator. There is no emotional involvement. The client often lacks a personal investment in participating in positive leisure activities. Examples would include staring at the television without any real interest in the storyline or sitting outside watching the cars drive by. Dehn points out that our mind, body, and emotions can become fatigued and that the need to just do nothing (and not feel guilty about it) is a form of healthy participation. Although this level of participation is on the healthy side of leisure, it does not fulfill all of our leisure needs. Clients should be encouraged to strive for higher participation levels.
- *Level 2 (Involved Spectator)*: This level is described as being an involved spectator. The spectator is emotionally involved in the activity. The client is interested in the activity and expresses or experiences emotions related to the activity. This type of participation provides emotional and/or cognitive health benefits, but it does not fulfill all of our leisure needs. Examples would include attending an opera where the songs and acting move you or getting charged up over watching a football game on television.
- *Level 3 (Active Participation)*: This level is described as active participation. The client is a player rather than a spectator. Clients at this level think of recreation in terms of activity (there are instructions, rules, a plan, etc.) and it requires physical, cognitive, and/or social components for participation. The activities must reflect a

balance of physical, social, and cognitive components (not all have to be reflected in one activity but in the client's activity pattern as a whole).

- *Level 4 (Creative Participation)*: This level is described as creative participation. Emotions are expressed. Participation in the activity does not follow a plan, pattern, or instruction. The client puts a part of himself/herself into the activity and the finished activity reflects what the client has given (making a clay sculpture, writing music or poetry). Creativity can be learned and practiced, it is not solely an innate skill.
- *Cathartic level*: This level is described as the ultimate level of leisure participation. The client has a high level of emotional involvement in the activity and it acts as a catalyst for growth in the client's lifestyle. Not everyone reaches this level of participation.

Neutral Level

Level 0 (Preoccupied): This level is described as being preoccupied. It is neither positive nor negative. The client is present at the activity (goes through the motions) but is too preoccupied with other things to really experience the full activity. Examples would include going camping at a beautiful lake but being so preoccupied with a troubled relationship that the client doesn't truly experience the beauty of the lake. Participating in activities that are used as a therapeutic means to cope with a problem that is preoccupying the individual are also considered to fall into this level. Such examples include going for a walk when feeling angry or journaling to help express feelings of sorrow. Clients who participate at this level usually have high levels of stress, frustration, and/or depression.

At first glance, it looks like Level 0 might be the same as "attendance," but, in reality, each of the levels in Dehn's model requires attendance. Attendance only measures where the body is. To record what the client is experiencing, we must describe where the mind and emotions are, too.

Negative Levels

The three negative levels in the model describe the type of leisure participation that cause harm to the client and others.

- *Level –1 (Harm to Self)*: This level is described as causing harm to one's self. It is the first level

in the unhealthy direction of leisure participation. An activity at this level either puts the client at high risk of harm or causes actual physical, mental, or emotional damage. Examples include smoking, not getting enough sleep, not eating a well-balanced diet, talking down to one's self (e.g., "I look stupid", "I'll never do this right"), and participating in dangerous high risk activities without proper training and safety measures.

- *Level –2 (Harm to Others)*: This level is described as causing harm to others. The leisure actions of the person have inflicted physical, emotional, or mental harm to others (e.g., hurting animals, ignoring family, substance abuse, gambling, stealing, destroying property, and gossiping). People at this level may deny that these things are hurtful (just having fun). People at this level are often in need of developing basic social skills and an awareness of their risk to spiral downwards towards "Lost Freedom."
- *Lost Freedom*: People at this level have 1. been voluntarily or involuntarily committed to an institution that places constraints on the type and amount of leisure that is available (e.g., prison, mental health facility, juvenile delinquency facility) or 2. have lost their freedom (mentally and emotionally) because of trauma (e.g., a victim of rape or a person in profound mourning whose leisure activities are constrained by thoughts and feelings of rage, guilt, fear, depression). Participation at this level has a drastic effect on the person, as well as other people who are around the person. People at this level are often preoccupied with suicidal thoughts, suffer from extreme depression and loss of interest, or have a total disregard for the self and others (e.g., gang fighting with no concern for self or others, infecting others with HIV, suicide attempts). Clients at this level are in need of developing leisure patterns that promote health. Counseling by a variety of disciplines is often required for the client to begin moving in a positive direction.

References

burlingame, j. (2001). *Idyll Arbor's therapy dictionary, 2nd Edition*. Ravensdale, WA: Idyll Arbor.

Dehn, D. (1995). *Leisure step up*. Ravensdale, WA: Idyll Arbor.

Precautions

This topic looks at common precautions for clients.

Falls Precautions

A falls precaution order is written by the treating physician for a client who is at a high risk for falls. This can be a client who has had a history of falls or a client who has a high risk of falling given his/her current health situation (e.g., a client who lacks insight into limitations, moderately impaired balance). If a client has a falls precaution, particular measures are put into place to reduce the client's risk of falling (e.g., restraint, supervision, education).

Physicians and therapists must be aware of other issues that could cause a fall and address them accordingly (e.g., balance problems, vision problems, hearing problems, side effects from medications, changes to the home).

Falls prevention is also implemented through the following recommendations:

- Prescription of adaptive devices (e.g., self-care equipment, mobility equipment).
- Teaching clients how to modify their homes and other frequently used environments (e.g., garage, wood working room, worksite) to decrease falls. This may include removing throw rugs, keeping items off the stairs, picking up items that are left in pathways, eliminating furniture that is seldom used, removing stacks of things on the floor that could topple over or take up needed walking areas, eliminating or moving electrical cords and phone cords so they are not a tripping hazard, wearing flat shoes that neither grab nor slip, installing railings on staircases, installing tub and toilet grab bars, moving commonly used items to waist height to decrease bending and reaching, using brighter light bulbs in areas where there isn't much light or in places where the surface is uneven, and using nightlights especially in the bedroom, hallway, and bathroom.
- Subscribing to a home medical system in case the client falls so s/he can push a button that is worn around the neck to instantly call for assistance or, at the very least, have a lightweight cordless phone on hand at all times (wear an apron, a canvas tool pouch, or a waist pack when in the home and keep the phone there during the day and back in the charging cradle at night). Choose a phone that has large buttons that are easy to see and push and not so many buttons that they confuse the client.
- Recommending a cell phone for emergencies that occur in the community. Some counties have a senior program that gives out free cell phones to older adults through the police station or senior centers. They are used phones that are turned in by community members. When kept charged, a subscription service is not necessary because emergency numbers are free of charge. Choose a phone with a simple design and few buttons to limit confusion.

Hip Precautions

Hip precautions are used for a total hip replacement (THP) or hip fracture with a closed reduction. They are designed to protect the hip joint and avoid further injury, such as dislocation. The usual precautions include:

- Do not flex involved hip beyond 90°.
  - Will have to sit on elevated chairs or toilet seats to maintain precaution.
  - Cannot bend over from the hips to reach objects or tie shoes (use a reacher).
- Do not rotate the hip internally (do not turn leg inwards).
- Do not rotate the trunk in a way that may result in internal hip rotation.
- Do not turn the feet excessively inward or outward.
- Do not cross the legs at the ankles or knees.
- Do no lie or roll onto the uninvolved side.
- Place a pillow between the legs when lying on the involved side.

An abduction wedge pillow is used during waking hours to prevent internal rotation of the hip. The "V" shaped abduction pillow is placed between the legs and Velcroed around the thighs the hold it in place. Sometimes clients are initially instructed to wear it when sleeping to prevent breaking hip precautions.

For some clients, individualized precautions may be prescribed by the surgeon. Inpatient rehab therapists must be diligent about checking the client-specific THP set by the surgeon.

Weight Bearing

Typically, clients with cemented joint replacements can weight bear as tolerated (WBAT) unless the procedure involved a soft tissue repair or internal fixation of bone. Clients with cementless or ingrowth joint replacements are put on partial weight bearing (PWB) or toe-touch weight bearing (TTWB) for six weeks to allow maximum bony ingrowth to take place. Weight-bearing precautions may also be set for a variety of other conditions. such as fractures and sprains. Weight-bearing precautions include:

- *Non-weight bearing* (NWB): Unable to put any weight on the identified extremities. If the restriction involves both lower extremities, activity is limited to those completed while sitting or in bed. May complete transfers using a transfer board.
- *Touchdown weight bearing* (TDWB) or Toe-touch weight bearing (TTWB): The majority of the client's weight bearing must be through the client's arms on the walking device and the unaffected extremity. Physical therapists recommend strategies for safe walking and prescribe a mobility device to help clients adhere to weight-being precautions. Close collaboration between the physical therapist and other allied health professionals working with the client is essential so that the client is able to engage in functional activity safely and effectively while using the device. Weight bearing on the involved extremity is limited to using toes to make contact with floor, primarily to maintain balance. Note that toe-touch weight bearing is not as much weight as the client can carry on his/her toes.
- *Partial weight bearing* (PWB): This typically refers to bearing 50% of the client's body weight on the involved extremity. It is frequently estimated by the client and therapist and requires sustained effort and attention. Note that when walking, a normal gait puts 100% of the client's weight on the extremity when it is the only limb on the ground. This would not be allowed with partial weight bearing.
- *Weight bearing as tolerated* (WBAT): The amount of weight put on the extremity is left to the discretion of the client based on his/her level of comfort.
- *Full weight bearing* (FWB): No restrictions on amount of weight put on the extremity.

References

Crepeau, E., Cohn, E., Schell, B. (2003). *Willard and Spackman's occupational therapy, tenth edition.* Philadelphia, PA: Lippincott Williams & Wilkins.

Rasul, A. (2002). Total joint replacement rehabilitation. http://www.emedicine.com/pmr/topic221.htm on 3/23/04.

Psychoneuroimmunology

The connection between the mind and the body is not a new concept. The Greeks, more than two thousand years ago, "understood intuitively that emotions and health are one" (Sternberg, 2000, p. 3). Hippocrates, whose oath still underlies the principles of modern medicine, taught that health lay in a balance among a healthy diet, pure waters, exercise, and the support of friends and family, as well as soothing activities that calmed them such as music, sleep, and prayer. "So integral to the healing of the body was the mind that the god of medicine carried a staff with the symbols both intertwined: Asclepius carried in his left hand the caduceus, a wooden staff with a serpent curled around it, an ancient symbol of body and soul, and today the universally recognized symbol of medicine" (Sternberg, 2000, p. 2).

Many traditional and alternative health professionals witness the power of the mind in healing the body and many behavioral studies have documented the connection between mind, emotions, activity, and health. However, despite how convincing and exciting these studies have been, the medical community desires concrete biochemical evidence that such a connection exists. A relatively new discipline, psychoneuroimmunology (PNI), is now providing that evidence. PNI is the study of the interrelationships between the central nervous system and the immune system. PNI has shown that the brain and the immune system are a closed bi-directional circuit. They are in constant communication with each other. Simply put, emotions and demands from the immune system trigger certain hormonal and chemical changes in the body. These biological changes travel throughout the body and affect bodily processes, including the immune system, which directly influences the process of disease in a positive or negative direction. In one study, Candace Pert, a neuropharmacologist at the National Institute of Mental Health, found that individuals who were made to feel helpless (loud noise prevented concentration on a puzzle) had slower than usual macrophage movement (macrophages surround and consume infection and rebuild damaged tissues). Thus she speculated that the client who gives up hope might fare worse than the client who is optimistic. The client who is optimistic will keep the macrophages moving while the client who gives up will slow down macrophage movement. She goes on to say that, "The more I look, the more I'm convinced that emotions are running the show" (Weschsler, 1987, p. 55).

Although we don't expect the medical community to shift totally from a conventional approach to a holistic approach, we do expect that the practice of medicine will become more holistically focused, taking into consideration the client's emotional, social, and spiritual health, aspects that are already included in the ICF. For recreational therapists, this branch of research also adds more validity to what we do for our clients. Our focus on helping our clients achieve optimal emotional and social health does, indeed, have a direct influence on our clients' recovery and disease process. Not only does this focus improve the quality of their lives, but it also contributes to the biomedical approach to eradicating disease.

Thoughts, Feelings, and Emotions

Since we are now aware that thoughts, feelings, and emotions influence our physical health, we need to ask the question, "What is it, exactly, that influences our thoughts and feelings?" This is an important question since healthy emotional responses are optimal in the recovery process. Is it our perception and interpretation of a situation? Is it hormonal and chemical changes in the body as a result of disease? Is it activity that triggers hormonal and chemical changes? Is it life experiences? Yes, yes, yes, and yes. All of these influence our thoughts and feelings. Our world, as well as ourselves, are complex systems functioning within systems of systems. All are inter-related and interdependent. Why should our thoughts and feelings be judged any differently? As recreational therapists, we are keenly aware of the many interventions that can be implemented to optimize emotional health both directly and indirectly.

Perceptions and Interpretations

"Our thoughts create the context that determines our feelings. In thinking about health, and especially in trying to change the consequences of an illness or the behavior that leads to it, an awareness of context — or what I have come to call 'mindfulness' — is crucial" (Langer, 1989, p. 48). If one thinks negatively, one's emotional response will be fear and high anxiety. If one thinks positively and realistically, one's emotional response will be hopeful with a controlled sense of calm. Our "perceptions and interpretations influence the ways in which our bodies respond to information in the world. If we automatically — 'mindlessly' — accept preconceived notions of the context of a particular situation, we can jeopardize the body's ability to handle that situation, we can jeopardize the body's ability to need to place our perceptions intentionally, that is, mindfully in a different context" (Langer, 1989, p. 48). Recreational therapists can enhance their client's perceptions and interpretations of situations via a variety of counseling techniques. See "Education and Counseling" in the Techniques section.

Hormonal and Chemical Changes

As reviewed earlier, PNI research indicates that the brain and the immune system are bi-directional. Therefore, it is not a far stretch to think that the immune system could affect emotions controlled by the brain.

> Signals from the immune system may even reach the emotional and rational centers of the brain, which may explain why people get irritable when they're sick, and why mental capacity often deteriorates at the same time as resistance to infection (Weschsler, 1987, p. 53).

You have probably heard a family member of a client say, "I don't know why he's like that. That's not like him." Sometimes a client may even recognize the changes in himself and make the same observation. Chances are the family member and client are right. It's probably not the typical behavior or emotional response of the client, but the illness or disease process that is triggering the release of certain hormones and chemicals that are affecting his behavior and/or emotions. The recreational therapist may be able to influence this process indirectly by enhancing macrophage movement. By fostering the client's emotional health in a positive direction (locus of control, achievement, esteem), macrophage movement will hopefully increase, thus optimizing the body's defenses to consume disease and rebuild tissue. The therapist can also assist the client in developing skills for managing unwanted emotional responses (e.g., relaxation techniques for anxiety, thought stopping for negative thinking cycles).

However, if the illness or trauma directly affects the functioning of the brain (e.g., a stroke), the changes in the client's behavior and personality may be better attributed to brain damage. If the behavior and personality changes are believed to be a direct result of brain damage, consult the sections on "Neuroplasticity" and "Behavior Manipulation" in the Techniques section.

Activity

Activity, in and of itself, can cause the release of hormones and other chemicals that enhance mood. For example, a "runners high" is explained by the release of endorphins (the body's natural painkillers). After a run, people often report feeling uplifted,

relaxed, and recharged. Those who practice yoga report feelings of inner peace and strength and those who participate in an activity that highlights personal skills may exhibit increased self-esteem. All of these positive and healthy emotions result in hormonal and chemical changes in the body. One must question, however, if it is the activity, in and of itself, that is the primary cause of the emotional response or is it the secondary benefits of the activity. For example, was it the chance to appreciate the beauty of nature that invoked a sense of relaxation from the run, was it the music that generated feelings of strength from yoga exercises, or was it the recognition of one's personal skills that fostered a sense of self-esteem from the activity? How one achieves emotional change varies from person to person and it is difficult, if not impossible, to tease out the specific things that fostered change, because, chances are, it was a coming together of many complex systems, of which activity is a part.

Activities that have been shown to enhance a client's emotional state include meditation, prayer, popping bubble-wrap, hypnosis, biofeedback, placebos, imagery, relaxation techniques, friends, pets, music, art, humor, and anything that provides a "thrill" (a subtle nervous tremor caused by intense emotion or excitement — climatic music, great beauty in nature or art, sexual activity, watching emotional interactions between other people). Knowing this, therapists educate clients on the positive and negative influence of the immune system on mood and work with clients to determine what activities are realistic as part of the clients' activity patterns. See "Activity Pattern Development" in the Techniques section for more information.

Life Experiences

One's past and present life experiences shape beliefs, attitudes, opinions, and actions...all of which influence emotional health (thus positively or negatively affecting the immune system). If one experiences betrayal, then one may mistrust. If one experiences unconditional love, then one may feel accepted. Who we are and what we have become are shaped by many things in our lives: our family, our friends, our accomplishments, our failures, our hopes and dreams, as well as our disappointments and struggles. These experiences give shape to how we interpret situations, cope, and live our lives. Therapists should not be blind to a client's life experiences and focus only on the present situation, for in the past one may find answers. For example:

> A 32-year-old female client is angry and bitter since being diagnosed with cancer and is unable to move past these emotions affecting many of her life

activities. The client shares with you that her mother died when from cancer she was young. You learn that she swore to herself that she would never leave her children as her mother did and yet she now finds herself in the same situation. The anger from her mother's death has still not been resolved and her own promise to herself will now be broken. The recreational therapist makes a referral to counseling services and designs an RT treatment program that addresses the development of healthy coping strategies.

A client who has been diagnosed with multiple sclerosis for 10 years is exhibiting signs of depression. At least once a year, he experiences an exacerbation. Rehabilitation following each exacerbation has improved his functioning moderately, but the exacerbations continue like clockwork. In the beginning, he exercised regularly, controlled his stress level, ate a healthy diet, and did not push himself past fatigue. Over time, his efforts have not yielded the results he had hoped for, thus extinguishing his internal locus of control. He now comes to you, his 10th exacerbation, depressed, and in "learned helplessness" mode. He has no motivation or initiative and just wants to sit in front of the television. This client's past life experiences have reinforced that no matter what he does it doesn't matter, despite how unrealistic this interpretation is to another. The recreational therapist educates and counsels the client about the relation of activity to exacerbation management and helps the client to better understand what his past actions "have" done rather than what they "have not" done for his health.

Other considerations that influence the client's life experiences include cultural and religious beliefs and practices. For example, some cultures believe that it is unacceptable to share or show emotions, while other cultures belittle a man who is unable to fulfill the traditional male role of being the provider, and certain faiths promote the idea that one is afflicted with disease due to bad behavior. All of these influence the client's emotional state (thus positively or negatively affecting the immune system), as well as affecting the client's ability to develop healthy coping skills. Therapists must be aware of their client's life experiences as they affect his/her current situation in order to best understand the client's emotional state and implement appropriate interventions to enhance emotional health (e.g., psychotherapy, education, values clarification).

Conclusion

The mind and the body, our being, is an interrelated complex system where behavior, emotions, and health are constantly seeking a biological balance. No longer are one's emotions and beliefs secondary in the healing process. It has been validated via psychoneuroimmunology (PNI) that our emotions directly influence illness and disease processes. Recreational therapists should use this information to add professional validation for the field, as well as to educate clients on the value of emotional health on functioning and recovery. As Asclepius's staff symbolizes the coming together of body and soul, so should we, as health professionals, uphold this belief and instill it in our clients.

References

Langer, E. (1989). The mindset of health. *Psychology Today, 23*(4):48.

Sternberg, E. (2000). *The balance within: The science connecting health and emotions.* New York, NY: W. H. Freeman and Company.

Weschsler, R. (1987). A new prescription: Mind over malady. *Discover. 8*:50.

Social Skills Development

[6] Acceptance in social systems is based on behaviors that meet the expectations of that system. Deviations from social norms often result in social isolation. Without specific training in social skills, many clients with cognitive impairments do not demonstrate appropriate social behaviors and appropriate social interactions skills. Their lives may be void of positive social interactions.

The World Health Organization recognizes the critical role that interpersonal interactions play in quality of life. Activities and Participation Chapter 7 Interpersonal Interactions and Relationships covers this set of abilities. In this section we will provide an overview of the social problems of clients with cognitive and physical disabilities. Then we will look at the development of social skills throughout life. For a discussion of the cognitive abilities required to develop social skills, see "Basic Awareness of Self as Part of Socialization" in the Concepts section.

Social Problems of Clients with Cognitive Impairments

Clients with cognitive impairments face many difficulties when they try to be part of community life. Historically, therapists, other health care professionals, and educators have focused on medical intervention, vocational training, and special education. Trends of normalization and mainstreaming, as well as subsequent legislation, have emphasized that such training is not enough. Training in other behavioral dimensions is also necessary. One critical dimension is social skills development as illustrated by the following case study and research.

Pat is a 19-year-old female client who has been diagnosed as having an IQ of 65. She has received extensive training in independent living and vocational skills. Pat works in a school cafeteria helping to prepare food and has moved from a group home into a satellite apartment. She does her assigned tasks at work willingly and thoroughly, but often gets into arguments when she needs to work cooperatively. During breaks and lunchtime Pat sits by herself and occasionally talks to an imaginary friend. After work she usually watches her TV or listens to her radio. At other times she walks around looking in store windows or sits on park benches. Her former group home has a weekly activities night, which she is required to attend.

Although she has the leisure skills to participate in the activities, she often sits on the periphery of the group and refuses to participate. Pat, like many of her peers with similar disabilities, is in jeopardy of failing on the job or in the community because she lacks social skills. As her loneliness increases, she becomes more restless and irritable at work. Pat's unhappiness is interfering with her ability to adapt and to function in the community.

Despite these problems, Pat is more fortunate than many of her former classmates. Sixty percent of the 120 mild to moderately impaired students who graduated with her never go out with friends. Many of her peers spend the majority of their free time doing self-stimulatory and repetitive activities, such as rocking. Others are seen in the community doing age-inappropriate activities, such as playing with dolls. Given the opportunity to interact with individuals that they know, many remain in their own worlds, sitting apart, gazing into space, and doing nothing. When they do engage in activities, the activities are generally solitary in nature, such as crafts and collections. Their difficulty in sharing, taking turns, giving consideration to others, and general collaboration is evident in group situations.

This lack of social interaction is a recurring theme in the literature. A study of the time usage of residents in group homes in Washington State revealed a pattern similar to that of Pat and her former classmates (Ballard, 1976). Four hours each day (23% of the waking hours) were spent in unstructured activities such as watching TV; three hours (17%) were spent in low-level activity, such as simply sitting, waiting, or gazing into space; 0.8 hours (5%) were spent in organized activities such as games, hobbies, and sports; and 0.5 hours (3%) were spent simply leaving the house.

This inactive, solitary lifestyle is a pattern for many clients with cognitive impairments, not just clients with developmental disabilities. One of the most striking aspects seen in initial assessments of clients with cognitive impairments is the lack of friends, the small amount of time, if any, spent with friends, the inability to use friendships constructively, and the resultant social isolation. When clients are able to name friends, these friends are generally schoolmates, casual acquaintances, or relatives with whom they have very limited interaction. It is not unusual for the "friends" named to be fantasized friendships with people of high social desirability such as the popular recreation instructor, the cute next-door neighbor, or even the bus driver on the bus normally ridden. Neighborhood people identified as

[6] This section is written by Phyllis Coyne and is an updated version of her *Social Skills Training: A Three-Pronged Approach* originally published in 1980 and funded by a grant from the Developmental Disabilities Office, Region X, Grant No. 50-P-50368.

friends are generally considerably younger or older than the client. The socialization opportunities available to clients with cognitive impairments tend to be limited to segregated, large-group experiences that do not facilitate normalization or the development of social interaction skills (Coyne, 1980).

In addition to deficits in social interaction skills, clients with cognitive impairments often exhibit an array of inappropriate social behaviors. While the lack of social interaction skills may result in arguments, depression, and isolation, inappropriate social behaviors may result in arrests, physical harm, and further alienation from the mainstream. Many clients with cognitive impairments who manifest inappropriate social behaviors are referred to programs that offer social skills training. For example, one referral involved a young man who was so pleased to receive a compliment from a stranger that he hugged her and was arrested for molesting her. A common incident is the young person who looks in neighbors' windows out of curiosity and is thought to be a Peeping Tom or potential rapist. Several clients who were mentally retarded have been arrested for child abuse after taking down the pants of neighborhood children. Although motivated by curiosity rather than sexual drive, such "doctor play" is age inappropriate and in conflict with the social value system. These behaviors severely jeopardize community placement.

Other behaviors do not lead to arrests but make individuals vulnerable and/or undesirable. For example, females with cognitive impairments become victims of sexual abuse because they think that a man who acts friendly by smiling or saying hello is a boyfriend. Some clients with cognitive impairments hear locker room comments such as "Hey, Babe, nice tits," or "Hey, Fella, you're really hung" and inappropriately make these comments in mixed company.

Another problem is frequent referrals to community mental health clinics because of inappropriate social behaviors. A study of clients with mental retardation referred to the Clackamas County (Oregon) Community Mental Health Program found that behavioral problems rather than psychiatric diagnoses were the major factor impeding successful functioning of this population (Grim, 1979). Some of the problematic social behaviors identified were attention seeking, isolation, immaturity, high dependency, inactivity, lack of motivation, non-compliance, explosiveness, hostility, tantrums, aggression, open masturbation, and promiscuity. This study also found that adolescents and young adults who were developmentally disabled tended to fall through the cracks and remain dependent citizens with severe social problems.

Social Problems of Clients with Physical Impairments

Clients with cognitive impairments are not the only ones who have problems with interpersonal interactions. Clients with physical disabilities may also experience social deficiencies.

Not all clients with physical disabilities have the same needs or share the same problems. The removal of architectural barriers has been one of the priority needs identified for clients with physical disabilities. However, lack of social skills may present a greater barrier to community participation than concrete barriers. Clients with physical disabilities, whether congenital or acquired, share many obstacles to development of interpersonal skills with clients who have cognitive disabilities. Some of the major ones include:

- Overprotection from risks or uncomfortable situations.
- Limited opportunity to interact with peers.
- Continued dependency on others.
- Attitudinal barriers.
- Limited opportunity for role experimentation.
- Lowered expectations.

Berryman, James, and Trader (1991) cite numerous studies that found that clients with disabilities experienced social isolation:

- Individuals who are disabled congenitally (from birth) have fewer opportunities for play, are less socially active as they get older, and have overprotective parents: all limiting factors in socialization (Rinck et al., 1989; Zoerink, 1989).
- Twenty-five percent of individuals with spinal cord injuries live alone compared to the national average of 11% (Dew et al., 1983).
- Thirty-one percent of Georgians with spinal cord injuries leave home less than once a week; many of them not at all (Anson & Shepherd, 1990).
- Individuals with disabilities report a lower marital rate (52% compared to 70%) and higher divorce rate than their non-disabled peers (Dew et al., 1983).

Problems with socialization are also found in other countries. A study in Sweden revealed that although 88% of children with physical disabilities were integrated into normal classrooms, at least one fourth of the integrated children still had no friends. Even those who developed friendships with non-disabled classmates often lost these friendships from seven to nine years of age and during the stressful period of adolescence (Paulsson, 1980). Another Swedish study found that the general attitude of non-disabled peers towards clients with mental retardation was one of accepting indifference. There was no systematic harassment, but there was a poverty of positive interactions (Soder, 1990). These findings emphasize that physical integration does not ensure social interaction.

Clients with physical disabilities have some unique characteristics. Many are of normal or above normal intelligence. Unlike clients with cognitive impairments whose limited ability for abstract thought makes it difficult to appropriately use peers as role models, people with physical limitations can often learn social skills through the normal process of social experiences. They are generally aware if they have had limited social exposure and consequent lack of social skills. Self-concept is also commonly affected by growing up "disabled" or "different." Speech and hearing impairments may create additional difficulties in interaction. Clients in this situation will sometimes avoid or refuse to be placed in a social situation, regardless of the desire to participate, because of a fear of rejection and/or poor self-concept. Brier and Demb (1980) found that many physically disabled adolescents rejected peers and held the belief that they would find older, more mature individuals who would understand them.

Adolescents with physical disabilities interviewed by Brier and Demb had a number of excuses for not socializing, such as too much homework, no one interesting in school, or more important things to do. They were poorly prepared to deal with interpersonal situations and tended to lack proficiency in having a conversation, joining a group, making decisions, and understanding others. Difficulty with sharing, responding to teasing, and dealing with interpersonal conflict were also evident. Their annoying and self-effacing behaviors in relationships that did develop often resulted in the early demise of these friendships. The unremediated deficits in the skills and behaviors that are needed to lead effective and satisfying interpersonal lives often result in adults with physical disabilities beginning to date in their late 20s, if at all.

Development of Interpersonal Skills

Social skills have a normal sequence of development through play and recreation. Babies initially interact with themselves by playing with fingers and toes. This play has been called solitary-self or intra-individual. Then they begin to reach out and play with toys, such as mobiles or rattles. This is the solitary-object or extra-individual stage. The toddler starts to play with toys next to others without interacting; the parallel or aggregate stage. Interaction and cooperation with others in associative and cooperative play in these early stages is in small groups, ranging from one to four others. This stage of developing cooperation in a dyadic situation is ongoing and critical to establishing future close relationships (e.g., friendships, marriage). The child begins to learn skills that are appropriate for competitive interaction.

As competitive skills emerge, the young child is very "I" oriented or egocentric and likes competitive one-to-one or inter-individual activities of the "I can do it better than you" nature. When competitive activities involve more than one other child, there is generally one child against the group or an "It" (e.g., tag). This is called the competitive antagonist or unilateral stage. Then the child plays in games where everyone is against everyone else: competitive mutual goal, cooperative team, or intra-group. This requires cohesion, compromise, and the expression of positive feelings for one another. Finally, the child learns to compete on a team against other teams in the competitive team or inter-group stage. There is increasing evidence that social skills at one level need to be mastered before skills at the next level can be acquired.

Understanding this progression is important in programming for clients with cognitive impairments because training in social interaction skills needs to start at the level where the client is presently functioning. Although the end goal is interaction, it is sometimes necessary to start at non-interactive levels. An individual who only rocks, gazes into space, or does autoerotic behaviors[7] needs to be assisted in developing an interest in objects and manipulating these objects. Then manipulation of objects next to others, parallel (aggregate) activities, can be encouraged. When interaction skills begin to emerge, the individual will initially have difficulty relating to more than one person at a time. Gradually, skills to interact with up to four others emerge. Studies of group process for individuals of normal intelligence have indicated that the optimum number for effective group interaction is between six and twelve. Therefore, large groups or other inappropriate social structures can actually hinder interaction and social skill development.

Therapists who work with clients who have lost social skills because of a disease, disorder, or injury later in life will use many of the same intervention principles described in this section. In all cases, the delivery of the intervention should match the

---

[7] Self-initiated behaviors that have sexual elements often done in socially inappropriate contexts or settings.

individual client's assessed needs and underlying skills.

Therapists can additionally refer to "Social Skills Training" and "Interpersonal Relationship Activities" in the Techniques section, Activities and Participation Chapter 7 Interpersonal Interactions and Relationships, "Basic Awareness of Self as Part of Socialization" in the Concepts section, and *Leisure and Social/Sexual Assessment* in the Assessment section.

Issues in Adolescence

Adolescence is a turbulent and confusing period of change and growth. In school and in the community, with peers, family members, and authority figures, clients with developmental disabilities must cope with and master increasingly complex personal and interpersonal skills. These include (Brier and Demb, 1980):

- The attainment of emotional independence from parents.
- The establishment of a meaningful and stable identity.
- The development of a personal value system.
- The development of the capacity for lasting relationships and for both tender and genital love.

These steps toward adult functioning are closely related to interpersonal relationships. For instance, the adolescent usually becomes less emotionally dependent on parents by establishing an outside support system comprised of best friends and a peer group. This peer group forms a highly complex social structure and testing ground for exploring both personal and interpersonal values and identity. In this transition the adolescent develops an ability to be close to and to participate in a special, exclusive relationship (Brier and Demb, 1980). The development of a sense of intimacy that results from the relationship with a best friend is a prerequisite for a mature adult love relationship, and an adult love relationship may not be truly attainable without this experience. Adolescent clients with cognitive impairments tend to lack both a best friend and a peer group creating more obstacles to mastering the tasks of adolescence.

Feelings of inadequacy, characterized by helplessness and dependency, often increase during this period. In addition to dramatic physical changes, such as the onset of menses and the development of breasts in females, the emergence of wet dreams in males, and the growth of pubic hair in both, the adolescent encounters unfamiliar feelings toward the opposite sex and other physiologically triggered emotions. The body changes of pubescence may seem particularly strange and frightening to those who do not understand the changes or have a poor body image. Clients with physical disabilities, in particular, may feel ashamed of their bodies and withdraw further from social contacts. Without intervention in the problems of social interactions and social behaviors encountered at this stage, there may be prolonged social immaturity.

Social Roles and Tasks: Stages of Family Life Cycles

Clients who become cognitively impaired during adulthood tend to have, to some degree, obtained success in social skills. Many of these social skills are related to families and have allowed the client to move through numerous stages of his/her family life cycle. Clients with new cognitive impairments have the dual task of re-learning old social skills while trying to learn the personal interaction skills necessary for continuing to move through the family life cycle. Duvall (1971) lists six stages of family development, which are described below with the interpersonal skills necessary for each level.

- *Stage 1 (Between Families; the Unattached Young Adult)*: For the parent of a young adult this requires the acceptance of role changes from being in charge of a child to allowing the child to make his/her own decisions. For the young adult this requires the ability to make one's own decisions and live through the consequences of those decisions. This requires a change of "boundaries," accepting a different definition of oneself and one's relationship to the family unit.
- *Stage 2 (Marriage; the Joining of Families)*: This stage requires the ability to transfer the emphasis of allegiances from one's family of origin to a new union. Flexibility in blending with someone else's social patterns is needed to realign interpersonal relationships with spouse, friends, and family.
- *Stage 3 (Family with Young Children)*: This stage requires additional skills in accepting others into one's close circle of relationships, the realignment of personal relationships, and being able to put someone else's needs before one's own needs, even more so than with spouse.
- *Stage 4 (Family with Adolescents)*: This stage requires the ability to allow adolescents to increase their independence while setting limits and still providing support. It is common for other relationship realignments to take place at this time including potential career changes and the increased need to take care of one's own aging parents.

- *Stage 5 (Launching Children)*: This stage is often referred to as the "empty nest" stage. Realignment of the "family" relationship to a stronger emphasis on a dyad relationship with spouse, establishing an adult-to-adult relationship with one's children, and integrating in-laws and grandchildren into one's circle of relationships.
- *Stage 6 (Family in Later Life)*: This stage involves the increased stress of declining health and abilities, greater reliance on the younger generations, and potential loss of spouse.

References

Anson, C. & Shepherd, C. (1990). A survey of post-acute spinal cord patients: Medical, psychological and social characteristics. *Trends: Research News from Shepard Spinal Center*, March 1990.

Ballard Jr., K. B. (1976). *Work and Training Release Program Evaluation*. Olympia, WA: Washington Department of Social and Health Services.

Berryman, D., James, A., & Trader, B. (1991). The benefits of therapeutic recreation in physical medicine. In C. P. Coyle, W. B. Kinney, B. Riley, & J. W. Shank (Eds.), *Benefits of therapeutic recreation: A consensus view*. Ravensdale, WA: Idyll Arbor.

Brier, N. M. & Demb, H. B. (1980). Psychotherapy with the developmentally disabled adolescent. *J Dev Behav Pediatr*; *1*(1):19-23.

Coyne, P. (1980). *Social skills training: A three-pronged approach*. Portland, OR: Crippled Children's Division University of Oregon Health Sciences Center.

Dew, M. A., Lynch, K. A., Ernst, J., & Rosenthal, R. (1983). Reaction and adjustments to spinal cord injury: A descriptive study. *Journal of Applied Rehabilitation Counseling, 14*:32-39.

Duvall, E. (1971), *Family development, 4th ed.* Philadelphia: Lippincott.

Grim, N. (1979). Falling through the cracks: characteristics of a community mental health population with both mental-emotional disturbances and mental retardation. Paper presented at Northwest Pacific Society of Neurology and Psychiatry, Harrison Hot Springs, BC, Canada. June 1, 1979.

Paulsson, K. (1980). *Varför integrering av rörelsehindrade ibland »misslyckas«*. Institutionen för praktisk pedagogik, Göteborgs universitet.

Rinck, C., Berg, J., & Hafeman, C., (1989). The adolescent with myelomeningocele: A review of parent experiences and expectations. *Adolescent, 24*(95):699-710.

Soder, M. (1990). Prejudice or ambivalence? Attitudes towards persons with disabilities. *Disability, Handicap and Society, 5*(3):227.

Zoerink, D. (1989). Activity choices: Exploring perceptions of persons with physical disabilities. *Therapeutic Recreation Journal, 23*(1):17-23.

Techniques

This section reviews recreational therapy techniques mentioned in the Diagnosis section and in treatments associated with the ICF.

Acclimatizing Clients to a Communal Living Arrangement

Rationale

In the United-States, 41% of women and 18% of men over 60 live alone making transition to a communal living arrangement such as a nursing home difficult (Administration on Aging, 2006). In addition, symptoms of depression have been identified in 8-20% of older adults living in the community (Office of the Surgeon General, 2006), further impacting a person's ability to cope with a change in living arrangements.

In order to facilitate the transition to a long-term care facility, opportunities for both friendships and privacy need to be created. Petrowsky (1976) found that interactions with friends in older adulthood can promote high morale. The presence of friendship can also have a buffering effect against social losses (Teaff, 1994). Conversely, in an institutional setting, shared bedrooms create little opportunity for patients to control their living space or ever have privacy. Therefore, a balance must be struck between how a geriatric center will accommodate friendships and human connections while maintaining possibilities for personal time and privacy.

Referrals

Clients who will be referred to the program include:
1. Any client newly admitted to the group living facility, including those who are readmitted (e.g., returning from an inpatient rehabilitation admission). Clients who are readmitted must be re-acclimated through this program to allow the therapist an opportunity to re-assess the client's abilities and limitations that may affect the re-integration process (e.g., exhibits signs of depression; new communication problems from a stroke now impedes the client's ability to socialize in the same manner as before and he is beginning to isolate himself; client exhibits new deficits in the area of orientation).
2. Clients admitted from isolated living conditions (to be determined through the admissions process).
3. Clients recently having gone through isolation protocol for MRSA or VRE infections, for which they were in a private room.
4. Acute care clients having been in hospital for over twelve weeks.

This treatment protocol was written by Magdalena Blaise (2004). Royal-Victoria Hospital, Montreal, Quebec, Canada.

5. Clients displaying symptoms of depression.
6. Clients having had conflict situations with roommates.

Risk Management

Prior to commencing the program, any contraindications pertaining to each client will be evaluated especially with regards to diet and behavior. Clients with special dietary needs will be clearly identified before integration in socially oriented programs where food can be an element. Clients displaying severe behavioral disturbance where they are putting themselves or others at risk will not be eligible for the program.

Professional Preparation

The therapist will display active listening skills, good analysis skills, and an aptitude for leisure education.

Structure Criteria

The program is composed of an individual and a group component. Individual interventions will be conducted at least three times weekly for 10-30 minutes, with attendance at the group occurring once a week for 75-90 minutes.

Process Criteria

The recreational therapist will ensure that contraindications are known for each client. S/he will also gather information regarding clients' interests, background etc. in order to open areas of commonality in group discussions. Cultural elements will also be identified.

Individual component

Individual interventions will address clients' specific needs regarding becoming accustomed to a communal living arrangement.

The therapist will:
1. Indicate areas where privacy can be obtained on unit, taking into account any wandering risks or orientation problems.
2. Teach clients methods of obtaining privacy in their room.
3. Teach clients self-initiated leisure that can be done individually or in small groups.
4. Provide opportunities for friendship via pertinent introductions to clients of similar culture, background, or presenting like interests.
5. Address any conflicts that arise between clients.

The client will:
1. Demonstrate knowledge of areas of privacy on unit.
2. Display understanding of methods of obtaining privacy in room.
3. Engage in self-directed leisure outside of scheduled therapist assisted time.
4. Initiate social interaction between clients.
5. Report any problems or conflicts to the therapist.

Group Component

Each group intervention will discuss common problems, issues, etc. related by clients. In addition, it will also have an open forum section in which clients can share current areas of concern.

The therapist will:
1. Introduce clients to each other.
2. Validate clients' concerns.
3. Indicate appropriate social reactions towards clients' concerns.
4. Identify similarities between clients based on group discussion.
5. Encourage acceptance and trust between clients.

The client will:
1. Be able to identify fellow group members.
2. Exhibit supportive attitudes towards fellow group members' concerns.
3. Identify commonalities in each other's situations.
4. All engage in discussion actively.

References

Administration on Aging. (2006). US Department of Human Services. www.aoa.gov.

Office of the Surgeon General. (2006). US Department of Human Services. www.surgeongeneral.gov.

Petrowsky, M. (1976). Marital status, sex, and the social network of the elderly. *Journal of Marriage and the Family 38*:20-31.

Teaff, G. (1994). *Coaching in the classroom.* Waco, TX: Cord Communications.

Activity and Task Analysis

This section will look at analyzing activities for your clients and the tasks that are required to perform the activities. To understand the difference between activity analysis and task analysis, let's begin by defining the terms "activity" and "task." Activity is defined as a specific pursuit a client participates in, whereas a task is defined as a part of the activity or a specific piece of work (or play) to be done. Activities are specific pursuits such as checkers, gardening, kite flying, or weight training and tasks as components within an activity such as setting up a checkerboard, repotting a seedling, winding up kite string, or performing one specific weight training exercise. Now that you understand these concepts, it is easy to understand that activity analysis "is a procedure for breaking down and examining an activity" (Peterson and Gunn, 1984, p. 180) and task analysis is a procedure for breaking down and examining a specific task within an activity.

Activity Analysis

Conducting an activity analysis is one of the first steps in choosing appropriate activities to meet the specific objectives of an individual or target population. Evaluation of activity components and inherent characteristics gives the therapist information s/he needs to make appropriate clinical activity prescriptions. It is not enough to choose an activity because it is available and the client agrees to participate. The therapist should prescribe an activity that s/he knows will address particular needs of the client. This is the difference between providing activities and providing therapy.

In addition to choosing activities based on the match between inherent characteristics and client objectives, activities are chosen on the likelihood of carryover for health promotion after discharge. Is the client able to afford this activity, have access to needed supplies and equipment, have available assistance, have transportation, etc.? For more information on choosing appropriate activities, see the "Assessment" section.

Peterson and Gunn (1984, p. 182) re-cap the primary benefits of activity analysis that still stand true today. It provides:

1. a better comprehension of the expected outcomes of participation;
2. a greater understanding of the complexity of activity components, which can then be compared to the functional level of an individual or group to determine the appropriateness of the activity;
3. information about whether the activity will contribute to the desired behavioral outcome when specific behavioral goals or objectives are being used;
4. direction for the modification or adaptation of an activity for individuals with limitations;
5. useful information for selecting an intervention, instructions, or leadership technique; and
6. a rationale or explanation for the therapeutic benefits of activity involvement.

When conducting an activity analysis, therapists should use a common activity analysis form. The analysis may need to be very detailed in identifying the key components and characteristics of the activity. Also note that the activity analysis should reflect the ICF categories (e.g., mental functions, mobility) rather than the common domain categories that many therapists are familiar with (e.g., cognitive, physical). Although the latter terms are still commonly used in practice, it is believed that with the increased use of the ICF, the use of domains will decrease and ICF categories will be the new standard.

Task Analysis

Task analysis is the evaluation of a specific task within an activity. This is different from activity analysis that evaluates the activity as a whole. Task analysis lists the steps *one* person takes to complete an action or a series of related actions. Task analysis is required for any evaluation a therapist does of client ability related to activity and participation. A task analysis allows a therapist to break down a task into specific components in order to compare the client's functional abilities to each component. This assists the therapist in identifying deficits for goal and objective setting.

The field of recreational therapy has a rich history of outstanding tools that analyze activities and tasks. However, these tools go beyond what is internationally recognized as task analysis. Many of the recreational therapy methods include affective aspects of the activity (e.g., anger, fear, frustration, guilt), social interaction patterns required for the activity (e.g., aggregate, inter-individual, multi-lateral), and administrative aspects (e.g., leadership style required).

As the world becomes more interconnected and standards of performance span international borders, the field of recreational therapy would benefit from following international practices. This does not mean that the therapist should not consider the social or emotional impact of activity or the practical aspects of administering an activity. Each of these elements is important, but they are separate from task analysis. The overall goal of task analysis is to standardize the analysis of activity across cultures and regions. This allows the therapist practicing in a country that emphasizes "community" (the action that increases the joy of the whole is more important than the ability of the individual to experience joy) to achieve the same results as the therapist working in a country that emphasizes "individualism" (the individual has the right to excel and be personally happy even if some of the people impacted are not pleased). Task analysis typically evaluates the observable physical actions and the anticipated cognitive processing skills necessary to carry out a task.

Task analysis is a breakdown of what one individual is *required* to do to achieve a task. The actions required include physical actions and cognitive processes required to successfully achieve a task.

When a therapist is analyzing the physical actions needed to complete a task, s/he answers the question, "What are the physical and/or cognitive steps that the client must go through to complete the task?" The physical actions needed to complete a task are linear in nature, one step logically following the one before it.

To do a task analysis, follow these steps:

1. Identify the task to be analyzed. For example, potting a seedling.
2. Break down the task into four to ten actions. If the task selected has more than fifteen subtasks (actions), the therapist has selected too global of a task. If the action has less than four subtasks it may not be a truly independent action. In the task of potting a seedling all the steps required to grow the seedling in the first place belong to another task or set of tasks.
3. Write down all the equipment needed to complete the task. Because the therapist will be required to "ground truth" the task analysis by performing the action as written, s/he should have all the equipment assembled.
   o   Seedling
   o   Fresh Soil
   o   Small hand shovel
   o   Empty pot
   o   Watering can (filled)
4. Write out the physical steps in a linear fashion (in the order that the task is completed) for repotting a plant. The easiest way to do this is for the therapist to actually write down each step while completing the task. Be sure to concentrate on a single task. If the client needs to gather his/her own equipment as part of the activity, it should be written up as a separate task.

   o   Scoop soil into pot until it is one inch from the top.
   o   Make a hole in the soil with fingers big enough to contain the root ball of the seedling.
   o   Pick up the seedling.
   o   Place the seedling into the hole.
   o   Cover roots of seedling with soil.
   o   Gently press the soil around the seedling.
   o   Water seedling so soil is damp, but not soaked.
   o   Place pot onto a tray to catch excess water.
5. Once the therapist feels that s/he has all the required steps listed, s/he should complete the task again by taking *only* the actions that are written down.
6. Any actions that are written down on the therapist's list that are not essential to completing the task should be eliminated from the list.
7. If the therapist feels that s/he has all the required physical actions listed, then s/he should give the sequential task list to another person and see if the other person can complete the activity taking only the actions that are written down. While the other person is sequentially working through the actions for the task the therapist should observe every movement taken to see if s/he forgot something or to note potential problems or acceptable variations.
8. At some point in the process, the therapist needs to look back at the purpose of the task, specifically at the setting in which the task will be performed, to see if there are any other requirements for completing the task successfully. In the example of potting a seedling, the timing of removing the seedling from where it was started is important. Having the seedling exposed too long will let the seedling's roots dry out and the seedling will die. For a group it may be possible to prepare the seedlings before the activity as a separate task. If the seedlings are being repotted one at a time, "Remove the seedling from the starting soil" should be substituted for "Pick up the seedling."
9. If (or when) a client has trouble with any specific step of the actions required to complete a task, the therapist should ask if the inability to complete the step is due to 1. physical impairment, 2. cognitive processing impairment, 3. social issue, 4. cultural issue, 5. affective (emotional) issue, 6. environmental issue, or 7. some other skill or variable that is affecting performance. The therapist will also want to evaluate the effectiveness and efficiency of the client's actions. If breakdown within a step

occurs and the specific problem is identified, objectives and an individually tailored treatment plan are established to restore the skill, modify the skill, or develop the skill. If success in restoring, developing, or modifying the skill is unlikely, the therapist evaluates the appropriateness of substituting one activity for another (e.g., taking a taxicab instead of a bus).

When the therapist writes up the individual steps associated with the task, there are many different formats s/he can follow. One format, an adaptation of Peabody's (2001) Task Outliner, is described below.

- The title of the task should be at the top of the page. The title of the task, because it is an action, should always start with a word that ends in "ing." For example, potting a seedling, paying the fare on a city bus, baking corn bread.
- The second part of the form should provide a short, one sentence description of the activity to help define the scope of the task.
- A list of the equipment needed should be clearly written out.
- A description of what action or activity typically causes someone to initiate the activity should be written. Peabody calls this a "trigger." For example, the trigger for paying the fare on a city bus would be, "The client steps into the correct bus at the bus stop."
- A description of the desired outcome against which performance will be measured is written down. For example, the outcome of paying the fare on a city bus would be to pay the correct amount of bus fare at the correct time.
- Therapists often practice tasks with clients in the clinical setting before they are practiced in the setting in which they normally occur. To help clients, each therapist should use the same lead-in phrase. For example, "When you step up into the city bus you will be expected to pay bus fare."
- The next part of the task analysis form includes the actual analysis of the specific actions required to execute the task. These steps are numbered and always start with a verb because each step is a physical or cognitive action.
- It would be appropriate to include an area for special considerations for each numbered step.

If the task has more than ten steps the therapist should see if the task can be broken down into subtasks and then have the client chain the subtasks together to complete the full activity. For example, paying bus fare is one task, looking for and occupying an appropriate place on the bus is another task, watching/listening for the correct bus stop to

---

Task: **Paying Fare on a City Bus**

Description: People must either pay bus fare or show a bus pass when they board public transportation. This task outline is for paying bus fare (not showing a bus pass).

Equipment Needed: The off peak fare for the city bus is $1.00 and the peak fare is $1.50. The client will need to have six quarters or other equivalent coin/paper money combinations (to ensure adequate fare during peak hours).

Trigger: The client steps into the correct bus at the bus stop.

Desired Outcome: The client pays the correct amount of fare.

Lead-In Phrase: When you step up into the city bus, you will be expected to pay bus fare.

Task Analysis:

#	Verb	Description of Action
1	**Walk up**	to fare box located next to the bus driver.
	Special Considerations	*If the client is in a wheelchair or scooter this process may be different (environmental factors; e120 transportation).*
2	**Read**	the posted amount of fare required.
	Special Considerations	*If the client has difficulty with this step determine if the client is able to read (d166) or has poor vision (b2100 visual acuity functions).*
3	**Count**	out correct change.
	Special Considerations	*If the client has difficulty with this step determine if the client is able to recognize the value of each coin or can add up coins (d860 basic economic transactions).*
4	**Place**	correct fare in fare box.
	Special Considerations	*If the client has difficulty with this step determine if the client has problems with simple voluntary movements (b7600).*
5	**Watch**	to make sure fare went into fare box.
	Special Considerations	*If the client has difficulty with this step determine if the client has the ability to attend to a task until completed (d160 focusing attention).*
6	**Take**	ticket from bus driver.
	Special Considerations	*Depending on the transportation system's procedures the bus rider may receive a bus ticket or a transfer pass to use on a connecting route.*

depart is another task, departing from the bus (including seeing if anything is left behind on the bus seat) is another task. Once the client has overlearned one task, then the therapist and client can work on the next task associated with riding the bus. Overlearning the task is not the same thing as being able to independently complete the task. The ability to complete the task means that the client is able to do the task. However, the client may complete all the steps but do them slowly because s/he needs to think about each step. Overlearning the task means that the client is practiced enough to do the task without spending undo time or thought on the process.

Complexity of the Task

In addition to having the steps (actions) required to complete a task the therapist will need at least two other skills:

1. The ability to break the skill down to the right level of detail, allowing identification of specific actions that the client needs to improve.
2. The ability to identify other dependent and independent tasks.

Level of Detail of Tasks

The actions needed to complete a task should be written at the correct level of difficulty, using increments that match a client's ability. The therapist will need to know the level of prerequisite skills (the skills that a client has already overlearned) his/her clients are likely to have. For therapists working with clients with severe cognitive impairment, the analysis of tasks to dress for gardening outside on a brisk fall afternoon may be made up of twenty or more subtasks as the client lacks many of the prerequisite skills to complete the overall task. As an example, the client may need to learn how to put on shoes, gardening gloves, gardening apron, and coat in addition to the skills required to determine how to

select the appropriate clothing. Each of these actions would have at least one task analyzed to compare performance. A client recovering from a heart attack without cognitive impairment is likely to have many more of the prerequisite skills intact, so the task analysis for this client may be very short.

Dependent versus Independent Tasks

There may be times that a client is able to demonstrate all the skills required for a specific task, such as riding the city bus, but still not be able to independently ride the bus. Tasks have dependent or independent subsets of skills. For many clients, learning the specific tasks associated with determining which bus to use, following the payment procedures for riding the bus, and knowing when to get off the bus may be challenging but doable. However, other skills (tasks) must also be integrated with the task at hand. For example, a client who is using a wheelchair for the first time not only needs to learn how to use the bus but will also need to learn mobility skills associated with riding a bus.

Task analysis is the basis of most of the assessments and objectives that a therapist does as part of treatment. One of the easiest ways to determine a client's needs is to compare the client's skills against a task analysis. If the therapist has a good collection of tasks already analyzed at the appropriate level for his/her clientele, then the therapist will find it easier to determine a client's functional level and to develop treatment objectives.

References

Peabody, L. (2001). *How to write policies, procedures, and task outlines: Sending clear signals in written directions.* Lacy, WA: Writing Services.

Peterson, C. & Gunn, S. (1984). *Therapeutic recreation program design: Principles and procedures, 2nd edition.* Englewood Cliffs, NJ: Prentice-Hall, Inc.

Activity Pattern Development

The goal of activity pattern development is to modify a client's activity pattern so that it is more healthy and/or therapeutic. Some of the issues involved include understanding the concepts of a leisure repertoire and balanced leisure lifestyle, determining the client's leisure interests, and developing appropriate activity patterns.

Leisure Repertoire vs. Balanced Leisure Lifestyle

The ability to carry out a daily routine (d230) requires that a client have many different skills and a relatively broad knowledge base of potential actions from which to build a daily routine. If the therapist and client identify the need to increase the number and diversity of leisure activities available to a client, the therapist will want to first help the client identify the activities in the client's leisure repertoire (see Interest Exploration below). Mobily, Lemke, and Gisin (1991) define leisure repertoire as the activities that the person feels s/he can do with competence. These authors propose that the more activities the person perceives competence in, the greater the client's ability to adjust to life's challenges.

One of the more common terms used in recreational therapy is "balanced leisure lifestyle." A balanced leisure lifestyle is generally considered to be a state in which the different facets in a person's leisure are equalized, allowing physical, mental, social, and emotional well-being. Edginton, Jordan, DeGraaf, & Edginton (1995) help define the purpose of a balanced leisure lifestyle.

> Contemporary society often views leisure as a way of bringing balance into one's life. Leisure is sought not only for the opportunity for relaxation, self-improvement, cultural and family stability and interaction, but also for escape, novelty, complexity, excitement, and fantasy. In many societies, people use leisure as a way of counter-balancing stresses that result from living and working in a technologically oriented, competitive, rapidly changing society that requires attention to a high degree of stimulation in the form of information, media, communications, and human interaction (p. 33).

When the therapist is working on activity pattern development, it is important to make sure that the client has a sufficient leisure repertoire and that the patterns that are being developed allow for balanced leisure.

Interest Exploration

When the therapist is trying to develop appropriate activity patterns, it is important to look at what the client is interested in doing. Even the best program will fail if it doesn't match the client's preferences for leisure. An understanding of a person's leisure repertoire is required prior to exploring the development of a balanced leisure lifestyle to be put into an activity pattern.

There are many different assessment tools for exploring leisure interests that assist the therapist in identifying specific activities or characteristics of activities that appeal to the client. The *Leisure Interest Measure*, part of the *Idyll Arbor Leisure Battery* reviewed in the Assessments chapter is a good measure to consider. Other possibilities include the *Leisurescope Plus* or the *Leisure Assessment Inventory*. The therapist can also opt for a more informal exploration by looking at the client's past interests, future goals, and interests of those who are close to him/her (e.g., spouse, friend). It is also helpful if the therapist is aware of current activity trends, popular activities in the area, and popular activities by demographics. The more experience a clinician has, the more skilled s/he becomes at "reading" the characteristics of clients and finding attractive activities for the client (e.g., a retired executive with strong work ethic may tend to gravitate toward more intellectual activities). However, therapists should also be very careful not to stereotype clients and assume that because of their age or resources that certain activities would not be a consideration (e.g., 75-year-old frail woman who loves hiking). The therapist should also remember that recreation is subjective. What is recreation for one person may be work for another (e.g., mowing the grass, washing the car). Interest exploration will be a springboard for developing a treatment plan. A treatment plan and functional goals should directly relate to a person's interests.

If a formal assessment tool is used, the name of the tool should be included in your documentation along with the results. The therapist explains the purpose of the assessment and how the information will be used to develop a healthy activity pattern and treatment plan for the client (e.g., "Client seen for assessment of activities that client finds desirable for participation. Post brainstorming, client was able to identify a possible interest in aquatics at the local YMCA. Client/therapist decided that involvement in an aquatic exercise program post d/c would be a good health maintenance activity to help with managing rheumatoid arthritis, as well as help decrease CVA risk. RT and client to further explore issues related to this task"). This would be scored in the ICF under the appropriate categories. (For this example the categories might include parts of d4 Mobility, d570 Looking after One's Health, and d920 Recreation and Leisure.)

Developing Activity Patterns

Developing an activity pattern means creating a coherent, integrated habit of participating in a variety of leisure activities that, as a whole, allow the client to be healthier and happier. One of the therapist's jobs is to help the client develop an activity pattern that is realistic given the circumstances, balanced given the client's needs, and that is enjoyable to increase the likelihood that it will become habit.

Once a client determines how s/he currently spends his/her time using the Pie of Life activity (see "Pie of Life" in the Techniques section), s/he can begin to explore modifications to be able to achieve a realistic activity pattern. The client may be familiar with the activities in his/her leisure repertoire but may need help from the therapist to broaden his/her options with suggestions of other activities that s/he may find enjoyable, that s/he is likely capable of doing, and that help create a better balance between leisure and other activities.

Activity patterns are developed to encourage health and growth using activities. A realistic, healthy activity pattern can increase the positive outcomes of therapy. There are many ways to design an activity pattern. Most of them involve the therapist working with the client and writing down the plan, allowing the client to work on integrating the activities into his/her normal routine. It should be designed and written in a way that maximizes the client's ability to use it as a recovery and health promotion tool. Here is a general idea of how to put together an activity pattern.

The therapist and client begin by making a list of all of the activities that need to fit into the client's daily life. It is helpful to identify and write down broad categories to guide the client in identifying activities prior to making this list (e.g., chores, school, work, recreation, exercise, meals, and therapy). This is to include lifestyle changes (e.g., reflection of an altered routine to help the client quit smoking, exercise program, activity precautions, extra time for preparing healthier meals, individual quiet time for stress reduction). Next to each activity, the client is to write down all of the things that s/he is to remember related to each task (e.g., aquatics: 3x/week, fill out and send in scholarship application; gardening: purchase self-coiling hose, garden in 15

minute increments). This allows the client an opportunity to reflect on his/her lifestyle and the changes to be made. It also gives the therapist an opportunity to evaluate how much the client is able to remember from therapy sessions and how realistic the client is in planning.

If the client's cognitive limitations prevent the client from taking an active role in the development of this list, the therapist puts together this list without the client or develops it with caregivers. Either way, the therapist must discuss this with the caregivers to promote carryover and follow through.

The client and therapist work from this list with the goal of transferring all of the data into a daily, weekly, or monthly schedule (most typically a week). This resembles a doctor's office scheduling book. The days of the week are listed across the top of the page and underneath each day are half-hour increments (e.g., 8:00, 8:30, 9:00, etc.). The client fills in a time slot with the name of the activity and then draws a line down to the time increment that reflects the end of the activity (e.g., 9:00-9:30 stretching program, 9:30-10:00 shower, 10:00-11:00 dress and breakfast, 11:00-11:15 make brown bag lunch, 11:15 leave for work, and so on).

Some clients find this very frustrating because what they are writing down to happen on a Monday is not necessarily something that will happen every Monday. Clients are told that this is a mock schedule. It is an opportunity to put together a tentative lifestyle plan that allows the client to apply and integrate all of the activities and tasks that are to become part of his/her lifestyle. Clients can use highlighters or different color pens to note activities that will occur regularly on specific days and times. It gives the therapist a clear picture of the client's ability to fully appreciate the role of activity in recovery and health, recall specifics related to each activity (e.g., techniques, resources, transportation needs, equipment needs, references, contacts, follow-up responsibilities, techniques utilized, adaptations, any special concerns, precautions and parameters relevant to the activity, relation of activity to personal health needs), allow opportunities to problem solve (e.g., client's medication schedule falls during the YMCA aquatic class), and evaluate his/her ability to incorporate all of the functional skills training, education, counseling, and integration training provided into a comprehensive lifestyle pattern.

If the client is not able to follow through with an activity pattern independently, other people need to be involved. This may include the client's family or caregiver. If the client is going to be discharged to a skilled care facility that employs an activity director, a call should be placed by the therapist to the activity director to discuss activities available, how they relate to the client's interests and needs, and any special accommodations (e.g., activity adaptations needed, cueing). A copy of the activity pattern should be given to the client/family, as well as sent directly to the activity director for reference.

The term "activity pattern" encompasses many different types of activities and does not fall into just one general category. The ability to integrate many different tasks required as a result of the demands in one's life falls under the general category of carrying out daily routine (d230). The activities necessary to put together a daily routine come from many areas including self-care (d5), domestic life (d6), interpersonal interactions (d7), major life areas (d8), and community, social, and civic life (d9). Therapists help clients narrow down what activities to put into an activity pattern by choosing those that are most

necessary for health. Having an activity pattern that is realistic and geared toward promoting health and happiness can have a significant impact on preventing illness and secondary complications (health promotion focus). Clients who have difficulty being aware of and selecting healthy activities would be noted as having a difficulty with d5702 Maintaining One's Health.

References

Edginton, C., Jordan, D. DeGraff, D. & Edginton, S. (1995). *Leisure and life satisfaction: Foundational perspectives*. Dubuque, IA: Brown & Benchmark Publishers.

Mobily, K. E., Lemke, J. H., & Gisin, G. J. (1991). The idea of leisure repertoire. *Journal of Applied Gerontology, 10*:208-223.

Adjustment to Disability

Psychosocial adjustment to disability is an essential component of successful community integration and ongoing quality of life. It is an individually defined and subjective process influenced by many variables. Psychosocial adjustment is a process of emotional growth that requires the development of healthy coping mechanisms to forge a new lifestyle that optimizes assets and health. The recreational therapist helps guide a client's adjustment, which is an outcome that ultimately impacts the client's ability to enjoy life and improve health.

Mary is a 32-year-old female who was in a motor vehicle accident. Fortunately, the accident did not result in brain injury. However, she did sustain a complete T-12 spinal cord injury. As she sits in a wheelchair, waiting for her next therapy appointment, she is consumed with anxiety and fear. She worries about how she is going to be able to care for her three young children (3, 5, and 7), especially since she is a single mom with no other family in the area. She is also fearful of losing her independence, her career as a flight attendant, and her relationship with her boyfriend of three years.

Sally is a 34-year-old female who fell while rock climbing. She also sustained a T-12 complete spinal cord injury. Sally is a single woman with a high-power career. She is a take-control and fix-it type of individual who thrives on stress and deadlines. As she sits in a wheelchair, waiting for her next therapy appointment, she is thinking about all the things that need to be done so that she can get back on track. She needs to call a contractor to have modifications made to her home, she needs to contact her employer to talk about needed changes, and she needs to set up an appointment with adaptive driving. She is overwhelmed by the multitude of tasks that she now needs to accomplish, yet she appears to be in control and organized.

Although both Mary and Sally sustained the same disability, they exhibited different initial responses to their disability. Why? Is it because of their different lifestyles, because of their different personalities, or because of their level of family responsibilities and relationships? Can one make the assumption that one will adjust better in the community than the other? The answer is no. There is no way to know how a person will react to a situation, nor can a client's initial reactions to disability predict his/her level of successful community integration. There are too many internal and external variables (e.g., past experiences, mental health, resource availability, coping mechanisms, belief structure, support, flexibility, accommodation) and they all interact in unpredictable ways. Therapists need to realize that each response is unique to the individual. It is not appropriate to tell a client s/he should feel a certain way. The therapist guides the client through the emotional hurdles to reach optimal emotional health.

Optimal emotional health is a primary component of the recreational therapist's job because it affects so many areas of a client's life, including the rehabilitation process. The client may have difficulty engaging in life activities, seeking out resources, or overcoming barriers. Disability may also affect the client's self-identity, life routine, leisure, relationships, self-esteem, confidence, and independence. In the rehabilitation process, a client may fail to make the most of his/her assets if depression, regression, and passivity persist. Likewise, a client who is aggressive, angry, and rigid may not be open-minded to new ideas and techniques. In a nutshell, disability (whether temporary, permanent, chronic, or life-threatening) disrupts a client's lifestyle. The ability to accommodate to disability affects the ability to be healthy.

Measuring adjustment can be a tricky process. A client can state that he is adjusting well, but his actions may not be consistent with his statement (e.g., social isolation, poor hygiene) or vice versa, a client may appear to be adjusting well to her disability (back to work, social outings with friends), yet verbally she expresses lack of identity and feelings of inadequacy. So, have these clients achieved psychosocial adjustment? The client, who is socially isolated and practices poor hygiene, may in fact be satisfied and content with his life. The client who verbalizes a lack of self-identity and adequacy may view these issues as a work-in-progress as they have been long-time issues unrelated to her current disability. Thus, psychosocial adjustment is subjective and complex. It requires attention to both actions and words, as well as how these relate to the client's belief system.

It [is] an evolutionary, changing, and highly individualized process rather than a stable state. The problems faced by the newly disabled person are those of coping with physical and psychological loss; changes in body image, social status, and earning capacity; the anxiety and grief which often accompany these changes; and the need to learn new behaviors and make concrete plans for an uncertain future. Each individual will seek personal solutions to these problems and thus define his own adjustment to disability (Stolov & Clowers, 1981, p. 14).

Therapists who understand the factors that influence psychosocial adjustment and how a client's actions can influence those factors will be equipped to help clients along their personal journeys.

Premorbid Factors that Influence Psychosocial Adjustment

There are many factors that help determine how and how well a client will adjust to a loss. One of the therapist's tasks is to assess factors impeding a client's adjustment to loss and to help develop a treatment program of emotional recovery. This section discusses some of the issues that may have already been part of the client's life before the loss.

Mental health: Depending upon the severity of the disability and how well it is being managed (e.g., medications, use of behavioral techniques) mental illness may affect a client's ability to adjust to disability. If a client has a history of mental illness, his/her emotional and behavioral health should be evaluated to determine a baseline. Psychotropic medications can affect a client's emotions and behavior. The team evaluates whether the client's current medications are adequate or need changing. New medications may also interact with prior medications resulting in emotional and behavioral changes leading to an impaired ability to develop functional coping skills.

Substance abuse: A client may have had a substance abuse problem prior to his/her current disability. This information is not always provided by the client or the client's family for a multitude of reasons (e.g., embarrassment, ignorance to the impact that substance abuse has on the client's current situation, fear of being arrested). Substance abuse does have a profound impact on a client's ability to cope and adjust to new situations. For many, substance abuse starts with soft drugs (e.g., marijuana, alcohol) and advances to more serious drugs (e.g., heroin, cocaine, ecstasy). The drugs are often used in the beginning for a variety of reasons (acceptance, relaxation, diminishing painful feelings, calming nerves, increasing social competence). However this initial "problem-solver" often leads to dependence or abuse and an inability to develop healthy coping styles. Obtaining an addictive drug may become the primary goal of each day, impacting every other area of the person's life. The client who is in a rehabilitation facility without access to his/her substance of choice experiences withdrawal symptoms. Some of the client's unproductive

behavior may be due to drugs or drug withdrawal and not the current disability. Clients with substance abuse as a secondary diagnosis should be encouraged to develop healthy coping strategies, become involved in a self-help group, or possibly receive further rehabilitation after physical rehabilitation to deal with the drug problem (e.g., inpatient drug rehab). Individuals who have a disability, whether or not they had a history of substance abuse, are at a higher risk for substance abuse. As Trombly (1989) says,

> Reasons predisposing disabled individuals to substance abuse problems can include a family and personal history, frustration and anxieties about being disabled; experiences with unproductive, unsatisfying, and dependent roles; functional inability to release tension; attendant motor and sensory deficits that accentuate the effects of alcohol; increased isolation; a lack of a sense of the ability to control events in their lives or to reach personal goals; and rejection experiences and other stressors related to loss and life-style changes. In addition, abuse of substances provides a way of avoiding the difficult and painful work of remediation" (p. 14).

Prior medical history: Prior medical history can also affect the client's ability to cope with the current disability. For example, an individual who has been living with a chronic disease (e.g., rheumatoid arthritis) might find it difficult to achieve a sense of control over the new disability (e.g., fractured hip). The client's experience with adjusting to prior disabilities may set a tone for adjusting to the current disability whether the prior adjustment strategies were healthy or not (e.g., "If I don't move around a whole lot my arthritis doesn't flare up, so I intend to do the same thing when I'm at home recovering from my hip replacement. I'm just going to stay in the house and wait until I feel better."). Education should be provided on the impact of different types of coping strategies. The therapist assists the individual in developing healthy lifestyle strategies to improve adjustment to disability.

Coping strategies: Everyone has different coping strategies (healthy and unhealthy) for dealing with problems. To cope some people exercise. Others talk with someone, withdraw, shop, yell, or bury themselves in work. Prior coping strategies are not always effective in dealing with new problems (e.g., used to go out for a run, but now having difficulty just walking; used to withdraw from the problems, but current problem can't be ignored). Coping strategies, even if they were effective before, may need to be changed. Learning and practicing healthy alternatives should be incorporated into the treatment plan.

Personality style: Many people have identified different types of personalities. Personality styles have been described as Type A and B, social/outgoing/extrovert, shy/quiet/introvert, just to name a few. Personality style will affect the client's ability to adjust to disability. A person who is outgoing and assertive prior to disability may find it much easier to access resources and meet needs compared to the individual who is quiet and reserved. Personality styles, although fairly consistent throughout one's life, can be modified. Individuals can learn assertiveness and social skills. Helping the client to understand why it is important to use a different coping strategy is an important step in the learning process. People cannot be changed, unless they want to change. Therapists are the catalysts for making change happen through education, modeling, shaping, and counseling.

Preferred patterns of life: People like to live certain ways. Some people can't envision their life outside of familiar patterns (e.g., going to work every day, going sailing, living in a cabin in the mountains). Unfortunately, there are many reasons why preferences can't be continued after a disability (finances, accessibility, functional abilities, support). Alternatives and adaptations (e.g., equipment, activity modification, resources) can be explored to continue with prior life patterns, and new alternatives can be suggested. A client's ability to accommodate to changes will affect his/her ability to adjust to the loss.

Developmental life stage: Each life stage has specific developmental tasks and roles that influence the client's ability to adjust to situations. Erikson (1968) outlines eight stages of development that are divided by chronological age, however he is careful to stipulate that the developmental process is affected by life experiences and events, hindering or enhancing the developmental process. Therefore, a client's chronological age does not necessarily reflect his/her psychological, social, emotional, behavioral, cognitive, or physical functional level. In addition, current situations can affect a client's developmental performance. Regression often occurs when the client does not have enough challenges or too many new challenges. The disability may move the client to a lower developmental stage due to physiological changes (e.g., traumatic brain injury) or the emotional demands of coping with the current situation (e.g., premorbid coping strategies are not effective for the current situation). In the assessment process the therapist compares the client's chronological age to the client's current functional age. Part of the assessment is to try to figure out how the client's premorbid health status, current disability, environment, and developmental stage,

impact his/her current development stage. A client's emotional and behavior level will provide a baseline to assist the therapist in developing a plan to enhance the client's psychosocial adjustment. For example, a teenager who is currently struggling with developing his own identity and autonomy may require a different approach than a 32-year-old client who is struggling with issues related to balancing her own needs with that of loved ones.

Culture: The client's culture affects his/her adjustment to disability, especially if there are strong gender roles (man provides for family and is now unable to do so) or religious beliefs related to disability (disability is the result of being possessed). Certain cultures also place high value on being reserved and not expressing emotions, which may also affect the adjustment process. Language is another cultural issue to consider. Does the client understand the spoken language of the hospital? Is an interpreter needed? Does the communication reflect the client's beliefs (e.g., never encourage women to make decisions)? If a client does not fully understand what the physician is saying, if beliefs reflect a negative connotation of the situation, or if the culture does not value the client's new role, the adjustment process will be difficult. The therapist should not jump to the conclusion that cultural beliefs cannot be changed, nor should the therapist ignore cultural values and beliefs. An awareness of culture and the impact it may have on adjustment will provide the therapist with a better frame of reference for addressing adjustment issues.

Educational level: The educational level of the client impacts psychosocial adjustment. If a client has less than a high-school education, s/he may not fully understand written material or medical discussions, resulting in an inadequate understanding of the situation. Material and discussions should be tailored to the individual's educational level, including those who have a higher level of education. In most cases the written material provided to the client and family members should be written at the eighth grade level. Microsoft Word comes with a tool that evaluates the reading level of the written material. This is usually located under "Tools: Spelling and Grammar." Clients should not feel as though they are being talked down to, nor should they feel talked-over. If a client feels disrespected or uninformed, adjustment to disability may be hampered.

Phases of Adjustment to Disability

Just as there are stages of grief, phases of adjustment to disability have also been proposed. Shontz (1965), as reviewed by Stolov & Clowers (1981), believes that there are five phases of adjustment to disability: 1. shock, 2. realization, 3. defensive retreat, 4. acknowledgement, and 5. adaptation. These stages are not sequential for everyone, nor do they occur only one time. For some, this process can take weeks; others may take months to years. The following is a discussion of the stages adapted from Stolov & Clowers (1981, pp 14-16):

- *Shock*: Shock occurs during the first few hours or days after the injury. The client is typically withdrawn and quiet and may not have a full understanding of the extent of the situation. During this phase the therapist begins to establish a relationship with the client. The client will be much easier to approach now rather than later at the next stage when anger, depression, and fear typically develop. Developing a relationship will lay the foundation for effective therapy later.

- *Realization*: The client's awareness of the situation and the extent of his/her disability as it applies to participation in life tasks are realized. The client may become anxious, angry, and fearful. Thoughts about death, losses, level of independence, and unpredictable change often precipitate these feelings. The therapist shows empathy to the client by acknowledging the client's fears. Empathy expressed through sincere reassurance is the best way to support a client at this stage. If the therapist was able to develop a relationship with the client in the "shock" stage, this type of support is usually well received.

- *Defensive retreat*: A primary defensive mechanism for coping is denial (denying the existence or seriousness of the disability). Denial may persist or disappear and then reappear long after the onset of the disability. Denial can be manifested in the client's verbalizations (e.g., "I am going to walk again.") or behavior (e.g., not participating in therapy, not making reasonable or realistic accommodations for the disability, refusing to adhere to specific recommendations of the therapist). The therapist realizes that the client's expression of denial is a way for the client to control the situation or avoid feelings of anxiety. Therefore, the therapist does not challenge the client (e.g., "The neurosurgeon's report says that you have a complete spinal cord injury, so you are not going to walk again.") because it will hurt the therapeutic relationship at a time when the client really needs the support. The therapist does not agree with the client either, because this would only reinforce the denial. Although the denial is a common coping strategy for loss, it is not a healthy long-term coping mechanism. The therapist encourages the client to take one day at a time and focus on the

here and now. For example, if a client with a complete spinal cord injury says, "I am going to walk again so I don't have to learn how to push this wheelchair outside." The therapist replies, "Well, let's focus on where we are today. Today you are not walking, so it is my job to teach you a new way to get around. And, if function does begin to come back in your legs, you will start out using a walker that will require a lot of upper arm strength and cardiovascular endurance…both of which we will be addressing when we work on pushing the wheelchair outside." The therapist is not to lie to the client, but to convey understanding of the client's hope. Hope is an appropriate and healthy emotion. All people hope for better things and therapists are not to extinguish a client's hope. Instead, help the client to develop a healthy balance between hope and reality.

- *Acknowledgement*: The client has a full understanding of his/her disability and the impact that it has, or will have, on life tasks. A natural reaction to acknowledgement is depression. Depression may be brought on by feelings of resignation, lack of knowledge on how to make adaptation for the disability, or poor initiation skills (e.g., "Well, here I am. What can I do about it?"). The therapist focuses on developing the client's internal locus of control by teaching the client disability adaptations (e.g., adaptive equipment, resources, solutions to common problems) and teaching healthy coping mechanisms for feelings of depression. The therapist does not pay special attention to the depression (e.g., sympathizing with the client) because s/he may inadvertently strengthen poor coping strategies that will not serve the client well in the long run.

- *Adaptation*: The client adopts healthy coping strategies, is realistic about his/her abilities and limitations, and exhibits motivation and confidence to participate in life tasks. This does not imply that the client happily accepts his/her disability and its resultant limitations, but rather accepts the limitations with the goal of maximizing assets.

Approaches to Encourage Adjustment

This section looks at how a therapist can assist a client's psychosocial adjustment. A therapist must first remember that each client is an individual and that a "cookie-cutter" approach does not work. Clients come from a variety of backgrounds; they experience different needs and respond differently to interventions. The information on different types of interventions for psychosocial adjustment listed below may be used as ideas to adapt and modify to meet the needs of the client.

Working on integration: Integrating clients back into the community is a vital step in their adjustment to a disability. A client's readiness level will determine the environment and level of challenge of the outing. For example, a client may not find a trip to his home very threatening, yet he may consider a trip to the mall or to his place of work much harder. Do not force a client to go on an outing that s/he is not ready for, otherwise it may increase the client's anxiety and fear of the community environment. Some clients are receptive to sequential outings consisting of small steps (travel training using a van, then bus, then train), while other clients want to jump right in and learn how to function in a challenging environment (travel training using a train). The therapist can also consider the use of groups for outings to provide added support for the client. Occasionally it may be appropriate for the therapist to use the same equipment as the client during the outing (e.g., use a wheelchair alongside the client). Family and friends should also be included on integration outings for family training, as well as to provide support for the client. They should be instructed on how to assist the client to integrate back into the community after s/he is discharged from the facility, as the full integration process can take weeks to months to years. For the client in denial who refuses to acknowledge deficits and limitations to the point where safety is a concern, the team may consider setting up a structured failure. In this situation the client will be faced with the direct results of his/her actions (e.g., client refuses to make phone calls to find out level of accessibility and the therapist purposely allows the client to plan an outing to a non-accessible facility). Integration can also be enhanced by allowing day or weekend passes with family and friends that have been adequately trained to assist the client (as long as these are approved by the physician and relevant insuring agency). Be aware that some health insurance policies will no longer pay for inpatient care if a client leaves the facility for more than a set number of hours.

Teaching relaxation techniques: Learning different techniques to relax assists with identification and awareness of stressors. Learning how to incorporate relaxation-training techniques as a problem solving technique is an important skill that helps decrease anxiety and panic. For more on this topic see "Relaxation and Stress Reduction" in the Techniques section.

Clarifying and expressing emotions or feelings in healthy ways: Allow opportunities for expression of excessive emotion. Clients may project anger, hostility, and frustration in negative ways (outbursts, stares, and attitude). Reflect the client's behavior (e.g., "Your stare makes me feel like you're angry. Is something upsetting you?"). Open the door to communication rather that allowing negative behavior to continue. Assist the client in understanding feelings (e.g., "It must be really hard to deal with people like me asking you to do things when you're used to doing things on your own schedule."). Model good communication of feelings. Negative behavior will distance relationships resulting in alienation rather than meeting the client's need of support. Allow opportunities for alternative modes of expression (e.g., writing, propelling wheelchair around outdoor track, weight training).

Fostering internal locus of control: Individuals who experience a disability are faced with the reality that there are things in their life that they are unable to control. Many of life's activities are controlled by others when a client is hospitalized (e.g., mealtime, appointments, assistance to use the bathroom, making decisions, privacy). Motivation and initiative are enhanced when internal locus of control is maximized. Allow as many opportunities for control as possible (e.g., therapy at 10 A.M. or 1 P.M., this activity or that activity, therapy inside or outside). Also allow opportunities for control that are outside of typical client parameters as appropriate to diminish "patient" role (e.g., eat in staff cafeteria, open time in gym to work on weight training, research on the internet in the evening).

Encouraging independence: As with the problems in locus of control, hospital settings, where staff can have a multitude of time sensitive responsibilities, often tend to provide the client with assistance to accomplish tasks rather than waiting a longer time for the client to complete the task alone or with assistance (e.g., it's quicker to put on the client's shoes rather than to wait for the client to put on his shoes, quicker to push the client to the next therapy than to walk alongside the client while s/he pushes himself/herself to the next therapy appointment). Hospital situations often foster dependence. The client's treatment plan should include the goal of independence as appropriate throughout his/her whole day, not just in therapy (e.g., responsible to get to own therapies, set alarm clock in the morning so has enough time to dress independently).

Providing active listening: Allow the client to express fears, concerns, anxieties, wishes, needs, and ideas with your full attention. Reflect back to the client what you are hearing and convey understanding. Understanding means that you understand what the client is saying; it does not mean that you agree with it. Gently offer guidance as appropriate. Listening, however, is therapy in and of itself. This does not mean that the therapist must abandon the treatment plan for the session and actively listen to the client. The therapist can sensitively redirect the client to the task at hand and encourage continuation of the discussion while completing the task. If the task is inappropriate given the situation, care should be given to change the focus of the treatment session (e.g., making phone calls for outing next week changed to outdoor wheelchair propulsion since it lends itself better to conversation with the therapist).

Accenting abilities and accomplishments: The rehabilitation process is fraught with attention to dysfunction. Although therapists highlight achievement over dysfunction, clients benefit from a focus on assets outside of dysfunction (e.g., intelligence, creativity, stamina). Individuals who are praised, acknowledged, cared for, and respected will develop a good sense of self (image, confidence, esteem). One of the ways this is achieved is by accenting the client's strengths, abilities, and accomplishments; not only in the physical realm, but the emotional, cognitive, and social realms as well (coping skills, providing support to another, problem solving abilities).

Clarifying values and attitudes: Helping a client to explore values and attitudes will focus on his/her belief structure. A belief structure forms the foundation of actions. What does the client value in life: family, work, leisure, sitting in the yard? What attitudes does the client have about life tasks (e.g., strong work ethic, strong gender role identity, negative leisure attitudes)? Understanding what the client values and the attitudes behind each value will assist the therapist in identifying a healthy activity pattern for the client. For example, if the client has a strong work ethic, then alternatives to work could be explored (e.g., enrolling for vocational rehab, finding volunteer work, exploring career alternatives). Clients who are able to return to prior life roles and activities are more likely to successfully adjust to a disability. Clarifying values and attitudes will also open the door to changing past values and attitudes and possibly open the door to new ideas and thoughts that will positively influence the client's adjustment. For example, a middle-aged adult who has been focused on obtaining external rewards from work and career may be in the process of reviewing past choices. Clarifying values and attitudes may assist the client in re-evaluating paths and highlight new paths that will meet needs, thus assisting the client to move on to meet goals.

Enhancing a positive self-image: Disability often has a negative connotation, including unproductiveness, helplessness, and poor appearance. Although health care professionals know differently, individuals who are disabled may fall into the trap of

viewing themselves negatively due to the disability and not evaluating themselves on who they really are. A positive self-image needs to be strengthened and stereotypes and myths need to be broken. Opportunities for attention to physical appearance (e.g., hairstyle/color, makeup, toenail polish, new outfit, teeth whitening) need to be provided, as well as opportunities to be independent and productive (e.g., help in designing accessible changes to home, organizing home care schedule).

Developing communication and interaction skills: Clients who are having difficulty expressing themselves in a healthy and appropriate manner benefit from learning how to communicate and interact with others effectively. In addition, clients who are newly disabled will need to assert and interact with people in new situations (e.g., inquiring about accessibility, requesting assistance with retrieving items, asking a store employee to alert others that there is someone of the opposite sex in the bathroom helping the client). Clients need to be instructed on the various styles of conflict resolution (passive, aggressive, assertive) and understand the outcomes of each style, as well as how to use new interaction and communication styles. Those that adopt assertion will be able to obtain resources and meet needs, thus impacting adjustment issues.

Engaging in problem solving: Initially the client's family and loved ones make the majority of the decisions for the client (e.g., choose the rehab, choose which clothes to pack), thus also impacting the client's involvement in problem solving. The therapist will also make decisions and problem solve for many situations without the assistance of the client (e.g., client is having an emotionally challenging day, so therapist changes treatment session focus). This type of behavior contributes to the client's lack of control and learned helplessness. Allowing the client to make decisions and solve problems contributes to internal locus of control, which directly contributes to psychosocial adjustment. The therapist should challenge clients to solve simple to complex issues (e.g., let me know on Tuesday where you want to go for our outing on Friday, draw a picture of the layout of your woodshop and come up with some adaptations that you think would work well for you). These skills must be enhanced as soon as possible, otherwise the client may fall into the trap of learned helplessness (I can't do it anymore, someone else needs to do it for me.).

Exploring new lifestyle options: "The patient's ability to adapt to disability is more certain when valued work, family and community roles, favorite activities, and membership in prized groups can be continued. Too great a variance between the premorbid and present life-styles may not be acceptable to the patient and will thus reduce intrinsic motivation to identify acceptable alternative roles and to retain belief in personal competence. These are generalizations, and much depends on the patient's range of interests, skills, past experiences, intelligence, and adaptability" (Trombly, 1989, p. 14). It can be difficult to accept that lifestyle changes are needed (e.g., housing, work, life pace). Every effort should be made to integrate the client back into his/her premorbid lifestyle as long as it is healthy. Sometimes changes are necessary. For example, the client's wife files for divorce when the client is in rehab and now the client must find an accessible place to live prior to discharge: a place in which the client can function independently. Accepting this is not always an easy task for the client. It can be equally difficult for the client to view his/her lifestyle any differently from what s/he already knows. Options should be discussed and available for the client to explore (e.g., integration outing to accessible apartment complex, research new career options). If a new lifestyle is needed and realistic options are identified with resourceful professionals, the client will be better prepared for the transition.

Opportunities for emotional support: Therapists and family provide the client with emotional support. However, support from someone who can personally relate to the client's situation can often be more helpful. Therapists and family can try to understand what the client is going through (empathy) but they may have never experienced what the client is going through. A client may express this by saying, "You don't know what it's like," or "You say you understand, but you really don't." People who mean well when they offer encouragement and a positive outlook can be met with sarcasm and anger. Sometimes clients just needs someone to sit in the mess with them, someone who can wallow in the mud hole, but also knows how to pull himself out. Clients, however, are not always receptive to meeting with someone who has a disability, especially if they are trying to "run away" from the disability or they have a negative view of the disabled and think, "I am not like them." Do not push the client into a support group or force a meeting with a past client. Gently suggest that you know someone (preferably someone who is the same age as the client, who has been recovering for more than two years, who can relate to what the client is going through, and who can offer some ideas about how s/he handles certain problems). An informal approach can also be taken, where a "mentor" just stops by or happens to be visiting with the therapist at the time of the client's appointment or shows up on an outing. Explain to the client that it is good to know someone who is in the same boat. One

way to explain this is to say something like, "It's good to have a guy friend to talk with about guy stuff, right? Well, it can also be good to have a guy friend who has a spinal cord injury, so you can talk about guy spinal cord stuff."

Setting appropriately sized goals: Long-term goals can seem like they take forever to accomplish. Identification of short, concrete, realistic goals provides more immediate feedback of progress, enhancing a client's self-esteem and confidence in task accomplishment and ultimately impacting adjustment.

Providing different approaches to treatment: Each therapist has his/her own personality, some more serious, others more flexible. Therapists should be open to changing their approach (despite how comfortable the approach is for the therapist) to meet the needs of the client. Some clients will respond better to a sensitive and quiet therapist while others may respond to a straightforward and confident therapist. Some clients relate better to therapists that they can identify with on some level. Some clients prefer an easy-going therapist while others like a stick-to-the-textbook approach. Although clients will be thrust out into a world of many different personalities, in the rehabilitation process the therapist should make every attempt to adapt his/her approach to meet the needs of the client so as to bring out the best in the client. Therapists should be careful, however, not to accommodate the client so much that treatment goals are not reached (e.g., therapist's flexibility allows client to ignore certain tasks such as cathing in public restrooms).

Encouraging healthy responses by family and friends: Family and friends are also in a period of adjustment. It can be difficult to know what to say to loved ones, as well as how to say it. Sometimes, people want to help so much that they help too much, thus perpetuating learned helplessness. Sometimes family and friends become angry with the client due to the client's denial or lack of motivation or initiation, thus distancing their relationship at a time when the client needs them most. Family (and friends as appropriate) should be made aware of the adjustment process and ways to respond to the client to enhance adjustment. Counseling services should also be made available to the family and friends.

The primary category for documenting a client's psychosocial adjustment to disability is d2401 Handling Stress with a descriptor to the right of the scoring area (e.g., "Impacted by psychosocial adjustment").

References

Erikson, E. H. (1968). *Identity: youth and crisis*. New York: Norton.

Stolov, W., & Clowers, M. (1981). *Handbook of severe disability*. Washington, DC: US Department of Education.

Trombly, C. (1989). *Occupational therapy for physical dysfunction, 3rd edition*. Baltimore, MD: Williams & Wilkins.

Americans with Disabilities Act Education

The Americans with Disabilities Act (ADA) is a civil rights law that was enacted in 1990. The ADA made it illegal to discriminate on the basis of disability in the areas of employment, public services, public accommodations, transportation, and telecommunications. The ADA applies to people who have a physical or mental impairment that substantially limits one or more major life activities (e.g., dressing, bathing, working, shopping). People who are currently using illegal drugs are not covered under the ADA. People who have HIV or AIDS are covered.

Therapists need to be very familiar with the ADA to facilitate successful community integration and empower and educate clients about their civil rights. Clients are usually very interested in the ADA because it addresses their ability to participate in life tasks such as work and recreation (e.g., Is my employer supposed to let me work a flexible workweek? Is the YMCA supposed to have a ramp out front? Is it reasonable for the grocery market to provide me with assistance in getting my groceries into the car? Is the city bus supposed to have a wheelchair lift?). Therapists should know the answers to these questions or know how to find out the answers to help facilitate positive changes and compliance with the ADA (e.g., calling the grocery store about available assistance, calling the YMCA to inquire about putting a ramp out front).

Therapists should have copies of the ADA technical manuals (I, II, III) and information on specific modes of transportation and telecommunications related to ADA compliance. Therapists must have a copy of the "Americans with Disabilities Act Accessibility Guidelines" and the "Uniform Federal Accessibility Standards." Both of these come in a checklist format and make assessment of facilities quite easy. Additionally, therapists should have copies of "A Guide to ADA Accessibility for Play Areas" and "Recommendations for Accessibility Guidelines for Recreational Facilities and Outdoor Developed Areas." Both are very helpful in clinical practice. All of these resources are discussed and contact information is provided later in the "ADA Resources" section.

Educating clients and/or caregivers about the ADA increases their insight into changes that have been made in our society. People who have a new disability are often not aware of this federal law that protects their civil rights and prohibits discrimination against them in regards to employment, transportation, telecommunication, and accessibility to buildings and programs. Knowledge of the ADA is a tool that can leverage change. It can expand a client's perception about what s/he can do in the community (work, recreation, travel), dispel disability myths (there are more opportunities and access than people usually expect), and empower the client to seek needed changes in his/her own life tasks (e.g., contact employer to discuss accommodations). This knowledge may also aid in decreasing anxiety (e.g., knowing that an employer needs to make reasonable accommodations lessens anxiety over what the client is going to do about a job), lifting feelings of depression (e.g., knowing that many places in the community are now wheelchair accessible and provide services to help someone who has a disability), and fostering an internal locus of control (e.g., knowing what s/he is entitled to under the ADA gives the client a knowledge base to assert change in his/her community). ADA education is one of many interventions that can increase the activity level of the client. Maintaining a healthy activity level decreases the client's risk for developing secondary complications from inactivity.

Indications: Any client who has a new disability needs to be educated about the ADA.

Contraindications: A client who has significant cognitive impairments that impact his/her ability to recall, retain, or apply verbal education. If significant cognitive impairments are evident, the therapist will need to educate the client's caregivers since they will be the ones to facilitate community activities.

Education

The length and frequency of ADA training sessions will vary depending on the identified needs and abilities of the client. On average, ADA training takes about one hour (one half hour to review the titles of the ADA and another half hour to practice applying the information through role-playing and phone calls). This is not to say that a client will be fully proficient in knowledge and application of the ADA in one hour, but the client who does not have cognitive impairments should be able to obtain a basic understanding of the law and its application.

Education should take place in a quiet/non-distracting environment to promote concentration, consideration of the implications of the act, and retention of information.

The therapist should have relevant materials (e.g., ADA booklet from the Paralyzed Veterans Association, paper/pen to write down barriers and identified solutions).

Additional sessions should be scheduled to allow for evaluation of activity performance (ability to apply learned information in a real-life environment). This is typically done in the form of community integration training on scheduled outings into the community.

The general process of ADA education is reflected in the outline below. Therapists should alter this process as needed to best meet the needs of the client.

1. *What is it?* Tell the client that there is a law called the Americans with Disabilities Act that protects their civil rights and prohibits discrimination on the basis of disability.

2. *How does it affect the client?* Tell the client, the ADA prohibits employers from discriminating against you because you have a disability and it requires them to make reasonable accommodations so that you can work. It also requires public facilities to be accessible so that you can get into libraries, police stations, banks, recreation facilities, and so on. The ADA also covers transportation. So if you need to use a taxi, train, plane, bus, or subway, you know what accommodations you can expect. If you find it hard to use the telephone due to hearing or speech problems, you also have access to a device that will allow you to type your message into the phone and an operator will tell the person on the other line what you are saying. Being aware of what is supposed to be available is very important so that you can make plans to do things without running into problems. Unfortunately, despite the many changes that have already been made, barriers still exist and you will undoubtedly encounter them. When these occur you will need to problem solve and talk with people to come up with a solution. The more you know, the better you will be able to problem solve for these situations.

3. *Review the ADA*: Educate the client about his/her rights under the ADA. Use the descriptions in this section as a guide. Following this outline is a description of each of the four titles under the ADA, which can also be used as a guide for educating clients.

4. *Problems*: Ask the client what problems s/he foresees and help the client problem solve (e.g., worksite is not accessible, can't get into the bathroom at the gym, no accessible parking spots at the local store).

5. *Questions and manuals*: If the therapist does not know the answer to a particular problem or question, call the EEOC if it is an employment issue or call the Office of the ADA if it has to do with any other ADA issue. The person at the office will be able to answer your questions or guide you to the appropriate resource. Clients

should also call these offices and ask for a copy of the technical assistance manuals. The EEOC can give you a copy of the ADA Title I (employment) and the ADA office can give you a copy of the technical assistance manuals, ADA Title II and III that cover public services and accommodations. The US Architectural and Transportation Barriers Compliance Board is responsible for the transportation component of the ADA (found under Title II and III) and can provide you with the specific ADA guidelines regarding all forms of transportation. They also publish a number of other helpful ADA manuals including "A Guide to ADA Accessibility for Play Areas" (information on designing accessible playgrounds) and "Recommendations for Accessibility Guidelines for Recreational Facilities and Outdoor Developed Areas" (sports facilities, places of amusement, play settings, golf, boating and fishing facilities, developed outdoor recreation facilities). Both of these publications are free. Finally, the Federal Communications Commission is responsible for Title IV of the ADA that covers Telecommunications and can provide you with information on the ADA guidelines regarding telecommunications and provide any needed assistance in this area. Once the information is received it can be put into a binder for later reference.

6. *Application*: Therapists help clients apply the information that they have learned about the ADA. This is usually done through phone calls and outings. The therapist may ask the client to identify a place in the community where s/he wishes to go and needs to know its level of accessibility and the services it offers to someone who has a disability. Draw up a list of questions to ask before the phone call is placed. The amount of assistance a client needs with this task will vary. Set a realistic goal for applying the ADA and re-explain the purpose of setting this goal, if needed. A possible goal might be. "Client to require minimal verbal cues to apply ADA information through telephone inquiries." Next, plan an outing to that site (or another site as appropriate) with the plan of working on the application of the ADA in a community environment (e.g., find out where the accessible bathroom is located, evaluate the bathroom to determine if it truly meets accessibility guidelines, identify the bathroom challenges for the client and then problem solve for a solution). Clients should be encouraged to identify problem areas, seek out assistance to overcome a specific barrier (client to ask store employee for assistance), and identify architectural or service

changes that could increase his/her function. Challenge the client further with "what if" questions (e.g., What would you do if you were told there was an accessible bathroom and when you got here you found out that it was a low toilet instead of a high toilet and now you require assistance? What would you do if the elevator was broken and you were on the second floor?). Challenging practical problem solving skills is important for successful community transitioning. See "Community Accessibility Training" and "Community Problem Solving" in the Techniques section.

The therapist documents the specific education provided and the client's ability to recall the information, verbally apply information to proposed situations, and demonstrate application of learned material in a real-life environment (activity performance).

Example: Client educated on the ADA. Client able to recall 75% of ADA material at modified independence (increased time and use of written reference — PVA booklet). Client able to contact a community facility via telephone and explore their level of accessibility and disability services offered with minimal assistance. During community integration session to Home Depot, client independently requested assistance from an employee to retrieve and carry large items.

The therapist can score d940 Human Rights when classifying the client's level of difficulty with enjoying human rights and/or the therapist may opt to score the specific problems that make it difficult for the client to enjoy human rights (e.g., b1266 Confidence, d166 Reading).

ADA Titles

You can use this material to help you explain the ADA to clients. This is a very brief description of the law. It is not a full account of all compliance requirements. Therapists and clients should consult the ADA technical assistance manuals and contact the appropriate organizations when more information is needed. How to obtain these manuals and the organizations that can assist you in understanding the ADA are provided below. A booklet that we have found to be particularly helpful is "The Americans with Disabilities Act: Your Personal Guide to the Law." It is a free booklet put out by the Paralyzed Veterans of America. Sometimes, the amount that they can send to an individual or organization is limited. Therapists can require the client to call and request their own free copy or the therapist (in anticipation of reviewing this information with the

client) can call on behalf of the client and have it mailed to the facility in time to review it with the client. See the references below for contact information.

Title I: Employment

If a person with a disability is qualified for the position and can perform the job requirements with or without reasonable accommodations, the employer cannot deny the person employment solely based on the fact that s/he has a disability. Employers who have 15 or more employees must abide by this law and make reasonable accommodations unless it is a proven hardship for the company. An undue hardship means that the accommodations would be unduly costly, disruptive, or extensive or would fundamentally alter the nature or operation of the business. In this situation, the person with the disability should be allowed to provide the accommodation (e.g., will supply the desk) and/or pay for the portion of the accommodation that is above the employer's ability. Tax incentives are available for employers who make accommodations for a person with a disability (tax credits and deductions). Reasonable accommodations could include job restructuring, modified work schedules, acquisition or modification of equipment, the provision of readers or interpreters, and any other accommodation that is deemed as being reasonable. Employees with disabilities are held to employment standards and termination could occur if they are not met (e.g., use of illegal drugs, inability to perform job even with accommodations). Employers who have less than 15 employees are not required to comply with this law (exception: state and local government employers with less than 15 employees must comply with the ADA). They are not required to comply because they will often lack the resources to make reasonable accommodations (e.g., lack of funds to build a ramp or purchase adaptive equipment).

Title II: Public Services

Any state or local government service, program, activity, or building must comply with the ADA. This includes the courts, town meeting halls, police and fire departments, voting locations and machines, emergency assistance (e.g., 911) and motor vehicle licensing. The person who has a disability cannot be denied access to a service, program, or activity because of disability. Integrated services must be implemented unless separate services are needed to ensure equal opportunity. Programs must be held in accessible locations in the building (e.g., held on the first floor rather than the second floor when there is no elevator). Public entities may choose between two technical standards for accessible design: the Uniform Federal Accessibility Standards (UFAS) or the Americans with Disabilities Act Accessibility Guidelines (ADAAG). Free copies of both of these guides can be obtained from the US Architectural and Transportation Barriers Compliance Board. Public entities are required to provide alternative forms of communication (e.g., interpreter, large print materials) when needed.

Title III: Public Accommodations

A public accommodation is defined as a facility operated by a private entity that affects interstate commerce and falls within at least one of these categories:

- Places of lodging, such as inns, hotels, and motels, except establishments in which the proprietor resides and rents out no more than five rooms.
- Establishments serving food or drink, such as restaurants and bars.
- Places of exhibition or entertainment, such as theaters, auditoriums, and stadiums.
- Places of public gatherings, such as auditoriums, convention centers, and lecture halls.
- Sales or rental establishments, such as grocery stores, bakeries, clothing stores, and shopping centers.
- Service establishments, such as dry cleaners, banks, beauty shops, hospitals, and offices of health-care professionals, lawyers, and accountants.
- Stations used for specified public transportation, such as terminals and depots.
- Places of public display, such as museums, libraries, and galleries.
- Places of recreation, such as parks, zoos, and amusement parks.
- Places of education, such as nursery, elementary, secondary, undergraduate, and postgraduate private schools.
- Social service centers, such as day-care or senior citizen centers, adoption programs, food banks, and homeless shelters.
- Places of exercise or recreation, such as gymnasiums, health spas, bowling alleys, and golf courses.

Private clubs and religious organizations are exempt from public accommodation requirements.

Such accommodations include making any new construction accessible (e.g., when remodeling the bathroom), providing accessible parking spaces, a ramp at the entrance, accessible seating, access to elevators, Braille markings, note takers, and interpreters.

Transportation Regulations

Transportation regulations fall under both Title II and Title III of the ADA, although the technical manual for transportation is kept separate. The ADA provides specific requirements for city buses, taxis, paratransit services, trains, airplanes, over-the-road buses (e.g., Greyhound bus service), university bus systems, vanpools, and subways. There are different regulations for each mode of travel depending on whether or not they are private or public, the number of people who are able to be seated in the mode of transportation, and the type of system it is (e.g., fixed route, demand responsive). Therapists consult the various technical assistance manuals from the US Architectural and Transportation Barriers Compliance Board. There is a manual for each mode of transportation.

Title IV: Telecommunications

Telecommunication relay services: A nationwide telephone relay service has been established through the use of Telecommunications Devices for the Deaf (TDDs). This allows people who have hearing or speech impairments to carry on a conversation with another person who is not using a TDD. An intermediate person or relay operator conveys the messages from the person using the TDD to the receiver and conveys messages from the receiver back to the person using the TDD. A TDD is a device with a keyboard and a message display that connects to a specially equipped telephone. Some TDDs have printers that print out the message as it is received rather than a screen. Sometimes they are referred to a Text Typewriters (TTs) or Teletypewriters (TTYs).

Before the ADA, a person with a hearing or speech impairment typed a message into the TDD and the message appeared on the TDD screen of the person s/he was calling. This meant that the other person also had to have a TDD. Now (because of the ADA) there is a nationwide telephone relay service so the other person does not have to have a TDD. The person who has a hearing or speech impairment types a message into the TDD and it is sent to a relay operator. The relay operator reads the message to the other party. The person responds to the message verbally (speaks to the relay operator). The relay operator sends the response to the person with the hearing or speech impairment through the TDD. This exchange continues for as long as the two parties wish to communicate and there are no restrictions on the content of the messages. Relay operators are not allowed to intentionally alter any part of the communication and they are prohibited from disclosing the content or nature of the calls. TDD calls cannot be limited or refused by the phone carrier. Service is available 24 hours a day. Therapists who are interested in acquiring a TDD for a client should contact their local phone company for further information.

Closed-captioning: All public service announcements that are federally funded or produced must have closed-captioning on the television screen. Closed-captioning is text on the bottom of the television screen similar to movie subtitles that allows a person to read what is being said on the television. All television sets that have screens larger than 13" have a built-in decoder chip to enable the set to display the captioning. Televisions that have this chip can be programmed to show closed-captioning on the screen when it is provided. Most programs now provide closed captioning.

ADA Complaints and Enforcement

If an accommodation is not provided and the client wishes to file a complaint, s/he is to contact the organization that is affiliated with the problem (e.g., if it is a problem with transportation contact the US Architectural and Transportation Barriers Compliance Board). They will assist you with solving the problem and/or filing a complaint.

ADA References

Equal Employment Opportunity Commission (EEOC)
1801 L Street NW
Washington, DC 20507
1-800-669-EEOC (Voice/TDD)
www.eeoc.gov

Provides free copies of the technical manual for Title I of the ADA (employment), provides assistance understanding and interpreting this title.

US Department of Justice
Civil Rights Division
Office on the Americans with Disabilities Act
PO Box 66738
Washington, DC 20035-6738
1-800-514-0301 (Voice)
1-800-514-0383 (TDD)
www.usdoj.gov

Provides free copies of the technical manuals for Title II (public services) and Title III (public accommodations) of the ADA, provides assistance with understanding and interpreting these titles.

US Architectural and Transportation Barriers Compliance Board
1331 F Street NW, Suite 1000
Washington, DC 20004-1111
1-800-872-2253 (Voice)
1-800-993-2822 (TDD)
www.access-board.gov

Provides free copies of the "Americans with Disabilities Act Accessibility Guidelines," the "Uniform Federal Accessibility Standards," technical assistance manuals for each mode of transportation, "A Guide to ADA Accessibility for Play Areas" (information on designing accessible playgrounds), and "Recommendations for Accessibility Guidelines for Recreational Facilities and Outdoor Developed Areas" (sports facilities, places of amusement, play settings, golf, boating and fishing facilities, developed outdoor recreation facilities).

Federal Communications Commission
Common Carrier Bureau
TRS Complaints
1919 M Street, NW
Washington, DC 20554
202-418-0500 (Voice)
202-632-6999 (TDD)

Provides information on telecommunication regulations and is responsible for the enforcement of Title IV of the ADA (Telecommunications).

Paralyzed Veterans of America
801 18th St., NW
Washington, DC 20006
1-800-424-8200 (Voice)
1-800-795-4327 (TDD)

Provides "The Americans with Disabilities Act: Your Personal Guide to the Law."

Anger Management

Anger is an emotion. Emotions are usually considered to be products of thoughts (the way things are interpreted and perceived). However, emotions are also controlled biologically through the release of hormones and chemicals within the body. Sometimes this biological process occurs without a precipitating external stressor. For example a client with a frontal lobe tumor may complain of feeling easily irritated and angered although the associated events were not perceived as stressors in the past. ("It never used to bother me when the dog barked, but now it infuriates me.") In this example, the frontal lobe tumor is affecting the client's brain centers for personality and emotion, heightening the client's sensitivity to sensations.

The emotion of anger is healthy and normal. When handled in a positive manner (e.g., talking out the problem, going for a walk to calm down), it can move people toward a positive result (e.g., solve a problem, learn something new). Anger is unhealthy when it becomes destructive to the person (e.g., anger is turned inward and induces feelings of depression, self-mutilation) or causes harm to other people (e.g., physical violence, rage attacks, verbal assaults, hostility, belligerence). It is important to note that aggression is different from anger. Anger is a strong feeling of displeasure or hostility, whereas aggression is the act of initiating hostility. When aggression is extreme, it is often referred to as rage (or a rage attack). Rage is best defined as a violent explosive anger with furious intensity.

Causes of Anger

Prior to addressing feelings of anger or acts of aggression or rage the therapist and the treatment team identify the root cause of the behavior so that it can be addressed appropriately. Some of the most important causes of anger are listed below. For many causes of anger there are appropriate treatments besides basic anger management. These are listed with each cause. Many are discussed in other parts of the Techniques section. In addition to the treatments listed in each cause, consider using the techniques specifically designed for anger management described later in this section.

Medical Illness

Any medical condition that affects the brain may cause anger. Illnesses that are known to affect emotions include brain tumors, other cancers (including reactions to chemotherapy), traumatic brain injury, stroke, influenza, syphilis, encephalitis, multiple sclerosis, hyperthyroidism, Cushing's disease, bipolar disorder, substance-induced mood disorder, and intermittent explosive disorder. The approach to dealing with anger will depend on the specific problem. Management of medical conditions should help to diminish or extinguish expressions of anger. Working with patients who have had trauma to the brain (TBI, stroke) includes stress reduction and lifestyle changes.

Additionally, Boshes and Gibbs (1972) report that feelings of irritability, rage, and fear can be symptoms (precursors) of an upcoming seizure attack. This origin of irritability may not be controllable since it is a result of neurological changes in the brain that are initiated by pre-seizure activity. Clients who have uncontrolled epilepsy may benefit from increased awareness of their irritable mood to help identify pre-seizure activity and take appropriate actions.

Medication Side Effect

There are many medications that can have a side effect of aggression. Zuckerman (2000) includes neurological medications, nonsteroidal anti-inflammatory drugs, anticancer medications, anesthetic medication, antibiotic medication, penicillin, procaine, heavy metals and toxins such as organic tin (can cause unprovoked rage attacks), amphetamines, bromides, cocaine, corticosteroids, levodopa, MAOI, tricyclic antidepressants, methylphenidate, over-the-counter stimulants and appetite suppressants, vitamin deficiencies, excess of fat-soluble vitamins, phenobarbital, anticonvulsant medication, and methamphetamines. If appropriate, medications can be changed and adjusted to help extinguish or diminish aggressive behavior. If this is not appropriate (e.g., other and more severe symptoms or consequences could occur), other interventions may be tried (e.g., stress management and relaxation training, behavior modification, and the techniques described below).

Task-Related Anxiety

When anxiety levels are raised beyond a client's coping ability, anger towards the task, self, or others can occur in some instances. Common techniques used to treat task-related anxiety include cognitive behavior therapy (combating distorted thinking patterns), stress management and relaxation training, progressive desensitization to the anxiety provoking task, and improved problem solving strategies.

Inability to Express Needs

Clients can have difficulty expressing needs for a variety of reasons including speech impairments (e.g., expressive aphasia) and poor communication styles (e.g., passive aggressive). Specific impairments related to needs expression are identified and appropriate interventions are implemented (e.g., use of alternative forms of communication such as an augmentative communication device, writing, gestures, sign language, and body language). If the issue is with communication style, the functions discussed in Body Functions Chapter 3, especially b355 Discussion, should be considered.

Obtaining Positive Reinforcers

Some clients may act out to fulfill an immediate need for attention or other positive reinforcers. For example, a client may receive immediate attention whenever he acts out behaviorally. Treatment for this cause of anger is behavior modification. See "Behavior Manipulation" in the Techniques section.

Escape or Avoidance Behavior

Some clients may use anger to avoid or escape something. For example, when a client feels vulnerable, she becomes aggressive to gain control and escape the situation. Teaching clients healthy coping mechanisms for stressors can be helpful (see "Coping with Stress," "Relaxation and Stress Reduction," and "Education and Counseling" in the Techniques section).

Normal Anger

Almost everyone has things that trigger their anger. These can be irritating situations or people anywhere in the person's life. In these cases there is no "underlying cause" that needs to be dealt with. The person needs to deal with the current situation, here and now. Some ways to deal with this normal anger in healthy ways are described below.

Anger Management Techniques

Anger management is training in techniques to control anger. It usually includes identification of triggers, re-assessment of values, relaxation techniques, and coping techniques. The range and cause of anger, irritability, or rage can be vast as described above. This part will look at the anger itself, rather than as a physiological or mental illness, and suggest appropriate ways for the client to manage the anger.

The first responsibility of the clinician is to reduce any underlying causes. Sometimes this can't be done completely, so the client may still need help to seal with anger.

Anger, like grief, does not follow a set schedule. However, failure to address feelings of anger may cause a barrier/block to further progress. For example, a client may be so angry at his current situation that it impedes his ability to concentrate and learn new skills. It may also affect his social relationships with others and his ability to problem solve for barriers (because "life just stinks and I'm too angry to deal with it"). Anger can also lead to adjustment problems (e.g., depression, anxiety, inability to work with caregivers).

Strong feelings of anger affect a client's health. When a person becomes angry, blood pressure increases, breathing can become labored, and muscles contract. For almost everyone, this can be contraindicated for good health. Prolonged stress on the cardiovascular system may increase the chances for illness (e.g., prolonged stress is a risk factor for stroke). For others, muscular contraction can become disabling when trying to complete a functional task (e.g., increased muscular tone in an arm that already has increased tone can result in a temporary inability to reach for an item). The role of the therapist is to guide the client in a positive direction towards understanding and coping with anger. There are many ways to do this and there is no cookie cutter approach to providing such guidance. However, some suggestions are provided below as a springboard for developing an individualized plan for a client.

- Assist the client in identifying "triggers" of anger (e.g., when client's friends come to visit him at the rehab and they are talking about all the fun they had over the weekend, the client begins to feel angry because he "knows" he will no longer be able to do those things). The first step to learning how to manage/resolve anger is to identify the root cause of the anger. Often it is fear. If you can't name it, you can't claim it.

- Critically evaluate the identified triggers and look for any faulty/distorted thinking patterns (e.g., is the client correct when he "knows" that he can't do the things that he used to do?). Teach the client the premise of the A-B-C Theory of Personality of REBT. (See "Education and Counseling" in the Techniques section for information on REBT.) The belief is that an event (friends talking about fun things they did over the weekend) does not cause an emotional/behavioral response (anger). It is the person's belief (fear) that he can no longer do those things that affects how he responds to the event. Review info on REBT for techniques that can be applied by the therapist to combat distorted thinking.

- Some clients may find it difficult to know when they are angry. They are not aware of the internal and external warning signs of becoming angry (e.g., clenches teeth, feels need to escape, becomes distracted). If a client is able to identify signs of anger, then the client will be able to identify the need to initiate a coping strategy (e.g., "I'm clenching my teeth again. Ok, just take a deep breath....1...2...3...4...5...").
- Some clients may not show anger in a manner that the therapist expects (e.g., client becomes quiet and withdraws). These clients may not feel as if they have a right to feel angry or it may not be acceptable within their family or culture to display feelings of anger. Help clients to understand that anger is a natural emotion that needs to be addressed. Otherwise it will manifest itself in other forms (e.g., ill health).
- Identify and provide healthy opportunities to vent feelings of anger (e.g., journal, physical activity, art, formal relaxation techniques).
- Help the client to "see" how anger can affect physical health, social relationships, and ultimately quality of life, as well as the current situation.

Whole books are written about how to manage anger. If a therapist is dealing with many cases of anger, s/he should investigate appropriate resources for the particular set of clients s/he is working with.

Documentation

Anger can be measured and documented in several ways:

- *Frequency*: Percent of angry verbalizations or gestures in a given time frame.
- *Identification of issues*: Current and resolved sources of anger.
- *Coping mechanisms*: Identification and utilization of coping mechanisms for anger (use percentage or level of assistance required, name of technique, and whether identified and/or utilized).
- *Statements*: Documentation of direct statements/comments of the client related to anger ("I hate this wheelchair. It makes me so angry!").

The ICF includes anger in b1522 Range of Emotion. Therapists teaching clients that it is all right to appropriately express anger should document the intervention by referring to this code. Therapists working other anger issues will probably be using d2402 Handling Stress with a notation to the right of the scoring area about anger management. Anger that is not a result of stress (e.g., frontal lobe tumor) would by scored using b1263 Psychic Stability with a notation to the right of the scoring area about anger, aggression, irritability, or rage.

References

Boshes, L. & Gibbs, F. (1972). *Epilepsy handbook, 2nd ed.* Springfield, IL: Charles C. Thomas.

Pary, R., Sikla, V., & Blaha, S. (1995). *Manual of clinical hospital psychiatry*. (Thienhaus, O., Ed.). Washington, DC: American Psychiatric Press.

Zuckerman, E. (2000). *Clinician's thesaurus, 5th edition.* New York, New York: The Guilford Press.

Balance

The ability to maintain a balanced position, any position, during activity is one of the main, underlying skills required to engage in almost any activity. It is so basic that it is often overlooked during the intervention process. The inability to remain balanced should be one of the first impairments addressed because without balance a client is not likely to gain independence in activity. Without some independence related to balance a client is less likely to initiate and engage in activity. Lack of activity increases sensory deprivation, deconditioning, and dysfunction: a vicious downward spiral.

Balance is a dynamic process in which the body maintains its center of gravity over its base of support so it can hold a position against gravity. For example, when skiing, the skier tries to keep his/her weight balanced over the center of the skis in such a manner that gravity does not cause a fall. The center of gravity for a typical skier versus a skier who has an above the knee amputation is different and requires different positions and strategies to keep from falling. (One of the strategies for skiers who have had amputations is to use ski poles with short skis on the end of the pole instead of a spike and basket.)

There are a number of important concepts associated with a client's ability to maintain balance during activities. The physical therapist and occupational therapist are often the first members of the treatment team to address balance. The recreational therapist begins to address balance as s/he expands the client's movements and actions beyond the basic skills and equipment taught by PT and OT. For example, the physical therapist may have prescribed a walker and grabber for the client to use after discharge. However, the client has always been an avid gardener and these two pieces of equipment do not allow the client to continue to garden. It is the recreational therapist's task to determine further adapted equipment and transfer procedures that allow the client to garden again. To do this, the therapist must have a solid understanding of balance in different positions and using different adapted equipment. Rose (2003) describes the basic concepts as center of mass (center of gravity), balance, posture, anticipatory postural control, reactive postural control, stability limits, and mobility.

- *Posture*: Good posture is the positioning of the body so that the individual is able to complete activities with the least amount of internal energy and the least amount of wear and tear on the body. When standing with good posture the individual's ears are generally aligned with the center of the hips, the front of the kneecaps, and the front of the ankle. When sitting, an individual's ears are still aligned with the center of the hips. For best support the knees are also aligned with ankles.

- *Anticipatory postural control*: Anticipatory postural control refers to learned actions that a client makes to ensure that his/her postural balance remains stable even when the environment changes. A client is able to increase functional balance through instruction and practice. For example, a recreational therapist, working with a client who uses a wheelchair, teaches how to balance on the back two wheels of the wheelchair in anticipation of using this skill to drop down from a curb that has no curb cut. Another example is teaching a client how to balance with both crutches in one hand while opening a door. Anticipated postural control is always a planned action.

- *Reactive postural control*: Reactive postural control is the quick action that must be taken to maintain postural balance in response to an unexpected challenge in the environment. One example of reactive postural control is grabbing onto the stair railing when your foot does not quite clear the step and you fall forward. Another example is when you put your hands on the seat in front of you to stop forward movement when the city bus on which you are riding makes a sudden stop. Reactive postural control is a reaction to an event and not a planned action.

- *Stability limits*: Stability limits are the greatest distance in any direction the client is able to (or feels comfortable to) move without changing his/her base of support, while still maintaining balance. Stability limits tend to shrink as an individual ages or develops sensory losses. Stability limits are part of engaging in many activities such as preparing a meal, gardening, arts and crafts, and sports. Even playing bingo (leaning forward to mark a number on the bingo sheet) involves a client's consciously or unconsciously moving within stability limits. Just as with range of motion, stability limits shrink with inactivity. Engaging in regular activity that moves a person safely to the edges of his/her stability should be a daily occurrence. For, just like cardiovascular endurance, stability limits are maintained or increased only through regular and ongoing activity.

- *Sway envelope*: Sway envelope is the common range of movement that an individual stays within during activity without changing his/her base of support. It is not unusual for people to have a smaller sway envelope than their stability limits. Sway envelopes are often "lopsided" as individuals lose function, favor one side due to pain, or lose function through neurological or musculoskeletal degeneration. For clients who seldom venture outside of their sway envelope or have a restricted sway envelope, the therapist will want to ensure that activities are offered that help "exercise" the stability limits beyond the sway envelope. For clients who have impairments that often cause them to venture outside of their sway envelope and outside their stability limits, balance safety should be taught.

Depending on the type of facility that the recreational therapist is working in and the make-up of his/her team members, the responsibilities for working on specific interventions related to improving posture, postural control, stability limits, and sway envelopes will vary. When clients are medically cleared to participate in activities, ensure that the activities offered have a variety of movements helping maintain or improve posture and stability. The types of movements the therapist will want to ensure (Rose, 2003) are

- Moving from different positions back to good standing posture. (Also, practice this with eyes closed.) For clients with significant limitations, lateral weight shifts in different directions may be a good place to begin. For clients with greater skill, leaning over and reaching for something on the ground and then returning to a good postural position may be appropriate.
- Moving from different positions (forward to backward and diagonal forward to backward) to reach a balanced seated position. (Also, practice this with eyes closed.)
- Maintaining balance while slowly raising each arm over the head, one at a time and together. If possible, the arm should be relatively straight and the elbow should be above the client's ear. Not only does this movement help with range of motion and stability, but it also helps expand the lungs and increases lung capacity.
- Moving the arms in an "airplane" movement. In an airplane movement the arms are stretched horizontally out to the client's side with palms down. As one arm is raised the other one drops as if the two arms together make up the wings of an airplane. (Also, practice this with eyes closed.)

- Turning the head and shoulders in a slow, lateral trunk rotation while the hips remain in the same place. This is the movement made when you look behind you as you are driving to see if anything is in the way of your backing up.
- Alternatively lifting one foot off the ground, then the other while standing and while seated. The therapist must ensure that the client is safe during these activities, spotting the client and ready to stop any fall. An intermediate step may be just lifting either the heel or the toe off the ground while leaving part of the foot still on the ground. For clients with less stability, seated "marches" or single leg raises may be appropriate.

Except for the first exercise, all of the exercises can be done in a sitting or standing position. The sitting position may be on a stool, but it is often better to use a balance ball. Balance balls are rubber balls of various sizes that are strong enough for clients to sit on for balance training. The therapist must use the right size ball for the client. The size of ball used is based on the client's standing height. Rose (2003, p. 95) provides the following rule of thumb for selecting ball sizes.

Height of Client	Size of Balance Ball
Below 5'5"	45-cm ball
5'5" to 5'8"	55-cm ball
5'9" to 6'3"	65-cm ball
6'4" to 6'9"	75-cm ball
6'10" and taller	85-cm ball

If there is not a physical therapist or occupational therapist specifically assigned to work on stability maintenance or enhancement with a client, the task may fall to the recreational therapist. Rose (2003) has an excellent set of exercise protocols described in her book *Fallproof! A Comprehensive Balance and Mobility Training Program* that the recreational therapist can use. (All of the exercises described above, and more, are included in the book.) The types of settings where stability training may fall within the recreational therapist's job responsibilities include nursing homes and assisted living facilities, community programs, and special education programs.

Balance is an important part of b755 Involuntary Movement Reaction Functions and all of the physical activities in Activities and Participation.

References

Rose, D. (2003). *Fallproof! A comprehensive balance and mobility training program*. Champaign, IL: Human Kinetics.

Behavior Manipulation

Behavior is a general term that describes any action that an individual makes that can be seen and measured by someone else. This includes actions reactions, responses, activities, and patterns of movement. When a client's behavior is hindering functioning, activity performance, independence, quality of life, safety of self or others, or negatively affecting any other aspect of health, interventions are sought and applied to promote positive change. Some of the most common interventions for manipulating behavior are cueing, structuring the environment, structuring expectations, and behavior modification. See "Lifestyle Alteration Education" for information on how to change lifestyle behaviors (e.g., smoking, exercise patterns).

Cueing

Cueing is the process of prompting someone to take a specific action (burlingame, 2001). Prompting includes not only words or gestures (including role modeling) but also visual cues in the environment, hand-over-hand direction, and other physical assistance. Cueing is one of the more basic methods of modifying a client's performance and is used most often with clients with cognitive impairments such as traumatic brain injury, dementia, and mental retardation. Cueing is similar to, but not the same as, behavior modification, which is covered later. Cueing is a forward process that does not necessarily give the person feedback about his/her actions; it reminds the client of the next action. Behavior modification involves providing feedback for actions already taken.

Used in therapy or in the community to facilitate participation in leisure activities, cueing is the graduated assistance used by a therapist to help clients perform desired actions or tasks. Cueing is not a haphazard way to remind a client to do something; it is a clinical technique used to influence the client's actions with a targeted outcome in mind.

Basic Concepts

There are some basic concepts and terms that are important to understand before trying to implement cueing techniques. Those terms are

- *Baseline*: When related to documenting the level of cueing a client requires, a baseline is the initial skill level that a client is able to demonstrate without cueing. The documentation for a baseline includes the command given, the actions completed by the client, and the point at which the client was no longer able to perform inde-

pendently. The point at which the client is no longer able to progress independently is likely the point that the therapist will address in treatment.

- *Chaining*: The sequencing of actions that, as a whole, make up the complete activity. For clients with severe cognitive impairments it is common for the therapist to work on one step of a task at a time until a client is able to successfully complete the different steps. At that point, the therapist works with the client to chain the steps together to make up a full task.

- *Command*: A command is the set of initial verbal instructions given to a client to begin a task. While very formal (and almost "bossy") sounding, the word command does not mean a military type order given to the client. The term command is used to mean the clear, simple, and short instructions given to the client about a task to be undertaken. It helps clients with cognitive impairments if the therapist (or treatment team) gives the same command each time. An example of a command is "Daryl, please find the phone number of the Dynasty Theater in the phone book."

- *Gesture*: Any visual cue initiated by the therapist physically moving his/her body to help the client complete the task. Gestures include modeling, motioning, nodding head, and pointing. An example of a gesture is the therapist pointing to a quarter in a pile of coins when the task is for the client to take all the quarters out of the pile.

- *Hand-over-hand technique*: When a client is unable to mentally process the movement needed, the therapist may use the hand-over-hand technique. The therapist stands slightly behind the client at the 8 o'clock or 4 o'clock position putting his/her hand over the hand of the client. Holding the client's hand, the therapist helps the client initiate and complete the task. At any point during the hand-over-hand technique, if it seems like the client is able to complete the task himself/herself, the therapist removes his/her hand. Less desirable, but still appropriate, the therapist positions himself/herself in front of the client and initiates the hand-over-hand technique. An example of a hand-over-hand technique is assisting the client in picking up a paintbrush to begin painting.

- *Independent*: After one verbal command, the client performs the task without any actions from the therapist to help the client correctly complete the task. For example, the therapist asks the client to create a grocery-shopping list for a picnic and the client does so without further intervention from the therapist.

- *Manipulation*: After one verbal command, the therapist provides complete physical guidance as the client is not able to complete the movement or that portion of the task himself/herself. Manipulation includes using a hand-over-hand technique and/or full physical assistance. An example of manipulation is the therapist helping a client put on a coat because the client is not able to cognitively process the steps required to put on the coat. It is important to always give a command before using a manipulation. Beginning an intervention using manipulation techniques without first giving a command takes away the client's opportunity to demonstrate some level of independence and initiation. By regularly initiating manipulation without a command the therapist is increasing the client's dependence on staff (often called institutionalization). For example, a client is sitting up in her wheelchair that has a tray attached to the arms of the chair. There is an open book on the client's tray but the client is not attending to the book and the therapist would like to work with the client using a xylophone. The therapist should first ask (verbal cue) the client to close the book, progress to touching the client's hand (prompt), then use a hand-over-hand technique (manipulative cue) to help the client complete the task.

- *No response*: Despite the therapist providing progressively more supportive cueing, the client is unable to initiate the task even with teaching cues. This is different from refusal to participate. An example of no response is a client being handed a beach ball (as the first step toward learning to throw the ball) and the client has no cognitive understanding that s/he is to hold the ball. Each try, regardless of the type of cueing, ends up with the ball being in the hands of the client for less than one second after the therapist removes his/her hands using hand-over-hand techniques.

- *Prompt*: Any cue that involves the therapist touching the client but the client is still responsible for some of the movement or part of the task himself/herself. Prompts are partial physical cues. Some examples include the therapist touching the side of the head for a client who has visual neglect cueing him to turn the head toward that side, touching a client's hand and saying "this is the hand that should push the elevator button," or touching a client's wrist and saying "it is easier if you hold your hands still."

- *Resistance to cueing*: Resistance to cueing is when the client actively blocks the therapist's attempts to cue the client to initiate a task or to implement the next step of the task. Resistance to cueing may have multiple origins including a client's hypersensitivity to touch, over-stimulation, dislike of the activity, dislike of the therapist, fatigue, and many other reasons. When a client resists cueing for a task that is part of the treatment plan, it is important for the therapist to determine the reason for the resistance.

- *Session*: An uninterrupted period of time in which the client and therapist work on a task, often repeating the task numerous times working toward greater independence. There may be one or many trials during a session.

- *Teaching cues*: Generally, teaching cues are a graduated system of assistance provided to a client to help complete a task. Specifically, after one verbal command, they are any type of action that you do to help ensure that the client will do what you want. The four types of teaching cues are (from least invasive to most invasive) gesture, verbal, prompt, and manipulation.

- *Trial*: A trial is one complete sequence of the task completed, regardless of the amount of assistance and cueing required by the client.

- *Verbal cue*: A verbal cue is the short, verbal assistance given to the client to help move to the next step of the task.

Cueing Guidelines

The underlying basis for cueing is task analysis. The therapist uses knowledge of the discrete steps and the action required for any specific portion of the activity and uses the appropriate level of cueing to help the client complete the task. For example, let us say that a client with moderate mental retardation is participating in a basic horticulture project of filling pots with soil and then placing the pots in a flat. To help the client gain greater independence in the activity, the therapist would use instruction, repetition of activity, and cueing to help the client master the activity. A sample breakdown of the steps required (task analysis) to complete this task is shown in Figure 4 (from Melwood, 1980, p. 195). The therapist demonstrates how s/he wants the task completed and then gives the client a command to start.

There are many ways to document how many and what type of cues were required by the client during the trial. The sample shown in Figure 5 is one method.

It is normal for any client who is learning a new activity or task to require some level of cueing in the

---

Basic Horticulture

Project A-1: Fill pots with soil and fill flats with pots.

Conditions: 1. Soil premixed and at potting bench, 2. 20 three-inch square pots at bench, 3. Plastic flat that holds 20 pots at bench, 4. trowel optional.

Standard for Independent Functioning: The normal *time* needed to complete successfully this task is 83 seconds for 20 pots or 4.2 seconds per pot. The standard for *accuracy* is 95% accuracy (19 out of the 20 pots done correctly) within the normal time. Any time needed to correct an incorrectly filled pot adds to the total time.

Process (Task Analysis):
1. Pick up pot.
2. Fill with soil (trowel optional).
3. Shake off excess (1/4 inch below top of pot).
4. Place in flat.
5. Repeat 19 times.

Figure 4: Basic Horticulture Task

beginning. It is beneficial for the therapist to document the level of cueing a client required and the length of time or the number of trials it took the client to become independent in the activity. Most of the clients who require cueing to engage regularly in any type of task are the ones with cognitive impairments. These clients benefit from an environment that provides consistency. There are a couple of guidelines for therapists working with clients who require cueing. These guidelines are important for all the team members to follow so the client will be provided with a consistent environment. It also ensures that when a therapist reports the level of cueing required by a client, the rest of the team has the same results. Some of the guidelines include:

- Wait five seconds after giving the command or five seconds between each cue to allow the client time to take action or correct action. Obviously, if the action that a client is about to take is unsafe, the therapist should intervene immediately.
- The therapist must have "quiet hands" so that random movement does not distract the client. Gestured cues should have an economy of motion.
- The therapist must ensure that the client is able to see any gesture made. This means that the therapist is in a position that allows the client to see the gestures. Having to ask the client to stop the activity and verbally command the client to

Task ↓ / Type of Cues →	Gesture	Verbal	Prompt	Manipulate
Pick up pot	11	8	5	0
Fill with soil	15	9	9	0
Shake off excess	20	4	0	0
Place in flat	12	5	0	0
Repeat 19 times	10	5	0	0

Figure 5: : Cueing Summary Trial #1

look at the therapist's hand is an inappropriate cue in almost all situations. If the client is being non-attentive, the first cue should be for the client to attend to the appropriate task. Then a second cue is given to work on the task. For example, if the task is to put puzzle pieces together and the client is blankly looking off into space, the first cue the therapist gives would be a verbal cue redirecting the client to the puzzle (attending to task). If, after the client's attention is back on the puzzle, the client does not initiate putting the next puzzle piece together, after five seconds the therapist cues the client to put the puzzle together (initiation of activity).

- The therapist must be disciplined to provide only one type of cue at a time. Otherwise, the therapist cannot know which cue the client was responding to. For example, if the therapist both asks the client to take his turn at cards (verbal cue) and points to the card draw pile (gesture cue), the therapist cannot be sure which cue was the one that the client responded to.
- The therapist uses cues in a progressively more invasive sequence, offering the lowest level of assistance first.

Cues in the Environment

Cues in the environment help clients be as independent as possible. This is a less formal type of cueing and can be a normal part of the environment. For example, we have street signs on our roads letting us know the speed limit, when a school crossing is coming up, or the name of the street. Environmental cues are also in the community recreation center (women's restroom, gym, location of golf tee, fast food menu on the wall) and the health care unit (client's name outside of client's bedroom; activity room; cafeteria; activity schedule posted on the wall; orientation board with the day's date, the month, the name of the facility). In health care facilities, the number of environmental cues should be as close to "normal" (e.g., those found in the community) as possible while still providing support for residents based on their functional needs.

Sometimes environmental cues are purposefully misleading to help ensure the safety of clients. An example of this type of cueing exists on units that have clients with dementia who are mobile. Often clients with dementia will wander off the unit and get lost, unable to remember how to get back (or even that they need to get back). The doors that lead off the unit have a picture of a bookcase full of books painted on the doors. Clients with dementia are unable to distinguish between the painting and a real bookcase. Since they remember (to some degree) that they never could walk through a bookcase, they do not try to exit the doors. Even if the client with dementia walks up to the painting and tries to remove a book, the client still does not seem to realize that the painting is really a doorway. Another technique that seems to work is to stretch yellow ribbon across a doorway attached to the doorframe with Velcro. Clients with dementia who perpetually wander, often going into other client's rooms and through their belongings, seem to avoid openings with yellow ribbon across the door about three feet off the ground.

Structuring the Environment

You walk into a facility. The doors to the unit are locked and it takes you 15 minutes to find someone to let you in. The walls are painted in bright industrial white. Clients are in their rooms or are sitting in wheelchairs littered along the hallway. There are no activities going on and it smells like urine. Staff aren't interacting with each other or clients. They are seated at their desks performing paperwork and they do not acknowledge your presence. There are beeping and alarm noises and several clients are yelling profanities. How does this scenario make you feel? What influence do you think it has on the clients?

The environment of a facility is very important. It can have a profound influence on client behavior and their achievements. Compare the stark facility described above with another facility. There is carpet on the floor and the walls are painted a soft green. Flowers are abundant and a sweet floral smell perfumes the halls. The clients are dressed nicely. They are chatting with others, engaged in activity, or smiling as you walk by. The staff look happy and make direct eye contact with you and say "hello." Does this scenario make you feel any differently than the first scenario? When compared to the first scenario, do you think that this environment provides the client with any added health benefits? If you were

choosing a facility for your mother, which one would you choose?

Designing an environment (a "milieu") that promotes health and wellness in all domains of health is ideal. "Milieu" is a term that refers to the treatment environment including the physical environment, the social environment, and general rules that define expectations and consequences for violating rules. Not all therapeutic milieus are the same and not every environmental intervention is appropriate. Each is specially designed to meet the needs of the clients served. For example, a therapeutic milieu for adolescent urban boys in rehab recovering from drug abuse will be different from a therapeutic milieu for older adults with Alzheimer's disease in a long-term care facility. In a rehabilitation or acute hospital setting, treatment teams modify the environment to make it easier for clients to learn skills that improve their likelihood of success when they move to a less restrictive environment. In a long-term care facility, milieus are designed to promote social interaction, enhance comfort, control specific behaviors, and promote an optimal quality of life. Creating a therapeutic milieu is an important part of the treatment process. The environment, in addition to the direct interventions given by staff, provides clients with extra support while they learn and incorporate new skills into their general patterns of behavior.

So, how do you go about designing a therapeutic milieu? Therapists begin by evaluating the needs of the population being served. What is it that this particular population needs from the environment to thrive? The answer will be different for different populations (it can also be different for different individuals) and it will be different for different facilities. Therapists learn what works best by talking to other professionals who are experienced in designing therapeutic milieus for the specific populations and doing research to find out what has worked and what has not worked (e.g., journal articles). And, as simple as it may sound, just plain observation of behaviors and good analytical skills can lead the therapist to a greater awareness and understanding of the environment.

A few broad concepts to consider when designing a milieu are provided below to get you on your way (Schwartz, 1957). However, it must be noted again that some of these components are not appropriate for all milieus (e.g., it would not be appropriate to design a milieu that increases insight on an Alzheimer's unit, although it would be an appropriate consideration for designing a milieu in a drug and alcohol recovery program):

- Provide experiences that minimize distortions of reality.
- Facilitate realistic and communicative exchange with others.
- Facilitate participation with others to derive greater satisfaction and security.
- Reduce anxiety and increase comfort.
- Increase self-esteem.
- Provide insight into the courses and manifestations of illness/disability.
- Mobilize initiative and motivate the client to realize more fully his/her potential for creativity and productivity.

As for specifics, Table 24 is provided to give you an idea of some of the differences in a standard treatment environment and a therapeutic milieu. Keep in mind that these are merely ideas and not a standard for creating a therapeutic milieu.

The Eden Alternative™ is one of the primary examples of a formally organized effort to create a therapeutic milieu. The Eden Alternative was started by Billy and Judy Thomas in the early 1990s to help create a healthier, more holistic nursing home environment. The mission of the Eden Alternative is to "improve the well-being of Elders and those who care for them by transforming the communities in

Table 24: Comparison of Environments

Standard treatment environment	Therapeutic milieu
Bed trays for dining/eating in room	Group dining to foster natural conversation, socialization, and support
Hospital gowns	Regular clothing
Hospital employees have control over most treatment activities (fosters external control)	Clients have control over appropriate aspects of treatment (fosters internal control)
Client is primarily in a "sick role" (can foster dependence and learned helplessness)	Client is encouraged to lead a "well role" (be proactive within recovery)
Lack of privacy	Privacy maintained (e.g., closed doors, private conversation)
Strange and unfamiliar equipment and language	Uses familiar equipment whenever possible, explains unfamiliar equipment, uses common language
Strange sights, sounds, and smells	Environment is transformed to imitate familiar sights, sounds, and smells (e.g., indirect lighting instead of fluorescent lighting, walls painted in warm home colors instead of industrial bright white, carpeting instead of hard floors, floral smelling cleaning supplies instead of ammonia)
Unvarying routines	Varying routines
Expectations of submissiveness to hospital staff	Graduated responsibility for own medical care (active participant in progression to health)
Random and undirected opportunities to talk with other clients	Purposefully directed interactions with other clients for mutual support
Individual treatment	Group treatment (helps clients to learn how to be the "helper" and to be "helped" — an important aspect of independence and an essential component of adjustment to chronic illness; promotes sharing and learning from others; helps put individual situations in perspective)
Schedules are made for clients	Clients responsible for creating and maintaining their own schedules
Roommates by chance	Roommates by planned intervention
Orientation by staff	Orientation by another client: A client is appointed as a patient representative to welcome new clients, show them around, introduce them to other people and activities, etc.
Limited family involvement	Active family involvement
No or limited opportunities for engagement in community activities	Therapeutic community passes and integration training are common

which they live and work" (Eden, 2006a). The Thomases identified three recurring problems in nursing homes: loneliness, helplessness, and boredom and created a vision to eliminate these by creating a milieu that recognized the nursing home as a habitat that needed to be balanced versus a facility providing services for individuals who could not take care of themselves. By following the rules of balance and interaction found in Mother Nature a "vibrant, vigorous habitat" (Eden, 2006b) is created. The Eden Alternative has ten basic principles (Eden, 2006c):

1. The three plagues of loneliness, helplessness, and boredom account for the bulk of suffering among our Elders.
2. An Elder-centered community commits to creating a Human Habitat where life revolves around close and continuing contact with plants, animals, and children. It is these relationships that provide the young and old alike with a pathway to a life worth living.
3. Loving companionship is the antidote to loneliness. Elders deserve easy access to human and animal companionship.
4. An Elder-centered community creates opportunity to give as well as receive care. This is the antidote to helplessness.
5. An Elder-centered community imbues daily life with variety and spontaneity by creating an environment in which unexpected and unpredictable interactions and happenings can take place. This is the antidote to boredom.
6. Meaningless activity corrodes the human spirit. The opportunity to do things that we find meaningful is essential to human health.
7. Medical treatment should be the servant of genuine human caring, never its master.
8. An Elder-centered community honors its Elders by de-emphasizing top-down bureaucratic authority, seeking instead to place the maximum possible decision-making authority into the hands of the Elders or into the hands of those closest to them.
9. Creating an Elder-centered community is a never-ending process. Human growth must never be separated from human life.
10. Wise leadership is the lifeblood of any struggle against the three plagues. For it, there can be no substitute.

The importance of creating a healthy, client-centered milieu is critical for client and staff well-being. Thomas points out that people in the United States who are over 65 years of age have a 50% chance of spending a significant amount of time in a nursing home. The only population that has a larger percentage of its group institutionalized are criminals (Public Broadcasting System, 2002).

Structuring Expectations

In addition to structuring the environment to reduce behavior problems, the therapist can also structure the expectations of clients and staff to reduce confrontation. Ito (1997) discusses techniques initiated by the therapist to avoid confrontation and prevent a build-up of inappropriate behaviors. Implementing the techniques reduces problematic behaviors in almost any setting with clients who have moderate to high cognitive function. They are likely to work the best in settings with length of stays of at least one week and if the entire team implements them. The techniques are

Activity Reinforcement

Set up the expectation that clients are expected to tackle, with assistance when needed, the less pleasurable tasks associated with therapy before the more rewarding tasks. This is the "Grandma's Law" technique. You need to eat your spinach before you can have your ice cream.

Antiseptic Bouncing

This technique has the therapist anticipating a developing behavioral outburst before it happens by recognizing the precursor activities. For example, the therapist knows that the client does not deal with frustration very well, usually resulting in a show of aggression toward an inanimate object. When frustrated the client throws his work against the wall or rips up his paper. Antiseptic bouncing is a technique where the therapist directs the client to another, short-term task, avoiding behavior problem by interrupting the buildup with a change of pace. An example of antiseptic bouncing is asking the client to take a note to the nursing station. If this intervention technique is used by the whole team, staff may develop a coding system for such notes so that the team member receiving the note realizes that the main purpose of the note is to offer the client an opportunity to take a break before his/her behavior became a problem.

Contract

Behavioral contracts are written agreements between a therapist (or treatment team) and a client that outline specific agreements, rules, and consequences to which they have mutually agreed. Contracts need to have reasonable expectations with short-term goals. One of the most common contracts is the one used on psychiatric units in which the client agrees not to harm himself/herself. Some of the terms of the contract are that the client does not cause harm to himself/herself and, in exchange, staff make time to help the client through specifically defined challenges. By seeking out help when needed and not harming himself/herself, the client earns privileges such as a daily walk around the block with a favorite staff person. However, less dramatic contracts are also used such as a client with developmental delays earning the right to walk with staff to get a latté from the corner Starbucks if s/he participates in the current events discussion with staff three days in a row.

Direct Appeal

The use of a direct appeal is meant to appeal to the client's sense of fairness. In a direct appeal, the therapist quietly and non-judgmentally asks the client to stop the behavior because of its consequences on others. For example, the therapist may approach a client on the spinal cord injury unit whose CD is too loud for another client to hear what his family member is trying to say. The therapist may say, "Mr. Henry cannot hear what his son is saying because your music is too loud. Could you please turn it down or go into your room and shut the door?"

Hurdle Helping

Unlike the antiseptic bouncing, hurdle helping does not try to remove the client from a stressful situation that often leads to behavior problems but "offers encouragement, support, and assistance" (Ito, 1997) to prevent the client from passing the threshold from acceptable to problematic behaviors. For example, a client newly admitted to rehab with a CVA (stroke) who now has paralysis in her left arm is having trouble drawing. The client is obviously very frustrated and looks like she is about to lose her temper. The therapist goes over and acknowledges that it is hard to draw when the paper is moving all around (because the non-dominant hand cannot hold the paper still). The therapist then offers a couple of ways to solve the problem including taping down the edges or using the other arm, physically placing the paralyzed arm on top of the edge of the paper to have the weight of the arm hold the paper down.

I Messages

A standard therapy technique is to express how someone's behavior is affecting you (making "I" statements) instead of "naming" the other person's behavior (making "you" statements). Ito offers this basic format for "I" statements: *When you _____ (behavior) I feel _____ (feeling) because I _____ (reason).* For example, say the therapist works with a veteran admitted for posttraumatic stress disorder.

The client is severely depressed and is exhibiting anhedonia (an inability to derive pleasure from life or appreciate the pleasures that most people enjoy). "When you say that you cannot enjoy any activity, I feel saddened because I know that many clients with posttraumatic stress disorder do start to feel better after joining the group." A "you" statement would be "You should come to the group because you will feel better if you do." The I-Message technique works best with clients who are calm and not exhibiting problem behaviors. Clients who are already well on their way to fully expressing the problematic behavior need other techniques.

Interest Boosting

This technique is used as a "nudge" to encourage a client to continue an activity the client has stopped, potentially because s/he was bored or lost interest. Interest is a curious concept. While the term is used freely in discussions, such as in "leisure interest," from a clinical standpoint a lack of interest is often a secondary psychological/medical problem associated with the disease process. Reber (1985) defines interest as "attention, curiosity, motivation, focus, concern, goal-directedness, awareness, worthiness, and desire" (p. 367). Many of the listed attributes of interest can be diminished due to fatigue, cognitive impairment, or other medical problems. By praising the client for work already done, by offering help, and/or encouraging the client to continue, the therapist is helping the client increase interest in the task.

Make-A-Date

In this technique the therapist realizes that the client's participation and behavior would probably be better if s/he were able to meet separately from the rest of the group to problem solve what is bothering him/her. The therapist quietly and privately agrees to meet later that day (or early the next day) with the client to discuss the client's issue. This technique works with clients who are able to reason and to wait for things to happen. The time set aside to discuss the client's issue can be a good time for the therapist to role model problem solving techniques.

Modeling

Modeling is a technique that uses someone (or a group) that the client respects to demonstrate (through a written story, a video, or live demonstration) the desired behavior and receive praise or positive reinforcement. Ito states that "the client with the challenging behavior must have regard for the model (a school leaders or athlete), share a common characteristic (age or sex), and be capable of performing the target behavior. It is important for the student to observe the model and receive positive reinforcement, as well as aversive consequences."

Monitor Sheet

A monitor sheet is a sheet of paper that lists the client's target behaviors, daily schedule, and spaces for staff to sign off if the desired behavior is demonstrated during different parts of the client's day. The client carries this sheet with him/her throughout the day. In every therapy session or activity where the client demonstrates the desired, positive behaviors, a staff person signs off on the monitor sheet. This technique works best with children and youth or clients with moderate cognitive impairment.

Peer Mediation

In some clinical settings, such as chemical dependency units, the "unit" is treated as a large household in which the clients help set the rules of behavior. With role modeling and other training from staff, clients may be able to use positive peer mediation techniques to help modify the client's behaviors. On some psychiatric units, even units with three to twelve day stays, the clients have a "resident council" that meets for a short time each night. They discuss how things went on the unit that day and what might need to be changed to help create a better living situation. A classic example of peer mediation can be found in Alcoholics Anonymous in which a member is selected to be a mentor to another client trying to abstain from alcohol. Peer mediation works best when the environment offers clients opportunities for increasing mentoring skills so that the interactions between peers remain healthy.

Physical Interactions

Physical interactions can be both positive and negative. While it might seem obvious, the expectation that staff and clients are not to pinch, push, pull, kick, strike, or otherwise touch clients in an aggressive manner needs to be clearly stated. Other physical interactions with clients, however, can be positively influential. For example, when a client does something well or exhibits an ability to extinguish a behavior (e.g., doesn't yell a profanity when angry), a pat on the back or a high-five can provide an external reward to encourage repeated appropriate behavior.

When a client's behavior is so out of control that someone is going to get hurt and other interventions do not work (e.g., deescalating techniques), a "show of force" or "take down" technique may need to be implemented. Shows of force are planned actions taken by staff when a client is out of control and a danger to himself/herself or others. A show of force is "called" and all staff assigned to respond in a crisis meet in the proximity of the client who is out of control. A team leader is identified and each staff person is assigned a body part to hold. Other staff are assigned to the task of applying any restraint (physical and/or medical) that is to be used. The team leader informs the client that s/he is going to be taken down and restrained for his/her own protection (or the protection of others). On the command of the leader, all staff execute their roles, whether it is to grab and hold a body part or to apply a restraint. It cannot be overstated how overwhelming taking part in or observing a show of force can be, or how dangerous it can be to both staff and client. A show of force will frequently use as many as eight staff to take down one client. This is an extremely frightening event for other clients to watch. Many clients are already afraid that they will "lose it," but to see someone else taken down in such a fashion only adds to the other clients' anxiety. Loss of control and safety are often big issues. Safety of the staff should also be considered throughout the entire process. Staff will need to glove up (in case of bleeding) and staff at the client's head risk being bitten. A client who is extremely strong and violent can hurt staff as they try to hold and take him/her down. Show of force practice should be a regular event for all staff just like fire drills and other emergency training (burlingame, 2001).

Proximity Control

If a client is beginning to exhibit problematic behaviors, and the client is cognitively able to exert some control over that behavior, having the therapist stand or sit in close proximity to the client often helps the client make the decision to change his/her behavior.

Reinforcing the Positive

Clients, especially clients with cognitive impairments who have trouble retaining new information, benefit from regular positive feedback about behaviors and actions that meet or exceed expectations. This should be done in a gentle, honest manner that is part of the normal conversation. When an environment has more positive than negative, most clients find it easier to perform well.

Removal of Distracting Objects

Sometimes annoying or distracting behaviors can best be dealt with by simply removing the object of distraction. The removal should be considered only a temporary solution, as clients who are easily distracted benefit from developing skills related to attending to task and impulse control.

Reprimand

A reprimand is a neutral but clearly delivered statement that helps halt a behavior that is about to harm or is harming the client, another person, or property. Ito (1997) states: "Establish eye contact. Deliver your words firmly, immediately, privately, clearly, specifically, calmly, and swiftly. Be sure to include the expected behavior and consequences of continuing the inappropriate behavior" (pp. 3-4).

Confrontation

In some cases, but not most, confrontation can be a beneficial part of the therapy process. Confrontation is a specific technique in cognitive therapy used to bring to the attention of the client something that s/he is not paying attention to and would benefit from. With clients who are able to cognitively process abstract thoughts, approach confrontation in a respectful manner. The goal of confrontation is to help a client face an issue or idea without raising the client's defenses or eliciting a hostile response. An example of a confrontation technique would be with a client who is in a community recreation program for clients with brain injuries functioning at a Ranchos Los Amigos Level Five and above. (See "Traumatic Brain Injury" in the diagnosis section for an explanation of the Rancho Los Amigos Scale.) Previously the client had been using street drugs and this use was a direct cause of his accident and resulting brain injury. The therapist running the group used the *CERT-Psych/R* assessment after each session to monitor each client's functional ability in groups. During the last two weeks, the therapist noticed a significant change (drop) in the client's scores. Suspecting that the client had started to use street drugs again, the therapist carefully selected an opportunity to have a private conversation with the client. The therapist first calmly reminded the client of an earlier conversation in which the client stated that street drugs were not a good thing in his life. The therapist then asked the client, "I noticed that your ability to get along with the rest of the group seems a little more difficult for you. Is there a chance that you are having problems with street drugs?"

Summary

Structuring expectations, as these examples have shown, takes many forms. It is best to try the positive approaches first, but a therapist must realize when a situation is getting out of hand — there is a danger to self, others, or property — and use more invasive techniques to ensure a safe environment.

Behavior Modification

Behavior is the set of observable actions that are a direct result of internal or external forces. Often behavior is a learned pattern of actions that, once learned, continue even when the situation changes. Behavior modification is a purposeful attempt to change abnormal or maladaptive behavior patterns using planned, systematic interactions with a client and structuring the client's environment to produce a desired change in behavior.

As Dattilo & Murphy (1987) say

> The development of behavior modification originates from the belief that behaviors are learned, rather than inherent, and can thus be altered or modified by additional learning. Whatever the behavior and whatever its cause, the behavior is present in an environment and is influenced and shaped by that environment. Behavior modification focuses on individuals' behaviors. It is the behavior that is the concern and it is behavior that can be changed (p. 1).

Behavior modification is used after all the underlying causes of the behavior have been evaluated. Behavior modification using negative reinforcers is an invasive technique, so staff need to clearly state that they believe it would be helpful in correcting poor behaviors and that other, less invasive methods have not been effective.

Dattilo & Murphy (1987) caution the therapist to identify overt behaviors (those that mean the same thing to everyone else, e.g., smile, laugh) rather than covert behaviors (those that do not mean the same thing to other people, e.g., upset, depressed) for behavior modification. Using overt behaviors ensures accurate identification and description of the behavior for the behavior modification process. They recommend recording counts of the behaviors by one of these methods:

1. *Frequency* (how often the behavior occurs within a particular time frame, e.g., smiled 4x in a 30 minute session), duration (how long the behavior lasted, e.g., attended to the activity without redirection for 8 minutes).
2. *Interval recording* (the number of intervals the behavior appeared in, e.g., within four 15-minute intervals that make up an hour, the behavior was exhibited during two of them — observer present for entire hour session).
3. *Instantaneous time sampling* (e.g., within four 15-minute intervals that make up an hour, the behavior was observed at the end of 3 intervals [last 5 minutes of interval] — observer present to make observations of behavior during last 5 minutes of each interval; observer not present for entire one-hour session).

Observation of behavior without any intervention to establish baseline behavior is a key element of behavior modification. A baseline measurement related to behavior modification measures *all occurrences* of specific behaviors seen during a predetermined time instead of *how long* a client is able to perform a task before cueing. With behavior modification, the therapist observes the identified behavior and records a baseline measurement. Measure in terms of description (pulled hair, yelled profanities, withdrew from contact, smiled, cried, etc.), percent of behavior (e.g., verbal outbursts in therapy occur for 50% of a 30-minute session), level of assistance (requires minimal verbal cues for reassurance of safety), or impact on task. The baseline measurement provides the therapist with information that helps to determine if the treatment interventions are resulting in a change.

Dattilo & Murphy (1987) are quick to point out that behaviors do not occur in isolation; the environment affects them. "Recognition and understanding of environmental events that influence the target behavior is extremely helpful. Because manipulation of environmental events is a fundamental aspect of behavior modification, knowledge of which events or conditions to manipulate is necessary for success. Thus, assessment of events that occur prior to (antecedent) and following (consequence) the target behavior is as important as accurate description and observation of the target behavior itself" (p. 41).

Modifying behavior to help clients improve their function and quality of life is one of the basic interventions used by therapists. There are a variety of standardized methods used in behavior modification. Some of the more common methods are described below. Also see the behavior modification discussion in "Social Skills Training."

Extinction

Withhold reinforcers of behavior and behavior will decrease; be sure that alternative positive reinforcers of behavior do not surface (e.g., Even if the therapist withholds attention for rude remarks in group session, the client may still receive reinforcement from the attention of other group members). Use positive reinforcement in conjunction with extinction to encourage desired behavior. Sometime there is an "extinction burst" where the client's undesired behavior increases when extinction is first used. The explanation is that, for example, one rude remark did not get the therapist's usual attention, so the client makes several remarks to try to gain the expected attention of the therapist. This

"extinction burst" usually subsides. However, the behavior may temporarily reappear from time to time (spontaneous recovery).

Negative Reinforcement

Removes or postpones an aversive antecedent, contingent on the occurrence of the behavior; the undesired antecedent is removed once the target behavior is exhibited (escape) or the individual will not have to experience the undesired antecedent (avoidance) if the target behavior is exhibited. This technique should not be used if the same goals can be obtained via positive reinforcement.

Positive Reinforcement

Most common; presentation of positive reinforcer after display of desired behavior (target behavior) results in an increase in target behavior. Positive reinforcers may include basic needs (e.g., food), social rewards (e.g., praise, smile), activity reward (e.g., allowed to participate in an event or activity), or token rewards (e.g., tokens received can be used to purchase desired items or tasks). Will only work if the reinforcer is valued by the client.

Punishment

The presentation of an aversive event or consequence immediately following an instance of inappropriate behavior that leads to a decrease in the occurrence of that behavior. Should always be used in conjunction with positive reinforcement of desired behavior.

Withdrawal of Reinforcement

Two types of withdrawal of reinforcement are "response cost" and "time-out from positive reinforcement." Response cost means taking away positive reinforcers an individual has accumulated (e.g., tokens). Should be used in conjunction with positive reinforcement of desired behavior. Time-out from positive reinforcement means removal of a reinforcer that results in a decreased rate of behavior; client is removed from positive environment for a fixed period of time (e.g., a child who sits in a time-out chair in another room for three minutes) or reinforcers from a positive environment are removed for a fixed period of time (e.g., a toy is taken away from a child for five minutes).

Documentation

To measure the effectiveness of the behavior modification program, use the same kind of observations used in creating the baseline. Behavior observations are typically represented in graph form in terms of frequency (how often), duration (how long), percentage (of time), and rate (of behavior). If the intervention is successful, the graph will show a change in the target behavior. Successful interventions will show more of a positive behavior and less of a negative behavior. Typically, behavior change is described as 1. maintained (unchanged), 2. accelerated (increased), or 3. decelerated (decreased).

Observe behavior in various situations and environments to see if the change has generalized. It may be necessary to expand the behavior modification program to other situations before the target behavior is brought to the desired level in the client's life.

References

burlingame, j. (2001). *Idyll Arbor's therapy dictionary*, (2ⁿᵈ ed.). Ravensdale, WA: Idyll Arbor, Inc.

Dattilo, J. & Murphy, W. (1987). *Behavior modification in therapeutic recreation.* Venture Publishing, Inc: State College, PA.

Eden, (2006a). www.edenalt.com/mission.htm.

Eden, (2006b). www.edenalt.com/about.htm.

Eden. (2006c). www.edenalt.com/10.htm.

Ito, C. (1997). Managing challenging behavior in the classroom. Presentation, Eastern Virginia, William and Mary, January 23, 1997.

Melwood. (1980). *The Melwood manual: A planting and operations manual for horticultural training and work co-op programs.* Author.

Public Broadcasting System. (2002). & thou shalt honor: The Eden Alternative. Author.

Reber, A. S. (1985). *Dictionary of psychology.* New York: Penguin Books.

Redford, W., Overlan, E., Ryzewski, J., Beach, M., & Willard, H. (1970). The use of a therapeutic milieu on a continuing care unit in general hospital. *Annals of Internal Medicine, 73*:957-962.

Schwartz, M. (1957). What is the therapeutic milieu? In M. Greenblat, D. Levinson, &. R. Williams (Eds.), *The patient and the mental hospital.* pp 130-144. Glencoe, Illinois: The Free Press.

Body Mechanics and Ergonomics

Body mechanics describe the efficient use of one's body to complete tasks and is closely tied with mechanical engineering principles. Ergonomics is the study of how to position the body and objects in the environment to maximize performance and decrease injury. This discussion takes into account physiology, psychology, and mechanical engineering.

There are seven basic elements that play a part in body mechanics. The therapist needs to know them for two reasons:

1. Often clients with impairments will have poor body mechanics. To help the client problem solve barriers to participation the therapist often needs to address at least one of the elements of body mechanics.
2. Other members of the treatment team discuss these elements during team meetings to describe impairments and precautions necessary for each client. To function as a member of the treatment team and to reduce potential risks to clients the recreational therapist will need to understand the elements of body mechanics.

Timbly and Lewis (1992) list the seven elements of body mechanics as:

1. *Gravity*: The force that holds us on the earth and causes everything to move to the lowest possible level. It defines up and down.
2. *Energy*: The capacity for action. Energy is required to move things from one place to another, including the client moving his/her body. Energy is required to handle gravity, but the amount of energy required is less with good body mechanics.
3. *Balance*: A position of equilibrium or stability. To stay in balance, a person must keep the center of gravity over the base of support. Larger bases of support make it easier to move and stay in balance.
4. *Center of gravity*: The central point of the mass of an object. The center of gravity for a standing person is about two inches below the belly button, halfway from front to back and in the middle from side to side. Obesity tends to move the center of gravity forward from the place where the body structures are best able to handle weight.
5. *Line of gravity*: An imaginary line defined by the pull of gravity to go straight up and down through the center of gravity. Good body mechanics requires other structures, such as the head, to also be on the line for lowest energy requirements.
6. *Base of support*: The part of an object in contact with the ground. Interactions with the center of gravity affect balance. The feet are the base of support when a person is in a standing position.
7. *Alignment*: The position of the parts of the body in relation to each other. We call the best body alignment good posture.

Often, using good body mechanics is based on common sense tempered with self-discipline about how you move your body. Trombly makes the point by stating:

> Use of correct body mechanics is absolutely necessary for anyone with chronic low back pain, but it is also recommended for all persons engaged in physical work inside or outside the home. The principles of good body mechanics elaborate on the ideas of joint alignment, use of large muscles instead of small, and working in harmony with gravity. Specifically, the principles are keep the head aligned with the trunk (tuck the chin); keep the shoulders and hips parallel (don't twist the trunk); maintain pelvic tilt (tuck the buttocks or keep one foot raised on a low stool while standing); maintain good balance (position the feet shoulder distance apart, one foot forward); keep the back straight (bend at the hip and knees simultaneously rather than bend over at the waist); and push before pulling and pull before lifting. If the person must lift and carry, he should keep the object close to the body to reduce the length of the resistance lever arm and subsequently the strain on trunk muscles and spinal ligaments (p. 412).

These principles can be applied not only in a static position (e.g., standing), but also in dynamic activity. For example, if you are walking past an item that you wish to retrieve, you should fully turn your feet, legs, hips, trunk, and shoulders to face the item rather than twisting your trunk.

One of the most common injuries due to poor body mechanics is lower back pain. However, muscle strains and sprains due to poor body mechanics are not limited to the lower back. The biggest risk factors for injury due to poor body mechanics include poor posture, being out of shape or overweight, and moving the body incorrectly. Individuals with physical disabilities may be at a higher risk of injury due to poor body mechanics because: 1. center of gravity, line of gravity, base of support, and alignment may be changed and compromised as a direct result of the impairment; 2. the client may lack knowledge or cognitive ability to understand good body mechanics based on the modified body structure; and 3. staff working with clients may not take into account a change in energy level, balance, center of gravity, line of gravity, base of support, or alignment when teaching the client new skills. Some of the basics of good body mechanics, appropriate for both clients and therapists, are presented next.

Bending and leaning: Even though bending and leaning usually brings up the mental picture of someone bending over and touching his/her toes, proper bending and leaning involves the hips, knees, feet, and stomach muscles more than the back.

- When bending to pick something up that is further away than the length of your arms, the first action should be to step closer to the item so that it is within arm's length. If this is not possible, widen your base of support. This means standing with your feet shoulder-width apart with one foot slightly ahead of the other. Use (tighten) your stomach and thigh muscles as you lean forward. This helps your body maintain balance as it moves out of optimal alignment and is pulled forward.

- When bending to pick up something that is lower than your hands, bend at the knees and hips instead of your back (squat down). Lower yourself using the strength in your thigh muscles. This helps maintain an alignment between your line of gravity and the body structures that are best suited to bear weight.

- If seated in a wheelchair, the task of bending and leaning will vary depending on the abilities and limitations of the client. A client may have mobility limitations that restrict trunk flexion or rotation due to paralysis (e.g., tetraplegia), surgery (e.g., short-term back surgery parameters of limited trunk flexion and rotation, total hip precautions that prohibit bending more than 90°), or injury (e.g., back injury that causes pain with flexion or rotation). If a client sitting in a wheelchair is able to bend at the trunk to pick up an item from the floor, the first thing that s/he should do is to propel the wheelchair past the item and then back up so that the item is now on the side of the wheelchair. The reason for doing this is twofold:
  - It properly aligns the caster wheels so that the front of the wheelchair is supported and does not tip forward when the client leans to pick up the item (when you back up the wheelchair, the caster wheels spin around so that the majority of the wheel is in front of the caster arm).
  - Reaching to the side to retrieve an item from the floor is safer than reaching forward because it minimizes the chance of the wheelchair tipping forward. Added supports for

bending and leaning include the use of a reacher (see Equipment section) and other sturdy objects to assist with balance when bending and leaning (e.g., hooking one arm around the wheelchair armrest to provide balance support, especially for people who have high level paraplegia).

Lifting objects: Lifting incorrectly is the most common cause of back injury in health care workers (Coastal Healthcare, 1993). Health care workers lift as much weight as construction workers. Usually the best lifting technique involves keeping the object being lifted close to your body with your feet straddling the object. Bend with your knees and hips. It is important to keep your head in alignment with your back (don't lean forward) and your shoulders in alignment with your hips (don't twist). If you need to lift a heavy object above your waist try to lift it to waist level, place it on a secure table, change your grip, and lift again maintaining good alignment with an adequate base of support to maintain your balance. Remember that when you hold an object your center of gravity shifts to the center of mass for you and what you are holding.

These techniques can also be used for clients who do not have lifting or movement restrictions. Lifting techniques will need to be modified for those who have restrictions such as weight limits (e.g., related to cardiac problems), range of motion impairments (e.g., upper extremity injury, contracture), paralysis (e.g., from stroke), or joint protection precautions (e.g., for rheumatoid arthritis).

Client transfers: In this case, client transfer refers to a therapist or caregiver physically moving a client from one location to another, not a transfer done by a client. Communication is the most critical element. You must make sure that you use the correct transfer for the client (check the medical chart) because using the wrong transfer technique may injure both you and the client. Communicate with the client to determine how much the client will be able to help you with the transfer. (Does the client understand what to do? Does the client have the skills or strength to help out?). And, if you are doing a two-person transfer, communicate with the other person to make sure that the transfer goes smoothly.

If you are moving a client in bed, point your feet in the direction that you plan to move the client. It is common for clients who need assistance with bed mobility to have a "draw sheet" under their torso. A draw sheet is a stout piece of fabric that usually measures two to three feet by five to six feet. If you put a sheet of plastic under the draw sheet, the sheet will slide more easily. Talk with the client and other staff who may be helping you to coordinate efforts.

If you are helping a client go from sitting on the side of the bed to standing, make sure that your knees are braced against the client's knees. This provides a counter balance, brings your mutual line of gravity closer to the muscles that need to support the weight, and dynamically provides a wider dynamic base of support for you as you lift the client. These dynamics only work well when the client has slip-resistant foot coverings.

Whenever possible (and if you are trained in its use) use a mechanical lifting device such as a Hoyer lift.

Posture: Having good posture for the back is the basis of good body mechanics. The back normally has three gentle curves that help distribute stress throughout the vertebra and discs. The three gentle curves in the back are at the neck (slight curve forward), the shoulders (slight curve backward), and the lower back (slight curve forward). Maintaining these curves through most activities will reduce strain on the back.

Pushing and pulling: Whenever possible push an item instead of pulling. People can usually push twice as much weight as they can pull before musculoskeletal damage occurs. When pushing an object, make sure to stay close to the weight of the load without leaning forward. Use arm, stomach, and leg muscles to move items.

Repetitive motion: Repetitive motions can cause damage to the moving body parts unless precautions are taken. Try to take breaks, vary the movements, move light loads, and turn the entire body instead of twisting at the waist when possible.

Sitting: Sitting is almost twice as hard on back muscles as standing (Coast Healthcare, 1993). Part of the reason for this is the beneficial curves in the spine are straightened out by sitting in some chairs. The lumbar curve is especially at risk to be reduced. This reduction in the curve modifies the center of gravity, line of gravity, and base of support. Chair height is also important in helping maintain beneficial spinal curves, base of support, and line of gravity. When sitting, your knees should be at the same height as your hips. If someone has a loss of sensation and sits in a way that reduces the lumbar spinal curve, base of support, or unbalances the line of gravity, accumulative damage may be occurring to the spine and associated muscles without the typical "warning" signs of lower back pain.

Standing: Standing, especially static (not moving around) standing, increases the stress on back muscles. To help relieve some of the stress it is a good idea to stand with one foot in front of the other and supported on a slightly raised footstool. Switch the forward foot every five or ten minutes.

Transfer belts: In a treatment setting almost all types of transfers should be done with the client wearing a transfer belt. A transfer belt is a cotton or nylon belt that is about three inches wide and five feet long. This is placed around the client's waist on top of all clothing and tightened so that the therapist's hand has room to comfortably hold firmly onto the belt with only a little extra slack. Transfer belts are for both the therapist's and the client's safety. If the client were to start falling, the therapist does not have to catch the client to stop the fall. S/he can use the belt to safely guide the client to the floor bending at the hips and knees and not the back.

If the client becomes slightly off balance the therapist can help the client regain balance by providing a steadying pull on the transfer belt.

Ergonomic Risk Factors

burlingame (2001) discusses seven risk factors that increase damage to the body and should be considered when evaluating clients' activities to ensure that no further harm is done. The seven risk factors are

- *Duration*: Duration refers to the length of time that the body is exposed to a stress in the environment. Increased length of exposure can lead to increased impact on the immediate area of exposure and increased general fatigue response. Generally, the greater the duration of exposure to a stressful risk factor, the greater the length of time it takes the body to revert to its baseline function.
- *Force*: The greater the force needed to complete the task, the greater the physiological stress to the body (muscles, tendons, and joints).
- *Mechanical compression or contact stress*: Mechanical compression refers to pressure points created when an object places uneven pressure on the body such as a garden shovel would place extra stress on the tissue in the palm of the hand at the points that the handle of the shovel contacts the hand. Mechanical compression can impede blood flow and interfere with nerve function.
- *Posture*: Awkward postures place stress on joints and surrounding tissue. This leads to extra muscle and tendon fatigue and joint soreness. The added stress is thought to contribute to an increased likelihood of musculoskeletal disorders.
- *Repetition*: A repetitive motion is an action that is repeated many times with a cycle time of less than 30 seconds or when the basic cycle accounts for 50% or more of the total work cycle (OSHA, 1995). This repetitive action can lead to acceler-

ated muscle fatigue and increased risk of muscle-tendon damage. Tasks that are very repetitive do not allow time for adequate tissue recovery.

- *Temperature*: The lower a temperature goes, the greater the loss of dexterity, sensitivity, and grip force. Also, a lower temperature can make the impact of vibration worse. OSHA (1995) recommends that metal surfaces be above 59°F as temperatures below this point decrease dexterity. Metal surfaces below 44.6°F may lead to numbness. The American Conference of Governmental Industrial Hygienists (1995) recommends the following exposure limits: for sedentary work, 60°F; for light work, 40°F; and for moderate work (fine motor dexterity not required), 20°F.

- *Vibration*: Vibration types can be impact, oscillation, or combined impact and oscillation. Vibration can also be categorized as localized (e.g., vibration of the hand) or whole body (e.g., riding on a motorcycle). National vibration threshold standards have been set for some aspects of the work place to limit the neurological and fatigue factors associated with vibration.

Documenting Ergonomic Skills

Many clients need education on correct body mechanics. Therapists document the specific problem that the client is having with body mechanics or ergonomics (e.g., client's computer station setup is not ergonomically correct contributing to lower back and neck pain), recommendations (e.g., recommended to raise computer monitor to eye height), ability to apply proper body mechanics and ergonomics (usually measured as a percentage), and areas where the client needs assistance (e.g., requires moderate verbal cues to maintain good body posture during table games).

Clients increase their skills for using good body mechanics through observing the therapist role modeling the desired skills, education, and practice. If a client has difficulty performing proper body mechanics because of a specific disability (e.g., kyphosis), the therapist encourages the client to come as close as possible to good body mechanics (e.g., stand as upright as possible). Activities can also be modified to increase a client's ability to maintain good posture (e.g., placing a box on top of the table and placing the activity on top of the box raises the height of the activity and encourages the client to stand upright).

References

American Conference of Governmental Industrial Hygienists. (1995). *Threshold limits for chemical substances and physical agents and biological exposure indices.* Cincinnati, OH: ACGIH.

burlingame, j. (2001). *Idyll Arbor's therapy dictionary*, (2nd ed.). Ravensdale, WA: Idyll Arbor, Inc.

Coastal Healthcare. (1993). *Protecting your back.* Virginia Beach, VA: author.

Occupational Safety and Health Administration. (1995). *Ergonomic protection standard* (draft). Washington, DC: Government Printing Office.

Timbly, B. & Lewis, L. (1992). *Fundamental skills and concepts in patient care* (5th ed.). Philadelphia, PA: Lippincott Company.

Boundaries

Many of us have a general understanding of what a boundary is. One of the easiest to understand examples of a boundary is a property line, which is the line between one person's property and his/her neighbor's property. Psychology and counseling have adopted the term "boundaries" to describe the invisible line between responsibilities that "belong" to a client and responsibilities that belong to others. When talking about the line that divides responsibilities, the word boundaries is plural to convey the idea that clients have multiple boundaries for which they are responsible. Boundaries are the skeleton on which all of our relationship skills are built.

Another word for boundaries could be personal limits, although "boundaries" is the term most often used in treatment. An example of a boundary may make the concept clearer. A teenager makes a pizza but leaves all of the dirty dishes for mom to clean. Developmentally a teenager is expected to be able to clean up after himself/herself. By leaving the dirty dishes for mom the teen has not assumed the responsibility for picking up after himself/herself. The consequences of not doing the dishes will help form the teen's understanding of his/her boundaries. If mom regularly cleans up the dirty dishes instead of ensuring that the teen cleans them, the teen learns that s/he can manipulate his/her responsibilities and boundaries and passively cause someone else to take on his/her responsibility. If mom sees the dirty dishes, asks the teen to clean the dishes, and some negative consequences are implied or explicit, then the teen learns that the dirty dishes are his/her responsibility.

People are not born with boundaries. We learn boundaries based on the environment in which we are raised and within our cultural understandings. Boundaries are skills that are like building blocks helping us to continually define "right" and "wrong" while working toward healthy relationships. A good foundation of boundary skills is required before social and/or intimate relationships can be healthy ones. Developmentally clients learn sets of skills as they go through a series of levels of personal boundaries. An infant has little awareness that s/he is a separate person from mom. As a toddler the child learns that all that s/he sees does not belong to him/her; in fact, quite a bit may be off limits. Hopefully, as a child grows his/her caregivers are slowly allowing the child to assume more responsibility. Once a client is an adult, the developmental process of changing personal boundaries does not stop. At first, when the adult has his/her own children, the adult is fully responsible for

the child and must learn along with the child the ever-changing line between what is the adult's responsibility and what is the developing child's responsibility. The adult's responsibilities associated with his/her parent(s) also continue to change with the adult child often taking over the caretaker role for aging parents.

Much of the literature related to boundaries and health care emphasizes the importance of maintaining professional boundaries between the therapist and the client. This section does not address that specific type of boundary but explores the various elements of personal boundaries that clients will need to learn to interact with their community.

Cloud and Townsend (1992) talk about boundaries as property lines. Most people are aware of when they are standing on their own property and when they cross over onto their neighbor's lawn. Cloud and Townsend list different types of boundaries for which we are personally responsible. If any of these boundaries are drawn in the wrong place, the client's relationship with others may be impaired. Some of the boundaries listed by Cloud and Townsend that frequently cause impaired relationships are 1. feelings, 2. attitudes and beliefs, 3. behaviors, 4. limits, and 5. desires.

Feelings

Feelings are emotions that originate because of what is going on around a person and because of chemical changes in the body. The client's feelings belong to the client. When a person takes responsibility for feelings the person has the ability to 1. identify the feeling and 2. realize that the origin of the feeling is within himself/herself. Owning a feeling is the first step in taking purposeful and productive actions within his/her feelings boundaries. Let's go back to the case of the teenager who left the dirty pizza dishes. Walking into the kitchen the mom becomes furious that dirty dishes are all around. With healthy boundaries the mom would:

- recognize that she is very angry (identifying her feelings),
- recognize that her teenager did not force her to have angry feelings but that she chose to be angry ("owning" her feelings),
- evaluate what exactly made her angry (identifying what upset her; such as being angry that her teen was inconsiderate of her feelings, that she was experiencing PMS emotional fluctuations, and/or she was having trouble balancing her checkbook and was already frustrated), and then

- evaluate the most productive actions for her to reduce her anger.

Owning your feelings allows you to *act* in a purposeful manner instead of *reacting*. Related ICF codes include b156 Emotional Functions and much of d7 Interpersonal Interactions and Relationships.

Attitudes and Beliefs

Attitudes are the cognitive position that one has in relationship to a situation and beliefs are things that someone accepts as "true." For example, a sixty-five-year-old woman believes that it is important to exercise every day and she has a positive attitude about herself because she manages to exercise almost every day. People tend to act or react to situations based on their attitudes, which are based on what they believe to be true. If a client believes something that is not true, then the actions that s/he takes because of attitudes can impair relationships. For example, one of the diagnostic criteria for anorexia nervosa is that the client *believes* that s/he is overweight when objective analysis would indicate that s/he is significantly below a healthy weight. As a result, the client with anorexia nervosa spends much of the day working hard to not gain weight. When the parents of the person with anorexia nervosa (or friends, or treatment team) tell the client that s/he is underweight, the client usually reacts with a pushback type response. The person's beliefs and attitudes are within his/her own personal boundaries. Regardless of the fact that the person with anorexia nervosa is wrong about his/her weight, s/he is right in trying to protect personal boundaries. While anorexia nervosa has one of the highest mortality rates of all psychological disorders, from a therapy standpoint it does not necessarily make good sense to teach the client that it is okay for the treatment team to violate personal boundaries except in the most extreme situations. Clients with anorexia nervosa often have very poor personal boundaries. Treatment for clients with anorexia nervosa should work with the client, helping him/her learn healthy personal boundaries while also working to modify the client's incorrect belief about being overweight. From a therapy approach this would look like educational opportunities and games that allow the person with anorexia nervosa to begin internalizing what normal weight looks like. The therapist would let the client know that s/he believes that the client is too thin ("To me it seems like your weight is so low that it is dangerous.") versus just telling the client and expecting the client to automatically change his/her belief ("You are too skinny."). This is similar to the I Messages discussed in "Behavior Manipulation."

A subset of boundaries associated with beliefs is the ability to recognize that one's thoughts are one's responsibility. Developmentally teenagers and adults have the responsibility to evaluate the ideas that others present to them or ideas that they think up themselves and to make the decision whether to accept them (believe them) or not. To have healthy thought boundaries it is important to examine thoughts for potential distortions, learn more, and take "ownership" for thoughts. A therapist may find that an appropriate intervention is to teach the client specific steps to evaluate the quality and accuracy of his/her thoughts. ICF codes b160 Thought Functions or one of the sub-codes under b164 Higher Level Cognitive Functions and d177 Making Decisions could be used to document a client's level of difficulty with boundaries.

Behaviors

Behaviors are visible actions that can be seen by others. All behaviors have consequences: cause and effect consequences. For example, a client gets really angry with a fellow client during a group therapy arts and crafts project. To show the other client how angry s/he is, the person who is angry grabs the other client's craft project and destroys it.

The other client's craft project was not the property of the person who was angry and by destroying someone else's property a boundary line was crossed. By crossing that boundary line not only does the person who is angry still have an issue that needs to be addressed, but now also should have the responsibility for "making right" the boundary that was crossed. A therapist has two directions to take to address skill development in this situation. First, clients need to learn that other people's property is off limits, period. This may require practice (maybe even game-type activities) to help the client more clearly define what is "his/hers" and what is "others." Second, working on identifying and owning one's feelings is an important skill to nurture.

People choose the actions they take, and healthy choices (behaviors or actions) are ones that are made because it seems right to take that action, not because others have pushed for that choice. Owning up to the responsibilities that are created by the choices one makes is a learned skill. See the treatment section at the end for possible ways to score an intervention in this area.

Limits

Limits are the boundaries to the *exposure* that people are willing to accept from different situations and people. A client recovering from alcohol dependence who decides not to include bars or other areas that serve alcoholic beverages in his/her free time activities is an example of someone who is exercising a healthy boundary related to limiting exposure. The "Just Say NO" anti-drug program for teenagers is another example of an exposure boundary. There are other exposure boundaries that are harder to define and identify. For example, an adult who is newly in a wheelchair after an automobile accident may find that his/her friends try "helping" by pushing the wheelchair around when the client is very capable of doing so himself/herself. For those who violate this boundary the client may need to learn appropriate assertiveness skills, starting with words, to re-establish his/her boundary. If words do not cause the "helpers" to limit their "help," then the client may decide to limit his/her exposure to those people. In many situations it is an appropriate use of boundaries for clients to use the skills/talents that they have without undo interference from others. Learning skills related to appropriate assertiveness training is important not only when the client is protecting his/her boundaries but also for general communication with others. ICF code b1266 Confidence is an appropriate place to score a client's level of difficulty with setting limits. It is also discussed in d240 Handling Stress and Other Psychological Demands,

Desire

Desire is another type of boundary. Wanting something or to control something that "belongs" to another person or is "within" the other person's boundaries is a common type of boundary violation. Clients need to learn not only what "things" are within their boundaries but also what "things" belong to others. This is a skill that usually starts developing around the age of two but it seems that even elderly adults still work on fine-tuning this boundary. People who are sex offenders desire others and lack good boundaries as to what is "theirs" versus "others." A lack of skills related to desire boundaries is often a deficit in victims of abuse and clients with a history of drug dependence or sociopathy. ICF codes under b130 Energy and Drive Functions look at these issues.

Treatment

A client's ability to establish and maintain healthy friendships and love relationships is tied very closely to his/her ability to exercise healthy boundaries. The development of skills related to boundaries must accompany the teaching of appropriate social skills.

When the client starts setting healthy personal boundaries, it disrupts his/her current relationships with family members, friends, coworkers, and peers. Chances are that if the client is seeing a recreational therapist, s/he has had a recent crisis or loss in his/her life. Cloud & Townsend (1992) point out that as clients learn to have healthy personal boundaries (or limits) one of two things happens: "1. we set limits and risk losing a relationship" or "2. we don't set limits and remain a prisoner to the wishes of another" (p. 64).

"Fixing" unhealthy boundary skills may further exacerbate the current crisis. The client will need a safe, welcoming, and healthy relation with at least one other person to feel comfortable using his/her new boundaries. A relationship that can provide consistency and caring is critical. The therapist cannot function as this support system as that might encourage co-dependency with the client. The therapist's job is to teach the skills necessary to improve personal boundaries, not to be the emotional anchor for the client.

It would be a violation of professional boundaries for the therapist to be this person. The therapist is in the role of teacher or therapist. Therapists may be friendly with clients but cannot be their friend (a mixing of roles that is in violation of professional ethics). The therapist needs to anticipate the potential stress on the client's current relationships as they work on developing healthier skills related to boundaries.

Codes that are especially relevant to boundary issues include b126 Temperament and Personality Functions, b152 Emotional Functions, b160 Thought Functions, and d155 Acquiring Skills. Understanding boundaries is also important for all of the relationship codes in Activities and Participation Chapter 7 Interpersonal Interactions and Relationships. Scoring in that chapter should be done by using the code for the particular relationship where the boundary issue comes up.

References

Cloud, H. & Townsend, J. (1992). *Boundaries*. Grand Rapids MI: Zondervan.

Community Accessibility Training

Community Accessibility Training (CAT) is the process of educating clients about community accessibility issues as they relate to architecture and services. This includes having an understanding of basic accessibility needs specific to the client's situation (e.g., ramp at front entrance that meets accessibility standards, someone to assist the client obtain groceries off of the shelves) and the ability to apply this information to real-life tasks and settings.

Community Accessibility Training increases the client's awareness of community barriers and encourages the development of skills for solving problems with barriers. Reducing architectural barriers may aid in conserving physical energy, as well as maximizing independence, functioning, and overall mental, emotional, physical, and social health. It also teaches the client activity analysis skills that assist with determining realistic community tasks. Engaging in tasks that meet the accessibility needs or expose the client to minimal barriers improves task performance that can affect self-esteem and confidence and increase the likelihood of community involvement after discharge.

Indications

The training is appropriate for:
1. A client who is new to using a wheelchair in a community setting.
2. A client who has been using a wheelchair in a community setting but is not fully aware of community accessibility issues.
3. A client who is using any other assistive device (e.g., walker, cane) or a client whose walking endurance is impaired. This client would also benefit from Energy Conservation Training (also in the Techniques section).

The more accessible a facility is, the less physical energy one has to expend (e.g., it takes less energy to enter a facility that has no steps than a place that has five steps, it takes less energy to walk on smooth surfaces than on surfaces that are uneven and bumpy).

Contraindications: A client who has significant cognitive impairments that impact his/her ability to recall, retain, or apply verbal education. If significant cognitive impairments are evident, the therapist will need to educate the client's caregivers since they will be the ones to facilitate community activities. This could be in the form of a face-to-face session, phone conversation, or in written form (giving the family a handout for review and encouraging them to contact you with any questions). A written handout should always be given to the client/family for future reference regardless of the form of education provided because often there are too many things to remember. The form should have a place for the therapist to fill in his/her name and phone number so that the client or family can ask questions at a later date. A sample handout is shown at the end of this topic.

Training Description

The length and frequency of Community Accessibility Training sessions will vary depending upon the identified needs and abilities of the client. On average, Community Accessibility Training takes about one hour (one half hour to review community accessibility issues and another half hour to practice applying the information through role-playing and phone calls). This is not to say that a client will be fully proficient in knowledge and application of community accessibility issues in one hour, but the client should be able to obtain a basic understanding of the information and be able to apply it to simple community activities.

Education should take place in a quiet/non-distracting environment to promote concentration and attention.

The therapist should have relevant materials (e.g., CAT handout, highlighter, pen).

Additional sessions should be scheduled to allow for evaluation of activity performance (ability to apply information in a real-life environment). This is typically done by planning a community outing. Clients are directed to determine the level of accessibility of a site prior to going to the site, as well as problem solve for perceived barriers. The amount of therapist assistance with this task will vary depending on the client's abilities and goals.

A general process of CAT training is reflected in the outline given below. Therapists should alter this process as needed to best meet the needs of the client.
1. The client is educated about the Americans with Disabilities Act (ADA) prior to being educated about specific community accessibility issues. (See "Americans with Disabilities Act Education" in this section.) This gives the client a foundation to better understand the compliance regulations for meeting accessibility and service needs.
2. The therapist reviews the importance of community involvement as it relates to all aspects of health. The therapist gives specific examples of how community involvement will directly affect the client's level of independence,

functioning, and quality of life. The therapist validates any reservations expressed by the client about participation in community activities and provides encouragement. If the client is saying "no" to community activities, then s/he is going to be resistant to CAT (e.g., listens to what the therapist is saying but blocks most of it out, refuses the session because he is not planning on going out of the house). Example: A client is afraid of going out into the community and expresses this fear to the therapist. The therapist validates the client's fear and reassures the client that feeling fear is normal because the situation is new and unfamiliar. The therapist stresses that they are a team and they will conquer the fear together. The therapist may also express faith in the client's ability to conquer the fear to reassure the client of his/her own inner strength (e.g., "Joe, I have faith in you. I've worked with lots of people who have had spinal cord injuries and I know you can do it. You are a strong and determined person. So, put some faith in me and trust that we can work through this together, ok?").

3. Once the client is ready to hear the information, the therapist explains the purpose of CAT (see the initial description of CAT at the beginning of this section). Explain to the client that employees who answer the client's questions about accessibility and services do not always know what accessibility entails. They may not be fully aware of what their responsibilities are for providing accessible services for people who have disabilities. Therefore, it is important to have specific questions that determine the level of accessibility of the facility and to learn how to think ahead (perform an activity analysis) of the outing to determine what assistance, if any, will be needed to access a facility.

4. The therapist reviews the handout shown below with the client, seeking to expand the client's knowledge about specific accessibility issues. It is a very basic worksheet that will not overwhelm the client. The therapist should make notations or changes to the worksheet to meet the client's individual accessibility needs (e.g., write down the width of a client's wheelchair if it is not a standard wheelchair). While reviewing the handout, the therapist expands on each issue by engaging the client in problem solving for "what ifs" (e.g., What if the bathroom is not wheelchair accessible? What if there are two steps to get into the building and it is a public facility?). Clients who are newly disabled can't be expected to know the answers to these questions because they probably haven't been exposed to these

issues. Therapists should actively engage the client in problem solving by asking leading questions and encouraging the client to identify solutions. For example:

Therapist: "Let's suppose that you are told that the place has a ramp at the entrance, but when you get there it is too steep and you are unable to push up the ramp. What would you do?" Give the client a moment to think about this barrier.

Client: "I guess I would go back home."

Therapist: "Under the ADA you are entitled to assistance that is reasonable. Knowing this, does this give you any other options instead of turning around and going back home?" Again, allow the client time to consider the problem.

Client: "I guess I could ask someone to give me a hand and help me push up the ramp, but I don't think I would do that."

Therapist: "No?" The question looks for a further response from the client.

Client: "No, it's too awkward, besides if I'm at the bottom of the ramp how would I get the attention of an employee unless I ask someone else to help me. Then what if they have trouble pushing me up the ramp and we both get hurt?"

Therapist: "That's a very good insight. I agree with you that you have to be careful in choosing whom to ask for assistance and you also have to feel comfortable turning down assistance if you don't feel safe letting that person help you. So, how do you think you could get an employee's attention?"

Client: "I guess I could ask someone who is going into the building to tell an employee that I need some assistance and to send someone out to give me a hand."

Therapist: "Good idea. Now let me pose this question. What if the employee comes out to help you and he is not helping you correctly? Let's say he tries to pull you up the ramp backwards instead of forwards, what would you do?"

Client: "Well, before he even started I would tell him exactly what I need him to do."

Therapist: "Excellent."

5. Once the therapist and client finish reviewing the handout, the therapist asks the client to go through each issue and repeat back what s/he has learned. This allows the therapist an opportunity to assess the client's understanding of the material and provide further education as needed

so that the client fully grasps the information. Clients can be additionally challenged to identify accessibility issues that relate solely to specific activities (e.g., "If you were planning to go swimming at a recreation center, what additional questions would you need to ask?" looking for issues related to the locker and pool area).

6. When the client has a good grasp of the information, the therapist asks the client to role-play a telephone call (e.g., "Let's pretend that I am an employee at the local hardware store and you need to find out if it is accessible and if they can provide you with the assistance that you might require. So, first tell me what questions you think are relevant to ask and then let's role-play how a telephone call to this place might sound."). The information in the handout at the end of this section is very basic. Therapists are encouraged to use the "Americans with Disabilities Act Accessibility Guidelines" and/or the "Uniform Federal Accessibility Standards" to help the client fine-tune his/her outline of questions so that it reflects the client's specific needs. For example, the questions that a client with a hearing impairment would ask will be very different from a client who has a complete spinal cord injury. Therapists may also find it helpful to make accessibility question sheets that relate to specific places and activities (e.g., a list of questions to ask a restaurant, a store, a state park).

Outcome Criteria

Ask the client to explain how s/he would handle particular situations, such as, "If you were invited to lunch at an unfamiliar restaurant, what questions would you need to ask to determine the level of accessibility?" Document the response in percentages (e.g., "Client able to verbally apply community accessibility issues to proposed community situations at 75%.") or level of assistance (e.g., "Client required moderate verbal cues to verbally apply community accessibility issues to proposed situations."). The client's ability to apply community accessibility issues to a "real-life" community setting or simulated community task should also be addressed and documented in the same manner (e.g., "Client contacted local restaurant via telephone to determine level of accessibility; required minimal verbal cues to fully identify level of accessibility."). CAT is not scored within the ICF. It is an intervention that is used to assist the client in problem solving (e.g., d175 Solving Problems), overcoming barriers (e150 Design, Construction, and Building Products and Technology of Buildings for Public Use), and

improving participation in specific activities (e.g., d910 Community Life).

Community Accessibility Training References

Therapists should consult the "Americans with Disabilities Act Accessibility Guidelines" and/or the "Uniform Federal Accessibility Standards" for specific measurements and dimensions required for accessibility. Therapists can request free copies of these documents. See "Americans with Disabilities Act Education" in this section for contact information. Therapists often consult these two documents to provide facilities and employers with accessibility dimensions when architectural changes need to be made. Private homes are not held to accessibility standards. For example, if a client needs to build a ramp to the entrance of his home, he does not have to build it to ADA specifications. However, if the ramp is too steep, the client may not be able to propel his/her wheelchair up or down the ramp safely. Clients are encouraged to build ramps and other structural changes as close to the guidelines as possible to maximize their ability to function in that space and ensure their safety. Therapists, therefore, also provide information on accessibility dimensions and codes to clients and their families. This information is often given in conjunction with a home, worksite, or community site evaluation. See "Integration" in this chapter for suggestions on completing these assessments.

Community Accessibility Handout

You will notice that the community accessibility handout (below) contains information on how to problem solve for each issue. This is incorporated into the handout to help the client consider other options if the ideal solution is not available. The client can make multiple copies of a generic sheet so that s/he has it handy for each place that s/he calls. To help the client remember the level of accessibility for each place and the services that are provided, the client can put them in a binder or store a copy on a PDA. When the client returns from the site, s/he can make additional notes about the facility (e.g., very steep ramp at front entrance, very helpful staff, tight bathroom but able to use it). Clients can also make up different sheets for different places (e.g., a form that contains questions that are specific for shopping centers, a form that contain specific questions related to going to outdoor recreation areas).

Accessibility Handout

When you are trying to determine the level of accessibility of a community facility (e.g., library, restaurant, or store), it is important to ask the specific questions that are relevant to your needs (e.g., the number of steps to enter the building, availability of handicapped parking). Calling the facility and asking these specific questions will not only increase your awareness of the obstacles that the facility may present, but it will also increase the likelihood of success and minimize frustration. It is important, however, to realize that a place may sound accessible and still not fully meet your needs when you arrive (e.g., step height is 10" and you are able to do 6", the manual doors are too heavy to open without assistance).

To use the handout, call the facility ahead of time, ask all of the relevant questions, and make notes in the right hand column. Here's a way to start the conversation, "Hello. I am considering coming to your theater to see a show. I have a disability and I (use a wheelchair, can't walk very far, use a walker, etc.). I was wondering about the level of accessibility at your facility. Are you accessible?"

If the person says that the facility is indeed handicap accessible, then say, "Ok, then I have a few specific questions that I need to ask you so that I don't get stuck when I'm there. Do you have a few minutes?"

Most people will say "sure." However, occasionally people will not want to help. If that happens, ask to speak with a supervisor.

If you have any questions concerning community accessibility while you are here or after you are discharged, please feel free to call your Recreational Therapist _____ at _____.

Accessibility Issue	Notes
Handicap parking *Preparation:* Did you apply for a handicap parking placard or tag? A placard can be moved from car to car because it is registered to you and not to a vehicle. You don't have to have a vehicle or a driver's license to get one. A tag is a license plate that stays on the car. You can apply for both. The placard is free and there is usually a fee for the license plate. *Questions:* Do you have handicap parking? Where is it? *Problem Solving:* If the facility does not provide handicap parking OR if there is no handicap parking available when you get there: 1. If it is safe, the driver can let you out of the vehicle at the front door. 2. If it is safe, the driver can pull halfway into a regular parking spot so that the car door still has enough room to open fully. Put the hazard lights on and allow the driver to assist you in getting out of the vehicle. Once you are out of the vehicle, the driver can pull the car the rest of the way into the parking spot. Reverse the procedure when you leave. 3. Park in the middle of two regular parking spots. Be sure to hang your handicap-parking placard if you do not have a handicap tag on the car. Place a sign in the car window, "I'm allowed to take up two spaces because there was no handicap parking space available." This sort of explanation will reduce the annoyance of others. Write the note on a piece of cardboard and keep it in the car at all times.	

Accessibility Issue	Notes
Entrance *Questions:* Is there a level entrance or a ramp? Where is it? How steep is it? If there are steps, how many steps are there and are there one or two handrails? How far apart are the handrails? *Problem Solving:* Consider the steepness and surface of the ramp, especially if you will be going to this facility by yourself. The suggested steepness is a one-inch rise for every 12" of distance (often described as one in twelve). So if there is a series of three steps that measure a total of 18" high, then the ramp should be 18' long). The level or ramped entrance may not be at the front door. Under the Americans with Disabilities Act (ADA) they are required to make "reasonable accommodations." It is reasonable to use a side or back door as an accessible entrance. Consider the number of steps. How many steps are you able to do at that time of the day (remember that energy level varies throughout the day)? If you need to hold onto two rails, remember to ask if the rails are close enough together that you can hold onto the right and left rail at the same time.	
Doors *Questions:* What type of doors do you have (electric, manual, revolving)? Are there doorsills or other access issues? *Problem Solving:* The issues you may encounter depend on the type of door: • Electric (only some of the doors may be automatic — find out where they are). • Manual (consider that you may need help due to weight of door). • Revolving (try to avoid these, if possible, because you can't control others who may push the revolving door too fast for you, and because the doors have limited space). Be aware of raised doorsills. Be sure to lift your foot and assistive device fully over the sill. If you are using a wheelchair, you may have to go through the door backwards because the front caster wheels may be too difficult to push over the sill.	
Interior Surfaces *Questions:* What is the flooring like (plush carpet, tile, concrete)? Is the surface flat throughout the facility, or will I need to go over bumps to move around? *Problem Solving:* Some surfaces can be more difficult than others. Moving on plush carpet requires more strength whether you are walking or propelling a wheelchair. Bumpy surfaces, such as doorsills, may require assistance.	

Accessibility Issue	Notes
Exterior Surfaces *Preparation:* You will need to consider how you plan to use the facility. At the very least, you will need to get to the front door from your transportation. If you are planning an activity such as going along a nature trail, you will also need to know about the specific paths you plan to use. *Questions:* What is the ground around the facility like (concrete, asphalt, gravel, packed dirt)? I will be arriving by _____ [car, bus], are there any breaks or obstacles in the surface that will make accessibility difficult? I'm planning to _____ [walk on the nature trail, use the changing room before going swimming], are there any accessibility concerns I should know about? *Problem Solving:* Packed dirt, grass, gravel, cobblestone, flagstone, bricks, hills, or tree roots can all be problems. Walking on uneven surfaces requires more energy and better balance than walking on smooth surfaces. If you are using a cane or walker on uneven surfaces, be sure that the assistive device is fully stable (not in a ditch or on a pebble) before you take a slow and careful step. If you are using a wheelchair, you may find it easier to pull the wheelchair over the uneven surfaces backwards so that the caster wheels do not get stuck in the depressions. Be sure to wear a seatbelt because if the wheelchair comes to an abrupt stop, you may not.	
Accessing Other Floors *Questions:* Is there an elevator? Is there an escalator? Where? *Problem Solving:* If you are using a wheelchair, enter elevators backwards so that you can easily see the floor numbers. Align yourself with the doors so that you can exit easily and not have to move around many people in a tight area. Escalators require a high degree of balance and quick reaction time. If you haven't had training in using escalators, it would be a good idea to get some before going to this facility. Use elevators when you can. If you are on a lower or upper floor and the elevator or escalator is not working, there are some things you can do: 1. Ask when it will be operational and wait. 2. Ask security if there is an alternate elevator (e.g., freight elevator) that is functional. 3. If repairs will not be completed in a timely manner and there is no other elevator, walk the stairs if you are able. If you are not able to walk the stairs, call emergency assistance and they will "blanket carry" you down the steps. 4. If you are using a wheelchair and are with people who are trained in this technique, they could bump you up or down the steps. If they are not trained, it could pose a great danger to you and those assisting you.	

Accessibility Issue	Notes

Bathroom
 	
Preparation: Know what kind of handicap stall you require. Usually there is a wide stall with a raised toilet seat set to the side of the stall so that a wheelchair can be placed beside the toilet. There should be a rail on the wall and another rail on the other side that flips up and down.
 	
Questions: Do you have a handicap bathroom that will meet my needs (raised toilet, rails, wide stall)? Where is it?
 	
Problem Solving: If you need assistance in the bathroom by someone of the opposite sex, ask if there is a family bathroom available or a bathroom with a locking door. If there is not, use the women's room. The men's room poses a greater threat to impinging on someone's privacy (urinals on the wall).
    If the bathroom does not meet all of your needs, you may need more assistance than usual to use the bathroom.
    Males should consider carrying a plastic bottle with a good screw-on, leak-proof lid (e.g., place it in a backpack or in a small bag on a cane or a walker) for situations where the bathroom is inaccessible (e.g., on the second floor of someone's home). Women, although it is not ideal, may want to consider wearing a protective pad designed for bladder control for situations in which the bathroom is inaccessible. Female urinals are available but they can be cumbersome. Knowing your bowel and bladder routine and designing your activities around it may also be helpful to minimize the chances of needing to use the bathroom when you are out.	

Telephone *Questions:* Do you have lowered public telephones available? Where? *Problem Solving:* Better yet, purchase a cell phone. It will be helpful in case of emergencies (e.g., car gets a flat tire, medical emergency, needing directions). There are many different types of cell phone plans that are relatively inexpensive.	
Water Fountain *Questions:* Do you have lowered public water fountains available? Where? *Problem Solving:* Better yet, keep a water bottle with you to keep yourself hydrated, as well as for taking any medication when in route to a facility.	
Aisle Width *Questions:* Are the main and side aisles wide enough to safely manipulate through using a wheelchair or walker? *Problem Solving:* Under the Americans with Disabilities Act (ADA) it is not unreasonable for an employee to move things out of your way (e.g., clothing rack on wheels) or assist you in obtaining items that are inaccessible (e.g., too high or low, aisle is too narrow to get to the item).	

Accessibility Issue	Notes
Rest Areas *Questions:* Are there rest areas available (e.g., benches along a park path)? *Problem Solving:* If your energy level is compromised, review Energy Conservation Techniques (ECT) with your therapist for ideas on how to conserve your energy and identify creative places to sit and rest. If you are using a wheelchair, be sure that long trips provide you with an opportunity to change positions.	
Special Services and Assistance *Questions:* What type of special services and assistance do you offer for someone with a disability? Ask about the specific needs that you foresee for the activity: This may include special seating, a key to use a private elevator, not having to stand in lines, discounts, specially designed rooms (handicap sleeping car on a train, handicap designed hotel room), assistance with obtaining items and getting them out to the car, availability of electric scooters, and much more. *Problem Solving:* You may be pleasantly surprised to find out the extent of services available to someone who has a disability. If there is something that you would like to do and you think that it would be too difficult, stop right there, call the place, explain your disability, and ask them what type of services they provide so that you can do it (e.g., deep-sea fishing, flying, snorkeling). Chances are that they have already considered your issues and have a solution. If they do not have a solution, propose some solutions of your own or call your recreational therapist for suggestions. As long as your requests are reasonable and easily accommodated, your ideas should be welcomed.	

Community Leisure Resource Awareness

Community leisure resource awareness is defined as identification of resources available in the community for leisure participation (e.g., transportation, facilities, programs). With this protocol the therapist can teach the client how to find leisure resources in the community that match his/her interests and allow greater participation.

Engaging in community leisure activities is recommended for health. Getting out of the house promotes exercise and socialization. Physical exercise and social support are vital components of good health (see d5701 Managing Diet and Fitness for information about benefits of exercise and Activities and Participation Chapter 7 Interpersonal Interactions and Relationships for information on the importance of friendship). Leisure in the community also exposes the client to new ideas and thoughts that can positively impact emotional and spiritual health (see d930 Religion and Spirituality). Involvement in community activities may also provide the client with an opportunity to contribute to his/her community (e.g., volunteer work). Giving time to help others can boost self-esteem and self-worth. It can contribute to feelings of productivity and make the person feel needed and wanted. All of which contribute to finding meaning in one's life as discussed in Existential Counseling in the "Education and Counseling" topic in the Techniques section.

Indications

Therapists routinely explore engagement in community leisure activities as part of the initial evaluation process of all clients. If the client's involvement in community activities meets the health needs of the client and the client does not desire to become involved in any other community activities, then community leisure resource awareness is not explored. Therapists address community leisure resource awareness if

- A client's community leisure activities do not meet the client's health needs.
- A client desires to become involved in additional community activities.
- A client is living in a new environment and is unaware of community leisure resources (e.g., recently moved into a new area or home or facility).
- There is a change in the client's abilities that will impact his/her ability to continue with prior community leisure activities.

Contraindications: If significant cognitive impairments are evident, the therapist will need to talk with the client's family member, guardian, caregiver, or activity director to ascertain if there is an indication for Community Leisure Resource Awareness. Therapists must remember that a client's interests can change with disability and that prior leisure involvement cannot be assumed to be a continued interest of the client. For clients who are unable to tell the therapist what they enjoy, the therapist should expose the client to various leisure activities and observe the client's reaction to each activity (behavior, level of participation, attitude, length of time engaged in the activity, etc.). Clients who have significant cognitive impairments will most likely respond positively to simple, physically based, repetitive activities (e.g., simple wood projects that require sanding and painting only).

If there is a positive indication, leisure interest exploration (see "Activity Pattern Development" in the Techniques section) will help determine the client's leisure attitudes, interests, and motivations to be able to match leisure desires to community resources.

Protocol

It typically takes 30 minutes or less to determine the community leisure interests and resources of the client.

A quiet and non-distracting environment is best to promote attention and concentration.

The therapist should have relevant materials (e.g., paper and pen to write down community leisure activities and resources).

Process

The therapist explores the following areas:

Community leisure places: The therapist asks the client if s/he engages in any leisure activities in the community (e.g., YMCA, teenager hangout, the park, tennis courts at the recreation center).

Frequency: For each activity noted, the therapist asks the client how often s/he participates in the activity (e.g., every Tuesday and Thursday) and the times that s/he participates (e.g., 1:00-2:00 P.M.).

Accessibility of community leisure places: If the client's functional abilities have changed since his/her last involvement in the community activity, the therapist asks the client if s/he is familiar with the level of accessibility of the place in the community. Clients who are not experienced in living with a disability will not understand this question, so the therapist will need to guide them through the thought process (e.g., is there a ramp or a level entrance to get in or are there steps, how many steps, is there a railing?). New clinicians will find it helpful to use the community accessibility worksheet as a guide for asking questions about each place (see "Community Accessibility Training" in the Techniques section). Clients may not know the answer to these questions if they have never had to pay attention to them. In this case, therapists will need to conduct "Community Accessibility Training" to teach the client about community accessibility and to find out if the places that they like to go in the community meet their needs.

Finding new community leisure places that meet the needs of the client: If a client needs to find places in his/her community for leisure, the best place to start is by finding the leisure interests and motivations of the client and matching them with the health needs of the client (see "Activity Pattern Development" in the Techniques section for information on leisure interest testing and exploration). Once the specific activity has been identified, the client and therapist explore places in the community that offer this activity (e.g., a recreation center, a senior center, a dance studio). Start out by asking the client if s/he knows of a place in his/her community that offers this activity. If the client does not know, use a phone book or a map tool on the Internet to find a place in the community. For example, click on a map tool, type in the client's home address, click on "find a business" (everything is called a business, even public recreation centers), and type in what you are looking for (e.g., recreation center, dance studio). A list of places will then appear in order of distance from the client's home. It provides you with the name of the facility, the address, the distance from the client's home, and even directions on how to get there. It helps to print this list out and then cross them off one by one if they do not offer the activity or are unable to accommodate the needs of the client. Keep searching until you find a place where the client can engage in the activity. If you are unable to find the activity using this method, call organizations (e.g., call the

Paralyzed Veterans Association or Special Olympics to help find an adaptive sporting program) and other recreational therapy professionals in the area who may be familiar with other programs that are not well advertised in the general community.

If possible, a community integration session to the place in the community should be scheduled to do a full assessment of the facility and the program as described in "Integration" in the Techniques section.

Outcomes

The recreational therapist documents the client's community activities on the initial evaluation form along with any relevant information that the client is able to provide (e.g., "Client attends a seated senior exercise program three times a week at Live Well Senior Center. The client believes that the center is fully wheelchair accessible. Therapist will place a phone call to the center to clarify their level of accessibility."). If a new community place for leisure is identified, it is documented along with its relevant information (e.g., "Identified a dance studio two miles from client's home that provides Tai Chi. Client was set up with her local paratransit service through social services to take her back and forth to the program. The dance studio is fully wheelchair accessible and is able to accommodate the needs of the client (Tai Chi from a seated position). Client plans to begin the program next month. Therapist to contact the client in three weeks to promote follow through, provide support and encouragement, and problem solve for any issues that have arisen.").

Community leisure resource awareness is an intervention, so it is not coded in the ICF. However, impaired community leisure resource awareness can affect the level of difficulty assigned to codes in many of the activities included in Activities and Participation Chapter 9 Community, Social, and Civic Life.

Special credentialing/training: There is no additional credentialing or training needed by a CTRS to implement this protocol.

Community Problem Solving

Community problem solving is the knowledge of, and ability to problem solve for, physical and non-physical barriers in a real-life setting (work, home, school, community). The client learns about anticipated barriers that may be experienced in a real-life setting and how to problem solve for such barriers. The specific material reviewed depends on the identified barriers of the task. This could include a combination of Community Accessibility Training (CAT), Americans with Disabilities Act (ADA) training, or a tailored focus on a specific problem (e.g., self-catheterizing in a public restroom). This protocol, although it incorporates the use of other forms of education and training, was included because it addresses the client's ability to integrate a variety of protocols for the task of community problem solving.

Therapists who address these issues proactively will maximize a client's problem solving skills, resource awareness, and functional application skills. Should a client encounter barriers that s/he is unable to solve, unhealthy consequences may occur. This could include the development of secondary disability (e.g., deconditioning due to decreased activity level), emotional adjustment issues, and decreased quality of life (e.g., does not pursue personal life goals because of perceived insurmountable barriers).

Indications

A client who 1. verbalizes concerns about his/her ability to function in a real-life environment, 2. exhibits difficulty identifying anticipated barriers, or 3. does not adequately solve for barriers resulting in undesirable outcomes (e.g., safety concerns).

Contraindications: A client who has significant cognitive impairments that impact his/her ability to recall, retain, or apply verbal, pictorial, or demonstrative education. If significant cognitive impairments are evident, the therapist will need to educate the client's caregivers since they will be the ones to facilitate community activities.

Protocol

The length and frequency of community problem-solving sessions will vary depending on the identified needs and abilities of the client. Barriers are identified through activity and systematic analysis of each task that will be a part of the client's activity pattern. There are three handouts contained in this protocol. A particular client may use one or all of them. Each one typically takes about 30 minutes for

review and verbal application to proposed situations for a client who does not exhibit cognitive impairments.

Education should take place in a quiet, non-distracting environment to promote concentration.

The therapist should have relevant materials (e.g., specific protocol handouts for review/reference after the session, paper and pen to write down barriers and identified solutions).

Additional sessions should be scheduled to allow for evaluation of activity performance (ability to apply information in a real-life environment). This is typically done in the form of community integration training. Please refer to "Integration" in the Techniques section for more information.

Process

The process for presenting information will vary depending upon the information reviewed. Typically, education is provided verbally along with a written handout that is given to the client for future reference. There are three handouts at the end of this protocol: Community Problem-Solving Techniques, Lower Extremity Amputation Community Problem Solving, and Spinal Cord Injury Problem Solving Worksheet.

The handouts are not meant to be complete, but a sample of some of the most common problems. We are unable to list community problem solving for every diagnosis, but the handouts should give you a good idea of what to look for and address. We encourage you to write specific community problems and possible solutions in a manner that is tailored to the needs of the individual client. Therapists are welcome to use the worksheets provided and alter them to meet the needs of their clients.

Therapists may also need to educate and train clients on other issues that could cause problems for the client in the community. Other issues may include, but are not limited to: "Wheelchair Mobility," "Walking Techniques," "Energy Conservation Training," "Anger Management," "Relaxation And Stress Reduction," "Emergency Response," "Americans With Disabilities Act," "Personal Leisure Resource Awareness" and "Community Leisure Resource Awareness." (all in the Techniques section); activities of daily living (see Activities and Participation Chapter 5 Self Care, Activities and Participation Chapter 6 Domestic Life, and the Equipment section); assertiveness training skills; dietary precautions management (see Body Functions Chapter 5 Functions of the Digestive, Metabolic, and Endocrine Systems); pain management (see b280 Sensation of Pain); anxiety management (see Generalized Anxiety Disorder); and "Social Skills Training" (in the Techniques section).

After education, the client is asked to verbally apply information and skills learned to proposed situations ("what would you do if..."). Following this intervention, clients are scheduled for community integration training to more fully evaluate the client's ability to apply the information and skills learned into a real-life environment.

Material should be presented carefully and gently to the client, especially the what-if questions. The therapist does not want to scare the client about possibilities, yet wants to educate and inform so that these barriers do not pose a threat to the client's continuing activity and community involvement and working towards his/her life goals.

Documentation

The therapist documents the specific education provided and the client's ability to verbally apply information to proposed situations as well as the client's ability to perform learned techniques in a real-life environment. *Example*: Post education on problem solving for weather conditions, the client was able to verbally apply information at modified independence secondary to increased time (capacity). However, in a community environment (performance), the client required minimal verbal cues to make adjustments for weather conditions because "I'm just not used to doing it."

In the ICF, therapists document a client's ability to problem solve for community barriers under d175 Solving Problems.

There is no additional credentialing or training needed by a CTRS to implement this protocol.

Community Problem-Solving Techniques

Carrying things

There are several ways to carry things if you are using a wheelchair, walker, or cane:

- *Backpack*: If you are using a wheelchair, hook each arm strap of the backpack over the back of the wheelchair. If you are using a walker or cane, wear the backpack. Here are several characteristics of a good backpack: waterproof, a dark color that won't show a lot of dirt, and several roomy compartments that are easy to open. A thin arm strap may be more comfortable to lean against if you are putting it on the back of a wheelchair. A thick arm strap may be more comfortable if you are wearing it.
- *Clothing*: Use clothing pockets, a waist pack, or a small pocketbook with a large strap that you can wear across your shoulders.
- *Custom bags and baskets*: You can make one or purchase one from a medical catalog. A small cloth bag or basket can be hung on the front bar of a walker. A small nylon bag can attach to a cane or crutch with Velcro. Small cloth bags can attach to a wheelchair armrest.
- *Shopping baskets*: If you are using a wheelchair, you can put a store basket on your lap. However there are several things that must be considered: 1. Sensation: If your sensation in your legs is impaired, you will not be able to feel the basket on your lap nor will you realize that it may be digging into your skin if it is overloaded with heavy items. This could cause skin breakdown. If you have poor sensation in your legs and want to use a basket, take a towel along with you (keep it in your backpack), lay it down on your lap, and then put the basket on top of the towel. Also, do not load it with heavy items. 2. Type of mobility device: If you are sitting in a wheelchair at a 90° angle, the basket may have a tendency to slide off your lap. If you are sitting on an angle that is less than 90°, your knees will be slightly higher than your hips. This position will keep the basket on your lap much more easily. If you are using a walker, you should not use a handheld basket at the same time. It is not safe. You need both hands on the walker handles. If you are using a cane, you can use a handheld basket provided you have enough strength in the other hand and arm to hold it, as well as the balance to compensate for the weight.
- *Store carts*: A standard store cart can be pushed with one hand while propelling the wheelchair with the other hand. It takes a bit of practice but it can be done provided you have enough upper body strength and endurance. If you are using a walker or a cane, do not put your device into a cart and push the cart. The cart handle is higher than your walker or cane, so the cart is only supporting your upper body, not your lower body. As a result you may find yourself leaning on the cart. This is not good. If you cannot walk upright while using the cart, you are not ready to use it.
- *Electric scooters*: Many stores have electric scooters for their customers to use. They are hand-operated. Ask at the customer service counter for a key and instructions. They are usually free and you do not have to prove that you have a disability to use them. After you transfer to the scooter, ask the customer service representative to take your assistive device back to the customer service counter and hold it for you. When you go through the checkout lane, ask the cashier to get a customer service representative to bring out your device and help you get your packages into the car.
- *Ask for help*: Under the Americans with Disabilities Act (ADA) you are entitled to have "reasonable accommodations." Asking for assistance to carry items it considered reasonable.

Rain

If it is raining outside and you are using a wheelchair:

- Choose your clothing carefully. If you are wearing good clothes and shoes (e.g., going to a wedding) and you don't want to get them wet, consider taking your good clothes with you and changing when you get there.
- When you are in the house (before you transfer into the wheelchair), waterproof the wheelchair cushion. This is very important. You do not want to wind up having to sit on a wet cushion (because it will get wet from the rain when loading the wheelchair into the car). Wet cushions are dangerous. If the water seeps out of the cushion, through your pants, and moistens your skin, you are at a higher risk for developing a skin breakdown. Skin is fragile when it is wet and is much more likely to break down, especially if you are putting pressure on the skin by sitting on it. To keep the cushion dry, slip the cushion into a clean kitchen trash bag. Slip the cushion (that is inside the kitchen trash bag) into a snug fitting cloth pillowcase. The plastic will

become a water barrier and the cloth pillowcase will keep you from slipping off the cushion when you sit on it. Transfer into the car. Pull the cushion into the car immediately. If the pillowcase is wet, take it off and put on a dry one. When transferring out of the car, quickly put the cushion onto the wheelchair and transfer onto it. If you are with someone, ask the person to hold an umbrella over the wheelchair to keep it as dry as possible. Once you enter the building, you can continue to sit on the pillowcase if it is not wet. If it is wet, have yet another pillowcase with you or simply take both the trash bag and the pillowcase off. Remember to repeat this process before you leave if it is still raining. Also, wear a poncho. A poncho will provide the most protection from the rain. Do not sit on the poncho. Put the back part over the back of the wheelchair. It will keep the wheelchair and backpack drier. An umbrella is not feasible. Even clip-on umbrellas have had limited success. Raincoats will not cover the back of your chair and they may be slippery to sit on.

If it is raining outside and you are walking:
- Choose your clothing carefully, as stated in the previous scenario.
- Wear a raincoat with a hood. The raincoat will not get in your way and will provide maximum protection from the rain. An umbrella is not feasible because you want both of your hands available to hold an assistive device or to assist with keeping your balance. A poncho is not feasible; it will get in your way when you are walking (too much material).

Clothing

Carefully consider the clothes that you wear when you go out. Here are some things to think about:
- Can you easily manipulate clothing for using the bathroom?
- Are they weather appropriate? If your sensation is impaired, it is very important to be aware of the weather. For example, you may not notice that your cotton pants aren't protecting your skin well on a very cold day.
- If you are using a wheelchair, you may want to purchase pants that are an inch or two longer than you normally would have purchased. The extra length will allow your pants to cover your ankles when you are in a seated position.
- If you are using a wheelchair, you may want to purchase shirts with a longer shirttail if you plan

on tucking them in, so that they do not work their way out of the back of your pants.

Parking

Do you have a handicap placard or tag? Do you need one? Talk with your therapist for more information on how to apply for one. Handicap parking spaces are not only close to the front door or accessible entrance but they are also wider to allow adequate room to get in and out of the car. If there are no handicap parking spaces available, you have several options:
- Park in the middle of two regular parking lot spaces and display your handicap parking placard or tag. Some people fear that other customers may become angry if you take up two parking spaces, so get a piece of poster board and write on it "I'm allowed to park here. There were no handicap parking spaces available. Thank you for understanding." This will usually avoid any confrontations.
- If someone else is driving 1. have the driver pull halfway into a regular parking spot and put on the hazard lights. Transfer out of the car and then have the driver pull the rest of the way into the spot. Vice versa for when you leave. 2. Have the driver let you off up front (if safe and appropriate).
- A word of caution: Do not enter/exit a car from a curb if at all possible. Getting in and out of the car by a curb can be very difficult because your wheelchair will be higher up making the transfer more difficult. If you are not using a wheelchair, your knees will be higher than your hips because you feet will have to be on the sidewalk making that transfer more difficult as well.

Social Posture

If you have poor sensation in your legs, you must be aware of your posture in relation to skin breakdown. It is very common for skin breakdown to occur in places besides your bottom.
- Knees (from resting ankle/foot on opposite knee).
- Ankles (from crossing ankles).

If your sensation is impaired, you will not be able to feel the discomfort that others feel from increased pressure. If you do rest your foot on your knee or cross your ankles, be aware of the length of time that you are in this position and vary your posture regularly. Remember to do a weight shift at least every 30 minutes. Some people have found it helpful to wear a watch and set it to beep every 30 minutes as a reminder.

Flat Tire

Most wheelchair tires have a solid insert so flats will not happen. However, if you do choose a tire that inflates with air, be sure to ask for instruction on how to change a tire. Be sure that you carry the repair supplies with you in your backpack. If you are unable to change the tire by yourself and you plan on being out by yourself a lot, you may want to choose a different type of tire.

Dead Battery

If you have a power wheelchair, make sure the battery is fully charged before you go out. You may wind up being out later than you anticipated, and use up more battery power than expected. If you do find yourself in a position where the battery is dead, change the wheelchair to manual mode. You will require assistance to push the chair. If you are by yourself, ask a passerby to push you to a safe area and call someone for help. This is a prime example of the importance of having a cell phone.

Emergency (Cell Phone, Road Assistance)

It is a very good idea to carry a cell phone with you at all times in case of an emergency (e.g., flat tire, a fall, car breaks down). It is also advisable to carry a 24-hour roadside assistance program just in case the car breaks down.

Medication

If you are taking medication on a regular basis, it would be a good idea to take it with you when you go out. This way, if you want to say out later, you can. If it is a narcotic, it must stay in its original prescription bottle to make it legal.

Bowel and Bladder

Using a public bathroom is not always an easy feat. It may not be accessible to your needs. Here are several things to consider.

If You Are Self-Catheterizing

- Make self-catheterization packs. Put everything that you need for one self-catheterization session into a plastic grocery bag, fold it over, and put it into your backpack. It is good to take a few extra packs just in case you stay out later or you drink more fluid. Remember, the more you drink, the more often you will need to self-catheterize.
- If it is feasible for you to learn how to self-catheterize from a seated position, you should do it. There are not many places to lie down and self-catheterize in a public environment. Inform your nurse and therapists of your desire to learn and practice this skill.
- If you are self-catheterizing in a public bathroom, pull up to the urinal or toilet, take out a self-catheterizing pack from your backpack, hook one of the plastic bag handles onto your chair, and let the other end of the bag hang open. Get yourself into the correct position to self-catheterize and then reach into the bag to get your supplies. A bungee cord works well to hold your pants open. Unzip your pants and hook one end of the bungee cord to the pant flap and then hook the other end to someplace on your wheelchair. Now you have both hands available for self-catheterizing. You could also use a bungee cord to keep the bathroom door shut. Sometimes there is not enough room to turn around to lock the door, so on your way in, hook the door somewhere (bottom, side) and then hook the other end somewhere else in the bathroom (toilet paper holder, wheelchair, side of stall).

If You Can Void on Your Own

- If you are male, keep a plastic bottle with a good leak-proof lid in your backpack. If you are unable to stand, you may still be able to sit to use the bottle, and then dump it in the urinal or toilet. It also comes in handy when bathrooms are on the second floor (e.g., private home). Find a private area to use the bottle and then ask someone to take it upstairs to dump it or you could put it back into your backpack and empty it at home. If you prefer to do this, you may want to pull a dark sock over the bottle. This way, anyone who goes into your backpack is none the wiser that the bottle contains urine.
- If you are female, you will want to call ahead to make sure the public bathroom meets your specific needs. If it does not, or there is no way to determine ahead of time if the bathroom is accessible, wear a protective pad especially made for holding urine just in case you can't get into the bathroom.

Bowel

- Know your bowel routine and try to be at home at that time.
- If you anticipate having to use the bathroom when you are out, call ahead to make sure it is accessible and have help with you to use the bathroom if necessary.
- Pack an extra change of clothes, as well as clean-up supplies and a Ziploc bag, in your backpack just in case of a bowel or bladder accident.

- When you are in the hospital, your nurse will set you up on a bowel program at a certain time of the day. This will help train your bowels to move at a particular time. Be sure to discuss your lifestyle with your nurse and set up a time that will work best with your lifestyle after discharge rather than your inpatient therapy routine.

Lower Extremity Amputation Community Problem Solving

Something Doesn't Feel Quite Right While You Are Walking

Stop what you're doing, sit down, take off the prosthetic, and inspect your skin and prosthetic.

- Is there any skin reddening? Some reddening is normal. It should resolve within 30 minutes. If it does not resolve, call your physician immediately as it may be a beginning sign of ulceration.
- Did the prosthetic shift position? Readjust the prosthetic.

You Find a Skin Opening

If there is a skin opening, you need to keep the prosthetic off. If you continue to wear it, it will make the opening worse. However, you also need to make it back to the car and into your house safely. Here are some ideas:

Wheelchair Available

- Is there a wheelchair for customers to use (e.g., at a store)? Ask your friend to get it for you. If you are by yourself, ask an employee to get it for you. If you are able, push the wheelchair yourself or request assistance to push the wheelchair back to the car.
- Once you arrive home you will need to exit the car and get into the house. Do you need to wear the prosthetic to get into the house? If you still have your walker or crutches in the home, can someone go inside the home and bring it out to you so that you can "hop" into the house? If you are by yourself or "hopping" is not safe for entering your home, put the prosthetic back on and enter your home as you did before. As soon as you get in the door, take the prosthetic off.

No Wheelchair

If no wheelchair is available:

- If you are using a walker or crutches, is it possible to "hop" back to the car?
- If you are not using a walker or crutches but you did in the past, is it possible to keep it in the trunk of your car in case of an emergency? Ask someone to go out to the car and get it for you.
- Is there some sort of transportation available to get you back to the car? For example, if you are at an arboretum, an employee may be able to drive you back to your car in one of their carts.
- If the previous options do not work, put the prosthetic back on and walk directly back to your car. Take the prosthetic off, drive home, and then

follow the previous suggestions for entering your home.

Walking on Uneven Surfaces

If you do a lot of walking on uneven surfaces (e.g., hiking), it is important to check your skin regularly for any irritation, since walking on uneven surfaces challenges the fit of the prosthetic. The prosthesis may also shift when you are walking, so it might need to be readjusted or repositioned periodically.

Sunburn

It is particularly important to avoid sunburn on your residual limb.

- Sunburn can cause blisters. Friction from the prosthetic may cause the blisters to open. Once the skin has an opening, you may be restricted from using the prosthetic until the skin heals. If you are diabetic, it could take quite some time for the opening to heal due to circulation problems.
- Sunburn makes your skin more sensitive. This can cause pain when wearing the prosthetic.
- Beware of using sunburn-soothing agents (e.g., aloe vera). Putting a wet substance on your residual limb will cause your skin to become more fragile and more prone to break down. Also, you do not want to use a sunburn-soothing agent on an open wound since it can cause an infection.
- If your residual limb becomes sunburned: Evaluate the severity of the burn. If it is just slightly pink and there are no blisters, you can try wearing your prosthetic. Check your skin frequently for irritation. If it causes any pain or discomfort, remove the prosthetic until the sunburn heals. If it is moderate to severe and there is a blister, it is recommended that you do not wear your prosthetic until the sunburn heals. You will have to problem solve for alternative ways to get around (e.g., crutches, wheelchair).

Water

It is important that the skin on your residual limb is totally dry before putting on the socks and prosthetic. Wet skin is fragile and can increase your risk of skin breakdown from the friction of wearing the prosthetic. Remember to fully dry your skin after showering, swimming, sitting in the sun (if the residual limb is sweaty), being out in the rain, etc. The correct procedure is to dry the limb with a towel and to let it air dry for at least 20 minutes. High periods of activity may cause your socks to become soaked with perspiration. Take extra socks with you at all times and change them regularly to prevent skin breakdown.

Socks

The volume (circumference) of your residual limb changes throughout the day so you will need to change your socks frequently to ensure a proper prosthetic fit. Because the number of plies you need will change, it is important to have a variety of sizes with you.

Traveling via Airplane

Some people report that their residual limb swells after flying due to air pressure changes and seems to take one full day to resolve. This may cause the prosthetic to not fit properly. Be prepared by taking thinner socks to wear with the prosthetic. Also, it might be helpful to consider light activities for your first day after flying (e.g., sedentary activities such as watching a show) which may provide you with easier alternatives for getting around if you are unable to use your prosthetic.

Kneeling

If you have a one-limb amputation (e.g., leg or arm), you may be able to kneel without much discomfort. However, it is important to make sure that you can do this in a safe manner and that it does not irritate the skin or the prosthetic. Work on this skill with your therapist. Do not attempt this for the first time on your own. Kneeling is not recommended for someone who has two or more limb amputations.

Spinal Cord Injury Problem Solving Worksheet

1. What would you do if you were out with two friends and you wanted to get into a building that had five steps? What if you were with one friend?

2. What would you do if you were up on the second floor and the elevator died?

3. What would you do if you couldn't open a heavy manual door at a store?

4. What would you do if you fell out of your wheelchair in the middle of the mall?

5. What would you do if there were no handicap parking spaces? What if someone who had no handicap tag or placard was parking in a handicap parking space?

6. What would you do if you were a passenger in a car and the passenger side of the car was parked along a curb? How would you get out of the car?

7. What would you do if there was no curb cut and you were with another person? What if you were by yourself?

8. How would get over a thick gravel driveway? If you still couldn't get over it, what could you do?

9. What would you do if your friends asked you to go on a deep-sea fishing trip and you were unsure as to how you would get on and off the boat? Let's say you really want to go along.

10. What would you do if you were out in the community and you got a flat tire?

11. How would you go out somewhere and not get wet if it was raining outside?

12. What would you do if you had to use the bathroom and the bathroom was not accessible? What would you do if you were at someone's house and the bathroom was on the second floor?

13. What would you do if your wheelchair would not fit between the clothing racks at the store and you wanted to look at a particular sweatshirt?

14. What would you do if something broke on your wheelchair (e.g., a hand rim)?

15. What should you put in your backpack?

16. What would you do if you experienced a dysreflexic episode in the community?

17. What would you do if you had to empty your Foley bag and there was no bathroom around?

18. What would you do if you realized that your Texas catheter has fallen off and you were in the middle of a store? What if you didn't realize that it fell off and you had a bladder accident?

19. What should you carry with you at all times in your backpack in regards to your bowel and bladder needs?

20. Come up with three other questions about things that could happen when you are out in the community. List possible solutions.

Spinal Cord Injury Problem Solving Worksheet Answers

1. If feasible, instruct them on how to bump you up and down the steps. Ask for assistance from security personnel. If no one is available to help or it is not safe for your friends to help, do not attempt the steps.

2. Ask how long it is going to be out of service. If you can wait, wait. If not, ask if there is another elevator (public, freight). If there is no other elevator, you will need to use the stairwell. Do not allow untrained people to bump you up and down the steps. If needed, call local emergency service and they will take you down the steps in a blanket carry.

3. Ask for assistance.

4. If you can, get back in the wheelchair. If you are unable to get back into the wheelchair, instruct someone to call the local emergency service for help. Do not allow untrained people to help you. If something seems "wrong" (e.g., broken leg, shooting pain), do not attempt to get into the wheelchair. Call the local emergency service.

5. Park in the middle of two standard parking spaces. Inform security or the store or office manager. The violators should be fined. Some people find satisfaction by making their own "tickets" and putting them on the windows of vehicles that are not legally parked in handicap spaces (e.g., "This is a warning. You are parked illegally in a handicap parking spot. Consider yourself lucky. Next time I will call the police and you will be ticketed.").

6. Look around for a parking garage or parking lot. If there isn't a parking garage, consider having the driver pull into a parking spot on an angle, put on the hazard lights, transfer out of the car into the street (between the car and the curb), bump up the curb, and then have the driver park the vehicle correctly. Avoid this situation by calling ahead to locate safe parking.

7. If feasible, instruct him/her on how to bump you up and down the curb. If you are unable to bump up and down the curb yourself, look for an alternative route (e.g., grassy incline). It is not safe to have an untrained person assist you. If there is no alternative route, you will not be able to access the building. This could possibly be avoided by calling ahead.

8. Pull the wheelchair over it backwards or look for an alternative route (e.g., grass on the side of the gravel driveway).

9. Call the charter boat company and ask them if they offer assistance getting on and off the boat. Do research on adaptive fishing to find out for

yourself a safe way to transfer on and off the boat. The main point: if you want to do something and you are not sure how to do it, explore it. Don't make assumptions. You could wind up denying yourself opportunities or you could put yourself in a dangerous situation.

10. Fix it. Ride on it if only for a short distance (e.g., to get home) and then fix it. Seek assistance (e.g., bike shop, garage). Call emergency number.

11. Poncho.

12. Find a private area and use a bottle (male). Plan ahead and wear a protective pad (female).

13. Ask a store employee to move the racks if possible (many are on wheels). If this is not possible, the store employee should get the sweatshirt and bring it to you. This is a reasonable accommodation under the Americans with Disabilities Act.

14. Call the wheelchair vendor. Get this information from your physical therapist. Do not attempt to fix the wheelchair yourself. It may void the warranty.

15. Bowel/bladder supplies; cell phone; medication; water bottle; and a medical card, with your physician name, phone number, your health history, and any allergies.

16. Call for emergency medical help. While you are waiting for help to arrive, you should try to resolve the problem yourself by checking for irritants such as a full bladder, full rectum, unrecognized injury, or tight clothing.

17. Use a bottle in a private area.

18. Immediately find a private area (e.g., bathroom) and put it back on. Change your clothes. Keep extra clothes in your backpack. If you don't have extra clothes, lay something over your lap (e.g., jacket, shirt, package) and head back home to change. You could also purchase clothes when you are out and change into them.

19. As it pertains to your situation: self-catheterizing supplies in packs, wipes, Ziploc plastic bag, and change of clothes.

20. Additional possible questions: What would you do if a child asked why you are using a wheelchair? What if a server makes assumptions about your intelligence because you are using a wheelchair and asks your companion what you want to order? What would you do if it was time to take your medication and you didn't have water (or, even worse, forgot to bring your medication)?

Coping with Stress

People cope with stress in many different ways. Some people may go for a run to release excess energy, while others may comfort themselves with food or talk with friends. The techniques that people use may be conscious decisions (e.g., I am under a lot of stress so I am going to take a long hot shower to help myself unwind) or unconscious decisions that are commonly engrained, learned behaviors (e.g., when under a lot of stress the person becomes very negative about everything).

The World Health Organization (1998) makes a clear distinction between coping and managing. Coping is currently defined as a capacity to respond and recover from something stressful. It implies that the individual has very little control over the situation, stressor, threat, or conflict. An example of coping would be eating less expensive food or using substances such as alcohol or illicit drugs. On the other hand managing implies that a person has no need to cope because s/he has the knowledge and resources to control the situation, stressor, threat, or conflict. Examples of managing would be dipping into one's savings account or asserting one's needs in a healthy manner.

The World Health Organization (1998) divides coping mechanisms into three categories. Although the categories were developed to describe coping mechanisms in the face of disaster (e.g., famine, village destruction, mass killings), it seems that they may be applicable to categorize the outcomes of the coping strategies employed by the individual.

1. *Non-erosive*: Non-erosive coping mechanisms result in little to no permanent damage (e.g., yoga, reducing meals, assertiveness).
2. *Erosive*: Erosive coping mechanisms result in harm or damage (e.g., illicit drug use, violence, anorexia nervosa).
3. *Failed*: Coping mechanisms employed fail and the person is overcome by the stressor. Damage and harm are irreversible. Dependence on external aid may be necessary. Examples include suicide, selling children, or prostitution.

Coping mechanisms are mostly learned behaviors. It is through experiences and observation of others that a person learns coping behavior. Clients who possess poor coping skills are therefore best taught new coping mechanisms through practical application of learned techniques (practice doing it; don't just talk about it) and observation of healthy role modeling (e.g., observing the therapist, community group, or sports team model healthy coping mechanisms).

Therapists, who work with diverse populations, including recent immigrants, are aware that the client's coping mechanisms may be influenced by cultural beliefs and upbringing and differ from the mainstream (for example, sacrifices, witchcraft, or avoidance of certain foods). Therapists do not assume that unfamiliar coping mechanisms are unhealthy, but rather determine the healthiness of these coping mechanisms, as well as any other coping mechanisms, by asking two questions 1. Is the mechanism employed causing harm to the client or others and 2. Is it effective, meaning is it resulting in better emotional, psychological, cognitive, physical, and social health? If the answer is no to either of these questions, alternative coping mechanisms should be taught through education and practical application.

Therapists who interact with clients on a regular basis (e.g., community recreation center, boys' and girls' club, residential facility) have the responsibility to foster and strengthen healthy coping mechanisms and to ensure continuity of, and support for, access to healthy coping mechanisms. Therapists foster and strengthen healthy coping strategies through:

Education: Clients are educated directly or indirectly about the consequences of specific coping mechanisms (e.g., assertiveness, drugs and alcohol, violence)

Providing opportunities to engage in healthy coping mechanisms: Activities that encourage teamwork (e.g., sports), relaxation (e.g., yoga), expression (e.g., art, dance, drama), and physical release of tension (e.g., martial arts, tennis, track) have inherent benefits to cope with stress. Therapists support the offering of such programs, articulate their benefits to others, and ensure access to such activities.

Provide support and encouragement: When high and unhealthy signs of stress are observed or a client confides his/her conflict with a therapist, support and encouragement are provided to help the client implement healthy coping mechanisms (e.g., refer client to counseling, encourage the client to be assertive).

The American Psychological Association (APA) supplies a more detailed description of some of the common coping styles that people use (referred to within the field of psychology as defense mechanisms). Defense mechanisms are automatic psychological processes (of which the person may or may not be aware) that protect the client from stress, anxiety, and psychological harm.

Many defense mechanisms can be both healthy and unhealthy depending on 1. the severity of the adaptation (e.g., a client uses the defense mechanism of humor to cope with stressors too often and it is now affecting his relationship with his spouse, "He never takes anything seriously."), 2. the psychological state of the client (e.g., the defense mechanism of anticipation is relatively a good coping strategy — looking ahead and planning a response — however, a client who has generalized anxiety disorder may heighten her anxiety with "anticipation"), and 3. the specific stressor involved (e.g., it may not be appropriate to assert one's feelings of frustration to a parent who has Alzheimer's disease). Although many defense mechanisms can be both healthy and unhealthy, some defense mechanisms are clearly healthy (e.g., asserting one's feelings in a non-confrontive style, provided that the other person is mentally and emotionally stable) and others clearly unhealthy (e.g., denial of stress).

Therapists are aware of defense mechanisms and are careful not to quickly attribute behavioral changes to biological changes (e.g., further progression of chronic cognitive disease). Attention to a client's defense mechanisms is helpful in measuring positive or negative changes in a client's coping abilities. When maladaptive defense mechanisms are suspected, the therapist attempts to identify the particular stressor, alleviate the stressor, and teaches the client healthier coping styles through counseling interventions (see "Education and Counseling" in the Techniques section). Common defense mechanisms observed include (American Psychiatric Association, 1994):

Acting out: The client responds to stressors or conflicts through actions instead of emotional reflection. Defensive acting out behavior is not necessarily bad, but it usually means that the client is not finding a way to deal with his stress by understanding it.

Affiliation: The client seeks assistance from others (e.g., advice, support), however the client does not necessarily seek to have others take responsibility for the problems.

Altruism: The client copes with stressors by seeking to negate the negative feelings through pleasing and helping others. This gives the client a sense of fulfillment and pleasure.

Anticipation: The client thoughtfully considers the possible stressors that may occur, the possible emotional feelings that could result, and the strategies that s/he could employ to minimize the stressor and its related emotional outcomes. For example, the mother of three young children anticipates the death of her husband due to terminal cancer and makes plans to ensure financial security and emotional support for the family.

Apathetic withdrawal: A pattern of behavior indicating indifference in which the person removes himself/herself and demonstrates an under-response or a lack of reactivity to a situation that should cause a response.

Autistic fantasy: When stressors and conflicts arise the client daydreams to avoid interaction with others, effective action, or problem solving.

Denial: The client does not acknowledge the emotional impact of a stressor even though it is apparent to others (e.g., a client lashes out at a co-worker for spilling his coffee yet later denies that it was upsetting).

Devaluation: The client overstates the negative qualities of himself/herself or others to manage stressful events (e.g., "She is always selfish. She never cares about anyone.").

Displacement: This is when a client transfers stressful feelings and thoughts to a less threatening source (e.g., a physically abused child displaces anger from the abusing parent to a sibling).

Dissociation: The client detaches himself/herself from reality to escape the stressor. This is a common coping mechanism for abuse. The client blocks out the situation and "goes somewhere else" ("I think about flying in the sky like a bird."). The client may not be able to recall the situation and may have a distorted perception of self, the environment, and sensory and motor behavior.

Help-rejecting complaining: The client deals with stressors or conflicts by complaining and continuing to ask for help. It disguises covert feelings of anger and blame. When assistance is given, the client rejects it. Complaints and requests for help can be related to a physical, emotional, or life task.

Humor: The client copes by accentuating the comical and ironic features of the stressor.

Idealization: The client overstates the positive qualities of others to manage stressful events (e.g., "He can't be causing me problems because he always does the right thing.").

Intellectualization: The client excessively intellectualizes the stressor or conflict to control the severity of the emotional impact (e.g., a client is upset with his father but rationalizes that his father is easily upset because of his upbringing, it was a hot and humid day, that his choice of words could have easily been misconstrued, and his father may not have heard his apology because he is hard of hearing).

Isolation of affect: The client emotionally separates from the event. The client is able to recall and describe the event in detail but it is void of emotional connection. For example, a client was terrified and anxious during a rape yet now describes the event in detail and feels no emotion about it. The client completely separated her emotions of terror and anxiety from the rape event.

Omnipotence: The client feels and acts as if s/he is better than everyone else and has special qualities that others do not possess (e.g., "She doesn't know what she is talking about. I know what's going on here and it is not about me.").

Passive-aggression: The client acts as is s/he is complying with what is requested, but the compliance masks covert resistance, resentment, or hostility. The resistance expresses itself in an indirect, nonviolent manner such as obstructionism, procrastination, inefficiency, stubbornness, and forgetfulness. It may be adaptive for individuals in subordinate positions who have no other way to express their feelings more overtly.

Projection: The client falsely attributes negative feelings and behavior caused by stress and conflict to another person or event rather than taking ownership for his/her feelings. For example, a client who is furious with his boss thinks about slashing his boss's car tires. The client does not like the thoughts he is having and therefore attributes the thoughts to his neighbor who was looking a little too carefully at his car tires this morning.

Projective identification: This is similar to "projection" except that the client reacts to the projected feelings, often leading the other person to actually experiencing the feelings that were projected. It can be confusing as to who is doing what to whom. For example, a client who says to someone, "You really don't like me." can lead to the person really not liking the client, if the client is insistent enough.

Rationalization: The client reassures himself/herself that actions, thoughts, and feelings are justified in order to conceal his/her real motivations. For example, a client runs a car off the side of the road because it was going too slow. The client justifies his actions by telling himself and others that he nudged the car to the side of the road because he thought the people were having car trouble.

Reaction formation: The client adopts behaviors, thoughts, or feelings that are utterly and completely opposite of his/her unacceptable thoughts or feelings. For example, a client may bend over backwards to please a boss that, objectively, should be reported to the police.

Repression: The client blocks stressful events from his/her conscious awareness. The client is unable to recall the event, yet is often conscious of the feelings and emotions resultant from the event. For example, the client feels angry but does not know where the anger originates (e.g., childhood trauma).

Self-assertion: The client asserts his/her thoughts and feelings appropriately.

Self-observation: The client reflects on his/her own actions, motivation, feelings, and thoughts about a specific conflict or stressor and carefully plans an appropriate course of action.

Splitting of self-image or image of others: The client deals with stressors or conflicts by splitting and alternating his/her self-image or the image of others into polar opposites of positive and negative qualities. Because the person is unable to simultaneously see (lacks emotional awareness of) both the positive and negative qualities of himself/herself or others, unrealistic views are held.

Sublimation: The client directs negative energy caused by conflict and stress into socially appropriate behavior or action (e.g., goes out for a walk, plays contact sports, works hard to change society).

Suppression: When stress and conflict become overwhelming, the client purposely chooses to ignore and avoid feelings or thoughts about the stressor or conflict.

Undoing: The client deals with conflict or external stress with actions intended to negate in part a previous action or communication. An example is a spouse who brings home flowers after having a lunchtime affair with another. It may be related to the magical thinking of childhood.

The most adaptive mechanisms are anticipation, affiliation, altruism, humor, self-assertion, self-observation, sublimation, and suppression. Some of the mechanisms make the client less aware of the stress. They include displacement, dissociation, intellectualization, isolation of affect, reaction formation, repression, and undoing. Minor distortions are found in devaluation, idealization, and omnipotence. At an even less insightful level, the stressors themselves may be kept out of awareness through denial, projection, and rationalization. Major distortions are found in autistic fantasy, projective identification, and splitting of self-image or image of others. Some mechanisms are active, although not in a healthy way. These include acting out, apathetic withdrawal, help-rejecting complaining, and passive aggression. At the most serious level, the stress may cause a break with reality. These mechanisms include delusional projection, psychotic denial, and psychotic distortion.

References

American Psychiatric Association. (1994). *Diagnostic and statistical manual of mental disorders, fourth edition.* Washington. DC: American Psychiatric Association

Education and Counseling

This section will look at the kinds of education and counseling that are part of recreational therapy practice.

To better understand the distinction between education and counseling it helps to review their definitions. Education is the process of acquiring skills and knowledge. It is largely based on information giving. Counseling is the process of facilitating growth and exploration. Although acquiring skills and knowledge can facilitate self-awareness, it is not the primary goal of education and, although personal growth and exploration can facilitate learning new skills, it is not the primary goal of counseling. We can agree that their common element is the desired outcome of positive change, that they do affect each other, and that they are commonly integrated, but they have two separate orientations.

In the past, the field of recreational therapy had a distinction between counseling and education. However, recent literature (Austin, 2004; Stumbo & Peterson, 2004) suggests that leisure counseling is part of the continuum of leisure education rather than a separate service. This debate is sure to continue and we urge recreational therapy researchers, professors, and authors to consider the impact of the ICF in our developing profession. Furthermore, we would like to note that becoming aware of leisure benefits and acquiring new leisure skills (education) and understanding personal values (counseling) does not always result in the client embracing and incorporating it into his/her way of living (leading a more healthy life). Saying it and doing it are two different things. Often the therapist does not know whether the client made changes because of the short-term nature of the therapist/client relationship. Defining and differentiating between education and counseling helps to develop better testing tools, making the impact of our services easier to measure.

The rest of this topic will look at some of the information communicated and techniques used for education and counseling.

Education

The kind of education most often practiced by recreational therapists is called "leisure education." Recreational therapists commonly use this term to describe any form of education that pertains to leisure activity such as resource education, benefits of leisure education, leisure appreciation education[8],

leisure skills education (e.g., rules of playing an adaptive sport), community skills education (e.g., teaching a client about accessibility rights under the Americans with Disabilities Act), and social skills education (e.g., how to respond in certain situations). This list could go on, but the basic idea is that the topic of education is broad and the context for which recreational therapists use the term leisure education encompasses a wide array of categories and topics. Note, also, that the kinds of information presented to clients go far beyond simple leisure skills and many of what appear to be leisure skills are also useful in other areas of the client's life. Recreational therapists would do well to keep this in mind when they are discussing the kind of work they do.

Because the terms "education" and "leisure education" are broad, it benefits the therapist, and those who read the therapist's notes, to clearly document the specific education needed, measured, and provided.

Education in the ICF

Education is an intervention. The ICF does not list interventions. Therefore the therapist must think about education from the following perspectives when deciding where to document issues related to education:

1. *Specific activity-related education*: The intervention of "education" is provided to assist a client in activity participation, therefore the therapist scores the specific activity for which the education is being provided. For example, if a client is having difficulty using public transportation because of a lack of knowledge about how to identity and utilize wheelchair accessible buses, then the therapist would code the level of difficulty that the client is having utilizing public transportation (d4702 Using Public Motorized Transportation). The therapist would then provide education to the client on how to identify and use wheelchair accessible buses as one of his/her interventions to assist the client in improving activity performance with using public buses. Using a specific activity code puts more of an emphasis on the activity, rather than a health behavior as described in #2.

---

[8] Leisure appreciation is the act of realistically estimating an activity's worth and the amount of enjoyment it causes. It involves

making a judgment and having a sensitive awareness of the emotional and physical benefits of an action, individual, group, or object. Nurturing leisure appreciation is the process of teaching clients about leisure and the health benefits of leisure participation and having the client apply the information by creating a healthy activity plan. Therefore education about the benefits of leisure and fostering leisure appreciation are often interlinked.

2. *Specific health-related education*: If education revolves around health practices, the therapist should consider using the relevant health code in the ICF including d570 Looking after One's Health, d5701 Managing Diet and Fitness, d5702 Maintaining One's Health, and d240 Handling Stress and Other Psychological Demands. Good questions to ask when deciding what code to use are "Why am I providing this specific education? What is the desired activity behavior that I wish to see in my client?" The specific activity behavior desired (e.g., d570 Looking after One's Health) would then be scored and education would be provided as an intervention to positively impact the specific activity behavior. Using a specific, health-related code puts more emphasis on the health behavior, rather than on a specific activity as described in #1.

3. *Leisure knowledge and application*: Another option available that will allow the therapist to more clearly note the skill of leisure knowledge and application is to use d198 Learning and Applying Knowledge, Other Specified. The therapist can specify "benefits of leisure," specific resource education such as "community resources for adaptive skiing," specific leisure activity skills such as "game rules for checkers," or any other type of educational topic and its application (e.g., identify and locate wheelchair accessible buses). The use of this code requires the therapist to clearly document the specific knowledge and application area. Using the general knowledge and application code puts more emphasis on the cognitive skill of knowledge and application of knowledge, compared to the emphasis on activity (described in #1) or health behavior (described in #2).

4. *Use of supporting e-codes*: Environmental codes, also called e-codes, can be used to reflect the extent that a particular resource is a barrier or facilitator for an activity. Changing the extent of a barrier or facilitator in a positive direction may require education. Using this approach, the specific education is not documented on the ICF. It is understood via the use of the e-code that education may be an approach to affect change. For example, if the therapist wishes to educate a client about adaptive equipment for a craft activity, s/he may choose the specific activity code of d9202 Arts and Culture and link the e-code e1401 Assistive Products and Technology for Culture, Recreation, and Sports. During the assessment process, this e-code may be scored as a barrier due to lack of knowledge, availability, or use of the adaptive piece of equipment. After educating the client about the piece of equip-

ment, ordering the equipment, and teaching her how to use it, the e-code optimally will become a facilitator for d9202 Arts and Culture. Using an e-code to imply an educational need is appropriate when the education revolves around a specific product or technology, natural environment and human made changes to environment, support and relationships, attitudes, or services, systems, and policies (the five chapters of Environmental Factors).

Counseling

As previously reviewed, counseling is different from education in that counseling is the process of facilitating growth and exploration, whereas education is the process of acquiring skills and knowledge. Many therapists use the term "leisure counseling" to denote a portion of the total scope of recreational therapy counseling. However recreational therapy practice expands past this term and utilizes a variety of counseling approaches and techniques to address a multitude of issues including psychosocial adjustment to disability and illness; clarification of values, beliefs, and attitudes; management of specific problems (e.g., anxiety, pain, anger); facilitation of personal growth and exploration that affect health practices and quality of life; relationship building; change in behaviors and thinking patterns; and understanding different perspectives.

Counseling can be provided in various formats (e.g., informal vs. formal, individual vs. group) and to various people by role or location (e.g., client, caregiver, support group, senior center). For example, in family training, attention is given to the needs of the caregivers to maximize compliance with recommendations. Some examples include:

1. A family may require counseling about the value of activity to understand its role in recovery and health promotion.

2. A mother of a disabled child who comes to a therapy session lacking sleep and breakfast may benefit from brief informal counseling on the importance of caring for herself related to her ability to help her child.

3. A caregiver that exhibits anxious behavior when learning how to assist her spouse in doing a car transfer may benefit from suspending the task for a moment and receiving counseling from the therapist on the value of relaxation training techniques in decreasing performance anxiety, thus maximizing her assistance.

Recreational therapists also expand counseling to people in the community. For example, a camp director may require counseling about reasonable accommodations under the Americans with Disabilities Act to be persuaded to make accommodations for a client. Recreational therapists may also provide counseling to community groups to promote health and optimal living (e.g., senior center).

To best understand the use of counseling in recreational therapy it is necessary to distinguish among forms of therapy, psychotherapy theory/approach, and counseling techniques. Forms of therapy refer to the broad therapy topic of practice (e.g., family therapy, drug and alcohol counseling, leisure counseling). Psychotherapy theory/approach refers to the specific orientations from which the therapist practices his/her form of therapy (e.g., cognitive behavioral therapy, existential therapy). Some therapists follow one specific theory or approach (e.g., a family therapist who only uses psychoanalytic therapy), whereas others use (and sometimes combine) a variety of theories and approaches (called an eclectic approach). Recreational therapists follow an eclectic approach. Lastly, counseling techniques refer to specific techniques or interventions that are used by therapists to promote change. Common counseling techniques can found across many different theories and approaches (e.g., techniques that help to build therapeutic relationships).

Psychotherapy Theories/Approaches

There are many psychotherapy theories and approaches. Entire textbooks are devoted to them. For the purpose of this section, we will review three of the most common found in recreational therapy practice: psychoanalytic therapy or supportive-expressive therapy, cognitive-behavioral therapy, and existential counseling.

Supportive-expressive therapy (SE): Psychoanalytic therapy is often referred to as supportive-expressive therapy. The therapist is "supportive" of the client's feelings and thoughts "so that the [client] will feel secure enough to venture to try to undo the restrictions in functioning" (Luborsky, 1984, p. 71). The therapist also encourages the client to "express" himself/herself by setting "the stage for the [client] to express thoughts and feelings and to listen and to reflect on them, with the aim of understanding and changing what needs to be changed" (p. 90).

The therapist gives support to the client by conveying (though words and manners) a sense of understanding, respect, acceptance, a we-bond (therapist and client are a team working towards a goal), and hope. Therapists highlight strengths of a client, give review and recognition of accomplishments (especially when the client applies learned

information), and encourage discussions (at times) about topics of interest other than exploratory topics to reflect genuine interest in the client.

To encourage the client to talk (express thoughts and feelings) the therapist first needs to employ active listening (eye contact, engaged body posturing, silence). Periods of silence can be very uncomfortable for new therapists, but it is within the silence that connections are made. Therefore, therapists should not be quick to fill in the empty space with talk. When the therapist understands in part or whole what the client is trying to convey, the therapist shares his/her insight with the client in terms that the client understands. The therapist then resumes active listening and listens for the client's reaction to the feedback in addition to new information shared.

Cognitive-behavioral therapy (CBT): Cognitive-Behavior Therapy (CBT) is also referred to as Rational Emotive Behavior Therapy (REBT). CBT stems from the premise that people's interpretations, reactions, and beliefs are a result of conditioning (learned behaviors). Working on thinking and acting rather than feelings and emotions changes these distorted thinking patterns. The client is taught new ways of thinking and behaving. Skills are taught and practiced until new and healthy thinking patterns overtake the previously held distorted thinking patterns (new learned behavior).

The A-B-C Theory of Personality is central to REBT. The belief is that an event does not cause an emotional/behavioral response. It is the person's belief that affects how the person responds to the event. The same event (e.g., traumatic spinal cord injury) does not result in the same emotional or behavior response (e.g., depression) for all individuals. The variable that influences the response is the person's belief system. If the person's beliefs are causing an unhealthy emotional or behavioral response, then the therapist will act by providing modalities that dispute the person's irrational belief system. For example, this may include education on quality of life for clients who sustain spinal cord injuries. The therapist will point out faults in client's belief system such as, "I will never be able to go skiing now that I have a spinal cord injury." This belief can be disputed by providing information on adaptive skiing, setting up a meeting with another person who has a spinal cord injury who skis, or viewing videos of adaptive skiing.

The therapist challenges the client's irrational beliefs by asking questions (e.g., "Why is it terrible or horrible if life is not the way you want it to be?"). "Through a series of refutations, therapists are instrumental in raising the consciousness of their clients to a more rational (self-helping) level" (Corey, 1996, p. 328). Other interventions include individual work (homework) in which clients are challenged to look at their beliefs rationally; replacing negative thoughts with positive thoughts; developing and participating in an action plan that refutes irrational beliefs; changing "should," "ought," and "must" language to preferences ("I would prefer if that didn't happen." or "It would be an inconvenience if …"); or using humor to "show absurdity of certain ideas that clients steadfastly maintain" (Corey, 1996, p. 330). Some of the techniques include role playing, relaxation techniques, modeling, systematic desensitization, self-management principles, and operant conditioning. The interventions provided will have an effect on the person's belief structure, thus resulting in a new feeling toward the current activating event. This is a very common technique used in recreational therapy, especially trying to change an individual's perspective on how his/her lifestyle has a direct effect on health, how s/he can still lead an optimal lifestyle, obtain personal goals, develop internal locus of control, and adjust to disability in a community setting. Disability, unfortunately, is fraught with many negative connotations and many of these must be tackled head on by the therapist in order to facilitate change and growth.

Existential counseling: Existential counseling is the process of searching for the value and meaning in life and encouraging clients to explore options for creating a meaningful existence. Clients are encouraged to become aware of their own power in making life changes rather than being a victim of circumstance. The client is the architect of his/her life. The choices that s/he makes not only determine the life that s/he leads but also the person that s/he becomes. To become aware of this power and make positive life changes based on this awareness is the focus of existential counseling.

There are no specific techniques that are well defined for existential counseling; however Corey (1996) outlines three phases in the therapeutic process:

- *Initial phase*: Therapists help clients to explore their assumptions about the world (What is life about?) and their perceived value and purpose in the world (Why am I here?). Clients are challenged to consider the validity of these beliefs. This can be difficult for some clients, especially those who have an external locus of control. Clients are encouraged to examine their own role in designing their life.
- *Middle phase*: Clients are encouraged to more fully examine their own role in designing their life (Who is really in control? Who has authority?) and what is truly valued as meaningful in their lives. This process typically leads to new

insights and some restructuring of attitudes and values. Clients begin to develop a clearer picture of the life they wish to lead.

- *Final phase*: The goal of this phase is to enable clients to concretely implement changes in their lives to reflect new insights and values, thus leading to more purposeful lives.

Education and Counseling Techniques

How the recreational therapist does education and counseling is as important as the kinds of education and counseling the therapist does. A therapist can have the perfect information or technique for a client, but it has no value if it is presented in a way that the client can't understand or if it is presented in a way that the client actively or passively resists. The next part of this topic will look at some of the ways a therapist can improve the client-therapist interaction.

Many of these techniques are common practice within the therapeutic milieu. They become almost second nature to the therapist who systemically addresses multiple issues in a treatment session. It is not uncommon for a therapist to delicately balance his/her relationship with the client while providing instruction and counseling around a particular issue. With experience, multi-tasking becomes easier and integrating these skills into a treatment session becomes instinctive — just as the therapist learns to adjust the client-therapist interaction into what the client needs to obtain maximal growth.

Some of the issues of counseling that are important to recreational therapists include relationship building, understanding actions and motivations, loss and crisis. Here are some techniques that are effective for dealing with these issues:

Relationship building

Interaction cannot be void of social-emotional contact, no matter what the basis of interaction. At the most basic level, pleasantries are shared (or not shared) and an attitude or perception of the person is formed. The therapist is judged on not only what was said or not said, but also how it was said, when it was said, who it was said to, and why it was said. The therapist is also judged on his/her appearance. Clients initially desire someone who looks professional, takes a genuine interest, is pleasant and friendly, and appears competent and trustworthy. How a client assesses a therapist is not consistent. Still, how the therapist is perceived has a great impact on the relationship.

The therapeutic relationship builds a foundation for treatment. It not only fosters the client's personal growth, but also directly influences physical and cognitive performance. For example, a client who perceives a therapist to be preoccupied and disinterested will be less likely to open up emotionally to the therapist. If this results in ill feelings towards the therapist, the client may in turn reflect his/her dislike for the therapist behaviorally (e.g., not perform a task at the level requested). This type of behavior will not only negatively affect the client's physical skill development, but also stunt the client's emotional growth and adjustment to disability. The client may also deal with cognitive challenges apathetically because s/he thinks the therapist doesn't care. The therapist must be constantly aware that the mind and body work together to form a sensitive and highly complex system that reacts to input in an integrated way. Consequently, the client-therapist relationship is much more than just an exchange of pleasantries. It is a catalyst for systemic change.

The employment of counseling techniques, along with a genuine and caring attitude, opens the door to growth. Luborsky (1984) recommends five steps for opening psychoanalytic therapy. These steps are also relevant for a variety of allied health professions. Incorporating these steps into the evaluation process will encourage the therapist to attend to relationship issues, which may otherwise be minimized because insuring agencies tend to focus attention on physical outcomes.

1. Listen in order to establish what the patient's problems are and let the patient try to cast these in terms of goals ordered in importance (client goals).
2. Explain and demonstrate to the patient what the therapist does (role of RT).
3. Make explicit arrangements about the treatment (time, place, etc.).
4. Allow a relationship of trust and rapport to be developed (genuine interest and concern).
5. Begin the process of formulating the basis for the main relationship, including problems and associated symptoms. This must be done because client-therapist relationship issues (e.g., client says that therapist doesn't understand his situation as a teenager) and manifestations of the issues in the client-therapist relationship (e.g., client is emotionally non-disclosing and repeats belief of therapist's lack of understanding) may allow the client to retreat from emotionally charged discussions.

A sixth step would be to form a relationship treatment plan. The therapist develops and implements planned interventions to enhance the client-therapist relationship, with the full understanding that positive relationship changes will enhance function within all domains, as well as contribute to the client's adjustment and integration.

Understanding actions and motivations

There are many things a therapist can do to improve the therapy interaction. One of the important ones is helping a client better understand his/her actions and motivations. Brammer (1988) identifies seven helping skills that the therapist can use to promote the client's understanding of himself/herself.

- *Listening skills*: The therapist actively attends to what is verbally and non-verbally expressed by the client (e.g., words, context, emotions, body language, mannerisms) to form a total perception of what the client is experiencing. This process is sometimes referred to as "listening with the third ear." Listening can be broken down into the following subcategories.
  - *Attending*: Genuine, warm eye contact is used to convey caring and understanding, as well as to hold the attention of the client and evaluate the nonverbal messages conveyed through the client's eyes (e.g., looking away, tearful, shut tight, hard stare). The therapist exhibits engaged social posture and gestures (leaning forward, arms uncrossed, etc.) and offers non-directional verbal comments (e.g., "I understand.") as appropriate to convey active attention.
  - *Paraphrasing*: The therapist reiterates (when there is an appropriate conversational pause) in concise terms what s/he is "hearing" verbally and non-verbally from the client (e.g., "Being here really makes you angry." or "You appreciate your mom's helpfulness, but I detect from your sarcasm that it bothers you sometimes." or "You say that you are fine but I detect that you are feeling a bit angry given that your arms and legs are crossed and folded tightly."). It is important to note whether the client confirms or denies what the therapist says.
  - *Clarifying*: The therapist poses questions to the client to clarify understanding (e.g., "I'm not sure I understand what you mean. Can you explain that to me again?") or states in more concise terms what s/he thinks the client is trying to communicate (e.g., "Are you trying to say that you are afraid?").
  - *Perception checking*: This is the process of determining if the perception that the therapist holds is correct. It is different from paraphrasing or clarifying because a perception reflects the therapist's awareness of a

large amount of material shared by the client rather than the last few sentences. For example, "I think I hear you saying two different things. On one hand you feel frustrated and yet on the other hand you feel relieved. Is this correct?"

- *Leading*: The therapist anticipants the direction of the client's thoughts and offers his/her insight to the direction.
  - o *Indirect leading*: Indirect leading encourages the client to talk (e.g., "What do you think that means?" or "How does that make you feel?"). It is a general question that is purposely vague. Following the question the therapist pauses in silence in anticipation of the client's response.
  - o *Direct leading*: Direct leading provides more direction for the client, yet it still encourages the client to assume responsibility for the conversation (e.g., "Tell me more about what you like about hiking." or "What do you mean by 'it makes you feel icky'?").
  - o *Focusing*: Focusing helps the client to explore a particular aspect of the conversation. Therapists challenge the client to focus when it behooves the client therapeutically (e.g., "You've been talking a lot about all of the things that scare you. Tell me, what makes you feel confident."). Therapists may also find it helpful to use just one word like "but?" or "so?" or "and?" to encourage the client to focus more on the particular aspect of the conversation.
  - o *Questioning*: Avoid the question "why?" because it comes across as being accusatory and often puts the client on the defensive. Ask open-ended questions (questions that require a client to answer through explanation rather than with a yes or no answer) to facilitate exploration of feelings or help the client to clarify thoughts (e.g., "How do you describe failure?").
- *Reflecting*: This expresses to the client that the therapist understands the client's frame of mind. The therapist reflects how s/he understands the feelings of the client, the experience of the client, and the content that the client is trying to express.
- *Summarizing*: Brammer (1988) says that summarizing gives the client a "feeling of movement in exploring ideas and feelings, as well as awareness of progress in learning and problem solving" (p.79). For example, "Let review what we have talked about so far." or "Let's take a look at the progress you have made."

- *Confronting*: Confronting a client may put the therapy at risk because the technique can result in a negative or defensive reaction from the client. It is a useful technique in certain circumstances, though, because it challenges the client and encourages open communication. Confronting the client allows the therapist to share with the client what s/he feels or thinks is going on (e.g., "I believe that you are underestimating yourself. Based on your performance in the clinic, I think that you will need very little physical assistance when you're out in the community.").
- *Interpreting*: This helps clients see their problems in new ways and encourages clients to explore new ways of looking at life problems on their own without the help of a therapist.
- *Informing*: This is part of the education process. Providing the client with information that impacts his/her ability to handle stress, maintain or improve health, or maximize functioning and independence is an essential component of helping skills.

Loss and crisis

Brammer (1988) explains that "dealing with people in crisis calls for flexibility of response, rapid and creative intervening with alternatives, and setting limited goals for getting the person functional" (p. 95). The client's ability to deal with stress and crisis depends on many factors including his/her values, beliefs, attitudes, culture, experiences, and personality. Examples of loss and crisis include death of a loved one, disaster, divorce, imprisonment, disability, and loss of a job.

Zuckerman (2000) recommends that therapists working with clients who are in crisis acknowledge and validate the client's distress, despite the therapist's own interpretation of the event, and encourage the client to express his/her feelings. The client and family should be reassured that the therapist and/or other identified health professionals are readily available and willing to help. When positive expressions are observed (e.g., a smile, verbalizing a positive feeling) the therapist is to acknowledge, support, and reinforce these responses. The availability and encouragement to engage in healthy coping activities is another helpful intervention (e.g., journaling, meditation, physical exercise). For clients who have a strong likelihood of making the current situation worse by making impulsive decisions clouded by stress (e.g., client says he is going to sell everything he owns and move into a shack in the mountains), written or verbal behavior contracts may be helpful. This also holds true for the client who has a strong likelihood to engage in unhealthy behaviors when feeling down and depressed (e.g., substance abuse, suicide). Finally, Zuckerman recommends that therapists provide ongoing support and reassurance until the crisis is resolved or able to be managed in a healthy way.

Singer (2001) proposes a different model for dealing with crisis. She suggests that the client should avoid thinking about or dealing with any aspect of the crisis until most of the details of normal life are restored. Some losses are so great (e.g., losing a home during a fire) that thinking about the loss can consume all of the survivor's limited energy. It is better to not think about the loss and concentrate that energy on getting life back together. She offers six tactics for survivors of emotional shock:

1. People who go through emotional shock need more than a bed for sleeping. Calm, uncluttered surroundings convey order and safety, which survivors need to mentally rest.
2. Return to basic routines as quickly as possible. This means regular mealtimes and bedtimes. In the first weeks, you should limit, if possible, unnecessary changes such as shuttling from one hotel to another.
3. Friends and helpers can give practical help with cleanup, food, telephone calls, and replacing survivor's toiletries with familiar brands and scents.
4. The anxiety triggered by emotional shock interferes with the survivor's ability to retain information. Let a helper take notes at meetings with FEMA, insurance adjusters, and bank officers.
5. Familiar faces of friends, neighbors, store clerks, and librarians stabilize and reassure survivors.
6. Steer away from replays of the fire, earthquake, or any other disturbing event as they can re-awaken impressions of the all-to-recent catastrophe and rekindle emotional distress. (p.18).

Lucas (2004) points out that there are two kinds of loss (or trauma) and that it is important to differentiate between them when deciding on a course of treatment. One kind of loss occurs in a way that is outside the client's control. This is most commonly seen in natural disasters such as fires, floods, and hurricanes. For this kind of loss, there is no reason for the client to spend any time or energy thinking about what happened. There is no way to change it, and other issues are more pressing. The second kind of loss occurs because of something that is in the client's control such as abuse of a child by an alcoholic partner. In this case the client can end the ongoing trauma by leaving the relationship. On-

going counseling to look at the bad relationship is appropriate in these cases because the client will need to think about the problem every day to avoid falling back into the old relationship or starting a new, equally destructive one.

While "processing" or "talking through" trauma is the generally accepted approach to all trauma cases, there are some situations where it makes the situation worse. The therapist needs to distinguish between the two kinds of loss or trauma and advise the client appropriately.

Experiential learning: Experiential learning is a counseling technique that can be applied in almost every situation. It is the process of learning through experiences. It relates to several old sayings, "I need to see it with my own eyes," "I need to experience it myself," and "seeing is believing." Therapists are wonderful educators, and they are also wonderful craftsmen and women. Therapists carefully design situations, environments, and events so that experiential learning opportunities are available. Such learning opportunities may be structured in a community environment where the client is challenged to carry over learned skills from the clinic or in a group situation where the client may be challenged to assert himself/herself in a healthy manner. Unless clients are challenged to actually practice and apply skills they have learned, they will be unlikely to do them on their own after discharge.

Common Psychotherapy Terms

Common psychotherapy terms often used in recreational therapy counseling literature are discussed below. Many of the issues discussed are not acknowledged in the ICF, because they are not universally accepted or defined in all cultures (e.g., one country may promote autonomy while another country does not). Consequently, if the therapist wants to note the extent of impairment of these functions within the ICF, it is recommended that therapists score the specific skill or activity that is being affected by the function and write a notation to the right of the scored code (e.g., d5702 Maintaining One's Health — affected by impaired self-efficacy). If the ICF does list a specific function described below, you will be directed to the correct code.

Autonomy: The extent to which a client feels free to make decisions and choices. Loss of autonomy is common for clients in health care settings commonly contributing to symptoms of depression. To maintain autonomy, clients should be given as many decisions and choices as possible (e.g., choose one of the two treatments modalities available for the session, contribute to therapy schedule development).

Self-efficacy: How well the person feels that s/he can perform a particular behavior/action within a defined setting given all of the probable constraints and facilitators. In other words, to what extent does the person feel that s/he can accomplish the task/behavior at hand? "Clients' expectations of themselves largely determine how willing they will be to deal with their problems, how much effort they will be willing to expend, and whether they will make a perseverant effort. Those who are self-doubters are likely to express little effort and will give up quickly if their initial efforts are not productive. Those with high efficacy expectations are apt to face their difficulties with determination, to exert maximum effort, and to persevere even when frustration is encountered" (Austin, 2004, p 409). Bandura (1986) identifies four sources of information that affect self-efficacy.

1. *Performance*: Successful (and repetitive) accomplishment of an action, task, or behavior that the client perceives to be successful. The concept of success is defined by the person's interpretation of his/her performance. Despite the interpretation of others, if the person does not view his/her performance as a success, it will not contribute to perceived self-efficacy. Recreational therapists provide clients with tasks that can be completed successfully and then gradually increase the complexity of the task as self-efficacy grows. For example, instead of the therapist asking a client with a newly acquired spinal cord injury to try to do a full wheelie, s/he shows the client how to pop the front caster wheels one inch off the ground and has the client perform this skill as a precursor skill to learning how to do a full wheelie.

2. *Vicarious experience*: Observing other people (who are similar to ourselves) succeed at a desired action, task, or behavior contributes to feelings of self-efficacy. It can be viewed as a source of motivation and a model of encouragement (e.g., "if he can do it, then I can do it"). In some cases, the recreational therapist is an appropriate model. However, in other instances a more similar peer would provide better self-efficacy outcomes. For example, the client may be somewhat motivated by watching her over-weight therapist exercise on her lunch hour. Observing a fellow client exercise during unstructured time who is more similar in age, injury, and abilities may instill a deeper feeling of self-efficacy. The use of peer counselors is another common intervention (e.g., asking a former client who has the same, or nearly the same, injury and life characteristics to meet with the current client who is experiencing a problem

or concern that the former client also experienced and worked through successfully).

3. *Verbal persuasion*: Positive remarks about performance from a respected and trusted person can affect perceived self-efficacy (e.g., "You are a strong person and I am proud of you. Keep going."). The best person to meet this need for the client will vary (e.g., peer, sister, parent). Therapists encourage positive remarks by modeling the behavior in front of the identified person (e.g., making positive remarks about the client in the presence of his parents). Therapists may also meet with the identified person separately and encourage the sharing of positive remarks with the client.

4. *Physiological arousal*: Some level of physiological arousal (e.g., anxiety) is helpful (e.g., "I was feeling a little nervous, but I did it." shows that the client's ability to work through feelings of anxiousness contributed to self-efficacy). If stress and anxiety are too high however, it can be detrimental to performance (e.g., "I'm too nervous to do it. There is no way I'm going to do that"). Finding a balance is key. Recreational therapists provide clients with tasks where success is expected and challenges are realistically achievable.

Self-awareness: The extent to which the client is aware of himself/herself (e.g., how much the client knows about his/her strengths, weaknesses, preferences, beliefs, attitudes, values). A realistic appraisal of oneself and some level of acceptance of one's attributes is a good foundation for developing a healthy leisure lifestyle. Austin (2004) defines education in leisure self-awareness as helping "clients examine their leisure lifestyles so that they may become aware of values, patterns, and behaviors reflected in their lifestyles, as well as barriers to achieving the leisure lifestyle they seek. Having such an understanding allows clients to plan and make alteration in their leisure lifestyle" (p.66). There is no comparable term in the ICF for self-awareness and at this time ICF does not contain this kind of category or component because it is not a concept that is universally held in all cultures. There are numerous categories in the ICF that relate to self-awareness including orientation to self (b11420), insight (b1644), experience of self (b1800), body image (b1801), ensuring one's physical comfort (d5700), managing one's health (d5702), and maintaining social space (d7204).

Self-esteem: The extent that a client feels good about his/her attributes. The amount of positive regard a client has for himself/herself. See "Self-

Esteem" in the Techniques section for more information.

Locus of control: Internal locus of control is the extent to which a client believes and behaves in a manner that reflects a feeling of control over his/her life, choices, and actions. The person feels like s/he is in control of himself/herself. External locus of control is the extent to which a client believes and behaves in a manner that reflects a feeling of lack of control over his/her life, choice, and actions. The person feels like s/he is being controlled by outside forces (e.g., family, relationships, work). Giving a client the kinds of experiences and choices discussed in the sections on self-determination, self-efficacy, and autonomy will allow the client to experience a more internal locus of control. The ICF does not have references to locus of control because cultures do not agree on which locus of control is most appropriate.

Self-determination: Being in control of behavior by acting based on values and beliefs instead of society's norms. Dattilo and Williams (2000) define self-determination as "being in control of the course a life takes" (p. 169). The concept of self-determination is one of the concepts used in recreation and leisure that has a cultural bias. Self-determination tends to be a strongly held belief in the United States, but it is not a universally accepted concept (Reber, 1995). Reber points out that self-determination tends to be supported by theorists with an existentialist orientation. Self-determination is not contained in the ICF model and probably falls under the heading of making decisions (d177). Austin (2004) reports that leisure self-determination is an attribute required for a person to experience leisure (e.g., "I create my own life; I choose my actions; I design my destiny"). Achieving self-determination and promoting control over his/her leisure lifestyle is a complex process that varies from client to client based on the client's current beliefs, experiences, and learned behaviors. Experiential learning (designing tasks in which the client experiences control), existential counseling, and cognitive-behavioral interventions (changing distorted thinking patterns) are common techniques used to promote and develop self-determination.

Attitude: A low intensity emotional state that is relatively short-lived (burlingame & Blaschko, 2002). Attitudes are often influenced by culture, religion, peers, life experiences, situations, and desired outcomes.

Attitudes are hard to measure because they are not visible actions. The measurement of attitudes relies heavily on the client's report through valid assessment tools. burlingame & Blaschko (2002) report that using a solid testing tool for measuring attitudes is important because "attitudes can clearly be barriers to developing and nurturing relationships,

being willing to risk new experiences to allow use of one's community, or even participating in treatment" (p.208). Additionally, attitudes help the therapist identify a direction of treatment (e.g., need for education, need for further assessment, doesn't need counseling on general benefits of leisure and can move on to assessment of leisure lifestyle). This is particularly important for the recreational therapist because attitudes and beliefs are typically assessed and addressed prior to implementation of other interventions. A full understanding of the benefits of leisure by the client along with the understanding by the therapist of the client's beliefs and attitudes forms the basis for developing a leisure lifestyle plan. burlingame & Blaschko (2002) discuss seven complete testing tools for attitudes. The most important ones are the *Cooperation and Trust Scale, Free Time Boredom,* the *Idyll Arbor Leisure Battery,* and the *Life Satisfaction Scale.* Brief summaries of the assessment tools can be found in the Assessment section.

Values: "Values are deeply held attitudes and beliefs we have about the truth, beauty, or worth of a person, object, action, or idea. One criterion of a 'true' value is that it has become a part of a pattern of a person's life. In other words, values must not only be identified, but embraced and expressed" (Purtilo & Haddad, 2002, p.5). Recreational therapists help clients explore what holds meaning in their lives, what holds importance, and what is cherished. It may be a specific action (e.g., spending time with grandchildren), a concept (e.g., peace and calm), a person (e.g., my sister), an attribute (e.g., honesty, health), or a variety of other things. Clients are asked to look closely at how they spend their time and lead their lives to evaluate the degree of expression of those things in their life. If they are reflected minimally or are absent from the client's lifestyle, the therapist and client explore ways for the client to experience and incorporate these ideals into his/her life, thus contributing to life satisfaction. Austin (2004) cautions therapists "not to impose a value or course of action on participants but to encourage them to look at alternatives and their consequences" (p. 70). Facilitating this insight is also educational. It highlights characteristics of activities, use of time, and personal values, all of which increase under-standing of leisure and heighten awareness of personal control (e.g., "Are you living and expressing your life in a way that you want to? What control do you have over changing it? How would you go about changing it?").

Beliefs: An emotional acceptance of a statement or position that cannot be supported by observable evidence (burlingame & Blaschko, 2002). Like values, beliefs are often influenced by culture, religion, and life experiences. It is the recreational therapist's responsibility to understand the client's beliefs. There are some serious ethical issues that arise when beliefs are involved, especially in the area of religion. Some religions believe that God is the only appropriate healer and that medical interventions are never appropriate. This leads to cases where parents refuse life-saving care for their children. Often the courts become involved to force the parents to allow the care. Whether it is appropriate for a therapist, a medical team, or the courts to try to change a client's beliefs or force a client to go against his/her beliefs is an issue we will not discuss in this book.

References

Austin, D. (2004). *Therapeutic recreation processes and techniques, 5th edition.* Champaign, IL: Sagamore Publishing.

Bandura, A. (1986). *Social foundations of thought and action: A social cognitive theory.* Englewood Cliffs, NJ: Prentice-Hall, Inc.

Brammer, L. (1988). *The helping relationship: Process and skills, 4th edition.* Englewood Cliffs, NJ: Prentice Hall.

burlingame, j. & Blaschko, T. M. (2002). *Assessment tools for recreational therapy and related fields, third edition.* Ravensdale, WA: Idyll Arbor.

Corey, G. (1996). *Theory and practice of counseling and psychotherapy, 5th edition.* Pacific Grove, CA: Books/Cole Publishing Company.

Dattilo, J., & Williams, R. (2000). Leisure education. In J. Dattilo (Ed.), *Facilitation techniques in therapeutic recreation.* State College, PA: Venture Publishing, Inc.

Luborsky, L. (1984). *Principles of psychoanalytic psychotherapy: A manual for supportive expressive treatment.* Basic Books.

Lucas, K. (2004). Private communication.

Purtilo, R., & Haddad, A. (2002). *Health professional and patient interaction (6th edition).* Philadelphia, PA: W. B. Saunders Company.

Reber, A. (1995*). Implicit learning and tacit knowledge: An essay on the cognitive unconscious.* New York, NY: Oxford University Press.

Singer, I. (2001). *Emotional recovery after natural disaster: How to get back to normal life.* Ravensdale, WA: Idyll Arbor, Inc.

Stumbo, N. & Peterson, C. (2004). *Therapeutic recreation program design: Principles and procedures.* (4th Ed.) San Francisco, CA: Pearson Benjamin Cummings.

UNESCO's International Standards Standard of Education ISCED-1997.

Zuckerman, E (2000). *Clinician's Thesaurus, 5th edition.* New York, New York: The Guilford Press.

Emergency Response

Emergency response is defined as recognizing a sudden, unexpected hazardous situation, and initiating action to reduce the threat to health and safety. This section describes a protocol to teach clients how to be more successful at emergency response.

Individuals who feel confident in their ability to handle unexpected events may feel less anxious in a community setting. Problem solving, in and of itself, can be empowering, as well as decrease or minimize the risk of injury or harm.

Indications

When working with clients who have disabilities, whether new or old, there may be a need to teach them how to deal with situations in the community that could endanger their health and safety. Just because an individual has had a spinal cord injury for five years does not mean that the therapist can assume the client knows what to do in case of an emergency. The client's ability to problem solve and act depends on many factors, including experience, knowledge, initiation, and functional abilities. Therapists assess the client's ability to verbally respond to proposed emergency situations while in the clinic (e.g., "What would you do if there was a fire in your home?", "What would you do if someone took your wallet when you were out at the store?", "What would you do if you were feeling symptoms of autonomic dysreflexia while at a friend's house?").

Knowing the client's medical history, ask the client if s/he has ever experienced an emergency in the community and how s/he handled the situation. The therapist should use this protocol if the therapist determines that the client is unable to quickly identify safe responses, is not able to identify emergency situations, or has not considered responses to emergency situations.

Contraindications: A client who has significant cognitive impairments that impact his/her ability to recall, retain, or apply verbal, pictorial, or demonstrative education is not appropriate for this protocol. If significant cognitive impairments are evident, the therapist will need to educate the client's caregivers and any other people that will be taking the client out into the community.

Protocol

The length and frequency of emergency response training will vary depending upon the identified needs and abilities of the client. Potential emergencies are identified through activity and systematic analysis of each task that will be part of the client's activity pattern.

Education should take place in a quiet, non-distracting environment to promote concentration.

The therapist should have relevant materials (e.g., specific worksheets developed by the therapist that reflect the potential emergencies that could occur and recommendations for handling such emergencies, paper/pen to write additional emergencies and suggested responses).

Additional sessions should be scheduled to evaluate performance (the ability to apply the information in a real-life environment). This is typically done as community integration training. Please refer to "Integration" and "Community Problem Solving" for more information on related issues.

Process

The therapist will need to:
1. *Identify the specific concerns relevant to the individual client*: There are too many emergencies to identify them all. However, the therapist can help the client to identify the most common emergencies for his/her situation and encourage the client to express his/her own community emergency fears (e.g., "I'm afraid that I might fall out of my wheelchair.", "I'm afraid I will have a bowel accident when I'm out in the community."). Once a list has been compiled, the client and therapist can move on to step two.
2. *Help the client identify possible responses*: There are many ways to respond to an emergency depending on the situation, the resources, and the client's abilities. For this protocol, one goal is to teach the client how to deal with a few common emergencies. A more important goal is to teach the client to respond to emergencies without panicking, so that s/he can figure out the best way to respond quickly and effectively, even to emergencies that s/he hasn't considered.

Start with one identified emergency such as, "I'm afraid I might fall out of my wheelchair when I'm out in the community."

Place the emergency into three or more contexts (e.g., falling out of the wheelchair at home, at the store, on the sidewalk).

Identify at least two different responses to each situation. Possible responses to falling at home are, "If I fall out of my wheelchair at home I can ask my wife to help me." and "If no one is home, I would have to lie on the floor until someone gets there since

I can't get into my wheelchair by myself. This could be a problem if I need to use the bathroom or answer the door or phone." Sometimes discussing emergencies will help the client figure out that there are things s/he could do to prepare for emergencies before they happen. (Sometimes the therapist needs to suggest looking for possibilities.) In this case the possibilities include keeping the cordless phone with the client so s/he can call someone to come and help. The phone would also give the client the ability to call an emergency center in case s/he is badly hurt and needs immediate care. Thinking about the possibilities might even convince the client to be more diligent about wearing a seatbelt to decrease the chances of falling out of the wheelchair.

3. *Practice implementing learned strategies*: Emergencies can be simulated. For example, let the air out of a wheelchair tire while at the mall and have the client fix the flat. Another common way to address emergency response is to ask the client during a community integration outing how s/he would respond to an emergency situation with the resources available. For example, when a client is getting ready to cross a busy intersection with a signal, ask the client what she would do if the light wasn't working and s/he needed to get across the street.

NOTE: If the client has significant cognitive impairments, the client will require supervision at all times in the community and caregivers will need to be educated on how to respond to community emergencies. If the client has mild cognitive impairments and supervision in a community setting will not be provided, the client will probably use a memory book (a bound notebook of written information such as things to do and contact numbers, as discussed in "Neuroplasticity" in the Techniques section). When identifying possible emergencies and responses, make a section in the memory book called "Emergencies" and write appropriate information in the memory book for reference. The information should be very simple and clearly written, including who to contact.

Documentation

The therapist documents the identified risks to the client's health and safety (e.g., disability-specific precautions, common community concerns, possible equipment failures). The therapist documents the education provided to the client and the client's ability to understand the information in theoretical situations. Every attempt should be made to have the client also implement responses, especially if the event is likely to occur. Documentation of the client's functional performance in a simulated or real emergency is also recorded. Emergency Response Training is an intervention, so it is not scored in the ICF. It is provided in response to identified difficulties such as b144 Memory Functions, d175 Solving Problems, d620 Acquisition of Goods and Services, d910 Community Life, and d920 Recreation and Leisure.

Special credentialing/training: There is no additional credentialing or training needed by a CTRS to implement this protocol.

Energy Conservation Training

Many clients seen in a rehabilitation setting fatigue easily during physical activity due to deconditioning, physical limitations (e.g., amputated lower extremity, knee replacement), and impaired body functions (e.g., poor cardiac or respiratory functions). Some clients may also have specific precautions or parameters that limit the amount of energy they are allowed to expend (e.g., cannot continue to engage in physical activity if blood pressure, pulse, or oxygen saturation reaches a particular level). This section discusses teaching clients how to participate in activities when they need to conserve their energy.

Keeping energy requirements within appropriate limits is very important. If the amount of physical energy spent goes beyond the client's limits, severe consequences can occur (e.g., heart attack, multiple sclerosis exacerbation, falls, fainting) impacting the client's level of independence, functioning, and quality of life. For example, a client with severe osteoporosis fell because she became fatigued when walking in a park that did not have park benches. As a result she fractured a vertebra and needs to wear a brace to stabilize her spine so that it can heal. Any activity that puts her at further risk of injury is now contraindicated until the vertebra heals. She now needs assistance with home and community activities and is unable to take her grandchildren to the park.

When the amount of physical energy that one is allowed to expend (or can expend) is limited, it poses great difficulty in completing activities, especially community activities that require a great deal of walking or wheelchair propulsion. Consequently, clients may avoid activities that require physical effort. This is often not the best choice since a sedentary lifestyle causes other complications (see "Consequences of Inactivity" in the Concepts section). Therapists must be careful, however, to teach clients a healthy balance between activity and rest. Both too much energy expenditure and too much energy conservation can be detrimental to health.

Energy conservation training is an intervention to teach clients how to conserve energy so that tasks can be accomplished without risk of injury or harm. It can also contribute to feelings of self-efficacy (e.g., I didn't think I could go to the mall because it requires a lot of walking, but now I can see how it is possible) and activity enjoyment (e.g., client enjoys the activity because he is not overwhelmed with feelings of fatigue and concern about breaking his cardiac precautions). In some instances, clients may need to be educated about why physical activity is needed prior to implementing this intervention.

Prior to implementing energy conservation training:
1. Therapists need to understand the client's limitations and precautions related to physical activity.
2. Therapists need to know the client's functional mobility skills (walking, wheelchair propulsion, transfers).
3. Therapists need to know the client's premorbid activity pattern (what the client's lifestyle looked like prior to injury) and have an idea of what the client's activity pattern will look like once s/he returns home (the activities and tasks the client desires to engage in after discharge).

Client Education

Educating clients involves explaining why energy conservation techniques are important and what steps to take to conserve energy.

The first step is to explain the purpose of energy conservation training as it relates to the client's health situation and the activities that s/he desires to perform.

Example: *"At our last session we talked about why it is important to stay active and get out of the house. My concern, however, is that you are currently walking only 150' with a rolling walker. This is a good distance for getting around the home, but when you are out in the community 150' won't get you that far. Do you know about how far 150' is? A standard grocery store aisle is about 100'. So, if you parked your car in a handicap parking spot and walked down one grocery store aisle you would be really tired. But...as we talked about before,...going to the grocery store is good because it gives you exercise, it gives you people to talk to, and it will help with your recovery because it helps you to become stronger. So, we have a dilemma...we know that is it good to go to the grocery store, but we also know that it is above what you can do. So let's talk about how you can do this."*

The second step is to let the client know how to conserve energy. One way is to think about energy conservation in terms of the five "Ps": Prioritize, Plan, Pace, Position, and Pounds.

Prioritize

Clients may put too many activities requiring a high amount of physical energy into one day. There is not only a risk of injury or harm, but it can also lead the client to feel frustrated when s/he is unable to complete the tasks. This can lead to depression or anxiety and giving up healthy activities (e.g., "It is too much work to go shopping, so I'll just let my husband do it.") leads to secondary complications from a less active lifestyle. Therapists encourage clients to:

- Make a list of all of the things that they want to accomplish in a day or week.
- Prioritize the activities based on their deadlines, needs, and desires.

When energy levels are compromised, many clients have a tendency to prioritize activities that have to be done (e.g., housecleaning, doctors' appointments, grocery shopping) and stop doing recreational activities. Clients must be educated about the importance of recreational activities for recovery and health promotion (e.g., It is very important that you continue to go to the senior center because that is where you get to be with all of your friends. You might not realize this now, but having people to talk to will help you get through tough times, and it is actually very good for you to laugh and have fun because when you laugh and have fun your body releases endorphins that actually help to reduce pain.). "Activity Pattern Development" in the Techniques section has more information on prioritizing.

Plan

Once a client is able to prioritize a healthy activity list for the day or week, the therapist talks to the client about planning techniques for each activity that can reduce the amount of energy expended to a level that is appropriate for the client. Some suggestions for planning include:

- Figuring out what time of day the client has the most energy. This is the best time to schedule activities that require a lot of energy. Although this is not always possible (e.g., client relies on her daughter to take her to the knitting shop and she is only available on Saturday afternoons), it is encouraged whenever possible.
- Doing an activity analysis of each activity and identifying techniques that can be used. For example:
  o Apply for and use a handicapped parking placard so that the client can park in a handicap parking space. This will reduce the amount of walking or wheelchair propulsion to the front door. Handicapped parking spaces are also wider (at least they are supposed to be) allowing the client extra room to open up the car door and easily exit the car.

o Plan a travel route. Where do you need to go in the building and what do you need to do when you are there? How far will you need to walk or propel the wheelchair? Are there places along the travel route to sit and rest? Planning out a travel route will reduce the chances of backtracking or spending unnecessary energy (e.g., walking down an aisle at the store that does not have an item). Clients are encouraged to use mall directories, aisle signs, and assistance from customer service whenever possible.

o Ask for assistance. Clients are encouraged to ask for assistance with tasks that are above their energy limits (e.g., carrying heavy bags, retrieving an item at the end of the aisle).

o Use adaptive equipment. Clients are encouraged to use electric store scooters if needed. They are available at many grocery stores, large store chains (e.g., Wal-Mart, Kmart, Sam's Club), malls, and even some amusement parks and other recreational spots. Explain the process of using a store scooter. Explore other personal adaptive equipment that the client may have to conserve energy (e.g., reacher, walker bag, backpack).

Pace

Rushing can put the client in a very dangerous situation that could lead to injury or harm. Common situations include trying to keep up with another person, trying to walk quickly across a parking lot so as not to hold up a car that is waiting, moving quickly in the home when trying to get ready for an outing, or not sitting and taking a rest because time is short or needing to rest is embarrassing. Therapists talk to clients about:

- *Build in extra time*: Clients are encouraged to build in extra time when getting ready to go out. Extra time is often needed to get ready due to limitations and impairments. It is also important to build in additional time to allow rest periods when getting ready. So, if a client currently requires one hour to get ready, then it would be best for the client to give herself an hour and a half to get ready.
- *Don't rush*: Clients are educated about the dangers of allowing their energy expenditure to be influenced by others (e.g., having to rush in line because of someone behind the client, not wanting to sit and take a rest because he knows that his shopping partner is in a rush to get home). It is often helpful to validate that these

feelings are normal, but that at this stage in the game the client needs to take care of himself/herself. Otherwise the resulting injury or harm may affect important and meaningful life activities even more negatively.

- *Sit before you are tired*: Clients are encouraged to sit before they feel tired. Once a client is tired, it is difficult to recoup and go on with the activity. Sitting without being tired can be a very hard thing to do, because it isn't natural to sit down and take a rest then. One technique is to encourage clients to look for places to sit while walking and when a place is spotted, perform a time check ("How long have I been walking?") and judge whether or not it would be beneficial to take advantage of the opportunity. Some places don't have many places to sit. Outside of the traditional chairs and benches, some creative places to sit and rest include the bathroom, stairwell, dressing room, shoe department, furniture department, sport department (e.g., open up a folding sport chair), or ledge. Tell the client if s/he has been looking for a place to sit and has not been successful in finding one, to be assertive and ask someone to bring him/her a chair or anything else that may be suitable to rest on. Encourage clients to explain the urgency of the situation so that action is taken immediately (e.g., "Excuse me. I am not feeling so great and I really need to sit down because I am afraid I am going to fall. Could you please get me something to sit down on?").

Position

The posture of the body, items being carried, and positions relative to the current task all have an impact on energy expenditure. See "Body Mechanics and Ergonomics" for more information. Common techniques include:

- *Posture*: Sitting or standing with good posture uses the least energy. It also opens up the lungs and allows for better oxygen intake for energy expenditure.
- *Objects*: Place objects in places where they are easy to reach (e.g., put coupons in a waist pack so they can be easily accessed instead of in a backpack).
- *Environment*: Design environments that reduce energy expenditure (e.g., organization reduces the amount of energy needed to find things, limited furnishings reduces the amount of energy needed to negotiate around things). When in environments that can't be manipulated, look for the best line of approach for the task to minimize energy expended (e.g., in an art class that

requires the client to get up and down multiple times to retrieve supplies, it would be best to choose a table that is close to the supplies to minimize the amount of walking).

Pounds

Carrying extra weight requires the client to expend more physical energy. Body weight and items being carried both add to energy expenditure. Common recommendations include:

- *Lose extra body weight*: Encourage clients who are overweight to strive for a healthy body weight.
- *Analyze extra weight carried*: Clients can place carried items on a scale to find out how much weight they are actually carrying.
- *Prioritize*: Prioritize what is needed such as limiting the number of things that are carried in a pocketbook or tote bag.
- *Exchange*: Exchange heavy items for lighter ones such as carrying a nylon jacket in a backpack instead of a heavy sweatshirt. Another common problem is using a heavy and cumbersome pocketbook. Not only is it in the way, making it more challenging to maintain balance, it also has a tendency to slide off the shoulder. Clients should opt for a smaller and lighter pocketbook that has a long strap so that it can be worn across the chest.
- *Carry/transport heavy items by different methods*: For example, carrying a five-pound item in a backpack puts less stress on the cardiovascular system than carrying it in the arms because the load is being carried through larger muscle groups and more efficient skeletal structures. Other examples include using a suitcase with wheels instead of one with a handle or going to the grocery store, picking out and paying for the groceries, and then requesting the items to be delivered to the home.

Documentation

Therapists commonly document ECT in three ways:

1. *Education given*: The therapist documents the education provided to the client. For example, "Client verbally educated about energy conservation techniques for community activities."
2. *Verbal application*: The therapist documents the client's ability to describe techniques for specific activities. To do this, the therapist identifies a place that the client will go after discharge (e.g., department store) and asks the client what s/he could do to decrease the amount of energy expended to complete the task. A typical note

might look like this, "After energy conservation education, client able to describe 75% of the appropriate energy conservation techniques for going to the department store."

3. *Direct application*: The therapist documents the client's ability to apply techniques in a specific activity. This can be done during a community integration session (e.g., trip to the mall) or on hospital grounds (e.g., trip to the hospital gift shop, walk around hospital grounds). A common approach is for the therapist to tell the client that s/he would like the client to apply energy conservation techniques. The therapist may review the techniques or test the client's recall by not making suggestions. The therapist then watches the client's actions and assesses his/her ability to perform the techniques throughout the activity. The amount of follow through is typically assessed in the percentage form. For example, if the therapist identified ten techniques that could be applied to the task and the client performed six of them, then the note might look something like this, "Independently performed 60% of energy conservation techniques during integration training at the mall."

Energy conservation training can be used to address deficits in many of the activities in Activities and Participation, especially the codes under d4 Mobility. Some other codes where energy conservation training may play a part in working on an impairment include d175 Solving Problems, d1551 Acquiring Complex Skills, d177 Making Decisions, and d220 Undertaking Multiple Tasks.

Exercise Basics

This section looks at the basics of providing an exercise program for clients. The most likely reasons for an exercise program are

- deficits in exercise tolerance (b455)
- deficits in b7 Neuromusculoskeletal and Movement-Related Functions
- other cardiovascular issues (b400-b499)
- rehabilitation from surgery
- rehabilitation after injury
- health promotion for maintenance of health or to prevent secondary complications

It is important that the therapist understands the reason for the exercise and the goals of the client and the medical team before any program is planned. This section will cover the basics of planning and carrying out an exercise program with a client.

Preparing for Physical Exercise

Obtain clearance from physician: Clearance must be obtained from the client's physician prior to engaging in an exercise program. For people who have health conditions, ask the physician or medical team for specific exercise recommendations (e.g., type of exercise such as aerobic, stretching, or weight training to meet desired goals; amount of time, intensity, and frequency of exercise to meet desired goals). The therapist will also need to understand precautions for the client's condition. These precautions will usually be stated as measurable physical parameters such as heart rate, blood pressure, or oxygen saturation levels. They may also include contraindication of certain body movements such as those required after a total hip replacement, restrictions on amount of weight to be lifted, or other limitations caused by the client's medical condition, such as immunological deficiencies.

Clearance to participate in an exercise program must be received from the client's treating physician prior to engagement in physical activity. Depending on the setting, the client may ask the physician directly for clearance (e.g., a client who desires to participate in a community exercise program) or a therapist may seek clearance for the client (e.g., therapist who is working with a client in an inpatient physical rehabilitation setting).

Choose specific forms of exercise: Once recommendations and specific orders from the physician are obtained, specific forms of exercise are chosen that are best matched with the client's interests and his/her precautions, parameters, and recommendations set by the physician (e.g., seated exercise video, walking, swimming, gardening, tennis, running).

Adaptations may need to be made to accommodate the client's abilities and limitations (e.g., adapting upper body exercises that are above the heart to exercise movements that are below the heart, walking instead of jogging, using a lighter piece of exercise equipment, or sitting instead of standing).

In a healthy adult, it is recommended that aerobic activity within one's target heart rate be maintained for 20 minutes. People who have particular health conditions, however, may not be able to sustain 20 minutes of cardiovascular activity, and it may not be safe for an individual to maintain aerobic activity for such a prolonged period of time (e.g., recovery from myocardial infarction). Depending on the client's medical condition, the physician may state a specific period of time that the client is allowed to participate in cardiovascular activity (e.g., no more than 10 minutes of sustained light cardiovascular activity). Physical measures other than heart rate may be required for assessing the safety of the physical activity in cases where the heart rate is controlled medically or mechanically. This may include blood pressure, respiration, and oxygen saturation level.

Strength training, resistance training, and weight lifting all refer to exercises that build muscle. Strength training helps the client to build muscle or to regain strength following an injury or surgery. Weight lifting is a typical way to build strength, but some clients may have conditions where weights are not appropriate. This should be covered in the physician's recommendations. If it is not, make sure you understand the client's limitations before you make a plan.

There are several important aspects of strength training that the therapist must consider when devising a program. Balance between muscle pairs must be maintained. Do not exercise one muscle (such as the quadriceps) without also exercising the other muscle in the pair (the hamstring) unless there are specific recommendations from the physician. Muscle strength is important, but studies have shown that the balance between muscle pairs is slightly more important for proper muscle function in regards to balance and the most efficient physical movements (Johnston, 1992; Rosenstein, 2002; Whitney et al, 2000). Regular strength training is important, especially in adulthood, because lean muscle mass is gradually lost through the aging process. Muscle also burns fat at a higher rate during aerobic activity, thus contributing to weight loss.

Educate the client about exercise and personal health: Prior to engagement in physical exercise, a client is educated (as appropriate) about:

1. The relation of exercise to the client's recovery and health promotion.
2. The specific precautions, parameters, and restrictions set by the physician.
3. Contraindications of particular forms of physical exercise (e.g., running as a form of regular physical exercise exceeds recommendations after a total joint replacement).
4. How to self-monitor vital signs (e.g., pulse, blood pressure).
5. Adaptations to assist the person in maintaining precautions, parameters, and recommendations (e.g., equipment, techniques).
6. Adaptations to maximize performance in physical activity (e.g., identification of accessible areas in the home to store exercise equipment, color coded play and stop VCR buttons to help a client with cognitive difficulties use an exercise video, workarounds for barriers to exercise participation).
7. Recommendations for the amount of time, frequency, and intensity of exercise.

Engaging in Physical Exercise

Warm-up: The therapist assesses the client's understanding of the information previously presented and establishes goals with the client (as appropriate) related to learning (e.g., client is able to independently locate, palpitate, and accurately count pulse rate; client can adapt exercise movements to stay within movement restrictions set by physician with minimal verbal cues).

Vital signs are taken before exercising to determine a resting baseline and to make sure that the client is within his/her precautions and parameters prior to engaging in physical activity. If appropriate, ask the client to measure his/her vital signs and check the client's accuracy (e.g., therapist assessed pulse at 77 beats per minute and client assessed pulse at 89 beats per minute) and re-teach the client alternative monitoring techniques as needed. One adaptation commonly used for taking a pulse is to hold the ears shut with the fingers and take an apical pulse by listening to the number of heartbeats while looking at the second hand on a wall clock.

If precautions and parameters are within the client's limits, a warm-up is initiated (five to ten minutes of light activity to increase heart and lung function and warm up muscles to prevent injury). Standard warm-up activities are light walking and/or range of motion exercises with the intent of lubricating joints and moving, but not stretching, ligaments and tendons. The latest recommendations are to postpone stretching exercises (where the client is trying to significantly increase the length of

muscles) until after warm-ups and usually after aerobic exercise.

Following the warm-up, vital signs are re-assessed to determine a post warm-up baseline and the safety of the client (e.g., maintenance of precautions/parameters).

Initiate cardiovascular activity: After the warm-up, increased cardiovascular activity is initiated. The amount of time that cardiovascular activity is sustained will vary based on the client's exercise functions, willingness to participate, and cognitive ability to sustain participation.

When the client is engaged in cardiovascular activity, the therapist closely monitors the client. Vital signs are taken every five to ten minutes. If vital signs become close to the client's limits or an unexpected change in vital signs is noted (e.g., irregular heart rhythm), the cool down portion of the exercise program should be initiated to bring the cardiorespiratory system back to a resting state. No further exercise should be done before the situation is reported to the medical team and the client's needs are re-evaluated.

In addition to vital signs, therapists monitor outward signs of fatigue including:

- *Shortness of breath* (e.g., difficulty doing the talk test, which is having enough breath to carry on a conversation while exercising).
- *Inability to perform exercise movements correctly* when they were performed correctly earlier (e.g., at the beginning of the program the client was able to perform large lateral arm circles and five minutes into the program the client is only able to perform medium size lateral arm circles).
- *Inability to maintain good posture.*
- *Difficulty maintaining the intensity* of the workout (e.g., able to do eight movements in a count at the beginning and ten minutes into the workout the client is only able to perform four movements within a count).
- *Difficulty maintaining prior level of balance* (e.g., able to maintain dynamic standing balance for a physical activity requiring moderate ranges independently and after 15 minutes of moderate intensity exercise the client requires minimal assistance to maintain dynamic standing balance for moderate ranges).

Initiate strength exercises: Strength exercises may be done before or after the cardiovascular exercises. Generally after is preferred because the body has a chance to warm up more. As with cardiovascular activity, the amount of effort put into approved strength exercises will depend on the client's willingness to participate and cognitive ability to sustain participation. One important consideration during strength exercises is the concept of sets and repetitions. Strength exercises are done in sets for a reason. A particular number of repetitions are required for the most efficient building of muscle tissue. Typically, six to 12 repetitions are used in a set. Because the muscles are being stressed by the strength exercise, they need a chance to recover slightly between sets for maximum benefit. Make sure the client pauses between sets to allow the muscles to relax slightly and to allow blood to restore the oxygen and nutrient levels in the muscles.

The therapist continues to closely monitor the client during these exercises. Vital signs are again taken every five to ten minutes. If vital signs become close to the client's limits or an unexpected change in vital signs is noted (e.g., irregular heart rhythm), the cool down portion of the exercise program is initiated to bring the cardiorespiratory system back to a resting state. Again, the therapist must report the conditions that limited the planned activity to the medical team before more exercise sessions are planned.

In addition to vital signs, therapists again monitor outward signs of fatigue including:
- shortness of breath.
- inability to perform exercise movements.
- inability to maintain good posture.
- difficulty maintaining the same number of repetitions.
- difficulty maintaining balance.

Initiate cool-down: Once the client's tolerance or allowance for cardiovascular exercise is exhausted, the cool-down portion of the exercise program is initiated. The purpose of the cool-down is to bring the body back to a resting state and reduce the stress on the body. It consists of light cardiovascular activity, range of motion exercises, breathing exercises, and stretching exercises.

Documentation

The therapist is responsible for documenting the physical activity the client accomplished in a way that the rest of the medical team can evaluate. It is also important for the documentation to be in a form that allows the client to see his/her progress in increasing fitness and abilities.
- Amount of time engaged in cardiovascular activity.
- The intensity of the cardiovascular activity. Objective measures should be recorded if possible such as exact distance walked in a stated amount of time or the number of repetitions of an exercise that are done during the aerobic activity.
- Exact amounts of weight and numbers of repetitions for every strength exercise.
- The client's ability to self-monitor vital signs and outward signs of fatigue.
- The client's ability to adapt exercises to meet needs (e.g., range restrictions, intensity alterations).
- The client's ability to perform the exercises correctly and safely.
- The client's reaction to participation in the exercise program.
- Vital sign measurements (see "Vital Signs" in the Techniques section for information on how to document vital signs).

References

Johnston, K. (1992). *The effects of exercise on standing balance, pain, and coping resources maintenance: A comparison of land and water exercise for arthritis patients.* Dissertation. Georgia State University, Atlanta, GA.

Rosenstein, A. (2002). *Water exercises for Parkinson's: Maintaining endurance, strength, flexibility, and balance.* Ravensdale, WA: Idyll Arbor, Inc.

Whitney, L., Deel, D., Marple, J., Metzger, S., Wilder, M., & Harrison, A. (2000, May). Balance, fear of falling, and quality of life in arthritic elders participating in an aquatic exercise program. *Physical Therapy*, 80:S36.

Fine Hand Use Ergonomics

This technique discusses issues relevant to fine hand use. How the environment is structured has an effect on the client's ability to perform tasks that require fine hand skills. It is the therapist's responsibility to create an environment that maximizes the client's potential.

Grandjean (1988) lists ten ways to improve a client's performance on tasks that require fine hand use skills. By setting up activities so that they comply with these ten principles the therapist ensures that a client's performance is based on the client's skill level and that the client is not handicapped by the environment. The ten principles are

1. *Elbow position*: The activity should be set up so that the client's elbows are generally slightly lower than the wrists with an angle of between 85° to 110° at the elbow.
2. *Visual distance*: For activities with small details that require good eye-hand coordination, bring the work closer to the client. The client's body position should be one of only a slight bend in the neck and head while leaning forward. The idea is to allow the activity to be placed close enough to the client to allow the client to see well while not requiring the client to assume an uncomfortable position that taxes the body's muscles. It is a good idea for the therapist to ask a client if s/he is able to see the object clearly. Often clients are admitted to facilities without their glasses or contact lenses or lose them once they are admitted. Adaptive devices for vision should be provided for the client so that s/he is able to work in an appropriate position.
3. *Limit muscle loading*: Muscle loading is increasing the amount of strength the muscles are required to exert to maintain the activity. Muscle loading can be holding a heavy load in an uncomfortable position or holding a heavy load in the same position longer than the muscles are able to maintain adequate strength. An example of muscle loading is holding a gallon of milk straight out in front of you, a position that tires the arm muscles fairly quickly. Holding the gallon of milk at rib height close to the body with the elbow lower than the wrist limits the muscle loading required to hold the milk. Muscles that have a heavy muscle load are difficult to control or to coordinate. Position both the client and the activity to reduce the amount of force that causes muscle loading. This may mean that the client uses slings, elbow supports, or lightweight equipment to help reduce muscle loading.

4. *Limit the diversity of fine motor activity required*: Performance on fine hand use tends to increase if the client is required to perform one fine hand use task at a time. An example of this principle is the old sewing machines versus the more modern ones. Older sewing machines required that one hand be used to start or stop the flywheel (that made the needle go up and down) while also guiding the fabric through the machine. Today's sewing machines tend to use foot peddles to start and stop the needle allowing both hands to move the fabric through the machine. Another example is in beading activities. If a client is stringing beads to make a necklace, it is not uncommon for the client to have to place a bead on the thread and then look around to select the next bead. Beading trays allow a client to select all the beads needed for the necklace, place them in the tray trough in the desired order, and then string the already selected beads. For clients with significant impairment of one hand and arm (e.g., after a stroke), taping drawing paper to the table instead of requiring the client to stabilize the paper while drawing also helps limit the amount of fine hand movement activity required at any one time.
5. *Activity setup*: The set up for the activity should help the activity flow from one step to the next and the materials selected should increase (instead of decrease) the client's chance of success. For example, in a painting activity the paper should be in front of the client, the paintbrush rinse water at two o'clock, the paper towel to help dry the brush (after cleaning) at one o'clock and the paints at twelve o'clock above the paper. (This placement is mirrored for a client who is left handed.) Fausek-Steinbach (2002) discusses how to select the materials for a drawing activity.

    The materials one selects to work with are just as important as the process they are used in. Drawing materials can vary from expensive colored pencils, to crayons. The way the materials are perceived, as well as how they perform, are very important when presenting them to your clients. I try to use oil pastels instead of wax crayons whenever possible only because crayons are perceived as "kid's toys" by teens and adults and quickly raise a red flag in the hesitant artist's mind. Avoid smudgy chalks or charcoal pencils for drawings, as the unintended smudges will frustrate your clients and give them an excuse to give up.

Opt for smudge free pencils or markers when asking them to draw (p. 73).

6. *Client-determined activity rhythm*: The speed and pace of an activity freely chosen by the client is, in most cases, preferable to a pace selected by the therapist. By being able to self-pace an activity, the client can concentrate on the activity at hand instead of being worried about complying with someone else's timing and pace. This principle does not usually apply to clients with severe or profound mental retardation, clients with dementia, or clients who have other significant cognitive impairments that interfere with activity initiation or carry through.

7. *Keep the activity in front of the client*: Fine hand function tends to improve if the activity is placed immediately in front of and close to the client. When the activity requires the use of both hands at once, the therapist should structure the activity so that each sequence begins with both hands working symmetrically when possible. For example, when fly-casting (fishing) and reeling in the fish line, the move should start with one hand on the base of the fly rod and the other on the rod near the reel. The fly is cast and then the two hands work together holding up the rod and reeling in the line.

8. *Arc of activity*: A client's fine hand function will be best if the activity takes place within the first two-thirds of the arm's range of motion arc. This arc extends both vertically and horizontally from the position of the elbows being at the side of the body. The further the arms extend from this

position, the more impaired the fine hand function will become.

9. *Horizontal versus vertical movement*: Horizontal and circular movements tend to allow better fine hand control than vertical or zigzag movements. For clients with fine hand movement impairments try to modify the activity to use horizontal or circular movements. As the client's ability increases add vertical or zigzag movements to expand capability.

10. *Handles and tools should fit the client's hands*: Handles to tools should fit easily within the client's hands without causing muscle loading and fatigue. This may require that the grips be modified to better fit the client's hands and ability. Gripping strength increases when the hand that is holding the tool is held in line with the client's forearm. For example, there are many gardening tools that have "trigger grips." These work well for clients with arthritis or weak grips.

This information is most appropriate for working with problems related to d440 Fine Hand Use and will probably be documented under that code. It may also documented using any skill code where fine hand use was a limiting issue.

References

Fausek-Steinbach, D. (2002). *Art activities for groups: Providing therapy, fun, and function*. Ravensdale, WA: Idyll Arbor, Inc.

Grandjean, E. (1988). *Fitting the task to the man: A textbook of occupational ergonomics*. New York: Taylor & Francis.

Integration

Integration training has always been a strong component of recreational therapy. The World Health Organization recognizes that clients show a difference in skill level between a standard environment and the real world by scoring Activities and Participation codes for both capacity (level of task difficulty in a standard environment, such as a clinic) and performance qualifiers (level of task difficulty in the client's real-life environment, such as the client's health club). This gives credence to the importance of integration training and supports underlying principles of recreational therapy practice.

There are many variables that influence the differences in level of difficulty for capacity and performance. The facilitators and barriers that are present in a standard environment can be very different from those in the client's real-life setting. In addition, in the community the client needs to deal with all of these variables at once. In a clinical setting the client may be able to handle (one at a time) a high curb or asking for assistance or a sudden rainstorm or a missed bus. In the real world the client may have to deal with them all at once and find that asking for assistance is much harder when everyone just wants to get out of the rain. Some of the important variables for integration are discussed here.

Emotional Connections

Real-life settings are often connected to specific emotions (fear, anxiety, distraction, frustration, discomfort, excitement) that affect activity performance. Emotional connections are difficult to simulate in a clinic setting. A client may be able to role-play a social interaction in a clinic (e.g., requesting movie tickets from a ticket window) without any need for assistance, yet when placed in the actual situation, the client's anxiety may increase to the point that s/he needs the therapist to provide cueing to decrease speech rate and volume.

Unpredictability

Community environments are less predictable than clinical settings and require a blending of skill sets. In a community setting, barriers and facilitators can change quickly and extremely. For example, in the clinic the curb is always 4" high. In the community however, each curb may be a different height varying from 1" to 12". In the clinic, there is always sufficient room at the top of the makeshift curb for the wheelchair. In the community, however, there may be a group of people standing on the corner that the client wishes to avoid or there may be a large pile of snow plowed up against it. The weather is pretty standard in a clinic. In the community there may be sudden, unexpected rainstorms.

Performing skills in a community environment requires better problem solving skills, faster reaction time, and more social skills, along with the use of blended skills (e.g., not just problem solving for how to bump a wheelchair up a curb that is twice as large as practiced in the clinic, but also to request assistance, look down the street to evaluate the accessibility level of the upcoming sidewalk, watch out for traffic, and cope with feelings of embarrassment or frustration). Consequently, a client's skill level is challenged more and may not be adequate for the problem solving required.

Support and Relationships

In a clinic therapists and other clients are usually available to give assistance. In a community setting, however, there are storekeepers, neighbors, friends, family, strangers, peers, schoolmates, workmates, bus drivers, etc. All of them have different skill sets and different amounts of desire to help the client. Therapists are trained in how to provide appropriate assistance to others. This cannot be assumed in a community environment. Consequently, assistance may not be available, not provided correctly, or provided to a much greater (perhaps inappropriate) extent than at the hospital.

Attitudes

Attitude of the client and attitudes of others change with many variables such as mood, situation, environment, previous events of the day, and current conflicts. Being in a community setting is one of those things that can affect a client's attitude in a positive or negative way. If the client is feeling pessimistic, embarrassed, frustrated, anxious, or in high spirits, his/her performance will be affected. The same is true regarding the attitudes of others. If the client is feeling negative attitudes from others (e.g., "Oh, man, I really don't want to drag that portable ramp up from the basement so this guy can get in here."), whether said or non-verbally relayed, the performance of the client will be affected. Attitudes, like the community environment as a whole, can change quickly and extremely, a variable that clients need to learn how to cope with and react to so as to maximize performance and quality of life.

Policies

In the hospital, the client has to deal with hospital policies such as only smoking in designated smoking areas. In the community the number and extent of policies that the client has to deal with are complex; some of which even the therapist may not know about. These can include policies that affect the level of accessibility of a restaurant, policies affecting the client's ability to return to work, or policies that limit or promote his/her participation in sports. These policies can be talked about in the clinic setting, but for the client to experience the policies firsthand and react to them in real-life situations is another skill altogether. For example, talking about how the ADA requires places to provide reasonable accommodations is different from dealing with a very busy store worker who is not providing the required accommodation.

Technology and Equipment

In the clinic, the client will have access to (or be given) particular pieces of equipment and technology to maximize his/her independence and functioning (e.g., cane, environmental controls). In a community setting, products and technology used by the client may not work (e.g., needs more support than a cane to walk on uneven surfaces, environmental controls are not available at the theater) or products and technology in the community may better facilitate performance and independence (e.g., electric scooters at the grocery store, chirping traffic lights for those with vision impairments).

Environment

In the clinic, the room temperature is set at a comfortable level, the flooring is flat and hard, the furnishings are simple with ample room to negotiate around, and there are buzzers and beeping noises, fluorescent lighting, and regulated air quality. In the community, however, things are much different. The weather, the flooring, the furnishings, the sounds, the lighting, and the air are all in constant flux.

A real-life community environment is so different from a clinic setting that it is negligent to not address these issues and skills. Clients must be integrated into their "real life" (actual performance, not just capacity) in order to make a significant impact on health. Therapists cannot assume that skills performed in a clinic will transfer into community life. Simulated environments are not a sufficient substitute for the real world.

Community Integration Training

Community integration has always been a strong component of recreational therapy. Typical places for community integration training include recreation locations (e.g., fishing creek, recreation center, senior center, roller-skating rink, tennis court, wheelchair sports game), store (e.g., department store, grocery store, drugstore, corner store), home (e.g., client's home, friend's home), worksite, school, neighborhood, restaurant, laundromat, bank, library, and transportation center (airport, bus terminal, subway, train station). Community integration training gives the therapist the opportunity to provide many services to the client. Some of the important ones are discussed here.

Assess Functioning

The therapist assesses the client's ability to integrate the skills s/he has learned into a real-life environment. It cannot be assumed that the client will be able to perform a skill or task in a community setting (performance), just because s/he is able to perform in the clinic (capacity). Different settings evoke different emotional responses that affect performance. Community environments are complex (many things go on at a time that affect each other), unstructured (variables in the community cannot be controlled), and unreliable (things in the community are always changing). Barriers cannot be fully anticipated and the client has to continue to respond to demands, unlike the clinic where the client can go back to his/her room if the frustration level gets too high.

Teach Skills

Therapists teach clients new skills during community integration sessions. The community is complex, unstructured, and unreliable, allowing therapists to take full advantage of these conditions to use them as teaching moments (e.g., client only knows how to bump up a four-inch curb and the curb in the community is six inches high, it begins to rain, something on the wheelchair breaks, a person flirts with the client). Learning is ongoing. There is always something new to learn. Although clients may obtain a good basic body of knowledge, they must also know to expect (and try to prepare for) unforeseen challenges.

Engage in Community Activity

Participation in community activities is necessary for health and participation in healthy activity is therapeutic, whether it is a planned intervention with specified goals or not. Recreational therapists who work in community centers may provide community outings for people with disabilities just because they are fun. Recreational therapists who work in inpatient rehabilitation centers take clients out in the community to address specific objectives (e.g., assessing function, teaching new skills). Even so, the therapists must be sure that the activity itself is enjoyable. The myriad variables around the activity need to be part of the experience.

Identify Needs

Community integration sessions allow the therapist to assess a client's functional skills in a real-life environment. Since we know that people perform differently in different environments, the client will perform differently in a community environment than in a clinic environment. Consequently, additional therapy needs may be observed during community integration sessions. For example, a therapist may find that a client has problems asserting her needs in the community even though she exhibited no signs of assertiveness problems in the clinic. As a rule, therapists should plan for the client to perform one level below the level demonstrated in the clinic. For example, if a client is able to walk 200' with minimal assistance with a single point cane on level indoor surfaces, the therapist should take a walker as a back-up (one step lower than a cane), plan for the client to be able to walk 100-150' on uneven outdoor surfaces, and be prepared to provide the client with moderate assistance when walking on uneven outdoor surfaces. Talking to the client prior to the outing about the difference in performance as it relates to the environment is helpful to minimize feelings of failure (e.g., "I was able to do this in the clinic. I don't understand why I am having so much trouble with it here at the store. I'm so disappointed in myself.").

Assess Accessibility

Recreational therapists assess the level of accessibility of places in the community as compared to the ADA Accessibility Guidelines and the Uniform Federal Accessibility Standards. See the "Americans with Disabilities Act" for information on how to obtain these documents. Therapists are aware of who does and who does not have to comply with accessibility guidelines and standards (e.g., a client's home, a private club, and employers with less than 15 employees do not have to comply). A client's home should come close to accessibility guidelines and standards to maximize the client's functional abilities in the environment. Private clubs and employers with less than 15 employees may still ask for recommendations and implement them out of a desire to keep the client as an employee or allow a club member access to their facilities.

Clarify Accommodations

Recreational therapists assess the service needs of the client in a specific community environment and make accommodation recommendations. Accommodations are reasonable changes that allow an individual to use a community service (e.g., helping a client to get his groceries into the car, carrying an awkward item from the back of the store to the cashier lane). If a service need is identified during a community integration session, the client is encouraged to ask for an accommodation rather than relying on the therapist for help. The therapist will not be there when the client goes out into the community after discharge, therefore helping the client could hinder his/her ability to ask for and receive accommodations. If the client has difficulty requesting assistance (e.g., speech impairment), the therapist can intervene as needed and assist the client in requesting the accommodation, although every attempt should be made to have the client do this by himself/herself (e.g., by writing the request down on a piece of paper).

For some clients, this is one of the hardest problems to overcome. It can be very difficult for clients to accept that they need help, much less ask someone whom they don't know. The therapist knows when to push a client and when not to. If a client is pushed too hard, s/he will be alienated, trust will be lost, and the therapeutic relationship damaged — all of which affects the outcomes of therapy. If the client is visibly upset or nervous, the therapist can talk with the facility employee or supervisor and design a plan of accommodation that is easy for the client. For example, if a client goes to the same grocery market every Wednesday and needs assistance taking the groceries out to the car, it may be helpful to introduce the client to the store manager and have the client hear, "Sure, its no problem. Just tell the cashier that you need some help and they will get someone to help you." After a few positive experiences of asking for and receiving accommodations, it will usually get easier for the client to ask for help.

Provide Caregiver Training

Community integration sessions provide an opportunity to train caregivers and friends on how to provide the client with assistance in the community (e.g., how to fold up the wheelchair and put it in the car trunk, how to de-escalate a client who becomes agitated). Usually, people learn best from hands-on experience. Taking caregivers on community integration outings provides this experience. Other people that the therapist might train during community integration sessions include activity directors and recreation leaders. For example, during a community integration session to the retirement community that the client is going to move into, the therapist may spend time showing the activity director how to adapt their woodworking equipment to meet the needs of the client.

Assess Safety Concerns

The client's performance during community integration sessions can be helpful in determining the safety needs of the client. For example, a therapist may recommend that a client have supervision at all times for community activities.

Suggest Adaptations

Along with assessing accessibility, the therapist may suggest adaptations that take into account the available space and finances of the client. Therapists need to be creative. Here are a few suggestions to help the client with integration back into the home.

Doors
- Community groups may build a ramp for the client free of charge or for a minor amount.
- Consider alternatives to a permanent outside ramp (outside elevator, portable aluminum ramp).
- If the doorsill presents a barrier, nail a small triangular piece of wood to either side of the lip so that the wheelchair rolls up and over the sill.
- If the door is too narrow, there are special door hinges (often called "swing away door hinges") that allow the door to open all the way so that the thickness of the door itself is out of the way. If the door is an inside door, the inside molding (called the doorstop) can be removed. This causes problems with having the door close properly, so most people remove the door completely and hang a curtain on rings that can be easily slid to the side.
- If the door opens and closes too quickly, posing a danger to the client, install a slow spring mechanism.
- If the client has difficulty turning the doorknob, change the handle of the door (e.g., thumb press latch, lever, automatic).
- If a door swings out onto a porch or hallway and there is not enough room for the client to back up to pull the door open or there is not enough room to get around the opened door, change the door hinges so that the door opens inwards. If it is an inside door, consider removing the door, hanging

a pleated folding door, hanging a curtain, or installing a pocket door.

Bathroom
- If the bathroom is too small to negotiate, consider removing the sink base cabinet (install a pedestal sink), remove freestanding towel racks, or change the large radiator to a baseboard radiator. Consider other options for toileting and hygiene if needed (e.g., commode in bedroom, installing a sink and/or a showering area in the bedroom).

Bedroom
- If the bed is too low, place blocks under the bed legs.
- Can't reach closet bar: lower the bar, hang fabric cubbies from the bar that can hold folded clothes, or make a hanger grabber from a wooden dowel with a hook on the end.

Furniture
- If the furniture is too low consider if it is safe to increase the height by doubling up the bottom cushions, raising the height of the furniture using blocks (a block with an indentation to cradle the furniture leg so that it does not slide off the block), or placing folded bathroom towels on the seat.
- If the furniture doesn't provide enough support to stand up (e.g., only has one sofa arm to push up from), consider purchasing a standing aid. This is a heavy piece of equipment that looks like a cane, which is placed on the floor and stands upright alongside a sofa or bed to provide additional support.

Operating lights/switches/fans
- Consider use of the "clapper," electronic devices/switches, or computer programs that operate home electronics. Specialty home automation catalogs, as well as local electronic stores (e.g., Radio Shack), have many options available.

Tables
- If the table is too high, consider shortening the table legs or installing a rollout table portion (like a rollout computer keyboard tray).
- If the table is too low, place blocks under the table legs.

Kitchen
- Change the refrigerator door hinges so it opens in the other direction.
- Lower appliances (e.g., microwave) to counter.

- Use a small cart on wheels to transport hot items.

Rugs
- Remove all throw rugs to reduce chances of tripping and falling.
- Hang bathroom floor mats on the side of the tub when not using the bathroom for bathing.

Community Integration Sessions

Recreational therapists have historically facilitated performance-based community integration sessions (e.g., taking a client to the local health club to assess his/her ability to perform skills, identifying further therapy needs, and making recommendations to the client, family, and facility as appropriate) and community recreation site evaluations (e.g., determining the level of accessibility of the health club and making recommendations to the facility and client to promote engagement in activities at the facility).

Recreational therapy's role in providing site evaluations has greatly expanded with the realization of our strong background in accessibility training and problem solving. Recreational therapists are now conducting home evaluations, work evaluations, and school evaluations with or without another allied health professional.

This role change has been facilitated by the increased demand on physical and occupational therapy to have more client contact hours (at most facilities physical and occupational therapy have to spend 85% of their day treating clients with only 15% of their time for documentation and miscellaneous tasks related to therapy). Not only are they required to spend more time treating clients, but the number of clients that they see within a treatment session has increased (e.g., it is not unusual for a therapist to see two or more clients at one time while supervising an aide who is also overseeing two or three clients). This trend is making it difficult for occupational and physical therapists to block out two or three hours of treatment time for only one client. Recreational therapists also have high percentage requirements of client contact (e.g., 75-80%). It is usually lower than OT or PT because recreational therapists often see more clients for less time thus creating a much larger caseload (an RT usually has a caseload of 15-18 clients compared to OTs and PTs who typically have caseloads of 6-8 clients). The more clients, the more documentation (e.g., writing 15 evaluations instead of 8), making the justification for a greater non-client time acceptable.

Recreational therapists have begun to add site evaluations to the client's community integration training. Since they are already in the community, the extra time to do an evaluation is not as large as the commitment required from other professionals who would need to make a separate trip into the community.

Community Integration Program

The Community Integration Program (CIP) developed by the Harborview Medical Center in Seattle, Washington recommends that clients participate in community integration covering specific types of outings as shown in Table 25. According to Armstrong and Lauzen (1994), "patients have reported that the most successful plans have included at least one transportation module and the environmental awareness evaluation" (p. 33). A pre-test, field-test, and post-test are administered to the client to assess integration skills. Therapists will find that a client's verbal application in a clinic situation and performance application in a community setting are not always consistent. Sometimes the added distractions in the community lower performance. Other times, the additional cues the client gets from a familiar environment improve performance. In addition, not all clients learn in the same manner. Some respond best to structured failures while others respond best to verbal instruction. Therefore, a post-test might not reflect what the therapist perceived the client to have learned during the outing. The CIP provides a variety of common community outings, along with issues to consider for each outing in the areas of:
- *Pre-arrangement*: The basic information that the patient should be able to answer prior to embarking on the outing.
- *Transportation*: How the patient will get to and from the activity.
- *Accessibility*: Special issues concerning architectural barriers and functional ability the patient will need to know about and problem solve.
- *Emergency/safety*: Mobility and health concerns that may come up during the activity.
- *Equipment*: Equipment the patient will need to bring along.

The authors note that changes in these areas may need to be made to meet the individualized needs of the clients.

Planning a Community Integration Session

A community integration training session requires a good deal of planning. The amount of planning will vary depending on the number of clients in the session, the complexity of the activity, and the complexity of the clients' conditions (e.g.,

Table 25: Community Integration Program Modules

Modules	Suggested Participation Requirement
Community Environment Environmental Safety Emergency Preparation Basic Survival Skills	• Environmental Safety — strongly recommended for each patient • Emergency Preparation — review formally or informally with each patient • Basic Survival — recommended for patients who are discharged to a less-than-stable residential environment (including those who may experience homelessness)
Cultural Activity Theater Restaurant Library Sporting Event	At least one of these
Community Activity Shopping Mall Grocery Store Downtown Bank Laundromat Community Skills	At least one of these
Transportation Personal Travel Taxi Train Air Travel City Bus Bus Station	At least one of these
Physical Activity Aquatics Wheelchair Sports Physical Leisure Activity	Only one activity is required; however, it is suggested that the patient attend the activity at least twice. Wheelchair sports is an introduction to possible future participation in the activity.
Individual Plan Leisure Activity	At least one group and one patient-directed outing

From Armstrong & Lauzen, 1994. Used with permission.

minimal medical issues versus complex medical issues, such as taking out a group of clients who are all ventilator dependent). In general however, there is a general planning flow:

1. Prior to discussing a community integration outing with the client, talk with the treatment team to identify any issues that may impact the planning process (e.g., the case manager may be aware of certain family issues that may affect the outing, the client may be receiving his new wheelchair in four days so it might be better to wait until it comes in, scheduled medical tests may interfere). If the plan is to take the client out for an extended period of time (e.g., greater than one hour), all team members need to be aware of the schedule. It is important to work with other therapists to pick the time of day that least interferes with other therapies. The best place to get input from the entire clinical team is at the team conference. Have a tentative idea of when you would like to take the client out and look at the therapy schedule before going to team so that

if you need to ask another therapist to change his/her therapy time for that day you can ask then.

2. Obtain a written medical order from the physician for community integration training. There must be an order written in the chart that allows the client to leave the facility for an integration outing. This can also be requested during team conference. Double-check the chart to make sure it was written. Sometimes doctors get busy and forget.

3. Discuss the integration outing with the client. Talk about the purpose, benefits, and objectives of the outing. Allow time to talk with the client about his/her fears, concerns, questions, or anxieties about going out. Identify a place to go. Choose a place that the client will actually go to after discharge (e.g., don't take the client to the grocery store when he doesn't do the grocery shopping; go to the specific place that the client frequents such as his local hardware store, not the one that is closest to the hospital). Taking a

client to his actual hardware store is not always possible due to time constraints and distance, but it is best to do this whenever possible. List things that the client needs to bring (e.g., coat, money, walker). Identify a tentative date and time (it may be difficult to identify a set day/time unless you have already talked to all of the therapies, asked family members who are coming along for training, and looked at the transportation schedule). Depending of the functional level of the client, have the client participate in planning the outing (e.g., phone calls, locating and reading bus schedules). Identify family, friends, or caregivers that need to be invited for community integration training.

4. Arrange transportation. This may be signing up for the hospital vehicle, finding out what time the public bus stops in front of the hospital, etc. If you are inviting family for training, be sure you tell them whether they will need to drive in their own vehicles or you can accommodate them in the planned transportation.

5. Now that you have talked with the family, therapists, and transportation scheduling, confirm the time for the outing and tell everyone involved.

6. Route the General Integration Note (shown below) to the client's primary physical therapist, occupational therapist, and speech therapist asking them to contribute to the objectives. Include other therapists as appropriate. Be sure to attach a routing slip that states the day that the form needs to be returned to the recreational therapist. This promotes teamwork and transdisciplinary care.

7. Make sure the integration backpack for the outing is fully equipped (e.g., cell phone, urinal, first-aid kit, towels, gloves, wipes, equipment tools).

8. Day of outing: Touch base with the client's primary nurse for the day to make sure that there are no issues that will affect the planned outing (e.g., fever, unscheduled test, client refusing), pick up the keys to the vehicle, make sure all the equipment is gathered (e.g., rolling walker, single point cane), and place the general integration note with the backpack (you will need to refer to the note for objectives and medical information). Finally, meet the client and go on the outing.

9. Upon return from the outing: Provide the client and family with feedback and recommendations (e.g., client will need close supervision at all times when out in a community setting), complete the integration note, make copies for each therapist who contributed to the integration note, and file the original copy in the client's chart.

To reduce the amount of work in planning community integration outings, therapists have found it helpful to schedule routine outings that tend to fit well within all constraints. For example, every Saturday morning, recreational therapy has the hospital van for community integration training sessions. Saturday is typically a light therapy day, which makes scheduling the vehicle and the client easier. It is also a very common day for family to be available for training. Therapists may also find it helpful to design community integration groups by disability. For example, every Tuesday morning a community outing is scheduled for clients with lower extremity amputations with a maximum of three clients. Recreational therapists, as well as other therapists, can refer clients to the group.

Documentation

Due to the number of clients that recreational therapists have on their caseload (about 15-18 clients), integration notes that have checkboxes, circles, and brief notes are often preferred. Therapists must be careful not to forsake quality with this type of note, therefore open box sections that allow the therapist to remark about behavior, verbalizations, adjustments, problem solving for a particular barrier, etc. are advantageous. The length and type of form used will vary depending on the purpose of the outing. For individual community integration sessions that are addressing skill performance, a performance-based note like the General Integration Note shown later in this topic would be best. If the therapist evaluates the accessibility of a site in relation to its impact on the client's performance, use a facility-specific note (see Home Evaluation, School Evaluation, Worksite Evaluation, and Recreation Facility Evaluation, also shown later in this topic).

Each code in the Activities and Participation section has a qualifier for "performance" (the client's ability to perform the skill in the client's real-life setting). Integration training addresses many different skills. In the ICF, therapists will need to identify what specific community integration skills were assessed and addressed, identify the related code, and then score the performance qualifier. Some codes in the Activities and Participation section are more skill specific such as d460 Moving Around in Different Locations or d7202 Regulating Behaviors within Interactions. Other codes are more task-specific such as d9292 Arts and Culture or d6200 Shopping. The choice of which codes to score is currently at the discretion of the therapist.

The rest of this section has several integration notes for your review. Feel free to adopt these forms for your own program, or use them as a springboard for developing your own forms. Please refer to the "Americans with Disabilities Act" for information on how to get a copy of accessibility guidelines. This will help you when you are making architectural recommendations for facilities.

References

Armstrong, M. & Lauzen, S. (1994). *Community integration program, 2ⁿᵈ edition.* Idyll Arbor, Inc: Ravensdale, WA.

General Integration Note

The general integration note is a transdisciplinary note in which the primary therapists working with the client document the client's current status for an outing and contribute to the objectives of the outing. It is primarily used for outings that evaluate a client's performance and is not an in-depth architectural evaluation of the outing location. The note is to be routed to the primary therapists (PT, OT, speech, psych, etc.) prior to the outing. Each therapist fills in the client's current functional status related to the outing (e.g., walking, transfers, use of compensatory strategies for speech production), as well as a related objective for the outing. The recreational therapist plans the outing to meet the objectives, evaluates the client's performance on the outing, and routes a copy of the form to each of the contributing therapists.

The top portion of the form provides an area to document who will be attending the training (Joan Smith, mother) and what training they have already received (e.g., car transfers). This helps eliminate repetitive education and gives the therapist an idea of the basic knowledge that the caregiver has received.

It also provides an area to document the client's medical status, as well as the current precautions and parameters to be followed. This information, along with the current equipment (e.g., platform walker), provides a quick reference for the therapist when preparing for the outing, as well as a reference while in the community. In case of an emergency, the therapist should also have the name of the client's doctors, medications, insurance, and phone numbers.

The note is designed for quick documentation. The therapist checks met or unmet for each outing objective. A space is provided in each objective so that the therapist can write notes about the client's performance. Further space is available in the additional comments section. In this area the therapist can document issues not easily described in the other sections (e.g., psychosocial adjustment, further descriptors of performance, family training, statements of client/family, further education/training required, recommendations by therapist). The therapist filling out the form checks the appropriate "report" box after a copy of the form is given to each therapist who provided objectives.

General Integration Note

Client name: _____   ID #: _____

Date of integration training: _____   Time of outing: _____

Location of outing: _____

Team Members		
Discipline	Name	Report
RT		☐
PT		☐
OT		☐
Speech		☐
		☐
		☐

Family/Caregivers		
Name of caregiver to attend outing for training	Training already received by caregiver prior to outing	Training on this outing

Client Information
Medical status

Precautions/parameters	Equipment needed

Integration objective	Discipline	Current status of client	Outcome/notes
1.			☐ Met ☐ Unmet
2.			☐ Met ☐ Unmet
3			☐ Met ☐ Unmet
4.			☐ Met ☐ Unmet
5.			☐ Met ☐ Unmet
6.			☐ Met ☐ Unmet
7.			☐ Met ☐ Unmet
8.			☐ Met ☐ Unmet
9.			☐ Met ☐ Unmet
10.			☐ Met ☐ Unmet

Additional comments from integration training session

Therapist signature/credentials/date: _____

Site Evaluations

The forms in this section cover evaluations of homes, schools, workplaces, and community recreation facilities. There are some basic areas that are evaluated for each site (bathrooms, parking, entrance). Other areas that need to be evaluated depend on the site (e.g., evaluating a lunchroom at a school, evaluating a craft room at a recreation center).

To reduce the length we have tried to modularize the forms. The evaluations described below suggest which forms you should use for particular types of evaluations. You may duplicate these forms for your use or use them as a springboard for developing your own forms.

The *Community Integration Program* (Armstrong & Lauzen, 1994) also has a set of 29 survey forms and nine summary forms that look at accessibility issues in much greater detail (e.g., ten pages on bathrooms with an additional seven pages on tub and shower facilities). If your practice includes a lot of integration where you are the primary therapist, we recommend you also have that book.

The rest of this section looks at the components of each of the evaluations.

Home Evaluation

The home evaluation looks at the accessibility of a client's home, as well as his/her functional abilities within the home. It is a rather lengthy evaluation, but the check boxes make it go rather quickly. A home evaluation should be done using the Site Evaluation sheet, the Basic Site Evaluation form, and the Home Evaluation form. These contain the following sections: heading, team members, family/caregivers, client information, layout, parking, entrance (evaluate two), bathroom, living room, dining room, kitchen, stairway, bedroom, hallway, basement, yard, specific activities, additional areas not listed, general safety, ability to perform other functional tasks not listed in the evaluation (e.g., computer workstation, garden, pool), additional comments and recommendation, and closing. As with the general integration note, other primary therapists may contribute concerns or suggest areas/tasks that they would like to have the therapist evaluate. A check box is provided so you can indicate who has received a copy of the report.

The therapist must be familiar with the ADA guidelines (see "Americans with Disabilities Act" for more information) to understand accessibility requirements. ADA guidelines, although they do not apply to a private home, should be followed whenever possible to maximize the client's functioning in the home.

School Evaluation

The school evaluation is complex because many areas need to be evaluated (e.g., auditorium, cafeteria, locker), along with the client's ability to participate in functional tasks in the school environment (clubs, nurse's office, hang-out areas, transport books, sit appropriately at desks). There also needs to be an evaluation of safety (e.g., accessible emergency exits, nursing availability). Psychosocial adjustment must also be critically evaluated and documented, as transitioning youth into a peer environment can be difficult due to the many life stage issues that this population faces (e.g., acceptance, desire to belong to a group, self-esteem and confidence issues). A typical school evaluation takes a few hours and must be coordinated with the school principal. Due to the many areas of evaluation, it is helpful to have more than one therapist for the evaluation (e.g., RT, OT, PT). The school evaluation should be done using the Site Evaluation sheet, the Basic Site Evaluation form, and the School Evaluation form. These typically encompass the following sections: heading, team members, family/caregivers, client information, layout, parking, entrance (evaluate two), mobility, bathroom (evaluate at least two), campus grounds, medical care, lunchroom, auditorium, sports field, library, additional areas not listed, specific activities, general safety, class schedule, class-schedule-locker-related issues, additional comments and recommendations, and closing.

Worksite Evaluation

The worksite evaluation is used as a comprehensive tool for evaluating the accessibility of the worksite, as well as the client's ability to perform in the environment. The evaluation should be done using the Site Evaluation sheet, the Basic Site Evaluation form, and the Workplace Evaluation form. These typically encompasses the following sections: heading, team members, client information, layout, parking, entrance, mobility, bathroom, campus grounds, stairway, hallway, lunchroom, additional areas not listed, specific activities, medical care, general safety, additional comments and recommendations, and closing.

Community Facility Evaluation

The community facility evaluation is used for evaluating the accessibility of a community facility, as well as the client's ability to perform in the environment (YMCA, community recreation center, veteran's center, etc.). The evaluation should be done using the Site Evaluation sheet, the Basic Site Evaluation form, and the Recreation Facility Evaluation form. These typically encompasses the following sections: heading, team members, client information, layout, parking, entrance, mobility, bathroom, campus grounds, stairway, hallway, additional areas not listed, specific activities, medical care, general safety, additional comments and recommendations, and closing.

Site Evaluation

Client name: _____ ID #: _____ Date:_____

Type of site: ☐ Home ☐ School ☐ Work ☐ Community facility _____ ☐ Other _____

Site location: _____

Site information: _____

_____

Family/Caregivers			
Name of caregiver	Training already received	Training during evaluation	Report
			☐
			☐
			☐
			☐

Health Care Staff			
Health care staff	Department	Concern	Report
			☐
			☐
			☐
			☐

Client Information	
Medical status	
Precautions/parameters	Equipment needed

Mobility	
Measures	Comments and recommendations
Is client independent with functional mobility skills (car transfer, walking, w/c propulsion)? ☐ Y ☐ N Is mobility assistance provided if needed? ☐ Y ☐ N	

Basic Site Information

Client name: _____   Site: _____

Layout
Layout: ☐ One-floor ☐ Multi-level ☐ Split-level
Elevator: ☐ Y ☐ N

Entrance	
Measures	**Comments and recommendations**
Location:	
Walkway surfaces from parking area to entrance: Client able to negotiate over surfaces? ☐ Y ☐ N	
Steps Number: _____ Step height _____ Step width _____ Number of rails _____ Height of rails _____ Width between rails _____ Ground to door sill height _____ Client able to negotiate steps? ☐ Y ☐ N	
Ramp Ramp pitch (inch to foot) _____ Ramp surface _____ Client able to negotiate ramp? ☐ Y ☐ N	
Platform at top of steps/ramp Length _____ Width _____ Adequate room on platform for client to safely open/enter/exit door? ☐ Y ☐ N	
Door Width of doorway _____ Client able to open/close/lock/unlock door?☐ Y ☐ N Client able to negotiate through doorway? ☐ Y ☐ N	

[Key: Y=Yes, N=No, S=Some]

Parking	
Measures	Comments and recommendations
Handicap parking available? ☐ Y ☐ N	
Does client have the endurance to walk or propel w/c from parking space to entrance? ☐ Y ☐ N	

Bathroom	
Measures	Comments and recommendations
Location:	
Access Can client negotiate to bathroom location? ☐ Y ☐ N Client able to operate lights? ☐ Y ☐ N Can client negotiate in bathroom? ☐ Y ☐ N	
Door Main bathroom door width _____ Can client open/close/lock/unlock door? ☐ Y ☐ N Can client negotiate through main door? ☐ Y ☐ N Sufficient room for client to close bathroom door? ☐ Y ☐ N	
Facilities Toilet height _____ Adequate room for client to transfer on/off toilet? ☐ Y ☐ N Client able to obtain toiletries? ☐ Y ☐ N Client able to transfer on/off toilet? ☐ Y ☐ N Client independent with toileting (including clothing management, hygiene, cathing, transfers)? ☐ Y ☐ N Can client operate faucets? ☐ Y ☐ N Is there a handheld shower? ☐ Y ☐ N Sink ☐ Y ☐ N Sink height _____ Can client operate sink faucets, soap, and paper towels? ☐ S ☐ Y ☐ N	

Additional comments and recommendations

Therapist signature/credentials/date: _____

Home Evaluation

Client name: _____   Site: _____

Layout
Type: ☐ Single ☐ Twin ☐ Duplex ☐ Complex ☐ Other: _____

Living Room	
Measures	**Comments and recommendations**
Width of doorway _____ Type of floor _____ Can client negotiate through doorways? ☐ S ☐ Y ☐ N Can client access and safely transfer on/off furniture? ☐ S ☐ Y ☐ N Client able to operate lights, switches, fans, etc.? ☐ S ☐ Y ☐ N Specific equipment/tasks that client desires to use/do in this area? Dimensions and assessment.	

Dining Room	
Measures	**Comments and recommendations**
Width of doorway _____ Type of floor _____ Can client negotiate through doorway? ☐ Y ☐ N Can client access and safely transfer on/off furniture? ☐ S ☐ Y ☐ N Client able to operate lights, switches, fans, etc.? ☐ S ☐ Y ☐ N Specific equipment/tasks that client desires to use/do in this area? Dimensions and assessment.	

Bathing Facilities	
Measures	**Comments and recommendations**
☐ Tub: Height _____ ☐ Shower Stall: Lip Height _____ Width _____ ☐ Shower curtain ☐ Shower doors Client able to transfer in/out of tub/stall? ☐ Y ☐ N	

Kitchen	
Measures	**Comments and recommendations**
Width of doorway _____ Type of floor _____ Can client negotiate through doorway?　　☐ Y ☐ N Client able to access cabinets?　　　☐ S ☐ Y ☐ N Client able to access table?　　　　　　☐ Y ☐ N Can client access and use appliances? (including stove knobs, refrigerator, freezer, microwave, coffee pot) 　　　　　　　　　　　　　　☐ S ☐ Y ☐ N Client able to negotiate throughout kitchen? 　　　　　　　　　　　　　　　　☐ Y ☐ N Client able to operate lights, switches, fans, windows, etc.?　　　　　　　　☐ S ☐ Y ☐ N Specific equipment/tasks that client desires to use/do in this area? Dimensions and assessment.	

Stairway	
Measures	**Comments and recommendations**
Steps Number _____　　Covering _____ Step height _____　　Step width _____	
Rails Rails on L or R (going up) _____ Number of rails _____ Height of rails _____ Width between rails _____	
Safety: Client able to negotiate steps?　　　☐ Y ☐ N Is stairway able to accommodate stairglide? Call professional for evaluation.　　　　☐ Y ☐ N Client able to operate lights, stairglide? 　　　　　　　　　　　☐ S ☐ Y ☐ N	

Hallway	
Measures	**Comments and recommendations**
Hallway width _____ Client able to negotiate up/down hallway? ☐ Y ☐ N	

Bedroom	
Measures	Comments and recommendations
Location/description Floor: _____ Primary occupant _____ Client's reason to access bedroom	
Door Width of doorway _____ Client able to open/close/lock/unlock door?☐ Y ☐ N Client able to negotiate through doorway? ☐ Y ☐ N	
Bed Size: ☐ King ☐ Queen ☐ Twin ☐ Cot ☐ Sofa Bed Height _____ Client able to transfer on/off bed? ☐ Y ☐ N Client able to perform safe bed mobility? ☐ Y ☐ N	
Furniture Client able to access and utilize furniture? ☐ S ☐ Y ☐ N	
Accessibility Type of floor _____ Client able to move throughout bedroom? ☐ Y ☐ N	
Windows Client able to operate windows and window treatments? ☐ S ☐ Y ☐ N	
Closets Client able to access closets? ☐ S ☐ Y ☐ N Client able to reach racks? ☐ S ☐ Y ☐ N Client able to reach shelves? ☐ S ☐ Y ☐ N	
Miscellaneous Client able to access and operate lights, fans, air conditioners, etc.? ☐ S ☐ Y ☐ N	

Basement	
Measures	Comments and recommendations
Steps and Rails Number _____ Covering _____ Step height _____ Step width _____ Rails on L or R (going up) _____ Number of rails _____ Height of rails _____ Width between rails _____ Client able to negotiate steps? ☐ Y ☐ N	
Appliances/Equipment Client able to access and operate appliances (washer, dryer, water heater, water shut off, etc.)? ☐ S ☐ Y ☐ N	

Yard	
Measures	Comments and recommendations
Type of surface _____ Client able to access yard? ☐ Y ☐ N Client able to negotiate over uneven surfaces (e.g., grass, flagstone)? ☐ S ☐ Y ☐ N Client able to access and operate yard equipment? ☐ S ☐ Y ☐ N Client able to perform yard tasks? ☐ S ☐ Y ☐ N	

Additional Areas Not Listed	
Measures	Comments and recommendations
Additional areas client desires to use in the home: Can client access the areas and all equipment/supplies? ☐ S ☐ Y ☐ N Can client safely and effectively use the areas? ☐ S ☐ Y ☐ N	

Specific Activities	
Measures	Comments and recommendations
What additional tasks does the client desire to perform in the home? Are there any concerns regarding access to activity and activity equipment/supplies? ☐ Y ☐ N Can client safely and effectively perform the activities? ☐ S ☐ Y ☐ N	

General Safety	
Measures	Comments and recommendations
Smoke detectors? ☐ Y ☐ N Fire extinguishers? ☐ Y ☐ N Adequate lighting? ☐ Y ☐ N Nightlights? ☐ Y ☐ N Cordless phone? ☐ Y ☐ N Safe flooring? ☐ Y ☐ N Police/fire department notified of person with disability living in the home ☐ Y ☐ N Are there any additional safety concerns (explain)? ☐ Y ☐ N	

Additional comments and recommendations

Therapist signature/credentials/date: _____

School Evaluation

Client name: _____   Site: _____

Lunchroom	
Measures	Comments and recommendations
Counter height _____ Can client reach countertops to retrieve food items? ☐ Y ☐ N Can client transport lunch items to table? ☐ Y ☐ N Does cafeteria offer appropriate food selections to meet client's needs? ☐ Y ☐ N Table height _____ Table height sufficient for client to sit at table safely? ☐ Y ☐ N Is there sufficient time for the client to purchase, consume, and clean up a meal? ☐ Y ☐ N	

Auditorium	
Measures	Comments and recommendations
Door Width of doorway _____ Client able to open/close door? ☐ Y ☐ N Client able to negotiate through doorway? ☐ Y ☐ N	
Aisles Aisle width _____ Client able to negotiate up/down aisles? ☐ Y ☐ N	
Seating Appropriate seating area for the client? ☐ Y ☐ N	

Sports Field	
Measures	Comments and recommendations
Are paths to sports field accessible to client? ☐ Y ☐ N Are there an appropriate seating area and a way for the client to get to the seating area? ☐ Y ☐ N	

Library	
Measures	Comments and recommendations
Door Width of doorway _____ Can client independently open/close door? ☐ Y ☐ N Can client independently negotiate through doorway? ☐ Y ☐ N	
Table Table height: _____ Table height sufficient for client to sit at table safely? ☐ Y ☐ N	
Resources Can client independently obtain books from shelves, index cards from files, and operate computer? ☐ Y ☐ N If no, are there accommodations? ☐ Y ☐ N	

Campus Grounds	
Measures	Comments and recommendations
Accessible paths? ☐ S ☐ Y ☐ N (describe routes)	

Restroom Stalls (primary)	
Measures	Comments and recommendations
Width of stall door _____ Can client open/close stall door? ☐ Y ☐ N Can client negotiate through bathroom stall door? ☐ Y ☐ N Sufficient room for client to close bathroom door? ☐ Y ☐ N	

Restroom Stalls (alternate)	
Measures	Comments and recommendations
Width of stall door _____ Can client open/close stall door? ☐ Y ☐ N Can client negotiate through bathroom stall door? ☐ Y ☐ N Sufficient room for client to close bathroom door? ☐ Y ☐ N	

General Safety	
Measures	Comments and recommendations
Are all designated emergency exits accessible? ☐ Y ☐ N Is there access to other floors (e.g., elevator)? ☐ Y ☐ N Is client able to operate elevator? ☐ Y ☐ N Are water fountains accessible to the client ☐ Y ☐ N	

Additional Areas Not Listed	
Measures	Comments and recommendations
Additional areas client desires to use at school: Can client access the areas and all equipment/supplies? ☐ S ☐ Y ☐ N Can client safely and effectively use the areas? ☐ S ☐ Y ☐ N	

Specific Activities	
Measures	Comments and recommendations
What additional tasks does the client desire to perform in school? Is access to activity and activity equipment/supplies available? ☐ Y ☐ N Can client safely and effectively perform the activities? ☐ S ☐ Y ☐ N	

Medical Care	
Measures	Comments and recommendations
Medical care client may require: Is adequate medical care available and accessible to client? ☐ S ☐ Y ☐ N Does office provide needed equipment (e.g., bed to lie down on to self-catheterize?) ☐ Y ☐ N Is client able to use equipment safely? ☐ Y ☐ N Name and qualifications of individual providing medical assistance: Are medical personnel familiar with and able to perform care needed? ☐ Y ☐ N Projected times when client will need medical care/area: Is office/area available at those times? ☐ Y ☐ N Are there any time conflicts with class schedule for medical needs? ☐ Y ☐ N Is client able to negotiate medical area? ☐ Y ☐ N	

Class Schedule

Time/date	Class	Distance	Seating	Classroom accessibility	Additional issues/ recommendations

Class/Schedule/Locker Related Issues	
Measures	Comments and recommendations
Client has good endurance for mobility to/from classes? ☐ Y ☐ N Sufficient locker time is available between classes in relation to amount of books client is able to handle at a given time? ☐ Y ☐ N Are lockers accessible (e.g., height, location, operation)? ☐ Y ☐ N Is client able to independently transport books? ☐ Y ☐ N Does the class schedule allow sufficient time for self-care/medical needs? ☐ Y ☐ N Is client able to independently perform all tasks required for class (e.g., gym, labs, taking notes)? ☐ Y ☐ N	

Additional comments and recommendations

Therapist signature/credentials/date: _____

Worksite Evaluation

Client name: _____   Site: _____

Lunchroom	
Measures	Comments and recommendations
Counter height _____ Can client reach countertops to retrieve food items? ☐ Y ☐ N Can client transport lunch items to table? ☐ Y ☐ N Does cafeteria offer appropriate food selections to meet client's needs? ☐ Y ☐ N Table height _____ Table height sufficient for client to sit at table safely? ☐ Y ☐ N Is there sufficient time for the client to purchase, consume, and clean up a meal? ☐ Y ☐ N	

Grounds	
Measures	Comments and recommendations
Accessible paths? ☐ S ☐ Y ☐ N (describe routes)	

Restroom Stalls (primary)	
Measures	Comments and recommendations
Width of stall door _____ Can client open/close stall door? ☐ Y ☐ N Can client negotiate through stall door? ☐ Y ☐ N Sufficient room for client to close door? ☐ Y ☐ N	

Restroom Stalls (alternative)	
Measures	Comments and recommendations
Width of stall door _____ Can client open/close stall door? ☐ Y ☐ N Can client negotiate through stall door? ☐ Y ☐ N Sufficient room for client to close door? ☐ Y ☐ N	

General Safety	
Measures	Comments and recommendations
Are all designated emergency exits accessible? ☐ Y ☐ N Is there access to other floors (e.g., elevator)? ☐ Y ☐ N Is client able to operate elevator? ☐ Y ☐ N Are water fountains accessible ? ☐ Y ☐ N	

Additional Areas Not Listed	
Measures	Comments and recommendations
Additional areas client desires to use in worksite: Can client access the areas and all equipment/supplies? □ S □ Y □ N Can client safely and effectively use the areas? □ S □ Y □ N	

Specific Activities	
Measures	Comments and recommendations
What additional tasks does the client desire to perform? Is access to activity and activity equipment/supplies available? □ Y □ N Can client safely and effectively perform responsibilities? □ S □ Y □ N	

Medical Care	
Measures	Comments and recommendations
Medical care client may require: Is adequate medical care available and accessible to client? □ S □ Y □ N Does office provide needed equipment? □ Y □ N Is client able to use equipment safely? □ Y □ N Name and qualifications of individual providing medical assistance: Are medical personnel familiar with and able to perform care needed? □ Y □ N Projected times when client will need medical care/area: Is office/area available at those times? □ Y □ N Is client able to negotiate throughout medical area to meet needs? □ Y □ N	

Additional comments and recommendations

Therapist signature/credentials/date: _____

Recreation Facility Evaluation

Client name: _____   Site: _____

Grounds	
Measures	Comments and recommendations
Accessible paths?　　　　☐ S ☐ Y ☐ N (describe routes)	

Restroom Stalls	
Measures	Comments and recommendations
Width of stall door _____ Can client open/close stall door?　　☐ Y ☐ N Can client negotiate through stall door?　☐ Y ☐ N Sufficient room for client to close door?　☐ Y ☐ N	

General Safety	
Measures	Comments and recommendations
Are all designated emergency exits accessible? 　　　　　　　　　　　　　☐ Y ☐ N Is there access to other floors (e.g., elevator)? 　　　　　　　　　　　　　☐ Y ☐ N Is client able to operate elevator?　☐ Y ☐ N Are water fountains accessible to the client (e.g., lowered)?　　　　　　　　　☐ Y ☐ N	

Recreation Areas	
Measures	Comments and recommendations
Areas client desires to use: Can client access the areas and all equipment/supplies?　　　☐ S ☐ Y ☐ N Can client safely and effectively use the areas? 　　　　　　　　　☐ S ☐ Y ☐ N	

Additional comments and recommendations

Therapist signature/credentials/date: _____

Interpersonal Relationship Activities

There are numerous activities that can be used to develop skills in interpersonal interactions and relationships. Sample activities that can be used to train clients with cognitive impairments in these skills are included in this section. Examples for all the social skills are not provided. Some social skills (such as adhering to rules) are inherent in most of the activities and, therefore, no specific activity is presented for the skill. In some cases several activities are presented for a particular skill. These may represent sub-objectives or merely ways to add variety to a program when needed.

Although there can be many reasons for participating in the activity, only the primary objectives of the activity relative to the three-pronged model described in "Social Skills Training" in the Techniques section are noted. These activities are presented in a developmental sequence. Many of these activities can and often should be done more than once. For instance, Dance a Name has been frequently requested by clients and has helped them become more aware of others.

A general procedure for each activity is given. Specific teaching and facilitation strategies must be determined by the therapist based on the needs of the clients. Clients with greater cognitive impairments may need a chaining process, physical assistance, verbal prompts, and demonstration, while clients with less impairment may be involved in more discussion. Similarly, the therapist must identify activity modifications needed. Some helpful suggestions are provided based on the types of clients on which this model was piloted.

There are many different methods to describe activities. The one used in this section was developed by the Workshop Planning Committee of the Portland Metropolitan Therapeutic Recreation Chapter. Where descriptors are provided, they are taken from the *Recreation Behavior Inventory* (Berryman & Lefebvre, 1979).

At the end of this section are some more complex activities. The lists of benefits for those activities have been adapted from materials by Bach and by Coyne. Two categories of benefits are identified: 1. those that are tangible and can be measured and 2. those that are intangible and are difficult to quantify. The adaptations presented are adjustments made to activities or equipment, which ensures that the activity is suited to the interest,

capacities, and limitations of clients with different types of impairments. These are categorical adaptation suggestions and, therefore, will not be appropriate to all of those in that category. Two examples of intervention activities with activity analysis, benefits, and adaptations follow. The use of a "double" is mentioned in several of these activities. A double is a person who stands beside the client during the activity and speaks for a client who is not sufficiently verbal or performs actions for a client with motor impairments.

(Other related sections of the book include "Social Skills Development" in the Concepts section, "Social Skills Training" in the Techniques section, and Activities and Participation Chapter 7 Interpersonal Interactions and Relationships for general information about using recreation as a means for developing skills in interpersonal interactions and relationships.)

Sharing and Taking Turns

Objectives:
- The client will share recreation equipment.
- The client will take turns when necessary.

Procedure:
- The therapist initiates a variety of games and activities that require the client to share or take turns (having fewer pairs of scissors than clients, playing catch).
- Client actively participates in the activity.

Materials: Varies by activity.

Therapist's Notes:
- Encourage the client who is not sharing and taking turns to do so.
- Praise the client for sharing and taking turns.
- Formalize sharing situation by giving partners one piece of recreation equipment and telling them they must share.

Double Stunts

Objective:
- The client will cooperatively perform a task with a partner.

Procedure:
- The therapist explains and demonstrates activity with another staff person or peer model.

The activities in this section are from Phyllis Coyne's *Social Skills Training: A Three-Pronged Approach* originally published in 1980 and funded by a grant from the Developmental Disabilities Office, Region X, Grant No. 50-P-50368.

- Client practices his/her part of the stunt with physical assistance, if necessary.
- Client does stunt with the therapist or peer model.
- Client does stunt with another client.

Therapist's Notes:
- The therapist should provide physical assistance, as needed.
- Provide double stunts in which both partners must perform their task for success. Some suggested stunts include holding each other's shoulders and standing on only one foot, both taking an end of a jump rope and swinging the rope together, folding a bed sheet together.
- Provide a spotter for all stunts.

Mirror

Objective:
- The client will work cooperatively with a partner and imitate his/her movements.

Procedure:
- The therapist explains and demonstrates the activity with another staff person or peer model.
- The therapist initiates movement and asks the client to follow his/her movements.
- The client initiates movement and the therapist follows.
- The client alternately initiates and follows movements with a partner.

Therapist's Notes:
- Give encouragement and feedback to the client.
- Stress that "Mirror" is not a competitive game.
- Stress that movement needs to be slow for others to follow.

Togeth-air Ball
(Collective Score Volleyball)

Objective:
- The client will work as a member of a group to keep a ball in the air.

Procedure:
- The therapist explains and demonstrates game with another staff person and/or a peer model.
- The client cooperatively plays the game.

Directions:
- Two teams are on either side of a line, rope, or net.

- The ball is batted back and forth in a continuous fashion.
- If a score is kept, it is a collective score. The goal is to see how long the ball can be kept in the air.

Materials: Ball, beach ball, Mylar balloon, string or net.

Therapist's Notes:
- Use a balloon or beach ball before going on to something more difficult, like a volleyball.
- Initially, count one point any time anyone hits the ball to provide greatest reinforcement.
- Lower or raise the string/net according to the skill level of the clients.
- Change rules for variety (players must use a part of the body other than the hand to get the ball over the net).

Adaptations:
- Mylar balloons may be used in place of a ball. Since they fall to the ground more slowly, they allow clients with motor retardation to get to the balloon. It is not recommended that therapists use rubber balloons because, if the balloon pops, the client may choke on the pieces.

Team Play (Volleyball)

Objective:
- The client will play competitively on a team.

Procedure:
- The therapist divides the clients into teams and discusses the concept of "team."
- The clients play volleyball as a member of a team.

Materials: Volleyball, net.

Therapist's Notes:
- Use color badges, tee shirts, etc. to identify team members.
- Once clients have the team concept, switch members of the teams often so that the clients get the opportunity to be a team member with all group members.
- Vary with other competitive team activities such as a relay race where the team is easily identified as opposed to intermixed team games like basketball.
- Modify the rules of the game when necessary.
- Encourage and praise team play and sportsmanship.

Non-Verbal Role-play

Objective:
- The client will role-play different ways of making contact and communicating different message through eye contact and facial expression.

Procedure:
- The therapist discusses messages communicated non-verbally.
- The therapist models use of facial expression to communicate a message.
- The client role-plays communicating messages upon request from the therapist.

Role-play Situations:
- Indicating yes and no.
- Showing someone that you are friendly (smile).
- "Saying" hello, e.g., shaking hands, slapping on shoulder.
- Showing someone that you like him or her; do not like him or her.
- Indicating that you will; you will not.
- Letting someone know that you are happy; sad.
- Letting someone know that you are pleased; angry.

Therapist's Notes:
- Use discretion in having the whole group do role-play situations simultaneously or having individuals do role-play in front of the whole group.
- If role-play is done in front of a group, start with clients who have the greatest capabilities to provide additional modeling for others.
- Use mirrors and make faces into the mirror with clients who have greater impairments who would not otherwise respond appropriately.

Role-Play Introducing Self

Objective:
- The client will introduce himself/herself to a peer using eye contact, appropriate verbalization, and handshake.

Procedure:
- The therapist introduces discussion on choosing the right time and place to introduce oneself as well as ways of introducing oneself.
- The therapist models greeting the other person and naming oneself while shaking hands (if appropriate).
- The therapist and client role-play appropriate behavior.

- The client practices behavior with a peer under supervision.
- The client practices behavior with peers independently.

Role-play Situation:
- Neighborhood: Introducing self to a new neighbor.
- Classroom: Introducing self to a new group member.

Therapist's Notes:
- Use physical or verbal prompts, as necessary, to keep the client looking at the other person. Prompt giver should be different from the person to whom the client is introducing himself/herself.
- For those with very limited verbal skills, initially use a double that stands next to the client and speaks for him/her.
- Reinforce appropriate introducing behaviors with physical gestures of approval and verbal praise.
- Have clients practice this behavior with guests who come to the program.

How Do You Do and Goodbye

Objectives:
- The client will appropriately introduce self.
- The client will learn the name of another person.

Procedure:
- This game is similar to musical chairs.
- The group forms a small circle with one person in the center.
- The therapist explains and demonstrates the activity.
- The therapist begins playing music while the client in the center starts walking around inside the circle.
- The client responds to introduction and gives his/her name.
- The client introduces himself/herself to another.
- The client continues to introduce himself/herself to the others in the circle.

Directions:
- The clients form a single circle facing the center, seated or standing.
- One extra person is in the center.
- The extra person walks around the inside of the circle until the therapist stops the music.
- When the music stops, the extra person halts and introduces himself/herself to the nearest person in the circle and learns his/her name.

- When the therapist starts the music again, the two join hands and walk around the inside of the circle while talking.
- When the therapist stops the music, the couple says "Goodbye" to each other.
- Each introduces himself or herself to the nearest person, and the two new couples walk and talk.
- New players are picked up each time the music stops until all are in couples, walking and talking.

Materials: CD player, CDs.

Therapist's Notes:
- Provide a high staff to client ratio for this activity.

Dance a Name

Objectives:
- The client will name each participant.
- The client will imitate movement during Dance a Name.

Procedure:
- The therapist explains and demonstrates the activity.
- The client participates in chanting as part of the group.
- The client does the activity as part of the group.

Directions:
- The group stands in a circle formation.
- Clients clap and chant, "Name, name, what's your name?"
- The first client says his/her name and does a movement with it (touch toes).
- Clients say the person's name while imitating the movement together three times.
- Continue until everyone in the circle has said his/her name with a movement.

Therapist's Notes:
- Position other staff and/or help(s) next to individuals who have low attention spans to prompt imitation.
- Use reinforcement, if needed. Generally this activity is reinforcing enough by itself.
- Provide verbal reminders for those who forget to do a movement with their name.

The Name Game

Objective:
- The client will accurately name other clients in the group.

Procedure:
- The therapist explains and demonstrates the game.
- The client plays the game with others.

Directions:
- The clients are in a circle.
- The first person states his name, e.g., Billy Boy.
- The second person repeats the preceding name and states her name, e.g., Nancy Nice.
- The third person repeats these names and supplies his own, e.g., Billy Boy, Nancy Nice, Jim Jones.
- This procedure continues until each person has at least two chances to name all participants.

Therapist's Notes:
- Require clients with greater impairments to name the person next to them and self only, at first.
- Have the clients change places around the circle to ensure that the client knows the name of other clients rather than their place in the circle.
- Encourage the client to look at the person s/he is naming.
- Provide verbal prompts of first two letters of the name, e.g., "Na" for Nancy, when needed.
- When the clients can name each other easily, have each client add something that s/he is good at or likes, e.g., basketball playing Billy, singing Nancy.

Name Catch

Objective:
- The client will use names to get the attention of others.

Procedure:
- The therapist explains and demonstrates the activity in a circle formation.
- The client gets attention of the person to whom the ball will be thrown by calling out his/her name and then throws.

Material: Ball

Therapist's Notes:
- Add saying something the person likes or is good at with his/her name after clients are good at naming people.
- Liven up the activity by having the clients go as fast as they can.
- Encourage clients to throw the ball to a variety of clients and not just the therapist.

- The therapist may need to cue the group on some of the client's names. For example, "Charlie, why don't you throw the ball this time to Claire?" while pointing to Claire.

Get Acquainted Musical Chairs

Objective:
- The client will accurately name seated players as they are passed.

Procedure:
- The therapist explains and demonstrates the activity.
- The client actively participates in the activity.

Directions:
- Chairs are arranged in a circle.
- Four clients are introduced to the group.
- Their four chairs are taken from the circle.
- Everyone else rises and the four without chairs find seats and sit down.
- As the music plays, the other players march around the circle.
- As they pass each of the seated four, they must call him/her by name.
- Anyone who forgets to speak to a seated player must sit down, too.
- When the music stops, everyone quickly finds a chair and sits down.
- The four left without chairs introduce themselves.
- The number marching keeps getting smaller, as everyone caught must remain seated.
- The marchers speak to each of those seated by saying, "Hello _____."

Materials: CD player, CDs, chairs.

Therapist's Notes:
- Introduce and seat clients with greater cognitive ability between clients with greater impairments.

This Is My Friend

Objective:
- The client will introduce a peer and tell something about that person to the group.

Procedure:
- The therapist explains and demonstrates activity.
- The client introduces self to partner; discovers partner's name and one activity that the partner likes.
- The client introduces the partner to the group and tells one thing that the partner likes to do.

Therapist's Notes:
- The therapist should have clients with greater cognitive ability lead off the activity.
- Provide verbal prompts as necessary. If the client needs more support than that, have staff work 1:1 with the client.

Guess Who I Am

Objective:
- The client will identify another client through a description of his/her hobbies, interests, etc.

Procedure:
- The therapist introduces the activity and gives an example, e.g., "I know that this person likes horseback riding."
- The therapist reads a description.
- The client guesses who has been described.

Therapist's Notes:
- Choose a descriptor that is unique to that individual.
- Later add descriptors that apply to several clients to highlight common interests that could be done together.
- Discuss interests.

Role-Play Starting a Conversation

Objective:
- The client will appropriately begin a conversation in a role-play situation.

Procedure:
- The therapist introduces a discussion on ways to start a conversation (telling something about yourself, commenting on something that you both have in common, asking a question).
- The therapist models telling or asking another person something to help start a conversation.
- The therapist and clients role-play starting a conversation.
- Clients role-play starting a conversation with a peer under supervision.
- Clients progress to the point of being able to independently role-play behavior with a peer.

Role-play Situations:
- Neighborhood: Starting a conversation with the person next door.
- Classroom: Starting a conservation with a peer during social lounge.

Therapist's Notes:
- For clients with very limited verbal skills initially use a double who stands in for him/her.
- Use verbal prompts to help the client whenever necessary.
- Reinforce with approval.
- Encourage clients to use these techniques in other parts of the program (social lounge, dining area).

Role-Play Listening

Objective:
- The client will demonstrate appropriate listening behavior in a role-play situation.

Procedure:
- The therapist discusses appropriate behaviors associated with listening, (looking at the person who is talking, nodding head, saying: "mm-hm," or phrases like "Is that right?", "I see.", "I know what you are saying.").
- The therapist models appropriate listening behavior while another staff or volunteer explains these listening behaviors during the conservation.
- The therapist and client role-play situations where the client is required to listen.
- The client practices listening to a peer while the therapist supervises.
- The client practices listening to a peer independently.

Role-play Situations:
- Classroom: The therapist explains an activity to the client.
- Home: Sister expresses sadness and the client listens.
- Neighborhood: Friends describes interesting TV program to the client.

Therapist's Notes:
- Use modeling, physical assistance, and verbal prompts whenever necessary to elicit appropriate listening behaviors.
- Reinforce appropriate behavior with approval.
- Practice listening behavior in the context of a conversation as much as possible.

Socialization

Objective:
- The client will socialize at appropriate times with group members.

Procedure:
- The therapist shows clients pictures from magazines and books that show people in social situations (talking, laughing, dancing, and eating).
- The therapist leads a discussion on appropriate times (social lounge period) and ways to socialize during the program.
- The client socially interacts with group members during social lounge.

Therapist's Notes:
- Encourage the client to visit with peers during social lounge.
- Encourage parents, friends, and significant others to include the client in a variety of social situations (picnics, going to movies, attending family parties).

Class Applause

Objective:
- The client will appropriately encourage and support other group members in role-play situations.

Procedure:
- The therapist discusses and demonstrates ways to support others (clap hands, give words of encouragement, give a hug or pat on the back).
- The client encourages and supports other participants in role-play situations.

Therapist's Notes:
- Encourage clients to sincerely give encouragement and support.
- Encourage clients to provide positive reinforcement in all parts of the program.

Mirror, Mirror

Objective:
- The client will compliment himself/herself while looking in a mirror.

Procedure:
- The therapist explains and models looking in a mirror and telling what s/he sees.
- The client looks at the mirror and says what s/he sees.

Materials: Full-length or hand-held mirror.

Therapist's Notes:
- The therapist facilitates the process by asking questions, e.g. what do you like best when you look in the mirror; what do you see first?
- If client cannot think of anything positive so say, point out assets.
- Vary activity by having the client give self a strength bombardment (see activity below).
- Use a double who stands next to the client and gives the client positive things to say about himself/herself whenever s/he is stuck.
- Allow client ample time to say something before assisting.

Bragging

Objective:
- The client will compliment himself/herself in front of the group.

Procedure:
- The therapist leads a discussion about personal strengths and pride.
- The therapist introduces the activity and models boasting about accomplishments, awards, skills, things s/he does well, etc.
- The client takes a turn naming something s/he is proud of.
- The therapist leads a discussion about the activity.

Therapist's Notes:
- Encourage clients to show recognition and positive support for each client's statement.
- Emphasize that the exercise is not a contest to see who is best.
- Give clients who have difficulty thinking of a compliment a hint, e.g. something you own, how you have earned some money, something you bought yesterday.

Sell-a-Fella

Objective:
- The client compliments a partner on his/her good characteristics.

Procedure:
- The therapist discusses giving compliments.
- The therapist models giving a compliment to a client.
- Client is instructed to "sell" his partner by pointing out all the good characteristics.
- Client tells the partner and the group why they might want the partner.

Therapist's Notes:
- Provide a double who stands next to the client to help clients to think of compliments.
- Have the client give only one compliment at first.

Strength Bombardment

Objective:
- The client will compliment each group member on strengths.

Procedure:
- The therapist discusses different kinds of strengths and develops a vocabulary of strength words.
- The client actively participates with other group members to bombard each client, one at a time, with his/her strengths.
- The therapist records strengths mentioned and gives a list to each client.

Materials: Pen, paper.

Therapist's Notes:
- Instruct clients that only positive assets are to be mentioned.

I Like You

Objective:
- The client will discuss and demonstrate ways to express affection.

Procedure:
- The therapist leads a discussion around: How did your family communicate, "I love you" or "I like you" to the client, friends, and relatives?
- The therapist leads a further discussion on appropriate and inappropriate ways of expressing affection in different types of relationships.
- Client acts out socially appropriate ways to touch affectionately.
- Client role-plays telling someone that s/he cares about them.

Role-play Situation:
- Home: expressing affections toward a parent.
- Neighborhood: letting a friend know you care about him/her.
- School/work: expressing liking for a teacher.
- Community: expressing affection for a date in a bowling alley or other public place.

Concepts:

- Hugging is a way to show affection for very special people, e.g. family, best friend, relatives. It is sometimes done when you have not seen a special person for a long time or are saying goodbye to someone you will not see for a long time.
- Expressions of strong feelings for a date are generally considered more socially appropriate when expressed in private places. Holding hands and putting an arm around a date's shoulders is an appropriate way to show affection in public.

Role-play Asking a Peer to Do Something.

Objective:

- The client will ask a peer to do something with him/her in a role-play situation using eye contact and appropriate verbalization.

Procedure:

- The therapist introduces a discussion on when and how to ask someone to do something.
- The therapist models asking someone to do something with him/her.
- The therapist and client role-play appropriate behavior.
- Client practices behavior with one peer under supervision.
- Client practices behavior with peers independently.

Role-play Situations:

- Neighborhood: Asking someone to go to the movies.
- Classroom: Asking someone to play Parcheesi in the social lounge.

Therapist's Notes:

- Use physical assistance, verbal prompts, and doubling if the client does not respond.
- Reinforce behavior with physical gestures of approval and verbal praise.
- Use language appropriate to the particular interpersonal situation.
- Encourage clients to use this approach in the social lounge.

Identification of Friends and Strangers

Objective:

- The client will identify individuals who are family members, friends, helpers, and strangers.

Procedure:

- The therapist introduces the concept of family, friends, helpers, and strangers.
- Client identifies family members and the therapist writes names on a blackboard.
- Client identifies two friends and how s/he knows these people.
- Client identifies two helpers, e.g. teacher, police officer.
- Client defines stranger.

Concepts:

- Stranger is someone who you do not know or who you have never met.
- Helper is a person who is paid to work with people or help them, e.g. teacher, police officer, doctor, nurse.

Materials:

- 5" x 8" cards with "Family," "Friend," "Helper," "Stranger."
- Blackboard.
- Chalk.

Making Friends

Objective:

- The client will discuss and role-play ways to enhance relationships with peers.

Procedure:

- The therapist leads discussions on ways people make friends.
- Client role-plays one of the best methods discussed.

Therapist's Notes:

- Facilitate discussion by asking questions, e.g., what is a friend; how do you make friends; when you first came to school, how did you make a friend?
- For those with limited verbal skills, initially use a double that stands next to the client and speaks for him/her.

Role-Play Dealing with an Approach by a Stranger

Objective:

- The client will appropriately deal with an unwanted approach by a stranger in a role-play situation.

Procedure:

- The therapist discusses how to deal with unwanted approaches.

- The therapist models dealing with an unwanted approach with a "stranger."
- Client role-plays ways to deal with a stranger under supervision.
- Client deals with a stranger in a non-structured part of the program, e.g. a real stranger comes in at social lounge time and invites client to go to movies.

Role-play Situations:
- Home: Dealing with a stranger who asks to come in.
- Neighborhood: Dealing with a stranger who offers a ride in a car.

Materials: Costume for stranger; props.

Therapist's Notes:
- Use a real stranger whenever possible. Many lower functioning people have difficulty with the concept of a stranger. This is even more confusing when the person playing a stranger is a teacher or friend.
- Use a double who stands next to the client to assist with non-verbal and verbal responses.
- Establish a stringent success criterion for this behavior. Many individuals have been trained to always do what someone else tells them and will have trouble refusing. Others are so pleased to be asked to do something that they will always want to say yes.

Dating Role-Play

Objective:
- The client will appropriately role-play: 1. asking for a date and 2. responding to an invitation for a date.

Procedure:
- The therapist asks clients to define a date and name activities that would be fun to do on a date.
- The therapist explains and models making a date while a co-therapist models accepting or rejecting a date.
- Client alternatively role-plays making a date and accepting or rejecting a date.

Therapist's Notes:
- Provide content guidelines for making a date, e.g. stating name, saying where and when the date would be.
- Encourage parents or other primary care providers to invite a friend of the opposite sex along on outings.

- Provide activities that require interaction between females and males, e.g. dancing.
- Provide information about when it is appropriate to reject a date (e.g., something else is happening at the same time, client would prefer not to be with the person asking).

Volleyball Variations

Objective:
- The client will actively participate in making a group decision to change volleyball rules.

Procedure:
- The therapist introduces concept of changing rules.
- The therapist suggests a variation of a volleyball rule, e.g. ball must be hit twice before being returned over the net.
- Client participates in group decision — changing one rule of the game, e.g. every time a team makes a point it can change one rule.
- Client plays the game with new rules.

Materials: Playground ball or volleyball; string or net.

Therapist's Notes:
- Divide team into sides with varying levels of cognitive abilities.
- Facilitate decision-making whatever ways are necessary.
- Allow clients to make impossible rules as part of the learning process; given an opportunity, they will generally change the impossible rule.

Visiting Friends Role-Play

Objective:
- The client will role-play appropriate behaviors for visiting friends.

Procedure:
- The therapist discusses good manners for visitors and develops a chart on manners with the group.
- The therapist models visiting a friend.
- Client role-plays visiting a friend.

Role-play Situations:
Neighborhood: Going to a friend's house to watch TV.

Materials: Magic marker, poster board, props.

Therapist's Notes:
- Encourage the client's parents or primary care provider to ask the client to accompany them when they visit relatives and friends.
- Tell parents to encourage the client to visit friends and relatives who live within walking distances of his/her home.

Appropriate/Inappropriate Behavior

Objective:
- The client will correctly identify 10 out of 13 behaviors as being appropriate or inappropriate.

Procedure:
- The therapist explains concepts of appropriate and inappropriate.
- The therapist shows slides of appropriate and inappropriate behavior to the entire class.
- Each client holds up a sheet of paper indicating if the behavior is appropriate or inappropriate.
- The therapist discusses why behavior is appropriate or inappropriate.
- Clients suggest alternative appropriate behaviors.

Concepts:
Appropriate: O.K., fine, ☺:
- Blowing nose in handkerchief.
- Cutting nails in bathroom.
- Wearing work uniform at work.
- Wearing best clothes to church.

Inappropriate: not O.K., ☹:
- Blowing nose on sleeve.
- Cutting toenails on bus.
- Wearing work uniform to dance.
- Wearing best clothes to play volleyball.

Reasons:
- Blowing nose is private behavior and covering nose with hanky makes it private.
- Cutting toenails is private behavior and should be done in private place.

Materials: 13 photographs with appropriate or inappropriate behaviors, slide projector, projection screen, (or use a PowerPoint presentation), sheets of paper with ☺ appropriate and ☹ inappropriate.

Therapist's Notes:
- Reinforce clients individually and as a group.
- Pair a co-therapist or higher functioning individual with those who have trouble paying attention and responding.

- Encourage clients to indicate appropriate and inappropriate behaviors to peers in other parts of the program.

The Face before Me

Objective:
- The client will touch partner's face gently.

Procedure:
- The therapist forms two lines facing each other.
- The therapist instructs players in row one how to explore portions of the face with a gentle touch.
- The therapist demonstrates carefully exploring the lips, eyebrows, eyelids, hair, and other parts of the face and head.
- Client in row one explores partner's face with a gentle touch.
- Client in row two repeats the process.

Therapist's Notes:
- Increase comfort level by having clients do more common touching first, e.g. shakes hands.
- Have clients explore partner's hands, progressing to wrists, forearms, elbows, upper arms, and shoulders.

Plaster Gauze Masks

Objective:
- The client will appropriately touch another client and work with a partner while making a plaster gauze mask.

Procedure:
- The therapist presents example of finished mask.
- The therapist simultaneously explains and demonstrates how to make a plaster gauze mask.
- Client makes a mask with a partner under close supervision.

Directions:
- Cut surgical gauze into 2" long strips.
- Put warm water in a bucket.
- Tie all hair back from face with a bandana.
- Put Vaseline all over face; make sure eyebrows, lids, and lashes are covered well.
- Dip surgical gauze in water, remove excess water, and place evenly on face of individual who is lying down.
- Cover face with three to four layers of plaster gauze.
- Allow mask to dry on face (approximately five minutes); the individual must keep eyes and mouth shut.

- Remove mask by having individual make faces behind the mask and lift it off.
- Remove Vaseline from the eyes of the client.
- Wipe off excess Vaseline from the back of the mask.

Materials: Vaseline, bandana, scissors, bucket, 1" surgical gauze, tissue, paper towels.

Therapist's Notes:
- Provide a high staff to participant ratio.
- Emphasize touching gently and helping each other.

Body Sculptures

Objective:
- The client will touch and move various parts of his/her partner's body into a sculpture.

Procedure:
- The therapist explains kneading and molding clay.
- The therapist demonstrates how to do this with a partner.
- Client takes turns with his/her partner as sculptor of clay.

Directions:
- Clients are paired. One player is the clay and his/her partner is the sculptor.
- Sculptor kneads torso, head, and limbs of clay and moves body parts to make a "sculpture."
- Clay holds body parts wherever sculptor puts them.

Therapist's Notes:
- Pair partners such that two lower functioning individuals are not together.
- Stress moving clay slowly and carefully.

Conversation Circle

Objective:
- The client will appropriately introduce self (and, for higher functioning clients, start a conversation) in a game situation on command.

Procedure:
- Therapist introduces rules of the game in a simplified manner.
- Therapist models desired game behavior with another staff or volunteer and/or peer models.
- The client actively participates in Conversation Circle.

Directions:
- Two circles facing each other. Gentlemen are on the inside facing out. Ladies are on the outside facing in.
- Both circles move to their right, in time with music.
- When the therapist stops the music, those facing each other shake hands and introduce themselves and talk about a topic assigned by the therapist until the music starts again.
- Anyone without a partner moves to the center of the circle to find one.
- The game continues until each player has met everyone in the group (or ten to twelve people if the activity is done with a larger group).

Therapists Notes:
- Demonstrate rather than explain as much as possible.
- Provide physical and verbal cues or prompts for clients as needed.
- Begin with introducing self, then progress to learning other person's name.
- For clients with greater cognitive impairments progress over time to a concrete conversation starter ("Tell your friend something that you like to do.").
- Have high staff/volunteer to client ratio for clients with greater impairments.

Activity Analysis for Conversation Circle
Descriptors:
- General category: Social mixer.
- Participants: Twenty or more (equal number of males and females).
- Activity structure: Structured, semi-active, simple roles, bi-lateral, short duration.
- Social structure: Cooperation, sociability, skill void of competition, creative expression, inclusion.
- Formation required: Circle.
- Levels of participation: One-to-one within group.
- Role: Equal participant, non-aggressive.
- Amount of physical contact: Frequent.
- Age appropriateness: High school, adult.

Benefits
- *Tangible* (measurable): Speaking, communicating
- *Intangible* (non-measurable): Cooperation, sharing, social interaction, interpersonal relations, awareness of others, self-concept enhancement

Adaptations:
- *Mental retardation*: Limit size of the group. Limit number of clients interacting simultaneously. Demonstrate rather than explain as much as possible. Provide physical and verbal cues or prompts for clients, as needed, and praise all efforts. Begin with introducing self and learning other person's name and progress over time to concrete subjects, ("Tell your friend how you got here today.") Have high staff to client contact.
- *Mental illness*: Limit size of group (8-14). For those in an acute psychotic episode focus on topics related to reality orientation and offer high staff-client contact. For clients who chronically and habitually engage in maladaptive behaviors (such as with schizophrenia) focus on using this to enhance communication skills (listening and speaking). For clients in residential settings the suggested guidelines listed above under mental retardation would also apply.
- *Physically disabled*: Place clients who cannot independently move about on the inside of the circle facing out and "move" to music. Have clients who can walk or push their own mobility devices around the outside of the circle. Adjust topic to cognitive level of clients. If clients cannot vocalize, focus on non-verbal communication, (how to let someone know you are friendly).
- *Geriatric populations*: No adaptations may be necessary. Some older clients would respond well to topics around the theme of "The Good Old Days." Others may benefit from topics related to reality orientation.

How Do You Like Your Neighbor?

Objective:
- The client will accurately name the other clients in a game situation.

Procedure:
- Therapist introduces rules of the game appropriate for the group.
- Therapist models desired game behavior with co-trainer and/or peer models.
- Client actively participates in How Do You Like Your Neighbor?

Directions:
- The players are seated in a circle with "it" standing in the center. There are just enough chairs for those seated and none for "it."
- "It" approaches one of the players and asks, "Who are your neighbors?"

- If the seated player cannot name them correctly before "it" counts to ten, s/he becomes "it."
- If the seated player does name them, "it" asks further, "How do you like _____?" naming one of the player's neighbors.
- If the reply is "all right," everyone shifts one seat to the right; if it is "all righteous," they all shift to the left; if the reply is "just fine," everyone shifts anywhere s/he pleases.
- If the answer is "Not at all," then the leader asks, "Whom do you like?"
- The seated player gives the names of any two people in the circle, for example, "I like Mary and Joe."
- Mary and Joe must then change places with those next to the player being questioned.
- "It" tries to get one of the chairs vacated by Mary and Joe during the shifting.

Therapist's Notes:
- Demonstrate rather than explain as much as possible.
- Provide verbal cues, as necessary.
- Increase the length of time allowed for response as needed.
- Therapist plays "It" until other clients can role-play.
- Play first just naming one or two neighbors.
- Progress, over time, to naming whole group.
- Add other components of game as clients are ready.

Activity Analysis for How Do You Like Your Neighbor?

Descriptors:
- General category: Social mixer.
- Participants: Six to twelve participants.
- Activity structure: Structured, semi-active, complex rules, time limits, short duration.
- Social structure: Cooperation, skill and chance, sociability, inclusion.
- Formation required: Circle.
- Levels of participation: One-to-others within group.
- Role: Leader/follower, non-aggressive.
- Amount of physical contact: None.
- Age appropriateness: Grade school, high school, adults.

Benefits:
- *Tangible* (Measurable): Attention span, self-control, spatial awareness, verbalization, memory retention.
- *Intangible* (Non-Measurable): Challenge, social interaction, body image enhancement, awareness of others, competition.

Adaptations:

- *Mental retardation*: Limit number of clients. In the beginning respondent may be required to name two neighbors. The length of time allowed for response should be increased. The therapist should be "it" until other clients can model the behavior. Play first just naming neighbors and add one rule as clients demonstrate understanding of the game.

- *Mental illness*: May be played with no adaptations depending on contact with reality, degree of confusion, etc. This activity may be too stimulating for some and increase tension levels. Clients with chronic mental illness may need many of the modifications listed above under mental retardation.

- *Physically disabled*: Individuals who can walk or push their own wheelchair could move from circles on the floor rather than from chairs. Individuals who cannot independently move, but have basic hand function, could pick up larger pegs or Nerf balls from a table that they are all seated around. Individuals who cannot vocalize can point to responses on a language board or other type of communication.

- *Geriatric populations*: May be played without adaptations depending on health problems. See above suggestions for ideas related to health problems.

References

Berryman, D. & Lefebvre, C. (1984). *The recreation behavior inventory manual*. State College, PA: Venture Publishing.

Coyne, P. (1980). *Social skills training: A three-pronged approach*. Portland, OR: Crippled Children's Division University of Oregon Health Sciences Center.

Lifestyle Alteration Education

Changing health behaviors is not an easy task. Think about your own life and how hard it has been to make healthy changes (e.g., quit smoking, exercise more, eat better, take time for self-nurturing and recreation). You might know that you need to exercise more but you don't (so from this we know that knowledge doesn't always equal action). Also, you may be really geared up to exercise more (e.g., you bought new workout clothes, you joined the local gym) but you find that the gym schedule doesn't work with your personal schedule (so from this we know that there are also barriers that hinder our ability to take care of ourselves). Additionally, if we don't believe in ourselves, the chances of following through with our newly planned behavior will most likely fail (e.g., would love to lose weight but in the back of our head we are telling ourselves that we really don't think it is possible). This is called self-efficacy.

Changing health-related behavior can be complex and there are many theories to help us understand and promote change (e.g., Health Belief Model; Theories of Reasoned Action and Planned Behavior Change; Transtheoretical Model and Stages of Change; Stress, Coping, and Health Behavior; Social Cognitive Theory; Theory of Gender and Power). Because there are so many aspects to the problem, a standard approach to changing health behaviors is not realistic. Therapists who are interested in theories of changing health behavior may find it helpful to read Glanz, K., Rimer, B., & Lewis, F. M. (2002). *Health behavior and health education: Theory, research, and practice, 3rd edition.* Josey-Bass: San Francisco, CA.

Health behavior change is also not a quick process. It is generally believed that a change in health behavior cannot be considered successful until it has been maintained for at least six months. The downside of this for recreational therapists is that we often do not have the luxury of working with clients for this length of time and we may see a client at the beginning, in the middle, or during maintenance of a changing health behavior. The following is a general outline of ideas that work well in an acute rehabilitation center.

Recreational Therapy Interventions in Acute Physical Rehabilitation

Changing health behavior can best be described as a process of changing a particular behavior in a positive direction to optimize health. Health is not only related to physical health, but also to social, emotional, cognitive, and spiritual health. Through the assessment process, recreational therapists evaluate the health of a client's lifestyle related to basic health needs, provide needed education, and implement recommendations. The following steps, although they may not be appropriate for all clients, can be a helpful guide.

Knowledge and Understanding

1. The therapist gains knowledge and understanding of the client's disability (e.g., diagnosis, prognosis, precautions, abilities, limitations, and disability or illness risk factors for the client's primary and secondary disabilities).

2. The therapist conducts an interview with the client and client's family to gain knowledge and understanding of the client's premorbid lifestyle with particular attention to lifestyle components that can be altered to promote positive change in health, functioning, and quality of life. Areas of exploration often include, but are not limited to the list shown in Table 26.

3. The therapist assesses the client's knowledge and understanding of his/her current health behaviors. Does the client know the benefits of positive health behaviors (e.g., engaging in regular physical activity for recovery and prevention of another stroke)? Does the client acknowledge the possible risks and severity of the consequences if behavior is not changed?

4. The therapist learns what the client values in his/her life (e.g., independence, socializing, spending time with grandchildren) so that recommended lifestyle changes are related to the impact that they will have on these activities. Some clients may be able to easily identify what is important and holds meaning in their lives. Others may find this to be a difficult task. Clients who have difficulty may benefit from attitudes and values exploration and/or existential counseling (see "Education and Counseling" in the Techniques section). Therapists working with clients who are cognitively intact will find it difficult to move on to the next step if this step is not accomplished.

5. The therapist then explores the level of knowledge that the client has about the risks and consequences of behaviors on his/her health. Education is not provided yet. At this stage, the therapist is only seeking knowledge and understanding. For example, does a client with multiple sclerosis realize that lack of exercise contributes to deconditioning and fatigue? Does she realize that if she does not increase her

---

Table 26: Aspects of Premorbid Lifestyle

Exercise: What form of exercise does the client do? How often? At what intensity? For how long at a time? How long has the client been following this exercise pattern? Does the client exercise alone or with others? What barriers or facilitators are influencing engagement at this time?

Diet: What is the client's typical eating pattern? What types of food are consumed? How much food is consumed? In what situations is food consumed? What triggers the client to consume food? What barriers and facilitators are influencing eating patterns at this time?

Smoking: What is smoked? How much? How often? What triggers the client to smoke? How long has the client smoked? Has the client ever tried to quit? What was tried? What barriers and facilitators are influencing smoking patterns?

Drug and Alcohol Use: What is used? How much? What triggers the client to use? How long has the client used? Has the client ever tried to quit? What was tried? What barriers and facilitators influence use patterns?

Leisure: How much time is allocated to leisure in a given day/week/month? What activities are engaged in during leisure time? What barriers and facilitators influence leisure behavior?

Social Environment: Who is a social support for the client? Who does the client interact with on a regular basis (family, friends, co-workers, neighbors)? How often does the client engage in activities with other people? What is typically shared with social supports? What barriers and facilitators are influencing social behavior?

Spiritual Environment: Does the client feel connected to a higher being or power? How does the client practice this belief? What barriers and facilitators are currently influencing spiritual health?

Emotional State: What is the client's current state of emotional health (e.g., feelings of depression, loss of control, anxiety, stress)? What is currently going on in the client's life that is presenting an emotional burden? What barriers or facilitators are currently influencing emotional health?

Cognitive Activity: To what extent is the client cognitively stimulated? By what activities? What barriers or facilitators are currently influencing cognitive health?

Sleep: How much sleep? When? How many hours at one time? What barriers and facilitators are currently influencing sleeping patterns?

---

physical activity level that it will impact her level of health, functioning, and independence (e.g., may need more physical assistance from others due to lost strength and endurance)?

6. The therapist learns about the client's available resources (e.g., finances, transportation, support) to make sure that recommended lifestyle changes are realistic given the client's available resources (e.g., therapist doesn't begin to explore going to a local YMCA when the client lives in a rural environment that doesn't provide transportation to and from the YMCA).

Education

Prior to educating the client about lifestyle changes the therapist needs to have a therapeutic relationship with the client. This is needed to build trust.

The therapist educates the client on components of his/her lifestyle that are seen as being clinically destructive to health, functioning, and quality of life. The approach used to educate the client will vary depending on the perceived receptiveness of the client. A very common approach is to 1. highlight the positives of the current situation, 2. convey a wish and hope for the client to continue to improve and not experience any further problems, and 3. share with the client lifestyle recommendations with genuine concern in the context of activities and tasks that hold value for the client. Activities that are valued (as identified in the "Knowledge and Understanding" section) are intrinsically motivating. Motivation must be present for the possibility of change to occur. For example, if a client said that she values family activities, then the therapist would relate how decreased physical functioning from lack of exercise could affect her ability to participate in family activities (e.g., "If you don't begin to participate in regular physical activity, you will continue to lose function due to deconditioning. If you lose strength and endurance it will make it that much harder to go to your son's baseball games and I know that this is something that is important for you to be able to do."). It is important to remember that people do not do something unless they get a benefit out of it.

Finding something that is truly meaningful to the client and tying it to the need to change the behavior provides motivation when "It would be good for you" just isn't motivation enough.

Implementation

Once the specific changes have been identified and the client buys into the importance of making these changes, a treatment plan is developed to achieve the desired changes in the context of tasks that hold value to the client. For example, if the client values friendship and being with others and needs to develop a regular exercise program, then the therapist explores exercise options that incorporate these qualities (e.g., walking clubs, aquatic exercise groups). Through involvement with the specific tasks self-efficacy is built (belief that s/he can do it), as well as functional skills (e.g., endurance, strength, assertiveness skills, social skills).

When the client is ready to be discharged from acute rehabilitation, the therapist assists the client in developing a healthy activity pattern that reflects the new behavior change. See "Activity Pattern Development" in the Techniques section.

Documentation

The ICF does not recognize the term "lifestyle alteration education" because it is an intervention rather than a function. Therapists provide lifestyle alteration education because it can have a significant impact on preventing secondary complications and illnesses (health promotion focus). Therefore, the therapist will commonly address lifestyle alteration as a means to work on the client's ability to d5702 Maintain One's Health,. Refer to this code for more information. The therapist can also document under any functional gain that is achieved through lifestyle change, such as b455 Endurance Tolerance Functions or d910 Community Life.

Discipline-specific documentation should reflect the specific health behavior change needed, the reason the health behavior change is recommended, the client's level of awareness about the health behavior change, the client's level of acceptance or rejection of the health behavior change, the level of assistance needed with the task, and discharge recommendations.

Motor Learning and Training Strategies

Clients who lack the ability to complete part or all of a motor task often need to have the task broken down into discrete steps. There are two, intertwined processes used to teach motor skills to clients. The first process is to conduct a task analysis of the activity so that both the client and the therapist are familiar with the discrete steps required to complete the activity. Task analysis can be found in this section. The second process is using information on how people learn to maximize skill development. O'Sullivan & Schmitz (1988) outlined a three-phase process that clients go through as they learn new motor skills. The three phases are 1. the cognitive phase, 2. the associated phase, and 3. the autonomous or final phase.

Cognitive Phase of Motor Learning

The first step in learning a new motor task is to develop an understanding of the task. To understand the task the client must be able to 1. know the specific steps and demands of the task, 2. compare his/her abilities against the skills required, 3. develop strategies to compensate for missing skills, and 4. organize his/her thought process to learn and complete elements of the task. Training strategies at this phase include:

- Therapist demonstrating the task at the ideal performance speed.
- Teaching individual components of the task and then the task as a whole.
- Asking the client to verbalize the components of the task.
- Manually guiding the client through the desired movement.
- Giving added attention to important elements of the task.
- Reinforcing the importance of performing a slow and controlled movement.
- Giving praise to reinforce good performance and limit verbal comments about errors.

The second stage is called the Associated Phase. At this stage the client practices movement patterns learned in the first stage. Through practice, skills become more refined and errors decrease. Training strategies at this stage include:

- Using visual feedback (e.g., use of a long mirror) as a direct modality for feedback.
- Having organized and consistent practice sessions.
- Identifying of consistent movement errors and intervening on only those movements (do not over-stimulate or frustrate the client by commenting on errors that are not consistent).
- Providing praise and constructive feedback.
- Encouraging the client to concentrate on each component of the movement.
- Practicing movements in a more real-life environment (e.g., walking in the hallways with other people instead of in the clinic) and gradually progressing to practicing movement patterns in an environment that is less predictable (e.g., walking outdoors).

The third stage is called the Autonomous or Final Phase. The client continues to refine his/her movement pattern skills and the need for cues from the therapist decrease. Training strategies include:

- Continuing practice sessions that are organized and consistent.
- Encouraging the client to strive for consistent performance.
- Promoting development of movement pattern skills in real-life environments that have fewer controls.
- Designing and causing distractions so the client can work on maintaining focus on movement patterns.

Sequence of Motor Return

Therapists need to be aware of the order in which motor functions return to best identify and stimulate the client's progress. The following can be used as a rule of thumb for the common order of motor return (O'Sullivan & Schmitz, 1988, p. 271):

- Gross motor control precedes the development of fine motor control.
- Return of function tends to occur in cephalo-caudal order (head to toe).
- Return of function tends to occur in proximal-distal directions (center of body to peripherals of body; shoulder to hand).
- Flexion and extension before rotation.
- Isometric movements (holding a posture) before isotonic control (moving in a posture).
- Symmetrical movement patterns before asymmetrical movement patterns.
- Discrete movements before continuous movement.
- Static control before dynamic control of posture.

References

O'Sullivan, S. & Schmitz, T. (1988). *Physical rehabilitation: Assessment and treatment*. Philadelphia, PA: F.A. Davis Company.

Neuroplasticity

This section describes the development of the brain as it relates to forming and shedding neural connections, defines the term neuroplasticity, and examines common therapeutic interventions to foster neuroplasticity (cognitive retraining, constraint induced movement therapy, weight suspended walking). A discussion about when neuroplasticity interventions are best used and other theories related to neurological recovery are also provided.

Neural Connections

At birth, a child's brain has most of the neurons that s/he will need for life. However, the neurons are not yet linked in the complex networks that are needed for mature thought processes. During the first few years of life, the child's brain develops these connections, known as synapses, very quickly. It is the interplay between the child's genes and his/her life experiences that stimulates the development of synapses. Positive interactions with caregivers, toys, exploratory objects, music, and reading are vital life experiences needed to develop and strengthen synapses. In adolescence, however, synapses are lost (connections are disconnected). Neurons die through a process called apoptosis in which neurons that do not receive or transmit information become damaged and die. Therefore, connections that have been used repeatedly are kept and those that are seldom used are shed.

The shedding of synapses is a natural process that appears to be necessary and beneficial for growing up. It helps to develop more efficient neural networks through better pathway organization, thus helping the person become better able to learn more difficult concepts and skills. Think of the brain as a tree. When the branches are pruned, each remaining leaf can get more sunlight. It is the same with the brain. The shedding of synapses makes the brain more efficient.

By adulthood, the brain is a "lean, mean machine." So, does this mean that an adult brain can never develop new neurons or synapses? No. The adult brain can change its structure (new or changed neural pathways and new synapses can form); however this is typically seen as an adaptation process after the brain has been damaged rather than a part of normal development.

The ability of the brain to change with learning, whether the brain is developing synapses during early childhood or adapting to an injury by reorganizing neural pathways after brain damage, is called neuroplasticity (also known as brain plasticity). New connections can form at an amazing speed, but in order to reconnect, the neurons need to be stimulated through activity. Rehabilitation attempts to stimulate particular neurons and pathways through repetition of a specific task.

Cognitive Retraining

As the saying goes, "use it or lose it." This holds true not only for physical skills such as muscle strength, but also for cognitive skills such as memory. The brain needs continuous challenges to develop, strengthen, and shed neural pathways. As discussed in the section above, brain development is not a one-time event. The brain continually changes its structure to meet the demands placed upon it.

The specific process involved in challenging the brain after injury is called cognitive retraining. Cognitive retraining is a descriptive therapy term, rather than a specific technique. It is a type of therapy used by many different disciplines, including recreational, physical, occupational, and speech therapy, to promote neuroplasticity. It is commonly used after brain damage (e.g., stroke, traumatic brain injury) to recover lost cognitive skills, throughout a progressive neurological disease (e.g., Alzheimer's disease, multiple sclerosis) to help promote maintenance of current cognitive skills, and to promote developmental growth of cognitive skills as in mental retardation. Therapists use a variety of approaches to promote neuroplasticity. They are best understood by dividing them into two types of interventions called recovery and compensation. Cognitive retraining that focuses on recovery aims to restore lost skills, while cognitive retraining that focuses on compensation aims to develop adaptations (or compensatory strategies) for the lost skills.

Recovery Approach

Cognitive retraining, although appearing easy in application, requires the clinician to integrate a variety of approaches and to continually manipulate the task, the environment, and the therapeutic input. The therapist needs to maintain a balance between tolerated, guided challenges and detrimental frustration of the client, all the while tracking the client's performance and reaction to the challenge. The steps to implement this process are described below.

1. *Identify the skills within a functional task and determine a baseline of functioning:*
   Restoring lost cognitive skills begins by identifying the specific cognitive skills that are lost (e.g., sequencing, short-term memory, problem solving)

and evaluating the client's current functional status (e.g., client requires moderate verbal cues to sequence five steps involved in staining a wood project; client is able to recall three of six grocery items after a five-minute delay; client requires minimal multi-modal cues to problem solve for issues related to using public transportation). Notice that the tasks in the examples are all functional tasks (woodworking, grocery shopping, public transportation). Generalizing cognitive skills from one task to another is a separate and distinct cognitive process and it can be very difficult for some clients to do, especially those who have had a traumatic brain injury. Therefore, it is recommended that the therapist address the specific deficit within a functional task that will be both familiar to the client and also part of the client's lifestyle after therapy. The therapist should also continue to use the same functional task throughout the course of cognitive retraining as much as possible. For example, if the therapist is using the task of repotting a plant to address the skill of sequencing and the client becomes proficient with the task, the therapist would then need to increase the complexity of the task to further challenge the client (e.g., tending a flower garden). When tasks are changed, the therapist still must be attentive to choosing a task that is going to be part of the client's activity pattern after discharge.

2. *Once a baseline for a deficit skill in a functional task has been determined, the therapist implements cognitive retraining using these strategies:*

   a. *Manipulate the environment.*

   The therapist begins by treating the client in a quiet, non-distracting environment and gradually increases the complexity of the environment. The environment can be manipulated by increasing or decreasing the number of supplies, the type and degree of distractions (e.g., people, pictures on the wall, a ringing telephone, an open door to a busy hallway), and paying special consideration to the type of environment chosen and the emotional reaction of the client to the environment (e.g., non-threatening, exciting, calming). Clients do not all perceive environments the same way. For example, one client may enjoy the peacefulness of a private therapy room while another client becomes anxious in such a setting. A quiet, non-distracting environment can enhance a client's attention and concentration on the skill being addressed thus maximizing neuroplasticity. However this type of environment is not always found in the real world. Therefore, the therapist begins with a quiet, non-distracting environment with the goal of increasing the complexity of the environment to match the client's anticipated real-life

setting or to reach a level of functioning that can be reasonably accommodated.

   b. *Graduated stepping.*

   Graduated stepping refers to small and progressive changes in the challenges presented to the client. The therapist can either increase or decrease the steps presented as long as they reflect a positive change (e.g., gradually decrease the verbal cues given to the client, gradually increase the complexity of the task). Negative stepping is not desirable, yet it is necessary at times (e.g., increasing the verbal cues given to the client, decreasing the complexity of the task) if the task presented is too difficult or there is a change in the status of the client (e.g., a medical issue that results in further deterioration of the client's cognitive skills). The goal is to increase the neuroplasticity of the brain through cognitive retraining. Therefore, the therapist wants to always present a challenge slightly above the client's current level of cognitive functioning. Examples of what a therapist can change include the amount of cueing provided, the type of assistance provided (e.g., decrease from a hand-over-hand assist to a verbal cue, decrease from moderate gestural cues to minimal gestural cues), the complexity of the activity (e.g., increase from a two-step activity to a three-step activity, increase from solving familiar problems to solving moderately familiar problems), and the environment (e.g., increase from a non-distracting environment to a minimally distracting environment).

   c. *Cueing.*

   The therapist provides the client with a variety of cues to help the client complete the task without the therapist doing the task for the client. Cues can include verbal cues, tactile cues, demonstrative cues, auditory cues, gestural cues, and/or visual cues. Cueing helps the client figure out the task. It does not give the client the answer (e.g., "What do we need next?" "It is on your right side" "It begins with the letter 's'." "You use it to scoop up soil.", "What do we have to do before we put in the seed?"). This is important to facilitate neuroplasticity as it challenges the brain to reorganize. Cueing is given in a graduated fashion and may need to be altered depending on the environment. For example, a client may require minimal verbal cues in a moderately distracting clinic (capacity qualifier in the ICF) and when in the community require moderate verbal cues (performance qualifier in the ICF).

   d. *Reinforced practice.*

   This refers to the need to practice the skill repetitively and consistently for facilitation of neuroplasticity. This means that the same skill is practiced at each therapy session with the client using the same activity. The skill does not need to be practiced for the duration of each session, thus hindering your ability to address other issues with the client, but it should be practiced for a specific duration in the treatment session. For example, if you are addressing problem solving for familiar tasks, ask the client one or two problem solving questions at the beginning of each therapy session. It is also important to be consistent in the approach taken with the client (cueing, level of assistance, task, environment), especially if the entire treatment team is focusing on the same skill. For example, if a client lacks insight about his impairments, the team may agree to jointly address this issue by 1. tying a laminated list of the client's five prominent impairments onto the side of her wheelchair, 2. asking the client at the beginning of each therapy session to name the five impairments without looking at the list and then record the results on a traveling documentation sheet on the back of the client's wheelchair, and 3. asking the client to refer to the list to identify deficits she didn't name.

Compensation Approach

Often there is not enough time to gradually increase the client's cognitive skills to achieve skill independence in the anticipated real-life environment or the client does not fully recover some cognitive skills, resulting in the need to adapt for the cognitive deficit. This would be a compensation approach. This approach, however, can be detrimental to the client in the long run if the activities are not also structured in a manner that promotes continued recovery of function. Brain function can be recovered over long periods of time, including after discharge from an inpatient rehabilitation facility. A compensation approach, while it can slow down the recovery process, may be required for two primary reasons:

- *Safety*: Without compensatory strategies the client has a high risk of harm to self or others (e.g., without a curtain hung in front of the main house door, the client would wander outside).
- *Activity participation restrictions*: Without compensatory strategies, the client's activity involvement would be restricted impacting health, functioning, independence, or productivity. For example, without a beeping watch that reminds the client to go outside to wait for the bus, the client would miss the school bus. This also includes a client's emotional health.

Recreational therapists understand the value of participating in recreative experiences for the pleasure they bring. Designing activities that require the assistance of another person, a special environment that is not typical of a real-life setting, and challenges that can be frustrating all limit the recreative benefits of participation. Consequently,

therapists often seek to balance both recovery and compensation. Therapists do this by 1. teaching the client's caregiver how to continue to facilitate neuroplasticity with activities after discharge (recovery approach) and 2. teaching the client and caregiver how to adapt the activity so that the client can participate in the activity with the greatest level of independence and pleasure (compensation approach).

Long-term and short-term memory deficits are common cognitive impairments. Some common compensatory strategies for cognitive deficits include the memory aids described here:

Memory books: The use of a memory book is a common compensatory strategy to help clients with their memory. A memory book is typically developed by a therapist to meet the needs of the client. The size and form of the book, the number of sections, the labeling of the book, the location where the book is kept, and the information in the book vary depending on the client's needs and abilities. For example, a memory book may be a binder that has four tabbed sections labeled "calendar," "people," "therapy schedule," "to do"). The calendar section has a copy of the current month. The client crosses off each day after dinner to help track the current day, month, and year. The people section may have two pages. One page is titled "therapists" and the other is "family and friends." On the appropriate page is a picture of each person (e.g., the client's recreational therapist, physical therapist, spouse, children). Under each picture is the person's name and relation to the client. This helps the client identify and remember common people in his/her life. The therapy schedule section is a printout of the client's therapy schedule for the day. Every morning the client puts in the new schedule and throws away the previous schedule. This is to keep the client aware of the schedule for the day and promote awareness of time. The to-do section has two sheets of blank or lined paper. It is a place for the client to write down things that s/he needs to remember to do for the day (e.g., call sister after lunch, ask nursing aid for an extra blanket). After each task is accomplished the client puts a line through it.

Memory books are typically used in a rehabilitation setting and caregivers are educated on how to continue the use of the book after discharge to help the client compensate for impaired memory. They are usually a large, white binder and clients either carry it or place it next to them on the wheelchair. Although memory books can be helpful, they can also be potentially bothersome, confusing, and disorienting to the client if they are not properly maintained and designed to fit the lifestyle of the client. For example, if a memory book is not cleaned out, too many pages can accumulate, confusing and disorienting the client further (e.g., client is looking at the wrong therapy schedule). Also, a large white binder that contains mostly therapy information can become cumbersome to transport and not correlate with the client's post-therapy lifestyle (e.g., client perceives the large, white memory book as embarrassing; it is difficult to carry when trying to carry a bag of groceries and use a cane at the same time).

Consequently memory books are often changed when planning for discharge (e.g., switching from a large, white binder to a small organizer) or the therapist helps the client identify adaptations for managing the book (e.g., carry it in a thin backpack). Changing the style and layout of a memory book can be problematic for some clients who may have difficulty generalizing information from one type of memory book to another. Therefore, the therapist who designs the memory book should be keenly aware of this issue and design a book that can transition from one setting to another with minimal changes.

Recorders: The use of a small recorder can be a helpful memory aid. The client can record bits of information that need to be recalled and pre-establish set times to review the recordings (e.g., listen to recordings at lunchtime and dinnertime). The client can write down recorded information and then attend to the information as appropriate (e.g., transfer notations onto the wall calendar in the kitchen, cross off items that are completed).

Signs: Another type of memory aid is the use of signs. Signs can be easily made on blank pieces of paper and posted in key locations to help the client remember specific things that occur in common locations. For example, on the inside of the front door a sign could be posted saying, "Remember keys?"

Lists: Lists are also a very common and helpful memory aid if they are placed in easily accessible and visible locations. Lists can be posted on the refrigerator (e.g., keep a running list on the refrigerator of food items that need to be purchased), in a computer (e.g., keep a list of items that need to be packed when going to the shore house, camping, or a simple day trip).

Alarms: Watches with alarms that can be preset for multiple times (e.g., alarm will sound at 9 A.M., noon, 3 P.M., and 6 P.M.) can be a helpful reminder for taking medicine, performing weight shifts, or trying to use the bathroom.

Placement of items: Strategic placement of items can be helpful. For example, if the client has to remember to put bills in the mailbox, she could place them on the table next to the front door.

There are many other memory aids available commercially (look in therapy catalogs), however the therapist should always remember to fit the aid to the client and not the other way around.

Education of the client's caregivers: Therapists train caregivers on how to provide the assistance needed (e.g., cues, environment, keeping memory book up to date) to continue to facilitate neuroplasticity post discharge through cognitive retraining. Changes in the brain can occur over an extended period of time; therefore the potential for further recovery is still there. This is why it is imperative to educate caregivers about the function of the brain and their role in assisting the client with further recovery. Failure to educate caregivers on this process can impede the client's recovery. Additionally, education helps the caregiver understand the importance of activity beyond the psychosocial benefits, thus promoting greater carryover of activities after discharge and greater assistance from the caregivers in helping the client to participate in activities. It helps when caregivers understand that what they do will continue to help the client get better.

Constraint Induced Movement Therapy

If the client's deficits are related to impaired motor skills (e.g., paralysis of the right upper extremity), a technique called *constraint induced movement therapy* or CIMT may be utilized. It is a common therapy technique used for stroke and brain injury rehabilitation. The initial CIMT program called for the non-affected upper extremity limb to be restrained (a soft web-like mitt placed over the hand and Velcroed around the wrist) to prevent the client from using the non-affected limb and to encourage use of the affected limb. The client is then challenged with graduated tasks to be completed by the affected upper extremity to facilitate neural pathway development. Since gross function returns prior to fine function (ability to bend elbow before ability to manipulate fingers) and proximal function returns before distal function (shoulder function before wrist function), graduated steps are presented in this order. When a client uses an upper extremity in an activity using gross function only, it is called gross assist (using arm as a weight to hold something down or as a blocker to keep something from sliding away). When a client uses his/her upper extremity in an activity using both gross and proximal function, it is called functional assist (grasping, manipulating).

One of the major problems with this technique is that the program required the client to wear a restraint 14 hours a day for a period of two weeks (ten consecutive weekdays) with six hours a day of direct care focused on having the client complete graded purposeful activities (Page, et al, 2001). Concerns that arose from this treatment included client safety outside of direct care, limited treatment hours available to address mobility (e.g., needing unaffected upper extremity to hold cane for safe walking), staffing ability to provide the required number of direct care hours, and client's compliance with the program requirements.

As a result, some facilities have adopted a modified CIMT program that consists of fewer restraint hours with positive results (e.g., five hours a day with directly supervised therapy). A study conducted by Page et al (2001) found that clients who received a modified CIMT program made "substantial improvement compared to those who received traditional or no therapy intervention."

Even the modified CIMT program is difficult for many rehabilitation centers to implement due to the number of therapy hours required. Consequently, the CIMT program has been further modified to feature non-restrained "forced use techniques" in therapy sessions. In this approach, restraints are not used. The therapist "forces" the client to use the affected limb in specially designed therapeutic activities. Use of the non-affected limb is limited (if allowed at all) in the activity to optimally promote neuroplasticity.

We do not recommend that therapists abandon compensatory skills training, as not all clients will fully recover and will need to develop compensatory strategies to enhance independence and function. However, we recommend that therapists incorporate forced use techniques into therapy sessions whenever possible and as appropriate.

Weight Suspended Walking

If the motor deficit lies in the lower extremities (e.g., paralysis of the right lower extremity) a technique often referred to as *weight suspended walking* may be utilized. It is typically implemented by physical therapists; although recreational therapists should be aware of this technique as part of the rehabilitation process.

To use weight suspended walking the client is placed in a harness that hangs over a treadmill. The height of the harness is adjusted so that the client's feet rest on the treadmill with a very slight knee flexion. Typically, two therapists or a therapist and an aide are needed. They stand on each side of the client. The treadmill is turned on at a very slow speed, which may be increased at the discretion of the therapist. The treadmill helps facilitate the gait cycle because the affected foot, which is resting on the treadmill, is passively moved backwards by the treadmill. The therapist standing on the client's affected side holds the client's leg and lifts it up to advance it forward. The treadmill then passively sends the foot and leg backwards again. The therapist

or aide on the unaffected side provides the client with support for balance. The repetition of the gait cycle helps to promote neural pathway development in the area of lower extremity motor function.

When to Implement Neuroplasticity Interventions

It is important to implement these techniques at the proper time. Stanford University's research center states that

> An important aspect of rehabilitation therapy is timing. If a person who has suffered from brain damage does not practice a lost movement, the damaged neurons — as well as surrounding neurons — are starved of stimulation and will be unable to reconnect. However, research on non-human animals indicates that if an injured limb is used immediately after the brain area has been damaged, damage to the brain actually increases. To be successful, rehabilitation must wait a week or two. By the second week, use of the injured limb stimulates damaged connections that would otherwise atrophy without input. Yet, a particular movement can be practiced too much. If practiced millions of times per month over years, for example, the pattern of connections can grow so much that it inhibits or "squeezes out" other patterns of connection, resulting in the inability to perform other movements. In short, rehabilitation therapy can indeed take advantage of the brain's natural flexibility for forming new neural connections; however, this is a delicate process that must be done carefully and under professional guidance (Hammond, 2002, p. 3).

Neuroplasticity does not always occur. The brain will not be able to reorganize itself if extensive damage to the area occurs. For example, Huntington's disease and other diseases that cause neuronal death may render the brain unable to reorganize itself, especially if the entire circuit is destroyed. However, the brain's ability to grow new neurons (called neurogenesis) can sometimes repair the damage.

Finally, from a maintenance perspective, active lifestyles maintain brain function. Therefore, therapists should be diligent in educating clients about the cognitive consequences of inactivity even when cognitive impairment is not evident. The spinal cord is similar to the brain in that it can repair some damage, but at a very slow rate. It seems to require extensive rehabilitation efforts to have even a small effect, but the possibilities of finding effective medical techniques are promising. Peripheral nerves can regenerate, usually getting close to the functionality of the original system. New nerve cells grow to replace the damaged cells and damaged axons regrow their connections.

Other Theories Related to Neurological Recovery

Neurological recovery cannot be attributed to one thing. It is most likely a variety of variables that all interplay to affect the recovery process. See the box to the right for descriptions of theories related to neurological recovery.

When talking about recovery, it is also important to clearly define recovery because it means different things to different people. One person may define recovery as restoration of lost skills (e.g., my right upper extremity was paralyzed and now it is not), while another may define recovery based on ability to perform specific tasks (e.g., was unable to use the computer and now is able to use the computer). Therefore, recovery can generally be described as progress towards a goal.

In the latter definition of recovery, recovery is described more as an adaptation process. Although individuals with progressive disabilities, such as multiple sclerosis or ALS, do experience some restoration of function at times, the primary goal of the rehabilitation process for these individuals would be to learn how to adapt and modify activities to maximize independence. Such adaptations may include equipment, alternative techniques, and adaptation of materials.

The client's level of motivation also plays a critical role in the recovery process

> Motivation plays a major role in functional recovery; without it, no recovery may occur, probably because functional recovery is actually a relearning process. Without motivation and active goal setting on the part of the learner, behavioral changes (learning) do not take place (Trombly, 1989, p. 78).

For clients who are cognitively intact, education about the usefulness of activity for recovery, independence, and quality of life can be an effective motivational tool. For clients who lack the required cognitive ability, education should be provided for the caregivers. Caregivers who will be the ones to initiate activity and provide care must fully understand their role not only as caregivers but also as "therapists" after the traditional rehabilitation process.

Theories of Neurological Recovery

The theories listed here are descriptions of how neuroplasticity may take place within the brain.

Diaschisis theory: Spontaneous recovery in the early weeks and months after brain injury due to a decrease in edema or bleeding.

Redundancy theory: When damage occurs to an area of the brain, other parts of the brain that are normally active in controlling the same function take over and assume greater responsibility in controlling the activity. Thus, the smaller the lesion, the greater the capacity for the remaining tissues in the area to assume functional control.

Vicarious function: This refers to the capacity of part of the brain to take on functions normally controlled by other areas. For example, speech is controlled by the left hemisphere in most individuals. If damage occurs to this area before speech patterns are firmly established, a child may develop speech using right hemisphere function.

Functional reorganization: This is when the structural organization of the brain changes. Neurons begin to grow (sprouting) and communication pathways reorganize.

Behavioral substitution: This refers to the ability of the brain to achieve the same goal by substituting an entirely different strategy. For example, a client with impaired proprioception may learn to position his/her body appropriately to achieve a stable sitting posture using vision and a long mirror.

Knowing that neurological recovery can take place over the course of years, it makes sense that the client's lifestyle and activity level can have a profound impact, whether positive or negative, on recovery.

References

Hammond, K. (2002). Neuroplasticity: The brain's natural reparatory ability. http://www.stanford.edu/group/hopes/treatmts/lifestyleandhd/u1.html. An educational product of HOPES (Huntington's Outreach Project for Education at Stanford). Stanford, CA: Stanford University.

Page, S., Sisto, S., Levine, P., Johnston, M., & Hughes, M. (2001). Modified constraint induced therapy: A randomized feasibility and efficacy study. *Journal of Rehabilitation Research and Development, 38*(5):583-590.

Trombly, C. (1989). *Occupational therapy for physical dysfunction, 3rd edition.* Baltimore, MD: Williams & Wilkins.

Oxygen

Recreational therapists are concerned about the oxygen their clients get because lack of oxygen will kill a patient faster and do more harm than any other problem. Oxygen is required for life. In first aid situations the order to check for problems is airway, breath, circulation.

Luckily, most recreational therapy situations are not as potentially life threatening as a complete lack of oxygen. It is usually enough to monitor the oxygen saturation in the client's blood during activities. The recreational therapist should have orders from the client's physician that specify the level of saturation required when the client is at rest and when the client is active.

Measuring Oxygen Saturation

There are two primary ways to measure oxygen saturation: an arterial blood sample and a pulse oximeter.

The most accurate test for measuring oxygen saturation is an arterial blood gas test. A small sample of blood is drawn directly out of an artery (instead of a vein). The blood is directly tested for its oxygen level. Other tests (such as the level of carbon dioxide and the pH of the blood) can be done at the same time. A recreational therapist will rarely be responsible for taking a blood sample, so this topic will concentrate on using an oximeter and observing other signs of too much or too little oxygen.

The pulse oximeter (PulseOx) measures the client's peripheral oxygen saturation. A small clip is placed at the end of the client's finger or on the client's earlobe. The clip usually has a pair of small light-emitting diodes (LEDs) on one side and a device to measure the amount of light received on the other side. One LED is red, with wavelength of 660 nm, the other is infrared at 910 nm. Hemoglobin (the part of the blood cell that carries oxygen) absorbs the light differently when it has oxygen and when it doesn't. From the difference in absorption, the oximeter can calculate the level of oxygen saturation. The latest generation of pulse oximeters use advanced digital signal processing to make accurate measurements in clinical conditions that used to be impossible, including when the patient is moving, when there is not much blood flowing, in bright ambient light, and when there is electrical interference. The devices are not perfect, however. Therapists need to make sure, among other things, that the client is not wearing red nail polish or something else that might block the light or affect the reading.

A normal blood saturation level is greater than 95%. If the saturation level is below the parameter set by the physician (e.g., client's level is 90 and the parameter set by the physician is >95), the therapist has the client stop the activity, close his/her mouth, and take slow deep breaths in and out of the nose to raise the saturation level. After a few minutes, the therapist takes the saturation level again. If the level does not rise, the therapist contacts the client's primary nurse and reports the situation to determine the next course of action (e.g., nurse instructs therapist to bump up oxygen by one liter, bring client back to nursing station, physician to be paged).

If the client's level is far below or above the parameter or if s/he is exhibiting signs of oxygen deprivation or toxicity (as discussed later), the therapist needs to call the client's primary nurse immediately. If the nurse is not available, the therapist needs to immediately call a physician.

If a client is on oxygen and will be engaging in a sedentary activity, the therapist is to take the oxygen saturation level of the client when the client enters the treatment room at the start of the session and then every 15 to 30 minutes throughout the duration of the session. If the client will be engaging in physical activity, the therapist is to take the saturation level prior to the start of the session and every five to ten minutes during the physical activity. Therapists who will be working with clients in a community setting that will not have immediate access to a physician, nurse, or respiratory therapist, must receive in-house training on changing oxygen tanks. An extra oxygen tank should be taken in case of an emergency (e.g., client requires oxygen level to be increased so the tank does not last as long as anticipated), along with an oximeter to monitor the client's oxygen saturation levels and a cell phone to contact the client's primary nurse, physician, or respiratory therapist should questions or concerns arise that do not warrant an emergency call to 911 and taking the client immediately to the closest emergency room.

In addition to the oximeter, there are other signs the recreational therapist can use to detect oxygen saturation that is too high (toxicity) or too low (deprivation).

Signs and Symptoms of Oxygen Toxicity

- *Chest pain*: with the pain generalized under the sternum.
- *Dry cough*: initially, with a moist cough developing as lung tissue is damaged by too much oxygen.
- *Nausea and vomiting.*

- *Restlessness*: "ants in the pants" restlessness; an inability to sit quietly.
- *Stuffiness of the nose*.

Symptoms of Oxygen Deprivation

- *Dyspnea*: shortness of breath; not being able to get enough oxygen into the blood to meet the body's need for oxygen. Dyspnea is not necessarily due to a disease process. When someone runs a mile faster than his/her physical condition is ready for, it is normal for the person to be "out of breath." The recreational therapist will want to watch for clients being more out of breath than would be expected given their current physical condition.
- *Hypoxia*: an inadequate saturation of oxygen at the cellular level.
- *Fatigue*: When the blood is not able to carry enough oxygen to meet the body's physical needs, the person becomes too tired to engage in normal activity.
- *Cyanosis*: bluish discoloration seen in the skin and lips.

Oxygen Therapy

For a variety of reasons clients will be using oxygen therapy equipment during leisure activities. The advent of more portable oxygen equipment allows clients to be more mobile and less constrained in where they can live and play. For that reason it is as likely that a recreational therapist will work with clients who use oxygen therapy equipment in the community.

Oxygen therapy is a physician-prescribed treatment that specifies the method of administration of the oxygen and the amount of oxygen to be given. Because the delivery of oxygen is a prescription, the recreational therapist should not change the delivery rate or method of delivery without written orders from the physician, nor should the therapist encourage the client to do so. (This is assuming that the recreational therapist is trained and approved to make changes with the physician's permission.) Too little oxygen can cause brain damage and too much oxygen can be toxic. Because clients may be more physically active during leisure, the therapist should watch for signs of low oxygenation and work closely with the client's physician to develop a regimen of oxygen therapy that describes when and how the flow of oxygen may be changed to accommodate activity.

Oxygen is prescribed in percentages but the flow meters for oxygen are often measured using liters of oxygen per minute. The type of equipment used to deliver the oxygen to the client makes a difference in the actual amount of oxygen received by the client.

For example, at 6 L/min (liters per minute) a nasal cannula delivers around 44% oxygen, a simple mask delivers around 50%, a partial re-breather mask delivers 35%, and a non-re-breather mask delivers 55-60% oxygen (Timbly & Lewis, 1992). Room air typically has about 20% oxygen.

Methods of Delivering Oxygen

There are numerous ways to deliver oxygen to the client. The most common methods that a recreational therapist will see are the nasal cannula, nasal catheter, oxygen mask, and direct delivery into a trachea. In rare cases the therapist may work with clients who are in oxygen tents.

- *Nasal cannula*: A nasal cannula is a narrow, clear plastic flexible tube that extends from the oxygen flow meter to the client. At the client end, the tube splits into a loop that lets the tubing be placed just below the client's nose, looped behind the client's head, with the tubing being tucked over each ear and then joined back together under the client's chin. At the portion of the tube that is placed under the nose there are two short stubs of tubing that are placed inside the nostrils. The nasal cannula allows the client the greatest freedom to engage in leisure activities of any of the oxygen delivery options. Its other advantage is that it is less visible and does not interfere with talking, eating, or drinking. The length of the tube from the flow meter to the client varies. If the length of the tube is too short for the client to engage in activities, the recreational therapist should ask the physician if it is medically appropriate for the client to have a longer tube. Some tubes can be ten feet or more in length. Tubes can also be too long, causing a tripping hazard. The recreational therapist can provide feedback to the physician as to appropriate tubing length.
- *Nasal catheter*: A nasal catheter is a flexible plastic tube that is inserted into the client's nose all the way to the nasopharynx (near the back of the throat). The nasal catheter is secured into place by taping it to the client's nose. This is a very efficient means of getting oxygen into the client's lungs while still allowing the client to eat, drink, and talk. However, it is fairly uncomfortable to have the tube placed up the client's nose and, unlike the nasal cannula, it is not easy to remove for short periods of time.
- *Oxygen mask*: There are many different types of oxygen masks. Oxygen masks cannot be used when eating or drinking and interfere with talking. They are used primarily when the client is very ill and needs to have high percentages of

oxygen delivered to the lungs. Clients often complain of feeling claustrophobic (fear of being closed in a small space). Clients may also develop skin problems where the mask touches the skin if masks are used for very long. Masks are often used with clients who have pneumonia, smoke inhalation, or carbon monoxide poisoning. When oxygen masks are taken off to eat, the client often needs to use a nasal cannula to ensure adequate oxygen saturation.

- *Transtracheal oxygen*: For clients with a long-term need to be on oxygen, some choose to have the oxygen delivered through a tracheal opening (an opening surgically cut into the throat at the trachea). The tube that is placed into the opening is called a catheter. The catheter is held in place by a thin chain that goes around the neck. Both the tracheal catheter and the necklace type chain can be hidden under a collar or scarf. Depending on the amount of mucus that the client has, the tracheal catheter may need to be replaced many times a day or only once or twice a week. A clogged tracheal catheter can be a life-threatening situation. Therapists who take clients with tracheal catheters into the community need to be trained in how to clean them out in case they become clogged.

- *Oxygen tent*: An oxygen tent is a portable, lightweight, clear plastic structure that fits over the client's head and chest while s/he is in bed. There is a motorized unit that provides oxygen at the desired rate while keeping the temperature in the tent comfortable for the client. Oxygen tents are seldom used anymore for adults but they may be used for young children or cognitively impaired adults who need humidified air and who tend to pick at and pull cannulas or catheters.

Activity and Oxygen Delivery

There are a few aspects of providing treatment and leisure activities for clients on oxygen that the therapist will need to take into account.

- *Infection control*: By far the most prevalent method of providing enhanced oxygen levels to clients is the cannula. Most people do not like to have a nasal cannula in their nostrils so they fiddle with them, sometimes taking them off for short periods of time. The stems on the nasal cannula from which the oxygen flow are placed inside the client's nose. That means that if the client takes the cannula off for a short period of time and places it on his/her lap while in bed, the germ-filled mucus on the cannula will deposit germs on the client's blankets. When the thera-

pist places a game board or other shared recreational equipment on the client's bed, the equipment itself becomes contaminated. If this equipment is used by other staff or clients before it is appropriately cleaned, it becomes a transmission source for germs. And, if the recreation equipment is not cleaned before being placed on the client's bed, the cannula will then pick up the germs when it is taken off. When the cannula is repositioned, it puts the germs into the client's nose and lungs, both excellent ways to transmit an infection.

- *Oxygen supply*: When the client is an inpatient, his/her oxygen tubing is likely to be hooked up to the oxygen port located in the wall of the room near the head of the client's bed. Occasionally the tubing becomes kinked when the client raises or lowers his/her bed. The therapist should check the integrity of the oxygen tubing each time the client repositions himself/herself or changes the position of the bed. Most recreational therapy activity rooms do not have oxygen in the wall. When the client goes to the activity room (or to the hospital cafeteria, outside the building, etc.) the client will be switched to a portable oxygen tank on a small cart. The portable oxygen tank has a gauge on the tank outlet that indicates how much oxygen remains in the tank. The therapist should watch the gauge and make sure that the client does not run out of oxygen. The recreational therapy department can usually work out an arrangement with respiratory therapy (the department that usually exchanges oxygen tanks) to replace the tank right in the activity room if enough notice is given.

- *Cognitively impaired clients*: Clients with cognitive impairments often fiddle with the oxygen gauges. It is a good policy for the recreational therapist to know what level of oxygen the client should be getting. This information should be written down in the recreational therapist's notes about the client and updated daily. When the therapist first greets a client who is on oxygen, s/he should read the level of oxygen being provided. If the level does not match what the therapist understood the prescribed level to be, she should immediately call the nurses' station to double check. The therapist should visually check the gauges once every ten to fifteen minutes throughout the activity, more often if the client is seen handling the gauge or is known to handle the gauge.

- *Open mouth*: With a nasal cannula, when the client's mouth is open (for talking, mouth breathing, or the mouth is positioned so that the lips do not seal), oxygen is lost out of the mouth.

In this case the client is not getting the prescribed amount of oxygen delivered to his/her lungs. A client may appear quiet and withdrawn in his/her room (as an inpatient) or in the doctor's office (as an outpatient having oxygen saturation measured) so that the percentage of oxygen prescribed only works when the client is in these situations. If the client becomes more physically active during recreational therapy, experiences increased activity levels at the community center, or has hours of conversation with friends, his/her oxygen saturation may drop to sub-therapeutic levels fairly quickly. If the therapist feels that the client's activities do not match the activity level that the oxygen percentage was set for, the therapist should work with the physician to get a more realistic oxygen therapy regime.

- *Increased restlessness and irritability*: Whenever a client, especially an elderly client, has increased in restlessness or irritability, the client's oxygen and carbon dioxide levels should be measured. Increased restlessness and irritability are signs of both oxygen deprivation and oxygen toxicity. Carbon dioxide narcosis is a cognitive state of being confused or disoriented because of high levels of carbon dioxide in the blood.

- *Anaerobic pathway by-products*: If there is not enough oxygen in the blood, the body starts pulling energy from a secondary (and less efficient) source, the anaerobic pathway. Normally, when a client breathes in oxygen, the body uses the oxygen and produces carbon dioxide as the by-product. When the cells are required to pull energy from the anaerobic pathway, a different set of by-products are produced. The parts of the body that are most susceptible to injury from the anaerobic pathway by-products are the brain, heart, pulmonary vessels, and the liver (Anderson, Anderson, & Glanze, 1994). If a client is receiving too high of a percentage of oxygen (oxygen toxicity), the brain decreases the respiratory stimulus and the client's breathing rate and volume decrease. With reduced respiration the client's body begins to retain carbon dioxide, causing the same symptoms as too little oxygen.

Precautions for Activities and Supplies

Oxygen enhances combustion of other material that can burn, so if it is exposed to spark, open flame, or lit cigarettes, there is a chance of an explosion. Here are some of the devices to watch out for:

- *Electrical devices*: Electrical devices, including hair dryers, electric saws, drills, and sanders,

may produce enough of a spark in their engines to ignite a fire.

- *Glue guns*: Many of the glue guns used in arts and crafts activities are low heat glue guns that require low heat glue. This type of hot glue gun is preferable to the higher temperature glue guns.

- *Open flames*: Open flames are inappropriate for clients using oxygen therapy. This includes being anywhere near the barbeque during picnics, use of candles, and campfires.

- *Petroleum products*: Petroleum products such as oil paints, rubbing alcohol, epoxy glues, oil-based face paints, and oil-based stains should not be used near oxygen.

- *Smoking*: There should be no smoking near clients with oxygen. In the United States almost every type of treatment facility and most recreation centers are now smoke free. However, there are places that a client can go and still be exposed to lit cigarettes. For example, if an inpatient on oxygen is going to sit outside of the hospital cafeteria with his family to enjoy the sunshine, he may end up sitting next to someone who is smoking. And, in fact, some clients on oxygen still smoke — a very dangerous situation.

- *Static electricity*: Static electricity from fabrics could cause an explosion. Some facilities have policies that prohibit staff from wearing uniforms or clothing made of materials that are highly susceptible to producing static electricity. When using fabrics for activities (even the use of parachutes for activities), the therapist will want to select fabrics that are less susceptible to producing static electricity. Cotton fabrics tend to not produce static electricity.

Equipment that is of special concern to therapists of clients on oxygen therapy includes:

- *Oxygen tanks*: When the client is receiving oxygen from a metal container, the therapist should ensure that the activities do not cause the tank to tip over or to be harmed. Tanks are usually secured in a carrying cart. Even without heat sources close by, if a tank tips over and the seal to the flow meter is broken, the therapist can have an explosive situation. The gas inside the tank is under a lot of pressure. The larger tanks will have internal pressures greater than 2000 pounds per square inch. When the cap or flow meter covering the tank outlet is cracked or broken off, the tank acts like a torpedo, propelled by the pressurized gas within the tank. It could very easily go through a brick wall.

- *Tubing integrity*: It is important that the tubing not be kinked or blocked during activity. The therapist should regularly check to make sure that the tank cart wheels are not on top of the tubing, that no one is standing on the tubing, that no books or other supplies are sitting on top of the tubing, and that no blockages are occurring. The clear tubing is often hard to see, especially for clients who have impaired vision, such as in nursing homes. The therapist should make sure that there is no room for anyone to walk between the client and his/her oxygen supply.

References

Anderson, K., Anderson, L., & Glanze, W. (Eds.). (1994). *Mosby's medical, nursing, and allied health dictionary.* (4th ed.). St. Louis, MO: Mosby.

Timbly, B. & Lewis, L. (1992). *fundamental skills and concepts in patient care* (5th ed.). Philadelphia, PA: Lippincott Company.

Personal Leisure Resource Awareness

Personal leisure resource awareness is the process of determining what resources are available in and around the client's home to engage in leisure.

The therapist explores the resources currently available to the client that will indirectly or directly influence his/her leisure involvement and choices. This list includes available equipment, space to do leisure, money and other ways to get leisure supplies, the availability of others to help with leisure activities, and the time available for leisure.

People tend to spend a significant amount of time in their homes. Although home leisure can be active (e.g., gardening, exercising, re-finishing large pieces of furniture), the majority of home leisure is passive or sedentary (television, computer, reading, talking on the phone, sewing, knitting). Passive leisure is a part of healthy leisure and many (but not all) of the choices need to be recognized for their cognitive and emotional health benefits (e.g., relaxation, learning, challenging cognition).

Before a therapist explores a healthy home leisure activity pattern for the client, the therapist needs to be aware of the resources available. The activities have to match the available resources. If resources are not available, the therapist needs assist the client in identifying ways to obtain resources so that activities can be successfully transitioned into the client's activity pattern (e.g., raising funds to purchase a DVD player so the client can watch exercise DVDs, re-designing the layout of the dining room to allow an area for making crafts).

Indications

Therapists routinely explore home leisure activities and resources as part of the initial evaluation process of all clients.

Therapists must remember that a client's interests can change with disability and that prior leisure involvement may no longer interest the client. For more information about exploring leisure choices, see "Activity Pattern Development" in the Techniques section.

Contraindications: If significant cognitive impairments are evident, the therapist will need to talk with the client's family member, guardian, caregiver, or activity director to obtain information about the client's personal leisure resources. For clients who are unable to tell the therapist what they enjoy, the therapist may be able to learn more by exposing the client to various leisure activities and observing the client's reaction to each activity (behavior, level of participation, attitude, length of time engaged in the activity). Clients who have significant cognitive impairments will most likely respond positively to simple, physically based, repetitive activities.

Protocol

It typically takes 30 minutes or less to determine the personal leisure resources of the client.

A quiet and non-distracting environment is best to promote attention and concentration.

The therapist should have relevant materials (e.g., paper and pen to write down home leisure activities and leisure resources).

Process

The therapist explores the following areas:
1. *Equipment and supplies*: Things required for leisure activities. The therapist asks the client what activities s/he does at home. If the therapist is unfamiliar with the activity, the therapist asks the client to describe the activity (how is it done, equipment used). If the therapist is familiar with the activity, but suspects that the client uses adaptive equipment or techniques, the therapist gets a description of special equipment or techniques. If there are specific pieces of leisure equipment that the client does not mention and the therapist perceives the piece of equipment to be helpful in meeting the health needs of the client, the therapist asks if it is available (e.g., do you have a computer, do you have a bicycle).
2. *Home and neighborhood*: Locations to engage in leisure activities. The therapist asks the client to describe his/her home to determine the amount of space for leisure and barriers to accessing areas (e.g., steps to enter the home; steps within the home; number and type of rooms; basement; are rooms packed tight with furniture or do they have a lot of open space; outdoor areas such as a garage, backyard, front yard, garden, pool, shed). The therapist also asks questions about the client's neighborhood (e.g., do you have sidewalks, is your neighborhood hilly, are you on a busy road, are there other kids on your block, do you talk with you neighbor). These questions help the therapist to be sure that adequate space is available for pursuing the client's leisure interests.
3. *Finances*: Ability to pay for leisure activities. If the client is an adult, the therapist asks the client if s/he is on a tight budget. This is a very general question that gives the therapist an idea of the client's finances. Activities have to fit within the

client's budget or alternative funding sources need to be identified. If the client is a child or teenager, this question will be best directed to the parents. Other ways to obtain supplies for leisure activities should also be explored such as the ability to get leisure supplies through donations and community programs where supplies are provided.

4. *Assistance*: Other people who are available to help the client with leisure activities. Find out who is available and the extent of their availability to help the client with leisure. Ask the client who lives with him/her and about other people the client spends time with. Relevant information includes their age, if they have any limitations in their ability to help him/her, do they work, what hours do they work, what do they usually do for leisure, do they have any common leisure interests with the client, do they think they would have the time and desire to help the client with leisure activities if needed? Finding out if there are common leisure interests and what the others enjoy is helpful, especially if the therapist perceives that assistance might be needed. Others are more likely to help if they enjoy the activity, too. It is not to say that others will only help a client engage in leisure activities if they like to do it, but it does make it more likely.

5. *Time*: Free time when enough energy is available to engage in leisure activities. Therapists ask clients to describe a typical workday and/or a typical non-work day. Therapists write this information down in the form of a time line. This not only gives the therapist an idea of the amount of leisure time spent but also the amount of leisure time available. It is also a good evaluation tool to determine the variety of leisure (physical, social, cognitive) and the value placed on leisure.

Taking a time line of daily tasks and activities also gives the therapist an opportunity to listen to how the client describes the day (does it sound hectic to the client, does it sound like the client is bored). There are many other subtle cues that a therapist can pick up from this discussion (e.g., no one is around, the client is by himself most of the day, the client has too many things to do in a day, the client is not adhering to the recommendations of his/her physician). A very brief example of taking a daily time line looks like this:

8:00 A.M. wake-up, shower, dress
9:00 A.M. leave for work
9:30 A.M. work that entails ...
Noon lunch at my desk
6:00 P.M. leave work
6:30 P.M. home and eat dinner
7:30-11:00 P.M. television

Outcomes

The recreational therapist documents all of these findings on the client's initial evaluation form. The information will be used later as part of the planning process for leisure activities.

Personal Leisure Resource Awareness is an intervention so it is not coded in the ICF. However, it can be used for difficulties in many parts of Activities and Participation Chapter 9 Community, Social, and Civic Life. If this protocol helps restore functionality to a particular activity, such as d9204 Hobbies, it may be documented in the chart notes as part of the treatment for that code.

Special Credentialing/Training: There is no additional credentialing or training needed by a CTRS to implement this protocol.

Pie of Life

Objectives:

- To help a client identify how s/he spends his/her time.
- To provide the client with a tool to make informed decisions about what to do with his/her time.

Materials:

- A piece of paper with each hour of a 24-hour day written down the left column with each hour on its own line. This paper should be labeled "How I spend my day."
- A circle that fills most of an 8½" x 11" piece of paper. The inside of the circle is divided into four equal quarter sections using dotted lines. Each quarter section represents six hours. This second paper can have numerous headings including "REAL" and "IDEAL."
- Something with which to write.
- Colored magic markers.

Procedure:

- The client is given two sheets of paper as described in the materials section and writing materials.
- Using the first paper (How I spend my day) the client writes down how each hour is spent. The therapist will need to give clear directions as to whether the client is to record a typical day (not necessarily what really happened on any one day, but what an average day would look like), what happened on a specific day, whether the client should select a specific day that includes time needed for health care issues and appointments, and whether the day is a work/school day or not.
- Have the client break down the activities into categories such as sleep, self-care/grooming, work, school, active recreation, reading, transportation, taking care of others, etc. Once the client has a group of activity categories s/he should add up the hours spent in each category.
- The client takes the total hours in each category and transfers this information to the pie chart.
- The six-hour quarters are there just to make it easier for clients to estimate how much of the pie any specific time period represents. For example, if the client spent three hours a day in the car, the client would divide one of the six-hour quarters in half to equal three hours.
- It is helpful if the therapist has the activity categories pre-determined and provides a different color magic marker for each category.

That way, if the group compares their pies, each client can judge how much more or less time s/he spends in any one category than others in the group. This can help spur discussions.

Variations:

- There are 168 hours in a week. The therapist may want to have a client look at a week as a time unit instead of a day. A week allows a better measurement of how one spends one's time. If a 168-hour time is used, each quarter of the pie represents 42 hours.
- The therapist can use two pies; one for "Real" and one "Ideal"; "While in Rehab" and "Once Discharged"; or "While Using Drugs/Alcohol" and "Not Using."
- The therapist can use different topics besides activities to show in a pie format. For example, Where my money goes; Where my energy goes; What portions of my day are creative? Interesting? Dull, Busy work? (St. Vincent Pallotti Center, 2004).

Questions for the Therapist to Ask:

After having the client look over his/her own pie and maybe talking about it with the people near him/her:

- Are you comfortable with the relative size of your slices?
- If you want to begin changing the size of any of the slices, what is realistic?
- The changes you have proposed require more/less energy. Is that realistic?

Every time a client decides to spend more time in one activity category, s/he is actively or passively deciding to spend less time in something else:

- When you make a commitment to do something, how often do you stop and ask yourself what you will cut out?
- Is this important to do?
- How would asking yourself this question change your life?

After a client has filled out the "Ideal" pie:

- Do you think that you will usually have enough energy to complete all the hours of activities that you have put down?

Most people find that the majority of their time is spent on work/school, sleep, and caring for self and others, leaving very little time for personal time or their spouse:

- How important is it for you to increase your time for individual interests or for time with your spouse?
- Many people have a certain image of themselves such as caring mother, athlete, or community activist. What does your pie say about you?
- Does it match your image of yourself, and, if not, why not?

Therapist Notes:

- This activity is a good lead in to time management discussions. It also lends itself to discussions about a client's physical needs such as self-care, sleep, and eating. Discussions about obligations and other demands on time are logical with this activity.
- Many people do not understand the difference between a *need* (the client needs something or else his/her health, significant relationships, or life will suffer serious consequences) and a *want* (the client wants something or else s/he will not be as happy, fulfill dreams, etc.). Once a client can be realistic about the difference between needs and wants, prioritization is easier.
- Often people learn better when taught using a multi-sensory approach. By having the client think, write down, color in, discuss, and re-configure, the therapist is having the client learn about how s/he spends his/her time using a multi-sensory approach.

References

St. Vincent Pallotti Center. (2004). The pie of life. www.pallotticenter.org/current/activityoftheweek/pie_of _life

Proverbs

The use of proverbs can be very helpful when treating clients who respond well to indirect communication, as well as those who use and value proverbs (e.g., Native Americans, Mexicans). Proverbs can also convey a therapeutic idea, thought, value, or attitude that challenges the client or strengthens a personal belief. Since proverbs are common methods of communication among ethnic groups, several ethnic proverbs are listed below (accessed from www.oneproverb.com). Be aware that ethnic proverbs are not limited in use to their specific origin. There are many more proverbs and sayings that therapists may find helpful when working with clients. See, for example, *The Little Words That Grew: A Guide to Using Proverbs in the Therapeutic Process* by Gary Beaulieu (1998) from Idyll Arbor.

Afganistani
- When an ant says "ocean," he's talking about a puddle.
- In the shop of the sightless jeweler, the ruby and pebble are one.
- Grumbling and carping are the muscles of the weak.

African
- Proverbs are the daughters of experience.
- Men fall only in order to rise.
- God conceals himself from the mind of man, but reveals himself to his heart.
- No one tests the depth of a river with both feet.
- He who asks questions cannot avoid the answers.
- To try and fail is not laziness.

Arabic
- All sunshine makes a desert.
- Ask the experienced rather than the learned.
- Do not stand in a place of danger trusting in miracles.
- Examine what is said, not him who speaks.

Bulgarian
- God promises a safe landing, but not a calm passage.

Chinese
- No wind, no waves.
- Only the man who crosses the river at night knows the value of the light of day.
- Better to light a candle, than to curse the darkness.
- The man who removes a mountain begins by carrying away small stones.

- Sour, sweet, bitter, pungent, all must be tasted.
- I was angered, for I had no shoes, then I met a man who had no feet.
- It is not the knowing that is difficult, but the doing.
- The wise adapt themselves to circumstances, as water molds itself to the pitcher.
- I dreamed a thousand new paths, I woke and walked my old one.

Haitian
- Behind the mountains, more mountains.

Inuit
- He that boasts of his own knowledge proclaims his ignorance.

Irish
- The seeking for one thing will find another.
- The stars make no noise.
- You must empty a box before you fill it again.
- You'll never plow a field by turning it over in your mind.
- The longest road out is the shortest road home.
- The older the fiddler the sweeter the tune.
- Even a tin knocker will shine on a dirty floor.
- You've got to do your own growing, no matter how tall your grandfather was.

Japanese
- The tongue is like a sharp knife, it kills without drawing blood.
- Beware the man of one book.

Kashmiri
- One plus one equals eleven.
- If it comes, it is golden; if it doesn't, it was made of grass.
- Eleven persons take eleven paths.
- A kick works as a treatment to a hunch-backed person.
- Unity is strength.
- Clean your heart and mind of negative thoughts.
- True religion is in one's heart.
- It doesn't take time to change one's destiny.
- The sufferer goes through hell till the truth comes out.

Mexican
- It is not enough to know how to ride, you must also know how to fall.

Native American
- The rain falls on the just and the unjust (Hopi).
- Those who have one foot in the canoe, and one foot in the boat, are going to fall into the river (Tuscarora).
- We will be known forever by the tracks we leave (Dakota).
- There is no death, only a change of worlds (Duwamish).
- It is easy to be brave from a distance (Omaha).
- Each person is his own judge (Shawnee).
- Tell me, and I'll forget. Show me, and I may not remember. Involve me, and I'll understand (tribe unknown).
- Man has responsibility, not power (Tuscarora).
- Listen or your tongue will keep you deaf (tribe unknown).
- If you see no reason for giving thanks, the fault lies in yourself (Minquass).
- Ask questions from your heart and you will be answered from the heart (Omaha).
- Don't let yesterday use up too much of today (Cherokee).
- Don't be afraid to cry. It will free your mind of sorrowful thoughts (Hopi).
- Wisdom comes only when you stop looking for it and start living the life the Creator intended for you (Hopi).
- The bird who has eaten cannot fly with the bird that is hungry (Omaha).
- One finger cannot lift a pebble (Hopi).
- Each bird loves to hear himself sing (Arapaho).
- Our first teacher is our own heart (Cheyenne).
- You already possess everything necessary to become great (Crow).
- God gives us each a song (Ute).
- They are not dead who live in the hearts they leave behind (Tuscarora).

Russian
- A man is judged by his deeds, not by his words.
- Every seed knows its time.
- All roads lead to Rome.
- All is not gold that glitters.
- As you cooked the porridge, so must you eat it.
- Better late than never.
- Take the bull by the horns.
- Idleness is the mother of all vices.
- The tongue speaks, but the head doesn't know.
- There is no evil without good.
- He who doesn't risk never gets to drink champagne.
- The hammer shatters glass but forges steel.
- One who sits between two chairs may easily fall down.
- A kind word is like a spring day.
- An enemy will agree, but a friend will argue.
- When you meet a man judge him by his clothes, when you leave a man judge him by his heart.
- The word is silver, the silence is gold.
- There are no bad ships at all, there are bad captains.

Tao Te Ching
- The more you know, the less you understand.

Yiddish
- One hand washes another.
- The eyes are the mirror of the soul.
- The whole world is a dream, and death the interpreter.
- He who puts up with insult invites injury.
- If you can't go over, you must go under.
- If you want your dreams to come true, don't sleep.
- Surrounding yourself with dwarfs does not make you a giant.
- If we all pulled in one direction, the world would keel over.
- He that can't endure the bad will not live to see the good.
- A half-truth is a whole lie.

Relaxation and Stress Reduction

There are many techniques that help reduce stress and increase relaxation. Some of the ones that are used by recreational therapists are described in this section.

Deep Breathing

When taking a breath, oxygen is sent to the lungs and then transported into the bloodstream to service vital organs and muscles. When oxygen is received by the cells they release carbon dioxide (a waste product that the body does not need). The carbon dioxide is carried back to the heart and then to the lungs to be exhaled and the cycle repeats.

Shallow breathing (also known as chest or thoracic breathing) does not allow for a good exchange of oxygen and carbon dioxide. Inadequate amounts of oxygen are taken in and not enough carbon dioxide is exported out. When the body does not receive enough oxygenated blood and carbon dioxide builds up in the bloodstream, muscles tighten and the heart rate increases to try to increase the transport of oxygenated blood. Over time, inadequate oxygen intake and carbon dioxide buildup can contribute to headaches, fatigue, and irritability.

Clients who experience anxiety (e.g., anxiety related to specific fear, generalized anxiety disorder), anger (e.g., conflict with spouse, intermittent explosive disorder), panic (e.g., panic attacks, panic disorder), or depressive symptoms (e.g., loss of energy, pleasure, motivation), psychosomatic or physiologically based chronic pain (e.g., chronic back pain) will benefit from learning how to breathe deeply (also known as abdominal or diaphragmatic breathing). People who lead sedentary or stressful lifestyles, are experiencing emotional events, or are wearing tight fitting clothes have also been found to breathe shallowly (Davis et al, 2000) and would benefit from diaphragmatic breathing. In addition, tight fitting clothes should be exchanged for more comfortable clothing.

Clients who have difficulty taking a deep breath (e.g., a client with tetraplegia or chronic obstructive pulmonary disease) should not be excluded from this technique. In fact, clients who are using oxygen through a nasal cannula (e.g., a client with obstructive pulmonary disease) or who do not have adequate upper body strength to maintain an erect posture to be able to take in a full deep breathe (e.g., a client with tetraplegia) can benefit greatly from learning how to breathe deeply. Although clients with chronic obstructive pulmonary disease may not be able to achieve the optimal level of deep breathing, breathing even a bit more deeply can be helpful in relieving some symptoms of thoracic breathing as well as increasing the client's oxygen saturation level. Clients with complete tetraplegia should be positioned in an upright, seated position (a chest strap may be needed) to help achieve the most ideal seated posture to improve breathing, as well as for a variety of other reasons (e.g., cough production, safety).

Clients are taught to breathe from the diaphragm by:

1. Teaching the difference between thoracic and diaphragmatic breathing. The client is instructed to place one hand on his/her chest (centered) and the other hand on his/her abdomen (centered) and told to breathe normally. Which hand moves or moves more? If the hand on the chest rises more, then thoracic breathing is evident. If the hand on the abdomen rises more, then diaphragmatic breathing is evident.

2. Educating clients about the symptoms of thoracic breathing as they contribute to the current problems of the clients. For example, when a client with chronic back pain breathes shallowly, muscles do not receive a good amount of oxygen causing them to contract and tighten. Muscles are already tight from inactivity due to pain. Muscles are now further tightened due to inadequate oxygen supply. When tightened muscles are stretched, pain results. The more pain, the less the client wants to move. The less the client moves, the tighter the muscles become and so the cycle continues affecting the client's ability to perform tasks, lead a quality life, and maintain independence. Deep breathing isn't a quick fix, but it does play a vital role in pain management.

3. Teaching technique of deep breathing:
   a. In a lying position, the client places one hand on his/her chest (centered) and the other hand on his/her abdomen (centered). If the supine position (lying on one's back) is not appropriate, another position can be substituted (e.g., seated, standing, reclining).
   b. Inhale slowly through the nose and pull the breath down into the abdomen. The hand on the abdomen should rise comfortably.
   c. Exhale through the mouth slowly. It is recommended that you allow the sound of the exhale to be heard (a whooshing sound). Making this noise brings more attention to the breath (a good thing) and frees the client from constraining the natural sound of an exhale. In some situations, however, the sound can be misinterpreted (e.g., a sigh of

frustration) or be inappropriate (e.g., at a quiet business meeting). The therapist explains this to the client and confirms that a quiet exhale is an appropriate adaptation to the technique for practical application.

Benefits of diaphragmatic breathing can be experienced immediately (e.g., muscles relax, blood pressure lowers) and learning how to breathe deeply only takes a matter of minutes, Davis et al (2000) note, however, that "profound effects of the exercise may not be fully appreciated until after months of persistent practice" (p. 22).

Progressive Muscle Relaxation

Progressive muscle relaxation reduces pulse rate, blood pressure, perspiration, and respiration rate and is commonly used in the treatment of muscular tension, anxiety, insomnia, depression, fatigue, irritable bowel, muscle spasms, neck and back pain, high blood pressure, mild phobias, and stuttering (Davis et al, 2000).

Clients are taught how to recognize muscle tension (e.g., sensation that shoulders are tight and shrugged up rather than relaxed) by progressively tightening and relaxing specific muscle groups. The client assumes a comfortable position (e.g., lying on the floor, sitting) in a quiet and non-distracting environment. Relaxing music can be used but it is not necessary. The client is instructed to tighten a specific muscle group for about five seconds (e.g., tighten the muscles in your forehead, wrinkle up your forehead, now hold it, keep it tight) and then the client shifts focus to relaxation of that same muscle group (now relax your forehead, it feels smooth and soft, there is no tension there, relax). The client focuses on the relaxation of the muscle group for 20 to 30 seconds (Davis et al, 2000). Many people do not have an awareness of where they hold muscle tension when stressed (e.g., neck, arms, hands), so every muscle group in the body is tightened and relaxed until the client increases his/her awareness of specific muscle groups that hold tension when s/he is under stress. The tightening and relaxing of muscles typically begins at the top or bottom of the body with the top of the body being the most common. Here is a list of muscle groups addressed in progressive muscle relaxation in top to bottom order. A brief description of how to tighten the muscle group is provided for some of the groupings that are less commonly known.

- Forehead (wrinkle forehead)
- Eyes (squint eyes shut tight)
- Jaw (clench teeth)
- Neck (pull in chin and squeeze muscles tight)

- Shoulders (shrug and tighten shoulder muscles)
- Arm (upper arm and forearm)
- Hands and wrists (make a fist and curl wrist in)
- Chest
- Upper back
- Stomach
- Lower back
- Buttocks (glutes)
- Upper legs
- Calves
- Feet (curl toes)

This process usually takes about 20 to 30 minutes to complete and it is recommended that clients do it at least once, if not twice, a day for a period of one to two weeks. Following the two weeks, clients will begin to become aware of where they hold tension in their bodies when under stress and should then be able to relax the area without having to go through the entire progressive muscle relaxation cycle (e.g., client experiences a stressor, client is aware that muscles of the shoulder are becoming tight, client relaxes tightened shoulder muscles). This is a very discreet relaxation training technique because once the client has a heightened awareness of muscle sensation, s/he can induce a relaxation response without other people noticing the intervention.

Progressive muscle relaxation will not cause harm to a client (contraindicated), however it is not appropriate to use with clients who have uncontrollable muscle dysfunction (e.g., tremors, spasms) or who have extensive paralysis (e.g., high tetraplegia). If a client has paraplegia or mild to moderate muscle dysfunction, the therapist can adapt progressive muscle relaxation to include only those muscle groups that are not affected. It is also not an appropriate intervention for clients who have difficulty following simple directions or attending to a 20-minute task.

Meditation

Meditation trains the mind to focus and in a sense open up the mind at the same time. The client chooses something to focus on such as a word (e.g., joy) or an object (e.g., candle flame, flower). The client finds a comfortable position in a quiet and non-distracting environment. The client can keep his/her eyes open to focus on the chosen object (e.g., a single flower in a bud vase) or close his/her eyes and focus on the specific word, phrase, or action chosen (e.g., "peace and comfort," focusing on one's breath). If a word is chosen, it can be said out-loud or internally (some people chant while meditating). Some people like to use instrumental music or soft nature sounds in the background while meditating although it is not necessary.

As thoughts other than the identified focus enter the mind, the client acknowledges the thought and then sends it away. The process of clearing the mind of distracting thoughts (e.g., "I have to remember to stop at the store.", "What am I going to wear tomorrow?", or "I so mad at her!") helps the mind to open itself to new thoughts, ideas, feelings, insights, and awareness that otherwise would not surface or develop due to the stimulation and crowding from typical patterns of thinking.

Being able to focus on one thing for an extended period of time can be very difficult to start with. It should not be a stressful task, so the client should meditate only for as long as s/he feels comfortable. With practice, mediation time will increase and feelings of relaxation will deepen. The client may even become able to focus for a few minutes on an object in his/her day-to-day environment (e.g., a picture on the wall at work) to induce feelings of calm.

Davis et al (2000) report that "meditation has been used successfully in the treatment and prevention of high blood pressure, heart disease, migraine headaches, and autoimmune diseases such as diabetes and arthritis. It has proved helpful in curtailing obsessive thinking, anxiety, depression, and hostility" (p.37).

Meditation is not an appropriate intervention to use with clients who have hallucinations or distorted thought processes (e.g., schizophrenia, paranoia) or clients who have difficulty attending to a task (e.g., severe brain injury).

Visualization/Guided Imagery

Imagination is a powerful tool. Emotions are affected by what we imagine and our body is affected by what we feel. If we imagine sad things (e.g., imagining what our life would be like without our spouse), feelings of sadness will arise and our body may respond with feelings of fatigue. If we imagine joyful things (e.g., imagining our wedding day), feelings of excitement, joy, and a few jitters will arise and our body may respond with a quickened heart and respiration rate. Emotions are tied to thoughts, thoughts affect our bodily functions, and thoughts are fueled by input whether real or imagined. Therefore it makes sense to harness that power and use it to our advantage to manage emotions and bodily processes.

When feelings and symptoms of stress surface, using imagination to take our thoughts to a happy, peaceful, and comfortable place will change our thought focus thus affecting the response of our body. Clients are asked to sit in a comfortable position in a quiet and non-distracting environment and think about a place or time that holds special meaning to them (e.g., swinging on tree swing at the age of six, sitting on the beach at sunrise, riding a roller coaster). The client is told to close his/her eyes and imagine himself/herself in the special place. The therapist poses sensory stimulation questions to heighten the experience and induce positive feelings of "really being there." For example, what do you see, smell, hear, taste, and feel? Other questions may be more specific to the place chosen by the client (e.g., How high is the swing going? Is someone pushing you? Who is there with you?).

Clients do not need to have an outside source such as a therapist to walk them through this process every time (this is called guided imagery). Clients, once educated on how to stimulate their imaginary senses, will be able to apply this intervention independently. Guided imagery, however, may be a preferred method for the client. There are many tapes and CDs that can be purchased at local music stores, bookstores, and self-help stores that provide guided imagery. For example, a CD mentally takes the person on a trip through a nature trail by offering enhanced auditory input (e.g., a person's voice describes sensory experiences, sounds of birds and running streams, etc.). Therapists can even make personalized tapes for the client.

Visualization and guided imagery are not appropriate for clients experiencing hallucinations (e.g., schizophrenia), clients who have difficulty attending to a task for a minimum of 20 minutes, clients who are paranoid, clients who have a strong tendency to dissociate from reality, or those who are unable to follow simple directions.

Visualization can be used to reduce many symptoms of stress, including feelings of anxiety, panic, and depression. Although outcomes are mixed, visualization research has been conducted with clients who have cancer and clients who have chronic pain (e.g., visualize cancer cells as green balls and a "Pac-man" like critter going around the body gobbling up the cancer cells or visualize special body chemicals flowing to pain sites to dissipate knots of pain).

Autogenics

Autogenics is the process of obtaining a relaxed state by imagining the body as being warm and heavy. The client finds a comfortable position in a quiet and non-distracting environment. The source of instruction can be a tape, CD, therapist, or the internal dialogue of the client. The client is instructed to take a few deep breaths and then to imagine specific body areas as being warm and heavy. Only one body area is focused on at a time. Body areas typically include the face, right and left arm and hand, chest, stomach, back, front and back of both right and left legs, and the right and left feet. Visualization is a commonly used method to induce this type of imagination. For example:

Imagine that you are on a raft in the water. Feel the water rise and fall under the raft. The sun is shining brightly and it is warm. The raft slowly floats to the right and your right arm is now in the sunlight. Feel the warmth of the sun on your right arm. The arm feels warm. Take a deep breath. With every breath you sink deeper into the raft. You feel heavy. Your right arm feels warm and heavy. (This continues with the various body parts entering the sunlight). Continue deep breathing, focusing on becoming heavier and sinking deeper into the raft and the body becoming warmer in the intensity of the sun.

Another example is for the client to dip his/her hand into the water. The water is to be imagined as a warm, orange liquid. The fingers draw the warm, orange liquid into the body as it gently swirls into each part of the body (e.g., up the arms, into the head, down into the chest) until it reaches the toes. The entire body feels warm and relaxed and heavy. Imagine the warm, orange water draining out the toes and back into the pool (e.g., feel the water draining out of the head, down past the shoulders). Feel the water rise and fall. With every breath the body sinks deeper into the raft. The body feels warm and heavy.

Davis et al (2000) report that autogenics "has been found to be effective in the treatment of muscle tension and various disorders of the respiratory tract (hyperventilation and bronchial asthma), the gastrointestinal tract (constipation, diarrhea, gastritis, ulcers, and spasms), the circulatory system (racing heart, irregular heartbeat, high blood pressure, cold extremities, and headaches), and the endocrine system (thyroid problems). Autogenics is also useful in reducing general anxiety, irritability, and fatigue. It can be employed to modify... reaction to pain, increase... resistance to stress, and reduce or eliminate sleeping disorders" (p. 84).

Autogenics is contraindicated for clients with high or low blood pressure, diabetes, or anyone with low blood sugar because of possible increases or sudden drops in blood pressure from this technique (Davis et al, 2000). It is also not appropriate for clients who experience hallucinations, illusions, or paranoia. As with any relaxation training exercise, if discomfort is experienced, the exercise should be stopped.

Some clients report immediate relief of stress-related symptoms following the first autogenics session and others will require extended practice (one to two times a day over a period of one or two months) to experience symptom relief. Eventually, the client will be able to feel warm and heavy upon the initial thought.

References

Davis, M., Eshelman, E. R., & McKay, M. (2000). *Relaxation & stress reduction workbook, 5ᵗʰ ed.* Oakland, CA: New Harbinger.

Self-Esteem

How a client feels about himself/herself can positively (or negatively) affect many life activities. Self-esteem that affects life activities in a negative manner can have a direct impact on health. For example, a client who has poor self-esteem may not give herself permission to care for her own needs ("I'm not worth it."). Lack of self-care could then impact her physical, emotional, social, spiritual, and mental health. Recreational therapists recognize that a basic sense of self-esteem is a fundamental building block to good health. For without self-esteem, optimal self-care will not happen. This section briefly explores theories of self-esteem, issues related to delinquent behavior, recreational therapy interventions, and documentation. Therapists may also find it helpful to refer to b1266 Confidence for additional information.

Theories of Self-Esteem

Self-esteem is a complicated topic. It is difficult to measure and there are several theories on its development. A popular theory of self-esteem, "perceived adequacy", as discussed by Feldman & Elliott (1990), is based on how adequately the person performs in domains that are considered important by the person. Therefore, success in areas judged unimportant by the person would have little impact on his/her self-esteem. It is the discrepancy between the person's expectations of himself/herself (the ideal self) and the person's perceived adequacy that affects self-esteem. So if the client doesn't place value on schoolwork, then poor academic scores would not affect his/her self-esteem. For a client who does value schoolwork poor academic scores would affect self-esteem. Although this is a very individualistic approach, the researchers did find common themes that affect self-esteem. The strongest influence on self-esteem from infancy through adulthood was how a person judges his/her physical appearance. The second strongest influence on self-esteem was social acceptance by peers. For children, however, parental attitudes have a greater impact on self-esteem than peers. In adolescence, attitudes of classmates are the greatest predictors of self-esteem although parental attitudes still weigh in at a heavy second. In the college years, peers far outweigh parental attitudes. Scholastic competence, athletic competence, and conduct follow behind.

Another theory ("the looking glass self") is that a person imitates the attitudes that significant others reflect about him or her. For example, a young child who receives negative verbal and non-verbal messages from his parents about himself takes on those negative attributes. The basic idea is that a person's self-esteem is defined by what is mirrored to him/her, hence the "looking glass" (the mirrored image). The client looks to others to define his/her self-esteem.

Self-Esteem and Delinquent Behavior

Feldman & Elliott (1990) makes some additional notes about self-esteem that are important for therapists to be aware of regarding the relation of self-esteem to depression and delinquent behavior. The risk of developing depression and suicidal ideation increases when the client fails to meet his/her standards in domains that the client judges as important (including domains that are important to the client's parents) and when peer support seems unattainable (especially when support is contingent on meeting parental expectations or conforming to peer demands). This can lead to feelings of hopelessness.

Another concern related to self-esteem is delinquent behavior in adolescents. Feldman & Elliott (1990) report that failure to meet the expectations of the dominant membership group (e.g., family, peers, club members) leads to negative self-attitudes. In turn the client seeks out adolescent groups where dominant standards are ignored and delinquent behaviors are admired. The client receives the benefit of increased self-esteem in this group (e.g., here is where I fit in) from engaging in anti-social actions. Adolescent boys with low self-esteem are at a larger risk than girls for delinquent behavior. In adult males, self-esteem is often measured by success, toughness, and sexual prowess.

Recreational Therapy Interventions

Combining these two thoughts on self-esteem helps to guide the therapist in developing a treatment plan. Recreational therapists can:
1. Design activities that encourage exploration of feelings about self-esteem (e.g., ask the client to make a picture frame and write all of the positive things that s/he feels about himself/herself on the frame and then place the client's picture inside; write the client's name down the side of a piece of paper and then ask the client to write a positive affirmation for each letter in his/her name such as "A" stands for "achieves good grades," "attractive," "athletic").
2. Explore alternative leisure activities with the objective of broadening the client's awareness of leisure options that could positively affect self-

esteem (e.g., Alphabet Leisure: write the letters of the alphabet down the right hand side of a sheet of paper hung on the wall. Clients shout out leisure activities that begin with each letter. The therapist writes the ideas next to the letter. Best done in a group to obtain a variety of ideas).

3. Involve the client in activities that will enhance positive feelings in areas that are important to the client (e.g., if a client values intellect and enjoys helping others, involve the client in a group that designs and implements community service projects).

4. Address precursor skills that inhibit the client's ability to achieve success in valued areas of self-esteem (e.g., social skills, teambuilding skills).

5. Consider who has the greatest impact on the client's self-esteem and implement a plan accordingly (e.g., if parental attitudes have the greatest impact on self-esteem, assess whether or not the parents would benefit from education about their role and what they can do to facilitate positive self-esteem in their child; if attitudes of peers have the greatest impact, steer the client towards positive peer groups that highlight competences of the client).

6. Provide opportunities for personal autonomy and freedom of choice to help enhance self-esteem.

Documentation

Self-esteem is a feeling about oneself that is not understood or recognized in all cultures, so it is not part of the ICF. However, b1266 Confidence is part of the ICF and is defined as "mental functions that produce a personal disposition that is self-assured, bold, and assertive, as contrasted to being timid, insecure, and self-effacing." Refer to b1266 Confidence for more information on how to assess, treat, document, and adapt for temperament and personality functions.

Setting measurable objectives for self-esteem can be difficult because it is not easily defined. Although it is an internal thought process rather than an external skill, it can still be measured through its reflection in specific behaviors such as positive self-statements, posture, tone of voice, interactions with others, initiation, communication (e.g., assertion versus passivity), self-care behaviors (e.g., taking time to care for self), acceptance of positive remarks made by others, and engagement in self-nurturing activities. To put this into practice, a goal for self-esteem may be a simple as "Improve self-esteem." The treatment objectives that fall under this goal could be: State three positive self-attributes within self-exploratory clinic activity; sit upright during group sessions with minimal cueing; verbally thank others independently for positive remarks about self made by others during group sessions; plan structured activities at rehab with moderate assistance within daily routine for self-nurturing; engage in planned self-nurturing activities at home independently.

References

Feldman, S. & Elliott, G. (1990). *At the threshold: The developing adolescent.* Cambridge, MA: Harvard University Press.

Sensory Stimulation

Often residents of nursing homes and other health care institutions are viewed as disoriented, agitated, or hostile. Health care providers often view these symptoms as irreversible even though research has proven this to not be the case in many situations. These individuals may be diagnosed with dementia, psychosis due to a general medical condition, or delirium. The characteristics are viewed as being a result of the aging process. According to Oster (1976), as the normal aging process continues, the absence of stimuli accentuates it. As a result, an increase in social isolation and a decrease in physical, cognitive, and emotional functioning occur.

There is more to disorientation and confusion than the aging process. Sensory deprivation is a factor relating to the psychological and physiological changes in elderly populations. Bower (1967) reported that dementia was only partially caused by pathological changes in the elderly. He found that the effects of sensory deprivation resemble the symptoms of dementia. Bower carried out his study by exposing 25 females diagnosed with dementia to intensive sensory stimulation treatment. When the experimental group was compared to the control group, the results supported Bower's hypothesis. He reported that dementia is a disease, but that it is only partially the result of changes in the brain. It is also influenced by the amount of sensory deprivation that is experienced by the individual.

Oster (1976) explained that sensory deprivation sped up the degenerative changes normally related to aging and that geriatric clients with different illnesses are particularly vulnerable to sensory deprivation. Kemp (1984) found physiological changes that occur in the body as a result of decreased sensory input to the central nervous system. These changes included a decrease in reflex response, metabolic changes, circulatory changes, a lower level of consciousness, a decrease in respiratory rate, an increase in heart rate, and low blood pressure.

Oster (1976) explains that because of these physiological changes in the body, the individuals display psychophysiological maladaptive behaviors. These behaviors were a decrease in learning, an inability to deal with stress, submissiveness, dependence, low sociability, low intellect, a decrease in conceptual ability, a lower attention span, hallucinations, and delusions. Because of these

---

The topic of Sensory Stimulation was written by Laura Eide with information from her Master's Thesis *The Design, Implementation, and Evaluation of a Sensory Stimulation Program for Elderly Individuals in a Nursing Home*, 1993.

changes taking place in the body and the mind, it can be seen why sensory deprivation is often mistaken for dementia and is not correctly treated.

Kemp (1984) believes that "the average person is in constant interaction with both the internal environment (body) and the external environment (surroundings) by means of the five senses" (p. 429). When an individual is placed in a nursing home, the environmental stimulus is often lost. The brain receives constant information from the muscles, joints, and senses (proprioception) (Okrey, 1986). If not enough stimuli are sent to the brain, normal functioning of the brain may not take place. If there is not enough environmental stimulation available to the individual, there may be losses in physical, cognitive, emotional, and social skills.

Clients who have experienced a stroke-related hemianopsia (blindness in one visual field) or visual neglect with pre-existing cognitive or hearing loss are often misdiagnosed as having depression instead of being correctly identified as having a sensory deprivation syndrome (Kelly, 1990). In fact, a client does not have to be elderly to develop functional impairments related to sensory deprivation. Numerous studies have been done on healthy, younger individuals in hospital or nursing home simulations. Just being placed on bed rest in these simulations was enough to create quantifiable loss of function.

> Bed rest has been compared to the experience of sensory deprivation... Performance on several intellectual tests deteriorated including verbal fluency, color discrimination, and reversible figures. In another sensory deprivation study, young subjects lay on a bed in an experimental hospital setting. Tapes played periodically simulated the effect of brief, disjointed conversations. The subjects' perception of time intervals became distorted during the brief three-hour test. In addition, several subjects described hallucinatory like experiences. Social isolation also made the subjects uncomfortable. Frequent complaints included feeling lonely and longing for some sign of recognition from the investigator. It is rather dramatic that these feelings occurred in perfectly healthy young people during only three hours of bed rest (Siebens, 1990, p. 179).

Atkinson (1985) found that the experimental studies done on environments with restricted sensory stimulation showed that clients reacted to inadequate sensory input by developing a reduced ability to think and reason, decreased coordination, a decrease in spontaneous movement, a decrease in mental alertness, and disorientation.

In another study done by Parent (1978), there were many changes found in individuals after they were exposed to a low stimulus environment and were deprived of necessary stimulation. Some major influences of the low stimulus environment on the individual were behavior changes, loss of skills, and a lower degree of gross motor skills than before exposure to this environment. The individuals had no desire to concentrate on anything while in this environment. Some individuals experienced disorientation during the study. Although this study was not done on an elderly group, the results can be generalized to the elderly population. The environment in which an elderly individual resides can definitely shape how s/he will act. Smith (1978) reports Kratz saying that an elderly individual may be better cared for in the bustle of a busy unit instead of dumped in a room.

Another aspect of sensory deprivation is the loss of one or more of the senses. Sensory loss can occur at any age. Because aging is an individual experience, it occurs at any age and at any time. An example, according to Zegeer (1986), is when an individual loses the hearing in one ear before the loss of hearing in the other ear. Another example is when an individual cannot identify a certain food by its smell, but the individual can identify the food by its taste.

Okrey (1986) believes that when an elderly individual loses one of the senses, the other senses must be stimulated to compensate for the sense that was lost. With this, the remaining senses can work together in identifying the individual's surroundings.

Often, for the elderly individual, the loss of a sense can be an embarrassment and prevent social interactions. The individual may become self-conscious and disregard any form of interaction. According to Kopac (1983), studies have shown a relationship between sensory loss and functional activity. Kopac referred to a study done by Heron (1961). Heron's study demonstrated that the subjects with sensory loss and deprivation experienced boredom, hallucinations, and experienced difficulty in thinking clearly.

Okrey (1986) felt that through planned sensory stimulation groups and with environmental modifications, these sensory losses or changes could be supported to facilitate self-sufficiency. With ongoing sensory stimulation treatment, the life of an elderly individual who suffered the loss can be more worthwhile and meaningful.

Sensory Stimulation

Isler (1975) reported that elderly patients who are disturbed can be rehabilitated, and many can function quite independently if they receive intensive treatment geared toward their needs. For elderly individuals experiencing sensory deprivation, sensory stimulation would be the treatment required.

A study by Bower (1967) showed the influence sensory stimulation had on 25 females. The condition of nearly half of the individuals in the group improved because of sensory stimulation training, while the others remained unchanged. No individuals were reported to have regressed during the training. Bower interpreted a "no change" as slowing down the dementia process.

A sensory stimulation study done by Richman (1969) showed the short-term effects that sensory stimulation had on some individuals with impairments. One individual, who was impaired before the sensory stimulation group, was seen after the groups helping other clients do their joint exercises. Another individual was engaging in a ball activity. These changes were caused by a few sensory stimulation sessions. One other reason for the effectiveness of the sessions was that the clients enjoyed participating in the session and did not find the sessions burdensome to attend. The sessions can be fun as well as stimulating, and they do not force the individual into something s/he does not want to do.

In a case study done by Rogers, Marcus, and Snow (1987), there was a significant change in the client's disposition following the sensory stimulation treatment. Before the treatment, the client was diagnosed with gout, dementia, and possible cancer. The client was also depressed. The client received intensive sensory stimulation treatment four days a week for five weeks. The outcomes were significant to the study. After three weeks of training, the client's hostility turned into open affection for the leader. By the fifth week, she could do all of the activities independently. Before the sensory stimulation treatment, the client was very disoriented to person, time, and place. She was totally dependent on staff for her self-care needs. After the treatment, the client became oriented to person, time, and place. She became self-feeding, cooperative, and had a good attention span. This change in the client was still evident in the one-year follow-up test.

In a sensory stimulation study done by Karney and Paire (1984), there were significant findings regarding the positive effects of sensory stimulation. This study was looking for changes in the reality orientation of the clients. The results, relating to the reality orientation for the individuals in the sensory stimulation group, were seen to be significant for all of the individuals involved in the program.

Norberg, Meli, and Asplund (1986) completed a study focusing on the effects of music, touch, and object presentation on the orientation of individuals in the final stage of dementia. The findings were such that both individuals reacted positively and differently to music than to touch or object presentation. One individual reacted by sitting up with her eyes open. This was a behavior the researchers interpreted as an orientating response. The other individual did not open her eyes while the music was being played. This behavior was interpreted as relaxation. It was the increase in the individuals' respiration rate, direct observation, and videotaped recordings that indicated these responses. A primary conclusion of this study was that clients in the final stages of dementia can be reached by music, through their auditory sense. Another conclusion was that individuals react differently to stimuli that are presented to them. This is important for a therapist to know before they begin a sensory stimulation program.

Smith (1988) completed a case study regarding the effects of sensory stimulation on the activities of daily living (ADL) performance of a 65-year-old woman with diabetes. Due to this woman's illness, she had lost some vision and had limited taste and smelling ability. The individual participated in the sensory stimulation sessions for thirty minutes, three times per week for four weeks. The results were to be based upon the accuracy and speed of the woman buttoning her shirt and completing telephone book tasks. The result indicated that after the completion of the program, the individual's ADL and self-care behaviors had increased in speed and accuracy. The findings of this study were consistent with those of Karney and Paire (1984).

Sensory Stimulation Programming

There are many studies that support the conclusion that regularly implemented sensory stimulation programs improve the functional ability of clients. Eide (1993) conducted a study of a sensory integration program that addressed five senses (1. visual, 2. olfactory, 3. tactile, 4. auditory, and 5. gustatory). Eide's sensory stimulation program provided beneficial outcomes for clients with mid-stage dementia. The program is described below. Therapists wanting to implement a sensory stimulation program may want to start with Eide's program, modifying the program based on client needs.

The therapist will need a variety of materials to implement a sensory stimulation program. Eide

(1993) suggests that equipment needed for the sessions includes a tape recorder or CD player, infection control cleaning supplies, and a cart to take materials from room to room. More specific materials needed for the session are

- *Vision*: a hoop about 8" across, colors on a beach ball, animal pictures, pictures of different types of food, kitchen utensils, a mirror.
- *Olfactory*: perfumes, peppermint extract, coffee, an onion, ammonia, strawberry jam.
- *Tactile*: shaving cream, warm and cold water, massage supplies, hand lotion, a pinecone, macaroni noodles.
- *Auditory*: a timer, a hand held vacuum, sounds of a storm, sounds of a car starting, coins to jingle in a glass, music to move to.
- *Gustatory*: applesauce, dill pickle (or juice), grapes, toothpaste, grapefruit juice, marshmallow.

Precautions need to be taken when choosing materials so averse effects do not occur. For example, foods appropriate for clients with diabetes need to be substituted as necessary.

Frequency is important in sensory stimulation programs. In Eide's program the sensory stimulation sessions were structured to occur during the morning hours four days a week for a minimum of eight weeks. Each session lasted approximately ten minutes. The sessions were conducted on a one-to-one basis in the client's room. Because this sensory stimulation program was based on frequent, intense, sequential building each day, the sensory stimulation activities were repeated throughout the week. The therapist attempted to focus on each client's senses. Repetition of the stimulus was used to reinforce learning and attention among the clients. Association of different stimuli was also encouraged for orientation purposes.

The order of the stimulation to the senses was based on the study done by Karney and Paire (1984). Olfactory was determined to be first, because of its more arousing characteristics. Vision was the next sense stimulated. Then there were touch, hearing, and taste.

Some items were used for stimulating vision, taste, and smell to reinforce learning. For example, first the client identified strawberry extracts with the olfactory sense. Then, the clients identified the strawberry by sight, and lastly, the client tasted strawberry Jell-O. This was done to reinforce the coordination of the senses.

When a therapist starts a program, s/he should use the first week to find a baseline of the client's responses. During this week all five senses are activated each day. Instead of working with the clients during this first week, the therapist presents the stimulus and records the client's response. No teaching takes place during the first week.

During the next six weeks the therapist presents the stimuli to the clients in a teaching/learning format. If the client does not identify an item, the therapist tells the client what it is. The therapist initiates conversation regarding the stimulus and its texture, size, and color. The therapist also tries to help the client reminisce about the item. During these six weeks the order of presenting the stimulus is the same for each client.

On even days of the week, the olfactory and visual senses are stimulated. These sessions start with an activity and intervention that stimulates the olfactory sense. If possible, while stimulating the olfactory sense, the therapist incorporates the activity and intervention to stimulate the visual sense, such as the example of strawberry jam above. Next the therapist begins reminiscing with the client about the jam. The therapist asks the client to look at the jam and identify its color. Before moving on to the next sense, the therapist asks the client to identify the jam by smelling it. By following this procedure the client can coordinate these two senses to identify the stimulus. Adequate response time (as long as the client is attending to the stimulus) is always given to the client after the presentation of each stimulus and intervention. Next, the visual stimulus is presented and the same procedure is followed. Depending on the client's attention span and willingness to participate, sessions are about ten minutes. After the ten minutes are up, the therapist allows about five minutes to record the scores and to move on to the next client's room. The same activities and interventions are followed with all clients following appropriate infection control measures (such as using a different spoon with each client for the jam and making sure that items that are touched by clients are cleaned before being presented to the next client). There is some natural variation to each session as each client's thought processes and reactions are different.

On odd days of the week the tactile, auditory, and gustatory senses are stimulated. The therapist begins by using an activity and intervention to stimulate the tactile sense. The client is instructed to feel the items and identify them. The therapist tells the client what the stimulus is called. At this point the therapist allows the client to look at the item. The therapist initiates a conversation about the item. After the conversation is concluded, the therapist asks the client to identify the stimulus one more time.

The auditory and gustatory senses are also stimulated on odd days of the week. At least one item should be used for each sense. Although the visual and the olfactory senses are not officially stimulated on these days, if possible, the therapist stimulates these senses with the items used to stimulate the tactile, auditory, and gustatory senses. For example, the client tastes a marshmallow and identifies it. (Small marshmallows may reduce the client's chance of choking. Check with the client's speech pathologist or nurse.) Then the therapist asks the client to look at the marshmallow and identify the color. This is done to stimulate the other senses not being addressed that day. This teaching method allows for coordination of the senses in hopes that the senses can be stimulated to work together. The sessions are implemented the same way each week during the teaching period.

No traditional reality orientation materials, such as a reality orientation board, are used during these sensory stimulation sessions. The goal of a sensory stimulation program is to improve client orientation through environmental awareness and not just through rote memorization of the date, time, etc.

Eide (1993) arrived at eight conclusions regarding the effectiveness of the overall functioning of the sensory stimulation program.

1. *The sensory stimulation program was effective.* First and foremost, the sensory stimulation program worked. This research found that the program was most effective with moderately lower functioning clients. For example, this sensory stimulation program is useful with clients who are considerably confused but had some ability to function physically. It is not recommended to use this program with clients who are verbally or physically unresponsive.

2. *No more than one day should pass between sensory stimulation treatments.* This conclusion is based on the observation that client scores were lower at the beginning of the week and higher at the end of the week. (The original research was run daily Monday through Thursday.) For example, many client scores on Monday were much lower than the scores attained on Thursday. The lower Monday scores probably occurred because there was too much time between the last day of the previous program week and the first day of the next week. Eide recommends that there is only one day between sensory stimulation programming, if any.

3. *Personal attention and social interaction helped increase the client's orientation.* The amount of attention and social interaction received by the client may have increased their overall orientation score. The clients were receiving an extra forty minutes of attention per week. It seems that attention alone, from individuals inside or

outside the facility, may encourage growth for clients living in nursing homes. Individuals from outside the nursing home who visit the clients may bring stimuli and memories to the client that s/he has lost touch with since entering the nursing home. Since this daily ten minutes seemed to be important to the clients, agencies should consider various methods for continuing such a service.

4. *Ten minutes was enough time for the therapist to interact socially with the client and present and discuss the stimuli presented and still have measurable change in clients' functional ability.* It was determined that ten minutes of social interaction with a client was adequate time to accomplish both stimulus identification and conversations relating to person, place, and time. Often nursing home personnel feel that each client needs a significant amount of time per day in order to orient the individual. Eide's study demonstrates that an individual needs only about ten minutes of sensory stimulation treatment per day over an extended period of time to help him/her better interact with the environment. There were occasions throughout Eide's study when the ten minutes of times spent with the individual was too much. Certain individual's attention spans and willingness to participate were low. In these cases it is up to the therapist to determine if the client should participate in the full ten minutes of programming.

5. *Common sense and appropriate individualizing is necessary for successful results of a sensory stimulation program.* It is up to the therapist implementing the sensory stimulation program to individualize the process to meet the needs of each client. The process described is a useful guideline yet does not preclude the use of common sense and appropriate individualizing. For example, a client may draw back in fear of the stimulus presented. The therapist should try to demonstrate that the stimulus will not cause harm. Another example is when it is clear that the client is familiar with, and can name, the stimulus presented. Asking the client over and over again for information that s/he has already easily presented may cause the client to feel insulted.

6. *The best time to conduct sensory stimulation programming is in the morning after breakfast.* Throughout Eide's eight-week program there were many factors that affected the responses of clients. One of these factors was the clients' alertness to the program and therapist. When meeting with some of the clients during mid-morning, the clients appeared tired from being

up so early and eating breakfast. This affected the clients' ability to stay awake during the ten-minute session. The inability to stay awake and on task greatly influenced the clients' overall orientation. Although during the research project this occurred most often during mid-morning sessions, the program was still implemented. Many clients living in nursing homes take naps in the afternoon making afternoons a poor option for many clients.

7. *Avoid program interruptions as much as possible.* Another factor influencing the effectiveness of a sensory stimulation program is the occurrence of other programs running while the sensory stimulation sessions were being implemented. Other employees may also interrupt the session. Often nursing assistants enter a client's room to work either with the client or his/her roommate. Sometimes nursing staff interrupt the session to take vital signs. The sensory stimulation program is likely to have greater (more beneficial) impact if it is not interrupted. The therapist may want to hang a sign on the client's door asking staff not to interrupt the session.

8. *When clients are tired, program implementation should be simplified.* At least two or three stimuli are typically presented to a client during each session. There will be times that clients are not alert and fully oriented to the program. When this is the case and two or three stimuli are presented back to back, the client is likely to become even more confused regarding what was presented. For example, during her research Eide presented macaroni noodles to a client. After the noodles were discussed, the sound of a car starting was presented. Being tired and confused, the client stated that the car starting sounded like macaroni noodles. Due to her not being fully alert, she completely confused the stimuli. This type of response is quite common in sensory stimulation programs and may be a sign that the client is actually being overstimulated at that moment. If the therapist feels that a client is not fully alert during any one session only one sense should be addressed.

In addition to demonstrating that regularly implemented sensory stimulation programs can improve a client's measurable functional level, Eide also developed recommendations for therapists who are implementing a sensory stimulation program.

• *Do not expect quick changes*: Frustration felt by staff does not imply that the sensory stimulation program is ineffective. As expected, when dealing with individuals for an extended period of time, many feelings will be reviewed during and after each session with a client. There are times when the therapist will become frustrated with the unresponsiveness of some clients. Some examples of unresponsiveness can be seen in such manners as "selective" hearing or uncooperative and resistive behaviors. Staff working with sensory stimulation programs should try not to be discouraged if the clients are sometimes unresponsive.

- *Sensory stimulation programs are best as a whole team approach*: It is good when all the nursing home staff respect and cooperate with sensory stimulation programming. Employees of a nursing home may not always recognize the benefit of a sensory stimulation program or accommodate the running of the program. Implementing a sensory stimulation program tends to be an intense process and disruptions by other staff can be frustrating. Working with, and getting the support of, the director of nursing services is a critical element in facilitating a successful program.

- *Clients appropriate for sensory stimulation programs tend to have complex, challenging needs, including social needs*: Successful sensory stimulation programs usually involve spending around ten minutes a day with each client in the program. While socialization is part of the sensory stimulation process, socialization is NOT the treatment goal. Many of the clients will desire more time from the therapist than is allotted. Many clients will ask (and even beg) the therapist to stay longer than the ten minutes required for the intervention, making it emotionally difficult for the therapist to move on to the next client. It is possible that some nursing home staff avoid short contact with clients because they find it difficult to leave when a client requests them to stay. This desire on the part of clients demonstrates a clear deprivation within the nursing home structure that is likely to negatively affect client health and well-being. This issue should be addressed but not with the expectation that the sensory stimulation program will be the answer to the problem. See information on the Eden Alternative (in "Behavior Manipulation" in the Techniques section) for more information.

- *Staff should receive training and support*: Since there are so many intense emotional responses that emerge during a sensory stimulation program, it is understandable why nursing home staff may avoid working with clients. The intensity of interactions and frequency of working with clients can contribute to staff members' emotional responses. Nursing homes

(staff and clients) benefit from training staff on how to cope with these feelings. This entails providing staff with the opportunity to process their days and receive emotional support when needed. With such support, clients with greater impairments may, in turn, receive more quality attention from nursing home staff.

Additional note from primary authors: Themed sensory stimulation programs are often implemented for a group of low functioning clients in residential facilities. Such themes may revolve around a particular place (e.g., beach), an activity (e.g., baseball games), a holiday (e.g., Christmas), an event (e.g., graduation), or a season (e.g., autumn). Although Eide's research was conducted only with individuals, sensory stimulation benefits can also be gained through group interventions. Additionally, a modified sensory stimulation program is often used with comatose clients to monitor progression from Rancho Los Amigos level I (coma stage) to Rancho Los Amigos level II (low arousal stage) (see Traumatic Brain Injury). It is unclear if sensory stimulation helps with progression from one stage to another or if it is only useful to monitor level progression. Gustatory stimulation (of course) would be contraindicated (can't feed a comatose client food or drink by mouth), but other senses can be stimulated. For example, auditory (e.g., music), tactile (e.g., washing face, massaging arm), visual (e.g., lights on and off), and olfactory (e.g., flowers, food) senses can be stimulated. Although clients at this stage will not be active participants in the sensory stimulation session as recommended by Eide, a modified sensory stimulation program can still be beneficial.

In the ICF, therapists can score b156 Perceptual Functions to reflect the client's level of difficulty with b1560 Auditory Perception, b1561 Visual Perception, b1562 Olfactory Perception, b1563 Gustatory Perception, and b1564 Tactile Perception. In discipline-specific documentation, therapists commonly document the amount of sensory stimuli identified correctly (e.g., able to identify 50% of auditory stimuli), ability to distinguish between or among stimuli (e.g., able to distinguish between two similar light tactile sensory stimulations independently), behaviors exhibited during the session (e.g., exhibited anxious behavior when challenged to identify visual stimuli), level of participation (e.g., required moderate verbal cues to participate in 10-minute sensory stimulation session), and ability to connect sensory stimuli to past events (e.g., able to reminiscence about past experiences related to sensory stimulation task with minimal cues).

References

Atkinson, L. (1985). *Fundamentals of nursing: A nursing process approach.* New York: Macmillan.

Bower, H. (1967). Sensory stimulation and the treatment of senile dementia. *The Medical Journal of Australia, 22*:1114-1119.

Eide, L. (1993). The design, implementation, and evaluation of a sensory stimulation program for elderly individuals in a nursing home. Masters Thesis.

Isler, C. (1975, June). Who says senile geriatric patients are untreatable? *RN Magazine.* 39-50.

Karney, R., & Paire, J. (1984). The effectiveness of sensory stimulation for geropyschiatric inpatients. *The American Journal of Occupational Therapy, 38*:505-509.

Kelly, J. (1990). Stroke rehabilitation for elderly patients. In *Geriatric rehabilitation.* (Kemp. B., Brummel-Smith, K. & Ramsdell, J. (Eds). Boston, MA: College-Hill Publication.

Kemp, B. (1984). *Fundamentals of nursing: A framework for practice.* Boston: MA: Little, Brown, and Company.

Kopac, C. (1983). Sensory loss in the aged: The role of the nurse and the family. *Nursing Clinics of North America, 18*:373-383.

Norberg, A., Melin, E., & Asplund, K. (1986). Reactions to music, touch, and object presentation in the final stages of dementia: An exploratory study.

International Journal of Nursing Studies. 23(4):315-323.

Okrey, C. (1986). [A sensory stimulation program]. Unpublished raw data.

Oster, C. (1976). Sensory deprivation in geriatric patients. *Journal of the American Geriatrics Society, 24*:461-463.

Parent, L. (1978). Effects of a low stimulus environment on behavior. *The American Journal of Occupational Therapy, 32*:19-25.

Richman, L. (1969). Sensory training for geriatrics patients. *The American Journal of Occupational Therapy, 23*:254-257.

Rogers, J., Marcus, C. & Snow, T. (1987). Maude: A case study of sensory deprivation. *The American Journal of Occupational Therapy, 41*:673-676.

Siebens, H. (1990). Deconditioning. In *Geriatric rehabilitation.* (Kemp. B., Brummel-Smith, K. & Ramsdell, J. (Eds). Boston, MA: College-Hill Publication.

Smith, C. (1988). Sensory stimulation and ADL performance: A case study approach. *The American Journal of Occupational Therapy, 23*:43-57.

Smith, J. (1978, August). Sensory deprivation: A primary concept of nursing. *Nursing Mirror.* p. 7.

Zegeer, L. (1986). The effects of sensory changes in older persons. *The Journal of Neuroscience Nursing, 18*:325-332.

Skin Breakdown

When a client stays in one body position for a prolonged period of time, increased pressure occurs on the skin that covers boney processes (areas that have little fat and muscle over boney prominences such as the buttocks, elbows, and heels). When pressure over a boney process is not relieved, blood circulation to the skin and its underlying body tissue is compromised. The circulation is cut off due to the pressure. Without a supply of fresh, oxygenated blood to the skin and underlying tissues, the cells become damaged and the skin begins to break down and die. Decubitus ulcers occur from the inside out. The increased pressure begins with the tissue pressing against the boney process. Cells at the innermost area begin to break down, eventually reaching the outside surface of the skin if the pressure is not relieved. The result is a hole in the skin (called a decubitus ulcer). The depth and size of the ulcer will vary depending on the length of time that the pressure continues and other reasons, including other trauma that has occurred, shear injuries, fever, amount of moisture, and infection. The longer the breakdown goes untreated, the worse it gets. Sometimes the damage goes clear to the bone as shown in Figure 6.

Other terms for skin breakdowns are decubitus ulcers, pressure sores, pressure ulcers, and bedsores.

Risk Factors

Clients who are unable to change body positions (e.g., a client with mobility restrictions) or who are unaware that body position needs to be changed (e.g., a client with a complete spinal cord injury) are at an increased risk for developing skin breakdown. Other risk factors include mental awareness, continence, mobility, activity, nutrition (including hydration), circulation, temperature, and medications (Shannon, 1984).

Affected Areas

The specific areas affected will depend on the body position that the client has been in for a prolonged period of time. For example, a client who has been in a sitting position for a long period of time is at an increased risk of developing decubitus ulcers on the shoulder blades (leaning against back of chair), spine (leaning against back of chair), hips (pressing against side of chair), buttocks (from sitting), back of the upper arm and lower arm (leaning against back of chair and leaning on armrests), hand, wrist, elbow (all from leaning on armrests), and feet (especially the heels and toes from

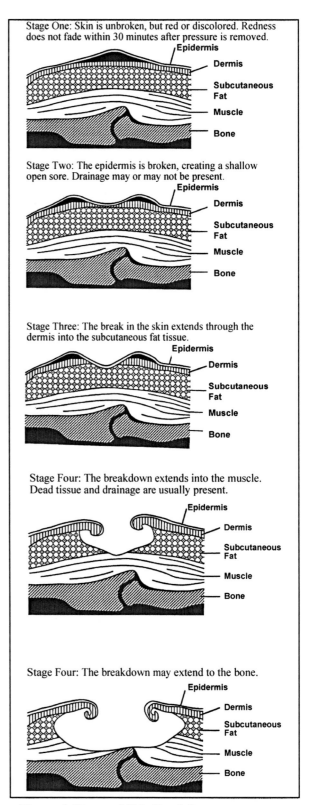

Figure 6: Stages of Skin Breakdown

leaning against wheelchair foot pedals). For a client who has been in a supine position for a prolonged period of time, decubitus ulcers are most likely to appear on the back of the head, shoulder blades, hip bones, elbows, spine, between the knees (especially when lying on the side), the hip, and anywhere the leg touches the bed (especially the heels). Devices such as casts, splints, braces, and prostheses can also cause skin breakdowns. Decubitus ulcers might also be seen in uncommon areas due to engagement in particular activities. For example, it is not uncommon for clients who have complete paraplegia from a spinal cord injury to pick up and rest the heel of one foot on the opposite knee to change their appearance. They may also carry heavy items on their lap for prolonged periods of time in order to use both hands to propel the wheelchair. In both of these situations, decubitus ulcers could occur on the top of the knees.

Treatment

Initial treatment is to relieve the pressure on the area by repositioning the body. For a client who is unable to move, the medical team is responsible for the repositioning. If this is not possible (e.g., client is restricted from moving), other methods to relieve pressure are sought (e.g., special mattress, automatic tilt beds). Antibiotic medications are prescribed to decrease risks of (or treat) infection from the open wound. If the wound continues to enlarge and the body is healing, surgery may be necessary. The procedure is called a skin flap. A piece of healthy skin that is adjacent to the ulcer is cut into a "V" shape. The top of the "V" is then pulled over the ulcer and sewn down. The hope is that the donor skin will knit together and help the ulcer to heal. Treatment for severe skin breakdowns is very difficult, often requiring six weeks of inpatient care after a surgery, so the medical team puts a large emphasis on prevention.

Prevention

Prevention of skin breakdowns involves some issues of general skin care and proper positioning (Armstrong & Lauzen, 1994).

General Skin Care

- Preventing long periods of pressure on any area of the skin, especially bony areas.
- Good nutrition from a daily diet that includes whole grain breads and cereals, meats, poultry, fish, milk products, fruits, and vegetables to promote healthy skin.
- Proper body weight for body build.

- Bathing to remove dirt, bacteria, and dead skin cells. Washing increases circulation, which increases the nutrition and oxygen supply to the skin. Be sure to remove all soap to avoid drying the skin.
- Use lotions and bath oil for especially dry skin.
- Keep toenails trimmed straight. Ingrown toenails cause irritation that can increase muscle spasms and the risk of infection.

Positioning

- Use as many different positions as possible; abdomen, back, sides, and sitting, standing if possible (use braces or standing table if needed).
- After each change of position, check for redness over bony areas.
- Skin tolerance in bed: The patient will usually start out with two-hour turns on both sides and on his/her back. Turn times are usually increased at 30 minute intervals as his/her skin tolerates the added time to a maximum of four hours per side or up to eight hours prone (on his/her abdomen).
- Allow a rest period of at least 60 minutes before resuming the same position. Only resume the same position for the same length of time if the patient's skin faded to normal color within 15 minutes.

Recreational Therapy Role

1. Recreational therapists promote an active and healthy lifestyle. Increased physical activity decreases a client's risk of developing skin breakdowns.
2. Clients are educated about skin breakdowns including graphic pictures of skin breakdowns, which can be very motivating.
3. Clients who are in a seated position for long periods of time and lack the sensation to recognize the need for body position change (especially those with a spinal cord injury), are taught how to perform weight shifts every 20-30 minutes. This relieves pressure from boney areas and allows fresh, oxygenated blood to reach and nourish the area. Weight shifts can be very difficult for clients to remember to do, especially when engaged in life activities. A watch that is set to beep every 30 minutes can be a helpful external reminder. The initiation and correct performance of weight shifts during activity is a common recreational therapy objective when working with clients who have a spinal cord injury (e.g., "Perform effective weight shifts every 30 minutes during activity in clinic without prompting"). The type of weight shifts

performed by the client will vary depending on the abilities and limitations of the client.

a. *Push up*: Lock the brakes if sitting in a wheelchair. Place both hands on the armrests. Push up with the arms so that the elbows are extended and the buttocks are lifted off the chair seat. Hold for 30 seconds.

b. *Side lean*: Sit upright in the chair. Hang one arm over the side of the chair and reach toward the floor until the opposite buttock is lifted off the chair. Hold for 30 seconds.

c. *Forward lean*: Lock brakes if sitting in a wheelchair. Lean forward (chest to knees) until back of buttocks is lifted off the chair. Hold for 30 seconds.

d. *Tilt*: This can be performed in three ways. For the client who is using a manual wheelchair and can independently perform a wheelie, a wheelie position is initiated and maintained for 30 seconds. For the client who has a manual wheelchair and is unable to independently perform a wheelie, another person tips the wheelchair backwards and maintains the balance point position for 30 seconds. For the client who is using a tilt-n-space power wheelchair, the client presses a button (or moves the joystick or performs a sip-n-puff sequence) so that the wheelchair moves into a tilt position. The position is held for at least 30 seconds.

4. Therapists teach clients how to evaluate the impact of activities on the development of skin breakdowns and problem solve on how to reduce their risks. This is commonly conducted with clients who have a spinal cord injury. For example, the therapist assists the client in problem solving for foreseen situations that could cause or contribute to the formation of skin breakdowns. For example, the therapist is working with a college student who has complete paraplegia from a spinal cord injury and desires to go back to school. The therapist foresees that the client will throw her heavy book bag on her lap so that she will have both hands free to propel the wheelchair. She also does her own grocery shopping and plans to place a handheld grocery basket on her lap and fill it with heavy items so that she has her hands free to propel the wheelchair. The therapist helps her to problem solve for these situations and identify alternative methods to decrease her risks of skin breakdowns. For example, the therapist could recommend the use of a backpack that hooks onto the wheelchair push handles and teach the client how to propel her wheelchair with one hand while pushing a grocery cart with the other hand.

5. Therapists, along with other clinical team members, remind clients to perform regular skin checks with a long handled mirror (so the clients can see all body areas) every day to increase awareness of beginning signs of skin breakdown. They are also reminded to keep their skin dry at all times. Moisture increases the fragility of the skin, quickening skin breakdown. If skin breakdown is treated during the beginning stages through the removal of pressure, the body can begin to heal. If the skin breakdown is allowed to continue, the client's health, level of independence, and functioning in life tasks can be severely affected.

References

Armstrong, M. & Lauzen, S. (1994). *Community integration program, 2nd ed.* Ravensdale, WA: Idyll Arbor.

Shannon, M. L. (1984). Five famous fallacies about pressure sores. *Nursing 84*(14):34-41.

Social Skills Training

There is a major thrust toward normalization of clients with disabilities to enable them to function within the mainstream of society. Social skills are essential to development, normalization, and independent adult functioning in the community. Social interaction skills, appropriate social behaviors, and adaptive social skills are all needed to enable acceptance as a member of the group, to make friends, and to participate in the mainstream of society.

Reduction of the present social isolation and maladaptive social behavior is not likely to occur without specific social skills training. There is increasing evidence that many clients with cognitive impairments will not develop social skills solely through the provision of opportunities to interact. Likewise, placing them in an integrated setting does not necessarily produce social interaction unless the social skills to interact according to society standards are present. Integration becomes meaningful only when it involves social interaction and acceptance within the social value system.

Many programs purport to develop social skills but lack a systematic approach to skill development. They frequently assume that grouping people together will result in social development and, therefore, do not actively facilitate this process. Specific intervention is generally programmed only for individuals that manifest negative social interactions or inappropriate social behaviors consistently. Although an individual's overall pattern of social interaction may appear adequate, deficits in special interaction skills or maladaptive social behaviors are likely to develop without intervention. The learning and internalizing of appropriate social patterns and values must be fostered over time to ensure community integration. The Competency-Deviancy Model (Gold, 1980) states that the more competencies a person has, the more deviancies are tolerated. Therefore, it is important to enable clients with cognitive impairments to obtain at least normative, if not super-normative, social interactive patterns and appropriate social behaviors. Socially integrated community involvement is only possible with these skills.

The approach to social skill training in this topic contains specific program strategies, assessment techniques, skills to be taught, and training activities.

The approach utilizes three interrelated techniques: behavior modification, didactic instruction with discussion, and experiential exercises. The need for a multifaceted approach is well documented. An individual with social interaction skills is more likely to become socially integrated; however, barriers may still exist because of a lack of other appropriate social behavior and lack of the ability to adapt to the demands of various social situations. Some individuals exhibit problem behaviors that interfere with socialization, but can be extinguished or managed by behavior modification techniques. Others exhibit inappropriate social behavior (e.g., blowing nose on sleeve, wearing work clothes to a dance) that results from a lack of knowledge about the appropriate behavior and can be corrected through instruction and external cues. Other clients may need intense practice in these skills so that behaviors become well established. A program that intervenes in both social interactive skills and social behaviors is most effective in preparing clients with cognitive impairments for social integration and fulfilling interpersonal relationships. Through the use of these three methodologies the client learns about appropriate social behaviors, is shown examples of such behaviors, is given opportunities to practice, is provided with systematic reinforcement, and is encouraged in a variety of ways to use these skills in the community.

The therapist is cautioned that this is not intended to be a specific set of protocols to be followed but rather an example of how social interaction skills and social behaviors can be taught. The importance of designing programs to meet individual needs in a systematic manner is stressed. Without this intervention, the social problems of clients with cognitive impairments can result in increased dependency, social isolation, and a lowered overall quality of life.

Three-Pronged Approach

Developmentally, social skills evolve slowly over time. Clients with cognitive impairments who lack these skills need systematic intervention. One of the biggest problems with social skills development programs is that behaviors that are developed and reinforced in one setting may not generalize or be reinforced in the individual's other settings (Walker, 1980). A truly effective approach must demonstrate social skills beyond the training setting and must prove to be enduring in the client's real-life situation. A combination of intervention procedures are

This section is written by Phyllis Coyne and is an updated version of her *Social Skills Training: A Three-Pronged Approach* originally published in 1980 and funded by a grant from the Developmental Disabilities Office, Region X, Grant No. 50-P-50368.

required to develop enduring social interaction skills and appropriate social behaviors.

The three-pronged intervention model for social skills development has been shown to be a particularly effective approach. This approach utilizes the interrelated techniques of behavior modification, instruction with discussion, and social practice through experiential exercises. In preparing for the program the therapist creates a series of Power Point slides or laminated pictures depicting individuals engaged in appropriate and inappropriate behaviors followed by discussion of the behavior. These slides should show people who are similar in age and cultural background to the client mix. Social interaction skills (e.g., introducing self) are modeled. The client is given considerable opportunity and encouragement to rehearse or practice the desired behaviors through role-playing, group exercises, and specific recreation activities. Positive feedback, approval, or praise is offered as the behaviors become more and more similar to those modeled and desired. Finally, the client is exposed to real-life situations that are designed to increase the likelihood that the newly learned behaviors will be applied consistently outside of the treatment situation.

Three particularly effective methods for social skill training: behavior modification, instruction with discussion, and experiential exercises are examined in detail in the following sections. The nature of each and techniques that maximize their impact are presented. Although described individually, it is the combination of these methods that increases the success of this approach.

Behavior Modification

Behavior modification techniques are a commonly applied method for changing behavior. Most individuals who work with clients with cognitive impairments are cognizant of these techniques. This section will provide a quick overview of the behavior modification techniques used in the Three-Pronged Approach. (See Behavior Modification in the Technique "Behavior Manipulation" for related information.)

Positive reinforcement is the primary means of performance feedback used for social skill development. Three types of reinforcement are used: 1. material reinforcement, such as food or money; 2. social reinforcement, such as praise or approval from others; and 3. self-reinforcement, which is a person's positive evaluation of his/her own behavior.

Social reinforcement is emphasized in this model because such reinforcement has been shown to be particularly potent in affecting behavior change. This type of reinforcement gives informative feedback and

also creates a positive feeling or affective feedback. It can be delivered without disrupting the behavior. In addition, attention, verbal praise, and physical gestures of approval are natural types of reinforcers. For instance, in real-life settings, helping a friend elicits "thanks" or approval. To be successful, social reinforcement needs to be genuine and expressive, not mater-of-fact.

Effective social skill training must attend to other reinforcers, because social reinforces alone do not always cause behavior change. For many, material reinforcement is a necessary base without which social reinforcement may be meaningless. In these cases, material reinforces are paired with social reinforcers and eventually eliminated. Clients also need to be assisted to become their own reinforcement suppliers, that is, they need to move from extrinsic to intrinsic motivation because many appropriate social behaviors and interactions go unnoticed, uncommented upon, and unappreciated by others. Clients who can evaluate and reward their own behaviors will be more likely to retain these behaviors in real-life settings. Thus, attention should be given to all three types of reinforcement.

In determining reinforcing events, it is important to be specific. Each person may respond differently to the three types of reinforcement outlined above. Certain types of reinforcers, such as approval, food, affection, and money have a high likelihood of being effective reinforcers, but are not rewarding to everyone. The individual's needs and past reinforcement history will affect the potency of intended reinforcers. It is vital to respond to current needs and past reinforcement histories to optimally influence motivation conditions in a behavior program.

A number of variables must be considered to maximize reinforcers. Several characteristics that enhance the effectiveness of reinforcers and permanence of the behavior include (Goldstein, et al, 1980):

- *Timing*: Behavior change occurs most effectively when the reinforcement follows immediately after the desired behavior.

- *Response contingency*: The contingent relationship or linkage between performance and reinforcement must be reflected in teaching and intervention procedures and made sufficiently clear to the client.

- *Partial (intermittent) reinforcement*: Behaviors that are intermittently reinforced (at fixed times, such as the end of each session; at a fixed number of responses, such as every fifth correct response) are more effective.

- *Amount of reinforcement*: With certain exceptions, the greater the amount of reinforcement, the greater the positive effect upon performance. (Excessive reinforcement, particularly of primary reinforcers such as food or liquid, can result in satiation — a dramatically reduced result or an ignoring of the stimulation because so much is received.)

- *Opportunity for reinforcement*: Behavior to be reinforced must occur with sufficient frequency that reinforcement can be provided. (Role-playing and other experiential activities provide an excellent opportunity to reinforce behavior.)

In programs with clients with cognitive impairments there are always some individuals who will not cooperate or manifest disruptive behaviors such as temper tantrums, violent anger outbursts, or bizarre forms of stereotypical behaviors (behaviors that remain the same even though they do not work in the current environment). During the pilot program of the model for this social skill development program, approximately 20% of the clients needed individualized behavior prescriptions. The following procedures were commonly utilized in the design and implementation of these programs:

- Identify and eliminate the causes of disruptive behavior.
- Withdraw social reinforcement for undesirable behavior by ignoring completely. (Not used with self-destructive or aggressive behaviors.)
- Interrupt the chain of events that lead to the situation so that the undesirable behavior does not occur.
- Condition an incompatible response or involve the client in an activity that competes with or does not allow the undesirable behavior to occur.
- Give a time out in a designated area for five to ten minutes.

Instruction with Discussion

Often clients with cognitive impairments do not acquire social skills because of a lack of opportunity to participate in social activities. Others have deficits in this area because they lack the abstract processes to learn by observing everyday social interactions. Therefore, concrete information is needed to help individuals understand basic concepts related to social behaviors and interactions. The instruction and discussion component of the training model for social skill development facilitates comprehension of the appropriateness of behaviors.

Basic social concepts must be presented in concrete behavioral terms before many clients with cognitive impairments can acquire appropriate behaviors. Therefore, the emphasis in the didactic approach is to develop a framework for social

behaviors through the presentation of basic concepts. Some individuals with limited cognitive functioning need individualized programs before they can begin to comprehend basic concepts and develop appropriate behaviors. Such prescriptive individualized programs consist of a behavioral objective, sequenced steps that are used to teach the objective specified, and ways to measure whether the objective has been reached.

To see how instruction with discussion can be used we will look at one of the most important of the basic interpersonal interaction skills: making friends or even recognizing who is a friend. Many clients with cognitive impairments will consider anyone who smiles or says "Hi" a friend. Others consider that their teachers, family members, bosses, or activity center/group home providers are their only friends. Therefore, teaching the concepts of family, friends, helpers, and strangers is important for establishing a basis for developing friendships. For teaching purposes, helpers are defined as people who develop a helping or serving relationship with the individual, such as a teacher, bus driver, police officer, group home provider, or a clerk in a store. Friends are generally peers and not family members, helpers, or strangers.

One method of teaching these concepts is to develop a picture packet for each client. Each packet is comprised of photographs of the client's family members, friends, helpers, and some photographs of people s/he does not know. Clients should be able to correctly identify the category of each photograph in one of these ways:

- By pointing to an appropriate photograph when asked to "Point to a family member, (or) friend, (or) helper, (or) stranger."
- By placing a picture under the appropriate label.
- By verbalizing who is a friend, family member, helper, or stranger. Other methods are discussed later in this section.

Another teaching method that is included in instruction with discussion is modeling or learning by imitation. The therapist models a certain set of behaviors allowing the clients to observe how they might appropriately handle a specific situation.

According to Goldstein et al (1980), certain circumstances significantly affect the degree to which learning by imitation occurs. These "modeling enhancers" include desirable characteristics of the model, the modeling display, and the client's perception of the value of following the behavior. More effective modeling will occur when the model:

- seems to be highly skilled or expert
- is of high status
- controls rewards desired by client

- is of the same sex, approximate age, and social status as the client
- is friendly and helpful
- is rewarded for the given behaviors.

More effective modeling will occur when the display shows the behaviors to be imitated:
- in a clear and detailed manner
- in the order from least to most difficult behaviors
- with enough repetition to make overlearning likely
- with as little irrelevant detail as possible
- with several different models, rather than a single model.

More effective modeling will occur when the person observing the model is:
- told to imitate the model
- similar to the model in background or in attitude toward skill
- friendly toward or likes the model
- rewarded for performing the modeled behavior.

Because of some of the above considerations, sometimes peer volunteers and siblings are useful as models in the program. Although Hutchison and Lord (1979) and others report that one of the most effective integration strategies is utilization of non-disabled as role models and tutors, a potential problem is that the non-disabled tend to socially interact with able peers and only interact with clients in the helping role. It is, therefore, important to provide orientation, training, and supervision to non-disabled peers that are used as models.

Experiential Exercises

According to Goldstein et al (1980), modeling alone is not sufficient for long-term change of behavior. Even though research has demonstrated the effectiveness of modeling, the positive effects are often short-lived. A number of other techniques must be used concurrently to maximize the potential for transfer to the community. As a tool for enhancing old behaviors as well as teaching new behaviors, modeling has been found to be most effective when the clients are given opportunities to rehearse what they have seen, are provided with systematic feedback, and are encouraged in a variety of ways to utilize their new skill in real-life situations. Modeling teaches the clients what to do, but they also need to practice how to do it and must understand why one should behave in a certain way through experiential exercises such as role-playing.

A large number of clients with cognitive impairments, when put in a social situation, do not interact on their own or interact inappropriately. Role-play enables clients who have not yet developed appropriate social skills to do so in a structured situation by practicing the modeled behavior under supervisions. Kempton (1975, Kempton & Kahn, 1991) points out many benefits of role-playing. Among them:
- It helps teach self-control.
- It promotes a better self-image because the client has an opportunity to be successful and receive social reinforcement for his/her performance.
- It allows opportunities for interaction with others.
- It helps to distinguish between reality and unreality.
- It is an effective tool for teaching responsibility.
- It can be used to reinforce socially acceptable behavior and to explore consequences of irresponsible and inappropriate behavior.

Role-playing is most effective when it is presented in a simple, concrete manner in the order from least to most difficult behaviors. Irrelevant detail should be minimized and repetition maximized to make overlearning likely. To insure success, role-playing should begin with very simple situations, such as one person introducing himself/herself to another person or one person paying a compliment to another person and that person responding by saying, "thank you." Each situation should be repeated until it is grasped by the client.

In the introduction to role-playing it is important to discuss what it means to pretend or to act the part of someone else and to make sure everyone understands the role-play situation and the part s/he is playing. The therapist should describe the role-play situation step by step and then check with the clients to make sure they understand who they are playing and what is supposed to happen in the scene. Props or costumes may be useful to make the role-playing situation more real and concrete. Concreteness is particularly important for clients with cognitive impairments.

Goldstein et al (1980) pointed out that these social interaction skills will occur and be lasting only if certain conditions or "role-playing enhancers" are met. Some of these are
- Choice on the part of the client regarding whether to take part in the role-playing.
- Reward, approval, or reinforcement for enacting the role-playing behaviors.

The opportunity to role-play and get attention or social approval from the group is often sufficient reinforcement for clients with less cognitive impairment while clients with greater impairment may need additional rewards.

Initially the situation should involve no more than two actors. First the therapist should model the situation demonstrating an appropriate social skill, such as introducing oneself to someone not known previously. Then a client should imitate the behavior with the therapist or another staff. Appropriate levels of support should be given to insure that the behavior is appropriate. The assistance may be in the form of:

- *Physical prompts*: Manually guiding the hand into a handshake or the head into a position so that eye contact is maintained when culturally appropriate.
- *Specific instructions or verbal prompts*: Verbally telling the client what s/he should be doing as s/he does the role-playing. The prompt giver should be different from the person to whom the client is introducing himself/herself.
- *Fading*: The gradual removal of physical or verbal guidance as in slowly removing the hand from the head when trying to establish good eye contact until the prompt giver is only pointing at the eyes or giving no prompt at all.
- *Doubling*: A double (another person) is used for clients with limited verbal skill. The extra person stands next to the client and speaks for him or her.
- *Reinforcement*: Physical gestures of approval or verbal praise should be provided contingent on successful approximations of the behavior.

For example, in order to teach an individual to have good eye contact when meeting and greeting someone, the therapist may have to manually guide the head into a position so that eye contact is maintained. A verbal cue (e.g., "look him in the eye") and praise may also be necessary for successful approximations of the behavior. As the individuals begin to maintain eye contact when shaking hands with someone, the therapist gradually lessens the physical contact to just barely touching the chin and then to pointing at the eyes. This is often combined with verbal instruction. Reinforcement should be awarded immediately, particularly when working with individuals who do not imitate readily.

After the client role-plays with a therapist, a more socially appropriate peer model can be used as the partner, with the therapist providing supervision. The following step would be for two clients to role-play the same situation. A step further would be to move the whole role-play situation into a real-life setting in the community to see if the clients can generalize from a structured environment to an unstructured one. To generalize the new skill to a real-life environment, it is helpful to have family members, caregivers, or others who live and work with the client to also model and reinforce the desired behavior. As the client exhibits the new behaviors, using the term "appropriate" is additionally reinforcing. Role-playing is particularly effective for certain goals, some of which are

- To increase interactive behavior skills.
- To increase interpersonal communication skills.
- To increase appropriate social behaviors.
- To decrease vulnerability to community risks.

Some examples of role-playing situations that can be used to meet the above objectives are

- Introducing oneself to someone else.
- Introducing two people to each other.
- Introducing someone to a group of people.
- Asking a friend to do something with you by telephone or in person.
- Asking someone on a date by telephone or in person.
- Asking someone to dance.
- Complimenting someone and s/he responds by saying "Thank you."
- Asking for the time at a bus stop.
- Asking for the location of a restroom.
- Asking for help when lost.
- Reacting appropriately when approached by a stranger on the street who says, "Would you like to come to my house?" and smiles.
- Reacting appropriately when a stranger says, "Hi, my name is Bill/Sue. I'll buy you something to eat."
- Additional role-playing situations can be found in the "Interpersonal Relationship Activities" in the Techniques Section.

Of the four goals listed above, the most difficult to meet is to decrease vulnerability to community risks. One of the words that most individuals have a hard time saying is the word "no." Individuals want people to be their friends and the concept of stranger is difficult to understand. A method of representing the concept of stranger is defining stranger as someone whose name is not known by the client and defining friend as someone whose name you have known for a long time. In a role-playing situation dealing with a stranger, it is important to reinforce that the client understands the meaning of pretending. Utilizing a real stranger is best whenever possible; however, in many cases one therapist will have to pretend to be a stranger. Costumes and props could be helpful in making the situation more real and believable. If a client responds inappropriately to an approach by a stranger, it is important that s/he repeat the role-playing situation until the appropriate response (e.g., ignoring the stranger) is demonstrated.

The following step, and a way to assess how well the behavior generalizes, is to arrange to have a person not known to the client approach the client in a real-life setting, such as a social gathering, and invite the client to leave with him/her.

If the clients are to gain insight from a role-playing situation, each scene must be discussed and evaluated. Therapist can demonstrate both appropriate and inappropriate behaviors to handle situations. The group can make decisions about the behaviors and discuss how the characters might be feeling in order to help the clients become more aware of their own and others' feelings. The behavior that the therapists role-play should relate to a behavior that one wishes to facilitate or inhibit in a client. Only therapists should act out inappropriate behaviors because role-playing a certain behavior reinforces that behavior.

Role-playing situations can become quite complex with clients who have less cognitive impairment. Discussing the situation provides clients with insights that can help clarify their values and provide them with an ability to make choices that lead to alternative ways of handling situations and to more responsible behavior. Some suggestions for role-play situations for clients with less cognitive impairment include:

- A man approaches a woman at a dance, asks her to dance, and then asks her to step outside and take a walk with him.
- On a first date, the boy wants to hold hands all the time and the girl feels uncomfortable about it.
- A girl is going steady and a male friend of hers asks her out on a date.
- A girl keeps approaching boys she doesn't know very well and calls them her "boyfriends."

Each of these situations should be role-played first by therapists and then enacted by a combination of therapists and clients with therapist supervision to make sure that the situation does not get out of hand. Discussion should concern various ways of handling each situation. The responsibility and feelings of the actors should be considered.

Interpersonal Relationship Skills

This section describes areas where the three-pronged approach may be used to develop interpersonal relationship skills that will enable the client to function in a manner that fits into the community's social system. It provides interventions in social interaction skills and appropriate social behaviors that have been identified as necessary for successful functioning in the community (including school and work settings). The social skills fall broadly into three categories: 1. interactive behavior skills, which are primarily non-verbal, 2. interpersonal communication skills, which require verbal interactions and 3. appropriate social behaviors, which are related to social norms. The order in which the skills are listed under each category reflect, as much as possible, a progression.

Interactive Behavior Skills

The client will:
- Independently engage in activities next to others.
- Share recreation equipment and take turns.
- Wait his/her turn whenever necessary.
- Engage in cooperative activities with others.
- Actively participate in competitive games.
- Work as a member of a group to accomplish tasks.
- Play as a member of a competitive team.
- Give assistance to others who may need or want it.
- Maintain eye contact during conservations.
- Participate in activities using pubic facilities, such as bowling, inline skating, and dances, as a member of a group.
- Participate in clubs, classes, and events sponsored by community groups such as scouts, 4-H, and garden clubs.

Interpersonal Communication Skills

The client will:
- Introduce himself/herself to others.
- Accurately name others in the group.
- Initiate interaction and activities with others.
- Introduce other people to one another.
- Start a conversation with appropriate social amenities.
- Compliment others on something about them or their activities.
- Express affection for those s/he cares about.
- Listen when someone is talking and try to understand what is being said.
- Talk to others about things of interest to both of them.
- Appropriately negotiate entry into an ongoing group or activity.
- Appropriately ask someone for a date by telephone or in person.
- Appropriately accept or reject social invitations by strangers and friends.
- Appropriately ignore an inappropriate approach by a stranger.
- Visit friends and relatives.
- Respond to teasing, rejection, and/or criticism without loss of control or aggression.
- Express negative feelings in a rational manner.

- Compromise when necessary, or otherwise deal with interpersonal conflict.
- Deal with losing with sportsmanship.
- Make effective decisions after considering possibilities.

Appropriate Social Behavior

The client will:
- Follow instructions and adhere to rules.
- Locate appropriate public restroom (male or female).
- Treat equipment appropriately and respectfully.
- Store equipment in assigned places.
- Dress appropriately for the activities and weather.
- Demonstrate situationally appropriate behaviors.
- Make situationally appropriate physical contact.
- Identify public and private places (living room vs. bedroom).
- Identify appropriate behaviors in public and private places (masturbation in bedroom).
- Identify inappropriate behaviors (hitchhiking, looking in windows).

Behavioral Goals

Since clients vary greatly in functional levels and abilities, the skills have been written in general terms. Therapists interested in fostering appropriate social behaviors and social interaction skills in clients with cognitive impairments must first decide where to begin with a client based on the list of social skills in the preceding section. Many social interactions require skills from all three categories. For instance, introducing himself/herself (interpersonal communication) also requires maintaining eye contact (interactive behavior) and, sometimes, physical contact by shaking hands (appropriate social behavior). The therapist must determine intervention strategies as well as short-term and long-term goals and objectives. Clients with greater cognitive impairment may need instruction in each of these skills before combining them, while some clients will already have one or more of these skills. It is important to have basic mastery of one skill before progressing to the next skill. It may take six weeks or more for some clients to learn to introduce another person.

Satisfactory performance can be measured when behavioral goals and objectives are established. The behavioral objectives should contain the kind of behavior that shows the objective has been met (terminal behavior), conditions under which the behavior is expected (conditions), and levels of acceptable performance (criteria). The following behavioral objective for maintaining eye contact was appropriate for Pat (a 19-year-old female client who has been diagnosed as having an IQ of 65 described in the "Social Skills Development" part of the Concepts section): "While introducing herself in a role-play situation, Pat will keep her head up and look directly at the face of the therapist four consecutive times." The criteria, condition, or behavior can represent various levels of mastery. For instance, "Pat will initiate asking someone to do something with her in four consecutive social lounge periods" is more difficult than, "Pat will appropriately ask someone to do something with her in four consecutive role-play situation." In the first example Pat is required to do something in an unstructured situation, while in the second, she is required to perform in a structured situation. The final goal would be for Pat to demonstrate this behavior independently in the community.

When determining the behavioral objective and intervention activities, it is important to carefully consider the essential characteristics of an activity, what skills are needed to participate, its potential benefits to clients, and modifications that might be necessary for clients to participate. Some social demands of an activity that should be examined are 1. the interaction pattern, 2. the number of clients, 3. the role of the clients, 4. the type of interaction (verbal or non-verbal), and 5. the level of sociability required. In addition, demands in the physical and cognitive domains must also be identified.

Program Organization

The organization of the intervention model will be explained in detail in this section. Selection and grouping of clients, skills of therapists, organization of session, and settings are presented.

Selection and Groupings of Clients

Each intervention group should consist of clients who are clearly deficient in the social skills to be taught. Homogenous groupings by functional ability and age, such as adolescents with head injuries functioning at the Rancho Los Amigos levels of V and VI, allow for some tailoring of the instructional methods to the shared characteristics of the group. The variance of abilities within such homogenous groups will also allow for the use of peers as role models and helpers. Since practice in as realistic a situation as possible is most beneficial, it is often useful to include clients of both sexes who have similar social worlds.

The optimal size of groups for effective social skills training varies from six to twelve, plus two therapists (or one therapist plus another staff person or well-trained volunteer to assist the therapist). In cases where it is necessary to apply the intervention techniques in a larger group, e.g., regular-sized school class, it is desirable to conduct role-playing and other experiential exercises in smaller groups. When there are two therapists, a teacher aide, student intern, or other adult who has been oriented to the procedures, the large group can be divided into appropriate sub-groups. Thus, the whole class would meet as a unit for the instruction and discussion and then break into smaller groups for experiential exercise.

Staffing

Because therapists must both lead and observe activities, a team of two therapists is the most effective way to facilitate sessions. Whenever possible there should be one male and one female trainer. One trainer can assist a client to enact the social skill, while the other attends to the remainder of the group. Some groups may require additional aides to assist clients with greater cognitive impairments. The therapist and others who help lead the social skills interventions should have the following skills:

* Flexibility and capacity for resourcefulness.
* Enthusiasm.
* Ability to work under pressure.
* Interpersonal sensitivity.
* Communication skills.
* Knowledge of the impact and functional ramifications of cognitive impairments.
* Ability to develop behavioral programs.
* Ability to plan and present live modeling displays.
* Ability to analyze and adapt activities.
* Ability to initiate and facilitate experiential exercises.
* Ability to present material in a concrete form.
* Ability to deal with problems effectively.

Number, Length, and Spacing of Sessions

If possible, interventions should occur at a rate of at least once, but preferably twice a week. Spacing between sessions is critical to provide the opportunity to try, in real life, the social skills learned in training. The program and clients should be evaluated after approximately twelve sessions to determine effectiveness and future directions.

Session length should be determined by a number of factors, such as attention span, impulsivity, verbal ability, and other characteristics of the clients. Sessions of forty-five to ninety minutes work best in most settings. However, if attention spans are very short, the session can be as brief as

twenty minutes. In such cases, more frequent sessions are advisable.

The Setting

One major principle for encouraging transfer from the treatment setting to the real-life setting is the rule of similar elements. Since not all elements can be identical to the real-life situation, available furniture and supplies should be used creatively. Several chairs can be pushed together to simulate a couch or a box can be a television set. Props and costumes make the experiential exercises more concrete for clients with cognitive impairments.

Arrangement of furniture can further enhance the learning experience. The horseshoe or semi-circle formation is an excellent way to arrange furniture for classroom instruction and role-play situations. It enables the therapists and role players to be seen by all clients while creating an inclusive environment. Some of the experiential exercises require a circle formation. In this case, the therapists are positioned as an integral part of the circle, preferably between clients who may need more assistance.

Experiential Exercises

Many different activities can be used to increase interpersonal interactions and relationships. This section provides an overview of how the activities should be run and some possible interaction opportunities.

Social interaction skills cannot be learned without experience and practice in these skills. However, the opportunity to interact is not enough. A social activity does not foster socialization if the clients do not have prerequisite skills. Pat, who was introduced earlier, is a wallflower at dances and parties. She just watches the others, eats, or gazes into space. She does not know how to participate or how to ask someone to dance with her. Like many of her peers, she needs activities that are specifically designed and facilitated to enhance the development of social interaction skills.

Group Games

Structured games often require and can teach interpersonal interaction skills. Because of this, they can be employed in an innovative intervention process. The group games used in this model were specifically designed or modified to facilitate the development of social interaction skills. This approach is described by Redl and Wineman (1952).

Practically all so-called social skills needed in any society can be translated into some game activities which combine the value of acculturation and socialization with the experience of happiness and fun in the process.

Thus, games can be played for enjoyment while offering a worthwhile learning experience. The skills are developed at the very moment a person is having all the fun and excitement playing a game has to offer.

The types of games used in this model are primarily social recreation activities, such as starters, icebreakers, mixers, warm-up exercises, and theater games. The games were created or adapted to meet goals, such as learning the names of the other clients, establishing trust in group members, developing group consciousness, and enhancing self-concept. The games for clients with cognitive impairments focus primarily on basic verbal and non-verbal interactions, whereas the exercises for individuals without cognitive impairments focuses more on self-concept, decision making, trust in others, and understanding others. The games are done in a small group or pairs, although learning is directed toward the individual in the group. Because the games are non-competitive, there are no individual winners or chance of failure. See "Interpersonal Relationship Activities" in the Techniques section for examples of the games.

To maximize the learning potential of the group games, the therapist must clearly present the game and facilitate interaction. Some clients need demonstrations and physical or verbal prompts, while others can independently engage in the games. Because the stimulation of the activity may not be adequate reinforcement for clients with greater cognitive impairments, individual reinforcement techniques outlined in the behavior modification section may be needed to maintain participation. Praise, acceptance, and a non-threatening environment create an atmosphere conducive to the development of social skills.

The games, themselves, have particular goals and are chosen based on the needs of the clients. Recreation and play provide a laboratory of learning for practicing and experiencing social interaction skills. Cooperative play behavior between individuals leads to learning acceptable modes of socialization such as sharing and taking turns. The role of recreation as a mediator of social development has been summarized by Luckey and Shapiro (1974):

> Games with increasingly complex rules and social demands further enhance children's social adaptation as they grow older and participation in clubs and organizations takes on increasing social importance during the school years… Organized sports additionally provide young adults opportunities for personal achievement. While

teaching rules of competition and the controlled expression of aggression.

In addition, recreation can foster adherence to set rules, collaboration, empathy, and competition. These social traits are necessary for successful adjustment in both vocational performance and integration into the community.

Recreation has additional benefits for clients with cognitive impairments. It can provide a means for overcoming or compensating for limitations. McDaniels (1971) found that greater participation in social activities can lead to increased social acceptance by non-disabled peers and more enduring friendships. Social recreation is also normalizing, in that the types of recreation most preferred by individuals who are not disabled involve affiliation (Neulinger & Raps, 1972). Thus, recreation provides a means for normalization and integration. Positive recreation experiences can create a feeling of well-being and increase self-concept so the participants want to interact with other people in the community. For those who are employed, recreation provides a worthwhile and necessary balance to work and work-related activities. In addition, recreation activities provide the stimulation needed to maintain an active interest in one's surroundings, in one's health, in social relationships, in work and life. Such interest, in turn, supports other maintenance, health, and rehabilitation services provided by educators and therapists. Most importantly, recreation can be creative, fun, and inspiring.

Unfortunately, socially inappropriate or unacceptable behavior is often propagated by the lack of appropriate skill training and outlets for recreation. When activities are taught or offered, clients often have problems with the activity, get into fights, or refuse to play because the social interaction skills required are too demanding for their current functional skills. Activities that require many social skills, such as competitive team sports, may be problematic for clients who lack these skills. Pat, the wallflower, also had difficulty with competitive team sports. Because Pat is very good in physical activities, she was enrolled in Special Olympics basketball. She had difficulty not only in cooperation and sportsmanship, but also in understanding the concept of group effort and accomplishment. After a successful game she would say, "I won," rather than "We won." Individuals like Pat need recreation experiences designed specifically to teach, facilitate, and reinforce social interaction skills and appropriate social behavior starting at their present level of social functioning. Such systematic and planned use of recreation can provide practice in a real-life situation that will also have carry-over value in the community.

Characteristics of the Recreation Activities

It is neither possible, nor desirable, to list all recreation activities appropriate for this model. All types of recreation activities are utilized, including physical activities, social activities, craft activities, and table games. Activities must be chosen based on individuals in the group. Some considerations for activity selection include:

- *Expressed or demonstrated interest*: Problems of motivating participation are minimized by this approach. In addition, activities of interest are most likely to continue and transfer into the community.
- *Compatibility*: The therapist should look for activities that are compatible with the client's cognitive, physical, and social functioning levels. In choosing activities, it is important to remember that the social component is only one part of what an activity demands from the client. For example, a client recovering from a stroke may have the social and physical skills to play checkers, but lack the decision-making, planning, and abstract thinking necessary for strategy. The client would be better able to play a game that relies more on chance (e.g., Parcheesi) than a strategy game. The therapist will want to use activity analysis to compare the client's abilities against the activity's requirements.
- *Age and cultural appropriateness*: Clients with cognitive impairments need to be taught recreation activities like those of their non-disabled peers. This includes an examination of the availability of the activity in the community and economic feasibility of continued client participation. Ceramics may be an age-appropriate activity, but is not a good selection unless it is available in the community at a price the client can afford. Selection based on these criteria will facilitate both normalization and integration.

The social progression of the activities needs to be taken into account. Examples of recreational activities that are appropriate for the normal social progression described in "Social Skills Development" in the Concepts section include:

- *Unoccupied behavior* (intra-individual with one client): Daydreaming, individual prayer, and meditation.
- *Solitary independent* (extra-individual with one client): Jogging, yoga, fishing, cooking, listening to music, playing instruments, reading, collections, arts and crafts, plant and animal care,

watching television alone, swimming, puzzles, sewing, solitaire, bicycling, kite flying.
- *Parallel* (aggregate two or more people): Bingo, watching a play, crafts class, going to sporting events.
- *Competitive one-to-one* (inter-individual, 1:1): Checkers, chess, tennis, badminton, racquetball.
- *Competitive one-to-others* (multi-lateral, two or more people): Swim match, target games (darts), table games (Parcheesi, lotto, dominoes, Monopoly), card games (war, poker, rummy).
- *Cooperative team* (intra-group with two or more people): Band and orchestra, choral groups, circle dances, group collage, theater groups, various clubs.
- *Competitive team* (inter-group with two or more people): Doubles tennis, bridge, team sports (e.g., volleyball, softball, and basketball).

Once the inherent social interaction pattern required by activities is understood, the therapist can superimpose higher levels of social interaction on the activity. Therefore, the same activity can be used to facilitate social interaction at different levels. For instance, craft activities, such as macramé, are usually done alone at home. However, an individual might be enrolled in a macramé class, creating a parallel (aggregate) activity that still does not require a true dyadic relationship. Scissors, beads, and other materials can be arranged so that sharing and taking turns are required. When the client is comfortable with this situation, the therapist may introduce social conversations between the client and the therapist, then gradually between the client and other individuals. Further cooperation (intra-group) may be introduced through a group macramé project to be hung on the multipurpose room wall. Competition (multi-lateral and intra-group) can be introduced through individual and group projects for a competitive art show. Another example is aerobic dance, which can be solitary in nature by "doing your own thing," parallel by following the leader, cooperative by dancing with a partner, or competitive by having a dance contest. For the optimal learning experience, the therapist needs to appropriately incorporate the behavior modification and teaching strategies previously outlined.

Recreation activities are particularly effective for the development of non-verbal interaction skills. Many recreation activities have components that lend themselves to teaching and practicing these skills. For instance, activities that require touching another person, such as making plaster gauze masks, emphasize appropriate touching. Helping others could also be fostered by this activity, if clients were required to cut gauze strips for each other.

Cooperation could be encouraged by changing the rules of volleyball so that the goal is to keep the ball going as long as possible resulting in a collective score. Verbal interaction skills, such as asking someone to do an activity, are required by many recreation activities. Other verbal interaction skills can be practiced by changing the rules of the game. For instance, if the group were playing catch in a circle, each client might be required to say the name of the person to whom the client was going to throw the ball. Thus, the use of carefully selected and modified recreation activities provides a way to enhance social interaction skills. See "Interpersonal Relationship Activities" in the Techniques section for more ideas about specific activities to teach specific skills.

The Social Lounge

Unstructured activities, such as a social lounge, are also an integral part of the model. Initiation, self-direction, and decision-making are social skills that are necessary for the independent pursuit of activities as well as relationships. Therefore, opportunities to choose activities and initiate asking another person to join in must be provided as much as possible. A social lounge situation, where socially oriented equipment and materials are available to allow a variety of simultaneous self-directed activities, can facilitate this process. Clients who do not lack basic social interaction skills often need to practice group decision-making, problem solving, planning, and other more advanced skills. The therapist can also foster these skills in the social lounge. In effect, the social lounge represents recreation areas found in the clients' home and assists transfer of learning.

The following guidelines are useful in skill development in social lounges:

- A variety of tasks, games, materials, or activities appropriate to home environments must be offered for the clients.
- The materials should include a variety of items that span the ability levels of all clients.
- Solitary materials, such as books, need to be minimized, while socially oriented equipment, such as table games, need to be maximized.
- Materials should be as durable as possible to withstand the wear and tear of client use. Lamination, taping, etc. can help.
- Therapists should introduce clients to every component of the lounge and demonstrate its use.
- The range of behavior or activity acceptable in the lounge should be established ahead of time to help alleviate inappropriate behaviors.

- Therapists must encourage and reinforce the choice of activities and social interaction unobtrusively, as well as be a positive role model.
- Lounges should be planned so that they can be successfully implemented within the available space and facilities.
- Some means for record keeping should be prepared for the lounge.

Transfer of Social Skills

The main interest of any intervention program is not in demonstrating the skills during treatment but in transferring the skills to real life. Transfer occurs when an individual learns a skill, concept, or behavior in one situation and is able to apply it in another situation. Research has identified a number of principles to maximize transfer benefits. Principles upon which this model is built are outlined below (Goldstein, et al, 1980; Mercer, 1979; Hutchinson, 1978):

- Transfer increases when individuals become competent and confident in tasks. Practiced behavior or behavior that has occurred most frequently in the past is likely to occur in the future when a similar situation arises. The higher the degree of original learning or overlearning, the greater the possibility of later transfer.
- Similarity of elements improves transfer from therapy settings to real-life application. Ideally, both the interpersonal and physical characteristics of the intervention and application settings should be similar. If possible, interventions should be done with others with whom clients will continue to interact in a real-life setting.
- Transfer increases when meaningful generalizations are developed. Positive transfer is greater when a variety of training stimuli, experiences, and tasks are employed. The concept, skill, or behavior to be transferred should be emphasized and verbalized.
- When the activities are meaningful and relevant for the clients, transfer is enhanced. Clients need to have opportunities to choose activities of interest to them that are age and skill appropriate.
- Entry into a new social situation is facilitated by the presence of a transition agent or person who can mediate the critical transition into the novel situation. To be effective, the transition agent must be an individual with whom the client has formed a relationship. Preferably, the agent should be established in the situation so that the agent can introduce the client to others, legitimize the client's presence, and support the

individual's efforts to function in the new situation.

References

Berryman, D. & Lefebvre, C. (1979). *Recreation behavior inventory.* Denton, TX: Leisure Learning. Systems.

Coyne, P. (1980). *Social skills training: A three-pronged approach.* Portland, OR: University of Oregon Health Science Center.

Gold, M. (1980). *"Did I say that?" Articles and commentary on the Try Another Way system.* Champaign, IL: Research Press Company.

Goldstein A., Sprafkin R., Gersham N.J., Klein P. (1980). *Skillstreaming the adolescent: A structured learning approach to teaching prosocial skills.* Champaign, IL: Research Press.

Hutchinson, P. & Lord, J. (1979). *Recreation integration.* Concord Ontario: Leisurability Publication.

Kempton, W. (1975). *Sex education for persons with disabilities that hinder learning.* Massachusetts: Duxbury Press.

Kempton, W. & Kahn, E. (1991). Sexuality and people with intellectual disabilities: A historical perspective. *Sexuality and Disability 9*(2):93-111.

Luckey, R., and Shapiro, I. G. (1974). Recreation: An essential aspect of habilitative programming. *Mental Retardation, 6:*150-151.

McDaniel, R.R., Jr. (1971, March-April). Tools of transmission of knowledge. *President's Bulletin Board,* 6-8. Division of Higher Education, Board of Education, The United Methodist Church, Nashville, Tennessee.

Mercer, J. (1979). *System of multicultural pluralistic assessment technical manual.* San Antonio, TX: Psychological Corporation.

Neulinger, J. & Raps, C. (1972). Leisure attitudes of an intellectual elite. *Journal of Leisure Research, 4:*196-207.

Redl, F., & Wineman, D. (1952). *Controls from within: Techniques for the treatment of the aggressive child.* New York: Free Press.

Walker, C. (1980). The learning assistance center in a selective institution. In K. V. Lauridsen (Ed.). *Examining the scope of learning centers.* (pp. 57-68). San Francisco: Jossey-Bass.

Transitioning a Client from Inpatient Rehabilitation to a Communal Environment

The purpose of this protocol is to help clients make a healthy transition from an inpatient rehabilitation setting to a group living environment (e.g., group home, skilled nursing facility).

Description

The recreational therapist develops a healthy activity pattern (see "Activity Pattern Development" in the Techniques section) for post-discharge participation for every client. This process requires the therapist to ensure that the activity pattern is realistic, meaning that it can be carried out given the activity limitations and participation restrictions of both the client and the client's environment. It must also reflect the interests of the client and provide a pattern of activity that optimizes health and prevents secondary complications/illness. For the client who will be transitioning to a group living environment, the therapist must consider the limitations and offerings of the setting and mesh those resources therapeutically into the development of the client's activity pattern. The premise is that direct communication with the activity director of the group facility enhances follow through with the client's activity pattern.

Rationale

Clients who are admitted to an inpatient rehabilitation setting may be discharged to an assisted care facility rather than a home environment. This occurs if the client's needs are greater than the client's support system (e.g., children work full time and are unable to provide care for the parent; client's finances are not adequate to pay for private care in his/her home). Clients may be returning to a previous group setting (e.g., client lived at a nursing home, was admitted to rehab for a hip replacement, and will be returning to the same nursing home after discharge), a client may be going to a new facility (e.g., client was living at an independent retirement community that does not provide skilled care, client was admitted to rehab for a stroke, and will be discharged to a skilled nursing facility that is able to provide the level of care that the client requires), or a client may be transitioning to a group living environment for the first time (e.g., client was living alone in her own home, was admitted to rehab for an exacerbation of multiple sclerosis, and will be discharged to an assisted care facility for the first time). Clients may live in a group environment for a short period of time (e.g., until the client progresses

to the point of being able to live alone) or the client may remain in a group environment long term (e.g., chronic condition that requires long-term care).

Indications and Contraindications

Any client who will be discharged from an inpatient rehabilitation facility to a communal living environment, whether it's a new or pre-existing placement.

If the client presents with behavioral or cognitive impairments that significantly impede participation in a portion of the program, the recreational therapist will complete that portion of the program independently without the client.

Structure Criteria

It is suggested that the therapist follow the five sessions and follow-up shown below. Each session is 30 minutes and is to take place in a quiet/non-distracting environment to promote concentration. The length and frequency of sessions may need to be varied depending on the identified needs and abilities of the client.

Process Criteria

The therapist will acquire the facility's contact information (name of facility, address, phone number). This is commonly communicated to the therapist via the case manager. Sometimes the facility is not known until a day or so before discharge (e.g., the family looks at and applies to three different facilities and waits to see which facility has an open bed for the client). Therefore, the therapist goes through sessions 1 and 2 whether or not the facility has been identified, and then conducts sessions 3 through 5 once the facility is known. If time is very limited, the therapist can conduct session 3 and 5 without the client present (therefore, only having to conduct session 4 with the client).

Outcome Criteria

The therapist documents the specific outcomes of each session as per facility protocol (e.g., daily notes). This includes documentation on education provided, client's ability to verbally apply newly learned information, contacts with facility and outcomes of conversations, level of assistance required to develop an activity pattern, etc.

Sessions	Therapist will...	Client will...
Session 1: Consequences of inactivity	Go through the information found in "Consequences of Inactivity" in the Concepts section.	Demonstrate understanding of the information in "Consequences of Inactivity" in the Concepts section.
Session 2: Interest exploration	See information on interest exploration in "Activity Pattern Development" in the Techniques section. Conduct interest exploration to identify leisure interests and motivation for leisure pursuits. *Note*: If the facility is not yet identified and there is adequate time for further treatment, the therapist is to address restoration and/or adaptation and modification of functional skills related to the client's ability to participate in activities identified from interest exploration (e.g., address fine motor skills).	Work with the therapist to develop a healthy, post-discharge activity pattern.
Session 3: Contact facility (once the facility is determined)	Once the facility is determined, the therapist contacts the activity director or equivalent at the facility. 1. The therapist obtains the contact information for the facility (name of facility, address, phone number). The case manager is typically the person who is first to know of the client's placement and has the contact information. 2. The therapist and client develop a list of questions to ask the activity director at the facility, including activities offered, times activities are offered, resources available in the facility — library, meditation room, gym, pool. *Note*: If the client has significant cognitive and/or physical impairments that impact his/her ability to complete this task (e.g., verbal communication deficits, unable to write down information), the therapist can make the phone call for the client. 3. See "client will" in next column. 4. Talk with the activity director to ask any further questions that the client may have missed Explore the department's ability to set-up the client for independent activity, provide supplies for independent work, make activity staff available to provide assistance to the client (e.g., Are there adequate staff to offer the client minimal assistance throughout a 30-minute art class?), and work with adaptive equipment that the client may need (e.g., if the staff are unfamiliar with the equipment, training will need to be provided). The therapist then thanks the activity director for his/her time and tells him/her that the therapist will be contacting him/her again once the client's activity pattern is developed. The purpose of this second contact is to relay, and jointly problem solve, on how to implement the client's activity pattern at the facility.	Place a phone call to the facility and ask to speak with the activity director. The client is to introduce himself or herself, explain the reason for the phone call (will be moving there, in process of developing a pattern of activity with his/her therapist), ask pre-developed questions, write down information provided by the activity director, request the activity director to fax a copy of their activity calendar to the rehab facility to use for a reference, and thank the director for his/her time. The client is then to ask the activity director to speak with the therapist.

Sessions	Therapist will...	Client will...
Session 4: Brainstorm how to mesh the facilities activities into the client's activity pattern	1. Compare the interests of the client with the offerings of the facility. Transcribe offerings that match the client's interests into the client's activity pattern (e.g., 2:00-3:00 P.M. Quilting club). 2. Problem solve with the client on how to incorporate interests not offered by the facility into the activity pattern (e.g., ask facility if they can offer a new activity not currently offered, explore independent set-up of the activity, explore possibility of joining a group outside of the facility). 3. Develop the activity pattern (see "Activity Pattern Development" in the Techniques section). *Note*: If the client has significant cognitive impairments that impact his/her ability to participate in this process, the therapist can complete this process independently.	Develop the activity pattern with the therapist (see "Activity Pattern Development" in the Techniques section).
Session 5: Contact activity director	1. The therapist is to call the activity director to review the client's activity pattern and problem solve for issues identified in session 4 (e.g., possibility of offering a new activity). The therapist tells the activity director about adaptive equipment the client uses for particular activities (e.g., universal cuff to hold paintbrush) and finds out if the facility has such equipment and has the knowledge to use the equipment. The therapist also informs the activity director on any adaptive techniques that the client requires (e.g., verbal cuing to follow multi-step directions). It is helpful for the therapist to type up this information and mail/fax/e-mail it to the activity director for reference. This information must include the therapist's name and phone number to encourage the activity director to contact the therapist with any questions. 2. The therapist is to review the outcomes of the phone call with the client.	
Follow-up	Contact the activity director of the facility and the client to assess the outcomes of transition process.	

(Also see "Acclimatizing Clients to a Communal Living Arrangement" in the Techniques Section).

Transfers

This section looks at several types of transfers. While each transfer has its specific techniques and protocols for implementation, there are some basic guidelines and common sense rules to follow. They are

- Before helping a client transfer, the therapist needs to know the transfer the client is going to use, how much assistance the client will need during the transfer, and any precautions necessary to safeguard both the client and the therapist.
- Look over the general area. Are there objects that need to be moved before the transfer can safely take place? Are the surfaces around the area safe or slippery?
- Mentally walk your way through the transfer. What are the good body mechanics that both the therapist and client need to use?
- Consider equipment needs. If the client is transferring out of a wheelchair, are the brakes on the wheelchair locked? If the client uses braces or splints to stabilize or safeguard the body, are they on? Can either of the surfaces be raised or lowered to make transferring easier?
- Consider the client's skin. How can shear be avoided during the transfer? (Shear is friction caused by rubbing the skin against another object while moving and may lead to skin breakdown and infection.)
- Communicate with the client. Are you both clear as to who is to do what and when?
- Consider using equipment to help make the transfer easier. Is the client too heavy or too unstable for the therapist to safely transfer alone? Timbly and Lewis (1992) point out that two female staff normally cannot safely move and carry a 250-pound patient by themselves. Special equipment and procedures are required.

There are a variety of transfer techniques that can be used. Choosing the best one depends on the client's abilities and limitations. This section provides a general review to familiarize the therapist with common transfer techniques. Clients may have specific cueing and assistance requirements identified by members of the treatment team. The recreational therapist should be able to find out about the client's specific needs by asking the client; checking in the medical chart; or asking the client's primary nurse, physical therapist, or occupational therapist.

Typically, recreational therapists perform transfers that require moderate assistance or less. If the physical or occupational therapist determines that the client requires more than moderate assistance, the recreational therapist seeks out the appropriate staff (primary PT, OT, or nurse) to determine the best technique. If the recreational therapist is new to transfers, s/he should obtain further training, usually from a PT or OT on the treatment team.

An overview of the most common transfer techniques is given below followed by detailed instructions for implementation.

- *Standing pivot transfer*: Client stands upright, pivots on lower extremities towards destination, and sits down.
- *Sit pivot transfer*: Same as standing pivot transfer except client does not reach full upright position in standing, but rather a half standing position.
- *Transfer board transfer*: A transfer board is placed underneath the client's buttocks while the client is in a sitting position. The other end of the board rests on the transfer destination (e.g., chair seat). The client, through a series of small buttocks lifts using upper and lower extremities, scoots over to the transfer destination. The client does not slide across the board because it causes too much friction and could cause damage to skin. There are a variety of transfer boards (sliding disc, long board, and short board) described in the Equipment section.
- *Hoyer lift*: Client is hoisted from one place to another using a piece of equipment called a Hoyer lift. The seat of the Hoyer lift is made out of a strong material that is placed around the client and buckled into place. The final outcome is the construction of a seat resembling a child's swing with a back. The swing is attached to a metal frame with wheels so that the client can be lifted up in the swing and then rolled to the next destination. The swing is then lowered onto the transfer surface and the buckles are undone.
- *Dependent lift of two*: For this lift the client is in a seated position. One person approaches the person from behind, places his/her arms underneath the armpits of the client and grasps the client's opposite wrist/forearm (e.g., therapists right hand grasps client's left wrist/forearm). The therapist pulls the client's arms under the client's chest for support when lifting. The second person approaches the client from the front. The therapist places both his/her hands underneath the client's knees. On the count of three, both therapists lift the client up and over to the transfer destination.

The PT or OT, as mentioned earlier, typically assesses transfers. The recreational therapist, depending on his/her competency with transfers, may or may not need to seek out the PT or OT to discuss the transfer techniques described here. Transfers are assessed through the amount of assistance required by the therapist (Functional Independence Measure), along with a description of cueing or assistance needed (e.g., moderate assistance for standing pivot transfer with minimal verbal cues to look up and straighten knees).

Transfer Training

The recreational therapist must be comfortable with transfer training, as s/he may need to help the client develop a technique to transfer onto an uncommon surface not typically reviewed in the clinic setting (for example, riding lawn mower, boat, movie seat with stationary arms, fourth seat over in a theater). If transfer ability is limiting the client's ability to perform activities being addressed by recreational therapy, then transfer goals should be established. Transfer training, depending upon the problems presented by the client, will vary. Some of the common techniques employed to enhance function include: repetition of task, guiding (for example, the therapist manually places the client's hand on the armchair before the client attempts to sit down), verbal cues, demonstration of desired skill, verbal review of steps in a transfer, positive feedback, and physical assistance (e.g., therapist helps client slide foot over to increase distance in stance).

Detailed instructions for the stand-pivot transfer and independent floor transfers follow. The authors suggest that student therapists borrow a wheelchair and practice each of these transfers. They can be harder than they seem and having experience trying each one will help the therapist be a better teacher.

Stand-Pivot Transfer (Wheelchair to Chair)

1. Position the wheelchair so that the wheelchair and the chair are at a 90° angle from each other ("L" form). This will minimize the amount of stepping/pivoting required for the client to reach the transfer destination. Whenever possible, the client should be positioned to transfer toward his/her stronger side.
2. Lock the brakes on the wheelchair.
3. Scoot forward to the end of the seat (walk buttocks one cheek at a time, hands on armrests and lift buttock to end of seat, client leans back against chair back and pushes buttocks forward). If the client is unable to scoot to the edge of the seat, the therapist may assist the client by

squatting in front of client, placing his/her hands around the client's buttocks, and pulling the buttocks forward.
4. Place feet flat on the floor and slightly flex (tuck) the feet behind the knees.
5. Place both hands on the armrests of the wheelchair.
6. On the count of three, stand up (lean forward, nose over toes, straighten knees and trunk, look straight ahead, straighten shoulders, tuck in buttock). If the client requires assistance with standing, the therapist stands on the affected side of the client. The therapist holds onto the client at the trunk in the back (grab hold of waistband of pants/belt) to assist with standing. Therapist places other hand on client's chest to provide support so that client does not go too far forward. Provide cueing and further assistance as needed. Should client require more assistance than this, therapist may need to stand in front of the client and instruct client to wrap his/her arms around the therapist's neck. Therapist (with knees bent) wraps both arms around client's trunk and grabs hold of the waistband/belt. On the count of three, the therapist lifts the client into a standing position.
7. Once the client is in an upright position, the client pivots his/her feet so that the buttocks are now in line with the transfer destination.
8. Client backs up to the transfer destination until the legs touch the transfer destination.
9. Client reaches back and places both hands on the armrest of transfer destination and slowly lowers himself/herself onto the chair seat (no plopping).

Independent Floor Transfers (Floor to/from Wheelchair)

Into a Kneeling Position from the Wheelchair to the Floor
1. Position the wheelchair so that it is ready for the transfer. Brakes are locked, casters are rotated in the most forward position, and the cushion is removed if necessary to decrease the height of the transfer.
2. Client scoots to the edge of the wheelchair.
3. Client places his/her feet on the floor and tucks them behind/underneath knees as tolerated (knee flexion).
4. Client places one hand on the seat of the wheelchair and flexes forward at the trunk slowly reaching with the other hand for the floor.
5. Client slowly lowers himself/herself toward the floor until s/he reaches the floor in a hands-and-knees position.

From a Kneeling Position from the Floor to the Wheelchair (This technique can be difficult with a wheelchair that does not have swing away leg rests.)

1. Position the wheelchair so that it is ready for the transfer. Brakes are locked, casters are rotated in the most forward position, and the cushion is removed if necessary to decrease the height of the transfer. It is replaced once the client is seated on the wheelchair seat.
2. With both knees bent to one side and buttocks on the floor, client places his/her hands on either side of seat/armrest.
3. Client lifts himself/herself into a tall kneeling position.
4. Client continues to lift the torso until the hips clear the edge of the seat.
5. Client rotates his/her hips to one side and moves one hand to the other armrest so that the buttocks are fully on wheelchair seat.

Into a Long Sitting Position from the Wheelchair to the Floor

1. Position the wheelchair so that it is ready for the transfer. Brakes are locked, casters are rotated in the most forward position, and the cushion is removed if necessary to decrease the height of the transfer.
2. Client scoots to edge of wheelchair seat and straightens his/her legs out to one side so that s/he is sitting at an angle in the wheelchair.
3. Client places one hand on the wheelchair seat/armrest and reaches towards the floor with the other hand.
4. Client slowly lowers himself/herself to the floor into a long sitting position.

From the Long Sitting Position on the Floor to the Wheelchair

1. Position the wheelchair so that it is ready for the transfer. Brakes are locked, casters are rotated in most forward position, and the cushion is removed if necessary to decrease the height of the transfer. It is replaced once the client is seated on the wheelchair seat.
2. Client positions himself/herself with his/her back to the wheelchair seat and legs straightened out in front of him/her on a diagonal away from his/her body.
3. Client reaches behind and finds two stable areas for his/her hands to lift himself/herself back into the wheelchair (e.g., one hand on the wheelchair seat and another on the lower part of the wheelchair frame).
4. Client pushes flexed elbows into extension and slides buttocks onto the wheelchair seat.
5. Client readjusts position on the wheelchair.

Back Approach for Long Leg Sitting Transfer from the Wheelchair to the Floor

1. Position the wheelchair so that it is ready for the transfer. Brakes are locked, casters are rotated in most forward position, and the cushion is removed if necessary to decrease the height of the transfer.
2. Client scoots forward on the wheelchair seat and extends his/her legs directly out in front.
3. Client places both hands on the wheelchair seat and slowly lower his/her buttocks onto the floor.
4. As the client begins to lower himself/herself to the floor his/her knees will bend up towards the chest.

Back Approach for Long Leg Sitting Transfer from the Floor to the Wheelchair

1. Position the wheelchair so that it is ready for the transfer. Brakes are locked, casters are rotated in most forward position, and the cushion is removed if necessary to decrease the height of the transfer. It is replaced once the client is seated on the wheelchair seat.
2. Client sits with his/her back to the wheelchair seat.
3. Knees are bent up towards chest.
4. Client positions both hands on the wheelchair seat and lift his/her buttocks onto the wheelchair seat.

Transfer training is not a cookie cutter approach. The instructions provided above are a general outline of the steps taken during the transfer. Techniques, cueing, and level of assistance vary depending on the abilities and limitations of the client and the transfer task itself. Here are some of considerations:

- *Proper height*: Transfers must be within the specific precautions or parameters of the client. For example, if a client has total hip precautions, it is contraindicated to do a floor transfer. It is also contraindicated to transfer onto another surface that breaks total hip precautions (e.g., transferring into to a car that flexes the hip more than 90°).
- *Proper support*: Therapists must be sure that the client is provided with the appropriate supports to ensure safe transfers (e.g., if a client requires the support of armrests to transfer, it is important to make sure that armrests are available or alternative techniques are taught, as in transferring onto or off of a sofa that only has one armrest).
- *Proper equipment*: Therapists make sure that transfer equipment is available and appropriate for the specific transfer (e.g., a client may be

able to independently transfer from a wheelchair to a bed using a transfer board, but the transfer board will not work to transfer from a boat dock into a boat. Physical assistance may be needed and the therapist will need to make sure that the assistance is available, safe, and appropriate).

- *Stability of transfer destination*: Clients should be instructed to check the stability of the items to be used during the transfer to make sure that they provide a safe transfer opportunity. For example, clients check chairs to make sure they will not slide or move because of a slippery tile floor or because the chair has wheels.
- *Secondary conditions that impact transfer technique*: It is not uncommon for clients to have a secondary condition that requires a modification in the transfer technique. For example, a client who has recently had a total knee replacement is expected to limit bending of the affected knee. The client may need to extend the affected leg when going from a standing to a sitting position.
- *Client's strength and endurance*: Therapists must consider whether the client has enough strength and endurance to complete the transfer safely. For example, a client who is deconditioned may have great difficulty in performing a floor transfer because it requires too much strength.
- *Client's available range of motion*: Therapists consider the available range of motion of the client and its impact on performing transfers. If range of motion is restricted, modifications of

transfer techniques may be required (e.g., left upper extremity paralysis requires the client to learn how to transfer using the support of only one hand).

- *Assistance needed is available*: For example, a client requires moderate assistance and his fishing buddy has a bad back. Because of this, his buddy is unable to help the client to transfer out of the car to go to the fishing dock. Consequently, the therapist will need to explore other transfer techniques (e.g., may be able to transfer with a transfer board with minimal assistance) or problem solve for other available resources (e.g., use of paratransit to get to the fishing dock).
- *Client's cognitive and perceptual skills to perform transfer techniques*: Therapists evaluate and problem solve for cognitive and perceptual problems that may interfere with a client's ability to perform a transfer (e.g., difficulty remembering the steps, poor awareness of body position).

See "Wheelchair Mobility Skills" in the Techniques section for information on car transfers and the Equipment section for more information about transfer equipment and its use. Therapists score the level of difficulty a client has with transfers using d420 Transferring Oneself.

References

Timbly, B. & Lewis, L. (1992). *Fundamental skills and concepts in patient care* (5th ed.). Philadelphia, PA: Lippincott Company.

Vital Signs

Vital signs consist of a person's temperature, pulse, respiration, and blood pressure. They are also called cardinal signs.

Vital sign changes indicate physiological changes within the body, so regular and consistent vital sign monitoring provides insight into a client's health. It is not within the practice of recreational therapists to determine the extent of a vital sign's impairment (e.g., coding Body Functions codes such as b4100 Heart Rate, b420 Blood Pressure Functions, b4400 Respiration Rate). However, recreational therapists do monitor vital signs. The contribution of the recreational therapist about a client's vital signs is valuable because it 1. monitors the client's physiological functioning in different environments, activities, and times; 2. ensures the safety of the client (e.g., making sure the client does not exceed blood pressure parameters during a strenuous physical activity), and 3. assists with identifying the effectiveness of treatment plans and the client's response to a specific intervention (e.g., client able to stay within pulse parameters during 15 minutes of cardiovascular activity compared to last week when client was only able to participate in eight minutes of cardiovascular activity prior to exceeding pulse parameters).

Vital signs have a standard range (e.g., normal blood pressure for an adult is below 120/80). However, depending on the age and health of the individual, the desired range may change (e.g., a physician desires a client to maintain a blood pressure that does not rise above 140/90 during exercise). Vital signs will also fluctuate. This is expected. Vital signs can change with time of day (e.g., pulse is quicker in the morning than in the evening), time of the month (e.g., body temperature rises with ovulation), exercise (vital signs rise with aerobic activity), age (e.g., a healthy resting pulse for a child is quicker than a healthy resting pulse for an adult), sex (e.g., males typically have fewer respirations per minute due to greater vital capacity), weight (e.g., weight increases blood pressure), metabolic conditions (e.g., any activity that increases metabolic rate increases vital signs), general health status (e.g., temperature rises when fighting infection), pain (e.g., pain increases heart rate and blood pressure), and medications/illegal drugs (e.g., cocaine increases blood pressure, specific medications can be prescribed that decrease blood pressure).

When documenting vital signs the following qualifiers are included: day, date, time of day, location, activity, and vital sign reading. If a response

to a vital sign was needed (e.g., client instructed to take deep breaths for several minutes), document the specific response taken and the outcomes of the action (e.g., O2Sat level increased from 89 to 94 after three minutes of deep breathing).

Body Temperature

Body temperature measures the internal temperature of the body. Humans are warm blooded. Unlike cold-blooded animals, such as reptiles, whose internal body temperature changes with the temperature of the environment, human beings regulate their internal body temperature. A constant body temperature optimizes cell and organ functioning. A normal body temperature is 98.6°F. Because of the various factors that influence body temperature, a slight deviation from the norm may be acceptable and appropriate.

Factors that Influence Body Temperature

- *Time of day*: Body temperatures are typically lower in the early morning and higher in the late afternoon and early evening.
- *Age*: Younger children typically have higher body temperatures because they 1. are more susceptible to temperature changes in the environment due to the immaturity of their thermoregulatory system and 2. have a higher level of physical activity and metabolic rate. Conversely, older adults typically have lower than normal body temperatures due to decreased physical activity and metabolic rates, as well as less subcutaneous tissue to provide insulation to protect against heat loss.
- *Emotions*: Extremes in emotion, whether joyous, sad, excited, or other, increase body temperature.
- *Exercise*: Exercise increases metabolic rates thus increasing body temperature.
- *Menstrual cycle*: During ovulation the body temperature rises slightly.
- *Pregnancy*: During pregnancy, the metabolic rate increases causing the body temperature to slightly elevate.
- *External environment*: On hot and humid days, the body temperature becomes slightly elevated. The outside temperature increases body temperature and the humidity impairs evaporation of sweat making it difficult for the body to cool down. On cold days the body temperature may be slightly lower due to the external environment cooling down the body.

- *Clothing*: Loose fitting cotton clothing allows the body temperature to cool down on warm days because it allows for the escape of body heat, compared to heavy layered clothing that traps body heat (optimal for cold days).
- *Location of measurement*: Rectal temperatures are slightly higher than oral temperatures and axillary temperatures (under the arm) are slightly lower than oral temperatures.
- *Ingestion of cold or warm foods and smoking*: Cold and warm foods, as well as smoking, can affect the recorded body temperature when taken orally. It is recommended that people refrain from the above 15-30 minutes prior to taking oral temperature readings. (O'Sullivan & Schmitz, 1988).

Measurement

- *Oral temperature*: Temperatures are commonly assessed in the hospital environment using an electronic thermometer. To take an oral body temperature, the thermometer is placed under the client's tongue in the back to the left or right of the frenulum (where the tongue connects to the bottom of the mouth). Ask the client to close his/her lips (not teeth) to hold it in place. The length of time will vary depending on the specific electronic thermometer (e.g., 10-45 seconds for a large hospital model, 2-4 minutes for a handheld battery operated unit). They will beep when the proper amount of time has elapsed.
- *Axillary temperature*: Axillary temperatures are less accurate than oral temperatures, so they are typically used only when oral temperatures are contraindicated. Contraindications include dyspnea (difficult or labored breathing), surgical procedures involving the mouth or throat, very young children, and delirious or irrational patients (O'Sullivan & Schmitz, 1988). Clinical glass thermometers are typically used. Pat the underside of the arm and the side of the trunk dry if needed (do not rub or it will increase body temperature). Place the thermometer between the upper arm and the trunk (about two inches down from the armpit) and ask the client to hold the thermometer in place by pulling the arm across his/her chest. In some instances the therapist may need to hold the thermometer in place (e.g., young child, poor upper arm control). When recording the temperature, note that it was an axillary temperature.
- *Rectal temperature*: Rectal temperatures are typically used only with young children and infants when an oral or axillary temperature

reading is difficult or contraindicated. Place the infant or child in a prone position (on stomach). Put a dab of Vaseline on the end of a digital thermometer and insert the tip of the thermometer into the anus about ¼ of an inch. When the digital thermometer beeps, remove it and record the reading.

Pulse

When the left ventricle contracts it sends a wave of blood through the arterial system. The measure of these waves it called a pulse. A newborn's pulse can range from 70-170 beats per minute (average is 120) and continues to slow down as a person grows older. In a healthy adult, a pulse of 70 beats per minute is average (range is 50-100).

Factors that Influence Pulse

Pulse rate is typically a bit lower in males than females. There are also external variables that affect pulse rate including emotions (e.g., anxiety, pain), exercise (to meet increased oxygen demands), and systemic or local heat (fever or the use of a hot pack causes vasodilatation of peripheral vessels to dissipate heat).

Measurement

The pulse can be palpated in several areas. Arteries that are close to the skin (superficial arteries) in front of a bony surface are the easiest to feel because the artery can be sandwiched between the fingers and the bony surface to feel the flow of blood. These areas are called pulse points. Guidelines for common pulse points are

- *Radial* (on the wrist at the base of the thumb): The radial pulse is the most frequently used for monitoring pulse.
- *Temporal* (top of the cheekbone, in front of the ear): The temporal pulse is used if the radial pulse is difficult to feel or if it is contraindicated (e.g., arm casts). It is the second most common pulse point for pulse monitoring.
- *Carotid* (on the side of the neck): The carotid pulse is used in cardiac arrest. It is also commonly used for infants due to the difficulty in feeling a radial pulse and for monitoring blood flow to the brain.
- *Brachial* (the inside bend of the arm): Although the brachial pulse can be used to monitor pulse rate, it is most commonly used as a pulse point to measure blood pressure.
- *Popliteal* (behind the knee, easier to palpate when the knee is slightly flexed): The popliteal pulse is used to monitor lower extremity circula-

tion. It can also be used for measuring blood pressure.

- *Pedal* (on top of the foot between the big toe and the second toe, about three inches from the toes): The pedal pulse is used to monitor lower extremity circulation.

To palpate a pulse point, place the tips of the first two or three fingers on the pulse point and press firmly enough to feel the pulse. If you press too firmly the artery will become occluded and a pulse will not be felt. Once the pulse is detected, look at a watch or clock with a second hand and count the number of beats felt for one full minute. This is the pulse rate (e.g., pulse 74). The therapist can also take the pulse for 15 seconds and multiply it by four or take it for 30 seconds and double it. Taking a pulse rate for the full minute is the most accurate.

If the pulse points are difficult to palpate or they are contraindicated for medical reasons, the therapist can listen to (instead of feeling) the pulse (called an apical pulse). A stethoscope is placed directly over the top portion of the heart. Count the number of beats heard in a minute to obtain the pulse rate.

When monitoring a client's pulse, a therapist feels for rate, rhythm, and volume. Rate is the number of beats per minute. Rhythm describes the regularity of the beats. If the amount of time between each beat is the same, it is said to be regular or constant, as contrasted with an irregular or erratic rhythm. Volume refers to the force of each beat. The force of each pulse beat should be equal. When feeling the pulse, pay attention to how easily the pulse can be halted by applying pressure. If blood volume is high it will be difficult to halt the pulse (a bounding or full pulse). If blood volume is low it will be easy to halt the pulse (a weak or thready pulse). Therapists may also note the quality or feel of the arterial wall. The vessel should feel soft, smooth, flexible, and elastic, compared to vessels that feel hard, rigid, patchy, or cordlike. Sclerotic changes of the vessels are common as part of the aging process resulting in decreased smoothness and elasticity of vessels.

Respiration

Respiration rate is the number of inhalations per minute. Baseline respiration rates are taken in a relaxed state. Respiration rates can also be taken during exercise to monitor levels of exertion.

Factors that Influence Respiration

- *Exercise/metabolic rate*: Exercise and any other event that increases the metabolic rate increases

respiration rate due to the increased oxygen demand.
- *Age*: The respiration rate for a newborn is between 30 and 60 per minute. It gradually slows down until adulthood when the average respiration rate reaches a minimum of 12 to 18 a minute. In older adults, the respiration rate may be slightly higher due to decreased lung functioning associated with the aging process (decreased elasticity of the lung, decreased efficiency of exchange).
- *Sex and body type*: Men, as well as people who are tall and thin, typically have a greater vital capacity (ability to hold more air in the lungs) than women or people who are short and overweight. People with greater vital capacity need fewer respirations per minute.
- *Emotions*: Extreme emotions (e.g., fear, anxiety) can raise respiratory rate.

Measurement

To measure the base respiration rate, the person should be in a relaxed and normal state. The person must not know that respiration rates are being counted. If the person is aware that respiration rate is being recorded, the person may inadvertently or purposefully alter his/her breathing resulting in a skewed measure. Typically, vital signs are taken one after another (temperature, blood pressure, pulse, and then respiration), so a common trick is to continue acting as if you are taking the pulse but count the respirations instead. It is recommended that the person's chest be exposed so the therapist can assess the depth of breath (shallow or deep) and easily see respirations by the rise and fall of the chest. If this is not possible, a technique that can be helpful is to take the client's pulse on the wrist that is furthest from you so that the client has to cross his/her arm across the chest. The person's arm will rise and fall to indicate respirations. Inhalations or exhalations are counted for a full minute or for 30 seconds and then doubled. If a 30-second measure seems irregular (e.g., faster or slower than expected), it indicates the need to do a full minute count. When monitoring respirations, the therapist assesses the depth of breathing (by looking at the chest for a full rise and fall to note whether breathing appears to be deep or shallow), the rhythm of breathing (same amount of time between each breath; regular or irregular rhythm), and the character of the respirations (the amount of effort and the sound of the respirations). Some common terms used to describe the character of respirations include (O'Sullivan & Schmitz, 1988):
- *Dyspnea*: labored or difficult breathing.

- *Wheezing*: a whistling sound produced by air passing through a narrowed bronchi or bronchiole. It may be heard on both inspiration and expiration but is more prominent on expiration. Apparent with emphysema and asthmatic patients.
- *Stridor*: a harsh, high-pitched, crowing sound that occurs with upper airway obstructions caused by narrowing of the glottis or trachea (e.g., tracheal stenosis, presence of a foreign object).
- *Rales*: rattling, bubbling, or crackling sounds which occur because of secretions in the air passages of the respiratory tract. They may be heard with the ear but are most accurately assessed by use of a stethoscope.
- *Sigh*: a deep inspiration followed by a prolonged, audible expiration. Occasional sighs are normal and function to expand alveoli. Frequent sighs are abnormal and may indicate emotional stress.
- *Stertorous sounds*: a snoring sound from secretions in the trachea and large bronchi.

Blood Pressure

Blood pressure is the force that the blood exerts against the wall of a vessel.

Factors that Influence Blood Pressure

- *Blood volume*: Blood loss will lower blood pressure (e.g., blood loss of traumatic injury) and increased blood volume will raise blood pressure (e.g., blood transfusion).
- *Exercise*: Physical activity raises systolic blood pressure because there is a greater cardiac output.
- *Body position*: If the person is in a position other than those reviewed, it must be reflected in the documentation because different body positions can affect blood pressure readings by as much as 20 mmHg. When taking a brachial blood pressure, the person is seated with the arm supported at heart level (about four inches higher than a standard chair armrest). This type of chair is common at a blood-testing lab but is not usually accessible in a standard therapy environment. Therapists typically rest a person's arm on a tabletop, counter, or adjustable rolling bed or therapy table to raise the arm into this position. When taking a popliteal blood pressure, the client is placed into a prone position with the knee slightly flexed.
- *Emotions*: Emotional stress such as fear, anxiety, anger, excitement, and upset can raise blood pressure.

Measurement

Blood pressure is measured using a sphygmomanometer, a blood pressure cuff, and a stethoscope.

- *Brachial blood pressure*: The cuff is wrapped around the upper arm about an inch above the bend of the arm. The correct cuff size must be used to get a proper reading (e.g., infant, pediatric, adult, extra wide for popliteal blood pressure or for a client who is morbidly obese). The cuff should fit snugly but comfortably. The center of the cuff is lined up with the brachial artery (the inside bend of the arm). Most cuffs have an arrow on the cuff to help identify the center of the cuff. Put on the stethoscope. With one hand, place the stethoscope on top of the brachial artery below the cuff. With the other hand, close the valve on the bulb of the blood pressure cuff and squeeze it continuously until the needle (or mercury) on the meter rises about 20 mmHg above the anticipated systolic pressure (e.g., if the anticipated blood pressure reading is 120/80, pump the needle up to 140). Very slowly open the valve on the bulb to release a little bit of air. The needle will begin to fall. Readjust the valve (tighten or loosen) if needed (e.g., the needle is falling too quickly to be able to accurately hear the heartbeat so the therapist closes the valve a bit more to slow down the fall of the needle). Listen for the first audible heartbeat through the stethoscope. The number that the needle is on when the first audible heartbeat is heard is the systolic blood pressure reading (highest pressure against the arterial wall). Continue listening until the heartbeat is no longer heard. The number that the needle is on when the last heartbeat is heard is the diastolic pressure reading (lowest pressure against the arterial wall). If there is difficulty hearing a heartbeat, readjust the stethoscope and/or re-tighten the bulb valve and gently give it a pump or two to raise the needle a bit higher past the point of uncertainty (e.g., if you are at 120 and are not sure if the heartbeat started at 125 or 130, close the valve, pump it back up to 140, gently loosen the valve and let to let out a small amount of air and re-listen for the heartbeat). Once the systolic and diastolic pressures are identified, fully open the valve of the bulb to totally deflate the blood pressure cuff. Remove the cuff and clean the stethoscope with an alcohol swab.
- *Popliteal blood pressure*: If taking a brachial blood pressure is contraindicated (e.g., surgery) or if a comparison of upper and lower blood pressures is needed (e.g., to monitor peripheral vascular disease), a popliteal blood pressure can

be taken (behind the knee). The person is placed into a prone position (on the stomach). A wide blood pressure cuff is wrapped around the lower third of the thigh and centered on the popliteal artery. The person is asked to slightly flex the knee of the leg to be used (raise foot about six inches). The stethoscope is placed on the popliteal artery below the cuff and the same measurement procedure is followed as in the brachial blood pressure above.

Reference

O'Sullivan, S. & Schmitz, T. (1988). *Physical rehabilitation: Assessment and treatment*. Philadelphia, PA: F.A. Davis Company.

Walking Techniques

This section looks at several aspects of walking techniques, starting with guarding techniques. After that there is a discussion of how to help the client to walk safely on uneven surfaces, followed by a discussion of how to safely use assistive devices in challenging situations. Because this is a text about the ICF, we have chosen to use their term, "walking," rather than the older term "ambulating."

Guarding Techniques

One of the tasks of the therapist is to help the client improve his/her ability to use the walking and moving skills learned on the unit in real-world situations. While the unit or the therapy gym offers a few challenges, normal environments offer greater challenges such as uneven terrain, ramps, curbs, elevators, escalators, doors and doorways, curb cuts, and stairs.

The physical therapist assesses and addresses gait training. Once the client develops a gait pattern, the physical therapist consults with the recreational therapist about helping the client use these walking and moving techniques in a community environment. The physical therapist will review the techniques employed, the amount of assistance needed, the type of equipment used, the client's endurance level, walking and moving distance, cueing techniques, and other concerns. Once the physical therapist clears the client for walking and moving outside physical therapy sessions, the recreational therapist can begin his/her work. Walking on uneven surfaces is much different that walking on smooth, level indoor flooring and requires practice, patience, and the problem-solving support and education offered by the recreational therapist.

Walking and moving outdoors offers greater physical and cognitive demand due to uneven surfaces, weather, and obstacles:

- Outdoor walking and moving requires more cardiopulmonary and muscular endurance.
- Barriers challenge problem-solving skills.
- Incorporation of a task (e.g., picking flowers) requires integration of many learned skills and the need to develop new skills that were not developed in a clinic setting.

Every client will present with different needs for walking and moving. Some may require only close supervision, while others may require a more hands-on approach (e.g., blocking the knee from buckling while walking or supporting the client who has a strong lean to the right to stand upright). The recreational therapist must be aware of the client's individual needs. The best way to do this is to talk with the physical therapist. If the recreational therapist is not familiar with the specific techniques employed by the PT, the recreational therapist should ask for instruction.

The general procedure has the therapist position himself/herself in the optimal position for assisting the client. One of the most common guarding techniques is described here:

1. A client is more prone to fall to his/her weaker side. The therapist stands on the client's weaker side slightly behind the client. If the front of client is 12 o'clock, the therapist stands on client's right side at 4 o'clock or left side at 8 o'clock.
2. The therapist holds onto the client's transfer belt/waistband with one hand and places the other hand in front of the client's shoulder. For example, if the therapist is standing on the client's right side, the therapist reaches around with his/her left hand and grasps the left side of the client's transfer belt/waistband and places his/her right hand in front of the client's right shoulder.

Even if the client is documented as being independent or requiring only supervision for walking, the recreational therapist should assume the guarding position described above when walking with the client (whether on level indoor surfaces or uneven outdoor surfaces) until the therapist is confident in the client's skills. It is normal for a client to be rated at a particular level of assistance in the clinic and then require a greater amount of assistance in a different environment. If the client begins to lose his/her balance while walking, the therapist (in the guarding position) can react as follows:

1. If the client begins to fall backwards, the therapist can stop the momentum of the fall, supporting the back of the client with the hand/arm that is extended along the back of the client to allow the client to move back into an upright position. If the client requires physical assistance to get back into an upright position, the therapist can push the client forward with the hand that is on the transfer belt/waistband. Pushing is ergonomically preferred to pulling and the dynamic between the therapist's base of support and strength help reduce the client's impaired line of gravity and balance. If the therapist is unable to support the client enough to regain an upright position, the therapist, because s/he is slightly behind the client, can place

his/her knee behind the client and lower the client onto the knee. The therapist needs to make sure that his/her foot is firmly on the ground for this technique and it is best if the foot is pointed toward the client. Placement of the foot on the ground and lowering the client onto the knee allow the therapist to use gravity, alignment, and base of support to work in his/her favor.

2. If the client begins to fall to his/her stronger side (which is unlikely because people tend to fall to the weaker side), the therapist, because s/he is standing slightly behind the client, can extend his/her arm from the transfer belt/waistband to the client's stronger side hip to provide support. This stops the momentum of the fall and allows the client to move back into an upright position with the therapist's assistance, as needed.

3. If the client begins to fall forward, the therapist's hand that is in front of the client's shoulder provides support. The arm can be extended across the chest, if needed, to provide extra support. This stops the forward momentum of the client to allow the client to move back into an upright position with the therapist's assistance, as needed.

4. If the client begins to fall to his/her weaker side, the therapist provides support with the hand that is in front of the shoulder by moving it to the outside of the shoulder to stop the momentum of the fall. This allows the client to move back into an upright position with the therapist's assistance, as needed. The therapist can also block the fall using the side of his/her body.

New therapists should practice these techniques until they are comfortable. The supervising therapist should imitate various clients and have the new therapist guard them for walking and moving. As part of the practice, the supervising therapist should imitate common types of loss of balance and falls allowing the new therapist to learn how to support and "catch" the client.

Walking on Uneven Surfaces

Walking on uneven surfaces presents challenges for clients who have deficits in their walking skills. This section looks at general guidelines and ways to handle specific circumstances.

General Guidelines

• *Go slow*: Walking on uneven surfaces challenges balance more than even indoor surfaces. Clients can compensate for increased challenges by decreasing speed. Guide the client to walk at his/her own pace and not be pressured to move at

a faster pace than s/he can safely move. For example, if a car is stopped and waiting for the client to cross the parking lot, the client should walk at a comfortable pace and not give in to the pressure of "hurrying-up."

• *Make sure that device and footing is secure*: Attention to outdoor surfaces is imperative for safety. Clients are to look at least five feet ahead of them at all times. Clients are not to look down at their feet. Because of divided attention challenges (e.g., looking at store windows and walking at the same time), the clients may not anticipate uneven surfaces ahead. For example, if the client does not recognize ahead of time that s/he is going to have to step over a section of buckled sidewalk, loss of balance may occur. Encourage clients to stay aware of outdoor surfaces when walking. The client can minimize loss of balance if consistent attention is given to things in the environment that challenge the stability of the mobility device or make footing less than optimal. This is especially true for clients with impaired gait and gait accommodation strategies.

• *If the client feels that s/he is losing balance, STOP*: Clients may have a tendency to step forward when losing balance in the hope of regaining balance. However when walking outdoors the next step forward could challenge the client's balance even more and increase the chances of falling. Encourage clients to be aware of their balance at all times and, if they feel as if they are losing their balance, they should STOP immediately, regain balance, and then proceed.

Grass, Cobblestone, Broken Sidewalk, Uneven Ground

• Educate the client about the common guidelines for walking and moving on uneven surfaces (described previously).

• When advancing the assistive device (e.g., cane or crutch), make sure that all points of the assistive device are stable (e.g., if one walker leg is in a ditch, the walker becomes unstable and increases the client's risk of falling). If advancing one foot, ensure that footing is secure (if a prosthetic leg is advanced, be sure that the client knows how to compensate visually for lack of sensation). If assistive device or footing is not secure, client repositions the assistive device and footing until stability is achieved.

• Once the assistive device is secure, the client can carefully take a step forward, making sure that footing is secure. The client should adjust footing as needed.

Hills and Inclines

- The client's gait pattern may need to be altered so that each sequenced step is halted rather than maintaining a smooth movement. This is done to control speed and balance (e.g., roll walker forward, STOP, advance one foot, STOP, advance other foot, STOP, advance walker, STOP).
- Practicing the correct methods should improve the client's skill level.

Curbs

Curbs can be major barriers for clients with impaired mobility. A common sequence of stepping up and down a curb is described below, but the recreational therapist needs to know the technique the physical therapist is using with the client, as techniques vary and clients need to have consistent techniques. See Device Specific Mobility below for information on specific techniques for going up and down curbs using a specific device.

Going up curbs: Walk close to the curb and place the assistive device on the sidewalk on top of the curb. Step up on the curb with the unaffected or stronger leg and then follow with the weaker leg. Clients with new impairments concentrate so much on walking that they often forget which leg goes first. A few mnemonics to help remember which leg goes up first are "Up with the good," "The good go to heaven," and "Up with the good things in life."

Going down curbs: Walk to the edge of the curb and place the assistive device in the street. Step down with affected or weaker leg and then follow with the stronger leg. Mnemonics to help remember which leg goes down first are "Down with the bad," "The bad go to hell," and "Down with the bad things in life."

Escalators

Discourage using escalators with clients who have balance problems or who use an assistive device. Encourage the use of elevators instead. Escalators require the client to have good reaction time. Trying to open or close devices on an escalator can be very difficult. If the client does lose his/her balance and fall, the injury could be severe. Escalator rails usually do not move at exactly the same pace as the footplates. This difference in speed may cause some clients to lose their balance.

Device Specific Mobility

This section reviews common techniques for moving around and overcoming barriers using specific walking devices (canes, crutches, and walkers). Refer to the Equipment section for more information about these pieces of equipment. Refer to "Wheelchair Mobility" in the Techniques section for information on wheelchair mobility skills.

Canes

Walking

During the gait cycle the client places full weight on the "good" leg. During the weight acceptance and limb support phase of the gait cycle on the weaker side the client distributes his/her weight between the weaker leg and the cane. To simplify this description, tell the seated client to place the cane in the hand that is on his/her stronger side (e.g., if the client has weakness in his left leg, he is to hold the cane in his right hand). Push up from the chair to get into a standing position.

1. Advance the cane 12-18" in front of the current position of the stronger leg.
2. Step forward with the leg opposite the cane until the foot is directly across from the cane. The cane and the opposite foot are now the same distance in front of the back foot.
3. Now advance the other leg (on the cane side). The leg should step forward past the cane and the opposite leg.
4. Go back to step 1 and repeat.

Steps or Curbs

Use a handrail if it is available. To help remember what foot to lead with when going up and down stairs you can remember the following saying, "Up with the good, down with the bad."

To go up steps (or up a curb):
1. Client is to hold the cane in the hand that correlates with his/her stronger side (e.g., if the client has weakness in his left leg, he is to hold the cane in his right hand).
2. Step up with the strong leg onto the first step.
3. Then bring the cane up onto the first step.
4. Now step up with the weaker leg onto the first step. Both legs and the cane are all on the first step. This is called a "step to step" pattern, rather than a "step over step" pattern.
5. Go back to step 2 and repeat the pattern.

To go down steps (or down a curb):
1. Client is to hold the cane in the hand that correlates with his/her stronger side (e.g., if the client has weakness in his left leg, he is to hold the cane in his right hand).
2. Lower the cane down onto the first step.
3. Lower the weaker leg down onto the first step.
4. Lower the stronger leg down onto the first step.
5. Go back to step two and repeat the pattern.

Crutches

Crutch Gaits

There are six different crutch gaits. They are described in the lowest to the highest energy requirements. A repertoire of crutch gaits is helpful because the client can use a slow or fast gait to meet the demands of a situation or preference. Also, each crutch gait uses different muscles so it allows the client to rest or exercise muscles as needed.

- *Drag-to gait*: This gait is used when the client has very limited control or weight-bearing ability in the lower extremity and good to strong strength in the upper extremity.
    1. The client begins by placing both crutches in front of the body. The crutches are slightly wider than shoulder width and placed between one and two feet in front of the client.
    2. The client leans into the crutches, placing most of his/her body weight on the crutches.
    3. The client then drags his/her feet forward until they are between the crutches.
- *Four-point alternate gait*: This is a low and stable gait that is used when a client is able to move each leg separately and bear considerable weight on each leg.
    1. Advance the right crutch forward to a comfortable reach (approximately 12").
    2. Advance the left foot forward so that it is even with the right crutch.
    3. Advance the left crutch forward past the right crutch (about 12").
    4. Advance the right foot so that it is even with the left crutch.
    5. Repeat step one through four.
- *Two-point alternate gait*: This gait is a little faster than the four-point gait and requires a bit more balance.
    1. Simultaneously advance the right crutch and the left leg a comfortable distance (about 12").
    2. Simultaneously advance the left crutch and the right leg a comfortable distance.
    3. Repeat steps one and two.
- *Three-point alternate gait*: This is a fairly quick gait that requires significant upper arm and body strength because the arms bear the majority of the weight. It also requires a moderate amount of balance.
    1. Simultaneously advance both crutches and the weaker leg a comfortable distance. The crutches and the weaker leg should be at the same distance in front of the back leg when landing.

2. Next, advance the strong leg so that it is even with the crutches and the weaker leg. To do this, most of the weight is born through the arm.
3. Repeat steps one and two.
- *Swing-to-gait*: This gait is faster than the three-point gait and it requires even more upper arm and body strength to support the entire body weight. This is a common crutch gait for axillary crutches.
    1. Weight bear on the good leg(s).
    2. Simultaneously advance both crutches forward a comfortable distance (about 12").
    3. Place all of the body weight through the crutches by leaning forward and then swinging both legs simultaneously forward to meet the crutches.
    4. Repeat steps one through three.
- *Swing-through-gait*: This is the fastest crutch gait and is commonly used by runners.
    1. Weight bear on the good leg(s).
    2. Simultaneously advance both crutches forward a comfortable distance (runners typically extend this reach as far as possible).
    3. Place all of the body weight through the crutches by leaning forward and then swinging both legs simultaneously past the crutches.
    4. Quickly advance the crutches past the landing area of the feet.
    5. Repeat steps one through four

Sit to Stand
- Scoot to the edge of the seat.
- Place both crutches in the hand that correlates with the stronger leg.
- Use the chair armrests to push up to a standing position.
- Move crutches to both hands.

Stand to Sit
- Back up until the chair touches the back of the legs.
- Transfer crutches into the hand the correlates with the stronger leg.
- Stretch injured leg forward so that the knee is straightened and the heel rests on the floor.
- Reach back for the chair armrests for support to sit back into the chair.

Stairs and Curbs

Going up and down stairs and curbs with crutches demands a lot of strength and balance. There are several possible techniques besides the one described here. The recreational therapist, like all health professionals, consults the other members of the treatment team to identify what technique is currently recommended for the client.

To go up stairs (or a curb):

• Step onto the first step with strongest leg. Then, step onto the step with the weaker leg and both crutches simultaneously. Repeat this pattern to the top of the stairs.

• If there is a handrail, tuck both crutches underneath one arm and use the handrail like it is the other crutch.

To go down the stairs without a handrail (or a curb):

• Simultaneously lower the weaker leg and both crutches down onto the first step. Then lower the stronger leg onto the first step. Repeat this pattern to the bottom of the stairs.

NOTE: If a client is non-weight-bearing on one leg, it is dangerous to go up and down steps. It is recommended that alternatives be identified (e.g., elevator, bumping up the stairs on the buttocks). To go up curbs, push up on the crutches to hop up onto the curb on the strong leg and then bring up the crutches. To go down a curb, lower the crutches down the curb and then hop down the curb on the strong leg.

Walkers

Walking

Using a standard walker: Advance the walker a comfortable arm's length and then step forward with the weaker leg first and then the stronger leg following. Advance the walker forward, and then step again. Do not step into the walker. The client's feet should be next to the back feet of the walker after the step is complete. Stepping too far into the walker will cause the client to lose balance. Advancing the walker too far ahead and taking small steps will cause the client to lean forward and not stand upright.

Using a hemi-walker: The hemi-walker is in the hand on the stronger side. During the gait cycle the client places full weight on the "good" leg. During the weight acceptance and limb support phase of the gait cycle on the weaker side the client distributes his/her weight between the weaker leg and the hemi-walker.

Using a rolling walker: There are two ways to use a rolling walker.

• *Continual pushing technique*: The client continually pushes the walker forward while stepping (a smooth walk). The client should maintain an upright position. The client should not step too far into the walker (see standard walker use above). Clients who use this technique need to be very aware of their surroundings so they can note changes in surfaces and lift the walker appropriately to transition from one surface to another (small walker wheels tend to get stuck easily on raised sidewalk blocks, pebbles, etc.).

• *Halting technique*: Clients who do not have the awareness discussed above (whether from a cognitive impairment or general anxiety with the task) should be instructed to push the walker forward until the back legs of the walker are just past the client's feet. Halt the walker and then step forward. Push the walker forward again, step again, and so on. This decreases the chances of the walker becoming stuck on an object and the client stepping before the walker has fully advanced, causing the client to step too far into the walker and risk loss of balance and a fall. This is also a good technique for client's to use when they are walking outside on uneven surfaces. For example, a rolling walker does not roll easily on grassy surfaces. So if a client wants to walk across a patch of grass, s/he will need to roll the walker slowly forward in halting motions as previously described. In some instances, the client may need to pick up the walker and advance it like a standard walker. The therapist should be aware of the added stress that lifting the walker puts on the client and assess whether or not this is an appropriate technique (short of breath, loss of balance, increased blood pressure or heart rate). The halting technique is also good for going up and down inclines because, when s/he is going down a hill, the client sometimes feels that the walker is starting to get away from him/her and, when going up the hill, the client often begins to push the walker too far forward and begins to lean forward as if pushing the walker up the hill. A halting technique will minimize these occurrences and increase the client's safety.

Curbs

To go up a curb:

1. Move up as close as possible to the curb.
2. Lift the walker up onto the sidewalk.
3. While holding onto the walker handgrips, step up with the stronger leg onto the sidewalk and then lift up the weaker leg onto the sidewalk.

To go down a curb:

1. Move to the edge of the curb.
2. Lower the walker down into the street.

3. While holding onto the walker handgrips, step down onto the street with the weaker leg and then lower down the stronger leg.

<u>Stairs</u>

It is not recommended for a client to go up and down stairs with a walker, but it is not impossible. Clients can be taught to use the folded walker like a crutch for going up and down stairs. This requires a moderate amount of skill, strength, and balance and is not a general recommendation. Therefore, if the client desires to learn this skill or if it is foreseen that this skill will be needed to access the client's real-life environment, the recreational therapist should consult with the physical therapist to decide who will instruct the client in this skill determine the best technique to use.

Wheelchair Mobility

This section looks at the basics of wheelchair mobility. It is divided into four sub-sections: an introduction to wheelchair mobility, dependent wheelchair skills with a manual wheelchair, independent wheelchair skills with a manual wheelchair, and power wheelchair and scooter skills. If a client requires the assistance of another to perform a specific wheelchair skill (e.g., requires total dependence on another person to bump the wheelchair up a curb), refer to dependent wheelchair skills. If a client is learning how to perform the skill independently (e.g., learning how to pop a wheelie), refer to independent wheelchair skills. If a client is using a power wheelchair or scooter, refer to power wheelchair and scooter skills. Therapists can also refer to the Equipment section for information about wheelchair components and how they work.

Introduction

It is very likely that the recreational therapist will be working with clients who use wheelchairs for mobility. Therapists expect to work with clients using wheelchairs in rehabilitation settings and possibly in residential facilities for clients with mental retardation or with older adults in nursing homes. In addition, a therapist in psychiatric settings or community settings may also have clients who use wheelchairs. Some of the clients that the therapist works with will be new to wheelchair mobility and others will be very skilled and involved in athletic competitions such as the Paralympics. In most situations the therapist will be expected to determine the client's level of skill for community mobility and help increase those skills as needed.

Moving from point "A" to point "B" in a wheelchair is more than the ability to roll forward or backward. A whole range of skills is necessary to move about in the community with a wheelchair. The recreational therapist will not only need to be competent in all these skills but also must have the ability to teach others how to become competent. The recreational therapist is often in the "train the trainer" position for teaching the skills associated with wheelchair mobility. In many cases the recreational therapist will be teaching wheelchair mobility skills to the client and the client's primary caretaker. They, in turn, will need to teach others to help as time goes by. For the recreational therapy student that may mean practicing the skill during therapy labs and then spending forty-eight hours in a wheelchair, practicing all the skills, experiencing the challenge of problem solving for physical barriers in real-life situations and dealing with well-intentioned but inappropriate

actions and comments of people in the community. Therapists who have not practiced these skills as part of their training should also spend the time to gain wheelchair skills so they will be more effective in teaching their clients.

There are many skills required to move around the community in a wheelchair. They include:

- *Basic maneuvering*: Stopping; turning; ascending and descending ramps, curbs, and curb cuts; moving over uneven terrain; moving through elevators, doors, and doorways.
- *Advanced skills for maneuvering*: Stairs, escalators, slopes that exceed 1:12 grade (for every one inch rise a ramp should extend 12" to meet ADA accessibility guidelines).
- *Weather related challenges*: Heavy rain, snow, ice, extreme wind.
- *Accessing pubic mobility devices*: Community scooters (such as the ones found at grocery stores for clients using mobility devices) and public transportation (bus, train, taxi).
- *Transfers into public transportation*: Using low pivot transfers, standing pivot transfers, one-man vs. two-man transfers. This may include using a step-up block or a transfer board and knowing how to accommodate for low car ceilings and door handles that are in the way.
- *Changing the wheelchair configuration*: Opening and closing the wheelchair, removing or folding footrests, removing armrests, and removing support braces.
- *Special precautions*: Head-in vs. buttocks-in first car transfers with trunk flexion precautions (such as after hip replacement surgery), modifying height of vehicle seat to meet total replacement hip or other precautions.
- *Strapping and tie down*: Procedures for securing the wheelchair into a vehicle with the client still in the chair or securing the client into one of the seats of the vehicle without the wheelchair.

The recreational therapist must work directly with the other primary therapists (PT, OT) prior to instructing the client on specific wheelchair techniques to provide a consistent message. Ask if there are any community mobility skills that the other therapists have discussed with or taught to the client before you begin training. Ask the therapist if there are any additional suggestions or recommendations that s/he might have.

The recreational therapist will likely be working with family members and friends of the client who may need to have some instruction. It is important to determine if the caregiver is physically and mentally capable of providing assistance. Ask if s/he has any physical limitations that would be a contraindication for assisting the client with wheelchair mobility. For example, some contraindications might be lifting restrictions, cardiac restrictions, feeling uncomfortable about helping, etc. If the caregiver has limitations, the therapist should not, under any circumstances, allow the caregiver to perform wheelchair skills that are contraindicated due to a limitation. The therapist must decide if s/he should train the caregiver on how to instruct another and transfer the training task to the caregiver or schedule another training session with the newly identified caregiver. This decision is based on availability of the other caregiver and time constraints.

A little preliminary work helps avoid this type of situation. Contact the caregiver ahead of time to discuss availability and limitations. Document conversations with caregivers and statements of health for the rest of the treatment team to consider. A sample chart note might be "(6/26/06) Mary Smith, the client's daughter, notified via phone about the community mobility skills training session scheduled for 6/28 at 4 P.M. Daughter states no restrictions or limitations to perform skills." or "Mary Smith, client's daughter, attended 4/12 RT tx session for training. Upon question, daughter reported a history of lower back pain but felt that she had no limitations or restrictions. Daughter was asked to get clearance from primary physician to perform physical tasks without restrictions, otherwise another caregiver will need to be identified to assist client with dependent community wheelchair skills. Daughter's availability for training is minimal; therefore daughter instructed on techniques but not allowed to perform the task. Daughter scheduled to attend 4/18 session for community integration training with client. If daughter receives clearance further training will occur at that time."

When conducting wheelchair skills training, it is important to evaluate the appropriateness of the wheelchair that the client is currently using. It is not uncommon for clients in a rehabilitation hospital to receive a standard inpatient wheelchair for moving from therapy to therapy. The type of wheelchair being used within the facility may not be the type of wheelchair that the client will be issued when going home (e.g., using a standard cross-brace wheelchair in the hospital while a rigid wheelchair is on order for discharge). It is also not uncommon for hospital wheelchairs to have "problems" that hinder wheelchair skills training. For instance, some facilities bolt the anti-tipper bars onto the wheelchairs so that they do not fall off or get misplaced. This might work well for the hospital setting, but it is not

appropriate for community and home life. A client will not bolt his/her anti-tipper bars at home. In fact, the client and caregiver will need to flip up or remove the anti-tipper bars to perform some of the wheelchair skills (e.g., to bump the wheelchair up a curb). Another common problem with standard hospital wheelchairs is that they are often a heavy-duty style so that they last (about 40-50 pounds) while clients are often prescribed a lightweight wheelchair for discharge (about 28-36 pounds). The added weight of a heavy-duty chair can be especially difficult for older caregivers (e.g., lifting a 50-pound wheelchair into a car trunk is more work than lifting a 28-pound wheelchair). We have also had the unfortunate problems of leg rests and armrests that are part of the wheelchair frame (can't be removed or are bolted on the wheelchair), rigid backrests that are bolted to the frame preventing the wheelchair from folding, and old, heavy-duty wheelchairs that have not been folded in years so that when we try to fold them, they seem to be almost rusted in a fixed position.

Consequently, it can be very frustrating, when you are ready to teach a caregiver how to perform specific community wheelchair skills, to discover that the wheelchair that the client is currently using is not appropriate for training. Prior to conducting a training session, the therapist evaluates the appropriateness of the wheelchair. Make sure it is similar to the type of wheelchair that the client is going to use after discharge and that all of the parts of the wheelchair are working. If it is not appropriate, the therapist identifies another wheelchair to use for the training session. This can typically be accomplished by talking to the physical therapist or wheelchair room mechanic to borrow a wheelchair that is appropriate for the training session.

Components of Wheelchair Skills Training

When teaching community wheelchair skills, the therapist will want to include:
1. Appropriate techniques for moving in the community.
2. Awareness of physical barriers in the community.
3. Awareness of social barriers in the community;
4. Problem-solving skills that address barriers for both the client and the caregiver.
5. Maximizing community independence and overall mental, emotional, physical, and social health through involvement in the community.
6. Decreasing chances of injury from impaired performance of mobility skills.

7. Improving task performance to increase self-esteem, confidence, and likelihood of community involvement.

Therapists will find it helpful to refer to other sections of this book to assist with wheelchair skills training including the "Americans with Disabilities Act," "Community Accessibility Training," and "Community Problem Solving" in the Techniques section, and "Wheelchairs, Scooters, and Wheelchair Accessories" in the Equipment section.

Learning Methods

There are several considerations that make learning wheelchair skills easier. They include:
1. *Real-life environment*: Skills should be evaluated in a realistic community setting. This usually requires the therapist, client, and caregiver to go out into the community. Although performance in the client's real-life environment is ideal, this is sometimes not possible due to time constraints or distance. If this is the case, the area neighboring the hospital (e.g., local store) or the immediate area around the hospital, residential facility, or community center typically offers enough different challenges to allow the evaluation to be done without having to use public or private transportation. If going out into the community is not possible and it is a bad weather day that makes it unsafe or impractical for practicing wheelchair skills outside, use available indoor equipment (e.g., practice curb in the clinic, ramp in the hallway, public bathroom in the hospital, lay a piece of carpet on the gym floor, position chairs or cones for obstacles, hospital elevators).
2. *Teach skills one at a time*: Most clients and caregivers learn new skills best when the therapist works on just one new skill at a time. If the client is unable to attend the session (e.g., not feeling well), but the caregiver is available, the therapist may want to consider training the caregiver without the client being present (especially if the caregiver's availability for training is limited).
3. *Emphasize proper body mechanics and techniques*: See "Body Mechanics and Ergonomics" in the Techniques section for more information.
4. *Use a long mirror*: A long mirror can be positioned so that the client can see what the therapist is doing as s/he helps maneuver the chair (e.g., position the long mirror next to the curb so that the client can see what the therapist/caregiver is doing to bump the wheelchair up the curb). This offers the client a visual

demonstration of the skill and acts as a teaching tool for the client. For clients who will be needing assistance with the skill, "seeing" the skill performed helps the client to better understand the steps involved, thus improving his/her ability to instruct another person on how to provide assistance. For the client who is learning how to perform the skill independently, a long mirror provides visual feedback of performance (e.g., is the client leaning far enough forward prior to backing down a two inch curb independently) Seeing his/her actions in conjunction with feeling the correct position is ideal for learning physical skills.
5. *Demonstrate before practice*: If the therapist is teaching a caregiver to perform a skill, demonstrate the skill several times and then ask the caregiver (and client as appropriate) to verbally repeat the steps involved. Once they are able to repeat the steps verbally, ask the caregiver to try the skill (and ask the client to practice verbally instructing the caregiver to perform the specific steps involved in the skill). The therapist stands close to the client and caregiver offering cueing and physical assistance as needed. The therapist may need to provide step-by-step instructions at first. The goal is to maximize the caregiver and client's ability to perform the skill without the therapist's help.

Once one skill is accomplished, the therapist moves on to the next skill until all of the skills have been addressed.

Documentation

The therapist documents performance in several ways:
- *Percentage* (e.g., "Client able to verbally sequence the steps involved in bumping a wheelchair up a curb with 75% accuracy").
- *Assistance* (e.g., "Mary Smith, client's daughter, able to bump wheelchair up/down four-inch curb with minimal assistance from therapist.", "Client able to instruct caregiver on dependent community wheelchair skills correctly with minimal verbal cues from therapist.").

Dependent Wheelchair Skills

If a client requires physical assistance to perform a wheelchair skill, refer to this section (e.g., requires assistance to go up a hill). Before training begins, the therapist establishes the client's baseline of skills and knowledge regarding community mobility and evaluates/discusses the specific mobility obstacles and challenges that the client will face in his/her real-life environment and activities. This usually involves getting performance information from the physical therapist and then meeting with the client to ask questions and evaluate skills.

Depending on the needs of the client, the therapist employs a variety of techniques. Demonstrating the skills, repetition and practicing skills, cueing, and providing positive feedback are typical techniques. Having pictures and videos of others using wheelchairs also are good techniques. Even after a skill is learned, an important next step is to work on some "what if" situations associated with that skill. This helps the client learn to incorporate problem solving into every skill. Therapists must be careful, however, not to overload the client with "what ifs" that could induce feelings of fear and anxiety. For example, after the client feels comfortable going down curbs, start working on "what ifs" such as "What if there is a three-inch deep puddle of water at the bottom of the curb?" "What if your chair tips sideways as you go down the curb and you fall out of your chair?" and "What if your wheels are really wet from the rain and you think that you will have a hard time controlling the descent of the chair because the wheel is slippery?"

If the client does not have a caregiver who is able to handle barriers in the community with advanced wheelchair skills and/or the client is unable to instruct another on wheelchair skills because of limitations, the therapist will need to identify alternatives. These include:

1. Identifying specific places in the client's community that are totally wheelchair accessible.
2. Identifying (in writing) services and other outside sources that provide assistance. This includes services that provide door-to-door transportation (e.g., paratransit) that includes dealing with barriers (e.g., if there is a curb that the client has to bump up to get to the door of the community center, the driver will bump the client up the curb because it is a "door-to-door" service).
3. Exploring the possibility of hiring a caregiver for community outings.
4. Exploring assistance available within a facility or program (e.g., assistance staff available to help a person in a wheelchair overcome barriers in getting from class to class).
5. Bringing identified problems that significantly impact the client's lifestyle to the attention of the treatment team for problem solving (e.g., if the client is unable to propel the wheelchair on a college campus due to endurance restrictions, the team may want to explore the possibility of a power wheelchair).

Specific techniques to using a wheelchair for a dependent client are discussed below. The information can be modified into a client/caregiver handout. Handouts are especially helpful as a reference when the client and caregiver are trying to remember the steps involved with each skill. It is also helpful for the client/caregiver when they train others on the skills. Although the techniques described below are the most common, it does not mean that they are universal. Careful attention must be given to the appropriate techniques recommended by the client's physical therapist. Be sure to take out, add, or modify information as needed to reduce the risk of performing incorrect or inappropriate techniques and causing injury or harm to the client or caregiver.

The caregiver must wear rubber-soled shoes for good traction, limit accessories that can get in the way, and be medically cleared, as appropriate, prior to performing any training in wheelchair skills.

Movement Techniques

This section describes how a caregiver should move a wheelchair throughout a community setting.

Pushing the Wheelchair
* When pushing a wheelchair, hold both handgrips, stand up straight, and look at least five to ten feet in front of the wheelchair to avoid obstacles.
* Keep the wheelchair a safe distance from the curb edge and other obstacles.

Stopping the Wheelchair
* To stop the wheelchair, hold the handgrips tightly and stop walking.

Turning
* To turn the wheelchair to the right, pull back on the right handgrip and push forward on the left handgrip.
* To turn the wheelchair to the left, pull back on the left handgrip and push forward on the right handgrip.

Uneven Surfaces
* When going over uneven terrain (e.g., broken sidewalk, gravel, cobblestone), it is advantageous to pull the wheelchair over the surface backward rather than push the wheelchair over the surface forward.
* Leading with the large back wheels will decrease the chance of the small front wheels getting stuck on small obstacles (ditches, cracks, bumps).
* If you choose to push the wheelchair forward over the uneven surface, raise the front end and

roll on the back wheels. If you do not, the small caster wheels in front may get stuck and bring the wheelchair to an abrupt stop. This is very dangerous, especially if the client is not wearing a seatbelt to keep the client from being thrown from the wheelchair.

Balance Point

This is a basic community mobility skill. It is the process of tipping the wheelchair back onto the large wheels with the front wheels in the air. There is a balance point where the weight of the wheelchair and client are resting directly over the back wheels. It will feel as if there is no pull for the wheelchair to tip either forward or backward. This skill is performed to get over many community obstacles (e.g., curbs, raised sidewalk squares).

- Tell the client that you are going to tip the wheelchair backwards.
- If the anti-tipper bars are turned down, turn them up or remove them completely to allow the wheelchair to be tipped backwards.
- Place one foot on a tipper bar.
- Hold on tightly to both handgrips.
- Push down on the tipper bar with your foot and simultaneously pull back on handgrips. Pull your hands back to your hips. Do not push down.
- Push with your foot and pull with your arms until the wheelchair is in full balance point position
- This will tip the person back in the wheelchair.

Curbs

To go up a curb:
- Stop the wheelchair about six inches away from the curb.
- Assume the balance point (refer to *Balance Point* for instructions).
- Roll the wheelchair forward until the back wheels hit the curb.
- Put your foot back on one of the tipper bars and slowly lower the caster wheels onto the sidewalk.
- Turn sideways, bend your knees, and place your hip against the back of the wheelchair.
- Using your hip and taking small side steps, "bump" the back wheels up over the curb.

To go down a curb:
- Back the wheelchair up to the edge of the curb.
- Stand sideways in the street with your hip facing the wheelchair.
- Roll the wheelchair backwards so that it rests against your hip.
- Bend your knees (and take small steps away from the curb as needed) to lower the back wheels onto the street.

- After the back wheels are on the street, face the wheelchair, push down on one of the tipper bars, and assume the balance point.
- Once in the balance point position, roll the wheelchair backwards until the caster wheels (and the leg rests) are clear of the curb.
- Place your foot back on the tipper bar for resistance and lower the caster wheels onto the ground.

Ramps

To go up a ramp:
- Approach the ramp
- If the ramp does not smoothly meet the sidewalk (e.g., there is a "lip"), assume the balance point to get the caster wheels over the lip.
- Once the caster wheels are on the ramp you can utilize one of two techniques:
- If it is a slight incline, you can push the wheelchair up the ramp facing forward. Be sure to keep a relatively straight back and use your legs to push the wheelchair up the ramp. *Do not use your back!*
- If it is a steep ramp, turn sideways and place your hip against the back of the wheelchair. Take small side steps. *Do not put your feet together!* Each time you step, be sure to leave a space between your two feet. This will give you a good base of support.

To go down a ramp use one of these two techniques:
- If it is a slight ramp and the person does not have any problems with trunk control, go down the ramp facing forward. It might be helpful to hold the curve of the handgrips (closer to the back of the wheelchair seat) for a better grip.
- If it is a steep ramp or the person does not have good trunk control, you may want to take the wheelchair down the ramp backwards. Place your hip against the back of the wheelchair and do side steps down the ramp. *Do not put your feet together!* Each time you step, be sure to leave a space between your two feet. This will give you a good base of support.

Escalators

Most escalators have a warning sign that prohibits strollers and wheelchairs. Elevators should always be your first choice for accessing other floors. However, in case of an emergency, it is good to know how to go up or down an escalator if it is your best option. Only consider this option:

- If you are on a lower or upper floor that does not have a formal or informal access (e.g., a service loading area) to the outside of the building.
- If the elevator is broken and it will not be repaired in an appropriate amount of time.
- If there are no elevators available (e.g., a service elevator).
- If it is determined that bumping the wheelchair up or down a stairwell is more dangerous than using the escalator (e.g., fire in stairwell, helpers lack strength or endurance to bump the wheelchair up or down the stairwell).
- If emergency personnel are not available (emergency personnel should be your first choice; they will either bump you up and down the stairs in the wheelchair or carry you up and down the stairs in a "blanket carry" and transport the wheelchair empty and folded).

Technique for going up an escalator:
- Measure the width of the escalator to make sure it can accommodate the width of the wheelchair.
- Remove anti-tipper bars and instruct the person in the wheelchair to lean forward.
- Roll the wheelchair onto the escalator (the first two steps are together and flat on the escalator).
- As the steps separate, the front caster wheels will be on the top step and back power wheels will rest on the lower step.
- The helper is behind the wheelchair providing support to the back of wheelchair to keep it from rolling backwards. Do not put the brakes on. The helper may find it best to place both hands flat against the back of the wheelchair rather than holding the handgrips.
- The person in the wheelchair can hold the escalator hand rims if the hand rims are going at the same speed as the escalator footplates (otherwise it is best to just lean forward with the hands on the lap).
- When approaching the top of the escalator, the helper pushes forward on the wheelchair to roll it off of the escalator.

Technique for going down an escalator:
- Measure the width of the escalator to make sure it can accommodate the width of the wheelchair.
- Remove the anti-tipper bars and instruct the person in the wheelchair to lean forward.
- The helper steps backwards onto the escalator and pulls the wheelchair backwards onto the escalator, supporting the back of the wheelchair to prevent it from rolling backwards.
- As the steps separate, the front caster wheels will be on the top step and the back power wheels will be on the lower step.

- Do not put the brakes on. The helper may find it best to place both hands flat against the back of the wheelchair rather than holding the handgrips.
- The person in the wheelchair can hold the escalator hand rims if the hand rims are going at the same speed as the escalator footplates (otherwise it is best to just lean forward with the hands on the lap).
- When approaching the bottom of the escalator, the helper steps off the escalator and then pulls backwards on the wheelchair to roll it off of the escalator.

Elevators
- It is best to pull the wheelchair into an elevator backwards and align the wheelchair with the door opening. This allows you and the client to easily see where you are when the doors open, view the floor numbers, and easily exit the elevator.

Stairs

Going up and down stairs is a difficult maneuver and always requires two people working together. One person alone should never attempt this. For going up or down stairs, the strongest person should be in the back.

To go up steps:
- Remove the leg rests.
- Back the wheelchair up until the large wheels rest against the bottom step.
- The person in back must be at least one step ahead of the wheelchair at all times. The back person holds the curve of the handgrips closest to the back seat of the wheelchair. The front person holds the front wheelchair frame.
- Slightly tip the wheelchair into a wheelie position. The greater the tilt, the harder it is to control the wheelchair on the steps. By tipping the wheelchair backwards, the individual's legs will swing slightly under the wheelchair seat so that they will not be in the way of the front person.
- The back person is the "counter." On the count of three, the back person rolls the wheelchair up onto the first step as the second person pushes the chair toward the step.
- The back person readjusts his foot location while the front person stabilizes the wheelchair by continually pushing the wheelchair into the step.
- Again, on the count of three they roll the wheelchair up another step and so on to the top of the stairs.

- When you reach the top landing, lower the front caster wheels onto the landing and replace the leg rests.

To go down steps:
- Use the reverse of going up steps. There are only a few differences: 1. instead of rolling up the step you roll down the step and 2. the person in back should have one foot on the same step as the wheelchair and one foot above it.

Narrow Doorways

If a doorways is too narrow to get through you can:
- Place a chair on the other side of the doorway and transfer through the door onto the chair. Fold up the wheelchair, roll it through the doorway, open it, and then transfer back onto the wheelchair.
- If the narrow door is in the client's home s/he should consider enlarging the door by removing the woodwork surrounding the door or installing swing away hinges that allow the door to swing completely open so that the width of the door is not an issue. These suggestions will provide an additional inch or so in width.

Manual Doors

Forward facing method (person using wheelchair is able to help)
- Approach the door normally.
- The individual in the wheelchair assists by pushing or pulling the door open with the arm closest to the door hinge.
- The helper can assist with holding the door open and pushing the wheelchair through the door.

Forward facing method (person using wheelchair is unable or limited in ability to assist)
- Approach the door normally.
- Helper opens the door and uses his/her back and feet to hold the door open.
- Helper grabs the side of the wheelchair and pulls the wheelchair through the doorway.

Backward facing method (This is a good choice if there is a raised doorsill.)
If the door opens away from you:
- Back up to the door.
- The helper pushes the door open with his/her back and legs and maintains the door opening with his/her foot while pulling the wheelchair through the doorway.

If the door opens towards you:
- The helper pulls the door open and maintains the opening with his/her foot.
- Push the wheelchair backwards through the doorways by holding the side/front of wheelchair OR walk backwards through the door while pulling the wheelchair through the doorway backwards (the person's arms are held inside the wheelchairs so that the door rubbing along the wheelchair does not hurt the person's hands and arms.

Car Transfers

Standing-pivot transfers and transfer board transfers are the most common transfer techniques for entering and exiting an automobile.

Standing Pivot Transfer
- A standing pivot transfer needs to have the car on a level surface (not up against a curb).
- Open the car door.
- Push the wheelchair up to the open car door and position it at a slight angle. The wheelchair should not be side by side with the seat of the car because the large back wheels and the armrest will be in the way of the person transferring.
- Remove the leg rests. You may need to reposition the wheelchair to remove the leg rests since they have to swing out to the side and the car would be in the way.
- Lock the brakes on the wheelchair.
- Remove the armrest that is closest to the car.
- The client scoots forward in the wheelchair and places his/her feet flat on the ground slightly behind the knees (slight flexion).
- The client leans forward and stands upright. If the client needs assistance with standing, the wheelchair may need to be positioned back further from the seat of the car to allow room for the caregiver to stand in front of the client and assist with the transfer. In some instances, the caregiver may be able to assist the client from behind the wheelchair by reaching over the back of the wheelchair seat.
- The client pivots on his/her feet and turns his/her body so that the back is lined up with the seat of the car.
- The client can hold the car dashboard or back of the seat for support; do not hold the car door because it moves and gives a false sense of security.
- Slowly lower buttocks onto the seat of the car.
- Swing legs into car.
- Buckle seatbelt.

Transfer Board
- Follow the first six steps listed in the standing pivot transfer instructions above.
- One end of the transfer board is placed under the person's buttocks and other end rests on the seat of the car (a long board is often preferable to a short board for car transfers).
- The client does a series of small lifts across the board until his/her buttocks are on the seat of the car.
- Lift legs into the car.
- The client then leans towards the middle of the car so that pressure is taken off of the buttocks and the board can be pulled out from underneath the buttocks.

Public Bathrooms

Maneuvering a wheelchair in a public bathroom can be difficult, especially if it is not fully wheelchair accessible. The height of the toilet, the availability of bathroom bars, and the width of the stall may not meet the client's needs and, therefore, the client may require more assistance in a public bathroom than at home.

Some wheelchairs have an option of a zipper back so that you can back into the bathroom stall, unzip the back of the wheelchair, and slide back onto the toilet. Some clients choose to transfer onto the toilet using a standing-pivot transfer or a transfer board. If the client chooses one of these transfers, it is important to practice it in a tight environment and evaluate the different positioning options that may be available to perform such a transfer.

Clients should become familiar with their bowel routine to reduce the need to transfer onto a toilet.

Refer to "Community Problem Solving" in the Techniques section for specific recommendations for using a public bathroom.

Folding a Manual Wheelchair

There are different procedures for reducing the bulk of a wheelchair depending on its design. The basic procedures for the most common types of chairs are presented below.

Cross-Brace Wheelchair
- Remove the leg rests.
- Remove the seat cushion.
- Remove any backpacks or bags on the back of wheelchair.
- Remove the back of the wheelchair (if hardback).
- The helper approaches the wheelchair at an angle, bends at the knees, and grabs the front and back of the wheelchair seat. Pulling up on the wheelchair seat will cause the wheelchair to fold.

Rigid Wheelchair
- Remove leg rests (if applicable), armrests, seat cushions, and any pouches or backpack from the wheelchair.
- Grab hold of the string that runs along the back of the wheelchair. Pull the string away from the chair and push the back of the wheelchair forward so that it collapses onto the wheelchair seat.
- Tilt the wheelchair on its side so that one wheel is off the ground.
- Stabilize the wheelchair with one hand while simultaneously pushing the wheel lock button found in the middle of the wheel with the other hand. This will release the wheel and it can be pulled off the wheelchair frame.
- Complete the same process to remove the other wheel.
- Remove or flip up the anti-tipper bars, if applicable.

Transporting a Wheelchair

Place a sofa-sized throw blanket over the open trunk so that half of it lies inside the trunk and the other half hangs outside the trunk. This will help keep the car paint from getting scratched and it will also help for getting the wheelchair out of the trunk. Having a blanket lining the floor of the trunk helps move the wheelchair in and out. When sliding the wheelchair into the trunk, the blanket may get wadded up under the wheelchair. Try to arrange the blanket so that it does not slide backwards into the trunk with the wheelchair. Instead of leaning far into the car trunk to pull the wheelchair out (which can hurt your back), grab the blanket and pull on it. The blanket will help guide the wheelchair up and out of the trunk so that you don't have to lean in so far.

In and out of the trunk (one-person lift):
- Fold the wheelchair according to previous directions. It is best to fold the wheelchair next to the trunk as everything taken off the wheelchair can be easily placed in the trunk. If the trunk is small, place the wheelchair parts into the trunk after the wheelchair is placed into the trunk so that the wheelchair can easily slide into the trunk without getting caught on the wheelchair parts.
- Lock the brakes on the wheelchair.
- Stand to the side of the wheelchair.
- Spread your feet apart for better balance and proper body mechanics. The width of the wheelchair is most desirable for the width of your stance.
- Bend your knees and tilt the wheelchair in towards your body so that it rests against you.

- Lean over the top of the wheelchair so that your arms hang over the other side of the wheelchair.
- Grab the wheelchair frame wherever you are most comfortable. Do not hold the wheels as they could become unlocked and move.
- Pull the wheelchair into your chest and, using your legs, lift the wheelchair up so that it juts out in front of you.
- Place the wheelchair in the trunk.
- Put all of the accessories that are not already in the trunk into the trunk (backpack, leg rests, cushion, etc.).

In and out of the trunk (two-person lift)
- Follow the first three steps in the previous directions.
- Stand on opposite sides of the wheelchair.
- Lock the brakes on the wheelchair.
- One person holds the handgrips and the tipper bars and the other person holds the front frame of the wheelchair.
- On the count of three, both people bend their knees and lift the wheelchair into the car trunk.

Alternatives: Wheelchairs can also be placed into the back of pick-up trucks and sport utility vehicles, as well as onto the floor of the back seat of a large two-door car. An overhead wheelchair carrier may be considered (see "Car Transfers" and "Wheelchair Loading" in the Independent Wheelchair Skills section below) or a car trailer (see "Transporting Wheelchairs" in the Power Wheelchair and Scooter section below).

Independent Wheelchair Skills

The treatment goal for many clients is to be independent in community wheelchair skills. In addition to having the physical strength, endurance, range of motion, and cognitive ability to be independent, there are other skills required. Some of the skills necessary for independent community wheelchair skills include:
- Demonstrating various methods for wheelchair propulsion, stopping, turning, and popping wheelies.
- Understanding the components of the wheelchair and how they work, including folding and opening the wheelchair.
- Problem solving physical barriers (curbs, ramps, curb cuts, uneven terrain, stairs, elevators, escalators, doors, and doorways).
- Transporting the wheelchair, including using public and private vehicles.
- Using community scooters.

Problems identified during recreational therapy sessions that impact the client's lifestyle should be brought to the attention of the treatment team. An example of a problem would be a client being unable to propel his wheelchair on a college campus due to endurance restrictions. The team may want to explore the possibility of a power wheelchair if this does not pose any additional problems such as a college campus that is not accessible to power wheelchairs, but is moderately accessible to manual wheelchairs.

Please refer to "Wheelchairs, Scooters, and Wheelchair Accessories" in the Equipment section for information on wheelchair components and accessories that affect independent community wheelchair skills (e.g., push gloves, tires, grade aids).

Movement Techniques

This next section describes how to move a wheelchair independently throughout a community setting.

Propelling the Wheelchair
There are two common techniques for propelling a wheelchair that assist with energy conservation and proper postural alignment. In general, the use of both upper extremities simultaneously is the most energy efficient.

Push and glide: Grip the hand rims slightly behind the trunk and simultaneously push the rims forward in a long stroke, releasing the hand rims while maintaining proper posture and allowing the wheels to glide freely.

Circular push: Grip the hand rims a little behind the top of the hand rim and continue to full extension of the arms and as far as body balance allows (forward and down). At full extension release the hand rims. The hands circle around back to the initial grip, re-grasping the hand rims, and pushing forward and down again. The arms should look like they are moving in a circular motion around the wheel.

Stopping the Wheelchair
To stop the wheelchair grip the hand rims tightly, stopping the motion of the wheels. When going down an incline, hold the hand rims loosely and let them slide through the hands. Tighten and loosen the grip as necessary to decrease or increase speed.

Turning
- To turn the wheelchair to the right pull backwards on the right hand rim while pushing forward with the left hand rim.

- To turn the wheelchair to the left pull backwards on the left hand rim while pushing forward with the right hand rim.

Rough Terrain

- When going over uneven surfaces, the client has the option of going forwards or backwards. The type of tires (large, pneumatic front casters compared to small, hard-plastic casters) will determine the method used.
- If the surface is not too uneven or bumpy and the client has large, pneumatic casters, the chair may easily go over the surface forward.
- Small, hard-plastic casters will not go over such surfaces as easily and could possibly get stuck in small cracks and divots. If this is the case, consider pulling the wheelchair over the surface backwards.
- Large power wheels will go over the surface much more easily and the front casters should follow.
- If the front casters become stuck (whether in forward or backwards motion), try turning the chair side to side to work the casters out of the rut.
- In addition to avoiding getting stuck, the correct technique will also reduce the chance of tipping over or falling out of the chair. If the chair stops abruptly, the client can be thrown from the chair, especially if s/he is not wearing a seatbelt.

Wheelies

This is a basic and fundamental skill for community mobility. This method is recommended for teaching this skill. It is a good idea for the client to wear a bicycle helmet or other head protection while learning how to do a wheelie. Refer to "Wheelchairs, Scooters, and Wheelchair Accessories" in the Equipment section for information on wheel positioning necessary to be able to perform wheelies.

To teach the appropriate wheelie position, the therapist tips the wheelchair backwards using the handgrips and the lever bars until the proper balance point is achieved (anti-tipper bars will need to be flipped up or removed). The client in the wheelchair focuses on maintaining the balance point through adjustment of the wheelchair and his/her body. It may be beneficial to instruct the client on a soft surface, such as a mat, until confidence is gained. Clients are never instructed to practice wheelie skills alone until the clinician feels the client is competent with the skills.

Once the client is comfortable and confident in maintaining the balance point, s/he works on initiating a wheelie as follows:

- Place the hands on the wheel rims slightly in front of the trunk.
- Gripping the rims tightly, push forward, leaning back in the wheelchair to get the front wheels of the chair off the ground.
- Maintain the wheelie position as practiced above.
- To return the wheelchair to a standard position lean forward and control the lowering of the wheelchair with body position and handgrip.
- Check to make sure feet are properly placed on the footrests.
- Work on movement wheelies. These are wheelies where the client moves the wheelchair forwards, backwards, to the left or right, and in a full circle while in a wheelie position. The client will need these skills for using a wheelchair for community mobility, such as rolling down a curb in the wheelie position.

Curbs

To go up a curb

From a static position:
- Roll the wheelchair up to within a few inches of the curb.
- Pop a wheelie and move forward until the casters are on the curb.
- To get the back wheels onto the curb, begin with the casters as close to the edge of the curb as possible. The client may need to back the wheelchair up a bit depending on the height of the curb. This will help to give the back wheels some room to gain momentum.
- Lean forward in the wheelchair and push forward on the tire/hand rims to roll the back wheels up onto the curb. Some people find it helpful to rock the back wheels up onto the curb (e.g., one... give a push... two... give a harder push... three... push with all your strength). Rocking also helps build momentum to get the back wheels up onto the curb.

In a dynamic position: This method requires much less strength but very good timing and skill.
- Roll towards the curb with all four wheels on the ground.
- Just before reaching the curb, pop into a wheelie position.
- Lower the caster wheels onto the curb BEFORE the back wheels hit the curb.
- Lean forward in the wheelchair and push hard on the hand rims to bring the back wheels up onto the curb in one smooth motion.

To go down a curb

From a static position:
- Back the wheelchair to the curb edge.
- Lean forward in wheelchair and place your hands on tires/hand rims.
- Slowly lower the back wheels onto the street in a controlled roll.
- To lower the caster wheels, place one hand forward on the tire/hand rim and the other hand slightly behind the torso on the tire/hand rim.
- Pull back with the forward hand and push forward with the back hand. This will cause the wheelchair to spin to one side.
- Spinning the caster wheels off of the curb to the side prevents the roller bar or footplates from becoming stuck on the curb.

In a dynamic position: This method is much quicker; however it does require good timing and skill.
- As you approach the curb in a forward direction, pop into a wheelie.
- While in the wheelie position, bump down the curb on the back wheels and then lower the caster wheels to the street.

Ramps
To go up a ramp:
- Pop a small wheelie if there is an edge/lip to the ramp. Not all ramps flow smoothly from one surface to the other.
- Lean forward in the wheelchair.
- Place both hands on the tire/hand rims of the wheelchair and push simultaneously.
- If the ramp is really steep (greater than a 1:12 ratio) and it has a decent width, try pushing up the ramp in a zigzag fashion. This will cut the grade of the ramp.

To go down a ramp:
Forwards: If the ramp does not have any obstacles that could pose a danger (e.g., holes, debris) and it is not too steep to handle, go down the ramp forwards.
- Place both hands on the tires/hand rims and lean back in the wheelchair.
- Slowly control the roll down the ramp by opening and closing the hands to loosen and tighten the grip as needed.

Backwards: If the ramp is too steep to handle or there are obstacles that could pose a danger (e.g., pebbles, sticks), go down the ramp backwards.
- Place both hands on the tires/hand rims and lean forward in the wheelchair.

- Slowly loosen and tighten the grasp to control the roll of the wheelchair down the ramp.

Stairs
Going up and down stairs independently with a wheelchair is very challenging and difficult. The client will need a lot of upper body strength and determination. People who are most likely able to perform these skills are young individuals with low paraplegia.

Ascending Stairs (going up stairs)

Ascending stairs on your buttocks:
- Transfer from the wheelchair to the second step.
- Tilt the wheelchair back onto the step (unfolded).
- Bump up one more step.
- Reposition the legs on next step.
- Pull wheelchair up one step and stabilize the wheelchair on the step while bumping up another step.
- If the wheelchair is difficult to stabilize while bumping up to the next step, try to hold the wheelchair with one hand and use the other hand to assist in raising the buttocks to the next step.

Ascending stairs in a wheelchair:
- Buckle seatbelt.
- Tilt wheelchair backwards so that the back of the wheelchair rests on the steps.
- Grab the rail with the closest hand (e.g., hold the right rail with the right hand).
- The other hand grabs the wheelchair tire/hand rim.
- Use the hand on the rail to pull the wheelchair up one step while the hand on the tire/hand rim also helps to roll the wheelchair up one step by pulling backwards on the tire/hand rim.
- Reposition the hands and continue.

Descending stairs (going down stairs)

Descending stairs in wheelchair backwards:
- Buckle seatbelt.
- Back wheelchair up to top step.
- Hold one rail with BOTH hands (one hand above the other) and slowly lower the wheelchair down the stairs one step at a time, repositioning hands as needed.

Descending stairs in wheelchair forwards:
- Buckle seatbelt.
- Initiate a wheelie position at the edge of the top step.
- Lower down the stairs in a wheelie position, using the tires/hand rims to control the descent.

- To assist in stabilizing the wheelchair, pull back on the tires/hand rims.

Doorways

It is important to know the width of the wheelchair, especially if it is a wide-width wheelchair or a wheelchair that has camber. To measure the width of a wheelchair measure from outer hand rim to outer hand rim. A standard doorway is 32" wide. A standard width wheelchair should fit through the majority of household and community doors. However, there will be times, even with a standard wheelchair, that a client will experience difficulty. Here are several ways to work around this.

Consider removing molding around the door, installing swing-away hinges, removing the door, using alternatives for doors (e.g., curtains, pocket doors), or expanding the doorway width through remodeling.

To transfer through the door:

- Place a chair on the other side of the doorway (e.g., side by side for transfer board transfer or at an angle for standing pivot transfer).
- Transfer from the wheelchair to the other chair through the doorway.
- Collapse or somewhat collapse the wheelchair and roll it through the doorway.
- Open the wheelchair and transfer from the chair to the wheelchair.

Manual Doors

If the door opens away from you (forward method):

- Approach the door.
- Push the door open as much as possible with one hand.
- While pushing the door open with the one hand, place the other hand on the tire or hand rim and push the wheelchair through the door. Chances are, if you don't have good momentum, you will be unable to complete this step smoothly. Typically, you will be able to get the leg rests of the wheelchair into the doorway before experiencing difficultly. The leg rests will help hold the door open while you give the door another push and propel yourself through the doorway. If the door is light enough, you may be able to give the door one more big push and then quickly push the wheelchair through the door with both hands on the tires/hand rims. It's a good idea to place your hands on top of the tires when pushing. This way, if the door swings back when you are pushing the wheelchair through the door, it will hit the outside of the hand rim and not your hands. You may also find it helpful to continue

pushing with just one hand when going through the door while maintaining contact with the door with the other hand to keep it open.

If the door opens away from you (backwards method):

- Back up to the door.
- Pull back on both tires/hand rims and push through the door. Using the tires instead of the hand rims may save you a scrape from the door.

If the door opens towards you:

- Approach the door in a forward position.
- Stay to the side of the door. For example, if the door handle is on the right hand side, align the wheelchair on the right side of the door so that the left hand can easily extend to pull the door open. This also positions the wheelchair farther away from the door hinge, which will make it easier when going through the doorway.
- When pulling the door open with the left hand, pull back on the right tire/hand rim to assist in opening the door.
- Push forward on the right tire/hand rim to spin the wheelchair forwards and to the left. This will help block the door open with the leg rests.
- If the door is very heavy and you cannot hold the door open to spin the leg rests into the door, this method might be helpful:
  a. When approaching the door, leave approximately a two-foot space between the door and the wheelchair. Put on the wheelchair brakes. Reach forward with the left hand and pull the door open.
  b. Since the brakes are on, the chair will not move. Reposition the left hand to the inside of the door.
  c. Release the right brake and spin the leg rests into the doorway. Release the left brake. Now you have successfully blocked the door open.
- Once the door is blocked open, push the door open further with the left hand and push the wheelchair through the door with the right tire/hand rim.
- If it is difficult to hold the door open with one hand and push with the other, give the door one big push open and then propel through the door using both hands. You can also plow through the door at an angle with power from both hands, using the force of the wheelchair to open the door.
- Place your hands on top of the tires when pushing through a door. If the door swings closed, it will hit the hand rim and not your hand.

<u>Escalators</u>

Refer to "Escalators" in the Dependent Wheelchair Skills section for forward information.

To go up or down an escalator in a wheelie position:

- Approach the step of the escalator and initiate a wheelie position.
- Hold the rails of the escalator while in a wheelie position for the descent or ascent.
- Use hands on the rails to assist with maintaining wheelie position.
- When approaching the end of the escalator, get ready to let go of the rails.
- There is usually a lip at the end of the escalator so you will have to be aware of maintaining the wheelie position long enough to clear the lip.
- When letting go of the rails, quickly place both hands on the tires and hand rims, lower the front wheels to the ground, and push the back wheels off of the last escalator step.

To go up or down an escalator in a non-wheelie position

- Refer to the methods described in the Dependent Wheelchair Skills section, minus the assistance.

Folding a Manual Wheelchair

See "Folding a Manual Wheelchair" in the Dependent Wheelchair Skills section. The steps are the same.

Car Transfers

The stand pivot transfer (SPT) and transfer board (TB) transfer are the most common techniques for entering or exiting an automobile. Refer to "Car Transfers" in the Dependent Community Wheelchair Skills section. The techniques are the same minus the physical assistance.

Clients who have lower extremity involvement (e.g., spinal cord injury) with no or minimal upper extremity involvement may be unable to stand upright for the standing pivot transfer or have difficulty controlling the position of the legs for transfer board transfers. They may find one of these techniques easier:

- Place one or both legs in the car before the transfer or during the transfer (e.g., place both legs on the floor in the front seat) and use a sit pivot to transfer to the seat of the car.
- Place one leg on the front seat floor and the other foot flat on the ground outside the car, complete two lifts across the transfer board, lift the other leg onto front seat floor, and then complete the

final lifts across the transfer board onto the seat of the car.

If the client is interested in driving, the physician may refer him/her to an adaptive driving program to fully evaluate his/her ability to drive. They will make recommendations for adaptive equipment (e.g., an elbow switch for turn signals, a knob on the steering wheels, push/pull levers for the gas and brake).

Wheelchair Loading

There are many different techniques for loading the manual wheelchair into the car:

<u>Rigid Wheelchair into Passenger Seat</u>

- Transfer into the driver seat.
- Fold the wheelchair outside of the vehicle. As you take off each component (wheel, armrest, etc.), place it on the floor of the opposite side of the car (e.g., if you are sitting in the driver seat, place the items on the floor of the front passenger seat).
- Slide the seat all the way back. If the steering wheel tilts, move it into a position that will interfere least with transferring the wheelchair into the vehicle. You may also need to recline the driver seat a bit to allow for extra room.
- Grab hold of the wheelchair, lift it, bring it across your body, and place it on the passenger seat.
- Strap the wheelchair in with the seatbelt (run it through the frame of the wheelchair).

<u>Cross-brace Wheelchair into Back Seat (You must have a large two-door car.)</u>

- Transfer into the driver seat.
- Fold the wheelchair outside of the vehicle.
- Place wheelchair parts on the floor of the passenger side (cushion, backpack, leg rests).
- Place both feet on the ground outside of the vehicle.
- Slide the driver seat all the way forward.
- Roll the wheelchair behind the front seat.
- Slide the driver side seat back into the correct position. The wheelchair will be stabilized by being "crushed" between front and back seat.

<u>Rigid or Cross-brace Wheelchair Pulled Across a Bench Seat (You must have a large two-door car with a bench seat.)</u>

- Transfer to the passenger side of the vehicle.
- Fold the wheelchair outside of the vehicle and place the wheelchair components (wheels, cushion, etc.) on the floor of the back seat.
- Grab hold of the wheelchair.

- Pull the wheelchair in as you scoot across to the driver side of the vehicle.
- Strap the wheelchair in with the seatbelt (run it through the wheelchair frame).

<u>Cross-brace Wheelchair into Overhead Wheelchair Carrier (cannot be used with a rigid wheelchair)</u>

A special overhead wheelchair carrier can be purchased and placed on the top of a car roof. (It looks like a luggage box.)

- Transfer into the driver seat.
- Fold the wheelchair. (See "Folding a Cross-brace Wheelchair" in Dependent Wheelchair Skills.)
- Place the wheelchair components on the floor of the passenger side (e.g., cushion, backpack).
- Place both legs back into the car.
- Push the special button installed inside the car that automatically lowers a strap from the carrier down by the side of the car.
- Hook the wheelchair frame to the straps.
- Push the button inside the car again. The straps automatically lift the wheelchair up, turn it sideways, and slide it into the overhead car carrier.

Power Wheelchairs or Scooters

Power wheelchairs are typically very heavy and pose some difficulty when the client is trying to overcome obstacles in the community. This section provides a general outline of community mobility skills for someone who will be using (or considering the use of) a power wheelchair in the community. Although power wheelchairs or scooters are battery operated and do not require the physical assistance of another person, there may be occasional instances when the power wheelchair or scooter will need to be placed into manual mode and require the physical assistance of another person. One of the most common reasons for needing help is when the battery runs out of power. This section not only addresses how to operate a power wheelchair in power mode but also in manual mode. This information is also helpful if the client is considering using a community scooter (e.g., has poor walking and moving endurance and will be using the electric scooter provided by the grocery store).

Accessibility Issues

Power wheelchairs cannot be placed in a balance-point position (tipped backwards onto back wheels with the front wheels in the air) because of the weight of the chair, the battery, and the positioning and type of wheels. Since power wheelchairs are unable to be tipped backwards, they can't be bumped up or down curbs and stairs, nor

should one ever consider taking a power wheelchair or scooter up or down an escalator. Therefore, it is very important to make sure that the places the client goes in the community are free of these obstacles. The recreational therapist should have handouts for clients about specific community accessibility issues. A handout about the Americans with Disabilities Act (ADA) is also appropriate. While many community locations are federally required to be accessible, others are not. Refer to the "Americans with Disabilities Act" and "Community Accessibility Training" in the Techniques section.

Movement Techniques

This section describes how to move a power wheelchair in a community setting.

<u>Pushing the Wheelchair</u>

Manual mode: Power wheelchairs can be placed into manual mode, allowing the caregiver to manually push the wheelchair. Typically, the wheelchair is turned from power to manual by releasing the wheel locks that are located in the center of the back wheels. Because of the weight of the wheelchair, plus the weight of the individual in the wheelchair, pushing a power wheelchair is not an easy task, especially on uneven outdoor surfaces.

- When pushing a wheelchair, hold both handgrips, stand up straight, and look at least five to ten feet in front of the wheelchair to avoid obstacles.
- Keep the wheelchair a safe distance from the curb edge and obstacles.

If the wheelchair is too heavy to push in this manner, try turning sideways. Take side steps and use your hip (the whole side of your body if needed) to push the wheelchair a short distance at a time. The power wheelchair is usually only placed in manual mode if there is a problem (e.g., the battery dies, the client isn't feeling well enough to operate the wheelchair). This should not be an everyday occurrence.

Power mode: Power wheelchairs can be operated by the individual in the wheelchair through a variety of modalities (e.g., joystick, sip and puff, head control). The right modality will be determined primarily by the physical and occupational therapists or through a referral to a power wheelchair clinic. Recreational therapists contribute to this process by providing feedback about the client's ability to utilize the modality in a functional setting. For example, if the client's hand continually slips off the joystick control on bumpy outdoor surfaces and the client requires assistance to reposition the hand, this suggests a different type of control may be needed — one that stabilizes the client's hand. A square control that the client's hand slips into rather than a "U" shaped control that the client's hand rests on may work better.

Stopping the Wheelchair
- *Manual mode*: To stop the wheelchair, hold the handgrips tightly and stop walking.
- *Power mode*: To stop the wheelchair, a specific function will need to be performed (e.g., lift hand off of joystick, one long blow on sip and puff).

Turning
- *Manual mode*: To turn the wheelchair to the right, pull back on the right handgrip and push forward on the left handgrip. To turn the wheelchair to the left, pull back on the left handgrip and push forward on the right handgrip.
- *Power mode*: To turn the wheelchair to the right or left a specific function will need to be performed (e.g., turn the head in the direction desired; push the joystick in the direction desired).

Uneven Surfaces
- *Manual mode*: In the Dependent Community Wheelchair Skills section, recommendations are made to pull the wheelchair backwards on uneven surface. Unfortunately, pulling a power wheelchair in manual mode is almost impossible due to the weight. Sometimes, the front wheels and the back wheels on a power wheelchair are the same size, thus allowing the caregiver to push the wheelchair forward over the uneven surface with the same ease (or difficulty) as going over the uneven surface backwards.
- *Power mode*: Power wheelchairs typically go over uneven surfaces such as grass, hills, and broken sidewalk with ease in forward motion. However, depending on the wheel size, alternative methods may need to be used.

Elevators
It is best to go onto an elevator backwards, aligning the front of the chair with the door opening. This allows the client to easily see where s/he is when the doors open, view the floor numbers, and easily exit the elevator. Usually the hallways outside of the elevators allow more room for turning around than the inside of the elevator does, especially if there are other people inside the elevator.

Ramps
- *Manual mode*: Ramps can be very difficult in manual mode due to the weight of the wheelchair. This can quickly turn into a very dangerous situation if the caregiver loses control. If it is necessary to push a power wheelchair up or down a ramp in manual mode, have a minimum of two people holding the back of the wheelchair (e.g., one hand on the handgrip and one hand clutching the top of the wheelchair back) for safety. The wheelchair should be pushed up a ramp forwards and guided down a ramp backwards. When you are going down a ramp, the caregivers are to stand sideways using their hips or side of the body to control the roll of the wheelchair.
- *Power mode*: Power wheelchairs should go up and down ramps easily. However, the client must use common sense when evaluating a ramp. If the ramp is full of debris (e.g., sticks, rocks, trash) or the surface does not seem secure/stable (e.g., loose gravel), the client should consider another route.

Manual Doors
Manual mode: Due to the weight of a power wheelchair it will be difficult for one person to push a power wheelchair through a manual door. The person assisting will need two hands to push the wheelchair and another person to hold the door open. Ask for assistance from a passerby to hold the door open and push the wheelchair forwards through the door.

Power mode: An individual using a power wheelchair typically has poor arm strength and function, therefore will need assistance to open manual doors. Look for automatic doors or doors with a handicap button that open the door automatically when pressed. If the client is unfamiliar with the door and it has a handicap button, press the button and watch to see how much time is allowed to get through the door. If the door opens and closes rather quickly, the client may still need to request assistance to hold the door open when s/he is going through.

Car Transfers

Standing pivot transfers and transfer board transfers are typical ways to get in and out of a car. However, individuals who typically use a power wheelchair may require much more assistance with transfers (e.g., maximum assistance of two people). It may be advantageous to explore vehicles that do not require the individual to transfer in and out of the wheelchair (e.g., a mini-van with a ramp and tie downs to stabilize the wheelchair inside the vehicle), especially if the caregiver is unable to provide the level of assistance needed (e.g., health limitations, age).

Another thing to consider is how the wheelchair will be transported. Some power wheelchairs fold or disassemble and others do not. Some power wheelchairs, although they are collapsible, do not fold easily despite their marketing promises. Therefore, it may not matter if the client can transfer in and out of the car if the car is unable to transport the wheelchair. The client who has a power wheelchair that does not fold (or does not fold easily) or whose caregiver is unable to disassemble the wheelchair should consider other alternatives for transporting the wheelchair. Examples of alternatives include vans with a lift or ramp, a car trailer for the wheelchair, or a trunk lift. Another option is using alternative transportation that provides van service with a lift (e.g., paratransit services).

Driving

If the client is interested in driving, his/her physician may refer him/her to an adaptive driving program. These programs evaluate the client's ability to drive and make recommendations for vehicle adaptations (e.g., knob on steering wheel, push/pull lever for gas and brake). Because the client is likely to be unable to load the power wheelchair or scooter by himself/herself, s/he may need to consider a van. There are many different types of vans to choose from and the professionals in the adaptive driving program will be able to provide the dimensions and specifications to meet the client's needs and recommend a particular style of vehicle.

Public Bathrooms

In addition to the comments on public bathrooms in the Dependent Community Skills section there are additional concerns for clients using power wheelchairs or scooters. Whether in power or manual mode, it can very difficult to maneuver a power wheelchair in a bathroom stall due to its size and poor turning radius. If the bathroom stall is wide enough to accommodate the power wheelchair or scooter, it may still be difficult to close the stall door.

An additional concern is the level of assistance that the client will need to use the bathroom. Many clients who have a power wheelchair require maximum assistance for transfers, therefore requiring the client to explore alternatives for bowel and bladder care (e.g., Texas catheter, incontinence pad). Refer to "Community Problem Solving" in the Techniques section and b6 Genitourinary and Reproductive Functions for further discussion. Individuals who use a scooter and are able to walk a short distance may opt to park the scooter outside of the stall and walk into the stall.

Wheelchair Breakdown in the Community

- If at any time there is a problem with the power wheelchair, call the technical assistance center.
- If the client is out in the community and a problem with the wheelchair can't be fixed quickly, put the wheelchair in manual mode and request the assistance of others to move to a safe location. Most times, a client who is using a power wheelchair is with or around other people who could offer assistance. If the client is by himself/herself or if the people with the client are not able to provide the assistance needed, call someone who can help. It is a good idea for the client to keep a cell phone with him/her at all times for such an emergency. Even if the client is unable to operate a cell phone, s/he can instruct another person to turn on the phone and dial the number. The worst-case scenario is that the client will be unable to get hold of someone by phone and the assistance available is not sufficient. In that case, the client can call or request another person to call the local emergency number (e.g., police or fire) and report a concern for safety. Request that the emergency operator remain on the line until help arrives. Although emergency personnel are trained professionals, the client cannot assume that they will know how to handle the specific situation. Teach the client how to be prepared to offer needed instruction (e.g., how to dismantle the wheelchair so they can transport the client and the wheelchair home, how to assist with transferring into and out of their vehicle).

Assessments

Descriptions of assessments are included to help therapists understand the purpose of the assessments and to point out why standardized assessments are important in the therapy process. Some of the descriptions are adapted from *Assessment Tools for Recreational Therapy and Related Fields. 3rd Edition,* by burlingame and Blaschko.

Bus Utilization Skills Assessment

Name: *Bus Utilization Skills Assessment*

Also Known As: *BUS*

Authors: joan burlingame and Johna Peterson

Time Needed to Administer: The *BUS* is best administered over a period of one to two weeks.

Time Needed to Score: The scoring takes about 15 minutes.

Recommended Group: Clients with cognitive and/or physical impairments.

Purpose of Assessment: To determine the breadth and depth of skills a client has related to the use of public transportation.

What Does the Assessment Measure?: The *BUS* is made up of two separate sections. Section One evaluates Functional Skills: 1. appearance, 2. getting ready, 3. waiting for the bus, 4. interaction with strangers, 5. pedestrian safety, 6. riding conduct, and 7. transfers. Section Two evaluates Maladaptive Behaviors: 1. anxiety, 2. depression, 3. hostility, 4. suspiciousness, 5. unusual thought content, 6. grandiosity, 7. hallucinations, 8. disorientation, 9. excitement, 10. blunted affect, 11. mannerisms and posturing, and 12. bizarre behavior.

Supplies Needed: 1. *BUS* Assessment Form (#A126), 2. phone book and telephone, 3. paper and pen for client, 4. enough change to pay for bus fare, 5. bus schedule, 6. some items to carry onto bus, 7. pictures for "Interactions with Strangers" section, and 8. transfer token.

Reliability/Validity: Initial validity studies were completed. Results may be found on the second page of the *BUS* instructions. Reliability not established.

Degree of Skill Required to Administer and Score: A recreational therapist, occupational therapist, or vocational trainer has the skills to administer, score, and interpret the results of this assessment.

Comments: The *BUS* is a detailed checklist that provides the therapist with a clear understanding of the client's actual ability to use public transportation. This assessment may be helpful to evaluate the level of difficulty that a client has with d4702 Using Public Motorized Transportation. It is also relevant for e1200 General Products and Technologies for Personal Indoor and Outdoor Mobility and Transportation.

Suggested Levels:
Rancho Los Amigos Level: 5-7
Developmental Level: 10 years and up
Reality Orientation Level: Moderate to No
    Impairment

Distributor: Idyll Arbor, Inc., 39128 264th Ave SE, Enumclaw, WA 98022, 360-825-7797 (voice), 360-825-5670 (fax), www.IdyllArbor.com.

Comprehensive Evaluation in Recreational Therapy — Psych/Behavioral, Revised

Name: *Comprehensive Evaluation in Recreational Therapy — Psych/Behavioral, Revised*

Also Known As: *CERT—Psych/R*

Authors: Robert A. Parker, Curtis H. Ellison, Thomas F. Kirby, and M. J. Short, MD

Time Needed to Administer: The *CERT—Psych/R* is scored after observing the client in a group activity. There is no administration time separate from the activity.

Time Needed to Score: The *CERT—Psych/R* takes approximately five minutes per client to score after the therapist observes the client in a group activity.

Recommended Group: Youth and adult clients with a developmental age of at least 10 years. This assessment works very well with both psychiatric and rehabilitation populations. The *School Social Behavior Scale* or the *Home and Community Social Behavior Scale* is developmentally more appropriate for youth from six to fifteen.

Purpose of Assessment: To identify, define, and evaluate behaviors relevant to a person's ability to successfully integrate into society using his/her social skills.

What Does the Assessment Measure?: The *CERT—Psych/R* measures three performance areas: General, Individual Performance, and Group Performance.

Supplies Needed: The therapist will need to provide the supplies s/he would normally supply for the activity. In addition, the therapist will need one *CERT—Psych/R* form for each client being evaluated. The Idyll Arbor version of this assessment has been designed to be used up to ten times with each client.

Reliability/Validity: Initial validity and reliability studies reported for the original version. The changes in the revised version should not change the original findings significantly.

Degree of Skill Required to Administer and Score: The professional using the *CERT—Psych/R* should have adequate and relevant training to score and interpret the client's measured functional level.

Comments: The *CERT—Psych/R* is one of the more usable assessment tools for many populations. It is a good tool to: 1. document client interactions after each treatment session, 2. measure changes that may be a result of medications, and 3. identify change over a period of time. The *CERT—Psych/R* is used with over 10,000 clients a year. This is a helpful assessment for several codes in Activities and Participation Chapter 7 Interpersonal Interactions and Relationships.

Suggested Levels:
Rancho Los Amigos Level 5 or above
Developmental Level: 10 or above
Reality Orientation Level: Severe and above

Distributor: Idyll Arbor, Inc., 39128 264th Ave SE, Enumclaw, WA 98022, 360-825-7797 (voice), 360-825-5670 (fax), www.IdyllArbor.com.

Coordination Tests

Coordination tests are divided into gross motor activities (e.g., walking, jumping) and fine motor activities (e.g., picking up objects with the hand). Coordination tests are further subdivided into equilibrium and non-equilibrium tests. Equilibrium tests assess a client's coordination while in a standing position in both static (still) and dynamic (movement) activities. Non-equilibrium tests assess a client's coordination when not in a standing position (e.g., sitting) in both static and dynamic activities.

O'Sullivan & Schmitz (1988, p.126-127) provide a list of questions that can help to direct the therapist's observations of the client's coordination:

* Are movements direct, precise, and easily reversed?
* Do movements occur within a reasonable or normal amount of time?
* Does increased speed of performance affect level (quality) of motor activity?
* Can continuous and appropriate motor adjustments be made if speed and direction are changed?
* Can a position or posture of the body or specific extremity be maintained without swaying, oscillations, or extraneous movements?
* Are placing movements of both upper and lower extremities exact?
* Does occluding vision alter the quality of motor activity?
* Is there greater involvement proximally or distally? On one side of body versus the other?
* Does the patient fatigue rapidly? Is there a consistency of motor response over time?

For all of the tests described below, the client is asked to perform the test first with his/her eyes open and then with his/her eyes closed. When the eyes are open, visual information helps the client maintain an appropriate position, whereas when the eyes are closed, the visual aid is extinguished. The therapist notes the level of deviation from the "holding" position in terms of level of impairment (normal performance, minimal impairment, moderate impairment, severe impairment, or dependent). Therapists may also note the amount of time needed to complete the test and any specific problems observed.

Equilibrium Coordination Tests

Below is a list of common equilibrium coordination tests described by O'Sullivan & Schmitz (1988, p. 126). If the client is able to maintain an upright balanced posture with eyes open but not with eyes closed, it indicates proprioceptive loss called a positive Romberg sign.

* Standing in a normal, comfortable posture.
* Standing, feet together (narrow base of support).
* Standing, with one foot directly in front of the other (toe of one foot touching heel of opposite foot).
* Standing on one foot.
* Arm position may be altered in each of the above posture (e.g., arms at side, over head, hands on waist, and so forth).
* Displacing balance unexpectedly (while carefully guarding patient).
* Standing, alternate between forward trunk flexion and return to neutral.
* Standing, laterally flex trunk to each side.
* Walking, placing the heel of one foot directly in front of the toe of the opposite foot.
* Walking along a straight line drawn or taped to the floor; or placing feet on floor markers while walking.
* Walking sideways and backwards.
* Marching in place.
* Altering speed of walking activities (increased speed will exaggerate coordination deficits).
* Stopping and starting abruptly while walking.
* Walking in a circle, alternate directions.
* Walking on heels or toes.

Non-Equilibrium Coordination Tests

Below is a list of common non-equilibrium tests described by O'Sullivan & Schmitz (1988, p.125):

* *Finger to nose*: The shoulder is abducted to 90° with the elbow extended. The client is asked to bring the tip of the index finger to the tip of the nose. Alterations may be made in the initial starting position to assess performance from different planes of motion.
* *Finger to therapist's finger*: The client and therapist sit opposite each other. The therapist's index finger is held in front of the client. The client is asked to touch the tip of his/her index finger to the therapist's index finger. The position of the therapist's finger may be altered during testing to assess ability to change distance, direction, and force of movement.
* *Finger to finger*: Both shoulders are abducted to 90° with the elbows extended. The client is asked to bring both hands toward the midline and touch the index fingers from opposing hands.
* *Alternate nose to finger*: The client alternately touches the tip of the nose and the tip of the therapist's finger with the index finger. The

position of the therapist's finger may be altered during testing to assess ability to change distance, direction, and force of movement.

- *Finger opposition*: The patient touches the tip of the thumb to the tip of each finger in sequence. Speed may be gradually increased.
- *Mass grasp*: An alternation is made between opening and closing fist (from finger flexion to full extension). Speed may be gradually increased.
- *Pronation/supination*: With elbows flexed to 90° and held close to body, the client alternately turns the palms up and down. This test also may be performed with shoulders flexed to 90° and elbows extended. Speed may be gradually increased. The ability to reverse movements between opposing muscle groups can be assessed at many joints. Examples include active alternation between flexion and extension of the knee, ankle, elbow, fingers, and so forth.
- *Rebound test*: The client is positioned with the elbow flexed. The therapist applies sufficient manual resistance to produce an isometric contraction of biceps. Resistance is suddenly released. Normally, the opposing muscle group (triceps) will contract and "check" movement of the limb. Many other muscle groups can be tested for this phenomenon, such as the shoulder abductors or flexors, elbow extensors, and so forth.
- *Tapping (hand)*: With the elbow flexed and the forearm pronated, the client is asked to "tap" the hand on the knee.
- *Tapping (foot)*: The patient is asked to "tap" the ball of one foot on the floor without raising the knee; heel maintains contact with floor.
- *Pointing and past pointing*: The client and therapist are opposite each other, either sitting or standing. Both client and therapist bring shoulders to a horizontal position of 90° of flexion with elbows extended. Index fingers are touching or the client's finger may rest lightly on the therapist's. The client is asked to fully flex the shoulder (fingers will be pointing toward ceiling) and then return to the horizontal position such that index fingers will again approximate. Both arms should be tested, either separately or simultaneously. A normal response consists of an accurate return to the starting position. In an abnormal response, there is typically a "past

pointing," or movement beyond the target. Several variations to this test include movements in other directions such as toward 90° of shoulder abduction or toward 0° of shoulder flexion (finger will point toward floor). Following each movement, the client is asked to return to the initial horizontal starting position.

- *Alternate heel to knee and heel to toe*: From a supine position, the client is asked to touch the knee and big toe alternately with the heel of the opposite leg.
- *Toe to examiner's finger*: From a supine position, the client is instructed to touch the great toe to the examiner's finger. The position of finger may be altered during testing to assess ability to change distance, direction, and force of movement.
- *Heel on shin*: From a supine position, the heel of one foot is slid up and down the shin of the opposite lower extremity.
- *Drawing a circle*: The client draws an imaginary circle in the air with either the upper or lower extremity (a table or the floor also may be used). This also may be done using a figure-eight pattern. This test may be performed in the supine position for lower extremity assessment.
- *Fixation or position holding*: To test upper extremities the client holds the arms horizontally in front. To test lower extremities the client is asked to hold the knee in an extended position.

To further test upper extremity coordination and dexterity, the therapist can administer the Jebsen-Taylor Hand Function Test, Minnesota Rate of Manipulation Test, Perdue Pegboard Test, and/or Crawford Small Parts Dexterity Test.

Coordination tests can be helpful in determining the level of difficulty with b7602 Coordination of Voluntary Movement Functions. It will also help in evaluating other movement and mobility functions that require coordination (e.g., d450 Walking) and activities that may be affected by coordination impairments (e.g., d920 Recreation and Leisure).

References

O'Sullivan, S. & Schmitz, T. (1988). *Physical rehabilitation: Assessment and treatment*. Philadelphia, PA: F.A. Davis Company.

Cooperation and Trust Scale

Name: *Cooperation and Trust Scale*

Also Known As: *CAT*

Authors: Jeff Witman, Ed. D.

Time Needed to Administer: Filling out the 15 statements of the *CAT* will take most participants under 10 minutes.

Time Needed to Score: Depending on the math skills of the individual scoring the assessment, the scoring process should take, on the average, another five minutes.

Recommended Group: Clients who are cognitively able to understand the questions.

Purpose of Assessment: To measure the participant's perceived level of trust and cooperation.

What Does the Assessment Measure?: Relative levels of perceived cooperation and trust. The test does not separate the scores for the two constructs (cooperation and trust) but combines the two constructs. The *CAT* is best used to measure changes in a client's attitudes about trusting others and cooperating with others. This is usually done through a pretest/treatment/posttest protocol. Because of psychometric difficulties inherent in trying to capture (measure) the construct of trust or cooperation, every client's score should be reviewed to see if it "fits" what the staff know about the client. The testing tool itself has good reliability and validity and can be used to assess trends in changing perceptions related to cooperation and trust. One of the greatest limitations to the *CAT* is the relativity small number of subjects used to establish reliability and validity and the lack of norm data.

Supplies Needed: Score sheet and manual.

Reliability/Validity: The initial testing on the *CAT* was reported in the *Therapeutic Recreation Journal*, Third Quarter, 1987 (p. 25). In that article, Jeff Witman reported the following:

> The CAT Scale was designed by the investigator to measure attitudes. It consists of 15 statements, which are rated for level of agreement. These statements were selected from a group of 25

statements of belief regarding cooperation and trust generated by participants (N = 96) in adventure programs who were asked their beliefs about cooperation and trust during initial program sessions. A group of adolescents (N = 26) involved in a summer adventure program offered by a school district rated these 25 statements. The statements that were correlated most highly with overall ratings (+.75 or -.75 or greater) were selected for the *CAT* Scale. Content validity of the scale was established through review by a panel of individuals involved with social skill development programming.

Idyll Arbor conducted additional testing on the *CAT* prior to releasing it commercially. Drawing from all four geographic regions of the United States, a series of test-retest trials were run to determine if it was likely that individuals would have similar scores if they took the *CAT* on different days. The participants (N = 115) were asked to fill out the *CAT*. The second time each participant filled out the *CAT* was between 24 and 72 hours later. The correlation of the test-retest was .725. The overall mean score of the first trial was 59.7 with the overall mean score on the second trial of 59.5.

Degree of Skill Required to Administer and Score: This tool is meant to be filled out and scored by adolescents. Basic reading skills are required.

Comments: The math skills required to score the *CAT* are approximately fourth grade math skills. This may be a helpful assessment for b1261 Agreeableness and b1267 Trustworthiness and Activities and Participation Chapter 7 Interpersonal Interactions and Relationships.

Suggested Levels: The Idyll Arbor, Inc. staff recommend the following guidelines to help determine if a patient is cognitively able to comprehend the statements used in the *CAT*:
Adapted IQ of 80 or above
Mental Age of 11 years or above
Rancho Los Amigos Level of 7 or above
Reality Orientation Level of "Mild to No Orientation Disability"

Distributor: Idyll Arbor, Inc., 39128 264th Ave SE, Enumclaw, WA 98022, 360-825-7797 (voice), 360-825-5670 (fax), www.IdyllArbor.com.

Fifty-Foot Walk Test

The Fifty-Foot Walk Test is a fairly simple test that can be used in the hospital or in the community. The test takes three measurements: 1. the speed the client walks normally (called the "preferred speed"), 2. the speed that the client walks when asked to walk fast, and 3. the number of steps the client uses to walk 50'. The therapist needs three supplies: 1. a stopwatch, 2. something to mark the floor or sidewalk with, and 3. a measuring tape that is at least 100' long.

The therapist measures the amount of time it takes the client to walk 50'. To measure the client's actual speed and not include the length of time it takes the client to start and stop, the therapist needs to have a seventy-foot long, straight, and flat surface. If the therapist is using chalk to mark the sidewalk four marks are made:

- One at zero (the starting point),
- One at 10' (the point to start timing the client and counting the number of steps taken by the client),
- One at 60' (the point to stop timing the client and stop counting the number of steps taken by the client), and
- One at 70' (the finishing point).

Standing near the zero mark, the therapist lets the client know that s/he wants to watch the client walk from the starting line to the finish line (the mark at 70'). This will be done twice, once at the walking speed that is comfortable for the client and once at a fast walk. The therapist makes sure that the client knows where the "start" and "finish" lines are located. The marks at 10' and 60' are not mentioned.

As the client is walking, the therapist walks just slightly behind the client (at about four o'clock or eight o'clock). This ensures that the client is choosing his/her own pace and not attempting to match the pace of the therapist. It is also provides a better vantage point for the therapist to count the number of steps the client takes between the 10' and 60' markers.

Dividing 50' by the number of steps the client took determines the client's stride length. To time the client's speed (both the preferred and fast) the therapist starts the stopwatch when the client passes the ten-foot mark and stops the stopwatch when the client passes the sixty-foot mark. The client's score is reported in feet per second and the average number of feet (and inches) per stride. The norms reported by Bohannon (1997) were taken from a relatively small sample and were obtained in a clinical setting and not

in the community. These norms are found in Table 27.

These norms provide the therapist with a benchmark, but further study is needed by recreational therapists to establish norms when using an outdoor course with a broader range of ages. An unexpected finding of these numbers is that participants in their seventies generally moved faster than participants in their sixties. This anomaly is probably due to the relatively small sample size.

In the standard testing situation the therapist does not talk to the client during the time the client is walking and being timed. A modification to the *Fifty-Foot Walk Test* is called the "Walkie-Talkie Test." This test measures whether the client can walk and talk at the same time. The functional ability to walk and talk at the same time is a mental function called "dividing attention" (b1402). As the therapist walks with the client along the 70-foot-long course the therapist asks the client an open-ended question that cannot be answered with either a "yes" or "no." If the client stops to answer the question the client receives a "positive" score on this test. A positive score means that the client needs assistance and may not be ready to enter groups or activities that require the client to perform multiple tasks. If the client is able to both walk and answer the question at the same time the client has a "negative" score. This means that the client is likely to function appropriately in tasks that require divided attention.

As a side note, the speed that a client walks may or may not be an issue affecting recreation, leisure, and community activities. Additionally, walking speed may be slowed purposely for safety. For example, a client who uses a walking device and/or has poor balance desires to water her flowers in the backyard. In this scenario, the client may be instructed to purposely slow down her walking speed to decrease her risk of falls and to increase attention to the placement of the walking device with each step to make sure it is stable. In an another example, a client who walks at a slow speed and needs to cross a busy road with a fast traffic light may need to work on increasing walking speed to ensure a timely street crossing. Consequently, therapists are not only aware

Table 27: Reference Values for the Fifty-Foot Walk Test

Age	Preferred Speed (feet per second)		Maximum (Fast) Speed (feet per second)	
	Men	Women	Men	Women
60s	4.46	4.25	6.34	5.82
70s	4.36	4.17	6.82	5.74

From Rose (2003), p.80.

of the distance, device, and level of assistance for walking, but the speed of walking as it pertains to a client's safety and optimal task participation.

The Fifty-Foot Walk Test may be helpful in determining the level of difficulty that a client has with d450-d469 Walking and Moving.

References

Bohannon, R. W. (1997). Comfortable and maximum walking speed of adults aged 20-79 years: reference values and determinants. *Age and Aging, 26*:15-19.

Rose, D. (2003). *Fallproof! A comprehensive balance and mobility training program*. Champaign, IL: Human Kinetics.

FOX

Name: *FOX*

Also Known As: This version of the assessment is known as "*The FOX.*" An earlier version is called "*The Activity Therapy Social Skills Baseline.*"

Author: Rodney Patterson and the treatment team that he worked with at the Fox Developmental Center. The questions from the *Fox Activity Therapy Social Skills Assessment* were reordered by Idyll Arbor after initial testing pointed out construct problems.

Time Needed to Administer: The *FOX* usually takes about twenty minutes or less per client.

Time Needed to Score: Scoring and interpretation of the results will usually take the therapist under 15 minutes per client.

Recommended Group: Individuals with a primary or secondary diagnosis of dementia, mental retardation, developmental disability, or brain injury.

Purpose of Assessment: To evaluate the client's relative level of skills in the social/affective domain. Most of the skills included in this assessment are important building blocks to the development of a mature leisure lifestyle.

What Does the Assessment Measure?: The *FOX* measures six areas in the social domain: 1. client's reaction to others, 2. client's reaction to objects, 3. client's seeking attention from others to manipulate the environment, 4. client's interaction with objects, 5. client's concept of self, and 6. client's interactions with others.

Supplies Needed: The therapist will need to determine which levels of the *FOX* to administer to ensure that all of the required objects are nearby. In addition, the therapist will need the *FOX* manual and score sheet #A106.

Reliability/Validity: The *FOX* was developed based on a task analysis of the discrete skills required in the six subscales. It was then administered to over 500 individuals to determine the tool's usability. When Idyll Arbor agreed with Patterson to distribute the test, making it available to a wider range of facilities and therapists, Idyll Arbor reviewed the constructs on which the tool was based and the scoring mechanism. Idyll Arbor staff found inconsistencies with the scoring using adaptive equipment. In some places when clients were required to use adaptive equipment (such as communication boards), the client received a higher score, and in other, similar situations, they received a lower score. Idyll Arbor corrected these inconsistencies of scoring but felt that the original developers of the testing tool had done a good job with the task analysis. The *FOX* has been used extensively and reports are that it is a very usable test. It has little, if any, formal psychometric analysis of its properties.

Degree of Skill Required to Administer and Score: Due to the lack of established validity and reliability this assessment is best scored and interpreted by a trained therapist.

Comments: While this is a very old testing tool, developed in the 1970s, it continues to be very useful for documenting small changes in a client's social skills. This may be a helpful assessment for d110-d129 Purposeful Sensory Experiences, b1800 Experience of Self, b1801 Body Image, b114 Orientation Functions, b122 Global Psychosocial Functions, and codes in Activities and Participation Chapter 7 Interpersonal Interactions and Relationships.

Suggested Levels:
Rancho Los Amigos: Level 2-5
Developmental Level: Birth to 5 years
Reality Orientation Level: Severe to Moderate

Distributor: Idyll Arbor, Inc., 39128 264th Ave SE, Enumclaw, WA 98022, 360-825-7797 (voice), 360-825-5670 (fax), www.IdyllArbor.com.

Free Time Boredom

Name: *Free Time Boredom*

Also Known As: FTB

Authors: *Authors of the testing tool*: Mounir G. Ragheb, Ph.D., Scott P. Merydith, Ph.D.

Time Needed to Administer: Most participants should be able to fill out the assessment form in approximately ten minutes.

Time Needed to Score: Five to ten minutes per test.

Recommended Group: The participant needs to read at the fourth grade level for the therapist to be sure that the participant understands the statements.

Purpose of Assessment: To identify the degree to which the participant is bored in the four components that make up boredom.

What Does the Assessment Measure?: The four aspects of boredom: *1. Meaningfulness*: The participant has a focus or purpose during his/her free time, *2. Mental Involvement*: The participant has enough to think about and finds these thoughts emotionally satisfying, *3. Speed of Time*: The participant has enough purposeful and satisfying activity to fill his/her time, and *4. Physical Involvement*: The participant has enough physical movement to satisfy him/her.

Supplies Needed: The therapist will need to have one test and one score sheet and the *Free Time Boredom* Manual. The participant will need to have a pen or pencil to write in his/her answers.

Reliability/Validity: The FTB has had extensive psychometric evaluation. Please see the Measurement and Item Development section in the manual.

Degree of Skill Required to Administer and Score: The actual supervision of the participant while

s/he fills out the score sheet may be done by a paraprofessional. In some cases the participant may be allowed to take the score sheet and fill it in without direct supervision. The scoring and interpretation of the participant's scores requires that the therapist be certified, registered, or licensed at the professional level.

Comments: The *FTB* may prove to be one of the more important tools related to recreational therapy treatment in the future. This tool has strong psychometric properties and, as such, should be able to predict behaviors, identify scoring patterns that indicate pathology, and provide treatment direction. The first step toward being able to predict, identify, and provide direction has been done — the tool has been developed. The next step is for this tool to be used with hundreds of participants and to compare their scores on the *FTB* with their diagnoses (especially psychiatric diagnoses). Clinical experience has shown that participants who have recently tried to commit suicide (or are on suicide precautions) tend to score a "1" on the mean-ingfulness scale. Collaborative research between clinicians and university faculty will only serve to strengthen this testing tool. This assessment may be helpful when addressing activity pattern development and scoring b130 Energy and Drive Functions, b1265 Optimism. See "Activity Pattern Development" in the Techniques section.

Suggested Levels: The Idyll Arbor, Inc. staff recommend the following guidelines to help de-termine if a patient is cognitively able to comprehend the statements used in the *Free Time Boredom*:
Adapted IQ of 80 or above
Mental Age of 11 years or above
Rancho Los Amigos Level of 7 or above
Reality Orientation Level of "Mild to No Orientation Disability"

Distributor: Idyll Arbor, Inc., 39128 264th Ave SE, Enumclaw, WA 98022, 360-825-7797 (voice), 360-825-5670 (fax), www.IdyllArbor.com.

Glasgow Coma Scale

This scale is used to measure the depth of a client's coma. It is scored by adding the scores for eye opening, best motor response, and verbal response. A score of 3-8 indicates a severe coma, 9-12 a moderate coma, and 13-15 mild to absent coma.

Function	Examiner	Patient Response	Score
Eye Opening (EO)	Spontaneous speech	Opens eyes on own	4
		Opens eyes when asked to in a loud voice	3
	Pain	Opens eyes when pinched	2
		Does not open eyes	1
Best Motor Response (BMR)	Commands	Follows simple commands	6
	Pain	Pulls examiner's hand away when pinched	5
		Pulls part of body away when examiner pinches patient	4
		Flexes body inappropriately to pain — decorticate posturing	3
		Body becomes rigid in an extended position when examiner pinches victim — decerebrate posturing	2
		Has no motor response to pinch	1
Verbal Response (VR)	Speech	Carries on a conversation correctly and tells examiner where he is, who he is, and the month and year	5
		Seems confused or disoriented	4
		Talks so examiner can understand victim but makes no sense	3
		Makes sound that examiner can't understand	2
		Makes no noise	1

Glasgow Coma Scale (accessed via website http://www.tbiinfo.com/scale.html on 6/1/02)

Home and Community Social Behavior Scales

Name: *Home and Community Social Behavior Scales*

Also Known As: *HCSBS*

Author: Kenneth W. Merrell and Paul Caldarella

Time Needed to Administer: Approximately 5 minutes for each client.

Time Needed to Score: After the therapist has read the entire manual (approximately 1.5 to 2 hours), the scoring time is around ten minutes.

Recommended Group: Youth between the ages of 5 years and 18 years

Purpose of Assessment: To measure the social competence and antisocial behavior patterns of youth. The *HCSBS* is designed to be completed by adult family members or other adults who interact with the youth in the community or home setting (including the recreational therapist). A comparison of the scores and norm data on a child using both the *SSBS* and the *HCSBS* may provide the treatment team with critical information about the differences in a youth's behavior based on the setting.

What Does the Assessment Measure?: The *HCSBS* measures Social Competence (peer relations and self-management/compliance) and Antisocial Behavior (defiant/disruptive and antisocial/aggressive).

Supplies Needed: Test manual and score sheets

Reliability/Validity: Well documented in test manuals. Good to outstanding psychometric properties.

Degree of Skill Required to Administer and Score: Moderate degree of observation skills and understanding behaviors. Parents and other adults who work with the youth should be able to be trained by the therapist to complete the *HCSBS* form. Scoring should be done by the therapist.

Comments: This testing tool is a great resource for therapists working with youth. This assessment may be helpful with codes in Activities and Participation Chapter 7 Interpersonal Interactions and Relationships and b126 Temperament and Personality Functions.

Suggested Levels: The clients assessed using the *HCSBS* should be cognitively or functionally between the ages of 5 years and 18 years of age.

Distributors:
Assessment-Intervention Resources, 2285 Elysium Avenue, Eugene, OR 97401. 541-338-8736.
or
Idyll Arbor, Inc., 39128 264th Ave SE, Enumclaw, WA 98022, 360-825-7797 (voice), 360-825-5670 (fax), www.IdyllArbor.com.

Idyll Arbor Leisure Battery

Name: *Idyll Arbor Leisure Battery*

Also Known As: *IALB* (*Leisure Interest Measure, Leisure Satisfaction Measure, Leisure Attitude Measurement,* and *Leisure Motivation Scale*).

Authors: Mounir Ragheb and Jacob Beard.

Time Needed to Administer: Approximately ten to thirty minutes per test.

Time Needed to Score: Approximately five to fifteen minutes per test.

Recommended Group: Clients with moderate to no cognitive impairment.

Purpose of Assessment: Each of the four testing tools measures a particular type of leisure attribute as shown on the next two pages.

What Does the Assessment Measure?: See the summaries, which follow, for more detail on each assessment.

Supplies Needed: Score sheet, manual for scoring formula, pen.

Reliability/Validity: The four tools have good to excellent reliability and validity.

Degree of Skill Required to Administer and Score: Basic reading and math skills are required.

Comments: The four testing tools in this battery may be administered separately or as one unit. The two authors are well known in the fields of leisure and recreation for the quality of work concerning the psychometric properties of the testing tools they develop. All four of these assessments may be helpful in understanding current recreation and leisure participation patterns that impact a client's level of difficulty with Activities and Participation Chapter 9 Community, Social, and Civic Life. They may also be helpful for leisure education/counseling and activity pattern development. See "Education and Counseling" and "Activity Pattern Development" in the Techniques section.

Suggested Levels: Idyll Arbor, Inc. recommends the following guidelines to help determine if a patient is cognitively able to comprehend the statements on the test sheets:

Adapted IQ of 80 or above
Mental Age of 12 years or above
Rancho Los Amigos Level of 7 or above
Reality Orientation Level of "Mild to No Orientation Disability"

Distributor: Idyll Arbor, Inc., 39128 264th Ave SE, Enumclaw, WA 98022, 360-825-7797 (voice), 360-825-5670 (fax), www.IdyllArbor.com.

Description of Instrument	Interpretation of Scores
Leisure Attitude Measurement	**Leisure Attitude Measurement**
The **Cognitive** component of leisure attitude gathers information in the following areas: a) general knowledge and beliefs about leisure, b) beliefs about leisure's relation to other concepts such as health, happiness, and work and c) beliefs about the qualities, virtues, characteristics, and benefits of leisure to individuals such as: developing friendship, renewing energy, helping one to relax, meeting needs, and self-improvement.	Score Intervention Cognitive — education about the need for leisure in society and one's life. Less than 2.5 Affective — provision of positive experiences related to interests, values, needs. Behavioral — education about the importance of leisure activities for improving quality of life.
The **Affective** component of leisure attitude is designed to take into account the individual's: a) evaluation of his/her leisure experiences and activities, b) liking of those experiences and activities, and c) immediate and direct feelings toward leisure experiences and activities. This component generally reflects the respondent's like or dislike of leisure activities.	
The **Behavioral** component of leisure attitude is based on the individual's: a) verbalized behavioral intentions toward leisure choices and activities, and on self-reports of current and past participation.	
Leisure Interest Measure	*Leisure Interest Measure*
Measures how much interest the client has in each of the eight domains of leisure interest. Areas Measured: 1. Physical 5. Service 2. Outdoor 6. Social 3. Mechanical 7. Cultural 4. Artistic 8. Reading	Score Intervention 4 or more High degree of interest. Ensure opportunity to participate in activities of interest. 2 or less Low interest. May need education, instruction. 2 Needs education and instruction in areas of interest and development of skill competence.

IDYLL ARBOR LEISURE BATTERY — EXECUTIVE SUMMARY

Description of Instrument	Interpretation of Scores
Leisure Satisfaction Measure	**Leisure Satisfaction Measure**
Measures which areas of leisure provide the most satisfaction for the individual. 1. **Psychological:** Psychological benefits such as: a sense of freedom, enjoyment, involvement, and intellectual challenge. 2. **Educational:** Intellectual stimulation and learning about self and his/her surroundings. 3. **Social:** Rewarding relationships with other people. 4. **Relaxation:** Relief from the stress and strain of life. 5. **Physiological:** A means to develop physical fitness, stay healthy, control weight, and otherwise promote well-being. 6. **Aesthetic:** Aesthetic rewards. Individuals scoring high on this part derive satisfaction from the places where they engage in their leisure activities because they find them pleasing, interesting, beautiful, and generally well-designed.	Score Intervention 4 or more High satisfaction. Ensure opportunities to participate in activities. 2 or less Low satisfaction. "2" Education/opportunities to increase satisfaction level. Review results of LAM, LIM, LMS. Determine if low score is having negative impact on client's ability to make progress on treatment objectives.
Leisure Motivation Scale	**Leisure Motivation Scale**

The **Intellectual** component of leisure motivation assesses the extent to which individuals are motivated to engage in leisure activities that involve mental activities such as learning, exploring, discovering, creating, or imagining.
 	
The **Social** component assesses the extent to which individuals engage in leisure activities for social reasons. This component measures two basic needs. The first is the need for friendship and interpersonal relationships, while the second is the need to be valued by others.
 	
The **Competence-Mastery** component assesses the extent to which individuals engage in leisure activities in order to achieve, master, challenge, and compete. These activities are usually physical in nature.
 	
The **Stimulus-Avoidance** component of leisure motivation assesses the need to escape and get away from overstimulating life situations. Some individuals need to avoid social contacts, to seek solitude and calm conditions, while others seek to rest and unwind.
	Score Intervention
	highest Primary motivating force.
	    • Ensure opportunity to participate in activities with motivating dimensions.
	    • Activity analysis modify/adapt.
	
	lowest Least motivating force.
	    • Provide choice.
	    • Avoidance behavior.
	    • Modify, adapt, adopt new activities.

Leisurescope Plus

Name: *Leisurescope Plus* and *Teen Leisurescope Plus*

Also Known As: Two instruments are available: *Leisurescope Plus* (adults) and *Teen Leisurescope Plus* (adolescents). The authors do not know of any other names for *Leisurescope Plus* or *Teen Leisurescope Plus*.

Author: Connie Nall Schenk

Time Needed to Administer: Depending on the format and clients, between fifteen and twenty minutes.

Time Needed to Score: Scoring takes place as the assessment tool is used. The only additional time needed is in reporting the summary. It rarely takes Idyll Arbor staff over ten minutes to develop the summary statement after administering the assessment.

Recommended Group: Adolescent and adult clients with little to no cognitive impairment.

Purpose of Assessment:
1. To identify areas of high leisure interest.
2. To identify the emotional motivation for participation.
3. To identify individuals who need higher arousal experiences (risk takers).

What Does the Assessment Measure?: The *Leisurescope Plus* measures the degree of interest that an individual has in ten areas of leisure, the feelings that the individual reports concerning involvement in a variety of activities, and the degree to which the individual seeks out high arousal (risk-taking) activities.

Supplies Needed: The *Leisurescope Plus* Kit.

Reliability/Validity: See reported reliability and validity in manual. Both are more than good enough to make the assessment valuable for individual testing.

Degree of Skill Required to Administer and Score: This test is usually self-administered and self-scored by adolescents and adults with little to no cognitive impairment. A professional trained as a therapist should be consulted if a client has barriers to his/her leisure.

Comments: Idyll Arbor staff have found that some clients interpret the pictures differently than intended. Some clients were found to select some cards because they thought that the cards represented "dating" or the clients liked the way the people in the pictures looked. If the therapist administering the test feels that this might true with some clients, it would be a good idea to ask the client to explain why s/he likes that specific card. This assessment may be helpful in understanding a client's current interest and motivation for recreational activities. This can in turn be helpful with understanding motivations in b1301 Motivation and participation pattern in Activities and Participation Chapter 9 Community, Social, and Civic Life; and assisting with activity pattern development. See "Activity Pattern Development" in the Techniques section.

Suggested Levels: Idyll Arbor, Inc. recommends the following guidelines:
   Mental Age of 6 years or above
   Rancho Los Amigos Level of 6 or above
   Reality Orientation Level of "Mild to No Orientation Disability"

Distributor: Idyll Arbor, Inc., 39128 264th Ave SE, Enumclaw, WA 98022, 360-825-7797 (voice), 360-825-5670 (fax), www.IdyllArbor.com.

Leisure Assessment Inventory

Name: *Leisure Assessment Inventory*

Also Known As: *LAI*

Authors: Barbara A. Hawkins, Re.D., Patricia Ardovino, Ph.D., CTRS, Nancy Brattain Rogers, Ph.D., Alice Foose, MA, Nils Ohlsen

Time Needed to Administer: 20-30 minutes.

Time Needed to Score: The test should take ten minutes or less to score and summarize.

Recommended Group: The *LAI* was originally developed for seniors and adults with developmental disabilities. The *LAI* is also appropriate for middle-aged and older adults with moderate to no cognitive disability.

Purpose of Assessment: The *LAI* was developed to measure the leisure behavior of adults.

What Does the Assessment Measure?: The *LAI* has four subscales:

The Leisure Activity Participation Index (LAP), which reflects the status of a person's leisure repertoire; thus, it presents a measure of activity involvement.

The L-PREF Index, which provides a measure of leisure activities in which the individual would like to increase participation. This index indicates a degree of preference for some activities over other activities.

Leisure Interest (L-INT) Index, which measures the degree of unmet leisure involvement based on the selection of activities in which the individual has an interest, but in which he or she is not participating or is prevented from participating.

The Leisure Constraints (L-CON) Index, which assesses the degree of internal and external constraints that inhibit participation in leisure activities.

Supplies Needed: The *LAI* picture cards and the various forms from the *Leisure Assessment Inventory* including:
- Participation Score Sheet
- Constraint Questions Score Sheet
- Summary and Recommendation Form
- Longitudinal Report

Reliability/Validity: Various measures of reliability and validity were run on the *LAI*. These studies are contained in the manual.

Degree of Skill Required to Administer and Score: Because the *LAI* requires clinical judgment related to probing questions used to better understand the client's reasoning for choices, a therapist is required to administer and interpret the *LAI*.

Comments: The *LAI* is one of the first standardized testing tools in recreational therapy that has pictures for clients who are fifty years old and older. Because many clients who are older have difficulty reading due to small type or have reading disabilities due to brain trauma, it is refreshing to have a testing tool that uses pictures as part of the testing process. This assessment may be helpful with understanding leisure participation patterns in Activities and Participation Chapter 9 Community, Social, and Civic Life; as well as assisting with activity pattern development. See "Activity Pattern Development" in the Techniques section.

Suggested Levels:
Rancho Los Amigos: 6 or above
Developmental Level: older adult
Reality Orientation Level: Moderate to No Impairment

Distributor: Idyll Arbor, Inc., 39128 264th Ave SE, Enumclaw, WA 98022, 360-825-7797 (voice), 360-825-5670 (fax), www.IdyllArbor.com.

Leisure and Social/Sexual Assessment

The purpose of the *Leisure and Social/Sexual Assessment* (*LS/SA*) is to provide a tool to assess the breadth and depth of a client's understanding of appropriate social and sexual roles. It was originally part of Coyne's *Social Skills Training: A Three-Pronged Approach.* The *LS/SA* was developed for adolescents with MR/DD. It may be used with other adolescents and adults when there are concerns about basic social or sexual issues. The *LS/SA* includes an interview and an observation section and typically takes an hour to complete.

Interview

The *LS/SA* is an example of a screening tool developed to obtain a basic profile of recreation and social skills for clients with cognitive impairments. It is used to develop objectives for teaching interpersonal interactions and relationships as covered by A&P Chapter 7 of the ICF.

The information needed to assess the individual and develop a profile must be kept in mind. When the necessary information cannot be gathered from the individual due to cognitive problems or a lack of expressive language, the interview can be adapted for use with a parent, teacher, or significant other. An interview with people familiar with the client's behavior is generally necessary for supplemental information and verification of data given by the client.

Interview Techniques

An environment characterized by privacy, freedom from interruptions, and a general atmosphere of calmness and warm acceptance helps establish rapport and carrying out an effective interview. The interview form suggests a format for collecting the necessary information during a direct interview with the individual. Generally, the natural flow of the interview will cause the interviewer to ask questions in a slightly different manner or different order than that presented in the interview form. One question may generate the answer to several others.

As a general rule, open-ended questions get the most spontaneous and extensive responses. However, as cognitive levels decrease, a shift to a multiple-choice format may be needed. Previous information about the individual's activities can be used as a base from which to ask questions. Yes and no questions should be avoided as much as possible.

The *LS/SA* is divided into three sections and takes approximately thirty to sixty minutes to administer. The sections include:

- Demographic Information: including orientation to person, time, and place.
- Activity and Socialization: including activities outside of work; friends and family; skills; leisure abilities and levels of participation; and leisure resources.
- Dating and Sexuality: including knowledge of sexuality as well as an examination of personal attitudes and interests related to social/sexual behavior, such as dating, marriage, and parenting.

Observation

Coyne's *Three-Pronged Approach* also includes a behavioral checklist to record observations of the client's social interaction skills. This checklist is included in the LS/SA because the therapist will find that having a behavioral checklist to compare against the client's verbal reports will help create a better understanding of the client's actual abilities and understanding. The following sections discuss the mechanics of conducting a checklist behavioral observation for clients in need of social skills training.

Direct Observation of Social Interactions

Behavioral observations have become an increasingly favored method for assessment of social behaviors and skills because these direct observational methods have the advantage of providing concrete and specific data. In addition, it indicates knowledge of both what the individual can do and what s/he chooses and initiates doing with some frequency. Social behaviors observed during free time are usually well learned and require no intervention. Therefore, baseline data on an individual's social level can be coded during several consecutive free periods in a large multipurpose area that allows for a variety of simultaneous, self-directed activities. This approach uses experiential exercises described below and allows individual assessment in a group setting. Thus, it can be easily integrated into the program and used from baseline to post-test provided that the conditions and procedures employed are identical. In order to show if a change in the client's behavior did or did not occur, materials, environment, peers, and observers should be constant.

Materials Used During Assessment

Materials and recreation equipment used should be age-appropriate and representative of those commonly found in school and home environments. There should be at least six different things to provide variety and an opportunity for all levels of social interaction. For example, where a magazine would provide an opportunity for solitary (extra-individual) activity, the presence of a rubber ball would complement that by providing the opportunity for cooperative interaction (inter-individual). The following are examples of materials utilized in the assessment of social skills:

- scissors
- crayons
- macramé cord
- Yahtzee
- cards
- screwdriver
- CD
- Nerf ball

- colored paper
- magazines
- Parcheesi
- checkers
- hammer
- nails, screws, boards
- CD player
- Frisbee

The social assessment may take place in groups as small as four clients with twelve clients being the largest desirable number of clients in the group for the purpose of assessment. Clients who are known to engage in cooperative activities should not be paired exclusively with peers who do not interact, because there would be no opportunity to demonstrate interactive skills.

Observing and Recording Social Skills

The therapist(s) who will be observing and coding the demonstrated social skills should introduce the free choice situation (group activity). The subsequent role of the therapist recording observed social skills is to avoid directive remarks while facilitating exploration and interaction. For clients with greater disabilities, facilitation involves describing what a client is doing, reinforcing appropriate behaviors with physical and verbal expressions of praise, and modeling. The therapist should avoid direct participation in an activity unless involvement is requested by a client.

The therapist who is recording the client's behaviors should be familiar with the use of the form. The best situation for recording social behaviors is for the therapist recording the observed skills to not be the individual supervising and role modeling the clients during the free time activity. But, in reality, staffing ratios do not usually allow the person running the activity to be different from the person recording the skills.

When the person recording observed social skills is not the person supervising the activity and s/he is approached by a client who is seeking attention, the observer should ignore and not make eye contact

with that client. Likewise, the observers should not alter the environment once the observation has started. It is important to use paired observers at least periodically, to check for observational reliability.

Coding Observations

Before beginning the observation period, the clients should be introduced to the setting and materials and given at least five minutes to adjust to the environment. Explanations should be given that this is a free period and that clients can choose to do whatever they would like to do. In addition, limits should be set for unacceptable behaviors. Observations of behaviors are recorded on the Social Behavioral Observation Sheet. The length of time of the observation to record the client's demonstrated level of social skills is twenty minutes divided into four, five-minute intervals. The Social Behavioral Observation Sheet has three areas: social level, social interactions, and activity involvement.

Social Level: Changes in social interaction levels occurring during any five-minute period are recorded by placing a check in the area provided for that interval. Check all of the levels demonstrated during that five-minute interval. They are coded as follows:
- *No Activity (Intra-Individual)*: The client demonstrates unoccupied behavior, such as staring into space, or self-stimulative activity such as rocking. Characterized by no contact with another person or external object.
- *Watches Others*: The client exhibits no behavior other than as an onlooker. The client is obviously aware of others and is observing them.
- *Plays Alone (Extra-Individual)*: The client plays alone and independently with an object that is different than those used by peers within speaking distance and does not interact. If physical manipulation is accompanied by eye contact, the behavior falls into this level.
- *Plays beside Peers (Aggregate)*: The client approximates the actions of one or more peers, but does not interact with them. The objects used may be identical, but there is no dependence on the action of others to sustain the activity.
- *Interacts with Staff but not Peers*: This area is peculiar to individuals with multiple disabilities who need more assistance interacting than a peer is able to provide. These clients generally play associatively and/or constructively with adults on a one-to-one basis. This category should be considered as a social level that precedes associative interactions with peers.
- *Interacts with Peers in Play (Associative)*: The client interacts with other clients concerning an

identical or similar activity. There is borrowing and loaning of equipment.

- *Cooperative Activity (Cooperative)*: The client mutually interacts with other peers in sustaining an activity. The activity cannot continue without cooperation between clients, e.g., playing catch or checkers. Activities can be inter-individual, unilateral, multilateral, intra-group, or inter-group.

Social Interactions: All social interactions during each five-minute interval are recorded in the area for that interval. It identifies whether the client interacts with adults and/or peers, initiates and/or responds to social interactions, and has brief interactions or continues to interact.

Activity Involvement: Behavioral anecdotal notes are recorded during each five-minute interval. The objects and other clients involved, where in the room being used for the observation the behavior occurred, and specific behaviors demonstrated are described in detail. This area supplements the information on social level and interactions and provides useful data for program development such as object preferences, peer preference, skill level, attention span, self-initiation, and inappropriate social behaviors. Five-minute intervals are necessary to identify activity intent. For instance, it would be easy to assume that a client who picks up a table game, such as checkers, takes it to a table, opens the box, and places the board on the table next to a peer is going to play checkers with the peer (inter-individual). However, during the five-minute period the client may ignore the peer and stack the checkers in different ways (extra-individual).

The data collected from successive sessions can accurately represent the social interaction level that the client has mastered, what skills are emerging, and the variables that facilitate the emerging skills for that particular client. Having the social lounge interfaced into the overall program can simultaneously provide ongoing assessment and social skill development.

LS/SA Summary Page

The summary page collects the information from the rest of the LS/SA on a single page that can be copied and placed in the medical chart. The following describes the information needed in each section of the summary page.

- *Leisure Activities*: A summary of activities the client participates in separated into domains. "Physical domain" refers to activities that emphasize functional skill development using gross motor activities, fine motor activities, or

cardiovascular activities. "Cognitive domain" refers to activities that emphasize problem solving, memory, receptive and expressive language, and thought processing. "Social domain" refers to activities that emphasize the ability to get along with others. "Sensory domain" refers to activities that emphasize development of our five senses (sensory stimulation): seeing, hearing, smelling, touching, and tasting. "Community domain" refers to activities that emphasize specific skills required to survive and function in the community (e.g., shopping).

- *Social/Sexual Summary*: This section provides the therapist with a quick summary of the client's social/sexual knowledge. A single check in the appropriate box and a one or two sentence summary is all that is expected for the four knowledge areas.

- *Social Behavioral Observation*: This section summarizes the social levels shown by the client during the observations. The range of actions and the predominant action should be described. Also summarizes the social interactions to describe how the actions came about, the range of interactions, and the predominant interaction.

- *Summary*: This space is provided for the therapist to compile the information from both the Leisure Activities Summary and the Social/Sexual Summary. It is extremely important to remember that the federal regulations require that the therapist both report the findings and clearly state in a measurable and meaningful way how the findings will impact the client's ability to perform.

- *Recommendations*: The intent of the federal regulations concerning clients in ICF-MRs is that no training objectives are to be developed until the interdisciplinary team can discuss (and approve) them at the appropriate care conferences. This section should list one to three possible program (training) ideas for the next one to three years.

The *LS/SA* is available from Idyll Arbor. To see a complete copy of the assessment, refer to burlingame and Blaschko (2002).

Reference

burlingame, j. & Blaschko, T. M. (2002). *Assessment tools for recreational therapy and related fields, third edition.* Ravensdale, WA: Idyll Arbor.

Coyne, P. (1980). *Social skills training: A three-pronged approach.* Portland, OR: Crippled Children's Division, University of Oregon Health Sciences Center.

Life Satisfaction Scale

Name: *Life Satisfaction Scale*

Also Known As: *LSS*

Authors: Variations of a *Life Satisfaction Scale* have been around for many years in many different forms. Some of the questions are similar to the *Philadelphia Geriatric Center Morale Scale*, the *Life Satisfaction Index*, and possibly the Oberleder Attitude Scale. Nancy Lohmann did research measuring the various questions against each other, and this *Life Satisfaction Scale* is a result of that research.

Time Needed to Administer: The *LSS* (either read by the client or to the client) should take no more than 20 minutes to administer.

Time Needed to Score: The *LSS* can be scored and summarized in approximately 5 minutes.

Recommended Group: Clients with moderate to no cognitive impairment.

Purpose of Assessment: To measure the client's perceived satisfaction with his/her life.

What Does the Assessment Measure?: The *LSS* measures the client's perceived satisfaction.

Supplies Needed: *Life Satisfaction Scale* Score Sheet and *LSS* Answer Sheet.

Reliability/Validity: Reliability and validity studies have been conducted on this assessment.

Degree of Skill Required to Administer and Score: As with all assessments used in treatment, it is best to have professionally trained staff interpret this assessment. However, the testing tool itself is meant to be self-administered.

Comments: The *LSS* is an assessment to help measure the client's degree of satisfaction. This type of assessment (and the accompanying care plan to improve low satisfaction) demonstrates that a facility is working to assure client rights. There are numerous testing tools that go by this same name. Dr. Lohmann's *Life Satisfaction Scale* is considered to be the best available. Subjective satisfaction is being considered as a fifth qualifier with Activities and Participation coding. This assessment may or may not prove to be helpful with this additional qualifier (if developed) because it looks broadly at the client's satisfaction with life rather than at a specific activity. This assessment may be more helpful with diagnosing depressive conditions (e.g., Major Depressive Disorder) and as an assessment tool to help gauge the level of life satisfaction in a long-term residential setting. See also "Education and Counseling" in the Techniques section.

Suggested Levels: Idyll Arbor, Inc. recommends the following guidelines:

Developmental Level: Due to the types of questions asked, client's who are chronologically 35 or over and cognitively 10 or above

Rancho Los Amigos Level of 7 or above

Reality Orientation Level of "Moderate to No Impairment"

Distributor: Dr. Nancy Lohmann, Interim Chairperson and Bachelor of Social Work Director, West Virginia University, 206 Stewart Hall, PO Box 6203, Morgantown, WV 26506-6203. The assessment may be used free of charge as long as the copyright notice appears on all materials.

Quality of Life Index

The Quality of Life Index (QLI) was developed by Robert S. Eliot, M.D. as a diagnostic and motivational tool for helping his patients evaluate their individual balance of stresses and strengths and then to make appropriate adjustments. With the permission of the Elliot Family Trust we are including the complete test in the Handbook for therapists to use both for themselves and for their clients. The goal of the index is to identify parts of a person's life that help them through life and the parts that cause ongoing stress.

High levels of stress may indicate difficulties handling stress (d2401) and help the therapist find the areas that are causing the stress (e.g., d7600 Parent-Child Relationship). Dr. Elliot notes that the average QLI score may also be a good indication of energy level (b1300).

Quality of Life Index

The Quality of Life Index (QLI) was developed as a diagnostic and motivational tool for helping my patients evaluate their individual balance of stresses and strengths and then to make the appropriate adjustments. Each of the items on the index represents issues my findings (as well as those of others) have shown will distinguish whether or not a specific lifestyle is high in stress. When the QLI is taken in good faith, it can provide remarkable insight into your individual stresses and strengths; and this knowledge can be the basis for your plan of stress control.

The QLI consists of forty categories that require you to evaluate and then rank, on a scale of 1 to 9, your perceptions of activities and situations within your environment. It's important to remember that this is a unique, individual, and personal tool to help you quickly gain insight — a stimulus for helping you categorize your own specific life circumstances. As such, there are neither right nor wrong answers, and it is not designed for you to compare yourself with anyone else.

These forty items will help you to identify the invisible, stressful weights you carry with you throughout your life wherever you go. When you know what they are and where they are, you can do something about them. You will also identify the parts of your life that already are helping you to lighten your load so that they can be strengthened.

Instructions

The following index asks you to evaluate your current perceptions of your life, family, work, and community. After reading each category statement, circle the number that most accurately reflects either your attitude or action.

Number 1 represents the most stressful response, and number 9 represents the least stressful response. Mark only one response per item. If a particular question does not pertain to you, mark it NA (not applicable). If you feel neutral about the category, circle the number 5.

The results will be most accurate if you answer quickly and honestly with the first gut-level response that comes to mind.

Many self-assessment tests are filled with tangential questions that are designed to corral a problem into a particular interpretation. The QLI is *not* such a test! It asks you to respond quickly and honestly for your own information. Of the thousands of people we have tested in this manner, we have reached a greater than 90 percent accuracy, as assessed by personal interviews.

1. GAME PLAN FOR CAREER/WORK
Often does not meet expectations   Usually meets expectations
1   2   3   4   5   6   7   8   9   NA

2. GAME PLAN FOR PERSONAL LONG-TERM/SHORT-TERM
    ASPIRATIONS AND DEVELOPMENTS
Have not reached many goals;   Have reached many goals;
often feel unsuccessful   usually feel successful
1   2   3   4   5   6   7   8   9   NA

3. HEALTH
Often ill   Usually well
1   2   3   4   5   6   7   8   9   NA

4. PRIMARY RELATIONSHIP (spouse, companion, significant other)
Not going well   Going well
1   2   3   4   5   6   7   8   9   NA

5. TIME SPENT WITH MY PRIMARY RELATIONSHIP
    (away from home, alone, and nonbusiness)
Rare (less than one per year)   Frequent (six or more per year)
1   2   3   4   5   6   7   8   9   NA

6. RELATIONSHIP(S) WITH CHILD(REN)
Unrewarding   Rewarding
1   2   3   4   5   6   7   8   9   NA

7. RELATIONSHIP(S) WITH PARENTS
Unrewarding   Rewarding
1   2   3   4   5   6   7   8   9   NA

8. RELATIONSHIPS AT WORK
    (with co-workers, boss, others)
Fraught with discord   Usually harmonious
1   2   3   4   5   6   7   8   9   NA

9. SOCIAL RELATIONSHIPS WITH FRIENDS, NEIGHBORS, GROUPS, AND
    OTHERS
Nonexistent   Strong
I feel distant   I feel close
1   2   3   4   5   6   7   8   9   NA

10. RELIGIOUS AND SPIRITUAL SUPPORT
Not relevant   Essential

1   2   3   4   5   6   7   8   9   NA

11. SOURCE OF APPROVAL/VALIDATION
External — people pleaser   Internal — self-assured

1   2   3   4   5   6   7   8   9   NA

12. PETS
Problematic   Either satisfying or I don't need them

1   2   3   4   5   6   7   8   9   NA

13. HOBBIES/OUTSIDE INTERESTS
Unsatisfactory or nonexistent   Satisfactory

1   2   3   4   5   6   7   8   9   NA

14. TIME MANAGEMENT/CIRCUIT OVERLOAD
Never enough hours in the day   Time well paced

1   2   3   4   5   6   7   8   9   NA

15. NEIGHBORHOOD
Unpleasant and dangerous   Comfortable and safe

1   2   3   4   5   6   7   8   9   NA

16. THE TELEPHONE
Often hampers my effectiveness   Not a problem

1   2   3   4   5   6   7   8   9   NA

17. COMMUTING/BUSINESS TRAVEL
Burdensome   Reasonably pleasant

1   2   3   4   5   6   7   8   9   NA

18. PHYSICAL WORK ENVIRONMENT
Noisy, hazardous, a nightmare   Safe and pleasant

1   2   3   4   5   6   7   8   9   NA

19. FINANCES
Out of control   Manageable

1   2   3   4   5   6   7   8   9   NA

20. MAJOR LIFE CRISES IN PAST SIX MONTHS
One or more devastating crises   Smooth sailing

1   2   3   4   5   6   7   8   9   NA

21. RELAXATION/MEDITATION
Not helpful   Beneficial
1   2   3   4   5   6   7   8   9   NA

22. CAREER/JOB MATCH
Mismatch   Good match
1   2   3   4   5   6   7   8   9   NA

23. HUMOR/PLAY/FUN
Who has time?   The staff of life
1   2   3   4   5   6   7   8   9   NA

24. INTERPERSONAL COMMUNICATION
I tend to talk more than I listen   I tend to listen more than I talk
1   2   3   4   5   6   7   8   9   NA

25. EXERCISE
Couch potato   Irregular   Regular
1   2   3   4   5   6   7   8   9   NA

26. SLEEP
Often a problem   Rarely a problem
1   2   3   4   5   6   7   8   9   NA

27. BODY WEIGHT
A problem   Not a problem
1   2   3   4   5   6   7   8   9   NA

28. ALCOHOL CONSUMPTION
More than eight ounces per day   Two ounces per day (two beers,
                                                     two glasses of wine) or less
1   2   3   4   5   6   7   8   9   NA

29. CAFFEINATED BEVERAGES (coffee, tea, cola)
More than five per day   Three per day   None
1   2   3   4   5   6   7   8   9   NA

30. TOBACCO
Ten or more cigarettes per day   Never smoked or have not
                                                     smoked for three or more years
1   2   3   4   5   6   7   8   9   NA

31. DEGREE OF CONTROL
I am invisibly entrapped   I have adequate options
1   2   3   4   5   6   7   8   9   NA

32. DECISION-MAKING
Can't make decisions easily   Make most decisions easily

1   2   3   4   5   6   7   8   9   NA

33. PERFECTIONISM
Things should always be done right   I do the best that I can

1   2   3   4   5   6   7   8   9   NA

34. TENDENCY TOWARD OPTIMISM/PESSIMISM
Whatever can go wrong, will   Most thing work out

1   2   3   4   5   6   7   8   9   NA

35. FEELINGS OF GUILT AND/OR SHAME
Frequently   Infrequently

1   2   3   4   5   6   7   8   9   NA

36. ASSERTIVENESS
I rarely say what I think   I usually say what I think

1   2   3   4   5   6   7   8   9   NA

37. ADAPTABILITY/FLEXIBILITY — PERSONAL/PROFESSIONAL
It's hard to change a plan   It's easy to change a plan

1   2   3   4   5   6   7   8   9   NA

38. ANGER
I am often angry   I take most things in stride

1   2   3   4   5   6   7   8   9   NA

39. SELF-ESTEEM
Often I feel unsure about myself   I feel good about who I am

1   2   3   4   5   6   7   8   9   NA

40. VALUES AND PRINCIPLES BY WHICH I LIVE
Not always clear   Very clear
Changeable   Stable

1   2   3   4   5   6   7   8   9   NA

Preliminary Interpretation

When you have responded to the list of 40 categories and feel that the scores represent your current perception of life, transfer the scores to the graph on the next page.

1. For each category, place a dot on the grid indicating the number (from 1 to 9) that you chose. Note that there is a separate line for NAs.
2. Now draw a line connecting the dots. You will probably see a zigzag pattern.
3. Next, compute an average score by adding all your scores and dividing the total by the number of categories that you completed. Do not count the categories you marked NA.
4. Now draw a straight line across the Quality of Life grid at the point of the average of your scores. For example, if your average is 6, draw a straight line from one 6 to the other.

This average is useful in two ways. First, the dots above the average line represent your strengths and your perception of the degree of your strengths. The scores below the average line represent your perception of the types and degrees of stress and struggle you currently face.

Second, we have found that the average line usually correlated with energy level. Respondents whose average is below 5 are often experiencing a low energy state such as burnout or depression. Higher averages often indicate high energy and optimism.

A word of caution: If all of your scores are high (in the 8 to 9 range), you may need to reevaluate the candor of your responses. Such scores usually turn out to be unrealistic. To consistently score 8s or 9s is to live in a Utopian world that does not exist. You also may have learned to deny pain or to internalize your stress by never complaining. Such a lifestyle pattern can be very destructive as unrecognized and unresolved stress merely builds in intensity. If you know you tend to me more stoic than others, you may obtain a more accurate assessment by lowering your scores by one or two points on each question.

As you examine your profile, remember this important point: *The numerical scores are not as significant as the position of the scores relative to one another.* Now look again at your highest and lowest scores. The highest identifies areas where your strengths and coping abilities can be found. These skills can cushion more negative areas of stress. The lowest scores need your greatest attention; they indicate areas of your life — the visible and invisible weights — that are most stressful to you. However, these areas also represent points at which change is possible and where opportunities abound to lighten your load.

Quality of Life Index
Summary Report

Name: _____

Date: _____

Column headers (left to right): 1 2 3 4 5 6 7 8 9 10 11 12 13 14 15 16 17 18 19 20 21 22 23 24 25 26 27 28 29 30 31 32 33 34 35 36 37 38 39 40 AVG

Row scale (top): 9 · 8 · 7 · 6 · 5 · 4 · 3 · 2 · 1 · NA

Row scale (bottom): 9 8 7 6 5 4 3 2 1 NA

Values	____
Self-Esteem	____
Anger	____
Adaptability	____
Assertiveness	____
Guilt/Shame	____
Optimism/Pessimism	____
Perfectionism	____
Decision-making	____
Degree of Control	____
Tobacco	____
Caffeine	____
Alcohol	____
Weight	____
Sleep	____
Exercise	____
Communication	____
Humor/Play/Fun	____
Career/Job Match	____
Relaxation/Meditation	____
Life Crises	____
Finances	____
Physical Work Environment	____
Commuting/Business Travel	____
Telephone	____
Neighborhood	____
Time Management/Overload	____
Hobbies/Outside Interests	____
Pets	____
Source of Approval/Validation	____
Spiritual Support	____
Social Relationships	____
Relationships at Work	____
Parents	____
Children	____
Time w/Primary Relationships	____
Primary Relationship	____
Health	____
Personal Aspirations	____
Career/Work	

Recreation Participation Data Sheet

Name: *Recreation Participation Data Sheet*

Also Known As: *RPD*

Authors: joan burlingame and Johna Peterson

Time Needed to Administer: The *RPD* is a data collection system. Experience has shown that it has taken aides (nursing aides and/or direct care staff) less than two minutes per client to fill out this form on a daily basis.

Time Needed to Score: The Idyll Arbor staff found that they were spending 30 to 45 minutes per client per quarter analyzing the data and comparing the changes from the previous quarter.

Recommended Group: All

Purpose of Assessment: To monitor a client's leisure activities to promote a balanced leisure lifestyle.

What Does the Assessment Measure?: The *RPD* helps the therapist keep track of the client's demonstrated functional ability in the following areas: 1. participation, 2. initiation, 3. independence, 4. physical output, 5. satisfaction, 6. average size of leisure groups, and 7. average time spent engaging in activities.

Supplies Needed: *RPD* sheets (the therapist may also use the supplemental physical activity sheet) and a calculator.

Reliability/Validity: No formal reliability or validity testing has been done. A clear correlation was found between the *RPD* findings and the *Leisurescope* with twelve clients whose primary diagnosis was Prader-Willi syndrome.

Degree of Skill Required to Administer and Score: The *RPD* was designed to be filled out by direct care staff and analyzed by a therapist. Because of the degree of professional judgment required in determining the appropriate balance of activities, a therapist who is familiar with the impairments and disabilities of any specific client is necessary.

Comments: The *RPD* has worked well in the six group homes it was developed for in 1985. This assessment may be helpful with evaluating the health of a client's activity pattern, as well as providing insight into participation patterns in Activities and Participation Chapter 9 Community, Social, and Civic Life. See "Activity Pattern Development" in the Techniques section and the MR/DD diagnosis.

Suggested Levels:
Rancho Los Amigos: 3 and up
Developmental Level: birth and up
Reality Orientation Level: severe and up

Distributor: Idyll Arbor, Inc., 39128 264th Ave SE, Enumclaw, WA 98022, 360-825-7797 (voice), 360-825-5670 (fax), www.IdyllArbor.com.

School Social Behavior Scales

Name: *School Social Behavior Scales*

Also Known As: *SSBS*

Author: Kenneth W. Merrell

Time Needed to Administer: Approximately 5 minutes for each client.

Time Needed to Score: After the therapist has read the entire manual (approximately 1.5 to 2 hours), the scoring time is around ten minutes.

Recommended Group: Youth between the ages of 5 years and 18 years

Purpose of Assessment: To measure the social competence and antisocial behavior patterns of youth. The *SSBS* is designed to be administered by professionals working with youth in a school or treatment setting. A comparison of the scores and norm data on a child using both the *SSBS* and the *HCSBS* may provide the treatment team with critical information about the differences in a youth's behavior based on the setting.

What Does the Assessment Measure?: The *SSBS* measures Social Competence (interpersonal skills, self-management skills, and academic skills) and Antisocial Behaviors (hostile-irritable, antisocial-aggressive, and disruptive-demanding).

Supplies Needed: Test manual and score sheets

Reliability/Validity: Well documented in test manuals. Good to outstanding psychometric properties.

Degree of Skill Required to Administer and Score: Moderate degree of observation skills and understanding behaviors. Scoring should be done by the therapist or teacher.

Comments: This testing tool is a great resource for therapists working with youth. This assessment may be helpful with Activities and Participation Chapter 7 Interpersonal Interactions and Relationships, as well as b126 Temperament and Personality Functions and d820 School Education.

Suggested Levels: The clients assessed using the *SSBS* should be cognitively or functionally between the ages of 5 years and 18 years of age.

Distributors:
Assessment-Intervention Resources, 2285 Elysium Avenue, Eugene, OR 97401. 541-338-8736.
or
Idyll Arbor, Inc., 39128 264th Ave SE, Enumclaw, WA 98022, 360-825-7797 (voice), 360-825-5670 (fax), www.IdyllArbor.com.

The Social Attributes Checklist
— Assessing Young Children's Social Competence

Name: *The Social Attributes Checklist — Assessing Young Children's Social Competence*

Also Known As: (no other name known)

Author: D W. McClellan and L. G. Katz

Time Needed to Administer: Based on observation of behavior over three to four weeks.

Time Needed to Score: 10 minutes

Recommended Group: Any group of children, disabled or not, who are preschool or elementary school aged.

Purpose of Assessment: To measure attributes of a child's social behavior related to developmentally appropriate social competence.

What Does the Assessment Measure?: Social attributes divided into three subareas: individual attributes, social skills attributes, and peer relationship attributes.

Supplies Needed: *Social Attributes Checklist*

Reliability/Validity: The set of items in the *Social Attributes Checklist* is based on research on elements of social competence in young children and on studies in which the behavior of well-liked children has been compared with that of less-liked children.

Degree of Skill Required to Administer and Score: Moderate skill in observation required. Does not necessarily require a credentialed professional.

Comments: The authors suggest that the child's demonstrated social skills be evaluated using an average of those skills over a period of at least three to four weeks. This assessment may be helpful for b126 Temperament and Personality Functions, Activities and Participation Chapter 7 Interpersonal Interactions and Relationships, and d9200 Play.

Suggested Levels:
Rancho Los Amigos: Level 5 and above
Developmental Level: preschool and elementary
    school aged children
Reality Orientation: not applicable

Distributor: Available from ERIC Clearinghouse on Elementary and Early Childhood Education, University of Illinois at Urbana-Champaign, Children's Research Center, 51 Gerty Drive, Champaign, IL 61820-7469. Phone: 800-583-4135, Fax: 217-333-3767, E-mail: ericeece@uiuc.edu, Web: ericeece.org

Vitality Through Leisure

Name: *Vitality Through Leisure*

Also Known As: *VTL*

Author: Mounir Ragheb

Time Needed to Administer: Most participants should be able to fill out the assessment form in approximately ten minutes.

Time Needed to Score: Five to ten minutes per test.

Recommended Group: The participant needs to read at the fourth grade level for the therapist to be sure that the participant understands the statements.

Purpose of Assessment: To identify the degree to which the participant gains vitality through his/her leisure pursuits.

What Does the Assessment Measure?: The *Vitality Through Leisure* Assessment measures how much vitality a person gets from leisure based on five components: Broaden-and-Build, Physical Condition, Relaxation and Stress Control, Optimal Arousal, and Personal Betterment/Restoration. It is intended to give therapists or participants insight into 1. the parts of leisure that currently increase vitality for the participant, 2. areas where leisure choices could be more effective, and 3. more understanding of the ways leisure can restore vitality.

Supplies Needed: The therapist will need to have one test and one score sheet and the *Vitality Through Leisure* Manual. The participant will need to have a pen or pencil to write in his/her answers.

Reliability/Validity: The VTL has had extensive psychometric evaluation. Please see the Measurement and Item Development section in the manual.

Degree of Skill Required to Administer and Score: The actual supervision of the participant while s/he fills out the score sheet may be done by a paraprofessional. In some cases the participant may be allowed to take the score sheet and fill it in without direct supervision. The scoring can be done by the participant and some interpretation is provided. Using the participant's scores to evaluate a therapeutic program requires that the therapist be certified, registered, or licensed at the professional level.

Comments: Although there is no norm data for this assessment, it is still reasonable to assume that scores of 4 and above on questions represent a participant's belief that the leisure activities s/he is doing are increasing his/her vitality. The absolute scores may be more important than norms because the ideal would be for every person to be receiving a great deal of vitality from his/her leisure. The most significant problem with not having norm data is that we do not know what scores indicate a problem that needs intervention. This assessment may be helpful with understanding a person's perception of positive attributes gained through leisure participation. This in turn can be helpful with understanding recreation and leisure participation patterns in Activities and Participation Chapter 7 Community, Social, and Civic Life, as well as in the development of a healthy activity pattern. It can be helpful in scoring b1300 Energy Level. Also see "Activity Pattern Development" in the Techniques section.

Suggested Levels: The Idyll Arbor, Inc. staff recommend the following guidelines to help determine if a patient is cognitively able to comprehend the statements used in the *Vitality Through Leisure*:
Adapted IQ of 80 or above
Mental Age of 11 years or above
Rancho Los Amigos Level of 7 or above
Reality Orientation Level of "Mild to No Orientation Disability"

Distributor: Idyll Arbor, Inc., 39128 264th Ave SE, Enumclaw, WA 98022, 360-825-7797 (voice), 360-825-5670 (fax), www.IdyllArbor.com.

Appendices

Appendix A: The ICF Model

Appendix B: Common Therapy Abbreviations

Mobility devices/terms
✓ = flexion
‖ = parallel bars
AAD = appropriate assistive device
HW = hemi walker
LBQC = large base quad cane
LOB = loss of balance
NWB = non-weight bearing
PW = platform walker
PWB = partial weight bearing
RW = rolling walker (some with seat and brakes)
SBQC = small base quad cane
SPC = single point cane
Std wlkr = standard walker
SW = standard walker
TTWB = toe-touch weight bearing
WBAT = weight bearing as tolerated
W/C = wheelchair

Mobility braces/orthotics
AFO = ankle foot orthosis
AS = air splint
KAFO = knee ankle foot orthosis
MAFO = modified or molded ankle foot orthosis

Extremities/Quadrants
(use R (right) or L (left) in front of single extremities to designate)
AE = above elbow
AK = above knee
Ⓑ = bilateral
B/L = bilateral
BE = below elbow
BK = below knee
BLE = bilateral lower extremity
BUE = bilateral upper extremity
LE = lower extremity
LLQ = left lower quadrant
LUQ = left upper quadrant
RLQ = right lower quadrant
RUQ = right upper quadrant
UE = upper extremity

Cognition
Attn = attention
LTM = long-term memory
STM = short-term memory

Body functions/movements
AROM = active range of motion
B & B = bowel and bladder
BM = bowel movement
BP = blood pressure
HR = heart rate
P = pulse
PROM = passive range of motion

Cues
dc = demonstrative cues
gc = gestural cues
tc = tactile cues
vc = verbal cues or visual cues

Level of assistance
From FIM
I = independent
Mod I = modified independent
S = supervision
Min A = minimal assistance
Mod A = moderate assistance
Max A = maximum assistance
D = dependent

A = assistance
CIS = close supervision
Ⓓ = dependent
DS = distance supervision
Ⓘ = independent
I'ly = independently
Ience = independence
Max = maximal
Min = minimal
Mod = moderate

Repetitions/Doses
Amt = amount
BID = twice a day
p.o. = orally
q = every
QID = four times a day
TID = three times a day
x1 = one time
x2 = two times
x3 = three times
and so on

Direction
↑ = increase
↓ = decrease
△ = change

Time
' = minutes or feet (e.g., 5')
$\overline{a}$ = before
$\overline{p}$ = after

Transfers/Walking
Amb = ambulation (obs.)
SBT = sliding board transfer
SPT = stand pivot transfer or sit pivot transfer
STS = sit to stand and stand to sit
Txfer = transfer

Other common abbreviations
- = negative
% = percent
? = question
+ = positive
1° = primary
2° = secondary
ADL = activities of daily living
$\overline{c}$ = with
c/o = complains of
cx = cancel
d/c = discharge
ELOS = estimated length of stay
eval = evaluation
F = female
f/u = follow up
hx = history
LOS = length of stay
LTG = long-term goal
M = male
N/A = non-applicable
NT = not tested
OOB = out of bed
PM&R = physical medicine and rehab
PMH = past medical history
PRN = as necessary
Rx = treatment, medication, prescription
$\overline{s}$ = without
SNF = skilled nursing facility
SOB = short of breath
STG = short-term goal
sx = surgery
Sxs = symptoms
TBA = to be assessed
TBD = to be determined
tx = treatment
WFL = within functional limits
y/n = yes/no

Appendix C: Anatomical Orientation/Positioning

In anatomy, certain terms are used to denote orientation. For example, a structure may be horizontal, as opposed to vertical. Anatomical positioning is defined by looking at a subject facing you with arms down by his/her side and palms facing forward. Some of the terms of anatomic orientation are as follows:

- Abduction: The process of moving a body part away from midline.

- Adduction: The process of moving a body part toward the midline.

- Anterior: The front, as opposed to the posterior.

- Anteroposterior: From front to back, as opposed to posteroanterior.

- Caudal: Toward the feet (or tail in embryology), as opposed to cranial.

- Cranial: Toward the head, as opposed to caudal.

- Deep: Away from the exterior surface or further into the body, as opposed to superficial.

- Distal: Further from the beginning, as opposed to proximal; further from the torso.

- Dorsal: The back, as opposed to ventral.

- Extension: Straightening or unbending a flexed limb. Moving two ends of a jointed part away from each other.

- Flexion: Moving two ends of a joint closer together.

- Horizontal: Parallel to the ground, as opposed to vertical.

- Inferior: Below, as opposed to superior; toward the feet.

- Lateral: Toward the left or right side of the body, as opposed to medial; away from the middle (medial).

- Medial: In the middle or inside, as opposed to lateral; towards the midline that divides left and right.

- Posterior: The back or behind, as opposed to the anterior.

- Posteroanterior: From back to front, as opposed to anteroposterior

- Pronation: Rotation of the forearm and hand so that the palm is down (and the corresponding movement of the foot and leg with the sole down), as opposed to supination.

- Prone: With the front or ventral surface downward (lying face down), as opposed to supine.

- Proximal: Toward the beginning, as opposed to distal; closer to the torso.

- Sagittal: A vertical plane passing through the standing body from front to back. The mid-sagittal, or median plane, splits the body into left and right halves.

- Superficial: On the surface or shallow, as opposed to deep.

- Superior: Above, as opposed to inferior; toward the head.

- Supination: Rotation of the forearm and hand so that the palm is upward (and the corresponding movement of the foot and leg), as opposed to pronation.

- Supine: With the back or dorsal surface downward (lying face up), as opposed to prone.

- Transverse: A horizontal plane passing through the standing body parallel to the ground.

- Ventral: Pertaining to the abdomen, as opposed to dorsal.

- Vertical: Upright, as opposed to horizontal.

Glossary

acalculia the inability to perform simple mathematical calculations (addition, subtraction, multiplication, division).

acetabulum a cup-shaped depression on the external surface of the hipbone, into which the head of the femur fits.

Adapin doxepin hydrochloride: a tricyclic antidepressant with numerous side effects.

advanced activities of daily living any of the seven categories of activities for being part of the community and interacting with other people.

afferent nervous system system of nerves that send messages from the environment of body systems to the brain.

ageusia having no sense of taste.

agnosia loss of ability to recognize sensory input without actual damage to the senses; usually associated with neurological illness or brain injury.

akinesia unusually limited physical activity often due to paralysis.

allergy a physiological disorder caused by the immune system as a result of hypersensitivity to a specific substance (such as pollen, dust, or type of food).

allodynia an extreme response to non-noxious stimuli in which a person with the disorder would feel pain or discomfort when a person without the disorder would feel no discomfort (such as the rubbing of clothing).

amblyopia (lazy eye) decreased acuity of vision (also referred to as a dimness of vision) in one eye; no physical defect or disease accounts for the impairment. Most people have a dominant eye. In amblyopia the non-dominant eye has become so much less dominant that the brain-eye connection has weakened enough to result in less visual acuity.

ambulate to move about; walk, including moving about using crutches; replaced with the term walking in the ICF.

amitriptyline a tricyclic antidepressant with serious side effects, most widely used for depression, but in smaller doses can also treat pain related to nerve damage.

amyloidosis a rare disease in which depositions of proteinaceous mass build up in tissues and organs causing damage to the tissue itself.

anarthria loss of articulate speech resulting from lesions of the central nervous system or damage to a peripheral motor nerve. Impairments of speech less severe than total loss are considered a dysarthria.

anemia a lower than normal number of red blood cells, either in a specific volume of blood or in the bloodstream as a whole, resulting in paleness and general lack of energy.

angiotensin-converting enzyme (ACE) a catalyst of the conversion of angiotensin I to angiotensin II—a vasoconstrictor. Due to this, ACE is targeted by treatments for high blood pressure and heart failure, among others.

anhedonia an inability to derive pleasure from life or appreciate the pleasures that most people enjoy.

anopsia blindness resulting from a defect or the absence of either or both eyes.

anosmia having no sense of smell.

anoxia deficiency of oxygen. After just a short time (three minutes) of anoxia the human body will start experiencing reduced functioning and death of cells.

anterograde post-traumatic amnesia an inability to recall events after the onset of amnesia with memory intact for events of long ago, in response to a traumatic experience.

antirheumatic treatment to prevent or relieve pain caused by rheumatism.

anxiolytic medications that cause a reduction in the patient's high level of anxiety. The therapist should be familiar with the side effects of the specific anxiolytic medication the patient is receiving, as restrictions in activity may be indicated.

aphasia the loss or decrease in the ability to speak, understand speech, read, or write.

aphonia inability to produce normal speech sounds from the larynx, due to paralysis, disease, overuse, or psychological causes. There is often a second word that describes the particular cause of the aphonia. For example, aphonia paralytica is aphonia caused by paralysis or disease of the laryngeal nerves.

apraxia inability to perform certain movements in the absence of loss of motor power, sensation, or coordination. In other words, the client has motor power, sensation, and coordination necessary to perform movement, but lacks the ability to perform these movements.

arachnoid membrane the middle of the three membranes protecting the brain and spinal cord.

areflexia a sign of nerve damage, shown through absence of reflexes.

arthroplasty the surgical reconstruction of a joint required because of trauma or ankylosis or to reduce excessive motion of the joint. A variety of materials may be used in this reconstruction including silicone, metal, or other types of implants.

articulation the quality of the production of speech sounds (e.g., the articulation of an "s" sound may be evaluated for the amount of lisping).

ascites accumulation of serous fluid in the peritoneal cavity most commonly due to cirrhosis.

astigmatism in the normal, healthy eye, light rays enter the eye and converge at a single point resulting in a clear picture. In astigmatism, the light rays that enter the eye do not converge at a single point because of distortion in the lens or the shape of the eyeball resulting in blurry picture.

ataxic dysarthria a dysarthria that results from damage to the cerebellar control circuit. The speech is described as being harsh and having a fluctuating voice volume that has an explosive quality. Increased effort to speak is evident. Equal stress is placed on all syllables spoken (a slow and pausing speech pattern). The slurring of the speech makes the person sound inebriated. It is the result of slowness and inaccuracy in range, force, timing, and direction of articulatory movements.

atelectasis the state in which either the whole or a part of the lung is collapsed or without air where the alveoli are deflated. Common causes are post-surgical splinting or blockage of the bronchiole or bronchus.

atheromas atherosclerotic plaque.

atherosclerotic plaque an abnormal buildup of cholesterol and other fatty substances on the walls of the arteries.

athetosis disorder characterized by the slow, involuntary, writhing movements of the extremities, occurring in 5% of people who have cerebral palsy. It is attributed to damage in the corpus striatum.

autoerotic behaviors self-initiated behaviors that have sexual elements often done in socially inappropriate contexts or settings; often associated with cognitive impairments.

autoimmune disease a condition where a person's immune system attacks parts of the person's own body, including rheumatoid arthritis and lupus; the cause is generally considered to be unknown, although some evidence may point to mycobacteria being present in the tissues being attacked and being the actual target of the immune system.

avocational referring to non-work related activities usually done for pleasure or hobby.

axillary crutch a medical tool that serves as a walking aide that is placed within the axilla (armpit). They have padding at the top to guard against axilla discomfort, and a hand grip near the middle for stability. These types of crutches are most often used for temporary disabilities or injuries.

axon the part of a nerve transmitting signals away from the nucleus.

Babinski sign (plantar reflex) a reflex in response to the stroking of a foot on the outer side from the heel to the metatarsal pads that causes the toes of infants or adults with spinal cord or brain injuries to extend upward. In uninjured adults, the toes curl downward.

banana cart a wheeled mobility device used for transporting a patient in a prone or supine position; patient looks like a banana on a rolling table.

bilirubin red pigment formed from hemoglobin during normal and abnormal destruction of red blood cells in the body.

body image disturbance a negative, subjective image of oneself; a negative perception of how others think about oneself; and/or an inability to adjust the perceived or real perceptions.

bradycardia an abnormally slow heart rate under 60 beats per minute, although not usually symptomatic until the heart rate drops below 50 beats per minute.

bradykinesia an abnormally slow reaction in spontaneous and voluntary movements. It is seen in Parkinson's Disease and other disorders of the basal ganglia.

bradylalia abnormally slow speech, usually due to a brain lesion or mental disorder.

brainstem the part of the brain responsible for many autonomic functions and integration of information.

cannula flexible tube inserted into the body to introduce medication or withdraw fluids into or from a duct or cavity. It can also refer to the tube used to administer oxygen to a patient's nose.

carcinoid syndrome the symptoms of individuals suffering from serotonin-secreting carcinoid tumors. Treatment includes surgical resection, if possible, and chemotherapy.

cardiomyopathy a dilation of the heart that leads to lessened efficiency and pumping power, a prime cause is alcohol and/or drug abuse.

cardiorespiratory referring to a process affecting both the cardiovascular system and the respiratory system.

central nervous system the brain and the spinal cord.

cerebellum the part of the brain responsible for coordination of voluntary movement.

cerebrum the largest part of the brain, responsible for interpreting sensation, thought, emotions, actions, decision making, etc.

chondrocyte cells only existing in cartilage that produce and maintain cartilage.

choreiform rapid jerky movements that resemble those associated with chorea.

circumduction one of the four basic movements of joints; the circular action of a joint, limb, or eye, as seen when the leg moves within the hip socket.

circumstantiality a speech pattern in which a patient has difficulty separating the important information from the unimportant while describing an event. While the patient describes the even, s/he becomes lost or sidetracked and may need to be redirected.

claudication pain caused by a lack of oxygen to the muscles that are being used that feels like cramping muscles. Because of the nature of some types of heart disease, a progressive conditioning program may do little more than increase the patient's tolerance of activity and decrease the occurrence of claudication. Patients may be encouraged to exercise through the use of activities multiple times a day to the point of discomfort (and not beyond).

clonus alternating and rapid involuntary contraction and relaxation of muscles.

cluttered speech erratic or dysrhythmic speech, consisting of rapid and jerky spurts; disfluency judged to be different from stammering.

comorbid two or more diseases or conditions that occur simultaneously in the same person.

concordance (in genetics) the traits shared by a set of twins.

congenital present at birth; originating during the development of the fetus.

contralateral on or from the opposite side. In injuries to the brain, the origin of the disability is on the opposite side of the body from where the trauma is located. For example, damage to the right side of the brain from a stroke will usually affect the left side of the body.

contralateral hemiplegia paralysis on one side of the body caused by damage to the opposite side of the brain.

contrecoup lesions caused by the brain's hitting the skull wall after its initial impact (counter bounce) due to a significant acceleration or deceleration of the head. Because the brain is encased but free-moving inside the skull, it will impact the skull initially when the head impacts an object and then rebound in the opposite direction to impact the opposite side of the skull. The lesions are caused by the impact of hitting the skull. These lesions may translate to reduced neurological functioning for months to years after the injury.

coprolalia also called coprophrasia; seen in some cases of schizophrenia Tourette's syndrome; involuntary swearing or use of derogatory remarks that commonly are taboo with possible references to excrement, genitals, or sexual acts. The statements do not necessarily reflect the opinion of the person.

corpus callosum the connection between the two hemispheres of the cerebrum.

Coumadin (warfarin) a blood thinning drug used to prevent and treat a thrombus or embolus. Also known as Jantoven®, Marevan®, and Waran®.

cyclothymic disorder a chronic low level form of bipolar disorder which must last a minimum of two years. It consists of short periods of depression alternated with hypomania.

deafferentation an impairment in the nerves that send information from the body to the central nervous system.

debridement removing foreign material or contaminated cells through cleansing, usually once every shift. Debridement is frequently extremely painful, especially when associated with "tubbing" for patients with burns.

decerebrate lacking a cerebrum or the neural connections between the brain and the lower portions of the CNS.

deconditioning a decrease in the combined functional ability of the circulatory system, cognition, neuromuscular movement, and metabolic system as a direct result of prolonged immobility and/or bed rest (usually two weeks or longer). This decrease is a direct result of inactivity and not a result of an injury or illness.

decubitus ulcer (pressure sore) a breakdown in the normally healthy condition of the skin due to pressure or shear. A Stage One pressure sore is a red mark that does not fade in 30 minutes after pressure has been relieved. A Stage Two pressure sore is a blister or an open sore which is just skin deep and caused, at least in part, by pressure or shear. A Stage Three pressure sore is an opening in the skin and into the muscle caused, at least in part, by pressure or shear. A Stage Four pressure sore is an opening in the skin and muscle down to the bone caused, at least in part, by pressure or shear.

dehydration loss of fluid (and usually electrolytes) from body tissues that can cause other serious physical problems. Restoring fluid volume and electrolytes should be done as quickly as possible.

delusions beliefs that are held regardless of the evidence against the belief including grandiose delusions and persecutory delusions.

demyelination the process of the breaking down, destruction, or loss of the myelin layer that surrounds nerves in the spinal cord and peripheral nervous system.

dendrite the part of a nerve receiving signals and transmitting them toward the nucleus.

depth perception problems the client has difficulty determining the distance of objects by using binocular vision.

detox (detoxification) the removal of toxic substances from the body either through medical treatment or changes in lifestyle.

diffuse occurring in a widespread area, with no central focal location.

diplopia (double vision) usually the result of decreased range of motion in one eye although it may also be related to amblyopia.

disfluency breaks in otherwise fluent speech that add no particular informational value to the conversation (phrases such as "er," "um," and "uh" as well as the more recent "like"). This also includes impediments such as stuttering and sentence repairs ("the car was going ea—um… north").

disinhibition the inability to suppress one's inner desires and feelings according to cultural norms and social regulations. This lack of inhibition may be due to brain damage or drugs, among other causes.

disruptable able to be disrupted or disturbed.

dissociative 1) disorders: a group of five psychiatric disorders that all share the feature of a break in normally integrated aspects of personality. With dissociative disorders an individual may demonstrate intermittent inability to act with one identity. In the past this set of disorders was referred to as multiple personality disorders; 2) drug: a drug that blocks signals to the conscious mind which can result in hallucinations and psychedelic mind states.

distal farther from the center.

diuresis increased excretion of urine; can be a symptom of diabetes mellitus.

donner a devise used to help put on articles of clothing.

dorsiflexion flexion of the food, hand, or digits backward towards the upper surface.

dura the outer of the three membranes of meninges that encase the brain and spinal cord.

dysarthria impairment in the articulation of speech, which results from damage to central or peripheral motor nerves. Speech intelligibility will vary depending of the extent of impairment. The ICF notes three types of dysarthria: spastic, ataxic, and flaccid.

dysdiadochokinesia impairment in ability to perform rapid alternating movements (e.g., rapid alternation between pronation and supination of the forearm). Movements are irregular, with a rapid loss of range and rhythm.

dysfluency see *disfluency*.

dyskinesia impairment in voluntary movement.

dysmetria an inability to measure distances involved in performing tasks; an inability to place the limbs correctly during voluntary movement using proprioceptive cues.

dysphagia difficulty swallowing due to impaired neurological functions to the muscles that control swallowing or obstruction of the esophagus such as an esophageal tumor. Obstructions generally allow swallowing liquids; impaired neurological function may prevent swallowing of both solids and liquids.

dysphonia any abnormality in the speaking voice. Hoarseness and changes in the speaking voice of adolescent boys (dysphonia puberum) are two possibilities. Any abnormality in the sound made by the vibration of vocal folds modified by the resonance of the vocal tract (phonation) is included.

dysphoria the opposite of euphoria characterized by feelings of depression and restlessness. Dysphoria is differentiated from depression by its feeling of agitation and is described as a "bad high" instead of a "low."

dyspnea labored or difficult breathing.

dyspraxia a loss of functional ability to perform voluntary movement not directly caused by a loss of motor or sensory input and function.

dysreflexia a serious medical problem that can occur in individuals with a spinal cord injury above the 7th thoracic level. Autonomic dysreflexia can be caused by many type of noxious stimuli below the level of the spinal cord injury and its symptoms may be mild or severe. Severe autonomic dysreflexia is a medical emergency, which, if not properly treated, can result

in a cerebrovascular hemorrhage (stroke) and possibly death. Common stimuli that cause autonomic dysreflexia include full or spastic bladders, a full rectum, tight or irritating clothing, a fracture, or another undiscovered, painful stimulus.

dysrhythmic having to do with a change in the normal rhythm. An abnormal change in the patient's speech rate due to illness or disability or a change in a patient's heartbeat due to illness or excessive activity are types of dysrhythmias.

dysthymia a type of mood disorder which has persisted for at least two years which decreases the individual's interest in activities because of a persistent feeling of sadness, of being "down in the dumps" or being "blue." The severity of the mood is not sufficient enough to warrant a diagnosis of depression but severe enough to impact activities. Individuals with dysthymic disorder tend to have low self-esteem, a feeling of hopelessness, and a tendency to self-criticize. This is a formal psychiatric disorder found in the DSM-IV.

dystonia muscle tone impairment.

dystonic movement a slow, gross motor movement with athetoid characteristics.

eccentric behavior literally, behavior that is off center. While society usually uses this term to describe someone who has been successful by taking a different route than others, in psychology it refers to behavior that is not quite typical *and* that is not functional to achieve goals.

echopraxia the abnormal and undesired imitation of another person.

efferent nervous system system of nerves that send messages from the brain to the rest of the body.

embolism a blockage in the circulatory system caused by a foreign body, including a blood clot that originates somewhere else in the vascular system, fat, and air; the result of the embolism depends on the location and completeness of the blockage.

endoscopic referring to looking inside a human body for medical purposes. This can be done with a camera or fiber optics through a small incision.

energy conservation techniques ways to conserve the amount of energy expended during activities to maximize safety and productivity.

enunciation the clearness and distinctness of speech regarded from the point of view of its intelligibility to the audience.

executive function high-level cognitive functions, including abstract reasoning, adapting to the environment, inhibition of inappropriate behavior, initiation skills, interpretation of social cues, judgment, planning skills, problem solving, and sequencing.

fine function movement and control of small muscles, as of the fingers.

flaccid dysarthria a dysarthria that occurs when muscles associated with voice production are paralyzed. The extent of voice impairment will vary depending upon the extent of damage. Damage can be unilateral (e.g., as a result of a cerebrovascular accident) or bilateral (e.g., as a result of a traumatic brain injury). In unilateral paralysis the affected side of the mouth droops, drooling occurs from the affected side of the mouth, the jaw deviates toward the weakened side, and the tongue moves towards the stronger side.

flavonoids compounds found in biological matter that are responsible for pigmentation. They have characteristics as anti-allergens and anti-inflammatories. They have been found to modify the body's reaction to allergens, viruses, and carcinogens.

focal occurring in a limited area.

functional assist using a body part to help with an action in a functional way, such as using the right hand to hold a piece of cloth while the left hand sews it with a needle; contrast with gross assist.

funiculi divisions of the spinal cord's white matter.

gait belt a wide belt worn at the waist that can be easily grabbed and held be a support person to assist with balance and physical guidance during walking or transfers; also known as a transfer belt.

gait cycle normal series of movements during walking or running; the time and actions required for one foot to touch the ground twice.

gastrocnemius the superficial muscle found in the posterior part of the leg (the calf).

geropyschiatric the study of the psychiatric aspects of aging and mental disorders suffered by elderly and the treatment thereof.

glaucoma a disease of the eye that increases intraocular fluid pressure. If left untreated over time, the optic disk becomes damaged, the eyeball can harden, and partial to complete loss of vision can occur, starting with a loss of peripheral vision, which should be noted in b2101 visual field functions.

glia the supporting tissues that help maintain and nourish the nervous system that are intermingled with essential elements of nervous tissue.

glucagon a hormone secreted by the pancreas that raises the level of glucose in the bloodstream, opposing the action of insulin by causing the release of stored carbohydrates.

glucocorticoids a type of steroid hormone. They affect carbohydrate metabolism and can reduce inflammation and raise blood sugar levels.

Glucometer a portable device used to measure blood glucose levels. It involves pricking the skin to obtain a drop of blood, which is then placed on the device's testing strip.

glucosamine a compound of amino sugar found in vertebrate tissues which is used in the formation of many parts of the body and is given as a treatment for osteoarthritis.

goniometer a device that measures geometric angles; usually used to measure range of motion.

gross assist using a body part to help with an action even though the body part has only gross motor function, such as using an arm as a weight to hold something down or as a blocker to keep something from sliding away; contrast with functional assist.

gross function large-muscle movements.

hallucination the perceived sensory impression that something exists without the normal sensory stimulus evoking the sensation.

handrim the circular tubing on the outside of the bigger wheels of a self-propelled wheelchair used for forward movement (both handrims used together) and side-to-side steering (handrims used independently).

Heberden's node hard or bony swellings in the fingers formed by calcific spurs of articular joint cartilage; a sign of osteoarthritis or other degenerative disease of the joints.

hematogenous infection an infection spread by the individual's own cardiovascular system.

hematoma an accumulation of blood within tissue as a result of trauma. As the trauma heals, the hematoma becomes a "black and blue mark."

hematuria the presence of blood in the urine that can be a sign of kidney or urinary tract diseases.

hemianopsia defective vision or blindness in half of the visual field. (Also called hemianopia.).

hemiparesis weakness of one side of the body.

hemiplegia paralysis of one side of the body.

hemorrhage a blood vessel that ruptures. It is often caused by a sustained increase in blood pressure.

hepatosplenomegaly simultaneous enlargement of the liver and spleen.

herniate cause a protrusion of part of the intestinal tract or other organ through a weak spot in the surrounding muscular wall.

Hib disease a disease caused by Haemophilus influenzae type b, the leading cause of pneumonia and bacterial meningitis. Usually it is acquired by exposure in daycare centers. A vaccine is given during infancy.

hyperadrenalism an over-active adrenal gland caused by excessive ACTH that is characterized by obesity.

hyperaesthesia a heightened sensitivity to stimuli.

hyperalert a state of extreme alertness.

hyperalgesia lowered threshold for and increased sensitivity to pain.

hypercalcemia excessive amounts of calcium in the blood resulting from dysfunction of the parathyroid gland, bone tumors and osteoporosis; causes abdominal pain, anorexia, apathy, muscle weakness, delirium, and personality and cognitive changes.

hyperflexion excessive flexion of a joint or joints.

hypergonadism a condition in which the testes or ovaries are overactive leading to an imbalance of hormones.

hyperkalemia the condition of having higher than normal amounts of potassium in one's bloodstream associated with kidney failure or diuretic drugs, can prove fatal if it causes a cardiac arrest.

hypermetria a condition that is characterized by the inability to control movement in such a way that all actions taken overreach their intended goal.

hypermetropia (farsightedness, longsightedness) a visual impairment caused by a defect in the eye, making sight for distant objects better than sight for near objects.

hypermobility a condition characterized by an abnormally large range of motion in joints.

hypernasality a speech disorder that occurs when the tissues of the palate and pharynx do not close properly, and air leaks from the nose during speech. Certain sounds such as "p," "b," "s," and "k" cause the most problems. In children, it can occur after surgery, from a deformation of the face, or from neurological problems.

hypernatraemia an electrolyte imbalance characterized by having higher than normal amounts of sodium in one's bloodstream; can be caused by lack of water, excessive sweating, diarrhea, or by an over-intake of sodium either orally or intravenously.

hyperopia (far sightedness) a person is able to see things at a distance but has difficulty seeing things that are close.

hyperosmolar a state of abnormally increased osmotic pressure of a solution.

hyperparathyroidism a condition in which too much parathyroid hormone is produced by the parathyroid gland; bones lose calcium, the calcium content of the bloodstream rises, and the amounts of calcium found in urine increase.

hyperpathia a condition in which the pain from a normally painful stimulus is increased, can also refer to an exaggerated patient response to painful stimuli.

hyperpituitarism excess activity of the pituitary gland leading to an excessive amount of growth hormones leading to abnormal growth of hands, feet, and internal organs.

hypersensitivity 1) allergy, or an enhanced response of the immune system to a foreign substance that leads to pathological changes 2) stronger reaction to a stimulus, usually tactile, than would normally be expected, perhaps even to the point where a light touch is experienced as pain 3) a psychological state where the emotional reaction is greater than would be expected from the situation.

hypersomnia a condition of excessive tiredness characterized by the inability to remain awake during a normal waking period.

hypertension the persistently elevated arterial blood pressure. It is the most common public health problem in developed countries. Emphasis on lifestyle modifications has given diet a prominent role for both the primary prevention and management of hypertension.

hyperthyroidism the excess production of thyroid hormones by the thyroid gland leading to weight loss, chest pains, cramps, and nervousness.

hypertonia a state of increased tension or tone in muscles.

hypoadrenalism (Addison's disease) the underproduction of hormones by the adrenal gland leading to anemia.

hypocalcemia deficient levels of calcium in the serum that may result from several causes including hypoparathyroidism, vitamin D deficiency, kidney failure, inadequate amounts of magnesium and protein, and acute pancreatitis; the deficiency may cause delirium and personality changes, formation of cataracts, seizures, cardiac arrhythmias, and intracranial pressure within the brain.

hypochondriasis a psychological condition in which the patient has imagined or highly exaggerated complaints of physical illness. The patient's concern about his/her heartbeat, sweating, breathing, or bowel/bladder functions interferes with normal day-to-day activities.

hypogeusia having a reduced sense of taste.

hypogonadism a condition in which the testes or ovaries are under-active leading to an imbalance of hormones.

hypokalemia inadequate amount of potassium in the blood that may cause weakness or flaccid paralysis.

hypometria a condition that is characterized by the inability to control movement in such a way that all actions taken fall short their intended goal.

hyponasality a deficit in the quality of voice that results from reduced nasal emission of air and lower nasal resonance. Speakers sound as if they have a cold.

hyponatremia an inadequate amount of sodium in the blood that may lead to confusion and memory problems, convulsions, and coma.

hypoparathyroidism a condition caused by the reduction or absence of secretions of the parathyroid gland.

hypophonia a condition characterized by softening (lowering) of volume during speech.

hypopituitarism a deficiency of one or more of the hormones produced by the pituitary gland.

hypoproteinemia an abnormally low amount of protein in the blood that tends to cause abdominal pain, diarrhea, edema, and nausea.

hyposmia having a reduced sense of smell.

hypotension blood pressure so low that the body has trouble getting oxygen to tissues.

hypothyroidism a disorder in which the thyroid activity is deficient causing a reduced basal metabolic rate, lethargy, and sensitivity to cold. In women (it affects a higher percentage of women), hypothyroidism may also lead to menstrual disturbances.

hypotonia the state of decreased muscular tone or tension.

hypovolemia a lack of blood volume causing life threatening shock.

ideomotor apraxia inability to demonstrate a physical movement when verbally asked to make the movement. Ideomotor apraxia is often associated with damage to the left hemisphere of the brain. Clients with ideomotor apraxia retain the neurological memory to perform the physical movements and can do so through habit.

idiopathic of unknown origin; related to an unknown cause.

ileostomy an ostomy placed in the ileum (small intestine).

immunological pertaining to the immune system.

incoordination lacking coordination of movements.

innervate 1) to supply nerves to a part of the body 2) to stimulate a part of the body (muscle, nerve, etc.) to movement or action.

innervation the conduction of nerve impulses to a muscle or gland.

intercochlear in the cochlea of the ear.

intermittent claudication pain caused by a lack of oxygen to the muscles that are being used that feels like cramping muscles. Because of the nature of some types of heart disease, a progressive conditioning program may do little more than increase the patient's tolerance of activity and decrease the occurrence of claudication. Patients may be encouraged to exercise through the use of activities multiple times a day to the point of discomfort (and not beyond). Pain subsides slowly with rest.

interphalangeal joints hinge-joints with a volar and two collateral ligaments. This type of joint only permits flexion and extension movements.

intervertebral referring to the space between two vertebrae.

intonation using pitch when speaking to convey syntactic information.

intracerebral referring to within the cerebrum.

intrapleural referring to within the pleural cavity.

intubation the insertion of a tube into a body structure; most commonly refers to the placement of a breathing tube in the trachea to aid with a patient's breathing.

ipsilateral on the same side of the body.

IQ a measurement of general cognitive processing abilities. In the early 1900's A. Binet, who developed one of the first testing tools to measure intelligence, felt that intelligence included the areas of adaptability, imagination, insight, judgment, and reasoning. Other researchers included skills associated with abstraction, learning dealing with novelty, and being able to function successfully within one's environments. Generally, testing tools that measure intelligence are used as predictors of scholastic success.

jejunostomy an ostomy placed in the jejunum section of the intestines.

jet lag a person's reaction to traveling across time zones, which forces a person to be awake and sleep at times that the person is not used to.

ketoacidosis a form of acidosis caused by the enhanced production of ketone bodies.

ketone the unusable acidic byproducts produced by the body during the breaking down of fats due to a lack of insulin.

kinesthesia the function of sensing the movement of body parts.

Korsakoff's syndrome an alcohol-induced disorder characterized by the presence of both anterograde and retrograde amnesia.

kyphosis a spinal deformity that causes the thoracic portion of the spine to curve forward causing rounded shoulders and impaired lung capacity.

lability inability to control emotions; typically crying or laughing unrelated to situation.

laminectomy surgical removal of the posterior aspect (the arch) of a vertebrae.

laryngectomy surgical removal of all or part of the larynx (voice box).

leisure appreciation the act of realistically estimating the worth of an activity and the amount of enjoyment it causes. It involves making a judgment and having a sensitive awareness of the emotional and physical benefits of an action, individual, group, or object. Nurturing leisure appreciation is the process of teaching clients about leisure and the health benefits of leisure participation and having the client apply the information by creating a healthy activity plan.

Likert scale a numerical scale developed by Rensis Likert which is usually used to measure attitudes and values. The scale, traditionally having five choices, runs from negative (usually "strongly disagree") through neutral ("uncertain") to positive ("strongly agree"). Less traditionally, scales with three, seven, or more choices are offered. The Likert scale allows the results of the individual's attitudes and values to be analyzed mathematically.

lisp using the th and *th* sounds in place of s and z; developmentally appropriate in young children and normal in some languages, such as Castilian Spanish.

locus of control a term used in social psychology to describe how much an individual perceives that s/he controls his/her own actions. A high internal locus of control implies that the client feels s/he is in control and responsible for his/her own actions. A high external locus of control implies that the client feels someone besides the client is in control of the client's actions.

logorrhea rapid speech associated with manic episodes and some types of schizophrenia, usually pressured with excessive volubility.

lordosis a spinal deformity that causes the lumbar spine to have an excessive curve backwards.

macular degeneration damage to the macula of the retina that causes blindness in the center of the visual field. It is caused by several different diseases. In severe cases complete loss of vision may occur in the macular region.

malaise a general sense of not feeling well.

mannerisms deep-seated, involuntary, and habitual movements such as continually stroking the jaw with the thumb.

Meniére's disease a disorder of the inner ear that can affect both balance and hearing. Is known to cause vertigo, tinnitus, and a feeling of fullness in the ear.

metabolism the physical and chemical processes continuously going on in cells that builds up tissue (anabolism) or tears down tissue and produces the energy cells use to function (catabolism).

metabolite any substance taking part in metabolism or produced during metabolism.

microvascular disease a disorder of the smaller blood vessels in the body. Individuals with diabetes may develop problems with nephropathy (disease of the kidneys), retinopathy (ongoing damage to the small vessels which provide blood to the eyes), and neuropathy (degenerative/pathological changes in the peripheral nervous system which decreases function).

mitral valve prolapse a common slight deformity of the mitral value in the heart causing it to bulge slightly into the left atrium when closed, allowing a small amount of blood to leak backward; can lead to palpitations, chest pain, and fatigue.

monoparesis paralysis affecting a single extremity or one part of the body.

monoplegia paralysis of one limb.

monotone an unchanging intonation.

morbidity occurrence rate of a disease or abnormal health condition.

mortality death rate.

mouthstick a device placed in the mouth used to steer wheelchairs, push buttons, or help in general life. It is usually only used with high level quadriplegics.

myeloma a type of cancer that is usually malignant, found in plasma cells in bone marrow.

myelomeningocele During the first 30 days of development, the fetus may experience an abnormal formation of his/her spinal cord, vertebra, and skin. Myelomeningocele is an abnormal opening in the spinal column, allowing a pouch of membranes containing both the meninges and the spinal cord to balloon out of the bony, protective covering of the spine. Manifestations include partial paralysis of the lower extremities with accompanying sensory deficits, bowel and bladder dysfunction, and a significant chance of hydrocephalus.

myocarditis inflammation of the heart muscle causing loss of efficiency which can lead to pain and possible heart failure, can be caused by viral infections or certain types of drugs or radiation.

myopathy diseases of the muscles that cause weakness, wasting, and histological changes within muscle tissue that is not the result of nerve dysfunction; seen in muscular dystrophies.

myopia (near sightedness) a person is able to see things up close but has difficulty seeing things that are at a distance.

neurogenesis the ability to grow new, functioning neurons in the brain.

neurogenic pertaining to origin in the nervous system or arising or stimulated by nerve tissues.

neuroplasticity the ability of the brain to form new connections to restore functions lost when a part of the brain is damaged.

neurotransmitter a chemical that transmits or inhibits a nerve impulse at a synapse.

noradrenaline catecholamine precursor of epinephrine released from the adrenal glands that serves as a neurotransmitter between nerve terminals.

norepinephrine a hormone produced by the adrenal glands acting as a neurotransmitter found in the parts of the brain that control autonomic behavior, attention, and the fight-or-flight response.

nosocomial infection infectious agents picked up in the hospital after admission with no evidence that the infection was already present or in incubation at the time.

nystagmus a rhythmic jerking or movement of the eyes.

oliguria problems with producing and passing urine causing the waste produced by the body to build up in the body.

opioid natural and synthetic chemicals that have opiate-like effects including endorphins and synthetic methadone.

orthosis type of brace which is applied externally to a deformed or compromised body part to provide control, correction, and support. When an orthosis provides control or provides correction, it does so by either putting extra stress or pressure on a body part or by reducing stress or pressure on a body part. To provide support the orthosis functions by reducing the weight bearing load of the body part and provides rigidity to reduce destabilizing motion. The material that the orthosis is made of is usually left up to the discretion of the orthotist unless the prescription specifically states the material to be used. Each prescription should include the type of orthosis to be made along with the type of control that is to be allowed by the orthosis. The three primary types of control provided by the orthosis are 1. free motion, 2. assisted motion, or 3. resisted motion.

orthostatic hypotension a sudden drop in blood pressure that may occur when a person stands.

osteoblasts cells that are responsible for the formation and development of bones.

osteoclasts cells responsible for the breaking down of and resorption of bone.

osteomyelitis a disease caused by infection or inflammation of the bone or bone marrow.

osteopenia a possible precursor to osteoporosis that is characterized by a decrease in bone mineral density because of a decrease in estrogen levels, for this reason it occurs most commonly in post-menopausal women.

osteophyte bone spur; outgrowths that form along joints caused by the body's response to damaged joints (by arthritis for example).

osteoporotic pertaining to or characterized by osteoporosis.

ostomy a surgically created passage that connects an internal organ to an artificial opening in the skin, usually used to bypass missing or damaged intestines.

overlearn to practice skills beyond initial mastery to the point that they become automatic.

over-stimulated subjected to an overwhelming amount of stimuli in the environment.

oximeter a monitoring device that measures the amount of oxygen in a person's blood in a painless and discrete way to ensure enough oxygen is flowing in the arteries.

paraesthesia (paresthesia) a burning or tingling sensation often described as "pins and needles" that seems to have no lasting or long-term effect (transient paraesthesia) unless associated with peripheral nerve damage (chronic paraesthesia).

paramnesia a disorder of memory in which reality is confused with events from dreams and fantasies.

paraparesis a weakness or slight paralysis of the low extremities.

paraphasic words unrelated to the current topic or unintelligible.

paratransit private or public transportation services that are more personalized than conventional for people with disabilities and special needs; instead of following a timetable, they are usually available whenever a need arises and offer door-to-door service.

paresthesia abnormal sensations such as burning, pricking, tickling, or tingling in an extremity.

pericarditis the inflammation or infection of the pericardium.

pericardium a double-walled sac that surrounds the heart and the major vessels around it.

perinatal trauma traumatic events during childbirth.

perineal pertaining to the perineum.

perioperative referring to the time between admittance to the hospital for surgery to the time of discharge.

peripheral nervous system the nerves not in the spinal cord and the brain, including the cranial nerves and the nerves exiting the spine (spinal nerves).

peripheral neuropathy degeneration or inflammation of the peripheral nerves; causes include lead poisoning and diabetes.

pertussis (whooping cough) a highly communicable, vaccine-preventable disease that lasts for many weeks and is typically manifested in children with paroxysmal spasms of severe coughing, whooping, and post-tussive vomiting. Transmission occurs through direct contact with discharges from respiratory mucous membranes of infected persons. Risk groups include children who are too young to be fully vaccinated and those who have not completed the primary vaccination series. Like measles, pertussis is highly contagious with up to 90% of susceptible household contacts developing clinical disease following exposure to an index case. Adolescents and adults become susceptible when immunity wanes.

phalangeal referring to the bones in the fingers and toes.

pleural effusions fluid buildup in the intrapleural spaces in the lungs causing dyspnea, chest pains, and non-productive cough.

polyneuropathy the simultaneous malfunctioning of many peripheral nerves at the same time. It is either acute or chronic, and give little or no warning before occurring.

polyradiculoneuropathy a disease of the peripheral nerves and spinal nerve roots.

polysubstance abuse the abuse of three or more drugs with the exception of caffeine and nicotine, which do not count as polysubstance abuse drugs.

polyuria an excessive volume of urine in any given period.

popliteal referring to the hollow point behind the knee joint.

postconcussional pertaining to the time after head trauma.

post-traumatic amnesia amnesia due to a concussion or other trauma to the brain.

postural hypotension orthostatic hypotension.

precox perceived inability of a therapist to establish an unrestrained and mutually-accepting relationship with clients with schizophrenia.

premorbid referring to the time before an injury/illness.

priapism an abnormal and persistent, painful erection of the penis that is seldom associated with sexual arousal.

prolapse referring to organs that "fall" or "slip" out of place, usually referring to the uterus or other organs protruding though the vagina, but can also refer to prolapses of the rectum and anus.

pronate in a prone position, lying flat with the face forward.

proprioception the conscious awareness of the position of a limb, or of the body in space.

proprioceptive function the ability to identify the location and action of a limb without using vision; it includes both position (statesthesia) and movement (kinesthesia).

proprioceptor a nerve that senses stretch and movement to provide information about the body's position.

proximal closer to the center.

psychometry study of mental measurement.

psychoneuroimmunology (PNI) a term that evolved during the 1980s to create an awareness and promote interdisciplinary focus to ascertain how emotional and cognitive functioning could affect immunological responses through traditional neurological connections.

ptosis drooping of the upper eyelids when the eyes are fully open due to nerve or muscle damage.

quadriparesis weakness in all four limbs.

rales rattling, bubbling, or crackling sounds which occur because of secretions in the air passages of the respiratory tract. They may be heard with the ear but are most accurately assessed by use of a stethoscope.

Rancho Los Amigos Level of Consciousness Scale an eight-point scale used to record impairment in cognitive functioning from Level I (coma or no response) to Level VIII (normal).

reacher adaptive device used to pick up objects that the client would not be able to get to, as items on the floor for a client who can't bend down or items on a shelf for a client in a wheelchair; usually has jaws for grasping objects, a stick, and a hand grip that can be moved to work the jaws.

rehydration the replenishment of water and electrolytes that were lost through dehydration either by oral or intravenous therapy.

reinfarction the reoccurrence of a infarction.

reinforcer a stimulus that increases the strength of a behavior; reinforcers can be either negative or positive.

remyelination a repair to damage of the myelin.

retractions respiratory distress characterized by the sinking in of the soft tissues of the chest between the ribs and cartilage; caused by increased inspiratory effort or an obstruction to breathing.

retrograde memory function ability to remember information that occurred before a traumatic experience (physical or emotional).

scleral icterus ("yellow eyes") yellowing of the whites of the eyes because of damage to the liver.

selective mutism a childhood disorder characterized by persistent lack of speech in at least one social situation, despite the ability to speak in other situations.

shear friction caused by rubbing the skin against another object while moving; damage caused by shear may lead to skin breakdown and infection.

sickling the development of sickle-shaped red blood cells, as seen with sickle cell anemia.

sigh a deep inspiration followed by a prolonged, audible expiration. Occasional sighs are normal and function to expand alveoli. Frequent sighs are abnormal and may indicate emotional stress.

somatization a disorder in which an individual has recurrent and multiple health complaints of a physical nature for which an organic cause cannot be found.

somatognosia body scheme disorders.

somatosensory referring to the sensory signals from all organs and tissues in the body.

spastic dysarthria a dysarthria caused by damage to the pyramidal tract resulting in increased muscle tone and incoordination that interferes with voice and speech functions. The vocal quality is harsh, strained, or strangled, pitch is predominantly low, bursts of loudness may occur, and there is a notable decrease in facial muscle range of movement, tongue strength,

and speech rate, as well as difficulty in phoneme-to-phoneme transitions.

spasticity hypertonic muscles with increased resistance to stretch; the stiffness is called hypertonia and produces a slowed response.

spinal cord the structure of nerves in the spinal column that transmits information between the brain and the rest of the body.

spirometer a device that measures the quantity and speed of inhaled and exhaled air to assess the workings of the lungs.

spondylitis inflammation of the spine or vertebrate bones due to injury, illness, or rheumatoid diseases.

stammer frequent repetition or prolongation of a sound or syllable, leading to markedly impaired speech fluency.

statesthesia the function of sensing the position of body parts relative to one another.

stenosis the abnormal narrowing of a blood vessel or other tube-like organ.

stereognosis the ability to identify an object through the sense of touch.

stereopsis the ability to perceive three dimensions through depth perception, used to judge distances.

stereotypical behavior behavior that remains the same even though it may not work in the current environment; usually inappropriate; often seem in clients with cognitive impairments.

stertorous sounds a snoring sound from secretions in the trachea and large bronchi.

stridor a harsh, high-pitched, crowing sound which occurs with upper airway obstructions caused by narrowing of the glottis or trachea (e.g., tracheal stenosis, presence of a foreign object).

stutter stammer.

synapse a connection between two nerves or a nerve and another cell, such as a muscle cell; sometimes referring to the space between the cells.

syncope a feeling of being light-headed followed by a short loss of consciousness; also known as "fainting." Syncope can be alleviated or avoided by placing one's head between the knees at the first sign of light-headedness.

tachycardia rapid beating of the heart, usually describing rates over 100 beats per minute.

tachylalia logorrhea.

tachypnea (hyperventilation) rapid breathing which reduces the carbon dioxide levels in the blood to below normal which can cause numbness or tingling, lightheadedness, headaches, chest pain, and fainting.

tardive dyskinesia a movement disorder characterized by involuntary movement of the tongue, lips, mouth, trunk, and/or limbs; usually results from long-term use of medications including antipsychotic drugs.

target heart rate the appropriate heart rate to maintain during aerobic activity to provide maximum benefit from the activity; typically 50-80% of the person's maximum heart rate (which is a function of age and condition). In health care settings there are many conditions that require special evaluation to set target heart rates, and in some cases they cannot be set. Extreme caution must be applied in exercise situations in these circumstances.

temporomandibular the hinge mechanism that connects the temporal bone at the base of the skill to the mandible (jaw) bone allowing the jaw to open and shut, move side to side, and in and out.

tenodesis an operation that sutures the end of a tendon to a bone; often done to provide the client with more stability at the cost of range of motion.

tetraparesis weakness in all four limbs.

tetraplegia paralysis in all four limbs.

therabands resistive exercise bands (tubing) used for building muscle endurance and strength after muscle or joint injuries.

thoracic orthosis a corset-like device that wraps around the trunk; commonly prescribed for clients who have had a vertebral fracture. It limits the movement of the spine to decrease the risks of fractures and provides support to the spine. There doesn't appear to be an established time frame for wearing the thoracic orthosis because it is helpful during the healing phase and the fracture prevention phase. However, it is known that prolonged immobilization results in bone demineralization.

threader a device used to thread a needle.

thrombosis a blood clot that originates in a brain vessel and blocks blood flow.

tics rapid, sudden, and non-rhythmic motor movements or vocalizations that the client has little control over.

transcutaneous pertaining to a procedure preformed through the skin.

transdisciplinary an approach to a problem that is not within the bounds of any specific academic discipline, and may cross over several.

transfer belt a wide belt worn at the waist that can be easily grabbed and held by a support person to assist with balance and physical guidance during walking or transfers; also known as a gait belt.

trauma 1) a bodily injury, wound, or shock caused physical force or a toxic substance 2) psychological injury or shock from a painful emotional experience.

tubbing removing foreign material or contaminated cells through cleansing, usually once every shift; mechanical removal for burns.

ureters the ducts that carry urine from the kidneys to the bladder, they propel urine along through muscular impulses.

Wernicke's encephalopathy an inflammatory disease of the brain caused by a deficiency of thiamine usually associated with chronic alcoholism; characterized by abnormal eye movements, confusion, and difficulties with coordination.

wheezing a whistling sound produced by air passing through a narrowed bronchi or bronchiole. It may be heard on both inspiration and expiration but is more prominent on expiration. Apparent with emphysema and asthmatic patients.

working memory the part of memory that holds information that was just presented until it is integrated into long-term memory.

Index

About the Authors

Heather R. Porter, CTRS, MS

Heather has been an adjunct instructor in the therapeutic recreation department at Temple University in Philadelphia for the past six years and has over 14 years of clinical recreational therapy experience in physical rehabilitation. She has two bachelor degrees in recreation and leisure studies (therapeutic recreation and sport/recreation management), an MS in counseling psychology with a certificate in marriage and family therapy, and is currently working on a Ph.D. in Health Studies. She is a field reviewer for the *Therapeutic Recreation Journal*, has spoken at local and national conferences, and serves on various professional committees, including ATRA's Public Health — WHO team.

joan burlingame, ABDA, HTR (formerly CTRS)

joan knew from a young age that she wanted to be a therapist. Her grandmother, Alice W. Burlingame, taught horticultural therapy at Michigan State University and would take joan along to nursing homes and hospitals to help run group therapy activities. joan studied community recreation at Northern Michigan University then transferred to the University of Colorado, Boulder, to add a second major in therapeutic recreation. After finishing her undergraduate degree, joan started on a PhD track at the University of Colorado, Denver, in Public Health Administration. Prior to finishing her PhD she left to accept a position at Children's Hospital in Seattle. In 1985 joan started Idyll Arbor, Inc., a consulting and publishing company.

joan has always had a passion for the natural environment and the challenge to protect the environment while promoting livable communities and ecologically sound recreation. In 2005 joan retired from health care to pursue a second career in land use and conservation.

CPSIA information can be obtained
at www.ICGtesting.com
Printed in the USA
LVOW09*1512011117

554604LV00017B/448/P